## Dr Jhodie R Duncan

Dr Jhodie R Duncan is a developmental and addiction neuroscientist with over 15 years of postdoctoral experience. She has been a CJ Martin Fellow at Boston Children's Hospital, ARC Future Fellow and Florey senior research fellow and lab head at the Florey Institute of Neuroscience and Mental Health.

## Professor Roger W Byard

Professor Roger W Byard is a forensic pathologist and professor of pathology at the University of Adelaide. He has written over 750 papers in peer-reviewed journals, has written/edited five texts (one in 3rd edition; one in 2nd), and has been the editor-in-chief of *Forensic Science Medicine and Pathology* since 2008.

This book is available as a free fully-searchable ebook from
**www.adelaide.edu.au/press**

# SIDS

## Sudden infant and early childhood death:

### The past, the present and the future

edited by

Jhodie R Duncan and Roger W Byard

THE UNIVERSITY
*of* ADELAIDE

UNIVERSITY OF
ADELAIDE PRESS

Published in Adelaide by

University of Adelaide Press
Barr Smith Library
The University of Adelaide
South Australia 5005
press@adelaide.edu.au
www.adelaide.edu.au/press

The University of Adelaide Press publishes peer reviewed scholarly books. It aims to maximise access to the best research by publishing works through the internet as free downloads and for sale as high quality printed volumes.

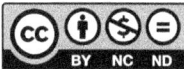

For the full Cataloguing-in-Publication data please contact the National Library of Australia: cip@nla.gov.au

ISBN (paperback) 978-1-925261-67-7
ISBN (ebook: pdf) 978-1-925261-68-4
DOI: http://dx.doi.org/10.20851/sids

Editor: Rebecca Burton
Editorial support: Julia Keller
Book design: Zoë Stokes
Cover design: Emma Spoehr
Cover image: iStockphoto

# Contents

*This book is dedicated to Professor Henry F Krous and Professor Torleiv O Rognum, two men who devoted their professional lives to understanding and eradicating SIDS, SUDI, and SUDC.*

# Acknowledgements

The editors of this volume would like to thank all authors for their contributions. We greatly acknowledge the financial assistance of Red Nose (Australia) and the very valued support they have given enumerable families over the years.

For Jhodie R Duncan's contributions, the Florey Institute of Neuroscience and Mental Health acknowledges the strong support from the Victorian Government and in particular the funding from the Operational Infrastructure Support Grant.

# Foreword

There has been a great need for a text such as this for some time now, with the last general book on sudden infant death syndrome (SIDS) published over a decade and a half ago, in 2001. Since that time many significant developments have occurred in our understanding of sudden and unexplained deaths in pediatrics, ranging from updated definitions with increased emphasis on mandatory death scene investigations to high-quality scientific work examining the role of neurotransmitter abnormalities in the brain. The issue of sudden death in toddlers over a year of age (SUDC) has also become an area of study, with a clearer understanding of the usefulness of the more general term sudden and unexpected death in infancy (SUDI). The Triple Risk Model has stood the test of time and has facilitated the integration of laboratory-based work with epidemiological risk factors. Many fringe theories have fortunately finally fallen into well-deserved historical obscurity along with odd entities such as status thymicolymphaticus.

As the reader will quickly realise, the text is an extremely eclectic mix of chapters written by experts in their respective fields. Important chapters deal with the history of SIDS, the role of parent organizations in promoting bereavement support, the very raw issue of parental grief, and research into the underlying mechanisms associated with SUDI. The later chapters focus variably on processes and locations, particularly within the brain, the roles of which in SUDI are being more clearly teased out and understood.

Of necessity there is some repetition in chapters, as SIDS and SUDI in general are a heterogeneous mix of mechanisms and processes that cannot be boxed into discrete areas. While this has sometimes led to different authors taking somewhat contradictory positions on certain subjects, it merely reflects the complexity and reality of the SIDS/SUDI arena today.

The editors hope that this text will have enabled experts from a variety of backgrounds to explain and elaborate on their particular areas of study and investigation. It will also serve as a summary of SIDS, SUDI, and SUDC as we know them today, and will lay the foundation for further exciting discoveries. As such, hopefully this book will provide an invaluable resource for individuals across many arenas, including parents, clinicians, medical examiners, and researchers. We are very close to understanding why SIDS/SUDI occurs: our next challenge is to prevent these tragic deaths from ever happening.

*Roger W Byard*, Adelaide
*Jhodie R Duncan*, Melbourne
August 2017

# 1

# Sudden Infant Death Syndrome: Definitions

Roger W Byard, MBBS, MD

*School of Medicine, The University of Adelaide, Adelaide, Australia and
Florey Institute of Neuroscience and Mental Health, Victoria, Australia*

*The beginning of wisdom is the definition of terms*
Socrates (470-399 BC)

## Introduction

Sudden infant death syndrome (SIDS), once known as "cot death", has been a somewhat controversial term that on one hand has been criticized for not being a proper diagnosis with pathognomonic features, contrasting on the other hand with situations where it has been uncritically and inconsistently applied to all manner of infant deaths. It has been argued that SIDS constitutes a disease with a single cause, an argument which is at odds with those who feel that it is instead a syndrome with common features, and probable heterogeneous and additive risk factors. For this reason it has been called a "diagnosis without a disease" (1). As will be evident from the following chapters, the debate continues.

The term "SIDS" is used when a sleeping infant, who has apparently been quite well, is found unexpectedly dead. Pathological evaluation, including ancillary testing, is unable to discern a cause of death (2-6). Despite the shortcomings of pathology, however, the SIDS story over the past several decades has been one of the great successes in infant healthcare. After specific environmental risk factors were identified in several large studies, awareness campaigns were initiated and promoted by SIDS organizations worldwide, which resulted in death rates from "SIDS" falling dramatically (7-10).

In the Australian context the number of SIDS deaths reduced from over 500 per year in 1988 to 134 per year in 1999 (11), which corresponded to a decrease in the average number of SIDS deaths per 100,000 livebirths from 196 in the 1980s to 52 deaths between 1997 and 2002. In California in the United States, the number of SIDS deaths per year fell from 110.5 deaths per 100,000 live births in 1990 to 47.2 deaths per 100,000 live births in 1998 (4). In more recent years SIDS death rates have levelled, although SIDS is still responsible for a large number of infant deaths globally (12-16).

It has become clear that the mechanisms of death in infants classified as SIDS involve a complex interaction of individual susceptibilities with developmental stages and environmental factors, rather than a convenient and simplistic "single cause" (17). This was first hypothesized by Bergman over half a century ago when he proposed that the multifactorial pathogenesis of this syndrome involved the interaction of a range of factors (18). This concept was expanded upon in 1972 by Wedgwood, who put forward a multiple contingency hypothesis in which he suggested that the risk of SIDS was increased when three overlapping factors coincided. These factors were [1] general, such as prematurity, sex, overcrowding, and poverty; [2] developmental; and [3] physiological (19). He emphasized that there needed to be an overlap of various risk factors, rather than one risk factor in isolation, and that death would only occur once the synergy of these factors exceeded the threshold for survival.

The next significant development was advanced by John Emery in 1983 when he suggested an "inter-related causal spheres of influence" model that was similar in philosophy to the Wedgewood model. Proposed risk factors included [1] subclinical tissue damage from infection; [2] environmental triggers, such as poor nutrition and medical care; and [3] poor postnatal development of reflexes and responses (20). Environmental triggers and a critical developmental period were considered vital, although individual variability was acknowledged.

The "fatal triangle" model subsequently proposed by Rognum and Saugstad used the same "three hit" framework but added possible roles for hypoxic and/or immunological events. Factors contributing to death were thought to involve [1] central nervous system vulnerability and altered mucosal immunity; [2] predisposing factors, including genetic polymorphisms and astrogliosis; and [3] triggering events, such as overstimulation of a developing immune system, possibly from viral infections (21).

These theories finally culminated in the 1994 "triple risk" model of SIDS advanced by Filiano and Kinney, in which the risk of SIDS was thought to be increased when a vulnerable infant was exposed to environmental stressors. Specifically, the three components of the model are: [1] a critical developmental period; [2] exposure to exogenous stressors: and [3] underlying susceptibilities (22). The critical developmental period is within the first six months, and specifically between two to four months, following birth. During this time the infant brain is undergoing rapid and extensive physiological changes, particularly in homeostatic control. Exogenous environmental stressors such as prone sleeping position, overheating with excessive bedding, and co-sleeping or soft bedding are now well recognized and will be discussed in much greater detail later in the text. Details of individual vulnerabilities involving brainstem control will also be the subject of later chapters. Although there has been criticism of this model, with suggestions that a more useful theoretical framework would give probabilities for a range of risk factors (23), it has provided a very useful conceptual framework to guide SIDS research over a number of years (17).

Despite the advances in our conceptual and actual understanding of SIDS deaths, and the development of definitions, numerous problems remain, not the least of which is the inadequate investigation of infant deaths in many jurisdictions. This has resulted in deaths being attributed to SIDS without even the most rudimentary of autopsies taking place (11, 24, 25). Single-cause theories of SIDS are often read about in the media without having been appropriately peer reviewed, a situation that causes considerable community confusion.

Research is also still being undertaken on cases that simply have not been investigated sufficiently for the conclusion of SIDS to be made. A study published in 2007 showed that 58% of randomly selected papers on SIDS from the literature either had not specified the definition that was being used or had used an idiosyncratic, not recognized definition. This study was repeated five years later and showed some improvement, although there were still one in three papers on SIDS which did not use a recognized definition (26, 27). Despite accepted definitions of SIDS specifying that the term cannot be used if significant or lethal disease is found at autopsy, authors have referred to "cardiovascular causes" of SIDS such as congenital heart disease, myocarditis, myocardial infarction, aortic stenosis, and rhabdomyomas. Idiosyncratic terms such as "SIDSplus" may be used to cover a range of deaths (28-30).

The quest to find a useful definition of SIDS continues; however, Emery's concerns that SIDS could become a "diagnostic dustbin" (31) still appear to be very much with us. This is exemplified in recent analyses of infant deaths where all deaths, including those in highly dangerous environments such as sofas (couches), are being lumped together under the rubric of "SIDS" (32, 33), despite the difference in sex ratios between infants who die while co-sleeping compared with infants who die alone, making it likely that these two groups are different (34, 35). It appears that every death in a cot may once again have become a "cot death".

## Recent Definitions

As was noted above, it is disappointing that standard definitions of SIDS are either being ignored or idiosyncratically modified to suit researchers' needs. The first major definition of SIDS to achieve some international acceptance was formulated in 1969. SIDS was defined as "the sudden death of any infant or young child, which is unexpected by history, and in which a thorough postmortem examination fails to demonstrate an adequate cause for death" (36). Issues that arose with the definition included a lack of positive features as well as difficulties that occurred in trying to define what was meant by "sudden", "unexpected", "thorough", and "adequate", as these terms were all quite subjective. It has been suggested that the definition was meant to have a requirement for death scene examination, but that this was inadvertently left out.

In 1991 the National Institute of Child Health and Human Development (NICHD) Group in the United States published the following definition, in which SIDS is referred to as "the sudden death of an infant under one year of age which remains unexplained after a thorough case investigation, including performance of a complete autopsy, examination of the death scene, and review of the clinical history" (37). The importance of this definition was that it built upon the previous 1969 definition but limited SIDS to infants under 1 year of age, and specified that the work-up of an unexpected infant death requires a case investigation, not merely an autopsy. Specifically, the authors correctly stated that review of the clinical history and formal investigation of the death scene were not optional extras, but were mandatory requirements that had to be undertaken before a conclusion of SIDS could be entertained.

It was slightly concerning that this definition was not immediately universally accepted, and that it was in fact criticized, with a number of alternative definitions being proposed. An example of a criticism of the requirement for a death scene examination was a paper by Becroft, which stated that, while the addition of a death scene examination to the definition initially seemed to be a good idea, "in retrospect it was not" (38). It is unclear why additional information would not be desirable, as it is well recognized that significant and serious errors may be made if a scene is not evaluated properly. The point is that an infant death cannot be attributed to SIDS until there has been an examination of the death scene by experienced personnel who can deal sensitively with bereaved parents as well as check for evidence of accidental or non-accidental injury (39, 40). Having death scene examination in the definition was, therefore, an excellent idea.

Concern was also expressed that the NICHD definition cut SIDS off at 1 year of age. However, this is not a problem, as it is recognized that 95% of SIDS deaths occur between 1 and 6 months of age, and unexpected deaths after the first year of life are rare (5).

A number of alternative definitions were published before and after the NICHD definition, all of which had different emphases on death scene investigations, history reviews, age range, associations with sleep, performance of ancillary testing, and the presence or absence of minor pathological findings (29, 41-43). These definitions did not greatly advance our understanding of the entity and have not stood the test of time. One suggestion that was made, however, to stratify cases into two or three categories in order to better define the requirements that have been fulfilled, or not, for diagnostic purposes (44, 45) led to the formulation of the San Diego definition.

# The San Diego Definition

In 2004 a panel was convened by the CJ Foundation (United States) whose mandate it was to re-evaluate the definition of SIDS and to attempt to provide a framework for diagnostic and research activities. It was intended that this definition should be continually updated as new information became available (46).

The panel met in San Diego and proposed a general definition for SIDS as "the sudden unexpected death of an infant <1 year of age, with onset of the fatal episode apparently occurring during sleep, that remains unexplained after a thorough investigation, including performance of a complete autopsy and review of the circumstances of death and the clinical history" (47). The definition added an apparent association with sleep to the NICHD definition and attempted to broaden the requirement for a death scene examination to include an evaluation of the entire circumstances of death in order to capture as much information about the infant's environment as possible.

In addition, a series of subcategories were formulated to assist with the assessment, classification and diagnosis of specific cases. The reason behind this was that it was hoped that the stratification of cases based on age groups and investigative information would enable researchers to identify the best cases for study. It was also hoped that application of this classification system would assist with identifying the most valid published data.

The general definition and subcategories were subsequently published in the journal *Pediatrics* (47) and are listed below:

## General definition

"[T]he sudden unexpected death of an infant <1 year of age, with onset of the fatal episode apparently occurring during sleep, that remains unexplained after a thorough investigation, including performance of a complete autopsy and review of the circumstances of death and the clinical history".

## Subcategories

### Category IA SIDS (classic features with complete investigation)

An infant death that meets the requirements of the general definition with all of the following:

*Clinical*: Older than 21 days and under 9 months; a normal clinical history, including term pregnancy (≥37 weeks gestational age); normal growth and development; no similar deaths in siblings, close genetic relatives (uncles, aunts and first-degree cousins), or other infants in the custody of the same caregiver.

*Circumstances*: Investigation of the various scenes where incidents leading to death may have occurred, and determination that they do not provide an explanation for death found in a safe sleeping environment with no evidence of accidental death.

*Autopsy*: Absence of potentially lethal pathological findings; minor respiratory system inflammatory infiltrates are acceptable; intrathoracic petechial hemorrhages are a supportive but not an obligatory or diagnostic finding; no evidence of unexplained trauma, abuse, neglect, or unintentional injury; no evidence of substantial thymic stress effect (i.e. thymic weight less than 15 g, and/or moderate to severe cortical lymphocyte depletion). Occasional "starry sky" macrophages or minor cortical depletion are acceptable; toxicology, microbiology, radiology studies, vitreous chemistry and metabolic screening studies are negative.

## Category IB SIDS (classic features with incomplete investigation)

An infant death that meets the requirements of the general definition and also meets all of the above criteria for Category IA except that: investigation of the various scenes where incidents leading to death may have occurred was not performed, and/or one or more of the following analyses was not performed: toxicology, microbiology, radiology, vitreous chemistry, and metabolic screening.

## Category II SIDS

An infant death that meets Category I criteria except for one or more of the following:

*Clinical*: Age range — outside Category IA or IB, i.e. 0 to 21 days or 270 to 365 days; similar deaths of siblings, close relatives, or other infants in the custody of the same caregiver that are not considered suspicious for infanticide or for recognized genetic disorders; neonatal and perinatal conditions (e.g. those resulting from preterm birth) that have resolved by the time of death.

*Circumstances of death*: Mechanical asphyxia or suffocation by overlaying not determined with certainty.

*Autopsy*: Abnormal growth and development not thought to have contributed to death; marked inflammatory changes or abnormalities not sufficient to be unequivocal causes of death.

## USID (unclassified sudden infant deaths)

This includes deaths that did not meet the criteria for Category I or II SIDS, but where alternative diagnoses of natural or unnatural conditions were equivocal (including cases where autopsies have not been performed).

## Post-resuscitation cases

Infants who are found in extremis and who are resuscitated but later die ("temporarily interrupted SIDS") may be included in the above categories, depending on the fulfillment of specific criteria (47).

As with the earlier definitions, the San Diego Definition provoked controversy and, for example, was not greeted with particular support when it was presented at the Eighth SIDS International Conference in Edmonton, Canada, in July 2004. However, despite quite vigorous discussion at the time there was no significant follow-up, and the definition has since proven useful in a number of different jurisdictions around the world (48, 49). Modification of the definition has, however, been requested because of difficulties in assessing some of the specified features such as failure to thrive and fever (50). It should also be mentioned that a mistake was probably made in replacing "death scene" with "circumstances of death". This was done in an attempt to broaden the capture of information from the death scene; however, it would have been more useful to word this as "circumstances of death, including death scene".

## Other Definitions

### SUDI

SUDI, or sudden unexpected death in infancy, is a useful term that refers to all sudden and unexpected infant deaths and not just to SIDS. It would be hoped that, by using this classification, all unexpected and sudden infant deaths would be captured for particular populations. This would mean that research and epidemiological analyses would not be hampered by loss of cases due to idiosyncratic or different classifications of infant death by different pathologists, coroners, or medical examiners, nor would they be influenced by diagnostic shifts; i.e. a case will fall under the umbrella of SUDI even if it has been classified as SIDS, undetermined/unclassified, or asphyxia.

Nothing is ever straightforward and so a problem has arisen due to the formulation of different definitions of SUDI. For example, while some jurisdictions will exclude accidents or homicides, others will include them. The author has found the CESDI (Confidential Enquiry into Stillbirths and Deaths in Infancy) study in the United Kingdom guidelines the most useful (51, 52). This definition has been published and has been trialed very successfully. A death is classified as a SUDI if it occurs between 7 and 365 completed days of life and fulfills the following criteria:

- deaths that were unexpected and unexplained at autopsy
- deaths during an acute illness that was not recognized as life-threatening
- deaths due to an acute illness of less than 24 hours' duration in a previously healthy infant (or death after this if life had only been prolonged by intensive medical care)
- deaths from a pre-existing occult condition
- deaths from any form of accident, trauma, or poisoning (51, 52).

Cases can be graded from Ia to III depending on the certainty with which a cause of death can be established. A "zero" classification can be added to identify certain cases which belong within SUDI, but in which information is missing, due to incomplete investigations, thus preventing them from being classified as explained or unexplained deaths (53).

If this definition of SUDI is being modified for local use, then this should be clearly specified. For example, certain jurisdictions prefer to include all deaths in infants aged from 0 to 365 days rather than to exclude the first week of life.

### SUDC

SUDC, or sudden unexplained death in children older than a year, is a rare event but is now being investigated as a separate entity from SIDS. The incidence in the United States in 2001 was 1.5 deaths per 100,000 live births, compared with 56 SIDS deaths per 100,000. The definition proposed by Krous and colleagues (54) is: "the sudden and unexpected death of a child older than one year of age which remains unexplained after a thorough investigation, including review of the clinical history and circumstances of death, and performance of a complete autopsy with appropriate ancillary testing".

## Conclusions

We now have a workable definition of SIDS with subcategories that should assist us in evaluating cases — but this will only work if definitions and criteria are applied consistently and uniformly. An example of a significant current problem is the labelling of certain cases of infant deaths in unsafe sleeping environments, such as on sofas, as "SIDS" without an acknowledgement of the possibility of other lethal mechanisms such as suffocation or positional/crush asphyxia (32, 33, 35, 55-57). So, having a definition is really only the first step in a long journey. It is very likely that Socrates would recognize that, although having a definition is the beginning of the wisdom, it is certainly not the end.

## References

1. Byard RW. Sudden infant death syndrome — A "diagnosis" in search of a disease. J Clin Forensic Med. 1995;2:121-8. https://doi.org/10.1016/1353-113 1(95)90079-9.

2. Beckwith JB. Discussion of terminology and definition of the sudden infant death syndrome. In: Sudden infant death syndrome. Eds Bergman AB, Beckwith JB, Ray CG. Seattle: University of Washington Press, 1970. p. 14-22.

3. Byard RW, Krous HF. Sudden infant death syndrome. Problems, progress and possibilities. London: Arnold, 2001.

4.   Byard RW, Krous HF. Sudden infant death syndrome: Overview and update. Pediatr Dev Pathol. 2003;6:112-27. https://doi.org/10.1007/s10024-002-0205-8.

5.   Byard RW. Sudden death in the young. 3rd ed. Cambridge, UK: Cambridge University Press, 2010. https://doi.org/10.1017/CBO9780511777783.

6.   Moon RY, Horne RSC, Hauck FR. Sudden infant death syndrome. Lancet. 2007;370:1578-87. https://doi.org/10.1016/S0140-6736(07)61662-6

7.   Henderson-Smart DJ, Ponsonby A-L, Murphy E. Reducing the risk of sudden infant death syndrome: A review of the scientific literature. J Paediatr Child Health. 1998;34:213-9. https://doi.org/10.1046/j.1440-1754.1998.00225.x.

8.   Moon RY, Fu L. Sudden infant death syndrome: An update. Pediatr Rev. 2012;33:314-20. https://doi.org/10.1542/pir.33-7-314.

9.   Salm Ward TC, Balfour GM. Infant safe sleep interventions, 1990-2015: A review. J Commun Health. 2016;41:180-96. https://doi.org/10.1007/s10900-015-0060-y.

10.  Vennemann MMT, Findeisen M, Butterfass-Bahloul T, Jorch G, Brinkmann B, Köpcke W, et al. Infection, health problems, and health car utilisation, and the risk of sudden infant death syndrome. Arch Dis Child. 2005;90:520-2. https://doi.org/10.1136/adc.2004.065581.

11.  Byard RW. Inaccurate classification of infant deaths in Australia: A persistent and pervasive problem. Med J Aust. 2001;175:5-7.

12.  Fleming PJ, Blair PS, Pease A. Sudden unexpected death in infancy: Aetiology, pathophysiology, epidemiology and prevention in 2015. Arch Dis Child. 2015;100:984-8https://doi.org/10.1136/archdischild-2014-306424.

13.  Heron M. Deaths: Leading causes for 2012. Nat Vital Stat Rep. 2015;64:1-93.

14.  Matthews TJ, MacDorman MF, Thoma ME. Infant mortality statistics from the 2013 period linked birth/infant death data det. Nat Vital Stat Rep. 2015;64:1-30.

15.  Moon RY. Task force on sudden infant death syndrome. SIDS and other sleep-related infant deaths: Expansion of recommendations for a safe infant sleeping environment. Pediatrics. 2011;128:1030-9. https://doi.org/10.1542/peds.2011-2284.

16.  Tursan d'Espaignet E, Bulsara M, Wolfenden L, Byard RW, Stanley FJ. Trends in sudden infant death syndrome in Australia from 1980-2002. Forensic Sci Med Pathol. 2008;4:83-90. https://doi.org/10.1007/s12024-007-9011-y.

17.  Spinelli J, Collins-Praino L, Van Den Heuvel C, Byard RW. The evolution and significance of the triple-risk model in sudden infant death syndrome (SIDS). J Paediatr Child Health. 2017;53:112-5. https://doi.org/10.1111/jpc.13429.

18. Bergman AB. Synthesis. In: Sudden infant death syndrome. Eds Bergman AB, Beckwith JB, Ray CG. Seattle, WA: University of Washington Press, 1970. p. 210-21.

19. Wedgwood RJ. Session 1. Sudden and unexpected death in infancy (cot deaths). In: Sudden and unexpected death in infancy (cot deaths). Eds Camps FE, Carpenter RG. Bristol, England: Wright, 1972. p. 22-8.

20. Emery JL. A way of looking at the causes of crib death. In: Sudden infant death syndrome. Eds Tildon JT, Roeder LM, Steinschneider A. New York: Academic Press, 1983. p. 123-32.

21. Rognum TO, Saugstad OD. Biochemical and immunological studies in SIDS victims. Clues to understanding the death mechanism. Acta Paediatr Suppl. 1993;82 Suppl 389:82-5. https://doi.org/10.1111/j.1651-2227.1993.tb12886.x.

22. Filiano JJ, Kinney HC. A perspective on neuropathologic findings in victims of the sudden infant death syndrome: The triple-risk model. Biol Neonate. 1994;65:194-7. https://doi.org/10.1159/000244052.

23. Guntheroth WG, Spiers PS. The triple risk hypothesis in sudden infant death syndrome. Pediatrics. 2002;110:e64. https://doi.org/10.1542/peds.110.5.e64.

24. Burnell RH, Byard RW. Are these really SIDS deaths?—Not by definition. J Paediatrics Child Health. 2002;38:623-4. https://doi.org/10.1046/j.1440-1754.2002.t01-2-00075.x.

25. L'Hoir MP, Engelberts AC, van Well GTJ, Westers P, Mellenbergh GJ, Wolters WH, et al. Case-control study of current validity of previously described risk factors for SIDS in the Netherlands. Arch Dis Child. 1998;79:386-93. https://doi.org/10.1136/adc.79.5.386.

26. Byard RW, Marshall D. An audit of the use of definitions of sudden infant death syndrome (SIDS). J Forensic Legal Med. 2007;14:453-5. https://doi.org/10.1016/j.jflm.2006.11.003.

27. Byard RW, Lee V. A re-audit of the use of definitions of sudden infant death syndrome (SIDS) in peer-reviewed journals. J Forensic Leg Med. 2012;19:455-6. https://doi.org/10.1016/j.jflm.2012.04.004.

28. Freemantle CJ, Read AW, de Klerk NH, McAullay D, Anderson IP, Stanley FJ. Sudden infant death syndrome and unascertainable deaths: Trends and disparities among Aboriginal and non-Aboriginal infants born in Western Australia from 1980 to 2001 inclusive. J Paediatr Child Health. 2006;42:445-51. https://doi.org/10.1111/j.1440-1754.2006.00895.x.

29. Rambaud C, Guilleminault C, Campbell PE. Definition of the sudden infant death syndrome. Brit Med J. 1994;308:1439. https://doi.org/10.1136/bmj.308.6941.1439.

30. Valdes-Dapena M, Gilbert-Barness E. Cardiovascular causes for sudden infant death. Pediatr Pathol Mol Med. 2002;21:195-211. https://doi.org/10.1080/pdp.21.2.195.211.

31. Emery JL. Is sudden infant death syndrome a diagnosis? Or is it just a diagnostic dustbin? Brit Med J. 1989;299:1240. https://doi.org/10.1136/bmj.299.6710.1240.

32. Carpenter R, McGarvey C, Mitchell EA, Tappin DM, Venneman MM, Smuk M, et al. Bed sharing when parents do not smoke: Is there a risk of SIDS? An individual level analysis of five major case-control studies. BMJ Open. 2013;3:e002299. https://doi.org/10.1136/bmjopen-2012-002299.

33. Vennemann MM, Hense H-W, Bajanowski T, Blair PS, Complojer C, Moon RY, et al. Bed sharing and the risk of sudden infant death syndrome: Can we resolve the debate? J Pediatr. 2012;160:44-8. https://doi.org/10.1016/j.jpeds.2011.06.052.

34. Byard RW, Elliott J, Vink R. Infant gender, cosleeping and sudden death. J Paediatr Child Health. 2012;48:517-9. https://doi.org/10.1111/j.1440-1754.2011.02226.x.

35. Byard RW. Bed sharing and sudden infant death syndrome. J Pediatr. 2012;160:1063. https://doi.org/10.1016/j.jpeds.2012.03.006.

36. Beckwith JB. The sudden infant death syndrome. Curr Prob Pediatr. 1973;3:1-36. https://doi.org/10.1016/S0045-9380(73)80020-9.

37. Willinger M, James LS, Catz C. Defining the sudden infant death syndrome (SIDS): Deliberations of an expert panel convened by the National Institute of Child Health and Human Development. Pediatr Pathol. 1991;11:677-84. https://doi.org/10.3109/15513819109065465.

38. Becroft DMO. An international perspective (Letter). Arch Pediatr Adol Med. 2003;157:292.

39. Byard RW. Hazardous infant and early childhood sleeping environments and death scene examination. J Clin Forensic Med. 1996;3:115-22. https://doi.org/10.1016/S1353-1131(96)90000-0.

40. Hanzlick R. Death scene investigation. In: Sudden infant death syndrome. Problems, progress and possibilities. Eds Byard RW, Krous HF. London: Arnold, 2001. p. 58-65.

41.  Cordner SM, Willinger M. The definition of the sudden infant death syndrome. In: Sudden infant death syndrome. New Trends in the nineties. Ed Rognum TO. Oslo: Scandinavian University Press, 1995. p. 17-20.

42.  Mitchell EA, Becroft DMP, Byard RW, Berry PJ, Krous HF, Helweg-Larsen K, et al. Definition of the sudden infant death syndrome. Brit Med J. 1994;309:607. https://doi.org/10.1136/bmj.309.6954.607.

43.  Sturner WQ. SIDS redux: Is it or isn't it? Am J Forensic Med Pathol. 1998;190:107-8. https://doi.org/10.1097/00000433-199806000-00001.

44.  Beckwith JB. A proposed new definition of sudden infant death syndrome. In: Second SIDS international conference. Eds Walker AM, McMillen C. Ithaca: Perinatology Press, 1993. p. 421-4.

45.  Beckwith JB. Defining the sudden infant death syndrome. Arch Pediatr Adol Med. 2003;157:286-90. https://doi.org/10.1001/archpedi.157.3.286.

46.  Mitchell EA, Krous HF. Sudden unexpected death in infancy: A historical perspective. J Paediatr Child Health. 2015;51:108-12. https://doi.org/10.1111/jpc.12818.

47.  Krous HF, Beckwith JB, Byard RW, Rognum TO, Bajanowski T, Corey T, et al. Sudden infant death syndrome and unclassified sudden infant deaths: A definitional and diagnostic approach. Pediatrics. 2004;114:234-8. https://doi.org/10.1542/peds.114.1.234.

48.  Bajanowski T, Brinkmann B, Vennemann M. The San Diego definition of SIDS: Practical application and comparison with the GeSID classification. Int J Leg Med. 2006;120:331-6. https://doi.org/10.1007/s00414-005-0043-0.

49.  Byard RW, Ranson D, Krous HF, & Workshop Participants. National Australian workshop consensus on the definition of SIDS and initiation of a uniform autopsy approach to unexpected infant and early childhood death. Forensic Sci Med Pathol. 2005;1:289-92. https://doi.org/10.1385/FSMP:1:4:289.

50.  Jensen LL, Rohde MC, Banner J, Byard RW. Reclassification of SIDS cases — A need for adjustment of the San Diego classification? Int J Leg Med. 2012;126:271-7. https://doi.org/10.1007/s00414-011-0624-z.

51.  Fleming P, Bacon C, Blair P, Berry PJ. Sudden unexpected deaths in infancy. The CESDI SUDI Studies 1993-1996. London: The Stationary Office, 2000.

52.  Blair PS, Byard RW, Fleming PJ. Sudden unexpected death in infancy (SUDI): Suggested classification and applications to facilitate research activity. Forensic Sci Med Pathol. 2012;8:312-5. https://doi.org/10.1007/s12024-011-9294-x.

53. Blair PS, Byard RW, Fleming PJ. Proposal for an international classification of SUDI. Scand J Forens Sci. 2009;15:6-9.

54. Krous HF, Chadwick AE, Crandall L, Nadeau-Manning JM. Sudden unexpected death in childhood: A report of 50 cases. Pediatr Develop Pathol. 2005;8:307-19. https://doi.org/10.1007/s10024-005-1155-8.

55. Horne RSC, Hauck FR, Moon RY. Sudden infant death syndrome and advice for safe sleeping. Brit Med J. 2015;350:h1989. https://doi.org/10.1136/bmj.h1989.

56. Byard RW. Sofa sleeping and infant death. Brit Med J. 2015;350:h1989. https://doi.org/10.1136/bmj.h1989.

57. Horne RSC, Hauck FR, Moon RY. Response to sofa sleeping and infant death by Prof Roger Byard. Brit Med J. 2015;350:h1989. https://doi.org/10.1136/bmj.h1989.

# 2 Sudden Infant Death Syndrome: An Overview

Jhodie R Duncan, PhD[1,2] and
Roger W Byard, MBBS, MD[1,2]

[1]*Florey Institute of Neuroscience and Mental Health, Victoria, Australia*
[2]*School of Medicine, The University of Adelaide, Adelaide, Australia*

## Introduction

The term sudden infant death syndrome (SIDS) was first proposed in 1969 in order to focus attention on a subgroup of infants with similar clinical features whose deaths occurred unexpectedly in the postnatal period (1). Today the definition of SIDS refers to death in a seemingly healthy infant younger than 1 year of age whose death remains unexplained after a thorough case investigation including a complete autopsy, review of medical and clinical history, and death scene investigation (2). SIDS is typically associated with a sleep period (3) with death presumed to have occurred during sleep itself or in the transition between sleep and waking (4). This led to application of the terms "cot" or "crib" death; however, these terms are rarely used today. Furthermore, while the definition is inclusive of infants up to 1 year of age, approximately 95% of SIDS deaths occur in the first six months of life with a peak incidence in infants aged between 2 to 4 months (5). While there are distinctive features associated with the syndrome there are no diagnostic features that can be attributed to a SIDS death. Indeed, application of the term relies on a process of elimination and when no known cause of death or contributing factors can be determined, the term SIDS is usually applied. Thus, while the debate continues regarding the definition and use of the term

SIDS, and no one definition has been universally accepted, one certainty persists, and that is that SIDS still remains a diagnosis of exclusion (1).

## History

Sudden death in a seemingly healthy infant during sleep is not a phenomenon of modern times, with cases being recorded throughout history for thousands of years. Indeed, one of the first cases is mentioned in the Bible (1 Kings 3:19). However, these deaths have generally been attributed to overlaying, as it was common practice to sleep in the same bed as a child. Indeed, the death of an infant by "overlay" was considered such an issue that by the seventh century the event was a punishable offence (6), with the introduction of a "protective" wooden arcuccio for infants to sleep in during the 18th century in Europe with severe penalties if the infant died in a co-sleeping arrangement and the frame was not used (7). By the 19th century the belief that the death of infants during sleep was due to overlaying was so entrenched that death was still attributed to this despite evidence suggesting otherwise (8), with calls for co-sleeping of parents and children to be illegal, especially if the parents were in an intoxicated state (9). This belief was maintained for the next 100 years (1). While fewer deaths are attributed to overlaying in modern times, it is often impossible to exclude this possibility when death has occurred in a bed-sharing situation, which often leads to a diagnosis of "undetermined".

As evidence built in the late 19th century that infants deaths were occurring without being associated with bed sharing (and thus overlaying), new theories of the factors mediating infant deaths began to arise. In 1830, Kopp's "thymic asthma" proposed that enlargement of the thymus in some infants resulted in a build-up of pressure leading to tracheal obstruction (10). Others suggested intrinsic asphyxial mechanisms (8), suffocation catarrh (11), superstition or the actions of witches and gods (12, 13) as the cause of sudden death. Although many theories have been discredited they have led to strong followings; the theory of status thymicolymphaticus, for example, was popular for over 30 years and resulted in over 800 publications, the most recent as late as 1959 (14). Even today, evidence is presented for numerous theories relating to the mechanisms mediating sudden death in infants (see below). Most recently a "wear and tear" hypothesis has been presented that suggests that "SIDS is the result of cumulative painful, stressful, or traumatic exposures that begin in utero and tax neonatal regulatory systems incompatible with allostasis" (15). The authors argue that SIDS will be highest in winter-born premature male infants who are circumcised due to increased vulnerability to seasonal illness and stimulation of nocioreceptors during removal of the foreskin. However, like many contradictory theories in the past, this prediction lacks conclusive evidence.

While explanation for sudden death in certain infants remains incomplete, the term SIDS was only accepted as an official diagnosis on death certificates in 1971, with the term "sudden infant death" being allocated a separate code (coding number 798.0) in the World Health Organization's International Classification of Diseases in 1979 (13).

## Incidence

There has been a dramatic decrease in the incidence of SIDS since the introduction of safe sleep campaigns, with a 30-83% reduction in the SIDS rate (16-18). While, historically, rates have been recorded as high as 2-6 per 1,000 live births (19), they currently stand at 0.2-0.5 per 1,000 live births in most countries (18), although this rate can be heavily influenced by factors such as geographical location, climate, and ethnicity, as discussed below.

While the rate of SIDS has decreased, it is also important to note that the use of the term SIDS is becoming increasingly controversial and there has been a diagnostic shift in recent years. This has resulted in a decrease in the application of the term as a diagnosis with many professionals classifying cases into other categories and employing terms such as "undetermined", "unknown", "unascertained" or "ill-defined" despite the fact that cases fulfil the criteria for SIDS (20). Thus it is possible that changes in terminology could be partially responsible for the reduction in SIDS rate, as opposed to there having been an actual reduction in the number of deaths.

## Diagnosis

One issue when applying the term "SIDS" is that there are no diagnostic features that can be attributed to a SIDS death, and thus application of the term relies on a process of elimination. When no known cause of death or contributing factors can be determined, the term SIDS is utilised. This leads the way to a large window of interpretation as to how the term can, and when it should, be used, especially considering that not all SIDS cases have the same characteristics. In the past, SIDS has been applied to cases even when the investigation does not fulfil the required definitions (21, 22) and an autopsy has not been performed (23). Indeed, it is estimated that an alternative diagnosis could have been made in up to 25% of SIDS cases or more (24, 25). Thus it is highly recommended that investigators use the Sudden Unexplained Infant Death Investigation (SUIDI) reporting forms devised by the Centers for Disease Control (26) in order to standardise data collection, increase uniformity across different medical examiners offices, and thus make the classification of the cause of death more uniform.

As stated above, the current definition of SIDS typically refers to an infant younger than 1 year of age whose death remains unexplained after a thorough case investigation including a death scene investigation, complete autopsy, and review of medical and clinical history (2). This definition also provides subcategories (as outlined in Chapter 1), which were introduced in an attempt to assist with classification and diagnosis.

The initial investigation of the death scene should combine the expertise of both law enforcement and medical personnel and should include, at a minimum, documentation of the sleep environment, the position that the infant was placed to sleep in, and the position in which he or she was found. This would preferably include photographic and video evidence and re-enactment using a doll of a similar size to the infant. In addition, information pertinent to understanding factors that may have contributed to the death — including (but not limited to) time and circumstances surrounding death, room temperature, details of household activities prior to the death, details regarding clothing and bedding, and any unusual features — should also be collected (27).

In combination with a full death scene investigation, a comprehensive autopsy utilising accepted protocols (25) such as the International Standardized Autopsy Protocol (ISAP) should be completed. Ideally, this would include full external and internal examinations, the latter complemented by radiology of internal structures, histological analysis for pathology of all major internal organs including the brain and liver, toxicology analysis, assessment for the presence of infectious agents, electrolyte and metabolic studies, and molecular/genetic studies. However, it should be noted that some facilities do not have access to all of these diagnostic techniques.

As part of a routine autopsy, and to complement the findings at autopsy, assessment of the infant's medical history should also be undertaken. This will aid in determining whether the infant had a history of potentially lethal conditions that may have contributed to death. This history should include details pertaining to the pregnancy and delivery (including type of delivery and any noted complications), method of feeding, and immunization status. Ideally, a full family history should also be reviewed to provide insight into parental illnesses and disorders, especially if a history of maternal drug use is present, including smoking habits, particularly of the mother during pregnancy. This history should also provide details as to whether there is a history of illness in siblings of the infant, including any previous deaths, as these may provide information relative to the presence of lethal inherited diseases or potential homicide. Therefore, without rigorous and in-depth investigation, there is a high potential that the cause of death could be labeled as SIDS based on incomplete or poor evaluation of the death instead of being labeled as a true "unknown" cause. It is also important to note that, despite fulfilling the requirements for a SIDS definition, some deaths may be listed as undetermined or ill-defined.

## Risk Factors for SIDS

The cause of sudden death in some infants has long been proposed to be multifactorial, involving interactions of a variety of factors (28); each factor alone is not sufficient to cause death, but may, when expressed or experienced in combination with one or more other factors, result in death. This theory was first presented as the multiple contingency hypothesis in 1972 by Wedgwood, who believed SIDS was most likely to occur when

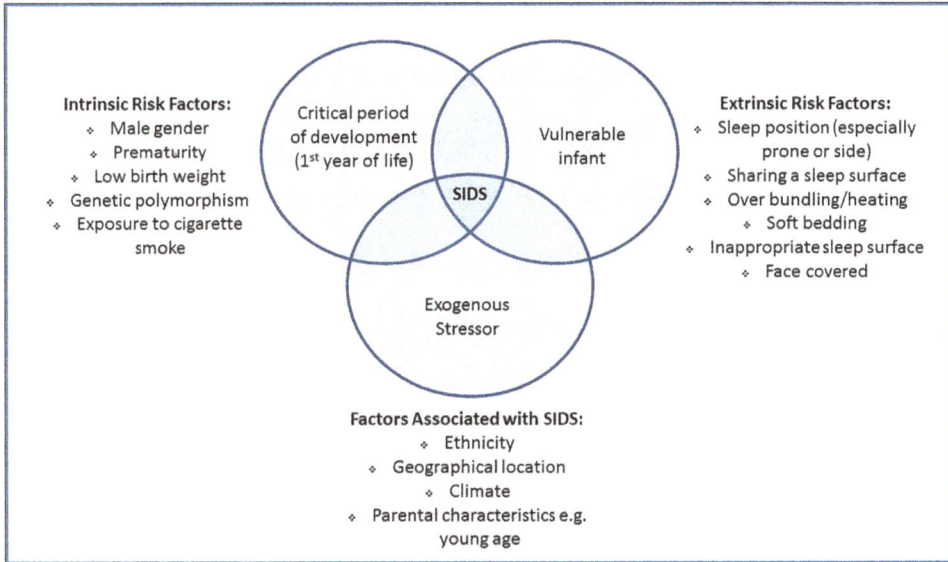

Figure 2.1: Triple Risk Model for SIDS proposed by Filiano and colleagues in 1994, highlighting the intrinsic, extrinsic and additional risk factors for SIDS. (Adapted from (32).)

three overlapping factors occurred simultaneously (29). This was shortly followed by Emery's interrelated causal spheres of influence model and Rognum and Saugstad's fatal triangle (30). While the emphasis varied, all placed the focus on a multifactorial cause of death.

In 1994, Filiano and Kinney proposed the "Triple Risk Model" for SIDS (31), which today stands as one of the most accepted models in the field. As with the previous theories, the Triple Risk Model proposes that SIDS is not due to a single common pathway but that interrelated and overlapping factors combine to increase risk. Specifically, Filiano and Kinney posit that SIDS results from the simultaneous occurrence in an infant of a critical developmental period (i.e. the first year of life), the presence of an underlying vulnerability that increases susceptibility (i.e. unrecognised pathology), and exposure to an exogenous stressor (i.e. being placed in a prone position for sleep) (Figure 2.1). When these factors align, the risk for SIDS is believed to be the greatest. The group further went on to propose that the risks for SIDS could be considered as either intrinsic or extrinsic, where intrinsic factors affect susceptibility and extrinsic factors represent physical stressors experienced around the time of death (see below) (32). While SIDS is not exclusive to infants with intrinsic or extrinsic risk factors, the importance of their role is demonstrated by the fact that at least one risk factor (and sometimes more) is present in approximately 90% of all SIDS cases, with very few SIDS cases reported where no extrinsic risk factors are present (32).

## Developmental period

By definition, for a death to be classified as SIDS it must occur in an infant some time before their first birthday. Sudden and unexpected death can occur after the age of 1, though these deaths would be classified as sudden and unexplained death in childhood (SUDC), which has a much lower incidence (currently 1.4 to 1.8 deaths per 100,000 children) (33, 34). While death can occur at any time during the first year, approximately 90% of cases happen in the first six months of life, and there is an increased incidence between 2 and 4 months of age, a period when the infant brain is undergoing dramatic neurodevelopmental changes, especially to systems controlling homeostatic control (5).

## Intrinsic risk factors

As mentioned above, intrinsic risk factors affect the vulnerability of the infant, increasing susceptibility to the influence of extrinsic risks. These factors include male sex, prematurity, low birth weight, genetic polymorphisms, and prenatal exposure to drugs, particularly nicotine (from cigarettes) and alcohol. Intrinsic risk factors are normally not modifiable, with the exception of exposure to maternal cigarette smoking or alcohol consumption during pregnancy. Although these could also be considered extrinsic risk factors (such as would occur via exposure to second-hand smoke after birth), as maternal exposure during pregnancy causes the highest risk for SIDS it will be presented in this section.

### Sex, prematurity, and low birth weight

There is clear evidence that the incidence of SIDS is higher in males than females (35), with a ratio of 60 to 40 respectively (5). While some suggest male vulnerability is influenced by sex differences in genetic and biological makeup, it is not clear why the incidence of SIDS is higher in males, and this may simply be a reflection of the fact that male infants are more vulnerable to illness and disease than females, with males having a generally greater mortality rate overall (36). Prematurity and low birth weight also increase the risk for SIDS fourfold (37, 38), the most likely reason being the associated increased vulnerability in these infants due to immature autonomic systems.

### Genetic polymorphisms

Unlike conditions such as Down Syndrome, where the presence of a third copy of chromosome 21 results in the phenotype, to date there has been no one gene identified in the etiology of SIDS. However, this does not exclude the possibility that some infants may carry unidentified genetic mutations or polymorphisms that interact with environmental or endogenous factors in complex ways, thus increasing their susceptibility to SIDS. A recent sequencing study of 161 SIDS infants by Neubauer et al. in 2017 identified potentially causative gene variants in 20% of their SIDS cases. These were associated with ion channelopathies (9%), cardiomyopathies (7%), and metabolic diseases (1%) (39). While it should be noted that the authors of this study focused specifically on genes associated with cardiovascular and metabolic diseases, mutations in cardiac ion channels, for example, could contribute to lethal arrhythmia and may explain sudden death in some infants. Others have reported differences in the expression of up to 17 genes in SIDS infants compared to controls, including three genes involved in mediating inflammatory responses (40). There have also been reports of polymorphisms in the promoter region of the serotonin transporter gene, which could result in altered serotonin uptake and regulation, supporting pathological and neurochemical studies reporting serotonergic dysfunction in SIDS (41, 42). Both Narita et al. (43) and Weese-Mayer et al. (44) reported an increase in the "L" allele in SIDS cases across different ethnic groups. The L allele is responsible for increasing the effectiveness of the promoter region of the serotonin transporter gene and thus an increased expression should lead to reduced serotonin concentrations. However, these findings have not been replicated in all studies (45, 46). In addition, findings of genetic abnormalities in SIDS vary across groups, with polymorphisms also being reported in genes for sodium channels, complement C4 and interleukin 10 (involved in immunity), and genes involved in the development of the autonomic nervous system, such as paired-like homeobox 2a and rearranged during transfection factor (RET) (47).

Two issues remain when trying to interpret the significance of gene mutations in SIDS. First, the rarity of multiple SIDS death in a family limits our ability to study the contribution of familial or inherited genetic abnormalities (see below). Second, many screening studies investigating genetic mutations in SIDS cases often identify several differences between groups in genes that have non-specific or heterogeneous functions; thus understanding the resultant consequences of changes to one or several genes becomes difficult.

## Prenatal exposure to drugs including maternal cigarette smoking

Maternal cigarette smoking increases the relative risk for SIDS up to fivefold, with additional risks from postnatal exposure (48, 49). Despite evidence that smoking during pregnancy can be harmful, approximately 13% of women continue to smoke during this period (50). These numbers may be as high as 75% in some high-risk and Indigenous populations (51). Furthermore, the prevalence of maternal smoking during pregnancy in SIDS mothers has increased from 50% to 80% (49), such that in the wake of reductions in prone sleeping, exposure to cigarette smoke is now considered the dominate modifiable risk factor for SIDS (49). In addition, exposure to second-hand cigarette smoke both prior to, and after, birth also impacts on infant wellbeing (52), so that recommendations now state that mothers should not smoke during pregnancy, and infants should be in a smoke-free environment in order to reduce the risk of SIDS.

While the exact mechanism of how maternal smoking increases SIDS risk is still to be fully elucidated, it has been hypothesised that nicotine (the major neurotoxic component in cigarette smoke) is able to cross the placenta into the fetal circulation where it binds to endogenous neuronal nicotinic acetylcholine receptors present in the fetal brain (53). These receptors are widely expressed in the fetal brain from as early as 4-5 weeks' gestation (54). Exogenous nicotine may bind to and inappropriately stimulate the function of these receptors. Indeed, there are several studies highlighting the impacts of prenatal cigarette smoking on fetal physiology including impaired arousability (55), changes to the apneic index for obstructive events during sleep (56), and altered parasympathetic control of heart rate (57) to name just a few. The processes by which this occurs are hypothesized to include the ability of nicotine (or other active ingredients in cigarette smoke) to control cell survival, affect neurite outgrowth, and regulate transmitter release (due to co-expression of these receptors on non-cholinergic neurons) (53) and synapse formation (see (58)). It has also been suggested that exposure to cigarette smoke in utero reduces lung capacity, thus resulting in chronic hypoxia after birth, or alternatively increases the risk of respiratory tract infection, both increasing infant vulnerability.

While the literature suggests that drug use, including cocaine and alcohol consumption, is associated with an increased risk for SIDS (59, 60), a direct relationship is often harder to determine due to the confounds of poly-drug use and environmental factors such as socioeconomic status. We do know that drug use, including cocaine and cigarettes, during pregnancy increases the risk of prematurity and low birth weight (61), themselves both associated with an increased risk for SIDS. Furthermore, infants born to mothers with a history of drug use are known to have altered physiology, including altered heart rate and fetal movements (62).

## Extrinsic risk factors

Extrinsic risk factors represent physical stressors experienced around the time of death and often relate to the environment that the infant faces. These factors include sleep position (especially prone sleep position), sharing a sleep surface, over-bundling/over-heating, soft bedding, inappropriate sleep surfaces, and having the infant's face covered.

### Sleep position

The majority of SIDS deaths occur in association with a sleep period, with infants most often found dead in their cots (63). However, there is no association with any particular sleep period, with deaths attributed to SIDS occurring at any time of the day (64). Thus it is not surprising that sleep position, especially prone sleep position, which places additional physiological stress on cardiorespiratory systems, is the most significant environmental or "extrinsic" risk factor for SIDS. Indeed, prone sleeping (whether the infant is placed in this position or they move into this position during their sleep period) is estimated to increase the risk of SIDS by up to 14-fold (65).

The mechanism of death attributed to prone sleeping is often suffocation, and while suffocation is a valid possibility in some cases, it does not account for all deaths. Therefore, there are numerous theories relating to the factors that contribute to death while an infant is in the prone position. These include, but are not limited to, the face-down position resulting in oxygen deprivation leading to hypoxia, rebreathing of carbon dioxide leading to hypercarbia, reduced arousal responses and increased waking thresholds (especially to exogenous stimuli), compromised cerebral blood flow, airway obstruction, splinting of the diaphragm, altered cardiovascular capacity, and increased body temperature (66-68).

Despite no clear mechanisms being identified, the recognition that prone sleeping position plays a role in infant death was first reported in 1944 (69), and in SIDS deaths some 20 years later. However, the recommendation to place infants on their stomachs to sleep continued until the late 1980s. It is estimated that during this period prone sleep recommendations may have contributed to the unnecessary deaths of an estimated 60,000 infants (70). Publications highlighting the association between prone sleep position and sudden death in infants saw a decrease in the number of infants being placed prone to sleep and this was closely mirrored by a fall in SIDS deaths, confirming the strong association (71). In the late 1980s and early 1990s this led to the initiation of "Reducing the Risk" and "Back to Sleep" campaigns, which saw a dramatic decrease in the number of SIDS deaths (72); in some countries this was as high as a 73-83% reduction in the average number of deaths per year (16, 17).

While the numbers of SIDS infants found prone has gone down by nearly 50% since safe sleep campaigns were introduced, there has been little decline in the incidence of SIDS since 2006, suggesting that other extrinsic factors may be present. Thus it is also not surprising that the number of deaths associated with other known risk factors such as prematurity and bed sharing have increased 18% and 9% respectively (32) since this time. It is also important to note that, even with the success of safe sleep messaging, some health workers continue to use non-supine positioning and promote incorrect sleep positions to parents (73). In the study by Patton et al., "fear of aspiration" during sleep was the primary reason given for not choosing supine positioning (73), despite the fact that the incidence of deaths associated with the aspiration of gastric contents has not changed since the recommendation of supine sleep position (74).

Side sleeping position also increases the risk for SIDS, some studies reporting this risk to be similar to that of the prone position (75). This is often attributed to the ease with which infants can roll onto their stomachs, as many SIDS infants who were placed on their side to sleep were subsequently found prone at the time of death. In addition, the risk for SIDS is increased by changing an infant's sleep position to one that they are not accustomed to, especially sleeping prone for the first time when an infant would normally sleep supine (76).

## Sharing a sleep surface

Evidence from over 20 years in the United Kingdom indicates a significant increase from 12% to 50% in the number of SIDS/unexpected deaths associated with a shared sleep environment (77). These data support the argument that sharing a sleep surface, primarily beds and couches/sofas, increases the risk for infant death (78) due to the proposed potential for overlaying, suffocation, or overheating. This risk increases more when there is a history of prematurity or low birth weight, when more than one adult is present on the sleep surface, or when additional factors are present such as obesity, sedation, intoxication, or cigarette smoking (especially maternal smoking during pregnancy) in the person sharing the sleeping space with the infant (79, 80), or when the infant shares the sleep space for the entire night, or is younger than 11 weeks of age (81). However, sharing sleep surfaces with an infant is not a phenomenon specific to modern times and remains a common practice in many communities worldwide, without an associated increase in SIDS/infant deaths (82). Thus it could be argued that contemporary practices — in particular, the use of soft bedding — make sharing a sleep surface dangerous. Furthermore, sharing a sleep surface facilitates breastfeeding (83), which is thought to reduce the risk of SIDS (84). Therefore, further studies in this area are needed in order to fully understand why these differences exist. While bed sharing increases the risk for SIDS/infant deaths, safe sleep recommendations advocate infants sleeping near their parents or caregivers, as this decreases risks (85). There is no increase in the risk for SIDS for sleeping infants held in bed with an awake caregiver.

## Soft bedding and inappropriate sleep surfaces

Sleep surfaces, and in particular soft bedding, also contribute to the risk of SIDS/unexpected infant death independent of sleep position; however, the risk is substantially higher again should the infant be placed prone (86). Soft surfaces, such as mattress and sheepskins, are thought to result in a potential "trough" when the surface depresses under the weight of the infant (87). In this situation, the infant may not be able to extricate themselves, resulting in the potential for suffocation, asphyxia, or overheating. Blankets and pillows may also constitute soft sleep surfaces, and may, in addition to the above, increase the risk of face covering (81). Importantly, the risk of infant death is greatly increased if infants are left to sleep on a couch or sofa, with an odds ratio as high as 66.9, especially if this occurs in association with sharing this surface with an adult (more so than bed sharing) (78).

## Overheating, over-bundling and covering of the face

A study by Kleemann et al. found that profuse sweating was present at the time of death in 36% of SIDS cases (88), suggesting that hyperthermia plays a role in some SIDS deaths. This has been attributed to endogenous factors including infections, immature central thermoregulatory centers, or increased amounts of brown adipose fat (89);

it suggests an additional intrinsic risk in these infants. However, overheating due to over-bundling, increased ambient room temperature, or covering of the face or head is most likely to be attributed to exogenous factors, thus serving as an extrinsic risk factor (88). These extrinsic risks have the highest incidence when ambient temperatures fall and there is overcompensation. Indeed, over-bundling and thus presumably overheating during a sleep period is considered an independent risk factor for SIDS (90). Understandably, covering of the face may not only increase the risk for overheating but may also contribute to the risk for SIDS due to the increased chance of suffocation, asphyxia, decreased respiratory function, hypoxia, and hypercapnia.

## Additional characteristics of SIDS cases

The above-mentioned risk factors are well documented to contribute to SIDS deaths; however, there are several additional factors that have also been shown to have an impact upon SIDS rates. Therefore, it is presumed that these factors influence the vulnerability of certain infants and could themselves be considered risks, though the means by which they impact on SIDS cases is not always evident. These factors include geographical location, climate, ethnicity, and certain parental characteristics. It is also worth discussing here the potential of altered sleep patterns in SIDS infants, and instances where there are multiple deaths of siblings in a single family, suggesting that the vulnerability may be inherited.

### Geographic location and climate

Geographical location has a considerable influence on the number of infant deaths, with SIDS rates varying considerably across the globe (27). SIDS is also more common in colder climates than in warmer climates; likewise, it is more common during winter months than at other, warmer times of the year (91, 92). This is not a reflection of age, as the month (and thus season) in which an infant is born per se has no effect on the rate of SIDS (91). It is possible that the same factors that cause an increase in numbers of cases in winter months will also act for a longer time in colder climates. However, it should also be noted that the incidence of SIDS during colder months has decreased since the introduction of risk campaigns; in some geographical locations, such as Alaska and Sweden, where winter temperatures are extremely low, there was no evidence of a winter peak even prior to the era of safe sleep campaigns (93). It is also possible that the influence of geographical location and climate is driven more by different childcare practices or diagnostic protocols than actual location, which should be considered when comparing rates across countries.

### Ethnicity

Ethnicity has been shown to be associated with the incidence of SIDS (94). The incidence of SIDS is lower in individuals with an Asian heritage (95), with a higher incidence reported in African-American (37) and Indigenous populations (96). For example, Native Americans of the Aberdeen Area of the Northern Plains have a rate of 3.5/1,000 live births, almost 7 times greater than the overall United States rate (96). However, these findings have not always been validated once socioeconomic factors, maternal history, and the presence of risk factors have been controlled for (97). In addition, the potential effects of ethnicity may be impacted by geographical location. For example, Californian infants with an Asian heritage have a higher rate of SIDS compared to Asian infants living in their country of ethnic origin (95). Again, consideration of different childcare practices should be made when interpreting the incidence of SIDS across different ethnic groups and assigning a potential genetic predisposition (98).

### Parental characteristics

Young paternal age (<20 years) is considered to increase the risk for SIDS, despite the fact that SIDS infants in younger parents are less likely to be the firstborn child (35). Single maternal marital status (99), complications during pregnancy, fewer prenatal examinations (35), multiple births (38), and admission for psychiatric treatment of either parent, especially drug-related disorders (100), have also been implicated in the etiology of SIDS.

### Sleep patterns

There is evidence to suggest that infants dying of SIDS have altered sleep patterns and altered responses to stressors while asleep. For example, in 1992 Schechtman and colleagues showed that SIDS infants have decreased waking time and therefore more sleep during the early morning period with more rapid eye movement (REM) periods throughout the night compared to controls (101). Abnormalities have also been noted in the organization, structure, and level of maturation of sleep in a group of "near-miss" SIDS infants (102). Furthermore, functions such as autoresuscitation and arousals during sleep are also altered in SIDS (101); these functions are especially vulnerable to the influence of maternal cigarette smoking during pregnancy (103). Thus it is possible that altered sleep states impact an infant's ability to respond to stressors, potentially increasing their vulnerability during sleep.

### Sibling deaths

The association of SIDS deaths amongst siblings is still debated. There have been reports of an increase in the incidence of SIDS of between two and ten times in infants who have had a sibling or twin death, including an increase risk based on the presence of SIDS in second- and third-degree relatives (104, 105). However, some of these outcomes have been explained once environmental and maternal factors have been controlled for and these families may only represent a small subgroup of individuals with increased vulnerability. There have also been reports of simultaneous sudden death in siblings supporting a genetic basis (106), although the importance of environmental factors should be taken into consideration under these circumstances. In addition, a report by Diamond et. al. indicated five consecutive sibling deaths in the same family (107), However, the authors feel that multiple deaths within the same family should raise concerns about other possible inherited conditions such as prolonged QT interval or metabolic disorders, homicide or potentially misclassified deaths of known cause. Thus, while multiple SIDS deaths in the one family may represent a genetic component in the etiology of SIDS, for 92% of families the risk of recurrence is considered small (105).

## Mechanisms Underlying SIDS Deaths

Based on the fact that the definition of SIDS is dependent on the elimination of known causes of death, it is not surprising that there are no identifiable mechanisms underlying these deaths. This has led to a vast number of theories on the mechanisms responsible for SIDS. Chapters throughout this book will provide in-depth discussions on the proposed causation of SIDS, but below is a short summary of some of the current theories, all of which, obviously, have yet to be fully substantiated. It is also worth noting that in many studies there is a lack of comparative "normal controls", which complicates our ability to interpret whether entities present in SIDS infants represent a primary cause of death or act as a secondary, or even an unrelated, phenomenon. Indeed, the authors of this chapter, along with others, are of the opinion that infant deaths attributed to SIDS are likely to represent a mixed population with various etiologies and disease entities contributing to one common endpoint (i.e. death) rather than all deaths being attributed to one single cause (108).

### Respiration and respiratory function

Respiratory failure has long been thought to contribute to sudden and unexpected infant deaths (109), especially considering that sleep heightens the possibility of airway obstruction and apparent life-threatening events such as apneas. Furthermore, SIDS infants are hypothesized to have defects in respiratory control resulting in altered respiratory function, prolonged periods of "breath holding", a failure of autoresuscitation, and defective arousal mechanisms (specifically, a failure to arouse to altered oxygen or carbon dioxide levels) (110-113). While some studies have reported mixed and obstructive respiratory events (114) or altered ventilatory control (115) prior to death in infants who subsequently died of SIDS, others have shown no difference in breathing patterns or respiratory rates (at least during regular breathing) (116), thus making integration of respiratory-related issues for SIDS difficult.

In SIDS cases there have been a number of anatomical abnormalities reported that are similar to those reported in obstructive sleep apnea/hypopnea syndromes (117), and thus it could be argued that these contribute to the respiratory issues hypothesised to exist in SIDS infants. These include retrognathic facial abnormalities such as retroposition of the maxilla, narrowing of the nasal passages, shallow temporomandibular joints, and enlargement of the tongue (117, 118). However, these abnormalities are not present in all cases and are not sufficient to enable a SIDS diagnosis to be made.

Siren recently postulated that SIDS occurs due to critical failure of the diaphragm (SIDS-critical diaphragm failure hypothesis) as a result of the increased respiratory workload following exposure to exogenous stressors leading to cessation of breathing and death (119). Others have suggested that abnormalities in peripheral airway stretch receptors, changes to peripheral sensory chemoreceptors including the carotid body, or dysfunction or immaturity in centrally located brainstem networks controlling upper airway functions could also contribute to respiratory issues, by increasing the risk for events such as apneas, or by reducing autonomic responses to airway obstruction during sleep (113).

Suggestions of respiratory-related mechanisms in SIDS have led to theories regarding an apparent protective effect of dummies/pacifiers, as supported by a recent meta-analysis by Alm and colleagues (120). It is thought that their use increases arousability, maintains airway patency and increases airway tone, and alters heart rate variability, thus improving autonomic tone (121). However, it should also be noted that there is contradictory evidence as to whether dummy or pacifier use interferes with the establishment of breastfeeding (itself thought to reduce the risk of SIDS) (122), and therefore caution should be given to the initiation of their use.

## Hypoxia and hypoventilation

Due to evidence of repetitive apneas and hypoxic gasping prior to death in some SIDS cases (123), it has long been proposed that SIDS infants succumb to death due to repeated episodes of hypoxic/ischemic injury. In support of this theory, studies have reported subtle morphological changes in the liver, adipose tissue, and heart and circulatory system, which could be attributed to a chronic hypoxic state (27), though the findings remain inconclusive. In contrast, others have not reported changes to markers that would be expected to be altered following chronic hypoventilation — such as serum erythropoietin levels, for example (124), and, with the exception of some reports, brainstem gliosis (125). There is also a lack of significant evidence at autopsy of hypoxic-related changes (126). Furthermore, our own studies have illustrated differences in neurochemical and enzymatic levels in the brainstem between infants who had chronic hypoxia-ischemia and those classified as SIDS (41), suggesting an alternative mechanism (or mechanisms) related to death other than impaired oxygenation.

## Cardiovascular function

It has been suggested that arrhythmia and cardiovascular changes are responsible for death in SIDS infants (127). This is driven by evidence proposing altered heart rate and heart rate variability; defects in centrally mediated cardiac control, primarily brainstem centers; autonomic imbalances and abnormal conduction pathways, including a left-handed His bundle (27, 128, 129); prolongation of the QT interval (the time from ventricular depolarization to repolarization) early in life (130); and severe bradycardia (with and without apnea) (131). While entities with known abnormalities of cardiac conduction are associated with sudden death, as with the issues around respiratory function mentioned above, there are considerable difficulties in proving a cardiac cause for SIDS, with some studies failing to report any differences in cardiovascular function (116). Furthermore, anatomical abnormalities related to cardiovascular function, if present, often exclude a diagnosis of SIDS, and in such cases, though they may be present, do not contribute to the cause of death (132).

## Gastrointestinal function

While aspiration of gastric contents into the lungs or airways has been proposed as a possible cause of sudden death, it does not appear to be a valid marker for SIDS and can often be explained as a secondary event that has occurred after death (133). It has been proposed that reflux of gastric contents into the upper aerodigestive tract without aspiration may contribute to SIDS, as infants who suffer gastroesophageal reflux also manifest respiratory issues (134, 135). Besides the potential of airway obstruction, it has been suggested that reflux may also result in stimulation of peripheral esophageal receptors resulting in vagally mediated fatal apnea or bradycardia (136), or that some infants may have altered laryngeal receptor function upon stimulation (137). However, signs of reflux have not been consistently observed in SIDS cases (138) and are common in early infancy.

## Nervous system abnormalities

There is a large body of literature suggesting that nervous system dysfunction plays a role in SIDS, especially in particular brainstem regions (41, 139, 140). These changes have been attributed to either abnormal development or to maturational delay, and are hypothesised to play a key role in SIDS due to their direct influence over homeostatic processes including cardiorespiratory control, sleep regulation, and arousal (41, 139-141). Furthermore, marked changes in neural control (including within brainstem regions) overlap the peak period for SIDS, i.e. 2 to 4 months of age (53). However, our ability to fully understand changes to nervous system processes in SIDS is often limited due to contradictory findings in the literature and our ability to apply histological and molecular techniques to examine post-mortem specimens (due to rapid deterioration of tissues after death).

### Central nervous system

Abnormalities in the brains of infants who have been classified as SIDS have been reported, including increased brain weight (142), and this is not attributed to simple edema or to cerebral anomalies. At the cellular level, studies have demonstrated focal granule cell bilamination in the dentate gyrus of the hippocampus (143), arcuate nucleus hypoplasia in the ventral medulla (144), altered development of the hypoglossal nucleus (145), altered neuronal cell number (140), changes to dendritic spines (141), and increased cerebral β-amyloid precursor protein (β-APP) expression (146). The latter study also showed that the expression of β-APP in SIDS cases was related to sleep environment, with a higher expression in infants sleeping alone compared to those bed sharing, possibly suggesting different mechanisms relating to death in these two populations. Periventricular and subcortical white matter changes (147) and brainstem gliosis in the nucleus of the solitary tract and inferior olive (141, 148) have also been reported. These changes have been attributed to ischemic damage, with ischemic necrosis also noted in these regions (149); however, many pathological findings overlap with observations from controls (150) and thus appear to have little diagnostic utility. Furthermore, while all of these abnormalities have the potential to alter brain function, it should be noted that the majority of these studies report findings in a subset of SIDS infants only (ranging from 20% to 94% across four publications alone) (141, 143, 146, 147), demonstrating that these changes are not present in all cases.

*Neurotransmitter abnormalities*

There are variable reports of altered neurotransmitter levels and changes to receptor systems in SIDS infants, with the majority of these focusing on brainstem regions. These have included changes to growth factors; cytokines; neuropeptides; and the catecholaminergic; cholinergic; and serotonergic systems (see (151) for an in-depth review). For example, Denoroy and colleagues reported a decrease in dopamine-β-hydroxylase and phenylethanolamine-N-methyltransferase in the medulla in SIDS infants, suggesting changes in the activity of central catecholaminergic neurons (152); however, Duncan and colleagues saw no difference in dopamine levels in the medulla (41). There have also been reports of increased levels of substance-P in the medulla (153), reduced gamma-aminobutyric acid (A) receptor binding and subunit protein expression (154), and subunit specific changes to nicotinic acetylcholine receptors (155). However, the reported differences in neurotransmitter or receptor expression between SIDS cases and control cases can further be influenced by factors such as maternal cigarette smoking during pregnancy (155), highlighting the importance of accounting for these factors when trying to interpret neurochemical changes.

There have also been reports of a number of differences in markers of the serotonergic system, suggesting that serotonergic abnormalities in the medullary network may play a key role in SIDS due to the fact that serotonergic pathways in this region impact on virtually all homeostatic processes (41, 140). These findings have been validated across four independent cohorts, which reported a reduction in the levels of serotonin 1A receptors in medullary nuclei containing serotonergic neurons and their projection sites in the same cases (140). These studies have also shown that SIDS infants have an increase in the number of serotonergic neurons in this region, though these neurons displayed an immature neuronal morphology (140) which may aid in the explanation of the observed reduction in the levels of serotonin in the raphe nucleus in these infants (41). SIDS infants also have reduced tryptophan hydroxylase2 (the key biosynthetic enzyme required for serotonin production) in the raphe obscurus, suggesting that SIDS infants may not be able to produce adequate serotonin levels (41); however the factors mediating reduced tryptophan hydroxylase2 levels remain undetermined.

While the literature on the central nervous system to date is heavily focused on the brainstem, more recent studies have reported changes to regions of the brain beyond the brainstem. Hunt and colleagues have shown a decrease in the immunoreactivity for orexin neurons, not only in the pons, but also in regions of the hypothalamus (156). Orexin plays a key role in the regulation of arousal and wakefulness, and thus changes to the levels of orexin are arguably well positioned to aid in the explanation of impaired arousal in SIDS.

Thus while limitations do exist with assessing changes in post-mortem tissues and the examples above are by no means all-inclusive, and numerous other pathological and neurochemical changes have been implicated in SIDS, they are suggestive of central nervous system abnormalities (particularly to brainstem regions) contributing to death in at least a subset of SIDS cases. However, due to the interrelated nature of central nervous system pathways, it is unlikely that changes to neurotransmitters system occur in isolation.

Peripheral nervous system

It is also possible that changes to peripheral nervous systems may impact on SIDS. Studies have reported histological changes such as a prominence of the dark variant of chief cells in the carotid bodies in SIDS cases (157). Changes such as this may suggest exposure to sustained hypoxemia and have the potential to impact the ability of chemoreceptors to respond adequately to changes in oxygen levels. However, interpretation of the role that changes to chemoreceptors play in SIDS is difficult, as conflicting outcomes regarding carotid body size, histological changes, and the number of neurosecretory granules and transmitter levels have been reported (157-159). As peripheral and central networks are highly integrated, it is likely that a change in one system may subsequently affect the other, and thus that both processes contribute to nervous system dysfunction in SIDS.

## Immune responses and infectious agents

Anecdotal evidence of "a mild cold" or upper respiratory infection (32) close to the time of death, the presence of markers of infection and inflammation, and a peak incidence in winter months in many SIDS infants has led to the hypothesis that SIDS infants are immunologically incompetent and that stimulation of the immune system may contribute to death (160). Indeed, increased levels of immunoglobulins (including IgG, IgM and IgA) have been reported in SIDS victims (161), while others have reported changes to the number of IgM positive cell numbers in the wall of the trachea compared to controls (162). This study concluded that the mucosal immune system is activated in SIDS; however, this was not to the same degree as infants where infection was known to contribute to, or cause, death. Others have suggested that SIDS infants have hypersensitive immune responses resulting in inappropriate allergic responses (163), though there is also evidence to support that this is not the case (11).

The argument for immune-mediated responses in the pathology of SIDS has been further strengthened by reports of the presence of viruses (164-166) including rhinovirus, cytomegalovirus, respiratory syncytial virus, *Bordetella pertussis*, enterovirus, and parvovirus, and also of the presence of bacteria including *Staphylococcus aureus*, *Clostridium difficile*, and *Escherichia coli* in the pathology of SIDS (167, 168). However, many of these are also present in control cases, suggesting that their presence may be more co-incidental than causative (167, 169). The hypothesis of immune-mediated mechanisms contributing to SIDS deaths was further fuelled when four infants died of SIDS in 1979 within 24 hours of receiving a diphtheria-tetanus-polio (DTP) vaccine (170). Although occasional studies today still suggest an association between vaccination and sudden infant death (171), no causal associations have been found (38, 172, 173); in fact, some studies suggest that immunization may actually reduce the incidence of SIDS (174).

Thus, while it is possible that the presence of one, or a combination of, infectious agents may increase the vulnerability of some infants to sudden death, especially should they be faced with additional stressors, there appears to be no conclusive evidence of a single infectious agent being responsible for death in SIDS infants. Indeed, the presence of infectious agents in some SIDS infants may represent no more than a mere coincidence. In addition, immune-based systems in infants within the peak age range for SIDS (i.e. 2 to 4 months) are often considered normal (175). Furthermore, SIDS cases display little evidence of sepsis (176), which, if present, would exclude the use of a SIDS diagnosis.

## Endocrine, metabolic and biochemical issues

Based on the pivotal role that the endocrine and metabolic systems play in regulating homeostatic functions, it is not surprising that abnormalities in these systems have been proposed to contribute to SIDS (177). Researchers have reported that SIDS infants have increased levels of tri-iodothyronine, which is released from the thyroid gland and affects nearly every physiological process in the body (178). Despite suggested changes to pancreatic (179) and pituitary gland pathology (180) or changes to cortisol and growth hormone levels (181), there is not sufficient evidence of endocrine system dysfunction. There has been some suggestion of pathological findings in the liver, spleen, and skeletal muscle, attributed to metabolic defects at autopsy (182, 183). However, the role of metabolic issues is hard to determine, as inherited metabolic disease can easily be missed if access to specialised units is not available. The identification of inborn errors of metabolism sufficient to result in sudden death would preclude a SIDS diagnosis.

Biochemical differences have also been reported, with significant differences in the concentration of vitreous levels of potassium, calcium, phosphorus, creatinine phosphokinase, and lactate dehydrogenase (among others) in SIDS infants (184); however, findings from this study have not being replicated (185). Thus, while it is possible that unrecognised metabolic and biochemical defects are present in some SIDS cases, there is no conclusive evidence. Furthermore, the most common metabolic abnormality, a deficiency of medium-chain acyl-coenzyme A dehydrogenase, has not consistently been reported to contribute to death in SIDS infants (186). Thus it would appear that the contribution these factors make to the number of SIDS cases is minimal.

### Nutrition and toxins

It is obvious that adequate nutrition is needed for development, both in utero and after birth. While breastfeeding is believed to reduce the risk of SIDS (120), there is no direct evidence that maternal diet can impact on SIDS, though inadequate or unbalanced diets may led to fetal compromise that does increase the SIDS risk, such as intrauterine growth restriction (37). Others have suggested that low levels of tryptophan, which is critical for serotonin production, as a result of either maternal diet or inefficient absorption from this diet, could result in lower brainstem serotonin levels and altered cardiorespiratory function in the offspring, as demonstrated using rodent studies (187). Changes to the levels of the trace metal magnesium have also been shown in SIDS infants (188), but these have not been substantiated, and there is no conclusive evidence to support an association between SIDS and vitamin (189) or thiamine (190) deficiencies. Thus the role of diet and nutrients remains to be determined. The same can be said for the possibility of accumulated toxins contributing to SIDS where there have been mixed findings on the levels of lead (191), cadmium, or chlorohydrocarbons (192). Furthermore, theories relating to sudden death due to inhalation of highly toxic trihydride gases from mattresses have never been proven (193, 194). SIDS infants show no evidence of poisoning by toxic gas, and the practice of wrapping mattresses, in an attempt to reduce the proposed toxic gas levels, has not affected the rate of SIDS deaths (195).

## Conclusions

Despite an increased understanding of why a seemingly healthy infant may die suddenly and unexpectedly with no discernible explanation, SIDS rates have plateaued in recent years and SIDS remains one of the leading causes of infant mortality in many countries (5). The mechanisms leading to sudden and unexpected death appear complex and multifactorial and require the alignment of several overlapping factors for death to occur. At present it is not possible to predict which combination of factors will result in a SIDS death for any one infant. However, one of the greatest issues faced by families, clinicians, medical examiners, and researchers is that SIDS itself is not a cause of death and remains a diagnosis of exclusion and, as there is no one standardized definition, the application of the term as a "cause of death" can be extremely subjective.

# References

1.  Beckwith JB, editor. Discussion of terminology and definition of the sudden infant death syndrome. In: Sudden infant death syndrome: Proceeding of the second international conference on the causes of sudden death in infants. Seattle: University of Washington Press, 1970.

2.  Willinger M, James LS, Catz C. Defining the sudden infant death syndrome (SIDS): Deliberations of an expert panel convened by the National Institute of Child Health and Human Development. Pediatr Pathol. 1991;11(5):677-84. https://doi.org/10.3109/15513819109065465.

3.  Krous HF, Beckwith JB, Byard RW, Rognum TO, Bajanowski T, Corey T, et al. Sudden infant death syndrome and unclassified sudden infant deaths: A definitional and diagnostic approach. Pediatrics. 2004;114(1):234-8. https://doi.org/10.1542/peds.114.1.234.

4.  Kinney HC, Thach BT. The sudden infant death syndrome. N Engl J Med. 2009;361(8):795-805. https://doi.org/10.1056/NEJMra0803836.

5.  Fleming PJ, Blair PS, Pease A. Sudden unexpected death in infancy: Aetiology, pathophysiology, epidemiology and prevention in 2015. Arch Dis Child. 2015;100(10):984-8. https://doi.org/10.1136/archdischild-2014-306424.

6.  Norvenius SG. Some medico-historic remarks on SIDS. Acta Paediatr Suppl. 1993;82 Suppl 389:3-9. https://doi.org/10.1111/j.1651-2227.1993.tb12863.x.

7.  Limerick SR. Sudden infant death in historical perspective. J Clin Pathol. 1992;45(11 Suppl):3-6.

8.  Feam SW. Sudden and unexplained death of children. Lancet. 1834;II:246.

9.  Templeman C. Two hundred and fifty-eight cases of suffocation of infants. Edinb Med J. 1892;38:322-9.

10. Krous HF. The pathology of sudden infant death syndrome: An overview. In: Sudden infant death syndrome: Medical aspects and psychological management. Eds Culbertson JL, Krous HF, Bendell RD. London: Edward Arnold, 1989. p. 18-47.

11. Golding J, Limerick S, Macfarlane A. Sudden infant death: Patterns, puzzles and problems. UK: Open Books, 1985.

12. Savitt TL. The social and medical history of crib death. J Fla Med Assoc. 1979;66(8):853-9.

13. Russell-Jones DL. Sudden infant death in history and literature. Arch Dis Child. 1985;60(3):278-81. https://doi.org/10.1136/adc.60.3.278.

14. Bailey H, Love M. A short practice of surgery. 11th ed. London: HK Lewis & Co., 1959.

15. Elhaik E. A "wear and tear" hypothesis to explain sudden infant death syndrome. Front Neurol. 2016;7:180. https://doi.org/10.3389/fneur.2016.00180.

16. Tursan d'Espaignet E, Bulsara M, Wolfenden L, Byard RW, Stanley FJ. Trends in sudden infant death syndrome in Australia from 1980 to 2002. Forensic Sci Med Pathol. 2008;4(2):83-90. https://doi.org/10.1007/s12024-007-9011-y.

17. Linacre S. Australia's babies: Australian social trends. Catalogue no. 4102.0. Canberra: Australian Bureau of Statistics, 2007.

18. Goldstein RD, Trachtenberg FL, Sens MA, Harty BJ, Kinney HC. Overall postneonatal mortality and rates of SIDS. Pediatrics. 2016;137(1):1-10. https://doi.org/10.1542/peds.2015-2298.

19. Alessandri LM, Read AW, Stanley FJ, Burton PR, Dawes VP. Sudden infant death syndrome in aboriginal and non-aboriginal infants. J Paediatr Child Health. 1994;30(3):234-41. https://doi.org/10.1111/j.1440-1754.1994.tb00625.x.

20. Malloy MH, MacDorman M. Changes in the classification of sudden unexpected infant deaths: United States, 1992-2001. Pediatrics. 2005;115(5):1247-53. https://doi.org/10.1542/peds.2004-2188.

21. Byard RW. Inaccurate classification of infant deaths in Australia: A persistent and pervasive problem. Med J Aust. 2001;175(1):5-7.

22. Burnell RH, Byard RW. Are these really sids deaths? Not by definition. J Paediatr Child Health. 2002;38(6):623-4; author reply 4-5. https://doi.org/10.1046/j.1440-1754.2002.t01-2-00075.x.

23. Kahn A, Wachholder A, Winkler M, Rebuffat E. Prospective study on the prevalence of sudden infant death and possible risk factors in Brussels: Preliminary results (1987-1988). Eur J Pediatr. 1990;149(4):284-6. https://doi.org/10.1007/BF02106296.

24. Byard RW, MacKenzie J, Beal SM. Formal retrospective case review and sudden infant death. Acta Paediatr. 1997;86(9):1011-12. https://doi.org/10.1111/j.1651-2227.1997.tb15191.x.

25. Mitchell E, Krous HF, Donald T, Byard RW. An analysis of the usefulness of specific stages in the pathologic investigation of sudden infant death. Am J Forensic Med Pathol. 2000;21(4):395-400. https://doi.org/10.1097/00000433-200012000-00020.

26. CDC Centers for Control and Prevention. The sudden, unexplained infant death investigation (SUIDI) 2016. [Available from: www.cdc.gov/SIDS/]. Accessed 12 September 2017.

27. Byard RW. Sudden infant death syndrome. In: Sudden death in the young. 3rd ed. UK: Cambridge University Press, 2010. p. 555-630. https://doi.org/10.1017/CBO9780511777783.016.

28. Bergman AB. Synthesis. In: Sudden infant death syndrome. Eds Bergman AB, Beckwith JB, Ray CG. Seattle: University of Washington Press, 1970. p. 210-21.

29. Wedgwood RJ. Session 1. In: Sudden and unexpected death in infancy (cot deaths). Eds Camps FE, Carpenter RG. Baltimore: Williams and Wilkins, 1972. p. 22-8.

30. Spinelli J, Collins-Praino L, Van Den Heuvel C, Byard RW. Evolution and significance of the triple risk model in sudden infant death syndrome. J Paediatr Child Health. 2017 Feb;53(2):112-15.

31. Filiano JJ, Kinney HC. A perspective on neuropathologic findings in victims of the sudden infant death syndrome: The triple-risk model. Biol Neonate. 1994;65(3-4):194-7. https://doi.org/10.1159/000244052.

32. Trachtenberg FL, Haas EA, Kinney HC, Stanley C, Krous HF. Risk factor changes for sudden infant death syndrome after initiation of Back-to-Sleep campaign. Pediatrics. 2012;129(4):630-8. https://doi.org/10.1542/peds.2011-1419.

33. McGarvey CM, O'Regan M, Cryan J, Treacy A, Hamilton K, Devaney D, et al. Sudden unexplained death in childhood (1-4 years) in Ireland: An epidemiological profile and comparison with SIDS. Arch Dis Child. 2012;97(8):692-7. https://doi.org/10.1136/archdischild-2011-301393.

34. SUDC Foundation. [Available from: www.SUDC.org]. Accessed 22 February 2017.

35. Jorgensen T, Biering-Sorensen F, Hilden J. Sudden infant death in Copenhagen 1956-1971. III. Perinatal and perimortal factors. Acta Paediatr Scand. 1979;68(1):11-22. https://doi.org/10.1111/j.1651-2227.1979.tb04423.x.

36. Pongou R. Why is infant mortality higher in boys than in girls? A new hypothesis based on preconception environment and evidence from a large sample of twins. Demography. 2013;50(2):421-44. https://doi.org/10.1007/s13524-012-0161-5.

37. Hakeem GF, Oddy L, Holcroft CA, Abenhaim HA. Incidence and determinants of sudden infant death syndrome: A population-based study on 37 million births. World J Pediatr. 2015;11(1):41-7. https://doi.org/10.1007/s12519-014-0530-9.

38. Jonville-Bera AP, Autret-Leca E, Barbeillon F, Paris-Llado J, & French Reference Centers for SIDS. Sudden unexpected death in infants under 3 months of age and vaccination status — A case-control study. Br J Clin Pharmacol. 2001;51(3):271-6. https://doi.org/10.1046/j.1365-2125.2001.00341.x.

39. Neubauer J, Lecca MR, Russo G, Bartsch C, Medeiros-Domingo A, Berger W, et al. Post-mortem whole-exome analysis in a large sudden infant death syndrome cohort with a focus on cardiovascular and metabolic genetic diseases. Eur J Hum Genet. 2017;25(4):404-9. https://doi.org/10.1038/ejhg.2016.199.

40. Ferrante L, Rognum TO, Vege A, Nygard S, Opdal SH. Altered gene expression and possible immunodeficiency in cases of sudden infant death syndrome. Pediatr Res. 2016;80(1):77-84. https://doi.org/10.1038/pr.2016.45.

41. Duncan JR, Paterson DS, Hoffman JM, Mokler DJ, Borenstein NS, Belliveau RA, et al. Brainstem serotonergic deficiency in sudden infant death syndrome. JAMA. 2010;303(5):430-7. https://doi.org/10.1001/jama.2010.45.

42. Paterson DS, Belliveau RA, Trachtenberg F, Kinney HC. Differential development of 5-HT receptor and the serotonin transporter binding in the human infant medulla. J Comp Neurol. 2004;472(2):221-31. https://doi.org/10.1002/cne.20105.

43. Narita N, Narita M, Takashima S, Nakayama M, Nagai T, Okado N. Serotonin transporter gene variation is a risk factor for sudden infant death syndrome in the Japanese population. Pediatrics. 2001;107(4):690-2. https://doi.org/10.1542/peds.107.4.690.

44. Weese-Mayer DE, Berry-Kravis EM, Maher BS, Silvestri JM, Curran ME, Marazita ML. Sudden infant death syndrome: Association with a promoter polymorphism of the serotonin transporter gene. Am J Med Genet A. 2003;117A(3):268-74. https://doi.org/10.1002/ajmg.a.20005.

45. Paterson DS, Rivera KD, Broadbelt KG, Trachtenberg FL, Belliveau RA, Holm IA, et al. Lack of association of the serotonin transporter polymorphism with the sudden infant death syndrome in the San Diego Dataset. Pediatr Res. 2010;68(5):409-13. https://doi.org/10.1203/PDR.0b013e3181f2edf0.

46. Opdal SH, Vege A, Rognum TO. Genetic variation in the monoamine oxidase A and serotonin transporter genes in sudden infant death syndrome. Acta Paediatr. 2014;103(4):393-7. https://doi.org/10.1111/apa.12526.

47. Hunt CE. Gene-environment interactions: Implications for sudden unexpected deaths in infancy. Arch Dis Child. 2005;90(1):48-53. https://doi.org/10.1136/adc.2004.051458.

48. Mitchell EA, Milerad J. Smoking and the sudden infant death syndrome. Rev Environ Health. 2006;21(2):81-103. https://doi.org/10.1515/REVEH.2006.21.2.81.

49. Fleming P, Blair PS. Sudden Infant Death Syndrome and parental smoking. Early Hum Dev. 2007;83(11):721-5. https://doi.org/10.1016/j.earlhumdev.2007.07.011.

50. Li Z, Zeki R, Hilder L, Sullivan E. Australia's mothers and babies 2010. Perinatal statistics series no. 27. Cat no. PER 57. Canberra: ANPEaS, Ed Unit, 2012.

51. Iyasu S, Randall LL, Welty TK, Hsia J, Kinney HC, Mandell F, et al. Risk factors for sudden infant death syndrome among northern plains Indians. JAMA. 2002;288(21):2717-23. https://doi.org/10.1001/jama.288.21.2717.

52. Treyster Z, Gitterman B. Second hand smoke exposure in children: Environmental factors, physiological effects, and interventions within pediatrics. Rev Environ Health. 2011;26(3):187-95. https://doi.org/10.1515/reveh.2011.026.

53. Duncan JR, Paterson DS, Kinney HC. The development of nicotinic receptors in the human medulla oblongata: Inter-relationship with the serotonergic system. Auton Neurosci. 2008;144(1-2):61-75. https://doi.org/10.1016/j.autneu.2008.09.006.

54. Hellstrom-Lindahl E, Gorbounova O, Seiger A, Mousavi M, Nordberg A. Regional distribution of nicotinic receptors during prenatal development of human brain and spinal cord. Brain Res Dev Brain Res. 1998;108(1-2):147-60. https://doi.org/10.1016/S0165-3806(98)00046-7.

55. Richardson HL, Walker AM, Horne RS. Maternal smoking impairs arousal patterns in sleeping infants. Sleep. 2009;32(4):515-21. https://doi.org/10.1093/sleep/32.4.515.

56. Sawnani H, Jackson T, Murphy T, Beckerman R, Simakajornboon N. The effect of maternal smoking on respiratory and arousal patterns in preterm infants during sleep. Am J Respir Crit Care Med. 2004;169(6):733-8. https://doi.org/10.1164/rccm.200305-692OC.

57. Duncan JR, Garland M, Myers MM, Fifer WP, Yang M, Kinney HC, et al. Prenatal nicotine-exposure alters fetal autonomic activity and medullary neurotransmitter receptors: Implications for sudden infant death syndrome. J Appl Physiol. 2009;107(5):1579-90. https://doi.org/10.1152/japplphysiol.91629.2008.

58. Dwyer JB, Broide RS, Leslie FM. Nicotine and brain development. Birth Defects Res C Embryo Today. 2008;84(1):30-44. https://doi.org/10.1002/bdrc.20118.

59. Kandall SR, Gaines J, Habel L, Davidson G, Jessop D. Relationship of maternal substance abuse to subsequent sudden infant death syndrome in offspring. J Pediatr. 1993;123(1):120-6. https://doi.org/10.1016/S0022-3476(05)81554-9.

60. Strandberg-Larsen K. Maternal alcohol-use disorder is associated with increased risk of sudden infant death syndrome and infant death from other causes. Evid Based Nurs. 2014;17(2):46-7. https://doi.org/10.1136/eb-2013-101376.

61. Bada HS, Das A, Bauer CR, Shankaran S, Lester BM, Gard CC, et al. Low birth weight and preterm births: Etiologic fraction attributable to prenatal drug exposure. J Perinatol. 2005;25(10):631-7. https://doi.org/10.1038/sj.jp.7211378.

62. Kopel E, Hill W. The effect of abused substances on antenatal and intrapartum fetal testing and well-being. Clin Obstet Gynecol. 2013;56:154-65. https://doi.org/10.1097/GRF.0b013e3182802cad.

63. Standfast SJ, Jereb S, Aliferis D, Janerich DT. Epidemiology of SIDS in upstate New York. In: Sudden infant death syndrome. Eds Tildon JA, Roeder LM, Steinschneider A. New York: Academic Press, 1983. p. 145-59.

64. Peterson DR. The epidemiology of sudden infant death syndrome. In: Sudden infant death syndrome: Medical aspects and psychological management. Eds Culbertson JL, Krous HF, Bendell RD. London: Edward Arnold, 1989. p. 3-16.

65. Mitchell EA, Freemantle J, Young J, Byard RW. Scientific consensus forum to review the evidence underpinning the recommendations of the Australian SIDS and Kids Safe Sleeping Health Promotion Programme-October 2010. J Paediatr Child Health. 2012;48(8):626-33. https://doi.org/10.1111/j.1440-1754.2011.02215.x.

66. Chong A, Murphy N, Matthews T. Effect of prone sleeping on circulatory control in infants. Arch Dis Child. 2000;82(3):253-6. https://doi.org/10.1136/adc.82.3.253.

67. Galland BC, Taylor BJ, Bolton DP. Prone versus supine sleep position: A review of the physiological studies in SIDS research. J Paediatr Child Health. 2002;38(4):332-8. https://doi.org/10.1046/j.1440-1754.2002.00002.x.

68. Horne RS, Ferens D, Watts AM, Vitkovic J, Lacey B, Andrew S, et al. The prone sleeping position impairs arousability in term infants. J Pediatr. 2001;138(6):811-16. https://doi.org/10.1067/mpd.2001.114475.

69. Abramson H. Accidental mechanical suffocation in infants. J Pediatr. 1944;25:404-13. https://doi.org/10.1016/S0022-3476(44)80005-1.

70. Gilbert R, Salanti G, Harden M, See S. Infant sleeping position and the sudden infant death syndrome: Systematic review of observational studies and historical review of recommendations from 1940 to 2002. Int J Epidemiol. 2005;34(4):874-87. https://doi.org/10.1093/ije/dyi088.

71. de Jonge GA, Engelberts AC. Cot deaths and sleeping position. Lancet. 1989;2(8672):1149-50. https://doi.org/10.1016/S0140-6736(89)91504-3.

72. Moon RY, & Task Force on Sudden Infant Death Syndrome. SIDS and other sleep-related infant deaths: Evidence base for 2016 updated recommendations for a safe infant sleeping environment. Pediatrics. 2016;138(5): e20153275. . https://doi.org/10.1542/peds.2016-2940.

73. Patton C, Stiltner D, Wright KB, Kautz DD. Do nurses provide a safe sleep environment for infants in the hospital setting? An integrative review. Adv Neonatal Care. 2015;15(1):8-22. https://doi.org/10.1097/ANC.0000000000000145.

74. Byard RW, Beal SM. Gastric aspiration and sleeping position in infancy and early childhood. J Paediatr Child Health. 2000;36(4):403-5. https://doi.org/10.1046/j.1440-1754.2000.00503.x.

75. Li DK, Petitti DB, Willinger M, McMahon R, Odouli R, Vu H, et al. Infant sleeping position and the risk of sudden infant death syndrome in California, 1997-2000. Am J Epidemiol. 2003;157(5):446-55. https://doi.org/10.1093/aje/kwf226.

76. Mitchell EA, Thach BT, Thompson JM, Williams S. Changing infants' sleep position increases risk of sudden infant death syndrome. New Zealand Cot Death Study. Arch Pediatr Adolesc Med. 1999;153(11):1136-41. https://doi.org/10.1001/archpedi.153.11.1136.

77. Blair PS, Sidebotham P, Berry PJ, Evans M, Fleming PJ. Major epidemiological changes in sudden infant death syndrome: A 20-year population-based study in the UK. Lancet. 2006;367(9507):314-19. https://doi.org/10.1016/S0140-6736(06)67968-3.

78. Tappin D, Ecob R, Brooke H. Bedsharing, roomsharing, and sudden infant death syndrome in Scotland: A case-control study. J Pediatr. 2005;147(1):32-7. https://doi.org/10.1016/j.jpeds.2005.01.035.

79. Byard RW. Is co-sleeping in infancy a desirable or dangerous practice? J Paediatr Child Health. 1994;30(3):198-9. https://doi.org/10.1111/j.1440-1754.1994.tb00618.x.

80. Byard RW, Hilton J. Overlaying, accidental suffocation, and sudden infant death. J Sud Infant Death Synd Infant Mort. 1997;2:161-5.

81. Carlin RF, Moon RY. Risk factors, protective factors, and current recommendations to reduce sudden infant death syndrome: A review. JAMA Pediatr. 2017;171(2):175-80. https://doi.org/10.1001/jamapediatrics.2016.3345.

82. Schluter PJ, Paterson J, Percival T. Infant care practices associated with sudden infant death syndrome: Findings from the Pacific Islands Families study. J Paediatr Child Health. 2007;43(5):388-93. https://doi.org/10.1111/j.1440-1754.2007.01085.x.

83. Huang Y, Hauck FR, Signore C, Yu A, Raju TN, Huang TT, et al. Influence of bedsharing activity on breastfeeding duration among US mothers. JAMA Pediatr. 2013;167(11):1038-44. https://doi.org/10.1001/jamapediatrics.2013.2632.

84. Hauck FR, Thompson JM, Tanabe KO, Moon RY, Vennemann MM. Breastfeeding and reduced risk of sudden infant death syndrome: A meta-analysis. Pediatrics. 2011;128(1):103-10. https://doi.org/10.1542/peds.2010-3000.

85. Mitchell EA, Thompson JMD. Co-sleeping increases the risk of SIDS, but sleeping in the parents' bedroom lowers it. In: Sudden infant death syndrome: New trends in the nineties. Ed Rognum TO. Oslo: Scandinavian University Press, 1995. p. 266-9.

86. Hauck FR, Herman SM, Donovan M, Iyasu S, Merrick Moore C, Donoghue E, et al. Sleep environment and the risk of sudden infant death syndrome in an urban population: The Chicago Infant Mortality Study. Pediatrics. 2003;111(5 Pt 2):1207-14.

87. Combrinck M, Byard RW. Infant asphyxia, soft mattresses, and the "trough" effect. Am J Forensic Med Pathol. 2011;32(3):213-14. https://doi.org/10.1097/PAF.0b013e31822abf68.

88. Kleemann WJ, Schlaud M, Poets CF, Rothamel T, Troger HD. Hyperthermia in sudden infant death. Int J Legal Med. 1996;109(3):139-42. https://doi.org/10.1007/BF01369674.

89. Lean ME, Jennings G. Brown adipose tissue activity in pyrexial cases of cot death. J Clin Pathol. 1989;42(11):1153-6. https://doi.org/10.1136/jcp.42.11.1153.

90. Fleming PJ, Gilbert R, Azaz Y, Berry PJ, Rudd PT, Stewart A, et al. Interaction between bedding and sleeping position in the sudden infant death syndrome: A population based case-control study. BMJ. 1990;301(6743):85-9. https://doi.org/10.1136/bmj.301.6743.85.

91. Ponsonby AL, Dwyer T, Jones ME. Sudden infant death syndrome: Seasonality and a biphasic model of pathogenesis. J Epidemiol Community Health. 1992;46(1):33-7. https://doi.org/10.1136/jech.46.1.33.

92. Beal S, Porter C. Sudden infant death syndrome related to climate. Acta Paediatr Scand. 1991;80(3):278-87. https://doi.org/10.1111/j.1651-2227.1991.tb11850.x.

93. Dwyer T, Ponsonby AL. Sudden infant death syndrome — Insights from epidemiological research. J Epidemiol Community Health. 1992;46(2):98-102. https://doi.org/10.1136/jech.46.2.98.

94. Davies DP, Gantley M. Ethnicity and the aetiology of sudden infant death syndrome. Arch Dis Child. 1994;70(4):349-53. https://doi.org/10.1136/adc.70.4.349.

95. Grether JK, Schulman J, Croen LA. Sudden infant death syndrome among Asians in California. J Pediatr. 1990;116(4):525-8. https://doi.org/10.1016/S0022-3476(05)81597-5.

96. Shalala DE, Trujillo MH, Hartz GJ, D'Angelo AJ. Regional differences in Indian health 1998-1999. Rockville, MD: US Department of Health and Human Services, 2000.97.

97. Irwin KL, Mannino S, Daling J. Sudden infant death syndrome in Washington State: Why are Native American infants at greater risk than white infants? J Pediatr. 1992;121(2):242-7. https://doi.org/10.1016/S0022-3476(05)81195-3.

98. Salm Ward TC, Robb SW, Kanu FA. Prevalence and characteristics of bed-sharing among black and white infants in Georgia. Maternal Child Health. 2016;20(2):347-62. https://doi.org/10.1007/s10995-015-1834-7.

99. Nelson EA, Williams SM, Taylor BJ, Morris B, Ford RP, Binney VM, et al. Prediction of possibly preventable death: A case-control study of postneonatal mortality in southern New Zealand. Paediatr Perinat Epidemiol. 1990;4(1):39-52. https://doi.org/10.1111/j.1365-3016.1990.tb00617.x.

100. King-Hele SA, Abel KM, Webb RT, Mortensen PB, Appleby L, Pickles AR. Risk of sudden infant death syndrome with parental mental illness. Arch Gen Psychiatry. 2007;64(11):1323-30. https://doi.org/10.1001/archpsyc.64.11.1323.

101. Schechtman VL, Harper RM, Wilson AJ, Southall DP. Sleep state organization in normal infants and victims of the sudden infant death syndrome. Pediatrics. 1992;89(5 Pt 1):865-70.

102. Guilleminault C, Coons S. Sleep states and maturation of sleep: A comparative study between full-term normal controls and near-miss SIDS infants. In: Sudden infant death syndrome. Eds Tildon JA, Roeder LM, Steinschneider A. New York: Academic Press, 1983. p. 401-11.

103. Richardson HL, Walker AM, Horne RS. Minimizing the risks of sudden infant death syndrome: To swaddle or not to swaddle? J Pediatr. 2009;155(4):475-81. https://doi.org/10.1016/j.jpeds.2009.03.043.

104. Beal S. Sudden infant death syndrome in twins. Pediatrics. 1989;84(6):1038-44.

105. Beal SM, Blundell HK. Recurrence incidence of sudden infant death syndrome. Arch Dis Child. 1988;63(8):924-30. https://doi.org/10.1136/adc.63.8.924.

106. Ladham S, Koehler SA, Shakir A, Wecht CH. Simultaneous sudden infant death syndrome: A case report. Am J Forensic Med Pathol. 2001;22(1):33-7. https://doi.org/10.1097/00000433-200103000-00005.

107. Diamond EF. Sudden infant death in five consecutive siblings. Illinois Med J. 1986;170(1):33-4.

108. Byard RW, Jensen LL. Is SIDS still a "diagnosis" in search of a disease? Australian J Forensic Sciences. 2008;40:85-92. https://doi.org/10.1080/00450610802047606.

109. Keens TG, Davidson Ward SL. Respiratory mechanisms and hypoxia. In: Sudden infant death syndrome: problems, progress and possibilities. Eds Byard RW, Krous HF. London: Edward Arnold, 2001. p. 66-82.

110. Read DJ. The aetiology of the sudden infant death syndrome: Current ideas on breathing and sleep and possible links to deranged thiamine neurochemistry. Aust N Z J Med. 1978;8(3):322-36. https://doi.org/10.1111/j.1445-5994.1978.tb04530.x.

111. Thach BT. Potential central nervous system involvement in sudden unexpected infant deaths and the sudden infant death syndrome. Compr Physiol. 2015;5(3):1061-8. https://doi.org/10.1002/cphy.c130052.

112. Kahn A, Blum D, Rebuffat E, Sottiaux M, Levitt J, Bochner A, et al. Polysomnographic studies of infants who subsequently died of sudden infant death syndrome. Pediatrics. 1988;82(5):721-7.

113. Franco P, Szliwowski H, Dramaix M, Kahn A. Decreased autonomic responses to obstructive sleep events in future victims of sudden infant death syndrome. Pediatr Res. 1999;46(1):33-9. https://doi.org/10.1203/00006450-199907000-00006.

114. Guilleminault C, Ariagno RL, Forno LS, Nagel L, Baldwin R, Owen M. Obstructive sleep apnea and near miss for SIDS: I. Report of an infant with sudden death. Pediatrics. 1979;63(6):837-43.

115. Shannon DC, Kelly DH, O'Connell K. Abnormal regulation of ventilation in infants at risk for sudden-infant-death syndrome. N Engl J Med. 1977;297(14):747-50. https://doi.org/10.1056/NEJM197710062971403.

116. Southall DP, Richards JM, Stebbens V, Wilson AJ, Taylor V, Alexander JR. Cardiorespiratory function in 16 full-term infants with sudden infant death syndrome. Pediatrics. 1986;78(5):787-96.

117. Rees K, Wright A, Keeling JW, Douglas NJ. Facial structure in the sudden infant death syndrome: Case-control study. BMJ. 1998;317(7152):179-80. https://doi.org/10.1136/bmj.317.7152.179.

118. Siebert JR, Haas JE. Enlargement of the tongue in sudden infant death syndrome. Pediatr Pathol. 1991;11(6):813-26. https://doi.org/10.3109/15513819109065479.

119. Siren PM. SIDS-CDF Hypothesis revisited: Cause vs contributing factors. Front Neurol. 2016;7:244.

120. Alm B, Wennergren G, Mollborg P, Lagercrantz H. Breastfeeding and dummy use have a protective effect on sudden infant death syndrome. Acta Paediatr. 2016;105(1):31-8. https://doi.org/10.1111/apa.13124.

121. Yiallourou SR, Poole H, Prathivadi P, Odoi A, Wong FY, Horne RS. The effects of dummy/pacifier use on infant blood pressure and autonomic activity during sleep. Sleep Med. 2014;15(12):1508-16. https://doi.org/10.1016/j.sleep.2014.07.011.

122. O'Connor NR, Tanabe KO, Siadaty MS, Hauck FR. Pacifiers and breastfeeding: A systematic review. Arch Pediatr Adolesc Med. 2009;163(4):378-82. https://doi.org/10.1001/archpediatrics.2008.578.

123. Sridhar R, Thach BT, Kelly DH, Henslee JA. Characterization of successful and failed autoresuscitation in human infants, including those dying of SIDS. Pediatr Pulmonol. 2003;36(2):113-22. https://doi.org/10.1002/ppul.10287.

124. Kozakewich H, Sytkowski A, Fisher J, Vawter G, Mandell F. Serum erythropoietin in infants with emphasis on sudden infant death syndrome. Laboratory Investigation. 1986;55:5.

125. Paine SM, Jacques TS, Sebire NJ. Review: Neuropathological features of unexplained sudden unexpected death in infancy: Current evidence and controversies. Neuropathol Appl Neurobiol. 2014;40(4):364-84. https://doi.org/10.1111/nan.12095.

126. Variend S, Howat AJ. Renal glomerular size in infants with congenital heart disease and in cases of sudden infant death syndrome. Eur J Pediatr. 1986;145(1-2):90-3. https://doi.org/10.1007/BF00441864.

127. Guilleminault C, Ariagno R, Coons S, Winkle R, Korobkin R, Baldwin R, et al. Near-miss sudden infant death syndrome in eight infants with sleep apnea-related cardiac arrhythmias. Pediatrics. 1985;76(2):236-42.

128. Bharati S, Krongrad E, Lev M. Study of the conduction system in a population of patients with sudden infant death syndrome. Pediatr Cardiol. 1985;6(1):29-40. https://doi.org/10.1007/BF02265405.

129. Schwartz PJ. The cardiac theory and sudden infant death syndrome. In: Sudden infant death syndrome: Medical aspects and psychological management. Eds Culbertson JL, Krous HF. London: Edward Arnold, 1989. p. 121-38.

130. Schwartz PJ, Stramba-Badiale M, Segantini A, Austoni P, Bosi G, Giorgetti R, et al. Prolongation of the QT interval and the sudden infant death

syndrome. N Engl J Med. 1998;338(24):1709-14. https://doi.org/10.1056/NEJM199806113382401.

131. Kelly DH, Pathak A, Meny R. Sudden severe bradycardia in infancy. Pediatr Pulmonol. 1991;10(3):199-204. https://doi.org/10.1002/ppul.1950100312.

132. Cohle SD, Lie JT. Cardiac conduction system in young adults. 12th World Triennial Meeting of the International Association of Forensic Sciences; 25-27 October; Adelaide, Australia, 1990.

133. Knight BH. The significance of the postmortem discovery of gastric contents in the air passages. Forensic Sci. 1975;6(3):229-34. https://doi.org/10.1016/0300-9432(75)90014-X.

134. Leape LL, Holder TM, Franklin JD, Amoury RA, Ashcraft KW. Respiratory arrest in infants secondary to gastroesophageal reflux. Pediatrics. 1977;60(6):924-8.

135. Jolley SG, Halpern LM, Tunell WP, Johnson DG, Sterling CE. The risk of sudden infant death from gastroesophageal reflux. J Pediatr Surg. 1991;26(6):691-6. https://doi.org/10.1016/0022-3468(91)90012-I.

136. de Bethmann O, Couchard M, de Ajuriaguerra M, Lucet V, Cheron G, Guillon G, et al. Role of gastro-oesophageal reflux and vagal overactivity in apparent life-threatening events: 160 cases. Acta Paediatr Suppl. 1993;82 Suppl 389:102-4. https://doi.org/10.1111/j.1651-2227.1993.tb12892.x.

137. Gomes H, Menanteau B, Motte J, Cymbalista M. Laryngospasm and sudden unexpected death syndrome. Ann Radiol (Paris). 1986;29(3-4):313-20.

138. Byard RW, Moore L. Gastroesophageal reflux and sudden infant death syndrome. Pediatr Pathol. 1993;13(1):53-7. https://doi.org/10.3109/15513819309048192.

139. Paterson DS, Thompson EG, Belliveau RA, Antalffy BA, Trachtenberg FL, Armstrong DD, et al. Serotonin transporter abnormality in the dorsal motor nucleus of the vagus in Rett syndrome: Potential implications for clinical autonomic dysfunction. J Neuropathol Exp Neurol. 2005;64(11):1018-27. https://doi.org/10.1097/01.jnen.0000187054.59018.f2.

140. Paterson DS, Trachtenberg FL, Thompson EG, Belliveau RA, Beggs AH, Darnall R, et al. Multiple serotonergic brainstem abnormalities in sudden infant death syndrome. JAMA. 2006;296(17):2124-32. https://doi.org/10.1001/jama.296.17.2124.

141. Takashima S, Becker LE. Developmental abnormalities of medullary "respiratory centers" in sudden infant death syndrome. Exp Neurol. 1985;90(3):580-7. https://doi.org/10.1016/0014-4886(85)90155-4.

142. Kadhim H, Sebire G, Khalifa M, Evrard P, Groswasser J, Franco P, et al. Incongruent cerebral growth in sudden infant death syndrome. J Child Neurol. 2005;20(3):244-6. https://doi.org/10.1177/088307380502000303.

143. Kinney HC, Cryan JB, Haynes RL, Paterson DS, Haas EA, Mena OJ, et al. Dentate gyrus abnormalities in sudden unexplained death in infants: Morphological marker of underlying brain vulnerability. Acta Neuropathol. 2015;129(1):65-80. https://doi.org/10.1007/s00401-014-1357-0.

144. Filiano JJ, Kinney HC. Arcuate nucleus hypoplasia in the sudden infant death syndrome. J Neuropathol Exp Neurol. 1992;51(4):394-403. https://doi.org/10.1097/00005072-199207000-00002.

145. O'Kusky JR, Norman MG. Sudden infant death syndrome: Postnatal changes in the numerical density and total number of neurons in the hypoglossal nucleus. J Neuropathol Exp Neurol. 1992;51(6):577-84. https://doi.org/10.1097/00005072-199211000-00002.

146. Jensen LL, Banner J, Byard RW. Does beta-APP staining of the brain in infant bed-sharing deaths differentiate these cases from sudden infant death syndrome? J Forensic Leg Med. 2014;27:46-9. https://doi.org/10.1016/j.jflm.2014.07.006.

147. Takashima S, Armstrong D, Becker LE, Huber J. Cerebral white matter lesions in sudden infant death syndrome. Pediatrics. 1978;62(2):155-9.

148. Kinney HC, Burger PC, Harrell FE Jr., Hudson RP Jr. "Reactive gliosis" in the medulla oblongata of victims of the sudden infant death syndrome. Pediatrics. 1983;72(2):181-7.

149. Atkinson JB, Evans OB, Ellison RS, Netsky MG. Ischemia of the brain stem as a cause of sudden infant death syndrome. Arch Pathol Lab Med. 1984;108(4):341-2.

150. Ambler MW, Neave C, Sturner WQ. Sudden and unexpected death in infancy and childhood: Neuropathological findings. Am J Forensic Med Pathol. 1981;2(1):23-30. https://doi.org/10.1097/00000433-198103000-00005.

151. Machaalani R, Waters KA. Neurochemical abnormalities in the brainstem of the sudden infant death syndrome (SIDS). Paediatr Respir Rev. 2014;15(4):293-300. https://doi.org/10.1016/j.prrv.2014.09.008.

152. Denoroy L, Gay N, Gilly R, Tayot J, Pasquier B, Kopp N. Catecholamine synthesizing enzyme activity in brainstem areas from victims of sudden infant death syndrome. Neuropediatrics. 1987;18(4):187-90. https://doi.org/10.1055/s-2008-1052477.

153. Bergstrom L, Lagercrantz H, Terenius L. Post-mortem analyses of neuropeptides in brains from sudden infant death victims. Brain Res. 1984;323(2):279-85. https://doi.org/10.1016/0006-8993(84)90298-1.

154. Broadbelt KG, Paterson DS, Belliveau RA, Trachtenberg FL, Haas EA, Stanley C, et al. Decreased GABAA receptor binding in the medullary serotonergic system in the sudden infant death syndrome. J Neuropathol Exp Neurol. 2011;70(9):799-810. https://doi.org/10.1097/NEN.0b013e31822c09bc.

155. Machaalani R, Say M, Waters KA. Effects of cigarette smoke exposure on nicotinic acetylcholine receptor subunits alpha7 and beta2 in the sudden infant death syndrome (SIDS) brainstem. Toxicol Appl Pharmacol. 2011;257(3):396-404. https://doi.org/10.1016/j.taap.2011.09.023.

156. Hunt NJ, Waters KA, Rodriguez ML, Machaalani R. Decreased orexin (hypocretin) immunoreactivity in the hypothalamus and pontine nuclei in sudden infant death syndrome. Acta Neuropathol. 2015;130(2):185-98. https://doi.org/10.1007/s00401-015-1437-9.

157. Heath D, Khan Q, Smith P. Histopathology of the carotid bodies in neonates and infants. Histopathology. 1990;17(6):511-19. https://doi.org/10.1111/j.1365-2559.1990.tb00790.x.

158. Lack EE, Perez-Atayde AR, Young JB. Carotid bodies in sudden infant death syndrome: A combined light microscopic, ultrastructural, and biochemical study. Pediatr Pathol. 1986;6(2-3):335-50. https://doi.org/10.3109/15513818609037724.

159. Naeye RL, Fisher R, Ryser M, Whalen P. Carotid body in the sudden infant death syndrome. Science. 1976;191(4227):567-9. https://doi.org/10.1126/science.1251191.

160. Goldwater PN. Infection: The neglected paradigm in SIDS research. Arch Dis Child. 2017. https://doi.org/10.1136/archdischild-2016-312327.

161. Forsyth KD, Weeks SC, Koh L, Skinner J, Bradley J. Lung immunoglobulins in the sudden infant death syndrome. BMJ. 1989;298(6665):23-6. https://doi.org/10.1136/bmj.298.6665.23.

162. Stoltenberg L, Saugstad OD, Rognum TO. Sudden infant death syndrome victims show local immunoglobulin M response in tracheal wall and immunoglobulin A response in duodenal mucosa. Pediatr Res. 1992;31(4 Pt 1):372-5. https://doi.org/10.1203/00006450-199204000-00013.

163. Coombs RRA, McLaughlan P. The modified anaphylactic hypothesis for sudden infant death syndrome. In: Sudden infant death syndrome. Eds Tildon JA, Roeder LM, Steinschneider A. New York: Academic Press, 1983. p. 531-8.

164. Samuels M. Viruses and sudden infant death. Paediatr Respir Rev. 2003;4(3):178-83. https://doi.org/10.1016/S1526-0542(03)00050-2.

165. Williams AL, Uren EC, Bretherton L. Respiratory viruses and sudden infant death. Br Med J (Clin Res Ed). 1984;288(6429):1491-3. https://doi.org/10.1136/bmj.288.6429.1491.

166. Dettmeyer R, Baasner A, Schlamann M, Padosch SA, Haag C, Kandolf R, et al. Role of virus-induced myocardial affections in sudden infant death syndrome: A prospective postmortem study. Pediatr Res. 2004;55(6):947-52. https://doi.org/10.1203/01.pdr.0000127022.45831.54.

167. Highet AR, Berry AM, Bettelheim KA, Goldwater PN. Gut microbiome in sudden infant death syndrome (SIDS) differs from that in healthy comparison babies and offers an explanation for the risk factor of prone position. Int J Med Microbiol. 2014;304(5-6):735-41. https://doi.org/10.1016/j.ijmm.2014.05.007.

168. Pearce JL, Bettelheim KA, Luke RK, Goldwater PN. Serotypes of Escherichia coli in sudden infant death syndrome. J Appl Microbiol. 2010;108(2):731-5. https://doi.org/10.1111/j.1365-2672.2009.04473.x.

169. Taylor BJ, Williams SM, Mitchell EA, Ford RP. Symptoms, sweating and reactivity of infants who die of SIDS compared with community controls. New Zealand National Cot Death Study Group. J Paediatr Child Health. 1996;32(4):316-22. https://doi.org/10.1111/j.1440-1754.1996.tb02561.x.

170. Centers for Disease Control and Prevention. DTP vaccination and sudden infant deaths: Tennessee. Morbidity and Mortality Weekly Report. 1979;28(131-2).

171. Huang WT, Chen RT, Hsu YC, Glasser JW, Rhodes PH. Vaccination and unexplained sudden death risk in Taiwanese infants. Pharmacoepidemiol Drug Saf. 2017;26(1):17-25. https://doi.org/10.1002/pds.4141.

172. Bernier RH, Frank JA Jr., Dondero TJ Jr., Turner P. Diphtheria-tetanus toxoids-pertussis vaccination and sudden infant deaths in Tennessee. J Pediatr. 1982;101(3):419-21. https://doi.org/10.1016/S0022-3476(82)80076-0.

173. Byard RW, Bourne AJ, Burnell RH, Roberton DM. No association between DTP vaccination and SIDS. Med J Aust. 1991;155(2):135-6.

174. Fleming PJ, Blair PS, Platt MW, Tripp J, Smith IJ, Golding J. The UK accelerated immunisation programme and sudden unexpected death in infancy: Case-control study. BMJ. 2001;322(7290):822. https://doi.org/10.1136/bmj.322.7290.822.

175. Huang SW. Infectious diseases, immunology and SIDS: An overview. In: Sudden infant death syndrome. Eds Tildon JA, Roeder LM, Steinschneider A. New York: Academic Press, 1983. p. 593-606.

176. Carmichael EM, Goldwater PN, Byard RW. Routine microbiological testing in sudden and unexpected infant death. J Paediatr Child Health. 1996;32(5):412-15. https://doi.org/10.1111/j.1440-1754.1996.tb00940.x.

177. Tildon JT, Chacon MA, Blair JD. Changes in hypothalamic-endocrine function as possible factor(s) in SIDS. In: Sudden infant death syndrome. Eds Tildon JA, Roeder LM, Steinschneider A. New York: Academic Press, 1983. p. 211-19.

178. Chacon MA, Tildon JT. Elevated values of tri-iodothyronine in victims of sudden infant death syndrome. J Pediatr. 1981;99(5):758-60. https://doi.org/10.1016/S0022-3476(81)80406-4.

179. Polak JM, Wigglesworth JS. Letter: Islet-cell hyperplasia and sudden infant death. Lancet. 1976;2(7985):570-1. https://doi.org/10.1016/S0140-6736(76)91814-6.

180. Reuss W, Saeger W, Bajanowski T. Morphological and immunohistochemical studies of the pituitary in sudden infant death syndrome (SIDS). Int J Legal Med. 1994;106(5):249-53. https://doi.org/10.1007/BF01225414.

181. Naeye RL, Fisher R, Rubin HR, Demers LM. Selected hormone levels in victims of the sudden infant death syndrome. Pediatrics. 1980;65(6):1134-6.

182. Bennett MJ, Hale DE, Coates PM, Stanley CA. Postmortem recognition of fatty acid oxidation disorders. Pediatr Pathol. 1991;11(3):365-70. https://doi.org/10.3109/15513819109064772.

183. Howat AJ, Bennett MJ, Variend S, Shaw L, Engel PC. Defects of metabolism of fatty acids in the sudden infant death syndrome. Br Med J (Clin Res Ed). 1985;290(6484):1771-3. https://doi.org/10.1136/bmj.290.6484.1771.

184. Richards RG, Fukumoto RI, Clardy DO. Sudden Infant Death Syndrome: A biochemical profile of postmortem vitreous humor. J Forensic Sci. 1983;28(2):404-14. https://doi.org/10.1520/JFS11522J.

185. Blumenfeld TA, Mantell CH, Catherman RL, Blanc WA. Postmortem vitreous humor chemistry in sudden infant death syndrome and in other causes of death in childhood. Am J Clin Pathol. 1979;71(2):219-23. https://doi.org/10.1093/ajcp/71.2.219.

186. Miller ME, Brooks JG, Forbes N, Insel R. Frequency of medium-chain acyl-CoA dehydrogenase deficiency G-985 mutation in sudden infant death syndrome. Pediatr Res. 1992;31(4 Pt 1):305-7. https://doi.org/10.1203/00006450-199204000-00001.

187. Penatti EM, Barina AE, Raju S, Li A, Kinney HC, Commons KG, et al. Maternal dietary tryptophan deficiency alters cardiorespiratory control in rat pups. J Appl Physiol. 2011;110(2):318-28. https://doi.org/10.1152/japplphysiol.00788.2010.

188. Caddell JL. Magnesium deprivation in sudden unexpected infant death. Lancet. 1972;2(7771):258-62. https://doi.org/10.1016/S0140-6736(72)91690-X.

189. Hillman LS, Erickson M, Haddad JG Jr. Serum 25-hydroxyvitamin D concentrations in sudden infant death syndrome. Pediatrics. 1980;65(6):1137-9.

190. Peterson DR, Labbe RF, van Belle G, Chinn NM. Erythrocyte transketolase activity and sudden infant death. Am J Clin Nutr. 1981;34(1):65-7.

191. Erickson MM, Poklis A, Gantner GE, Dickinson AW, Hillman LS. Tissue mineral levels in victims of sudden infant death syndrome I. Toxic metals-lead and cadmium. Pediatr Res. 1983;17(10):779-84. https://doi.org/10.1203/00006450-198310000-00002.

192. Kleemann WJ, Weller JP, Wolf M, Troger HD, Bluthgen A, Heeschen W. Heavy metals, chlorinated pesticides and polychlorinated biphenyls in sudden infant death syndrome (SIDS). Int J Legal Med. 1991;104(2):71-5. https://doi.org/10.1007/BF01626034.

193. Blair P, Fleming P, Bensley D, Smith I, Bacon C, Taylor E. Plastic mattresses and sudden infant death syndrome. Lancet. 1995;345(8951):720. https://doi.org/10.1016/S0140-6736(95)90891-9.

194. Warnock DW, Delves HT, Campell CK, Croudace IW, Davey KG, Johnson EM, et al. Toxic gas generation from plastic mattresses and sudden infant death syndrome. Lancet. 1995;346(8989):1516-20. https://doi.org/10.1016/S0140-6736(95)92051-X.

195. Mitchell EA. Wrapping a cot mattress in plastic does not explain the continuing fall in SIDS mortality. Eur J Pediatr. 2008;167(2):251-2. https://doi.org/10.1007/s00431-007-0526-8.

# 3  Sudden Unexplained Death in Childhood: An Overview

Elisabeth A Haas, MPH

*Rady Children's Hospital, San Diego, USA*

## Sudden Unexplained Death in Childhood Defined

Although many sudden deaths are unexpected, deaths that remain unexplained intensify anguish among family, friends, and the community at large, especially when the decedent is an infant or child. Sudden infant death syndrome (SIDS) and sudden unexplained death in childhood (SUDC) are assigned as "causes" of death after the exclusion of any other known reason (1). There are two main differences between SIDS and SUDC: [1] SIDS is much more common, with a rate of 38.7 deaths per 100,000 live births; this compares to the SUDC rate of 1.0-1.4 deaths per 100,000 of the population; and [2] SIDS affects infants up to the age of 1 year, and SUDC affects mostly toddlers, aged greater than 1 year (highest incidence in 1-4-year-olds). Also, risk factors for SIDS (tobacco smoke exposure, placed prone for sleep, bed sharing) have not been shown to be risk factors for SUDC. These deaths deserve extensive investigation and merit dedicated research in an attempt to uncover any potential cause(s) of death in the young child. In 2005, Krous and colleagues (2) provided the working definition of SUDC: "[t]he sudden and unexpected death of a child over the age of 1 year that remains unexplained after a review of the clinical history and circumstances of death and performance of a complete autopsy with appropriate ancillary testing". For the purposes of this chapter, discussion is limited to deaths that occurred during a sleep period.

## Global Perspective

Only one-third of 55 million global deaths per year are tracked in an established civil registry (3), and only one-quarter of the global population lives in a country that registers at least 90% of births and deaths (4). Globally speaking, performance of a complete autopsy, especially when supplemented by ancillary studies, is uncommon. The United Nations (UN) and World Health Organization (WHO) are proponents of Sample Vital Registration with Verbal Autopsy (SAVVY) (5) for most countries attempting to develop a system of Vital Records. A substantial amount of information available for mortality for children aged less than 5 years is based on the collection of birth histories, verbal autopsy, disease modeling, and other strategies in absence of a civil registration system.

Worldwide (6), the main causes of death of children under the age of 5 in 2015 included preterm birth complications (18%), pneumonia (16%), intrapartum-related complications (12%), diarrhea (9%), and sepsis/meningitis (9%). Importantly, almost half of all deaths in children under 5 are attributable to undernutrition (7). These causes of death account for essentially 100% of child deaths, underscoring the rarity of SUDC around the globe.

Even in the United States, with a well-established vital records registry, standards vary widely among the 2,300 medical examiner and coroner jurisdictions regarding which deceased individuals will be examined post-mortem, who performs the autopsy, concomitant toxicology and other ancillary testing, organ sampling, tissue retention, and duration of storage.

The National Center for Health Statistics (NCHS) through the Office of Analysis and Epidemiology (OAE) at the Centers for Disease Control and Prevention (CDC) produces statistics on a wide range of factors (birth, disease prevalence, morbidity, and mortality incidence). The CDC has compiled data from death certificates since 1968, using International Classification of Disease (ICD) codes and ICD-10-CM (version

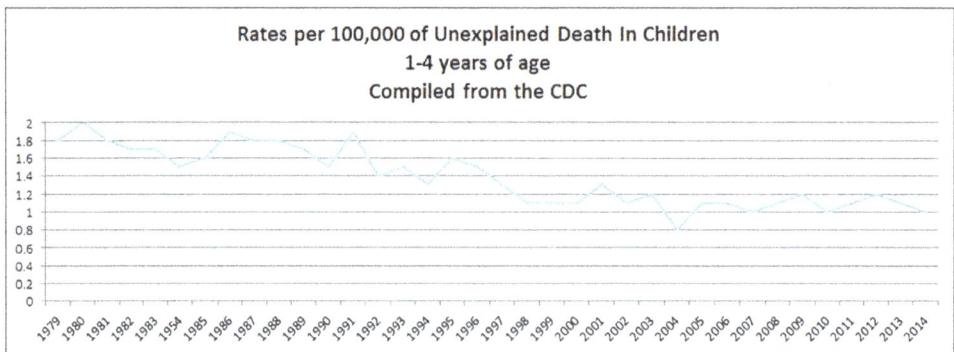

Figure 3.1: Rates of SUDC compiled from CDC. X-axis represents year; y-axis represents rate.

10 Clinical Modification, simplified and condensed for purposes of morbidity). The CDC categorizes children by age groups: the 1-4-year age group is most relevant for this overview. Using unexplained death codes from ICD-9 (798.1 and .2 and .9 as well as 799.9) and ICD-10-CM (R95-99), rates of sudden and unexplained death in the 1-4-year age group have ranged from 1.0-2.0/100,000 population for the nation, roughly 224 deaths per year (Figure 3.1) (8).

## Review of the Literature

At the time of the initial publication of Krous et al. on SUDC in 2005, there was a lack of literature on negative-autopsy deaths in children over 1 year of age. Molander (9), in 1982, published his review of 43 cases of sudden unexpected natural death (SUND) in a series of 389 child and adolescent (through age 20 years) deaths over a six-year period in Sweden. Molander found that some sudden deaths were nonetheless not unexpected due to chronic heart disease, or epilepsy, for example. In his cohort, there were only four cases for which the cause of death was unknown, a rate of 0.007 per 1,000 live births, substantially less than that of SIDS, which was 0.6 per 1,000 live births in Sweden at that time.

In 1985, Neuspiel and Kuller (10) reviewed 207 cases of SUND over nine years. The ages of their population were 1-21 years; ultimately, 15 of 62 deaths in the 1-4-year age group remained unexplained, and they found that "referral for medicolegal evaluation was inconsistent". Siboni and Simonsen (11) reviewed 1920 medicolegal autopsies of children and young adults (age range 2-30 years) over a 10.5-year period. SUND accounted for 78 (4%) of deaths and ultimately only one case (a 22-year-old female) was unexplained.

In 1987, Southall et al. (12) published their findings of SUD (sudden unexpected death) in a cohort of 9,856 infants followed from birth. They subsequently published their findings on cot death (death occurring in an infant while in a cot or crib during a sleep period) in this prospective study in a separate article in 1983 (13). There were 15 deaths between the ages of 1 and 5 years. Of these, five (33%) remained unexplained after post-mortem examination.

Hoffman et al. (14) published an article with their findings from a case-control study examining SIDS risk factors. The study population was aged 2 weeks through 2 years of age; 16 deaths occurred among toddlers between the ages of 52 and 103 weeks, that were classified as "definitely" or "probably" SIDS (the investigators used 103 weeks as the upper age limit for SIDS deaths). Eleven cases of unexplained death were found in an investigation by Keeling et al. (15) of SUND over a 20-year period. The cases ranged from 2 to 20 years; 169 out of 1,012 (17%) cases were SUND.

Since these publications and that of Krous et al. (2), multiple investigators from various countries have published their findings upon researching the phenomenon of sudden and unexplained death in childhood. Within the last five years, almost

200 different articles have addressed sudden death in childhood, although a majority focus on sudden cardiac death or sudden unexplained death in epilepsy (SUDEP).

Regarding unexplained deaths, researchers in New Zealand (16) published their results in 2011 from a prospective, population-based study constructed on a nationwide protocol of molecular autopsy when someone aged 1-40 years dies suddenly, with a negative post-mortem examination. Genetic investigation after autopsy confirmed that 15% of deaths were due to Long QT Syndrome, i.e. LQTS, an acquired or inherited condition affecting the heart rhythm, characterized by a prolonged QT interval on an electrocardiogram (17); while another 15% of subjects had a probable cause of death established due to the information gained from cardiac screening of family members of the proband (e.g. arrhythmogenic right ventricular cardiomyopathy). The study had four subjects aged 5 years and younger; all four were male, an 18-month-old, a 25-month-old and a 28-month-old were all asleep at the time of death; the 5-year-old child was "vomiting". Interestingly, although this study included ages up to 40 years, 55% of the study population were asleep when they died.

In June 2012, McGarvey et al. published a review of SUDC cases, along with a comparison to SIDS, in Ireland (18). This research supported findings of Kinney et al. (19) with male predominance, a high incidence of febrile seizures, and being found prone after a sleep period. Unlike SIDS in Ireland, maternal smoking was not associated with increased post-infancy risk of dying suddenly without explanation.

In December 2012, researchers in Denmark published their findings (20) of 44 cases of sudden unexplained death (subjects aged 1-35 years) with DNA available for cardiogenetic testing. Given that previous estimates of sudden cardiac death accounted for one-third of cases referred for testing in Denmark, the authors wanted to investigate the incidence of genes associated with LQTS and sudden cardiac death in a cohort from 2000 to 2006. They found that genopositive results explained death in only 11% of cases.

In March 2013, researchers in Ireland published their conclusions from an ambitious audit of SUDC cases autopsied in Ireland (21), utilizing a modified Rushton Scoring Method (22) (see Table 3.1). Using a Minimal Acceptable Score (MAS), chosen somewhat arbitrarily and representing 60% of total possible points, 300/500 points, they compared SUDC (defined as deaths ranging from 52-152 weeks of age) autopsies with SIDS autopsies, and found that the proportion reaching the MAS was 67% for SIDS cases and 58% for SUDC autopsies. When they analysed data by site, 19/21 (95%) of SUDC cases referred to a Specialist Center and autopsied by a pediatric pathologist achieved the MAS. Reasonably, they recommended that all cases of SUDC should be referred to specialist centers and that guidelines for investigation should meet the same protocols as followed in a SIDS investigation.

Researchers from Sydney, Australia, published their findings in 2014 of a comparison of conventional autopsy to magnetic resonance (MRI) and computer tomography (CT) imaging in sudden death cases up to age 35 years at death (23). Only three children less than 6 years of age at death met study criteria. All were male, two were found deceased in bed (the 5-year-old with intracranial tumor and 18-month-old with a history of "febrile convulsions" and unexplained death). A 4-year-old with gastrointestinal upset was taken to hospital but deteriorated. MRI and autopsy did not explain the cause of death; the CT diagnosis was intra-abdominal hemorrhage.

Table 3.1: Rushton Modified Scoring Method. (Reproduced with permission from Dr A Treacy.)

| Category | Total Score | Breakdown |
|---|---|---|
| Weights and measures | 80 | Body weight, Crown-rump length, Crown-heel length, Head circumference (20 each) |
| Normal organ weights | 20 | Heart, Lungs, Liver, Kidney, Brain (4 each) |
| Main organ weights | 40 | Heart, Lungs, Liver, Kidney, Brain (8 each) |
| Minor organ weights | 15 | Spleen, Adrenals, Thymus (5 each) |
| Histology main organ | 50 | Heart, Lungs, Liver, Kidney, Brain (10 each) |
| Histology minor organ | 30 | Spleen, Adrenals, Thymus (10 each) |
| Radiology | 100 | |
| Microbiology | 50 | Swabs (20), Blood cultures, CSF, PCR (10 each) |
| Biochemistry | 20 | |
| Toxicology | 35 | |
| Virology | 10 | |
| Metabolic investigations | 50 | Frozen tissue, Acyl carnitine screen, Organic acid screen, Skin fibroblast culture, Basic screen |
| Total Score | 500 | |

## Developments

### San Diego SUDC Research Project

As cited above, Krous et al. were the first to define SUDC (2) and they were also the first to accrue a large series of cases, albeit retrospectively. Krous began studying sudden infant death early in his career and authored nearly 100 articles on SIDS and other sudden unexpected deaths in infancy. Following an invited presentation on "post-infancy SIDS" at the 1999 SIDS Alliance Annual Conference, Krous was approached by several parents of toddlers who had died suddenly and unexpectedly, all with either a negative autopsy, or with questionably lethal findings (mild bronchiolitis, interstitial pneumonitis). He offered these families a second-opinion review of their child's case. From that point, the case load of families wanting a second review grew and two bereaved mothers founded the non-profit Sudden Unexplained Death in Childhood Foundation in 2001. The SUDC Foundation continues to this day with both a research component and an element offering family support, outreach, and fundraising.[1]

The individual consult appeals were the foundation for what would become the San Diego SUDC Research Project, an expansion of the San Diego SIDS Research Project based at Rady Children's Hospital. Krous accrued cases via the SUDC Foundation website, word-of-mouth among parents, and, occasionally, directly from coroners and medical examiners. The San Diego SUDC Research Project evolved over time with additional cases and collaborators, resulting in 11 articles published in peer reviewed medical journals, along with increasingly detailed and specific pathology findings, and the emergence of a phenotype.

A major weakness of the SUDC research population is that it was self-selected. Due to the rarity of sudden unexpected death in children, especially among toddlers, and the novelty of concerted investigation into these deaths when the San Diego SUDC Research Project was founded, there were no surveillance efforts, nor was there an organized community of afflicted families at that time. The fledgling project relied on families to self-enroll, and the resulting study population was predominantly white (82%), and college-educated (88% of mothers and 84.5% of fathers). The demographic homogeneity is striking, given that cases came from foreign countries (Australia, Canada, England, Germany, Ireland, New Zealand, Russia, and Scotland) as well as from 36 states and the District of Columbia. More than half (51%) of the San Diego SUDC research parent population had pregnancy complications and/or difficulty in conceiving. A number (16%) had conceived with the aid of fertility drugs; 38% had a history of miscarriage/stillbirth; and, with the SUDC child, many (36%) had complications prenatally (e.g. pre-eclampsia, gestational hypertension, gestational diabetes, vaginal bleeding, and premature labor).

While there are no legally mandated federal or international autopsy standards in such cases, some counties, states, and foreign countries have established guidelines for autopsy. A requirement for study participation was that microscopic slides from autopsy were available for review, and this resulted in a wide range of the number of organs sampled for histologic evaluation as well as considerable variation in the number and type of post-mortem ancillary studies. All available hospital and clinic medical records were obtained and reviewed, along with a lengthy family survey completed by the child's primary caretaker. None of the cases were being litigated in civil or criminal

---

1   See http://sudc.org for more information.

court. After review of all available materials, a study cause and manner of death was established for each case.

The initial publication of the San Diego SUDC Research Project was in 2005; it summarized the findings from the first 50 cases reviewed, 36 of which remained unexplained (2). Perhaps not surprisingly, aside from age, certain aspects of these cases' phenotype mirrored that of SIDS: male predominance and being found dead, prone, and face-down during an apparent sleep period. An unexpected and important observation was the association of SUDC with a personal and/or family history of seizures, especially those that were febrile, either in the toddler (32%), his/her immediate family (31%), or both (21%). The high incidence of febrile seizures was well in excess of the 2-5% incidence found among toddlers in the general population (24).

The next manuscript was published in 2007 (25) and included pediatric neuropathologist Hannah Kinney's observations of hippocampal gross asymmetry and a variety of microdysgenetic abnormalities among a subset of five unexplained toddler deaths. The abstract suggested a "potential entity" of microdysgenetic hippocampal and temporal lobe findings somehow associated with sudden death during a sleep period.

In a 2009 publication from the San Diego SUDC Research Project (19), Kinney et al. elaborated on the new entity of the 2007 publication and included stronger association with febrile seizures and the observation that some cases of SUDC resembled SUDEP via an unwitnessed seizure precipitating sudden death. An article from 2012 (26) examined potential genetic inheritance of sudden death among toddlers among three generations of family related to the toddler, which showed autosomal dominance in two-thirds (although in one family there was variable expression).

*Case reports of explained sudden unexpected deaths in toddlers and childhood*

Among the individual cases of sudden death in childhood, some novel pathologic findings were noted, which led to publication of five case reports. In 2005, a case of sudden unexpected death in a 13-year-old male with meningioangiomatosis detected at autopsy was summarized (27). The adolescent was found dead in bed, prone, with no medical history of any significance except for being medicated with methylphenidate for an attention deficit disorder. He had no seizure history and there was no family history of meningioangiomatosis.

In 2007, a case report of a unique expression of tuberous sclerosis in a 9-year-old female who died suddenly and unexpectedly was published. Autopsy findings were significant for a cardiac rhabdomyoma, cardiomegaly, involuting adrenal ganglioneuroma, and megalencephaly. The cause of death was assigned as a lethal cardiac arrhythmia arising from the tumor in the subendocardial conduction fibers on the right side of the posterior ventricular septum (28).

Another case report published in 2007 (29) presented two toddlers dying suddenly and unexpectedly with viral meningitis, leading to massive cerebral edema, neurogenic pulmonary edema, and hemorrhage. In 2008, a report of the sudden and unexpected death in a toddler with Williams syndrome was published (30). The final case report from the SUDC Research Project population was published in 2009 — a toddler death associated with laryngeotracheitis caused by human parainfluenza virus-1 (31).

NORD webpage

With the co-operation of the SUDC Foundation website, SUDC was added to the list of uncommon diseases and disorders provided by the National Organization for Rare Disorders (32).

## San Diego SUDC Research Project, phase II

Following Krous's retirement in 2012, his longtime collaborator and member of the SUDC team of investigators, Hannah Kinney, with Boston Children's Hospital, took over as Principal Investigator of the study. Kinney and her colleagues undertook a new review of all the cases in the San Diego SUDC research project dataset, the result of which led to a few cases having the cause of death assigned as SUDEP, given the personal and/or family seizure history. She also limited the dataset to children less than 7 years of age at the time of death.

Under Kinney's supervision, Hefti et al. distilled all the information and study findings from the cases into two manuscripts (33, 34). Part I summarized the pathological, phenotypic, and socioeconomic variables. The most salient observations included a statistically significant association with SUDC, and a personal and/or family history of febrile seizures and SUDC, and being found dead during a sleep period; hippocampal abnormalities were the most common neuropathologic finding in SUDC cases (almost 50% of those cases with neuropathological tissue available).

The companion manuscript, Part II, delineated the range of neuropathology discoveries among the cases for whom neuropathologic tissue was available to review. Not surprisingly, a hippocampal abnormality was more often found with an increase in number of microscopic slides of brain tissue available to review. Given that 55% of 83 cases with neuropathologic tissue available had an abnormality, one wonders about the brains of deceased children that were not sufficiently sectioned to determine a cause of death. This manuscript proposes a new category of SUDC: hippocampal malformation associated with sudden death (HMASD). Neuropathological defects were largely

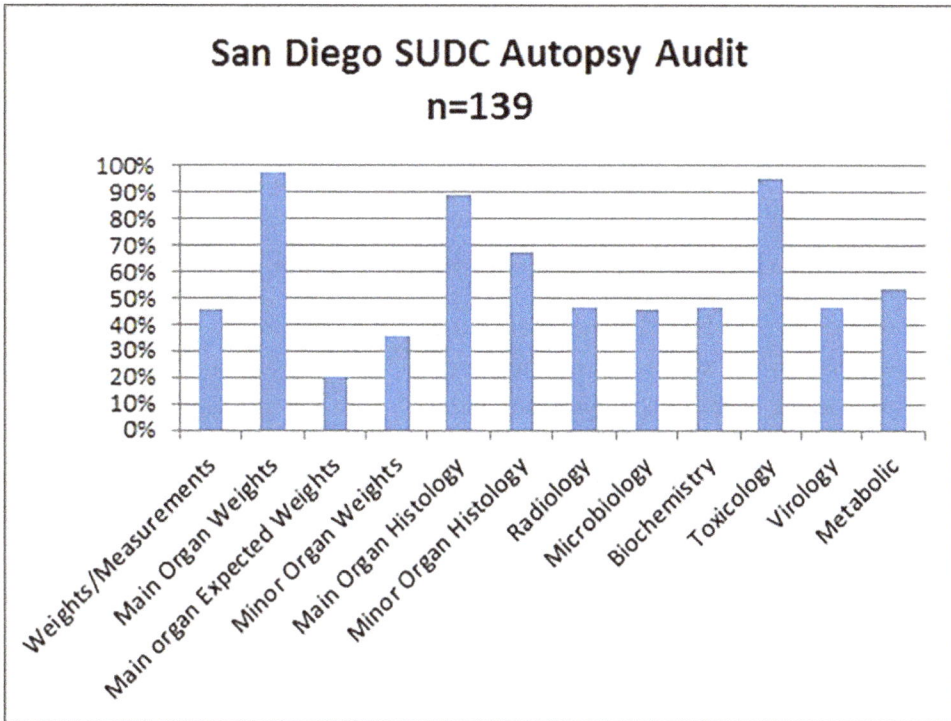

Figure 3.2: Results of audit of autopsies from the San Diego SUDC Research Project. (Format borrowed with permission from Jane Cryan and Ann Treacy.)

confined to the temporal lobe in this study population, excepting the commonality of hyper-eosinophilic acutely ischemic neurons found in all categories of cause of death.

Autopsy audits

The author is grateful to her colleague Dr Jane Cryan and fellow researchers (specifically Dr Ann Treacy) for permission to reproduce their modified Rushton scale to audit Krous's SUDC cases. Of 151 SUDC cases, 139 autopsy reports of children under 5 years of age were available to review. The original Rushton total maximum score is 500 points, with a Minimal Accepted Score of 300 points (60%) (Table 3.1). Measures of central tendency for the Krous cohort of SUDC cases include a mean of 330 ± 85.5 points, with a median of 325 and a mode of 270 (n=7) points. The range of scores was 142-490. Almost half (58 cases, i.e. 42%) of the autopsies did not attain the MAS of 300 points. The item missed most often was expected organ weights for the major organs. Figure 3.2 indicates the percentage fulfilling each criterion, except for microbiology, which shows the proportion of cases reaching at least 30 of 50 possible points.

Because these cases accumulated from around the globe, the specialty (or non-specialty) of the prosecting pathologist was often not readily discernible from the available paperwork, so comparisons cannot be made between the quality of autopsies by pathologists holding board certification in forensics and other prosecting physicians.

## Current Status

### Sudden unexplained death in pediatrics (SUDP)

As the San Diego SUDC Research Project could not transition to Boston Children's Hospital, Kinney and Goldstein continue research into SUDC and other unexplained pediatric deaths with a new program currently limited to families residing in Massachusetts. A comprehensive team of investigators with Harvard and Boston Children's Hospital collaborate with the Massachusetts Office of the Chief Medical Examiner (OCME) as well as the Massachusetts Center for Sudden Infant Death Syndrome and the Massachusetts Infant and Child Death Bereavement Program. In 2016, Kinney et al. (35) published a comprehensive review of their neuropathological findings and sudden death across all pediatric life stages.

### CDC Sudden death in the young

On 24 October 2013, the National Institutes of Health (NIH) (37) and the CDC announced an expansion of the registry for sudden unexpected infant deaths (up to age 1 year). The expanded Sudden Death in the Young Case Registry (SDY-CR) includes deaths under age 19 years and excludes deaths from homicide, suicide, or trauma. This effort formalizes surveillance of SUDEP and sudden cardiac death (SCD). Seven states (Delaware, Georgia, Minnesota, New Hampshire, New Jersey, Nevada and Tennessee) and three jurisdictions (San Francisco; Tidewater, Virginia; and selected counties in Wisconsin) applied for, and received, funding for their epidemiologic efforts in 2014. Deaths occurring in 2015 are the first to be included. Data collection began in April 2016. The SDY-CR provides autopsy guidelines, an autopsy summary document, a field guide, and family interview questions. The Registry includes a biorepository at the University of Michigan, which will store de-identified blood specimens indefinitely.

## Future Possibilities

The aim for future research and clinical efforts is to avert these tragic deaths in children, perhaps through early detection of genetic defects in utero or chromosomal analysis proceeding from a family member's heart condition, or prompted by a history of seizures in the family. Determining a cause of death may have implications for future pregnancy plans or siblings, or for both.

## Molecular autopsy

Molecular autopsies do not replace traditional autopsies, but are helpful after a negative gross autopsy with no conclusive findings from histology, microbiology, and toxicology studies. In 1997, the CDC established an Office of Public Health Genomics (OPHG), tasked with "identifying, evaluating, and implementing evidence-based genomics practices to prevent and control the country's leading chronic, infectious, environmental, and occupational diseases". As of 30 November 2016, there are 1495 publications from this office. The CDC examines the sensitivity and specificity of tests, the costs, extent of ease or invasiveness to obtain testing material, along with the disease or disorder incidence and prevalence in the population to be studied. They have established evidence-based guidelines on which genetic tests are useful and appropriate for specific populations.

According to the US National Library of Medicine National Institutes of Health website, PubMed[2], one of the first English-language articles in which genetics gave insight into autopsy findings was in 1987 by Tanzi, who described mapping a gene for β amyloid peptide precursor to chromosome 21 in an Alzheimer patient (38). In 2001, Ackerman published an account of determination of the cause of death following the negative autopsy of a 17-year-old male found dead in bed (39). An epinephrine challenge of the boy's mother indicated a defect encoded in the KVLQT1 gene. Ackerman was subsequently able to recover molecular material from the boy's paraffin-embedded heart tissue which revealed a 5-base pair deletion in the same gene as the mother. Importantly, he was able to establish a likely cause of death and demonstrate that necropsy tissue is viable for DNA investigations. To date, Ackerman has gone on to publish 16 articles on molecular autopsy, cardiomyopathy, and channelopathies.

Since then, several countries/states/institutions have published their findings with this approach to unexplained death. Whole exome sequencing (WES) is increasingly available, and at decreasing cost. Rady Children's Hospital, San Diego, unveiled their Institute for Genomic Medicine in 2016; at the time of this writing, they held the Guinness Book of Records for the fastest genetic diagnosis, by successfully diagnosing critically ill newborns in just 26 hours. The initial candidates at Rady are patients in the Neonatal Intensive Care Unit and Pediatric Intensive Care Unit, some acutely ill with an unknown cause. This institute will also incorporate epigenomics, proteomics, and metabolomics.

The office of the San Diego County Medical Examiner has partnered with Scripps Translational Science Institute (STSI) since 2014. This partnership offers no-cost genetic testing for suddenly deceased individuals less than 45 years of age at death with no obvious anatomic explanation for their death. STSI provides a report looking at whether the decedent was positive or negative for any genetic variants that may explain

---

2   See http://pubmed.gov for more information.

a sudden death. The range of positive findings includes "Likely Causal DNA Variants" and "Plausible Causal DNA Variants".

## Routine cardiogenetic testing

Genetic testing is not currently routine at autopsy. The cost would be prohibitive, and public health tenets mandate that effective screening tests account for prevalence of the disease (or gene) being studied, and also that prevention or treatment is available and affordable, concomitant with infrastructure to notify and follow up with the families of individuals with genopositive results.

The New York Office of the Chief Medical Examiner (40), however, has had its own molecular genetic laboratory since 2008. Since then, autopsy-negative SUD (sudden unexplained death) cases have been screened for the six genes most often associated with a cardiac channelopathy (*KCNQ1*, *KCNH2*, *SCN5A*, *KCNE1*, *KCNE2*, and *RyR2*). The results from testing a series of 274 ethnically diverse SUD cases revealed that 13.5% of infants and 19.5% of non-infants were positive for a total of 22 previously classified channelopathy-associated variants, along with 24 novel channelopathy variants. The *SCN5A* gene accounted for 68% of infant and 50% of non-infant positive results. The researchers concluded that molecular testing is valuable, especially for establishing a cause of death, and for providing potentially life-saving information to family members of the decedent.

Researchers in Australia (41) evaluated screening of autopsy-negative sudden arrhythmic death syndrome (SADS) and unexplained cardiac arrest (UCA). The targeted genetic testing of more than 100 SADS families had a diagnostic yield of 18%, while the yield of UCA families was 62%. The majority findings in both groups were LQTS and Brugada syndrome.

A literature search on PubMed reveals that the future of life-saving interventions is at the molecular level. In addition to the increasingly popularity of looking for a genetic link to LQTS, Short QT intervals have been noted to be perilous as well. Previously, family members of a decedent with putative cardiac cause would be subjected to exercise or epinephrine stress tests, wearing a heart monitor for 24 hours (or more), echocardiogram, and MRI for cardiac anatomical defects. Now, given the future in genomic medicine, those families may be able to obtain answers upon submitting a cheek swab.

## Globally expanded routine newborn screening
### Metabolic screening

Screening infants at birth for inherited and treatable disorders of hemoglobin (e.g. sickle cell), endocrinology (e.g. congenital adrenal hyperplasia), and metabolism (e.g. phenylketonuria (PKU)) is effective in the US because >98% of infants are born at a birthing center or hospital (42). In some developing countries, up to 80% of infants are not born in hospitals. Also, in some countries (e.g. the Philippines) newborn screening is not free (43). Screening at birth is crucial in preventing irreversible brain damage and other physical problems stemming from disrupted metabolism or hormonal disorders.

Although few of the cases reviewed in the SUDC research project were posthumously diagnosed with an inborn error of metabolism, increased screening for these and other disorders would undoubtedly save lives. In 1967, Guthrie (44) (a physician and also a microbiologist) was working with bacterial inhibition assays, which led to the invention of a card of filter paper and desiccant to enable collection of blood spots on newborns to screen for PKU (his niece was diagnosed with PKU). He also had a son with "mental retardation" and he was intent in finding ways to prevent the same condition in other children. He went on to develop a test for maple syrup urine disease and galactosemia.

The use of the newborn screening test became widespread in the United States in 1969-70 (45). Nationally, the Secretary's Advisory Committee on Heritable Disorders in Newborns and Children (SACHDNC) is charged with monitoring the Recommended Uniform Screening Panel (RUSP) of 31 core disorders and 26 secondary disorders for newborn screening tests. The recommendations are merely suggestions, and are not enforceable. Although there is a panel of standard tests suggested by the federal government, each state independently decides which diseases or disorders to test for based on the state budget, the established infrastructure for testing and follow-up of positive results, the prevalence of the disorder in the state, as well as treatment availability for the disease or condition being tested. Advances in polymerase chain reaction (PCR) have enabled additional tests to be done, using the same quantity of blood from a heel stick.

California currently screens for 58 conditions. Parents in California also have the option of signing a form to request that the state incinerate their child's blood spot after screening is completed. As another example, Alaska (46) partners with Northwest Regional Newborn Screening Program at the Oregon Public Health Laboratory (OPHL) and Oregon Health Sciences University (OHSU) for their newborn blood spot tests. In 2002, OHSU used a new technology (tandem mass spectrometry) that allowed additional screening tests for organic acid disorders, fatty acid oxidation disorders, and amino acid and urea cycle disorders but without the need for additional blood or heel sticks. Alaska agreed to test newborns for the OHSU expanded panel of metabolic diseases beginning in 2003. Table 3.2 has a list by state of tests in addition the RUSP.

Ireland has the highest prevalence of cystic fibrosis (CF) (47) of any country in the world but it was not until July 2011 that screening for CFAND carrier status was implemented. In addition to CF, Ireland also tests for PKU, congenital hypothyroidism, maple syrup urine disease, classical galactosemia, and homosystinuria. 2M Associates, Inc. is associated with the University of Colorado Health Sciences Center, and provides expanded newborn screening in the United States, India, the United Arab Emirates, and several other countries.

Dot "●" indicates that screening for the condition is universally required by Law or Rule and fully implemented
A = universally offered but not yet required, B = offered to select populations, or by request, C = testing required but not yet implemented
D = likely to be detected (and reported) as a by-product of MRM screening (MS/MS) targeted by Law or Rule

**25 RUSP Secondary Target Conditions [1]**

| STATE | Fatty Acid Disorders | | | | | | | | Organic Acid Disorders | | | | | | Amino Acid Disorders | | | | | | | | Other Metabolic | | Hb |
|---|---|---|---|---|---|---|---|---|---|---|---|---|---|---|---|---|---|---|---|---|---|---|---|---|---|
| | CACT | CPT-Ia | CPT-II | DE-RED. | GA-II | MCKAT | M/SCHAD | SC AD | 2M3HBA | 2MBG | 3MGA | Cbl-C,D | IBG | MAL | ARG | BIOPT-BS | BIOPT-RG | CIT-II | H-PHE | MET | TYR-II | TYR-III | GALE | GALK | Variant Hbs |
| Alabama | ● | | ● | | ● | | | | ● | ● | ● | ● | | | | ● | ● | ● | ● | ● | ● | ● | | | ● |
| Alaska | ● | ● | ● | | ● | | | ● | ● | ● | ● | ● | ● | ● | ● | B | B | ● | ● | ● | ● | D | B | B | ● |
| Arizona | D | D | D | | D | | | | D | | D | D | | | | | | D | D | | D | D | | | D |
| Arkansas | | | | | | | | | | | | | | | | | | | | | | | | | ● |
| California | ● | ● | ● | | ● | | ● | ● | ● | ● | ● | ● | ● | ● | ● | ● | ● | ● | ● | ● | ● | ● | | | ● |
| Colorado | ● | ● | ● | | ● | | ● | ● | | ● | ● | | ● | ● | | | | ● | ● | ● | ● | ● | | | ● |
| Connecticut | ● | ● | ● | ● | ● | | ● | ● | ● | ● | ● | ● | ● | ● | ● | ● | ● | ● | ● | ● | ● | ● | | | ● |
| D. of Columbia | ● | ● | ● | ● | ● | ● | ● | ● | ● | ● | ● | ● | ● | ● | ● | A | A | ● | ● | ● | ● | ● | ● | ● | ● |
| Delaware | ● | | ● | | ● | D | | ● | D | ● | D | ● | | ● | | D | D | ● | ● | ● | ● | ● | ● | ● | ● |
| Florida | ● | ● | ● | | ● | | | ● | D | D | D | D | D | | | D | | ● | D | ● | D | ● | | | ● |
| Georgia | D | D | D | | D | D | D | D | D | D | D | D | D | D | A | | | D | D | D | D | D | B | B | ● |
| Hawaii | ● | ● | ● | | ● | | | ● | ● | ● | ● | ● | ● | ● | ● | B | B | ● | ● | ● | ● | ● | B | B | ● |
| Idaho | ● | ● | ● | | ● | | | ● | ● | ● | ● | ● | ● | ● | ● | B | B | ● | ● | ● | ● | ● | B | B | ● |
| Illinois | ● | D | ● | D | ● | D | ● | ● | D | ● | ● | ● | ● | ● | ● | D | D | D | ● | ● | ● | ● | | | ● |
| Indiana | ● | ● | ● | ● | ● | ● | ● | ● | ● | ● | ● | ● | ● | ● | ● | ● | ● | ● | ● | ● | ● | ● | | | ● |
| Iowa | ● | ● | ● | | ● | | | ● | ● | ● | ● | ● | ● | ● | ● | ● | ● | ● | ● | ● | ● | ● | | | ● |
| Kansas | | | | | | | | | | | | | | | | | | | ● | | | | | | ● |
| Kentucky | A | A | A | | A | | | ● | A | A | A | A | A | A | A | D | D | A | ● | A | A | A | | | ● |
| Louisiana | | | | | | | | | | | | | | | | | | | ● | | | | | | ● |
| Maine | D | D | ● | | ● | | | ● | | D | D | ● | D | | ● | | | ● | ● | D | ● | D | ● | ● | ● |
| Maryland | ● | ● | ● | | ● | ● | ● | ● | ● | ● | ● | ● | ● | ● | ● | B | B | ● | ● | ● | ● | ● | ● | ● | ● |
| Massachusetts | D | D | A | A | D | D | A | D | D | D | D | D | | D | A | D | D | A | D | D | D | D | D | D | D |
| Michigan | ● | ● | ● | ● | ● | ● | ● | ● | ● | ● | ● | ● | ● | ● | D | ● | ● | ● | ● | ● | ● | ● | | | ● |
| Minnesota | ● | ● | ● | ● | ● | ● | ● | ● | ● | ● | ● | ● | ● | ● | ● | ● | ● | ● | ● | ● | ● | ● | ● | ● | ● |
| Mississippi | ● | ● | ● | A | ● | A | ● | ● | A | ● | ● | ● | ● | ● | ● | A | A | ● | ● | ● | ● | A | | | ● |
| Missouri | ● | ● | ● | ● | ● | ● | ● | ● | ● | ● | ● | ● | ● | ● | ● | ● | ● | ● | ● | ● | ● | ● | | | ● |
| Montana | D | | | | | | | | | | | D | | | | | | D | D | ● | D | D | | | ● |
| Nebraska | D | D | D | D | D | D | D | D | D | D | D | D | D | D | D | D | D | D | D | | D | D | ● | ● | ● |
| Nevada | ● | ● | ● | | ● | | | ● | ● | ● | ● | ● | ● | ● | ● | B | B | ● | ● | ● | ● | ● | B | B | A |
| NewHampshire | D | D | ● | | ● | | | ● | | D | D | D | | | ● | | D | D | D | ● | D | | ● | ● | ● |
| New Jersey | ● | ● | ● | ● | ● | ● | ● | ● | ● | ● | ● | ● | ● | ● | ● | ● | ● | ● | ● | ● | ● | ● | | | ● |
| New Mexico | A | D | A | | A | | | A | D | D | A | A | D | D | D | B | B | A | A | A | A | D | B | B | ● |
| New York | ● | ● | ● | ● | ● | ● | ● | ● | ● | ● | ● | ● | ● | ● | ● | ● | ● | ● | ● | ● | ● | ● | | | ● |
| North Carolina | ● | | ● | | ● | | | ● | | ● | | ● | ● | | | | | ● | ● | ● | ● | ● | | | ● |
| North Dakota | ● | ● | ● | | ● | ● | ● | ● | ● | ● | ● | ● | ● | ● | ● | ● | ● | ● | ● | ● | ● | ● | | | ● |
| Ohio | ● | ● | ● | | ● | | | ● | ● | ● | ● | ● | ● | ● | ● | ● | ● | ● | ● | ● | ● | ● | | | ● |
| Oklahoma | ● | ● | ● | | ● | D | | ● | ● | ● | ● | ● | ● | ● | ● | ● | ● | ● | ● | ● | ● | ● | | | ● |
| Oregon | ● | D | ● | | ● | | | ● | D | D | ● | ● | D | D | D | B | B | ● | ● | ● | ● | ● | D | B | B | ● |
| Pennsylvania | B | B | B | B | B | | B | B | B | B | B | B | B | B | B | B | B | B | ● | B | B | B | ● | ● | ● |
| Rhode Island | | D | | | | | | | | | | | | | | | | | ● | | | | ● | ● | ● |
| South Carolina | ● | ● | ● | ● | ● | ● | ● | ● | ● | ● | ● | ● | ● | ● | | ● | ● | ● | ● | ● | ● | ● | | | ● |
| South Dakota | ● | ● | ● | | ● | ● | ● | ● | ● | ● | ● | ● | ● | ● | ● | ● | ● | ● | ● | ● | ● | ● | | | ● |
| Tennessee | ● | ● | ● | ● | ● | ● | D | ● | ● | ● | ● | ● | ● | ● | ● | ● | ● | ● | ● | ● | ● | ● | ● | ● | ● |
| Texas | D | D | D | C | D | C | C | C | D | D | D | D | C | C | C | D | D | D | ● | D | D | D | | | ● |
| Utah | ● | ● | ● | | ● | D | | ● | ● | ● | ● | | ● | ● | D | | ● | ● | ● | ● | ● | ● | | | ● |
| Vermont | D | D | D | | D | | | | | D | D | ● | | | D | | | ● | ● | D | D | D | ● | ● | ● |
| Virginia | D | D | D | | D | D | | | D | D | D | D | | | | D | D | D | ● | D | D | D | D | D | ● |
| Washington | D | | D | | D | D | | | D | D | D | D | | | | D | D | ● | D | D | | | | | ● |
| West Virginia | D | D | D | D | D | D | D | D | D | D | D | D | D | D | D | D | D | D | ● | D | D | D | ● | ● | ● |
| Wisconsin | ● | | ● | ● | ● | ● | ● | ● | ● | ● | ● | ● | ● | ● | ● | | ● | ● | ● | ● | ● | ● | | | ● |
| Wyoming | ● | ● | ● | ● | ● | | | | | | | | | | ● | | | | | | | | | | ● |

[1] Terminology consistent with ACMG report - Newborn Screening: Towards a Uniform Screening Panel and System. Genet Med. 2006; 8(5) Suppl: S12-S252

### Deficiency/Disorder Abbreviations and Names (optional nomenclature)

| Abbrev | Name | Abbrev | Name | Abbrev | Name | Abbrev | Name |
|---|---|---|---|---|---|---|---|
| 2M3HBA | 2-Methyl-3-hydroxy butyric aciduria | CACT | Carnitine acylcarnitine translocase | GA-II | Glutaric acidemia Type II | MAL | Malonic acidemia (Malonyl-CoA decarboxylase) |
| 2MBG | 2-Methylbutyryl-CoA dehydrogenase | CBL-C,D | Methylmalonic acidemia (Cbl C,D) | GALE | Galactose epimerase | MCKAT | Medium-chain ketoacyl-CoA thiolase |
| 3MGA | 3-Methylglutaconic aciduria | CIT-II | Citrullinemia Type II | GALK | Galactokinase | MET | Hypermethioninemia |
| ARG | Argininemia (Arginase deficiency) | CPT-Ia | Carnitine palmitoyltransferase I | H-PHE | Benign hyperphenylalaninemia | SCAD | Short-chain acyl-CoA dehydrogenase |
| BIOPT-BS | Defects of biopterin cofactor biosynthesis | CPT-II | Carnitine palmitoyltransferase II | IBG | Isobutyryl-CoA dehydrogenase | TYR-II | Tyrosinemia type II |
| BIOPT-REG | Defects of biopterin cofactor regeneration | De-Red | Dienoyl-CoA reductase | M/SCHAD | Medium/Short chain L-3-hydroxy acyl-CoA dehydrogenase | TYR-III | Tyrosinemia type III |

Table 3.2: Newborn screening tests by American state. (Reproduced with permission from Dr Brad Therrell, Director, National Newborn Screening and Global Resource Center (NNSGRC).)

In 2011, the United States Secretary of Health and Human Services recommended adding pulse oximetry to the RUSP. Given that heart defects often lead to hypoxia, oximetry is a noninvasive way of ensuring that a newborn's blood is sufficiently oxygenated. The seven main disorders screened for with pulse oximetry are hypoplastic left heart syndrome, pulmonary atresia, tetralogy of Fallot, total anomalous pulmonary venous return, transposition of the great arteries, tricuspid atresia, and truncus arteriosus. Some birthing hospitals in the United States have already initiated screening for congenital heart defects via pulse oximetry (48). Pulse oximetry is more cost-effective with larger populations because of a greater yield of true positive results, and necessitates referral to a pediatric cardiologist for abnormal findings. The future may include routine MRIs or digital echocardiograms to ensure congenital heart and lung defects are diagnosed prior to the infant leaving the hospital.

## Infrastructure concerns

While it is encouraging that viable DNA can be obtained from either fresh-frozen or paraffin-embedded tissue, there are substantial system issues to be addressed to ensure that material is available for genetic testing. In some jurisdictions, the system for retaining and storing specimens and tissue blocks is chaotic and disorganized. Older medical examiner and coroner facilities are often smaller and may have outgrown their storage capacity. Local and state governments likely do not have funds available to hire an employee trained and dedicated to shipping specimens in compliance with United States federal guidelines. Some offices lack even a basic inventory of shipping supplies — for example, appropriately sized, insulated shipping containers, packing tape, and Dry Ice UN 1845 adhesive labels. Most medical examiner and coroner offices do not have dry ice for shipping frozen specimens because it is not a part of a daily forensic practice. Ideally, medical examiner and coroner offices would have a designated -40 °F (or colder) freezer for specimen storage. Another important component of sending specimens is that the freezer is sufficiently organized to enable retrieval of a specific case.

## Ethical considerations

In California, as in most of the United States, there is no right to privacy after death. With the United States Privacy Act, an individual's right to privacy terminates at death (49). However, under the United States Freedom of Information Act (FOIA), the privacy of a decedent's survivors may be considered and, in some landmark cases, families have prevailed (*Marzen v HHS* in 1987; *New York Times Co. v NASA* in 1991[3]). Also, as in other jurisdictions, death certificates, autopsy, and investigative reports are part of the

---

3  *Marzen v Department of Health and Human Services*, 825 F.2d 1148 (7th Cir, 1987); *New York Times Co. v NASA*, 782 F. Supp. 628 (DDC, 1991).

public record in California, unless sealed by law enforcement. Scientists in Houston, Texas, (50) have addressed ethical considerations of molecular autopsies, customarily done by a medical examiner or coroner without additional consent from next-of-kin in their purview to determine a cause and manner of death. Their recommendations include that genetic testing results should be treated as an "unwarranted invasion of privacy" and that the genetic results are exempt from disclosure and discovery under the FOIA. Other recommendations include guidelines for disclosure of results to first-degree relatives and the importance of underscoring the limitation of current knowledge in the case of negative findings for a genetic cause of death. Families of a decedent with a positive genetic finding associated with a sudden death should be referred to genetic counselors and specialists in the clinical condition accounting for death.

## Conclusions

In summary, this is an exciting and rewarding time to be researching causes of sudden death in childhood. Surveillance efforts in the United States are expanding; there is an established online support community for bereaved families; and DNA sampling technology is widespread and becoming more common, easier and affordable. There are also effective treatments for known disorders screened at birth. The sudden death of a child is always tragic, and grief is compounded when a cause of death cannot be ascertained. With an increase in successful determination of cause and manner of death, whether through genetic testing, advances in forensic science, or scientifically tenable prevention efforts, we can hope for a future with fewer deaths among toddlers.

## References

1. CDC. Sudden unexpected infant death and sudden infant death syndrome. [Available from: https://www.cdc.gov/sids/data.htm]. Accessed 13 September 2017.

2. Krous H, Chadwick A, Crandall L, Nadeau-Manning J. Sudden unexpected death in childhood: A report of 50 cases. Ped Dev Path. 2005;8(3):307-19. https://doi.org/10.1007/s10024-005-1155-8.

3. Mikkelsen L, Lopez A, Phillips D. Why birth and death registration really are "vital" statistics for development. 2015. [Available from: http://hdr.undp.org/en/content/why-birth-and-death-registration-really-are-%E2%80%9Cvital%E2%80%9D-statistics-development]. Accessed 13 September 2017.

4. United Nations. UN Stats. [Available from: http://unstats.un.org/unsd/vitalstatkb/ExportPDF50666.aspx]. Accessed 13 September 2017.

5.  UN. Sample Vital Registration with Verbal Autopsy. [Available from: http://unstats. un.org/unsd/vitalstatkb/ExportPDF50666.aspx]. Accessed 13 September 2017.

6.  World Health Organization. Monitoring the health goal — Indicators of overall progress. 2016. [Available from: http://www.who.int/gho/publications/ world_health_statistics/2016/EN_WHS2016_Chapter3.pdf?ua=1]. Accessed 13 September 2017.

7.  World Health Organization. Vital statistics. [Available from: http://www.who. int/gho/publications/world_health_statistics/2016/EN_WHS2016_Chapter3. pdf?ua=1]. Accessed 13 September 2017.

8.  CDC WONDER Online Database. Centers for Disease Control and Prevention, National Center for Health Statistics: Compressed Mortality File 1999-2013, Series 20 No. 2S, 2014, as compiled from data provided by the 57 vital statistics jurisdictions through the Vital Statistics Cooperative Program. [Available from: http://wonder.cdc.gov/cmf-icd10-archive2013.html]. Accessed 31 May 2017.

9.  Molander N. Sudden natural death in later childhood and adolescence. Arch Dis Child. 1982;57(8):572-6. https://doi.org/10.1136/adc.57.8.572.

10. Neuspiel DR, Kuller LH. Sudden and unexpected nautral death in childhood and adolescence. JAMA. 1985;254(10):1321-5. https://doi.org/10.1001/ jama.1985.03360100071016.

11. Siboni A, Simonsen J. Sudden unexpected natural death in young persons. Forensic Sci Int. 1986;31(3):159-66. https://doi.org/10.1016/0379-0738(86)90183-0.

12. Southall DP, Stebbens V, Shinebourne E. Sudden and unexpcted death between 1 and 5 years. Arch Dis Child. 1987;62(7):700-5. https://doi.org/10.1136/ adc.62.7.700.

13. Southall DP, Richards J, deSwict M, Arrowsmith WA, Cree JE, Fleming PJ, et al. Identification of infants destined to die unexpectedly during infancy: Evaluation of predictive importance of prolonged apnoea and disorders of cardiac rhythm or conduction. First report of a multicentred prospective study in to the sudden infant death. BMJ. 1983;286:1092-6. https://doi.org/10.1136/bmj.286.6371.1092.

14. Hoffman HJ, Damus K, Hillman L, Krongrad E. Risk factors for SIDS. Results of the National Institute of Child Health and Human Development SIDS cooperative epidemiological study. Ann NY Acad Sci. 1988;533:13-30. https:// doi.org/10.1111/j.1749-6632.1988.tb37230.x.

15. Keeling JW, Knowles S. Sudden death in childhood and adolescence. J Pathol. 1989;159(3):221-4. https://doi.org/10.1002/path.1711590308.

16. Skinner J, Crawford J, Smith W, Aitken A, Heaven D, Evans C, et al. Prospective, population-based long QT molecular autopsy study of postmortem negative sudden death in 1 to 40 year olds. Heart Rhythm. 2011;8(3):412-19. https://doi.org/10.1016/j.hrthm.2010.11.016.

17. Boston Children's Hospital. Long QT Syndrome symptoms & causes. [Available from: http://www.childrenshospital.org/conditions-and-treatments/conditions/long-qt-syndrome]. Accessed 12 January 2018.

18. McGarvey CM, O'Regan M, Cryan J, Treacy A, Hamilton K, Devaney D, et al. Sudden unexplained death in childhood (1-4 years) in Ireland: An epidemiological profile and comparison with SIDS. Arch Dis Child. 2012;97:692-7. https://doi.org/10.1136/archdischild-2011-301393.

19. Kinney HC, Chadwick AE, Crandall LA, Grafe M, Armstrong DL, Kupsky WJ, et al. Sudden death, febrile seizures, and hippocampal and temporal lobe maldevelopment in toddlers: A new entity. Pediatr Dev Pathol. 2009;12:455-63. https://doi.org/10.2350/08-09-0542.1.

20. Winkel BG, Larsen M, Berge K, Leren TP, Nissen PH, Olesen MS, et al. The prevalence of mutations in KCNQ1, KCNH2, and SCN5A in an unselected national cohort of young sudden unexplained death cases. J Cardiovasc Electrophysiol. 2012;23(10):1092-8. https://doi.org/10.1111/j.1540-8167.2012.02371.x.

21. Treacy A, Cryan J, McCarvey C, Devaney D, Matthews TG. Sudden unexplained death in childhood. An audit of the quality of autopsy reporting. Ir Med J. 2013;106(3):70-2.

22. Rushton DI. West Midlands perinatal mortality survey, 1987. An audit of 300 perinatal autopsies. BJOG. 1991;98:624-7. https://doi.org/10.1111/j.1471-0528.1991.tb13446.x.

23. Puranik R, Gray B, Lackey H, Yeates L, Parker G, Duflou J, et al. Comparison of conventional autopsy and magnetic resonance imaging in determing the cause of sudden death in the young. J Cardiovasc Magn Reson. 2014;16:44-53. https://doi.org/10.1186/1532-429X-16-44.

24. National Institute of Neurological Disorders and Stroke. Febrile seizures fact sheet. [Available from: www.ninds.nih.gov/Disorders/Patient-Caregiver-Education/Fact-Sheets/Febrile-Seizures-Fact-Sheet]. Accessed January 2018.

25. Kinney HC, Armstrong DL, Chadwick AE, Crandall LA, Hilbert C, Belliveau RA, et al. Sudden death in toddlers associated with developmental abnormalities of the hippocampus: A report of five cases. Pediatr Dev Pathol. 2007;10:208-23. https://doi.org/10.2350/06-08-0144.1.

26. Holm IA, Poduri A, Crandall L, Haas E, Grafe MR, Kinney HC, et al. Inheritance of febrile seizures in sudden unexplained death in toddlers. J Pediatr Neurol. 2012;46:235-9. https://doi.org/10.1016/j.pediatrneurol.2012.02.007.

27. Wixom C, Chadwick AE, Krous HF. Sudden, unexpected death associated with meningioangiomatosis: Case report. Pediatr Dev Pathol. 2005;8:240-4. https://doi.org/10.1007/s10024-004-9105-4.

28. Masoumi H, Kinney HC, Chadwick AE, Rubio A, Krous H. Sudden unexpected death in childhood associated with cardiac rhabdomyoma, involuting adrenal ganglioneuroma and megalencephaly: Another expression of tuberous sclerosis? Pediatr Dev Pathol. 2007;10:129-33. https://doi.org/10.2350/06-04-0081.1.

29. Krous HF, Chadwick AE, Miller DC, Crandall L, Kinney HC. Sudden death in toddlers with viral meningitis, massive cerebral edema, and neurogenic pulmonary edema and hemorrhage: Report of two cases. Pediatr Dev Pathol. 2007;10:463-9. https://doi.org/10.2350/06-08-0156.1.

30. Krous HF, Wahl C, Chadwick AE. Sudden unexpected death in a toddler with Williams syndrome. Forensic Sci Med Pathol. 2008;4:240-5. https://doi.org/10.1007/s12024-008-9035-y.

31. Lucas JR, Masoumi H, Krous HF. Sudden death in a toddler with laryngotracheitis caused by human parainfluenza virus-1. Pediatr Dev Pathol. 2009;12:165-8. https://doi.org/10.2350/08-06-0485.1.

32. National Organization for Rare Disorders. NORD. [Available from: rarediseases. org]. Accessed January 2018.

33. Hefti MM, Cryan J, Haas E, Chadwick, AE, Crandall LA, Trachtenberg, FL, et al. Hippocampal malformation associated with sudden death in early childhood: A neuropathologic study. Forensic Sci Med Pathol. 2016;12(1):14-25. https://doi.org/10.1007/s12024-015-9731-3.

34. Hefti MM, Cryan JB, Haas EA, Chadwick AE, Crandall LA, Trachtenberg FL, et al. Sudden unexpected death in early childhood: General observations in a series of 151 cases. Forensic Sci Med Pathol. 2016;12(1):4-13. https://doi.org/10.1007/s12024-015-9724-2.

35. Kinney HC, Poduri AH, Cryan JB, Haynes RL, Teot L, Sleeper LA, et al. Hippocampal formation maldevelopment and sudden unexpected death across the pediatric age spectrum. J Neuropathol Exp Neurol. 2016;75(10):981-97. https://doi.org/10.1093/jnen/nlw075.

36. Hesdorffer DC, Crandall LA, Friedman D, Devinsky O. Sudden unexplained death in childhood: A comparison of cases with and without a febrile seizure history. Epilepsia. 2015;56(8):1294-300. https://doi.org/10.1111/epi.13066.

37. NIH National Heart, Lung and Blood Institute. Frequently asked questions about the sudden death in the young case registry. [Available from: https://www.nhlbi.nih.gov/news/spotlight/fact-sheet/frequently-asked-questions-about-sudden-death-young-case-registry]. Accessed 13 September 2017.

38. Tanzi RE. Molecular genetics of Alzheimer's disease and the amyloid beta peptide precursor gene. Ann Med. 1989;21(2):91-4. https://doi.org/10.3109/07853898909149191.

39. Ackerman MJ, Tester DJ, Driscoll DJ. Molecular autopsy of sudden unexplained death in the young. Am J Forensic Med Pathol. 2001;22(2):105-11. https://doi.org/10.1097/00000433-200106000-00001.

40. Wang D, Shah K, Um S, Eng LS, Zhou B, Lin Y, et al. Cardiac channelopathy testing in 274 ethnically diverse sudden unexplained deaths. Forensic Sci Int. 2014;237:90-9. https://doi.org/10.1016/j.forsciint.2014.01.014.

41. Kumar S, Peters S, Thompson T, Morgan N, Maccicoca I, Trainer A, et al. Familial cardiological and targeted genetic evaluation: Low yield in sdden unexplained death and high yield in unexplained cardiac arrest syndromes. Heart Rhythm. 2013;10(11):1653-60. https://doi.org/10.1016/j.hrthm.2013.08.022.

42. CDC. Trends in out-of-hospital births in the United States, 1990-2012. [Available from: https://www.cdc.gov/nchs/products/databriefs/db144.htm]. Accessed 12 January 2018.

43. Raho J. The changing moral focus of newborn screening: An ethical analysis by the President's Council on Bioethics Appendix Newborn Screening: An international survey. [Available from: https://repository.library.georgetown.edu/bitstream/handle/10822/559379/thechangingmoralfocusofnewbornscreening-appendix-josephraho.pdf?sequence=1]. Accessed January 2017.

44. Newborn Screening Translational Research Network. Robert Guthrie, MD, PhD. [Available from: https://www.nbstrn.org/about/spotlight/Guthrie]. Accessed January 2017].

45. National Newborn Screening & Global Resource Center. National Newborn Screening Status Report. [Available from: genes-r-us.uthscsa.edu]. Accessed January 2017.

46. Alaska DHS. Newborn metabolic screening program. [Available from: http://dhss.alaska.gov]. Accessed January 2018.

47. CF Ireland. Newborn blood spot screening for cystic fibrosis. 2016. [Available from: https://www.cfireland.ie/newborn-screening-for-cf]. Accessed 12 January 2018.

48. CDC. New study findings: How cost-effective is screening for critical congenital heart defects? [Available from: https://www.cdc.gov/ncbddd/heartdefects/screening.html]. Accessed January 2018.

49. Herold R. Is there privacy beyond death? [Available from: http://www.privacyguidance.com/files/Privacy_Beyond_Death_Herold.pdf]. Accessed 13 September 2017.

50. McGuire A, Moore Q, Majuimder M, Walkiewicz M, Eng CM, Belmont JW, et al. The ethics of conduycting molecular autopsies in cases of sudden death in the young. Genome Res. 2016;26:1165-9. https://doi.org/10.1101/gr.192401.115.

# 4

# Sudden Infant Death Syndrome: History

Leanne Raven, MNS, BAppSc

*Faculty of Science, Health, Education and Engineering,*
*University of Sunshine Coast, Queensland, Australia*

## Introduction

Over the last century human life expectancy has increased in many countries throughout the world. After World War II it was still accepted by the medical and scientific community that an infant could die suddenly and unexpectedly from no known cause (1). In the 1960s, this view began to be challenged and in 1963 and 1969 two international conferences were held to focus on the etiology of sudden infant death syndrome (SIDS), and the first working definition of SIDS was established (1).

However, given the overall decline in perinatal mortality during the last century due to medical advancements and higher standards of living, our societal expectations have changed. It has now become the norm that children will thrive and grow to outlive their parents, when 100 years ago this was frequently not the case. With our increased knowledge about how the human body functions and about how to prevent childhood diseases, it has become unthinkable that in the 21st century a healthy child would die in their sleep from SIDS, and yet this still happens to many families. Indeed, SIDS remains the leading cause of infant mortality in Western countries, contributing to half of all post-neonatal deaths (2, 3).

For any parent there could be no greater nightmare than the silent tragedy of SIDS. When a child's death is attributed to SIDS, a diagnosis of exclusion, the infant's death remains unexplained even after a thorough investigation, including performance of a complete autopsy and review of the circumstances of death and clinical history (4). It has been estimated by Red Nose that, on average, at least 60 people are impacted by a child's death to SIDS. The parents, siblings, and extended family are at the core of this experience, with friends, work colleagues, first responders, coroners, and health professionals included in the network of those impacted. SIDS communities have formed in every country as a result of these tragedies, often through the significant leadership and unrelenting passion of the families and individuals who have lived through the experience of SIDS. These families have embarked on a quest for answers as to why this tragedy happened to them, with their journey often involving activities undertaken in honor and memory of their beloved children.

## Establishment of SIDS Organizations in Australia

In Australia these parent organizations were founded by individuals from families who experienced the death of a child from SIDS in the late 1970s, when the number of child deaths from SIDS was much higher than it is now. On average during 1980 to 1990 there were 195.6 deaths per 100,000 live births (5). The first of these organizations, called the "Sudden Infant Death Research Foundation Incorporated" (now known as Red Nose), was founded by Kaarene Fitzgerald in July 1977 in Melbourne, Victoria, following the death of her son Glenn to SIDS. Kaarene's vision was contagious and others soon followed, with parent organizations being established in each State and Territory of Australia. The founders of the parent organizations advocated for answers to many questions as they struggled with their own grief journeys; looked to help other families impacted by SIDS; and created local networks of supporters. They had many questions to pursue, such as:

- Why has this happened to my perfectly healthy infant?
- Who is to blame for these deaths?
- How could we have prevented this from happening?
- How can other families be saved from experiencing such a tragedy and loss?
- How can families who experience this tragedy be better supported and helped to build their lives again?

Parent organizations advocated for funds to invest in research to find answers to these questions. They worked with medical pathologists, police and coroners to see what could be learnt from death scene investigations and how best to define the phenomenon of SIDS. As prevention knowledge started to emerge from physiological and epidemiological studies, they developed health promotion campaigns with risk reduction messages that were implemented throughout the community. They focused on educating health professionals to communicate these messages to new parents, and introduced support services for impacted families by providing individual counseling, peer support programs, and group activities.

In order to create a cohesive national voice in Australia the parent organizations grouped together in 1986 to form a national company, the National SIDS Council of Australia, of which they became the founding members. This national organization formed strong relationships with a network of national and international scientists, medical researchers, health professionals, pediatricians, midwives, nurses, coroners, pathologists, bereaved families, and the community. Individuals in these networks and professional disciplines supported the SIDS cause by continuing to educate the community with risk reduction messages, by conducting research in search of a cause of death in a challenging field, sharing their expertise in bereavement care and supporting fundraising efforts such as Red Nose Day. This iconic fundraising event, introduced by Kaarene Fitzgerald in 1988, was the first signature charity day in Australia.

From my discussions with colleagues in other countries, it is clear that the development of parent organizations emerged in each country in different ways; however, the thrust of the movement began from those bereaved families' lived experiences and the concerns and interests of those in the vast network who were impacted by these child deaths. Thus the pathways of development, whilst different in many respects, have much in common across Western countries. Parent organization relationships extended across many countries in all continents and the international SIDS movement was formed with the establishment of SIDS Family International (SIDSFI) in 1987.

## International SIDS Community

The International Society for the Study and Prevention of Perinatal and Infant Death (ISPID), which I had the honor of chairing from 2012 to 2016, documents the history of the international SIDS movement on its website (5). In summary, following a meeting in Brussels in 1985 it was realized that benefits could be gained by countries working together, sharing ideas, and providing support for each other. A subsequent meeting, held at Lake Como Italy in 1987, formed the organization SIDSFI. The Chair of SIDSFI was Kaarene Fitzgerald. At a successive meeting the organization changed its name to SIDS International (SIDSI) to better reflect the professional services provided by its members.

The aims of SIDSI were to

- better understand the causes of, and thereby reduce the incidence of, SIDS and other sudden unexpected deaths in infancy (SUDI)
- act as an international voice and facilitate the international sharing of information on SIDS- and SUDI-related issues pertaining to statistical information, research, counseling, support, education, and service provision
- conduct an international conference every two years to facilitate the work.

ISPID was formed in 2008 in an amalgamation between the "first ISPID" and SIDSI. The first ISPID was formed in 2004 by a merger of the European Society for the Study and Prevention of Infant Death (ESPID) and the SIDS Global Strategy Task force (GSTF). ESPID was formed in 1990 and GSTF in 1992.

As an international leading body, ISPID is dedicated to the exchange of information among families, scientists, and other specialists in the field of perinatal and infant health, and to educating the global community on the prevention of infant death and stillbirth. The collective work of ISPID has brought together researchers from over 20 countries and has resulted worldwide in both information sharing of evidence-based preventative measures and the reduction of SIDS. ISPID has also been successful in implementing international standards and improved quality of care for bereaved parents. Its activities include co-operative workshops and studies; bestowing awards and travel grants to researchers, educators, and new investigators; and information sharing through meetings and biennial conferences which are usually hosted by member parent organizations (7). Since 2010, ISPID has held joint conferences with the International Stillbirth Alliance in recognition of the overlap in skills and expertise required to decrease the burden of stillbirth worldwide.

## Theories and Research Milestones

On the ISPID website you will find a list of peer reviewed references for all major SIDS case-control studies with parent contact (8). The list documented by Dr Peter Blair, the current Chair of ISPID, spans over 27 years from 1985. The most significant milestone in research into SIDS was identified over 25 years ago with a series of case-controlled studies, leading to a breakthrough in research which has saved over an estimated 9,000 babies' lives in Australia alone, and many more thousands of lives worldwide. This breakthrough identified that infants who slept on their backs were less likely to die from SIDS than those who slept on their stomachs (9). With the communication of this message through health promotion programs launched in many countries in the early 1990s, the number of deaths immediately decreased by 50% (9, 10). In Australia today we know that these deaths have decreased by some 80% since 1989 when risk reduction campaigns began (11).

The evidence base for risk factors, including both intrinsic (i.e. gender) and extrinsic (i.e. sleep position) factors, has been integrated in a "Triple Risk Model", found to be a useful framework for better understanding sudden infant death (9). The historical development of this model has been documented by Guntheroth and Spiers (12). In 1970, Bergman (13) argued that the phenomenon of SIDS was not dependant on a "single characteristic that ordains an infant for death, but on an interaction of risk factors with variable probabilities". Other researchers, including Wedgewood (14), Raring (15), and Rognum and Saugstad (16), developed the model that has evolved over time and is today applied by many scientists to guide research and development in the field (17).

The contemporary Triple Risk Model (1) proposes that when three conditions are present concurrently, a sudden infant death occurs. These conditions are: [1] the vulnerable infant (preterm birth, exposure to maternal smoking during pregnancy); [2] a critical development period (2-4 months of age); and [3] an exogenous stressor such as prone sleeping, head covering, co-sleeping, infection, or overheating.

## Prevention and "Reduce the Risk" Campaigns

In the search to find what causes SIDS, and ultimately how to prevent it, research breakthroughs have identified ways to reduce the risk of SIDS happening. The main breakthrough was to sleep the infant on its back; but in the early days of the program the message was both back and side sleeping. The messages contained in all of the SIDS health promotion programs have been drawn from the best available evidence. As a consequence, at times this has generated a lot of debate and there have been changes in messages over the years. Three examples spring to mind:

1.   the change to "back sleeping only" when "side sleeping" was dropped

2.   the inclusion of breastfeeding in the early campaigns, followed by breastfeeding not being emphasized for many years until it was found to be protective against SIDS; the inclusion of breastfeeding returned in 2011, following the publication of a meta-analysis of studies (18)

3.   the controversial home monitoring message, which is no longer advocated given insufficient evidence.

The first "Reduce the Risk/Back to Sleep" publication in English was produced by Cowan from the Canterbury Cot Death Society in New Zealand in May 1987. The first policy change recorded for health professionals was in July 1990, when Community Services Victoria in Australia informed all of the maternal and child health nurses to advise parents to place their babies on the back or side to sleep and to avoid overheating. A year later, a 12-page color brochure was produced in English and 10 other languages by the SIDS parent organization in Australia.

Following the SIDSI meeting in Sydney Australia in 1992, where papers focused on "Reduce the Risk/Back to sleep", campaigns began over the next few years in many countries. Further papers and discussions were held on reducing infant mortality at subsequent SIDSI/ ISPID meetings in Stavanger, Norway (1994); Washington DC, USA (1996); Rouen, France (1998); Auckland, New Zealand (2000); Florence, Italy (2002); Edmonton, Canada (2004); Yokohama, Japan (2006); Portsmouth, England (2008); Sydney, Australia (2010); Baltimore, USA (2012); Amsterdam, The Netherlands (2014); and most recently Montevideo, Uruguay (2016).

In many countries there have been multiple campaigns as the evidence base has changed over time. For example, in Australia there have been five campaigns: July 1990 was the start of the "Reduce the Risk" campaign in Victoria Australia; in June 1991 the

"Reducing the risk of SIDS" program was launched by the National SIDS Council of Australia; in June 1997 the "Three Ways to Reduce the Risk" program was launched; May 2002 saw the launch of the SIDS and Kids "Safe Sleeping Program"; and in 2011 the "Sleep Safe, My Baby" Program was launched by SIDS and Kids.

The success of the "Reduce the Risk/Back to Sleep" programs hinges on keeping up with the current research findings, and this is where the international SIDS community and the scientific committees of professional or parent organizations play a key role. The American Academy of Pediatrics produces recommendations for a safe sleeping environment in America and they keep these under review, having just released revised guidelines in 2016 (19). In some countries, parent organizations, such as the Lullaby Trust in the UK and Red Nose in Australia, produce guidelines and keep them under review through the establishment of networks of scientists or National Scientific Advisory Groups.

Results of these campaigns have been outstanding across the Western world, with many countries experiencing a significant reduction, between 50-80%, in infant mortality. However, these reductions have not been as great for the first peoples of many countries. Specific, culturally appropriate programs targeting these key groups have been implemented in an attempt to reduce the high rates of SIDS in Indigenous communities, as the rates in these groups are now often two or three times the rates in non-Indigenous groups (and have been much higher in previous years). The Reduce the Risk of SIDS in Aboriginal Communities (RROSIAC) program in Western Australia and the Pēpi-Pod® program in New Zealand and Australia are current examples of these targeted interventions.

Given that we cannot currently identify individual vulnerable babies at risk, the overall recommendations must focus on removing as many risk factors as possible during the first year of life, thereby minimizing the risks and reducing the likelihood of SIDS occurring. Concurrently, it is important to recognize that it is not possible to eliminate all risk without facing the negative consequences of disengagement from evidence-based messages by some groups or individuals (1). Innovative education programs need to be developed to target specific groups. Considerable success in educating health professionals has been obtained through online education programs based on competency assessments (20, 21).

## Grief and Loss Developments

Grief and loss support for parents, families, and individuals impacted by the death of a child has always been a key focus for the SIDS community at both international and local levels. In my experience the scientific and health professional community has always embraced the impact on families in a serious and respectful manner, recognizing the significant role played by parent organizations in raising awareness of the field and advocating for change and the advancement of knowledge.

We know that everyone will experience multiple losses in their lives and most people will not require bereavement counseling, as overtime they will make adjustments and adapt their life without their loved one/s. However, the loss experienced from the death of a child is a certain type of loss that is often more problematic. This loss becomes more challenging when it is sudden and unexpected, given that the parents and families can experience both the effects of trauma as well as profound grief. Similar types of losses include suicide and murder (22).

Grief can be overwhelming and parents can be confronted with intense, and often conflicting, experiences that can be challenging both for them personally and for their relationships. Petra den Hartog (23) identifies some of the hardest experiences that parents have to deal with, and these include: conflicting emotions of guilt, shame, anger, and blame; lowered confidence and self-esteem; feeling alone and isolated from friends and family; repression of feelings and masking grief; understanding there is no right or wrong way to grieve; different perceptions that test relationships; and the fear of relationship breakdowns.

Getting external help can be of benefit for many people, as the death of an infant is a tragic and devastating event. The grief journey is a process that takes time, understanding, empathy, and support. To enable families to normalize their grief, a strong support structure is essential. Bereavement support services provide choices for those impacted and assist in building resilience within the bereaved families' community (22). The range of services provided by parent organizations includes

- professional counseling for couples or individuals, which can be delivered face to face, via phone or email
- bereavement support helplines operating each day of the year, which are imperative for those needing support in order to enable them to make contact with someone at any time of the day
- peer support services, whereby trained bereaved parents can help in the healing process
- support groups allowing parents to share experiences and feelings, which are a part of the grief journey
- sibling programs, which are usually activity-based programs for children offered during school holidays
- internet support groups, which are moderated fora for bereaved parents and families
- memorial services or functions, which provide opportunities to remember those babies who have died.

Today most of these services have been expanded to embrace families and communities who have experienced the death of a child during pregnancy, birth, infancy, and childhood, regardless of the cause. Specific grief and loss online platforms have more recently been developed. These websites have expanded the reach of support for those with lived experience of child death, often through direct online chat facilities. They are also able to provide relevant and practical information for many groups impacted by these sudden and unexpected deaths.

## SIDS Community Today

Some 40 years on since Kaarene and Kevin Fitzgerald experienced the death of their son the question of what causes SIDS remains unanswered. Although we have seen a dramatic decrease in the incidence of SIDS through the success of safe sleeping health promotion programs and the increased knowledge of risk factors that increase the vulnerability to SIDS, SIDS still remains the leading cause of death for infants in Western countries (9).

We do today have an internationally agreed definition of SIDS; however, this term is not used in all cases and related classifications such as "unascertained" or "undetermined" are still being used in some jurisdictions. In Australia

- we do not have an agreed death scene investigation process in each state and territory, even though we now understand what constitutes best practice for death scene investigations.

- we are not creating new tissue banks for researchers to be used in Australian laboratories, although in the United States they continue to build on their tissue banks with parental consent.

- Red Nose (formally SIDS and Kids) does have an evidence-based health promotion program entitled "Sleep Safe, My Baby" which is used to inform parents and carers, and this program is kept under review and up to date by a National Scientific Advisory Group. However, there are mixed messages in the community, as each state and territory's Health Department develops their own modified guidelines. We are in desperate need of a National Health and Medical Research Council (NHMRC) Infant Safe Sleeping guideline in Australia.

Resources to tackle these problems are forever tight and we need to continue to strive for further knowledge to assist in targeting our endeavors. Even with the restructure of the parent organization groups in Australia, whereby seven of the ten SIDS and Kids organizations joined together as of April 2016 to form one national organization now known as Red Nose, there still remains an active SUDI agenda to address, with limited funds to pursue.

Parents and families are still living the SUDI experiences; healthy babies are still dying in their sleep; we have no way of understanding which individual babies are more vulnerable than others and why; and the rates of SUDI deaths are three times as high in Aboriginal and Torres Straight Islanders communities than in other communities. This agenda has also extended to the phenomenon of sudden unexplained death in childhood (SUDC), whereby a similar syndrome occurs in children aged over 12 months. In addition, the agenda now also includes stillbirth prevention, particularly late term stillbirth, given that many of the risk factors for SUDI and stillbirth are the same and some of the latest studies are focusing on maternal sleep position.

When birth numbers continue to increase and different carer groups, such as fathers and grandparents, emerge as playing a prominent role in infant care practices, then the community risk-minimization education remains of high importance. Indeed, targeted, innovative health promotion programs remain just as relevant today as they ever were. Furthermore, if the Red Nose aspirational goal of zero child deaths is to be achieved, then the existing research program must invest in new channels of investigation, exploring the different stages of a child's development to uncover why unexplained death occurs and how it can be prevented. Researchers are dedicated to finding the root causes of these death and this investment into cutting-edge research is critical in preventing the sudden and unexplained death of healthy children.

## SIDS Priorities in the Future

The recent international consensus project entitled Global Action and Prioritization of Sudden infant death (GAPS) aimed to strategically identify the top 10 research priorities in sudden unexpected infant death (SUID) in an effort to reduce these deaths worldwide (9). The author was a member of the multidisciplinary steering group for the project and the facilitator of the Australian workshop. The group recognized how vital it was, particularly given our limited resources, to identify where our best research efforts should be directed. The project aimed to harness the priorities from both lay and expert members of the SUID community. Three main themes emerged amongst the priorities in addressing the global SUID problem:

1. a better understanding of mechanisms underlying SUID

2. the importance of ensuring best practice in data collection, management, and sharing

3. a better understanding of target populations and more effective communication of risk.

Of the top 10 priorities, over half of the research priorities relate to the first theme — that is, the need for a better understanding of the mechanisms underlying SUID, in particular, the way that environmental factors interact with these mechanisms, the identification of associated biomarkers for cause of death determination by pathologists, and ultimately death prevention. Other related research priorities were the role of genetic factors in the risk of SUID; how the underlying mechanism of SUID risk differs with different ages; and the role of abnormal or immature brain anatomy and physiology. The priority in the second theme was enabling best practice processes and systematic data collection for accurate classification of SUID deaths in order to inform research and prevention. The final theme priorities related to better understanding of the behavior in target populations in order to inform new ways to make safe sleep campaigns more effective. Other priories include better understanding of cultural factors affecting parental choice in sleep practices and the practice of sharing a sleep surface with an infant, including how this interacts with other factors and its impact on risk.

## Conclusions

In my work with SIDS and Kids/Red Nose over the last 10 years, I have seen firsthand the untold and far-reaching devastation wrought by the sudden and unexpected death of a child. I have witnessed the importance of providing grief and loss support to these families and, as a result, have had parents thank me for our work at Red Nose because our wonderful counsellors have saved their lives. The death of a child from SIDS is something that no parent or family should ever have to experience. With the GAPS project identificating the list of shared research priorities, we have tremendous hope for an opportunity to emerge which will have maximum impact globally to tackle the problem of SUID. If policy makers, research funders and researchers working in the field of infant mortality implement these research priorities and continue to share this knowledge, we have good cause to be hopeful for a brighter future without SIDS.

## References

1.    Red Nose. Information statement: The Triple Risk Model. [Available from: https://rednose.com.au/downloads/Triple_Risk_Model_Information_Statement2017.pdf]. Accessed 22 September 2017.

2.    Carpenter RG, Irgens LM, Blair PS, England PD, Fleming P, Huber J, et al. Sudden unexplained infant death in 20 regions in Europe: Case control study. Lancet. 2004;363(9404):185-91. https://doi.org/10.1016/S0140-6736(03)15323-8.

3.    Byard RW, Krous HF. Sudden infant death syndrome: Overview and update. Pediatr Dev Pathol. 2003;6:112-27. https://doi.org/10.1007/s10024-002-0205-8.

4.    Krous HF, Beckwith BJ, Byard RW, Rognum TO, Bajanowski T, Corey T, et al. Sudden infant death syndrome and unclassified sudden infant deaths: A definitional and diagnostic approach. Pediatrics. 2004;114:234-8. https://doi.org/10.1542/peds.114.1.234.

5.    International Society for the Study and Prevention of Perinatal and Infant Death (ISPID). The history of ISPID. [Available from: https://www.ispid.org/ispid/history/]. Accessed 22 September 2017.

6.   Tursan d'Espaignet E, Bulsara M, Wolfenden L, Byard RW, Stanley FJ. Trends in sudden infant death syndrome in Australia from 1980 to 2002. Forensic Sci Med Pathol. 2008:4(2):83-90.

7.   International Society for the Study and Prevention of Perinatal and Infant Death (ISPID. ISPID's strategic directions and goals. [Available from: https://www.ispid.org/ispid/strategic/]. Accessed 22 September 2017.

8.   International Society for the Study and Prevention of Perinatal and Infant Death (ISPID. SIDS case-control studies. [Available from: https://www.ispid.org/infantdeath/id-pub/sidsccs/]. Accessed 22 September 2017.

9.   Hauck FR, McEntire BL, Raven LK, Bates FL, Lyus LA, Willett AM, et al. Research priorities in sudden unexpected infant death: An international consensus. Pediatrics. 2017;Epub(July):e20163514.

10.  Horne RD, Hauck FR, Moon RY. Sudden infant death syndrome and advice for safe sleeping. BMJ. 2015;350:h1989. https://doi.org/10.1136/bmj.h1989.

11.  Red Nose. Facts and figures. [Available from: https://rednose.com.au/page/facts-and-figures]. Accessed 22 September 2017.

12.  Guntheroth WG, Spiers PS. The triple risk hypotheses in sudden infant death syndrome. Pediatrics. 2002;110(5):e64. https://doi.org/10.1542/peds.110.5.e64.

13.  Bergman AB. Synthesis. In: Sudden infant death syndrome. Eds Bergman AB, Beckwith JB, Ray CG. Seattle, WA: University of Washington Press, 1970. p. 210-11.

14.  Wedgewood RJ. Review of the USA experience. In: Sudden and unexpected death in infancy (cot deaths). Eds Camps FE, Carpenter RG. Bristol: John Wright & Sons, 1972. p. 22-8.

15.  Raring RH. Crib death: Scourge of infants — Shame of society. Hicksville NY: Exposition Press, 1975. p. 93-7.

16.  Rognum TO, Saugstad OD. Biochemical and immunological studies in SIDS victims: Clues to understanding the death mechanism. Acta Paediatrica Suppl. 1993;Suppl 389:82-5. https://doi.org/10.1111/j.1651-2227.1993.tb12886.x.

17.  Spinelli J, Collins-Praino L, van den Heuval C, Byard RW. Evolution and significance of the triple risk model in sudden infant death syndrome. J Paediatr Child Health. 2017;53(2):112-15. https://doi.org/10.1111/jpc.13429.

18.  Hauck FR, Thompson JM, Tanabe KO, Moon RY, Venneman MM. Breastfeeding and reduced risk of sudden infant death syndrome: A meta-analysis. Pediatrics. 2011;128(1):103-10. https://doi.org/10.1542/peds.2010-3000.

19. Moon RY, & AAP Taskforce on Sudden Infant Death Syndrome. SIDS and other sleep-related infant deaths: Evidence base for 2016 updated recommendations for a safe infant sleeping environment. Pediatrics. 2016;138(5):e20162940. https://doi.org/10.1542/peds.2016-2940.

20. Young J, Higgins N, Raven LK, Watson M. Supporting nurses and midwives to promote a safe infant sleeping e-learning program. Aust Nurs J. 2013;21(2):41.

21. Young J, Higgins N, Raven L. Reach, effectiveness and sustainability of a safe infant sleeping e-learning program. Women and Birth. 2013;26(Supp 1):S21. https://doi.org/10.1016/j.wombi.2013.08.281.

22. Raven LK, Green J. Supporting parents through grief after a stillbirth or perinatal death. Australian Midwifery News. 2014;14:46-7 (spring).

23. den Hartog PN. Supporting parents following perinatal death. Grief Matters: Aust J Grief Bereavement. 2014;17(2):58-61 (winter).

# 5

# Responding to Unexpected Child Deaths

Peter Sidebotham, MBChB, PhD[1],
David Marshall, QPM, MSc[2] and
Joanna Garstang, MBChB, MSc, PhD[1]

[1]*Warwick Medical School, University of Warwick, Coventry, UK*
[2]*Dave Marshall Consultancy Ltd., London, UK*

## Introduction

> All hospital staff were very respectful of our wishes and explained everything well that they needed to do. We were given plenty of time and privacy with all our family after the baby died. (Bereaved parent)

> I was sat in the back of the police car and no-one spoke to me, I always remember the silence, it was awful, the silence was so bad. (Bereaved parent)

When a child dies suddenly and unexpectedly, we, as professionals, have a wide range of duties and obligations that must be fulfilled. Statutory requirements may place constraints on what we can do, when we need to do it, and how we can go about it. At the heart of it all, however, there remains a bereaved family, for whom the worst thing imaginable has just happened. As one bereaved mother put it: "Words may hurt me or make me angry, but I have lost my child, so don't flatter yourself — nothing that you say will actually make the situation worse".

Nevertheless, as the quotes at the start of this chapter highlight, parents' experiences following the death of their child vary enormously, and the way we respond to them can make a considerable difference. The way we respond can make a difference also to the outcome of an investigation. Identifying an unusual medical cause of death, or uncovering the circumstances of a tragic accident or a case of intentional filicide is more likely with a thorough, systematic investigation, conducted with sensitivity and respect, than with one carried out carelessly or in a haphazard or aggressive manner.

In most jurisdictions, the sudden unexpected death of an infant or child requires the case to be referred to a coroner, medical examiner, or procurator fiscal. In England, for example, a coroner is obliged to conduct an investigation into violent or unnatural deaths, deaths where the cause is unknown, and deaths which occur in custody or otherwise in state detention (1). Coroner's officers, or police officers acting on behalf of the coroner, will need to carry out an investigation into the causes and circumstances of the death. Where there are concerns about parenting, or the possibility of abuse or neglect, there may be other children in the family who need protection, necessitating the involvement of children's social care services.

Nevertheless, the reality is that in the majority of cases the child's death will be from natural causes, whether or not we are able to ascertain the actual cause. Therefore, health practitioners will need to carry out full investigations to look for possible medical causes, including infectious or genetic causes, which may have wider implications for the family or community. While infant mortality has fallen dramatically over the past decades, and continues to fall across the world, every death should still be seen as a tragedy, and we should do all we can to further reduce mortality rates and to reduce the risks of future child deaths. In order to do this effectively, we need to learn lessons — from each individual child's death, and from the patterns of children's deaths in any area — to identify potentially modifiable factors, and to take effective action to improve childcare, health and welfare services, and support for families. Through all this, all professionals will need to respond sensitively to the family in those awful, early stages of grief — in coming to terms with the reality of their child's death, in coping with the practical arrangements that need to be made, in breaking the news to family and friends.

Bearing in mind these varying and, at times, potentially conflicting obligations, five primary aims of our response to unexpected infant deaths can be defined (2, 3):

1.  to establish, as far as is possible, the cause or causes of the infant's death
2.  to identify any potential contributory or modifiable factors
3.  to provide ongoing support to the family
4.  to ensure that all statutory obligations are met
5.  to learn lessons, in order to reduce the risks of future infant deaths.

Underpinning this are three fundamental principles of practice which support a positive response: a thorough, systematic approach to investigation, a sensitive approach to supporting families, and an attitude of collaboration and learning (Figure 5.1).

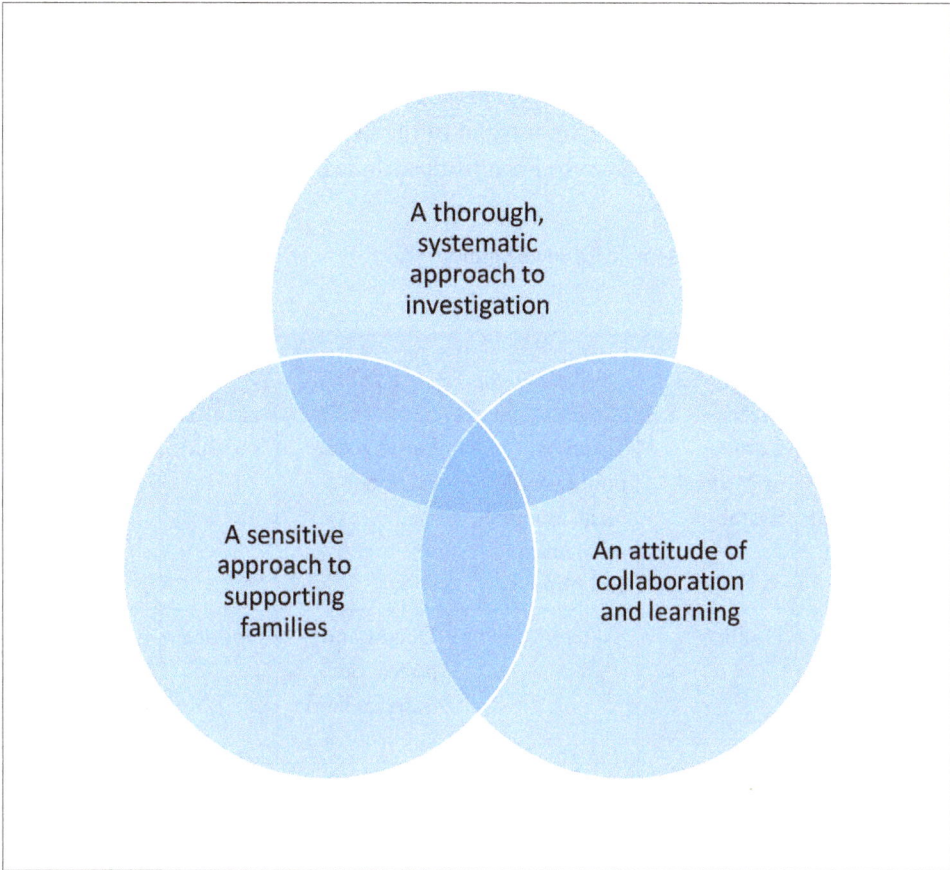

Figure 5.1: Principles of practice in responding to unexpected child deaths. (Authors' own work.)

## Models of Response

Every country has different ways of investigating unexpected child deaths; these may also differ widely within countries. The different models of response can be categorized as coroner- or medical examiner-led, police-led, healthcare-led or led by a joint agency approach (JAA); these are described in Table 5.1.

There is no internationally accepted standard for best practice management of sudden and unexpected death in infancy (SUDI), although the minimum standard could be considered as one that enables a diagnosis of sudden infant death syndrome (SIDS) to be made according to the 2004 San Diego definition; this relies on a detailed medical history, complete post-mortem examination, and a review of the circumstances of death (4). A more recent international consensus suggested that, in addition to the San Diego definition, a SIDS diagnosis requires a thorough scene examination by forensic medicine experts or specially trained police officers and a multi-professional meeting to classify the death (5). The joint agency approach, coroner- or medical examiner-led, and healthcare-led models all have the potential to meet this standard and have the potential to meet the five primary aims of SUDI investigation described previously, providing that care and support for families are integral to the investigative process and there is a robust child death review program to learn from such deaths.

Table 5.1: Different models of SUDI investigation (2).

| Model name | Lead Agency | Initial history from parents | Death scene examination | Autopsy | Individual case reviews |
|---|---|---|---|---|---|
| Coroner- or Medical Examiner-led investigation | Coroner or Medical Examiner | Taken by police, death scene examiner, or Medical Examiner | Death scene examiner | Variable | Variable |
| Healthcare-led investigation | Health | Taken by doctor | Doctor and police, but independently | Optional | Multi-disciplinary case review within health |
| Police-led investigation | Police | Police | Police and forensic team | Variable | None |
| Joint Agency Approach model | Health and police jointly | Taken by pediatrician and police | Jointly by police and pediatrician | Standard | Multi-agency case review |

Irrespective of the investigative model used, certain key factors promote effective investigation. These include close work between agencies; the integration, if possible, of SUDI investigations with any coronial or legal investigations rather than them running in parallel; and clear leadership from senior police and healthcare professionals. Ideally, detailed SUDI investigation should be mandatory; if not, many parents will decline them, limiting the learning from individual cases and for whole populations (6).

## The Structure of the Response

For the remainder of this chapter, we will outline the overall structure of the joint agency response as we understand it. This approach has been our practice over many years, and is embedded in national guidelines for England (3, 7-9). We describe our practice in England, recognizing that procedures and practices may well differ in different countries. Nevertheless, it is our view that the general principles underlying these

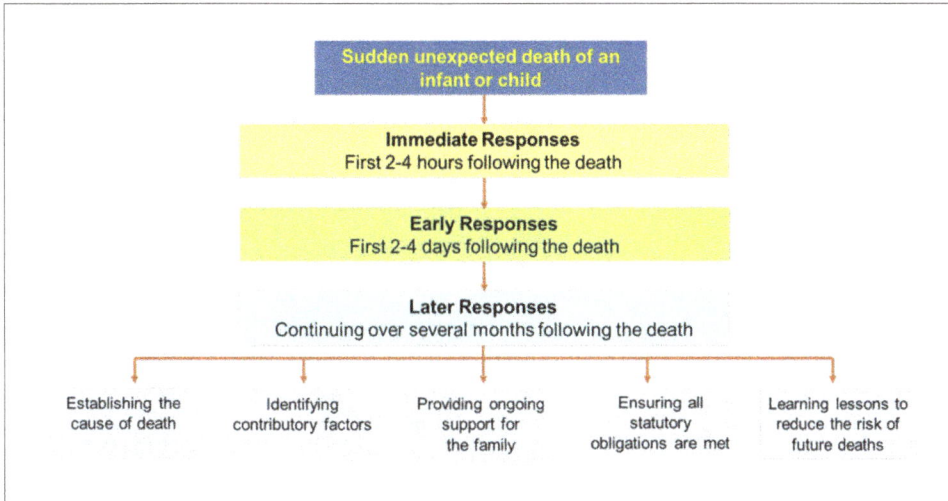

Figure 5.2: The structure of the joint agency response to an unexpected child death. (Authors' own work.)

responses are universally important. While the details of how this approach is worked out may vary between different areas, and according to the model in place, a number of core components can be identified (3):

1. careful multi-agency planning of the response

2. ongoing consideration of the psychological and emotional needs of the family,

3. including referral for bereavement support

4. initial assessment and management, including a detailed and careful history, examination of the infant, preliminary medical and forensic investigations, and immediate care of the family, including siblings

5. an assessment of the environment and circumstances of the death

6. a standardized and thorough post-mortem examination

7. a final multi-professional case discussion meeting.

The response can be divided into three overlapping phases, all of which contribute to meeting the overall aims (Figure 5.2). The different phases will be outlined in detail, although it must be emphasized that there is considerable overlap between the phases, and many of the procedures involved are ongoing processes rather than one-off events.

## Immediate responses

Under the heading of immediate responses, we are considering those activities that typically take place within a few hours of the child's death, including first responder

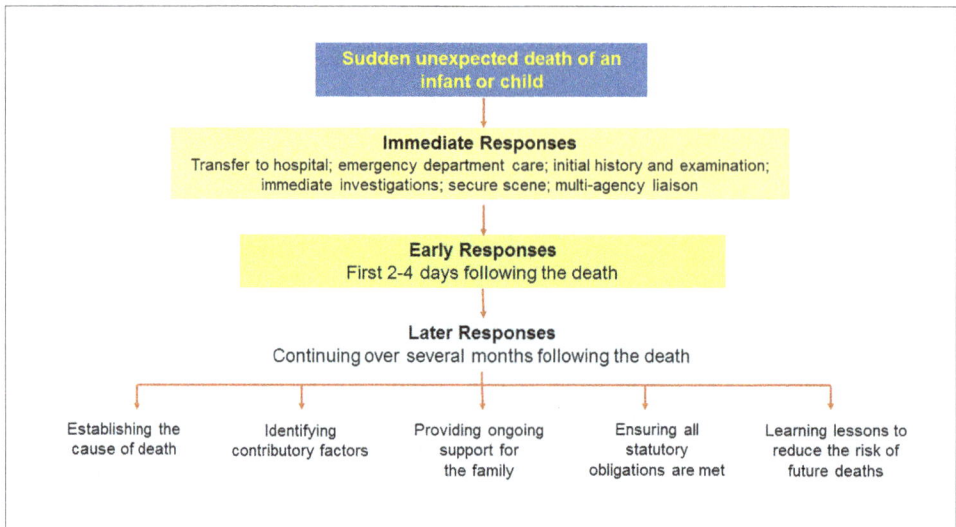

Figure 5.3: The immediate responses. (Authors' own work.)

and police actions at the scene of the death, transfer of the child and carer(s) to an emergency department, initial medical management and early information gathering, and initiating the joint agency components of the response (Figure 5.3).

When a child dies or collapses unexpectedly in the community, a family member or other person will usually call the emergency services promptly on discovering the child. The emergency services should despatch both an ambulance crew or first responder and a police officer. Ideally, the officer should be an appropriately qualified investigator, although it is recognized that this will not always be possible.

Immediate management at the scene of death

Unless it is clear that the infant has been dead for some time, for example with the onset of rigor mortis or signs of dependent livido, the ambulance crew will normally commence resuscitation according to appropriate pediatric guidelines. The ambulance crew may take an initial brief history from the parent while they are initiating resuscitation, particularly to establish the primary circumstances within which the child was discovered. They will also ascertain if there are any particular medical issues, such as a known ongoing or recent illness, or any drugs or medication (prescription or otherwise) that the infant may have received which may have a bearing on the resuscitation or understanding of the cause of death. They should note their initial impressions of the environment in which the child was found, along with the appearance of the child, and they should enquire as to any other children in the home, their welfare, and who will be looking after them.

The attending police officer will be able to help with arrangements to support the family, including considering the welfare of any other children, arrangements for the parents to attend the hospital, and notifying relatives or friends. The police officer should also make a note of their impressions and any immediate information they obtain on the circumstances and environment of the death.

## Transfer to hospital

Unless there are exceptional circumstances, such as clear signs of homicide, the infant will then normally be transferred to the nearest emergency department with pediatric facilities while continuing resuscitation. At the same time, arrangements should be made for the parent(s) or carer(s) to also attend the hospital, either in the ambulance or separately. Notifying the hospital of the child's anticipated arrival will enable the hospital team to prepare for their ongoing resuscitation. Transferring the infant to an emergency department serves a number of important purposes:

1. It ensures that all appropriate resuscitation can be continued, and that any decision to stop resuscitation is made in a considered way by an experienced team.

2. It provides immediate support for the parents by health personnel who are experienced in dealing with traumatic circumstances and bereavement.

3. The death of the child can be confirmed and documented by an appropriately qualified health professional.

4. It enables the initial history and examination of the child to be conducted by a pediatrician with appropriate skills and knowledge.

5. It enables immediate investigations to be carried out in a clinical setting.

6. It helps protect the environment where the child died until qualified investigators can review it.

7. It ensures that appropriate people are notified of the death and the joint agency response is initiated.

## Resuscitation and the decision to stop resuscitation

On arrival at hospital, resuscitation should be continued according to established guidelines for advanced pediatric life support, until it is clear that further resuscitation is futile, the child is confirmed dead, or a decision has been made to withdraw care. Also on arrival at the hospital, a member of the health team should be allocated to be with the parents to support them through the process, keep them informed of all that is happening, and help them with contacting other family members or sources of support. Consideration should be given to allowing the parents to be present during the resuscitation, and if so, they should be supported in that by the allocated member of the health staff.

There may be some situations where a child is successfully resuscitated and stabilized prior to transfer to an intensive care unit, only to have care withdrawn subsequently. In those circumstances, the timing and process of the joint agency response may need to be adapted, but consideration should still be given to the same underlying principles. The decision to stop resuscitation or withdraw care should be made by an experienced pediatrician, in consultation with the parents and the full healthcare team. Once resuscitation has been stopped, confirmation that the infant is dead should be made by a suitably qualified medical practitioner according to established guidelines. Confirmation of the infant's death, along with details of the resuscitation and of the joint agency management of the death, should be carefully documented in the child's medical records.

Once the infant has been confirmed dead, a senior medical practitioner should inform the family. This should ideally be carried out in a suitable, private, and quiet room, where the family can be with their infant if they so wish, and where they can be supported by the allocated member of staff. The family should be provided with time to take in the information and to ask any questions they may have, and a balance is required between sensitive, caring support and providing the family with space to be on their own.

Normally it will be appropriate for the family to hold and spend time with their infant, ideally after the infant has been examined by the pediatrician and all relevant immediate investigations have been completed. Even if there are suspicions of possible abuse or neglect, it may be appropriate for the family to spend time with their infant, following discussion with the lead police investigator, and with a discreet professional presence. If the family so wish, and following discussion with the lead police investigator, consideration should also be given to the taking of photographs, hand- or footprints or other mementos. If there are causes for concern with forensic implications that may be addressed during the post-mortem examination, it may be appropriate for some of these mementos to be taken after the post-mortem examination.

Early history taking

Taking a history is not a one-off event, but an evolving process that may require interviewing several people, and may involve going back over details to clarify points. However, repeated questioning by different professionals should be avoided, as it adds to the distress of parents and may contaminate evidence. Health staff, police officers, and social workers will need to work together on gathering the history, particularly where the death is unexplained, or there are potentially suspicious circumstances. An initial full history should be taken at the hospital jointly by a police officer and a pediatrician, with a pediatrician taking the lead due to the likely medical explanation for the death. It is crucial at this early stage to obtain as much information as possible to assess the circumstances of the death. This needs to be undertaken sensitively, but talking and contributing to the process of trying to establish how their child died can have a positive effect for the carer.

An outline of the key components of the history following a sudden infant death is provided in Box 1. A template or proforma may help in ensuring that all elements of the history are covered thoroughly.

## Box 1: The medical/forensic history following an unexpected infant death

- Detailed narrative account of events, particularly focusing on the 24 hours prior to death
- Circumstances of death, including place and position when put to sleep and when found
- Events following discovery of the death, including resuscitation and emergency responses
- Usual infant sleep arrangements
- Pregnancy and birth details
- Child's medical and developmental history, including feeding and growth, routine checks and immunizations, and health over previous weeks
- Household and family composition
- Family medical history, including previous miscarriages, stillbirths, and sibling deaths
- Parental health and use of medication, including mental health and disability
- Social history, including parental relationships, employment, social support, housing
- Parental smoking; antenatal and current smoking habits; alcohol consumption; use of illicit drugs
- Family involvement with social care

While history taking will start with the ambulance crew and be continued by the hospital medical staff, the full history from the main carer will often only be obtained at the home visit. A detailed narrative account of the events over the 24 (or more) hours leading to the death and discovery of the death is crucial to the investigation. This will often be far clearer when the parents are able to talk through the events in situ, jogging their memories and enabling details to be clarified directly.

Any discrepancies in the history, or changes, should be noted, although it is not uncommon for a history to change as it is retold and this does not necessarily imply anything suspicious. The process of taking a history provides an opportunity to make an assessment of the veracity, demeanor, and attitude of the parents. While one should take note of any inappropriate or unusual responses to the child's death (e.g. remoteness, insensitivity to circumstances, indifference to death, disposal of articles), it is also important to bear in mind that each person responds differently to grief and stress.

If there are significant suspicions which would give the police reasonable grounds to suspect the carer(s) of a criminal offence, the history taking may be bound by legal restrictions. For example, the *Police and Criminal Evidence Act 1984* (10) would put conditions on any conversation which could constitute an interview. However, even if there are suspicions, the police would be eager to establish whether there was any plausible explanation to explain these suspicions and also to allow factual questions regarding non-contentious areas such as the age of the child, and the names of parents or other siblings to be asked by medical staff. Where there are potential concerns, it may be considered appropriate to talk to the carers separately and with additional support for them if necessary. Talking to parents separately may, as well as highlighting possible inconsistencies in their accounts, also add credibility to what each of them is saying.

## Examining the child

Following confirmation of the death, the attending physician in the emergency department should carry out a thorough examination of the child, ideally in the presence of an investigating police officer. This will be followed up by an external examination by the pathologist at autopsy. However, the initial findings in the emergency department are important, as some signs may alter with the passage of time, and initial signs may alert the joint agency team to particular concerns that may require further investigation or management, such as the presence of a purpuric rash indicating the possibility of meningococcal sepsis, or a finding of injuries which may require specific police enquiries. It is important to be thorough and to document all findings clearly, using a body chart to demonstrate any external markings.

Ideally, all visible marks of possible significance should be photographed using a scale and then photographed again later, as marks may develop over a period of time and become clearer (e.g. bite marks or bruising). Some injuries may be clearer if photographed using alternative light sources such as UV light or a polarized filter. The police investigator will be able to advise on the appropriateness of this. Similar to the differential diagnosis excluding certain medical possibilities, many of the police inquiries are undertaken to establish what may have happened, which may rule factors out as well as discovering their presence.

Specific aspects of the examination are outlined in Box 2.

## Box 2: The examination of the child

The examining physician should take note of the following aspects:

- The child's overall appearance — noting any lividity, pallor, position, and tone of limbs; hygiene; any specific markers of disease or disability.

- Lividity (Figure 5.4) is usually deep purple in color, although the depth and degree may vary and may be influenced by underlying skin color. Livido develops due to gravity-assisted pooling of the blood so will take on a distribution corresponding to dependent parts of the child's body, often with sparing in areas of direct pressure. Typically it begins to develop during the first two hours of the child's death, but does not become fixed for 4-6 hours.

- Rigor mortis, a generalized stiffness of the muscles, again develops during the first 2 hours.

- Any blood/frothy fluid (Figure 5.5) or vomit around face, nose, mouth — in any death, frothy, blood-stained fluid can be forced out of the lungs. This is a normal terminal finding and does not indicate any particular cause or manner of death. Frank blood from the nose or mouth can arise from a number of medical or forensic causes and needs to be fully evaluated.

- Examination of the entire body for any rashes, abrasions, skin lesions, or injuries (recent or old); also noting the state of hygiene and any signs of neglect.

- Documenting all skin markings, lesions, and injuries on a body chart and consideration of photographs.

- Examination of the genitalia, and inside the mouth, including the lingual and labial frenae for any injuries or abnormalities.

- Retinal examination, where possible, looking for any evidence of bleeding or retinal pathology, bearing in mind that after death, the cornea quickly clouds over, which may preclude any detailed view of the retina. If any abnormalities are noted, or there are other indicators of concern, it may be appropriate to request an urgent review by an ophthalmologist.

- All interventions during resuscitation (e.g. sites of venepuncture) should be documented. Cannulae and endotracheal or nasogastric tubes may be removed, but their correct siting should be documented prior to removal (e.g. by direct laryngoscopy) by an independent observer.

- Documenting all growth parameters (weight, length, head circumference), marking these on appropriate centile charts, and also documenting markers of the state of nutrition.

- A core body temperature (low reading thermometer).

- Where there are any markers of injury or neglect, arrangements should be made for early photo-documentation by a police or medical photographer.

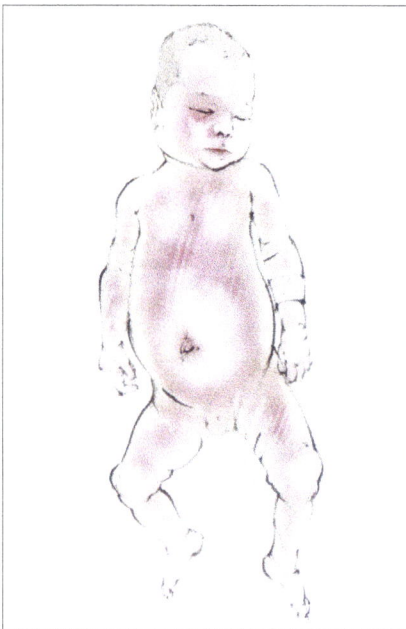

Figure 5.4: Post-mortem changes: Dependent lividity. (Reproduced with permission from the University of Warwick, UK.)

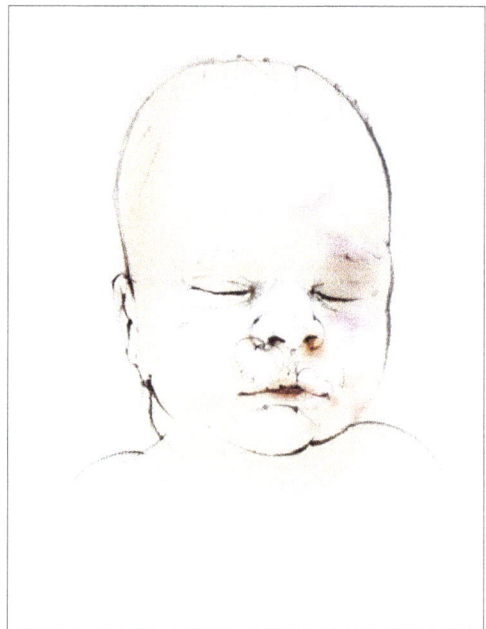

Figure 5.5: Post-mortem changes: Frothy, blood-stained mucus. (Reproduced with permission from the University of Warwick, UK.)

Following a sudden unexpected death in infancy, unless the cause of death is immediately apparent, a range of medical and forensic investigations are required to help ascertain the cause and any contributory factors (5). Samples may have been obtained during the course of any resuscitation; these should be carefully labeled and sent, along with any post-mortem samples obtained, for further analysis.

Following the resuscitation, consideration should be given to taking any further medical or forensic samples prior to the post-mortem examination; it may be necessary to seek consent from the coroner or police before doing so. If the post-mortem examination is to take place within 24 hours, sampling may be left to the pathologist. Blood samples should be taken from a single attempt at femoral artery puncture or cardiac aspiration; repeated attempts are best avoided, as they may compromise the post-mortem examination. Urine can be obtained by catheterization or supra-pubic aspiration, although the bladder is often empty in SIDS cases. A lumbar puncture should be attempted to obtain cerebro-spinal fluid, although this should not be undertaken if there is any suspicion of possible non-accidental head injury, as the autopsy findings could then be compromised. A skin biopsy should be taken from an unobtrusive area such as the back or inner arm or thigh. All sampling sites, whether successful or not, must be documented in the medical notes to avoid potential subsequent confusion with injuries or bruising. Emergency Departments can prepare a SUDI box with details of all specimens needed, sampling equipment, and paperwork to ease the process for medical teams dealing with such cases. Details of specimens required are listed in Table 5.2 (3).

Table 5.2: Details of specimens required immediately after death in SUDI cases.

| Specimen | Laboratory | Test |
| --- | --- | --- |
| Blood (culture bottles) | Microbiology | Aerobic and anaerobic culture for microscopy, culture, and sensitivities. If insufficient blood, aerobic only |
| Blood (serum) | Clinical Chemistry | Toxicology if indicated (spin and store serum at -20 °C) |
| Blood (from metabolic screening "Guthrie" card) | Clinical Chemistry | Amino acids, acyl carnitines |
| Blood (lithium heparin) | Cytogenetics | Karyotype and genetic testing if indicated |
| Urine | Microbiology | Culture for microscopy, culture, and sensitivities |
| Urine | Biochemistry | Metabolic testing, toxicology |

| Cerebro-spinal fluid | Microbiology | Culture for microscopy, culture, and sensitivities |
|---|---|---|
| Cerebro-spinal fluid | Virology | Polymerase chain reaction (PCR) |
| Skin biopsy | Histopathology | Fibroblast culture |
| Throat swab | Microbiology | Culture for microscopy, culture, and sensitivities |
| Throat swab | Virology | PCR, viral cultures, immunofluorescence |
| Naso-pharangeal aspirate | Virology | PCR, viral cultures, immunofluorescence |
| Skin swabs from any identifiable lesion | Microbiology | Culture for microscopy, culture, and sensitivities |

In addition to any medical samples obtained, any stool or urine passed by the infant, for example in a nappy or diaper, should be frozen and sent for analysis. Arrangements should be made for a full radiological skeletal survey and any other appropriate imaging. This requires a full set of films, as per a child protection investigation, and not merely a single "baby-gram". The images should be reported on by an experienced pediatric radiologist prior to the post-mortem examination.

Where there are no suspicions of abuse or homicide, the police will be conducting their input into the joint investigation on behalf of the coroner or medical examiner who is trying to establish who has died, and how, when, and where they have died. Where there is no indication of any criminal offences, samples are taken on the authority of the coroner to try and answer these questions. However, where there are grounds to suspect that a criminal act may have contributed to the death, the overall investigation will be led more by police than by medical personnel (although they will still work closely together). In these circumstances there may be particular legal frameworks, such as the *Police and Criminal Evidence Act 1984* (10), within which any samples must be taken and handled.

## Family support

After resuscitation has stopped, all medical equipment, such as intravenous lines and endotracheal tubes, should be documented and then removed, unless there are concerns that their use may have complicated the resuscitation. Endotracheal tubes may be removed after their correct placement in the trachea has been confirmed by independent direct laryngoscopy. Unless there are forensic concerns, the child's face can be washed, the nappy replaced, and the child wrapped in a clean blanket or dressed in clean clothes. The family should be offered the option of cleaning and dressing their infant if they wish; this may be particularly important in some cultures. All actions taken during and after resuscitation should be carefully documented in the child's medical notes.

It is important that families are then able to have time with their child to say goodbye. If parents are prevented from doing so, they may deeply regret this; however, for some families, seeing their child after death may not be important. Grandparents, siblings, and other family members can be invited to join parents; families may also wish for a faith leader to attend. Hospital staff should offer parents mementos such as hand- or footprints and a lock of hair; for very young babies, parents may wish to have photographs if they have not been able to obtain these in life. Families should not feel rushed through the process of saying goodbye; ideally, the child should be moved from the resuscitation room to somewhere more peaceful and private (11). However, as with any unexplained death, families need to be supervised by hospital staff or police officers while they remain with their child's body.

When the family are ready to leave the hospital, they need to have clear information, preferably in the form of a leaflet; this should include details of the process of SUDI investigations so that parents know what to expect next, telephone numbers for the key professionals involved, and details of bereavement services. Most parents will want to know where their child's body will be over the coming days and how to arrange to see them again. Families may need help arranging transport home. Hospital staff should ensure that family doctors and community health services are notified as soon as possible of the death, so that they can offer support to the family.

## Early multi-agency liaison

Early multi-agency liaison is central to the joint agency response following an unexpected child death. The team should aim to hold an information sharing and planning meeting at the earliest possible opportunity following the death, bearing in mind that important aspects of the immediate and early responses should not be delayed while waiting to meet together. This early multi-agency discussion ideally takes place in the emergency department within a few hours of presentation. The discussion should involve the police, pediatrician, emergency department staff, social worker, and other relevant staff, depending on the nature of the case. The initial discussion may need to be by telephone, but a more formal meeting should be arranged as soon as possible. There may need to be repeated meetings and telephone discussions depending on the nature of the case.

There are two key components of this first multi-agency meeting:

1.  *Information sharing*: Those present should share initial information known to any agencies, including the emergency department history, and reports from emergency services; they should identify what further information is required and where and how this will be obtained; they should specifically identify if there are any initial child protection concerns or implications for other children in the family.

2. *Planning the process of investigation and agreeing on roles and responsibilities*: This should include planning a joint scene visit; arranging the post-mortem examination; identifying any outstanding investigations; discussing what bereavement support can be offered to the family; ensuring all relevant services are notified; and considering what information can be shared with the family and how. It is particularly important to identify any statutory/ forensic requirements, including scene security and preservation of evidence prior to the scene visit.

## Police responses at the scene of death

The location where the child died or collapsed prior to its death and examination is an essential element of the investigation into why the child died and may help identify factors relating to the cause of death and the circumstances. It is also one of the key areas that are considered when deciding on the appropriateness of using the classification of SIDS.

The paramedics in their initial response will have noted the environment, but their focus will have been on the needs of the collapsed child and transferring them to a hospital with pediatric resuscitation facilities. The initial attending police officer should ideally be an appropriately qualified investigator in plain clothes. They should undertake a preliminary assessment of the premises including — as a priority — checking on the safety of any other persons in the home, including other children.

In order to maintain the integrity of the environment in a condition as close as possible to the time of the death or collapse, consideration should be given to temporarily moving any remaining family members or others in the home to an alternative location. This should also include pets such as dogs, whose presence may have an adverse impact on subsequent examinations.

To capture a "snap shot" of the environment at this early stage, it is good practice for the police officer to undertake a walk through the premises and record, photographically, images of the environment before any further actions are taken. This record of the environment as close as possible to the key time of collapse may prove invaluable to the multi-agency team responding to the death and in particular to the police, lead health professional, and pediatric or forensic pathologist. It will provide essential information that will assist in identifying or eliminating potential concerns that can feature in relation to the death of a child.

The premises should then be discreetly secured or supervised by the police, pending further developments. Unless there are urgent forensic or timing considerations, items of interest should be left in situ for the joint home visit but recorded, including photographs (360-degree photography is particularly useful and can be used to produce a 3D model which can be used to in effect "walk through" the premises and examine it from various angles without having to physically visit it).

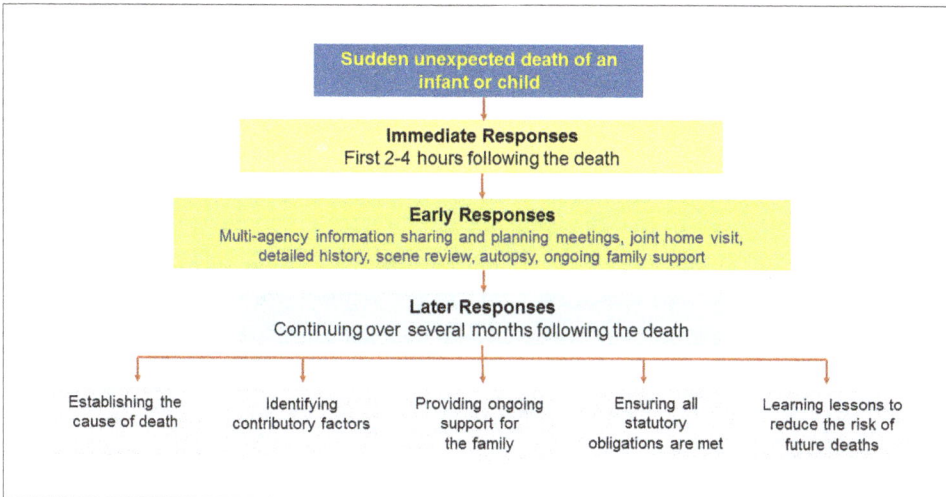

Figure 5.6: The early responses. (Authors' own work.)

The importance and rationale for preserving the integrity of the environment where the child collapsed should be explained to the parents and their consent obtained, although, as the police are acting on behalf of the coroner, general principles of law would justify them "searching not only the body, but the effects of the deceased, and the premises where the body is found, if there is reason to think that the search is likely to lead to the discovery of evidence bearing on the cause of death" (12). The statutory guidance in England regarding the joint agency response to an unexpected infant death clearly sets out the responsibility and expectation for the "[p]olice to consider appropriate scene security" (9). If the death is considered to be suspicious and a criminal offence(s) suspected, then control of the scene will be catered for under relevant legislation and guidance, and the police will take over the lead in what will still remain a joint agency investigation.

## Early responses

Following the initial management in the emergency department and the place where the child died, a process of further investigation and information gathering continues, along with ongoing support for the family (Figure 5.6). These next 24-48 hours present a golden window of opportunity for gathering important information and planning the ongoing investigation. They are also a crucial time of acute grief for the family, with particular emotional and practical needs arising. It is essential during this time that different professionals work together and maintain close communication; this may require further multi-agency meetings or discussions. A central part of these early responses is the joint home visit involving a police officer and health professional.

The visit to the home (or to the environment where the child died/collapsed) is a key element of the joint agency response and should be conducted as soon as possible after the infant's death and certainly within the first 24-48 hours, particularly if the environment is to be left secure and undisturbed. The purposes of the visit are to obtain further, more detailed information about the circumstances and environment in which the child died, including additional information from the family, as well as to provide further support to the family in these early stages. While there may be circumstances where the family do not wish, or are unable, to be present, wherever possible, this visit should include the parents or carers, so that full information can be obtained, and so that they can benefit from the process and support being offered.

The professionals would generally include the lead health professional, police investigator, family general practitioner or health visitor if possible, and another family member for support if required. Consideration should also be given to the presence of an appropriate member of police staff to record relevant sections of the visit, such as photographs of relevant items or locations, or a video of reconstructions.

We would normally begin the home visit in a neutral room, such as the kitchen or lounge, to introduce the members of the team and explain the reason for the visit and what it will involve. Parents may need a lot of reassurance over the purpose and process of the visit. This initial stage provides an opportunity to sensitively go over the history, clarifying any points, and filling in any earlier gaps. It enables the team to get to know more about the infant and family in a more familiar environment. When the family are ready, it is important for the police officer and lead health professional to examine the environment where the child died. This needs to be done sensitively and with support for the parents. Parents may have some concerns about going back to the room where their infant died, although often, doing so with a health professional or police officer present can be helpful. We find that usually one or other parent is keen to talk through the events and describe what had happened, although we would always respect a parent's wishes if they did not want to do so. Re-examining or clarifying the circumstances surrounding and leading up to the death in the actual environment can prove invaluable and can add support to explanations or accounts previously given, but great care is required to support the family during the process. The level of participation in the process and its emotional impact should be closely monitored but ultimately determined by the family members themselves.

There are a number of important considerations in the review of the environment where the child died (Box 3).

## Box 3: Review of the environment where the child died (13)

What is the general condition of the house?

- Is there evidence of smoking, alcohol, drug abuse?
- Is there any evidence of neglectful care?
- Is the room cramped? (Is there space for an adult to stand comfortably beside the cot/bed?)
- Is the room cluttered? (Is more than 50% of floor space visible, excluding fixed furniture? Is there at least one clear surface for placing things on/changing an infant?)
- Is the room dirty? (Is there rubbish or excrement on the floor/ surfaces? Is there uncleared food or nappies?)

What is the condition of the sleep environment?

- Is the sleeping space cluttered? (Is there space around where the child was lying?)
- Is the bedding dirty or worn?
- Is there adult-sized bedding, cushions or pillows?
- How many layers was the infant wrapped in?
- What was the temperature in the room? (Consider taking a drawer temperature to give an indication of the ambient temperature over the preceding hours; check any heating appliances and settings, and any ventilation.)

Are there any potential hazards?

- Are there any conditions that might have contributed to overheating?
- Are there any restrictions to ventilation or breathing (including risks of entrapment)?
- Are there any toxins?
- Are there any faulty appliances or fixings?

Are there any clues to causation?

- Is there any evidence of blood or vomit?
- Are there any medications or substances?

Some jurisdictions use carefully managed doll reconstructions of the final events. While this is not our usual practice, if done sensitively by appropriately trained investigators, it can add to the understanding of what happened and where and how the infant was found. This, or a very careful, detailed talk-through of the events in-situ, can aid the investigation enormously and may, for example, provide crucial pointers towards accidental asphyxiation as a possible or likely cause of death.

Some items may need to be taken for further examination in order to identify, or exclude, possible factors that could have had a bearing on the death. This may include a bottle containing the last feed, a nappy, or any medication or substances found. Before removing any items, however, careful thought should be given as to whether their removal will benefit the investigation. Often, a photograph or other form of recording would suffice, and at times removal of items such as bedding may impede the investigation if the investigating team have not been able to see them in situ. Routinely seizing bedding should no longer occur but it should be considered and taken only if necessary to do so, in instances such as in the presence of frank blood or vomit.

Once all relevant information from the history and examination of the home environment has been reviewed, time should be given to go through the findings with the parents, and to address any questions they may have. This provides a good opportunity for checking on any new or ongoing support needs the family may have and for informing them about the subsequent aspects of the investigation, including the post-mortem examination. All the findings from the home visit need to be carefully documented and included in a report that will go to the pathologist and the coroner.

## Causes for concern

> Every infant who dies deserves to be treated with respect and care. This includes the right, in an unexpected death, to have the death fully and sensitively investigated in order to identify, where possible, a cause of death and to learn lessons for the prevention of future infant deaths (3, p. 8).

While police investigators recognize that the majority of child deaths are not suspicious, they are also conscious that a minority of family members may deliberately harm their children. Even though there may be no initial indications of causes for concern at the outset of an investigation, that does not preclude the possibility that some may be identified as the investigation progresses. The police approach will be to maintain an open mind in a search for the truth (wherever that might lead) in order to try and establish the answers to four questions:

1.  Why did this child die?
2.  What was the cause of death and the circumstances?
3.  Are any criminal offences disclosed? (There may be no indication on current information, but police should keep it under review as the investigation

progresses — it is a question that must be considered, however briefly based, on available information even if the conclusion is "none".)

4.   If so — who was responsible for committing those offences?

This approach of professional curiosity, which applies equally to all members of the joint agency team is, in fact, grounded in respect for the rights of the child, as emphasized in the UK joint Royal Colleges report on sudden unexpected death in infancy and childhood (3). While it is essential that the family is supported and included as an essential constituent of the investigation, the ultimate primary focus should be on the deceased child, to ensure that the following poignant reminder from the Department of Education's 2015 report, "Working Together to Safeguard Children" (page 9, para 20) is heeded: "Effective safeguarding systems are child centred. Failings in safeguarding systems are too often the result of losing sight of the needs and views of the children within them, or placing the interests of adults ahead of the needs of children" (9).

An element of investigating any death involves looking at the circumstances and comparing them against the information provided in the accounts given. This process can confirm the accuracy of the initial picture of what has occurred and lower any level of concern; or, if contradictory information is evident, then the level of concern may be raised until resolved. If the level of concern reaches the threshold of the possibility of a criminal act being a contributory factor in the death, then the police may refer to the death as being "suspicious".

In this context "suspicious" could be defined as follows (14): "Although there is no direct evidence or grounds to suspect a specific criminal act there are, however, factors that raise the possibility that a criminal act may have contributed to the death and thereby merit a more detailed investigation of the circumstances of the death" (p. 127). The police will take into consideration, as part of their assessment, the presence or absence of a number of factors associated with abuse, including some specifically identified by research as being associated with child deaths or abuse where criminal offences were disclosed (15). While the presence of these factors may raise concerns, meriting a more detailed investigation of the circumstances to ensure a full, sensitive, and thorough investigation, they are not conclusive and may be incidental to the death. When collecting detailed information, a number of factors may, at this early stage of the investigation, raise the possibility of a non-natural cause, but it is important to stress that none of these factors, either alone or in combination, is direct evidence that the death is non-natural. Many of these factors are also commonly associated with an increased risk of death from natural causes.

For parents with significant learning difficulties, particular care is needed to ensure that they understand what is happening, as apparently inappropriate responses may be indicators of a lack of understanding rather than evidence of a non-natural cause.

These factors may be grouped into categories linked to the child or parent/carer, the circumstances of the death, or the wider context (Box 4).

## Box 4: Factors indicating possible cause for concern

1. Child-Related

History

- Previous atypical hospital visits or unusual or unexplained illnesses such as apparent life-threatening events (ALTE)
- Current or previous child protection concerns around the child or siblings, or family known to Social Services/Children's Social Care
- Previous sibling death

Physical features

- Child appears to have been dead longer than stated
- Atypical bruises or other injuries, particularly in pre-mobile infants
- Frank blood from the airways (as distinct from the pink frothy mucus regularly seen)
- Signs of neglect, including evidence of malnutrition or poor hygiene
- Foreign body in upper airway in the absence of a plausible history
- Evidence of internal injury (including fractures, intracranial hemorrhage, retinal hemorrhages) at post-mortem examination or on radiology
- Toxicology indicating drugs present in the child

2. Parent/Carer-Related

- History of violence to children
- Domestic violence and abuse, including aspects of coercive control
- Significant mental health issues, particularly where there is evidence of suicide attempts, or delusional thoughts about self or child
- History of alcohol or substance abuse
- Criminal record, particularly for violent crime
- Evidence of non-engagement with health and welfare services, such as persistently missing appointments for the child
- Cruelty to animals

3. Circumstances/Events related to death
  - Unexplained delays in seeking help
  - Unexplained inconsistencies or variability in the history or findings
  - Findings not in keeping with the child's abilities (such as reported rolling in a very young infant)
4. Environment
  - Extreme squalor
  - Home environment/conditions — evidence of drug or alcohol misuse
  - Dangerous sleeping environments
  - Family/household dynamics — interaction between parties (e.g. between parents and others)
  - Economic and neighborhood factors such as social isolation

## The post-mortem examination

The post-mortem examination or autopsy is a central component of any SUDI investigation. These examinations must be carried out as soon as possible after the child's death by an appropriately experienced pediatric pathologist. In some circumstances, where dual-trained pathologists are not available, it may be necessary to conduct a joint autopsy involving a pediatric and a forensic pathologist. Details of the autopsy procedure are covered in Chapter 24 and will not be considered here.

As a key part of the overall interagency response to an unexpected death, it is important that the pathologist is included in the ongoing information sharing and decision making. The pathologist should be provided with a preliminary report of the investigation by the lead police and health professionals. This should include details of the initial history and examination findings, any pre- or post-mortem investigations carried out prior to the autopsy, and findings on the home visit and review of the environment where the child died. All this information can be important in directing appropriate investigations as part of the post-mortem examination and in interpreting the findings.

It is essential that the family are informed of the need for, and the nature of, the autopsy. In an unexplained SUDI, it is the coroner who makes a decision about the need for an autopsy and the parents do not get an option to consent or not. Where there are particular parental concerns, or cultural or religious considerations, the coroner and pathologist will do their best to accommodate these concerns, but they do not remove the need for an appropriate and thorough post-mortem examination. Throughout the process, the child and family need to be treated with respect: parents understandably often feel very concerned about the autopsy, not wanting their child "to be put through even more". Simple measures such as referring to the child by name, explaining the process (with sensitivity and taking account of the parents' wishes), and introducing the pathologist to the parents may help reassure them. Similarly, the parents may be given choices, for example, over what their child will be dressed in following the autopsy, whether they want a particular cuddly toy to stay with their child, and whether or not they want to spend time with their infant after the examination. Where parents do want to see their child after the post-mortem examination, they should be informed of some of the likely changes in the appearance and feel of their child.

Parents need to be informed of any tissue or organ samples taken at autopsy and what will happen to those. Where appropriate, parental consent should be obtained for retention of any samples for future records, audit, or research, or for appropriate disposal of these samples. Our experience is that, when given the option, most parents would want small tissue samples to be retained and available for appropriate research or further investigation.

Once the initial results of the post-mortem examination are known, the joint agency team, with the agreement of the coroner, may meet with the family to update them on the progress of the investigation and the preliminary findings. It is important at this stage to stress that any findings are provisional and that the determination of the final assigned cause of death rests with the coroner, who will reach his or her conclusion based on all the available information.

## Later responses

The later stages of the response to a SUDI can be a confusing and distressing time for families. Often, after an initial flurry of activity, the family can be left feeling abandoned and forgotten, while some of the further aspects of the investigation can drag on for weeks or months. These later responses are primarily around pulling together and making sense of all the findings from the investigation, including any further investigations and enquiries; meeting all statutory obligations such as the coroner's inquiry and notification of the cause of death; and providing ongoing support to the family (Figure 5.7).

### Collating the information

As information from the investigation comes to light, it is important that those leading the investigation work together to collate and interpret this information. This is an ongoing process and may require regular meetings or discussions, particularly if there are unexpected findings which may alter the course of the investigation. Some key questions can help guide our interpretation of the information obtained (Box 5).

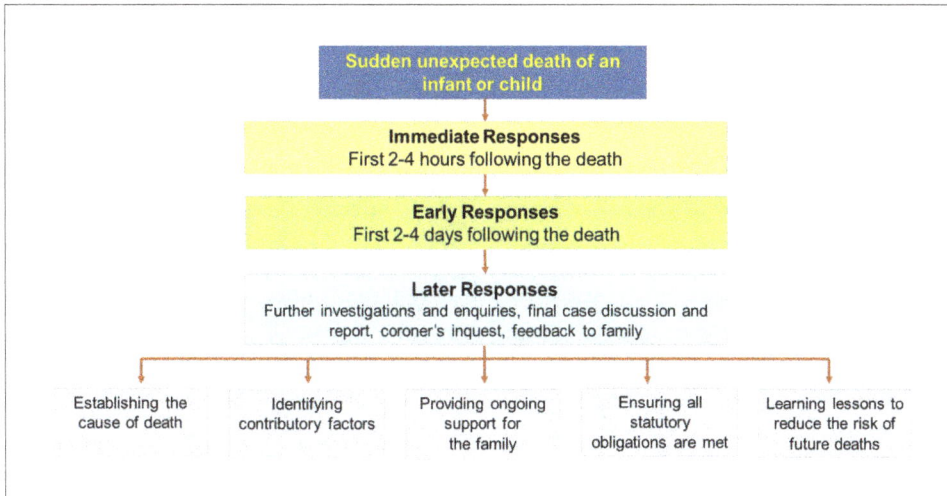

```
┌─────────────────────────────────┐
│  Sudden unexpected death of an  │
│          infant or child        │
└─────────────────────────────────┘
                 ↓
┌─────────────────────────────────┐
│       Immediate Responses       │
│  First 2-4 hours following the death │
└─────────────────────────────────┘
                 ↓
┌─────────────────────────────────┐
│        Early Responses          │
│  First 2-4 days following the death │
└─────────────────────────────────┘
                 ↓
          Later Responses
Further investigations and enquiries, final case discussion and
report, coroner's inquest, feedback to family
```

| Establishing the cause of death | Identifying contributory factors | Providing ongoing support for the family | Ensuring all statutory obligations are met | Learning lessons to reduce the risk of future deaths |

Figure 5.7: The later responses. (Authors' own work.)

## Box 5: Interpreting the information obtained

- What information have we gathered?
- What does it tell us about the possible cause of death?
- What does it tell us about any contributory factors?
- What further information do we need?

Following the early stages of the investigation, there may be a number of outcomes which will influence the course of the later responses (3, 13):

1. The post-mortem examination may provide a complete and sufficient natural cause of death, such as an overwhelming infection, a previously unrecognized lethal congenital anomaly, or a life-limiting metabolic disorder. In such circumstances, this should be given as the cause of death, the coroner may be able to conclude his investigation, and the family should be informed of the cause. It remains important to continue collating information about the circumstances of the death and any contributory factors so that the family can be appropriately informed and so that any wider lessons for prevention can be explored.

2. If the history, examination, scene review, and post-mortem examination point towards homicide, abuse, or neglect as the most likely explanation for

the death, the police will need to take the lead in any further investigations, involving social services and other agencies, and following any statutory frameworks for further investigation. The family will still need understanding and support, and this needs to be carefully managed alongside the need for police questioning or arrest of any suspects. Consideration must be given to the safety and wellbeing of any siblings or other vulnerable children in the family or their social network.

3.  In many cases, the cause of death may remain unclear, whether or not any contributory factors (including parenting factors) have been identified. In these circumstances the coroner should be informed and the family can normally also be informed that there is no clear explanation for their child's death, but that there will be further investigations.

## Final case discussion

Just as the initial information sharing and planning meeting is a crucial first step in initiating the joint agency response to an unexpected child death, the final case discussion provides a crucial focus for concluding the response. These two discussions provide essential anchors on which the whole of the response between the two steps rests.

This multi-agency discussion, usually held two to three months after the death, provides a framework for reviewing and interpreting all the information gathered through the investigation in order to clarify the cause or causes of the death and any contributory factors. It enables those working with the family to identify and respond to any continuing family support needs, including those of other or future children. It creates a safe place for debriefing and supporting the professionals involved. And it contributes to the ongoing learning arising from the child's death.

The final case discussion should be planned at an early stage so that people can schedule it in their diaries. Our practice is to hold the meetings at the GP clinic so that members of the primary care team can attend, but there are also advantages to holding them in the local hospital, which ensures engagement of the hospital teams. Those practitioners involved with any previous or ongoing care to the family should be invited, along with those involved in investigating the child's death (Box 6).

Different proformas may be used to collate and analyze the information arising from the investigation, including the Avon clinico-pathological classification (16) or the English Child Death Overview Panel form C.[1] These allow the information to be reviewed in a systematic manner, both ensuring that all issues are considered and enabling the participants to reflect on the likely significance of any contributory factors.

_____

1 Available at https://www.gov.uk/government/publications/child-death-reviews-forms-for-reporting-child-deaths.

The conclusions of the meeting need to be reported to the coroner and to any independent child death review team to inform further learning. Arrangements should be made for appropriate members of the multi-agency team to meet with the family following this meeting in order to feed back the outcome and address any questions or further support needs the family may have.

## Box 6: Final case discussion invitees

- General Practitioner
- Health Visitor or Midwife
- Pediatrician
- Emergency department staff
- Ambulance staff
- Other professionals who had worked with the child or family (e.g. nursery staff)
- Investigating police officer
- Lead SUDI health professional
- Pathologist
- Coroner's Officer

## Family Support

> You may never know the value of the support you give but don't let that stop you from giving it. (Bereaved parent)

The professional responses to an unexpected infant death, as outlined in this chapter, are varied and wide-ranging. There can be periods of intense activity interspersed with weeks or even months of waiting for results or further investigations. There are statutory requirements to be met and specific tasks that must be completed. In all of this, it is important that we do not lose sight of the child and family at the center. The death of their child is perhaps the worst thing any family could go through, and this fact does not get any less important as time goes on. It is essential, therefore, that throughout the response we treat the family with sensitivity and respect, and are attuned to their needs and what they are telling us.

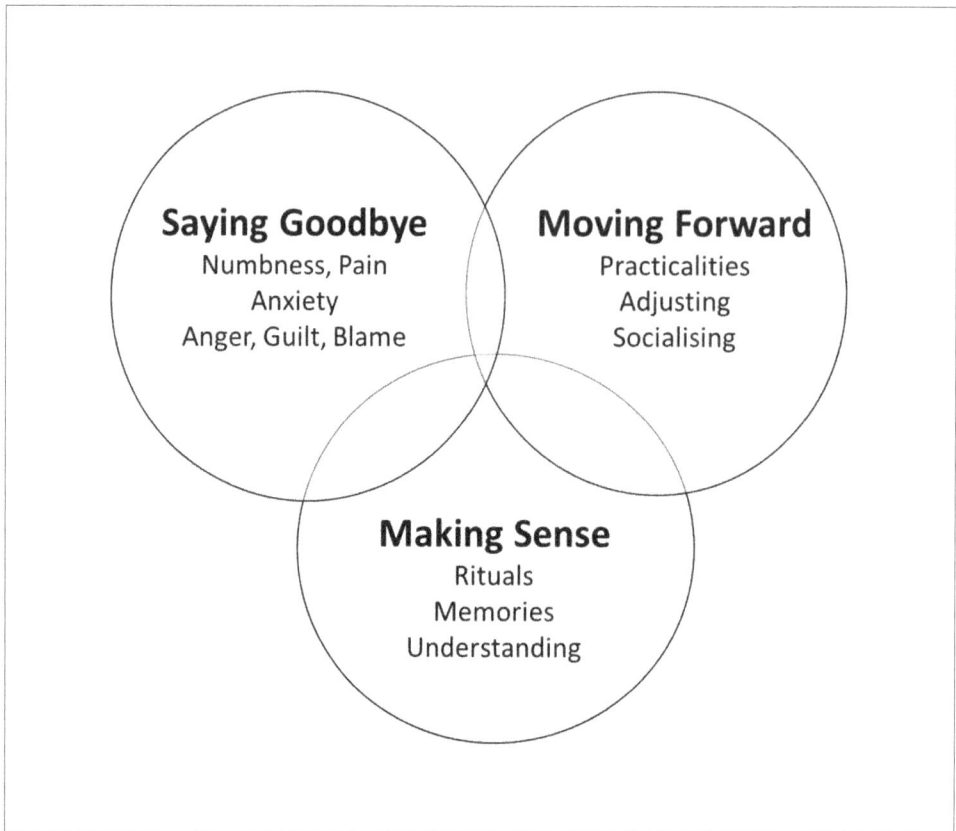

Figure 5.8: The family's response to the death of a child. (Authors' own work.)

Our work with bereaved families suggests that there are three core aspects to any family's grieving (Figure 5.8), although the manner in which these are expressed varies with each individual family. Further perspectives on the grieving process and the needs of families following the death of a child are covered in other chapters, so here we focus just on a few principles as they relate to the overall professional responses. In the words of one bereaved parent: "To be the greatest help to a newly bereaved family, you do not need to know about 'stages of grief', bereavement theory, child development, or have any qualification in counselling. You need only to carry out your normal clinical/professional role, of appropriate questioning, information giving and facilitating shared decision making, in a respectful, sensitive and straightforward manner".

The concept of "saying goodbye" encompasses much of the expressive side of grief. Parents, siblings, and grandparents will all approach this in their own individual ways. Two of the key lessons for practitioners, particularly in the early stages, are to provide time and space for the family to say goodbye, and not to pre-judge how they might want to do this. This may, at times, seem to conflict with the urgency of initiating the multi-agency investigation, but with careful thought, the parents' wishes can usually be accommodated.

After the family have left hospital, one of their key support needs will be for information; nearly all parents will want to try and understand why their child died (17). This is a central part of the parents' attempt to make sense of their child's death. In most cases the preliminary post-mortem results will be inconclusive; however, parents appreciate a telephone call or visit to inform them that the post-mortem examination has finished and to give them an idea of the length of time before the final results will be available. Once all investigations are concluded, the cause of death established, or the diagnosis of SIDS reached, an appointment should be made to discuss the findings with the family. This is likely to be some time after the death and gives the parents a chance to revisit earlier events and ask further questions. It is good practice to share all relevant information with parents, including those relating to risk factors for SIDS, such as parental smoking or sleep environments, although these are difficult conversations. Even where such discussions are difficult and raise questions about the parents' own practices, parents tend to appreciate honesty. Indeed, such discussions may help parents to work with the sense of blame that many feel (17).

Alongside the emotional responses that parents go through and their need to understand and make sense of their child's death, there are important practical aspects to moving forward. Life continues for the parents and the family, even though it is totally different and disrupted. It is important that they have clear information explaining the SUDI process to them and advising them about whom to contact if they have further questions. This may have been explained to them already, but, given the shock of the sudden loss of a child, many parents will need repeated explanations. There may be specific medical support needed, such as help with suppressing breastmilk production for breastfeeding mothers, or with managing anxiety, depression, or sleeplessness. Practical information and support may be needed around the funeral arrangements, as well as around specific issues in relation to employment, housing, or benefits. While the joint agency team may not be able to respond to all avenues of support, they should know where and how to signpost families to the right sources.

Parents may want help accessing bereavement services for themselves or their surviving children. Although many such services expect clients to self-refer, parents may need assistance to make initial contact, as they may find it too upsetting to explain their situation when arranging a first appointment. Often parents have questions about the grieving process for siblings and how to support them; pediatricians are well placed to provide this advice. Many parents find official support groups such as SIDS organizations very helpful; parents should be given details of these groups soon after the death. These organizations may provide local information leaflets for bereaved parents which can be kept in Emergency Departments to distribute to families.

## Conclusions

Responding effectively to an unexpected child death requires a co-ordinated response from police and health professionals working together with other agencies to investigate the cause and circumstances of the death, and to ensure that the family are appropriately supported through the grieving process. The precise manner in which this is achieved will vary between different areas and is dependent on certain statutory obligations. It is essential, however, that this is done in a thorough, systematic, and sensitive manner. In this chapter we have outlined a co-ordinated joint-agency response, as practiced in England, which we believe can meet current best standards for investigation and support.

The professional response to an unexpected infant death can be traumatic, adding to the sense of bewilderment already felt by a family, particularly when no specific cause of death is found. However, if carried out thoroughly and systematically, with an attitude of sympathy and respect, our responses can be an important part of helping families say goodbye to their child, make sense of what has happened to them, and move forward with their lives.

It is every family's right to have their baby's death properly investigated. (Baroness Helena Kennedy, QC (3))

## References

1. *Coroners and Justice Act 2009* (UK) c 25.

2. Garstang J, Ellis C, Sidebotham P. An evidence-based guide to the investigation of sudden unexpected death in infancy. Forensic Sci Med Pathol. 2015;11:345-57. https://doi.org/10.1007/s12024-015-9680-x.

3. Royal College of Pathologists, Royal College of Paediatrics and Child Health. Sudden unexpected death in infancy and childhood: Multi-agency guidelines for care and investigation. London: RCPath, 2016.

4. Krous HF, Beckwith JB, Byard RW, Rognum TO, Bajanowski T, Corey T, et al. Sudden infant death syndrome and unclassified sudden infant deaths: A definitional and diagnostic approach. Pediatrics. 2004;114(1):234-8. https://doi.org/10.1542/peds.114.1.234.

5. Bajanowski T, Vege A, Byard RW, Krous HF, Arnestad M, Bachs L, et al. Sudden infant death syndrome (SIDS) — Standardised investigations and classification: Recommendations. Forensic Sci Int. 2007;165(2-3):129-43. https://doi.org/10.1016/j.forsciint.2006.05.028.

6. Garstang J, Ellis C, Sidebotham P. An evidence-based guide to the investigation of sudden unexpected death in infancy. Forensic Sci Med Pathol. 2015;11(3):345-57. https://doi.org/10.1007/s12024-015-9680-x.

7. Sidebotham P, Fleming P. Unexpected death in childhood: A handbook for practitioners. Chichester: Wiley, 2007. https://doi.org/10.1002/9780470988176.

8. Sidebotham P, Pearson G. Responding to and learning from childhood deaths. BMJ. 2009;338:b531. https://doi.org/10.1136/bmj.b531.

9. HM Government. Working together to safeguard children. London: Department for Education, 2015.

10. *Police and Criminal Evidence Act 1984* (UK) c 60.

11. Garstang J, Griffiths F, Sidebotham P. What do bereaved parents want from professionals after the sudden death of their child: A systematic review of the literature. BMC pediatrics. 2014;14(1):269. https://doi.org/10.1186/1471-2431-14-269.

12. Home Office. Circular 68/1955 — Consolidated circular to coroners on matters other than deaths from industrial accidents and diseases. London: Home Office, 1955.

13. Sidebotham P, Fleming P. Responding to Unexpected Child Deaths. In: Unexpected death in childhood: A handbook for practitioners. Eds Sidebotham P, Fleming P. Chichester: Wiley, 2007. p. 97-131. https://doi.org/10.1002/9780470988176.ch7.

14. Marshall D. Effective investigation of child homicide and suspicious deaths. Oxford: Oxford University Press, 2012.

15. Mayes J, Brown A, Marshall D, Weber MA, Risdon A, Sebire NJ. Risk factors for intra-familial unlawful and suspicious child deaths: A retrospective study of cases in London. Journal of homicide and major incident investigation. 2010;6(1):77-95.

16. Fleming PJ, Blair PS, Sidebotham PD, Hayler T. Investigating sudden unexpected deaths in infancy and childhood and caring for bereaved families: An integrated multiagency approach. BMJ. 2004;328(7435):331-4. https://doi.org/10.1136/bmj.328.7435.331.

17. Garstang J, Griffiths F, Sidebotham P. Parental understanding and self-blame following sudden infant death: A mixed-methods study of bereaved parents' and professionals' experiences. BMJ Open. 2016;6(5):e011323. https://doi.org/10.1136/bmjopen-2016-011323.

# 6

# The Role of Death Review Committees

Sharyn Watts, PhD

*South Australian Child Death and Serious Injury Review Committee,*
*Department for Education and Child Development, Adelaide, Australia*

## Introduction

A 5-month-old infant placed to sleep in a partially inflated plastic bed was found, unresponsive, with her face pressed against the plastic in a trough created between the base and the side of the inflatable bed (1). The infant's death was attributed to suffocation. Byard (2006) reviewed the circumstances of this death and recommended assessment of these types of inflatable beds by product safety experts (1).

Details about the circumstances and cause of this death were also collected by the South Australian Child Death and Serious Injury Review Committee, which undertook its own in-depth review. The result of this review was to recommend to the South Australian government that it request the relevant national regulatory body to amend regulations about children's portable cots to incorporate the requirement that "no component of a portable folding cot be inflatable" (2). This change in national regulations was achieved three years after the infant's death.

## Child Death Review in South Australia

Since 2005, the Child Death and Serious Injury Review Committee ("the Committee") has been responsible for reviewing the circumstances and causes of all child deaths in the state of South Australia. Similar teams and committees are now well established in other states and territories in Australia and in other countries including Canada, New Zealand, the United Kingdom, and the United States.

In South Australia, the Committee consists of a multidisciplinary team with expertise in fields such as pediatrics, education, disability, psychology, social work, child protection, public health, and justice who come together to consider the information that has been gathered about an infant's death. This broad base of knowledge and experience leads to a comprehensive overview of the circumstances of the death and identification of systemic issues that may have contributed to the quality of service provision to that infant and their family. The review process can also identify the absence of particular services, or of regulatory or legislative mechanisms which, if present, may have resulted in a different outcome for the infant.

At the conclusion of a death review, the Committee can make recommendations to government about changes to legislation, policy, or practice which could potentially lead to a reduction in the risk of deaths occurring under similar circumstances, such as the change to portable cot regulations.

In addition to reviewing in-depth the death of infants, such as the 5-month-old child who suffocated when she was placed to sleep in a partially inflated plastic bed, the Committee also monitors the trends and patterns of all child deaths in its jurisdiction.

## The Functions of a Child Death Review Team

The ability of a child death review team to confidently make recommendations rests on the quality and depth of the information it collects about each sudden and unexpected infant death. Because a child death review team is interested in all aspects relevant to the prevention of child death, it collects information about the infant's socioeconomic circumstances and the mother's health and wellbeing, as well as information about records that detail provision of postnatal services and (if relevant) involvement with child protection services, welfare, and housing services.

To maximize the effectiveness of their recommendations, child death review teams develop working relationships with government and non-government agencies and organizations which have varying levels of responsibility for the safety, health, and wellbeing of children, including agencies that

- protect children from risk and harm — child protection, justice, law enforcement agencies
- improve their health and wellbeing — health agencies and agencies providing mental health services
- provide support to families — housing agencies and those providing welfare services

- prevent serious injury or death — injury surveillance and prevention organizations
- monitor child health and wellbeing — agencies collecting vital statistics
- advocate for children and young people — Commissioner for children or child advocates.

## Contributing to the Prevention of Sudden Unexpected Infant Deaths

The actions taken by the Committee to suggest and support the regulations limiting the sale of inflatable plastic beds, and the recommendations made about targeting the State's most vulnerable families, demonstrate some of the ways in which the information collected by a child death review team can contribute both to an understanding of sudden and unexpected infant death and to its prevention.

Police, pathologists, or coroners may not have the time or opportunity to scrutinize their data-gathering procedures. Garstang, Ellis and Sidebotham (2015) identified four different models for investigating sudden unexpected infant deaths. These authors concluded that the "police-led" model of investigation was the least likely to meet the minimum standards for investigation of sudden unexpected infant deaths, based on international consensus about those standards. New South Wales (NSW) was identified as using this model of investigation (3). Based on this information, and the results of its own reviews, the NSW child death review team recommended to the NSW government that it was critical that this model be improved to reflect best practice standards; it also recommended the adoption of a more consistent approach to the definition of sudden and unexpected infant death in that jurisdiction (4).

Through their review processes, child death review teams can influence systemic change in relation to the sudden and unexpected deaths by

- monitoring diagnostic changes in the ways pathologists attribute cause of death to sudden and unexpected cases of infant death
- identifying gaps in death scene investigation procedures
- monitoring the quality of death scene investigations
- identifying trends and patterns in rates of sudden and unexpected infant deaths
- monitoring changes in the occurrence of risk factors for sudden and unexpected infant deaths
- contributing to prevention efforts.

In 2011, New Zealand experienced a major earthquake that left many families homeless, and public health concerns were raised regarding the anticipated increased likelihood of infants co-sleeping with their parents. These concerns prompted the supply of portable infant sleeping spaces for earthquake-affected families. Initial evaluation showed that these portable sleeping spaces were well received and appropriately used (5). In 2013, the Child and Youth Mortality Review Committee in New Zealand concluded that "suffocation in place of sleep is the most common cause of death from unintentional injury in the first year of life in New Zealand and is largely preventable" (p. 24). The Committee made national policy and practice recommendations that included the provision of portable infant sleeping spaces to families that met an agreed threshold of need; a community campaign to increase awareness and education; and a national strategy for New Zealand's Indigenous population. It also made recommendations for government and non-government agencies about the development and implementation of safe sleeping policies and recommendations for best practice in community messaging (6).

Mitchell, Cowan and Tipene-Leach (2016) reported a 29% fall in post-perinatal mortality deaths in New Zealand between 2009 and 2015 (7). They attributed this fall to several factors including the provision of portable infant sleeping spaces to vulnerable families; agreement to, and adoption of, a set of clear, concise, evidence-based messages about safe sleeping; and training of professionals working with families in the provision of these messages. In the same year, the New Zealand government agreed to fund a safe sleeping program that included the provision of portable infant sleeping spaces (8).

## Monitoring Trends and Patterns in Sudden Unexpected Infant Deaths

The general population of South Australia is approximately 1.7 million people, and nearly 5% of this population are children aged 1 to 18 years (approximately 350,000 children). Between 2005 and 2015, the death rate for children in South Australia was 31.3 deaths per 100,000 children. On average, approximately 20,000 infants are born in this state every year. Between 2005 and 2015, the infant mortality rate was 3.2 deaths per 1,000 live births. In the same 11-year timeframe, the sudden and unexpected infant death rate was 0.7 deaths per 1,000 live births (9).

The Committee has been monitoring the sudden and unexpected infant death rate since 2005. Between this time and 2015, the rate has been declining in South Australia (on average by 7% per year) (9). Other jurisdictions in Australia also monitor sudden and unexpected infant death rates and also report that these rates have decreased. In the state of Victoria this reduction was most notable between 1985 and 1995, with no further significant decreases since then (10). In the state of New South Wales, the rate of sudden and unexpected infant death has declined since 2001, and the rate in 2015 was the lowest recorded since 2001 (4). In the state of Queensland, rates have fluctuated in the past decade but the 2014-15 rate was the lowest reported since 2004 (6). It is interesting to note that in South Australia the decline in the rate of sudden and unexpected infant deaths has been far greater than that of the general death rate for children (0-18 years) and of the infant mortality rate. These death rates have decreased by only 3% on average per year (9).

Sudden and unexpected infant deaths occur more often in South Australia's most disadvantaged areas (67% of infants who died lived in these areas). In the same 11-year period between 2005-15, the families of almost half of these infants had come in contact with the state's child protection agency in the three years before they died (9). A recent report from the New South Wales child death review team also noted the association between sudden and unexpected infant death and disadvantaged and vulnerable infants. The association of these deaths with indicators of vulnerability has given rise to recommendations by child death review teams, including the Committee, about prevention efforts that target these more vulnerable populations (4).

## Conclusions

Child death review teams have the capacity to consider sudden unexpected infant deaths in ways that encompass the cause of death and the infant's and family's circumstances, and to consider the ways in which systems designed to keep infants safe might be improved. In doing so, they can hold a system to account for its actions and advocate for the safety and wellbeing of infants, especially those who are most vulnerable. These teams can be powerful partners in any efforts to inform, support, and promote understanding and prevention of sudden unexpected infant deaths.

## References

1. Byard RW. Inflatable beds and accidental asphyxia in infancy. Scand J Forensic Sci. 2006;12(1):22-4.

2. *Fair Trading Amendment (Children's Portable Folding Cots) Regulation 2009* (NSW). [Available from: http://www.legislation.nsw.gov.au/regulations/2009-92.pdf]. Accessed 27 September 2017.

3. Garstang J, Ellis C, Sidebotham P. An evidence-based guide to the investigation of sudden unexpected death in infancy. Forensic Sci Med Pathol. 2015;11(3):345-57. https://doi.org/10.1007/s12024-015-9680-x.

4. NSW Child Death Review Team. Child death review report 2015. [Available from: https://www.ombo.nsw.gov.au/news-and-publications/publications/annual-reports/nsw-child-death-review/nsw-child-death-team-annual-report-2015]. Accessed 27 September 2017.

5.  Cowan S, Bennett S, Clarke J, Pease A. An evaluation of portable sleeping spaces for babies following the Christchurch earthquake of February 2011. J Paediatr Child Health. 2013;49(5):364-8. https://doi.org/10.1111/jpc.12196.

6.  Child and Youth Mortality Review Committee (Te ropu Arotake Mate o te Hunga Tamariki, Taihoi). Special report: Unintentional suffocation, foreign body inhalation and strangulation. [Available from: https://www.hqsc.govt.nz/assets/CYMRC/Publications/CMYRC-special-report-March-2013.pdf]. Accessed 27 September 2017.

7.  Mitchell EA, Cowan S, Tipene-Leach D. The recent fall in postperinatal mortality in New Zealand and the safe sleep programme. Acta Paediatr. 2016;105(11):1312-20. https://doi.org/10.1111/apa.13494.

8.  Carville O. Sleep pods to be funded as officials over-ruled. [Available from: http://www.nzherald.co.nz/nz/news/article.cfm?c_id=1&objectid=11686108]. Accessed 27 September 2017.

9.  Child Death and Serious Injury Review Committee South Australia. Annual report 2015-16. [Available from: http://www.cdsirc.sa.gov.au/wp-content/uploads/2017/07/2015-16_cdsirc_annual_report.pdf]. Accessed 10 January 2018.

10. Consultative council on obstetric and paediatric mortality and morbidity Victoria. 2012 and 2013: Victoria's mothers, babies and children. Section 1: Findings and recommendations. [Available from: https://www2.health.vic.gov.au/~/media/health/files/collections/research%20and%20reports/v/victorias%20mothers%20babies%20and%20children%202012%20and%202013%20%20section%201.pdf]. Accessed 27 September 2017.

11. Queensland Family and Child Commission. Annual report: Deaths of children and young people, Queensland, 2014-15. [Available from: https://www.qfcc.qld.gov.au/annual-report-deaths-children-and-young-people-queensland-2014%E2%80%9315]. Accessed 27 September 2017.

# 7 Parental Perspectives

Joanna Garstang, MBChB, MSc, PhD

*Warwick Medical School, University of Warwick, Coventry, UK*

## Introduction

"You can stop resuscitating; leave the notes on my desk."

Back in the early 2000s, when I was a junior pediatrician, this was the typical advice that I would receive from my seniors when I was dealing with a case of sudden unexpected death in infancy (SUDI) in the Emergency Department; it was considered appropriate for junior staff to manage SUDI without direct consultant support. Parents would usually be offered an outpatient appointment with a consultant pediatrician some weeks later to discuss the results of the post-mortem examination, but few families attended as they had never met the consultant beforehand. Bereaved parents described saying goodbye to their dead infant in the Emergency Department, leaving the hospital, and never receiving any further information from medical staff about the possible reasons for the death. As a junior doctor, I felt that this process was wrong and that families deserved better care; thankfully, during the next few years the management of SUDI changed dramatically in England.

In 2008, a new joint agency approach (JAA) to investigating SUDI was introduced in England (1); this approach aimed to establish the complete causes for death, including any risk factors, and to address the needs of the family, including the need to safeguard other children. Professionals therefore have to balance the need to forensically investigate the cause of death and offer appropriate support to bereaved families (2). The JAA has been described in detail in Chapter 5, but is summarized here. Police, health, and social care jointly investigate deaths following national statutory guidance (2). The investigation is led by experienced pediatricians and the police response is provided by specialist teams with particular expertise in managing child death and child safeguarding enquiries. Key elements include taking the deceased infant to an Emergency Department, a pediatrician (possibly accompanied by the police) taking a detailed medical history from the parents, a joint examination of the scene of death by police and pediatrician, and follow-up for the parents. There is inter-agency communication throughout the JAA with a case conference to discuss the full causes of death. The process of the JAA is shown in Figure 7.1. Despite statutory guidance, the practice of joint police and pediatric examination of the scene of death is still variable, and often police examine death scenes alone.

Many countries now have Child Death Review (CDR) programs, which may be similar to the JAA, to investigate SUDI. The aim of these programs is to identify the full reasons for each death to help prevent deaths in the future (3, 4). Frequently, CDR includes prospective investigation of unexpected deaths, with physicians obtaining detailed medical histories from parents, analysis of death scenes by police and healthcare professionals, and multi-agency case reviews (5). CDR has the potential to help bereaved parents, as one of their greatest needs is to understand as fully as possible why their child died. Parents may also want ongoing support and follow-up from medical staff who cared for their child (6).

Parental self-blame and feelings of guilt are common following sudden infant death syndrome (SIDS), and this may relate to the lack of explanation for the death (7-10). Detailed SUDI investigation may lead to increased parental understanding about the causes of death, thus alleviating some of these feelings, but self-blame is also a common feature of all types of bereavement (11). Understandably, there is concern that SIDS parents may blame themselves more for deaths, particularly when there are discussions about modifiable factors such as parental smoking. Previously, healthcare professionals were advised to reassure SIDS parents that their actions played no role in the death, thus potentially reducing self-blame, given that SIDS was neither predictable nor preventable (12, 13). Given our current understanding of SIDS, these explanations often seem inappropriate, as many SIDS deaths involve modifiable risk factors relating to unsafe sleep environments, parental smoking, or alcohol consumption and, as such, are within parents' direct control.

Parents may therefore find SUDI investigations supportive in providing them with a detailed understanding of why their child died, but conversely this information may cause them distress, leading them to question their actions and choices. The process of SUDI investigation itself also has the potential to be highly intrusive for bereaved families, who may prefer privacy during a very emotional period.

As I continued in my higher professional training as a pediatrician, I became involved in establishing the new JAA investigation of SUDI in the West Midlands

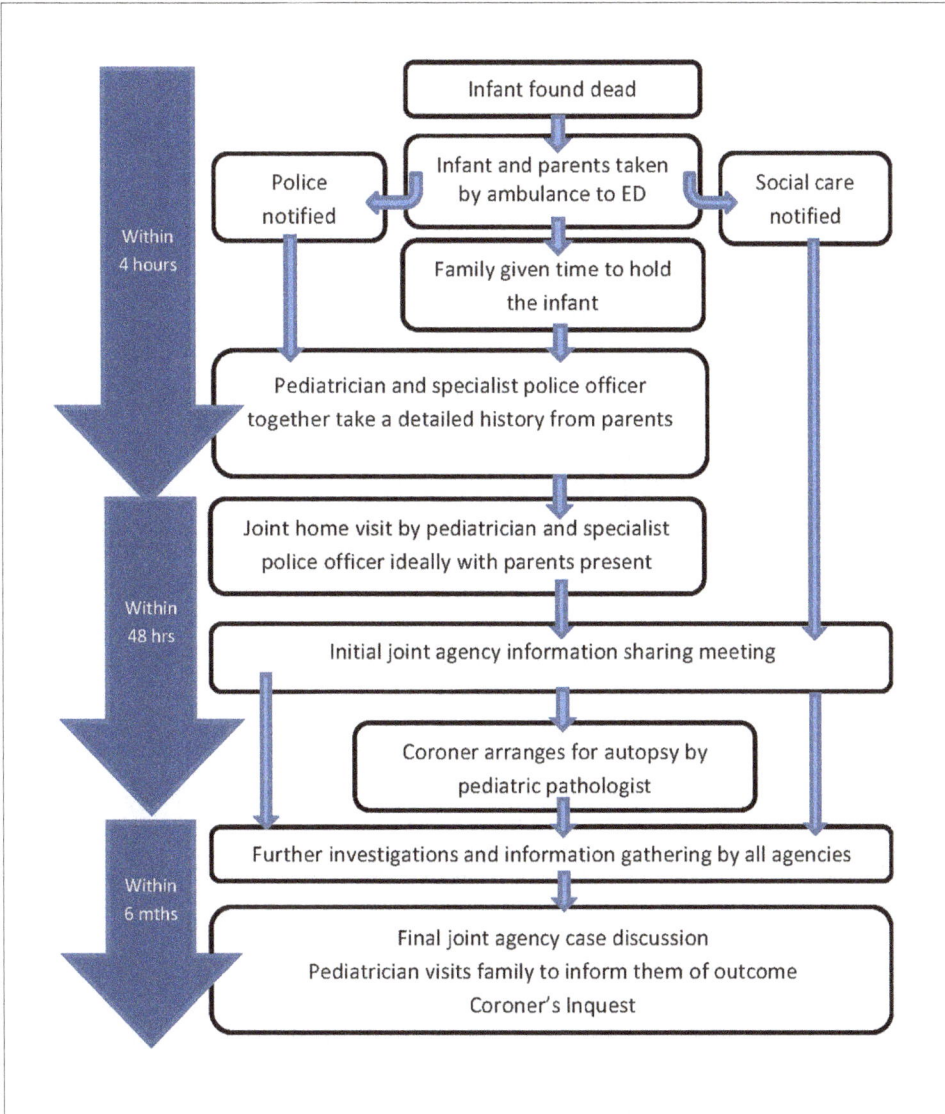

Figure 7.1: Flow chart of JAA (14).

region of England. This region has a population of 5.6 million and covers an area of 13,000 square kilometres. There are 14 hospitals, 11 different local government areas and 3 police forces. Given the uncertainties about how the JAA could impact on families, I decided to research this further. I embarked upon a mixed-methods study to evaluate the JAA with the overall aim of improving the wellbeing of bereaved parents; this research formed the basis of my PhD (14). I heard firsthand of many parents' experiences, and these are presented here along with suggestions for improving the care and support provided. These findings along with other results from my PhD have been published elsewhere (15, 16).

The research questions for the study were:

1. What are the experiences of bereaved parents whose infants died suddenly and unexpectedly and were investigated by a JAA?

2. What are the experiences of professionals, relating to bereaved parents, of using the JAA to investigate SUDI?

## Study Methods

### Inclusion and exclusion criteria

Bereaved parents were recruited after the conclusion of JAA investigations. For inclusion, deaths had to have presented as SUDI, according to the Confidential Enquiry into Stillbirths and Deaths in Infancy (CESDI) SUDI study definition (17). The infants had to be aged from 1 week to 1 year at death, and to have passed away between 1 September 2010 and 31 August 2013. Infants had to have lived and died in the West Midlands region of England. Cases were excluded if there were ongoing criminal enquiries.

### Identification and recruitment of cases

The regional perinatal pathology service performs all SUDI post-mortem examinations locally and they notified me of all eligible SUDI cases. Parents were informed of the study by local pediatricians. Participants gave written consent to take part in the study having been fully informed of all risks and benefits.

### Data collection

Parents could choose to participate in in-depth interviews or complete questionnaires about their experiences. All parents completed the Hospital Anxiety and Depression Scale (HADS) (18), which is a validated mental health screening tool. Parents were visited at home to conduct in-depth interviews between 6 and 18 months after the death, which was their first contact with me. Interviews were audio-recorded and field notes taken; they lasted between one and four hours and the recordings were transcribed in full. Parents who were recruited in the first two years of the study were invited to participate in a follow-up interview around two years after the death. Both interviews covered the parents' experiences of the entire JAA and their understandings of the causes for death. The interview schedule was developed with the advice of the Lullaby Trust, the UK support group for SIDS parents. The questionnaires covered the same range of subjects as the in-depth interviews but in less detail.

All parents gave consent for access to case records from health, police, social care, and coroners. Data were extracted using a standard template. Parents' primary healthcare records were examined for details of consultations in the year following the death.

Prior to initial interviews, I was unaware of any case details and so relied on listening to parents say what they thought was relevant. However, at follow-up interviews, having analyzed initial accounts and reviewed case documents, I was able to probe parents further about their experiences and understanding. After completion of each initial parental interview, I interviewed the professionals involved in each JAA investigation about their experiences, specifically in relation to the recruited SUDI case, with questions guided by analysis of parents' accounts.

## Qualitative data analysis

I analyzed all qualitative data using a Framework Approach (19) assisted by NVIVO 10 software, with data analysis concurrent with interviewing. Starting with the data from parents' accounts, I thematically analyzed their experiences of each stage of the JAA. After coding 10 parental interviews, I reviewed the codes with a wider study team including SUDI professionals and bereaved parents. Coding then continued, including data from follow-up and professional interviews. For each case I considered data from case records and professional interviews for corroboration and contrast with the parents' data and created a framework matrix. Quotes have been given to illustrate each theme; they are only identified as being from the mother, father or as a professional, and whether the death was SIDS or medically explained to ensure anonymity.

## Ethical issues

Parents were initially contacted by their own local pediatricians and given time to consider whether or not to take part. Participation was on the basis of fully informed consent. Parents were warned that if they disclosed information leading to concerns about child abuse further action would need to be taken, including possibly referring the matter to police and social care. Parents could stop interviews or withdraw from the study at any time. After interviews, parents were provided with details of relevant support agencies. The study received ethical approval from Solihull NHS Research Ethics Committee 12/WM/0211 and 10/H/1206/30.

# Results

## Recruitment

During the study period there were 113 SUDI cases, of which 104 were eligible for recruitment: 23/104 (22%) were recruited to the study; 32/104 (31%) families were not informed of the study by local pediatricians; 20/104 (19%) of families failed to attend

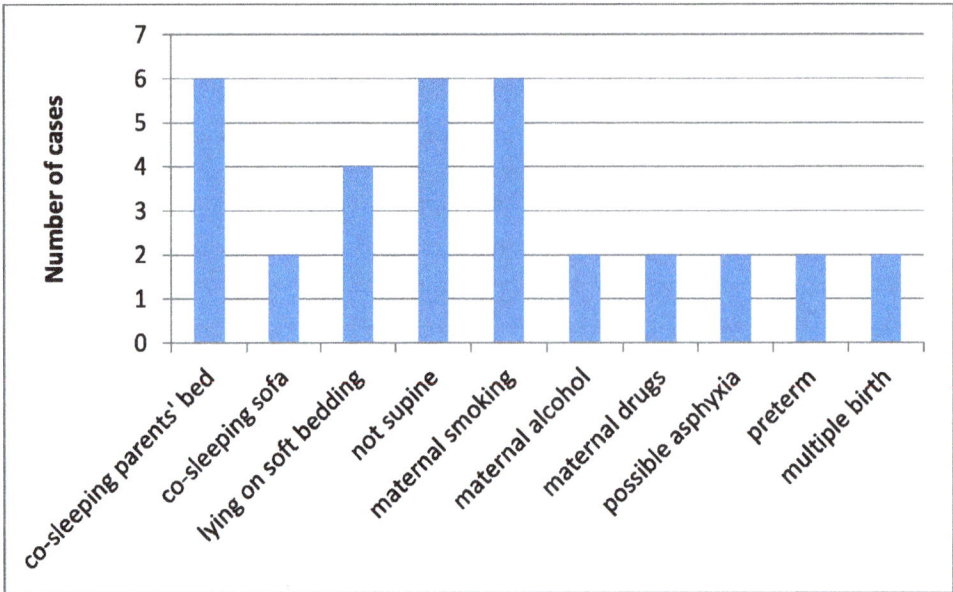

Figure 7.2: Profile of risk factors for SIDS cases (14).

follow-up appointments with pediatricians so could not be informed; 29/104 (28%) of families declined to participate in the study when asked. The results in this chapter are from the 21/23 recruited families who completed questionnaires or interviews and the 26 interviewed professionals (10 pediatricians, 3 specialist nurses, 2 social workers, and 11 police officers). All parents appeared to vividly recall the events of their children's deaths and their interaction with professionals despite the elapse of time; the Framework matrix enabled us to corroborate these accounts. Despite the low rates of recruitment, theoretical saturation of data was obtained; this was defined as the point when few new data emerged that were relevant to the developing theory (20). I compared social deprivation scores, based on postcodes, for both recruited and non-recruited cases. There was no statistical difference suggesting that recruited and non-recruited families were similarly socially deprived.

There were 14 SIDS deaths and 7 deaths due to fully explained medical causes. The mean age at death of recruited cases was 100 days (95% CI: 69-131 days). 13/14 SIDS cases had multiple modifiable risk factors including unsafe sleep environments, parental smoking, or parental alcohol consumption. Only two SIDS deaths occurred in infants sleeping in their own cots. The profile of risk factors is shown in Figure 7.2.

## Parents' experiences

Parental data related to two key themes: their need to understand why their child died and their experiences of the JAA investigation. These are considered separately, although many of the issues are interrelated. Analysis of parents' experiences revealed a clear conflict for professionals in the requirement to carry out a thorough investigation while remaining sensitive to the needs of bereaved families. Overall, despite the shock of the sudden death, most parents found the JAA a positive experience, particularly as it enabled them to know why their baby had died, which they felt was extremely important.

## Understanding the cause of death

In most interviews bereaved parents explained, without prompting, that they had an overwhelming need to understand why their baby had died; this was true for both SIDS and explained deaths. No parents said that the cause of death was unimportant to them. If there were medical reasons for the death, parents felt relieved, and this relief was often witnessed by the professionals working with them.

> Yes, I suppose I felt it was quite important really to hear what the findings were really because it was unexpected, she was such a healthy girl and it was such a shock. ... I really wanted to know and that was all really I guess. (Father, SIDS case)

> [F]or me that was amazing, seeing her the week after because she was just a totally different woman. This was a woman that didn't go outside, never smiled and she was up, she was dressed, she was, you know, smiling ... a totally, totally different woman from when we first saw her, it was just amazing, just the results of that just changed her completely. (Specialist nurse, medically explained death)

However, for SIDS parents the lack of complete explanation for death was a source of ongoing distress.

> It's just, not having an answer; I don't think it's fair like ... why? (Mother, SIDS case)

> I have days when I have really been beyond sad and I'm angry ... because you can't understand a healthy baby dying. You can understand a poorly baby dying but you can't understand a healthy baby dying. (Mother, SIDS case)

Usually, the cause of death is not immediately apparent at post-mortem examination and detailed metabolic and histological tests are required. There is typically a delay of at least three months for these investigations to be completed. Parents often became increasingly anxious about the cause of death during this long wait for information. One mother described even starting to question her own actions and creating theories for the death:

> ... [Y]ou turn it on yourself when you don't hear anything, then you make things up in your head. "It must have been this, it must have been this, it must have been this" ... because you don't know anything ... Which leaves me to sit there wondering what it was and thinking "we don't know anything about the toxicology" and I'm thinking "how could you possibly have poisoned ... how have you poisoned him?" Well you don't know, until that comes back, you don't know, and that was weeks. (Mother, SIDS case)

SIDS is potentially difficult to explain to families, but despite this, half of the SIDS parents were able to give accounts that showed that they understood the concept of SIDS as deaths remaining unexplained after complete investigation. Some parents' descriptions matched current physiological explanations.

> ... [T]hat was one of the things I asked the pediatrician, I said, "[W]hat is it?" and she said, "[T]hat's the whole point, we don't know". (Mother, SIDS case)

> ... [S]omething in his brain ... [H]e'd stopped breathing and his brain wasn't developed enough to sort of say ... "Baby, you're not breathing, breathe son". (Father, SIDS case)

Not all SIDS parents seemed to understand the concept of SIDS; others, while apparently understanding it, debated how SIDS could be a natural phenomenon.

> I know they are saying natural causes but what's natural about a healthy person dying? (Mother, SIDS case)

## SIDS parents' understanding of modifiable risk factors

In nearly half of SIDS families, parents spoke about hazardous sleep environments or their smoking habits and they seemed to understand the relevance of these issues. For other parents, it seemed that they had found discussing risk factors with their pediatrician difficult and it was similarly so at interview. These are clearly difficult issues, as for some parents accepting the role of modifiable risk factors in the death may lead to the realization that had they made different choices, the outcome may have been different, with their baby not dying.

> She clearly understands and I mean she did say to me when she was pregnant with the [next] baby ... [S]he said, "I'm going to be really, really, really clear this time, that this baby will be sleeping in their own crib and that as much as I might be tempted, I will not be co-sleeping". (Specialist nurse, SIDS case)

> Yes because my wife sort of listened to it [the pediatrician talking about risk factors] and thought, "[W]ell he was in our bed at the time when he died and should I have put him in there? ... [H]ad I put him in his cot, would things have turned out differently?" (Father, SIDS case)

During interviews, a few SIDS parents did not talk of relevant risk factors despite case records documenting conversations concerning these between parents and pediatricians. One parent described their baby's death as "straightforward SIDS" with no elaboration, although the professional interviews detailed discussions with the family about the impact of alcohol, drug consumption, and co-sleeping on the death. It is possible that parents may have been minimizing the significance of the risk factors, or denying them completely to protect themselves from the reality of the knowledge, or that they simply did not understand. Pediatricians and specialist nurses commented that explanations about risk factors were challenging and they were concerned that this could lead to the parents self-blaming; some professionals avoided these discussions altogether.

> ... So once the death has happened, we don't ... I don't think we dwell on the risk factors because I think, that's right, we're not trying ... [W]e don't want to apportion blame to parents. (Pediatrician, SIDS case)

## Self-blame

Due to the potential that greater understanding about risk factors could lead to increased parental self-blame, this aspect of the research was analyzed in some detail. The topic of blame often came up spontaneously at interview, although parents were not specifically asked about it. Self-blame was a major feature in six cases involving six mothers and one father: these parents blamed themselves partially or completely for the deaths. These mothers felt guilty because they had failed as mothers, as their children had died. These feelings occurred irrespective of cause of death: three cases were of SIDS in unsafe sleep environments and three were unpreventable deaths from medical causes.

> At this point I didn't have any idea how long I'd been asleep and then feeling this overwhelming guilt ... I've slept for hours and she's just died. (Mother, medically explained death)

> I blame myself, if I hadn't have gone back to work, he'd be fine. (Mother, medically explained death)

Three mothers blamed themselves completely for the deaths, and their feelings of overwhelming guilt dominated interviews; only one of these deaths was from SIDS and the other two were from medical causes. These feelings of guilt and self-blame may have been related to maternal mental health issues, as all three mothers had clinically significant scores for both anxiety and depression on HADS. Their scores were significantly higher than those of mothers showing no or moderate self-blame; these are shown in Table 7.1 and Figure 7.3.

Table 7.1: Comparison of HADS scores for mothers (14).

| | Mean (95% CI) HADS anxiety score | Independent t test for HADS anxiety score | Mean (95% CI) HADS depression score | Independent t test for HADS depression score |
|---|---|---|---|---|
| Over-whelming self-blame (n=3) | 17.0 (14.5-19.5) | $t(19)= -3.91$, $p<0.001$ | 18.3 (15.5-21.2) | $t(19)= -3.68$, $p<0.002$ |
| Moderate or no self-blame (n=18) | 9.9 (8.4-11.5) | | 8.8 (6.6-11.0) | |

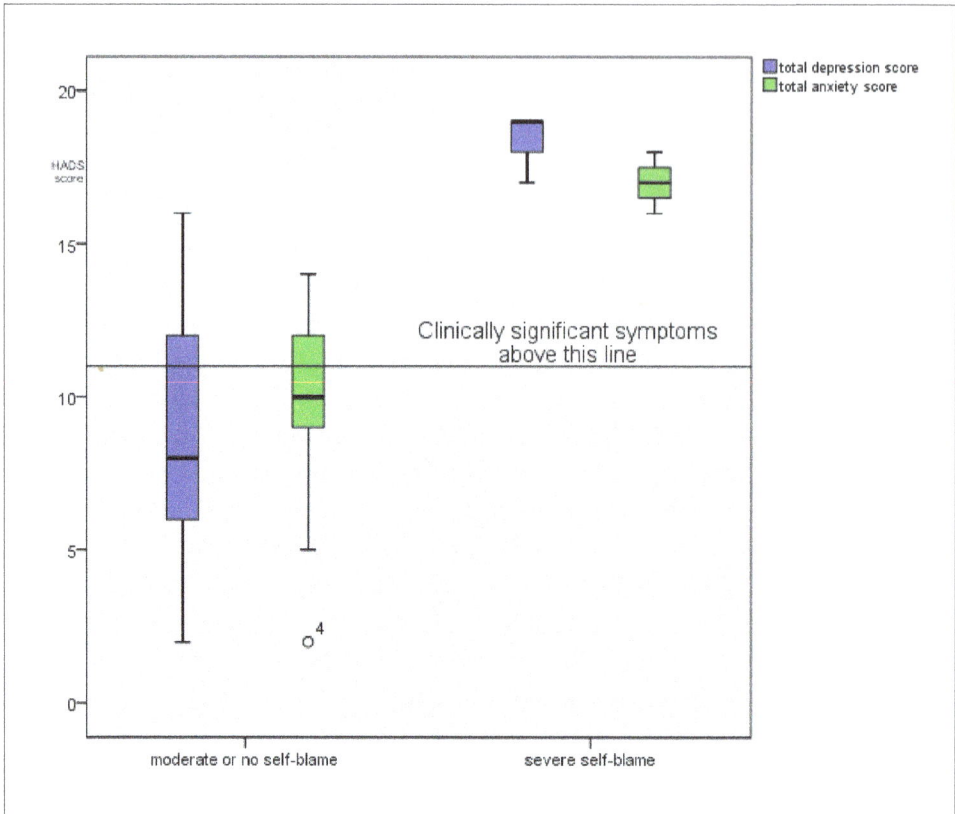

Figure 7.3: Box plots of HADS scores for mothers (14).

Some mothers explained that they had initially blamed themselves for the death but as time passed these feelings resolved. Other SIDS parents accepted responsibility for their choice of actions but not blame, viewing this as a negative option.

> And I could choose to let myself feel very guilty and that in a sense would kill your spirit … I'm happy to accept that I have some responsibility in his death and that's a different thing to being guilty. (Mother, SIDS case)

Some parents viewed the diagnosis of SIDS as one in which no blame could be attributed, despite the role that modifiable risk factors or their own actions may have played in the death. This lack of self-blame could be considered as a self-protection mechanism or even a denial of the issues surrounding the death.

> We've both always said we were quite glad when it came back that it was Sudden Infant Death …. [B]ecause it's been Sudden Infant Death, we sort of go, "[W]ell we couldn't have done anything, if it was going to happen, it was going to happen … "(Father, SIDS case)

## Parents' experiences of JAA investigation

Parents' experiences related to three sub-themes: the JAA investigation itself, follow-up after the investigation, and emotional support throughout the process; and parents described both positive and negative experiences for all three.

### The investigative process
### The Emergency Department (ED)

Most parents felt that they had been well cared for while in the ED, particularly by nursing staff. Parents were able to hold their baby to say goodbye without feeling rushed and they were not distressed by the need to give detailed accounts to pediatricians and specialist police. There were some issues with poor communication, particularly when parents had found their infants lifeless and correctly assumed that their baby was dead; they were then confused by reports from hospital staff that the baby was being resuscitated or to hurry to the hospital.

> The nurse that was on duty that morning, she was just amazing. She even sat and cried with us ... So you know, they were lovely, but they helped us so much ... [T]hey were fantastic. (Mother, medically explained death)

> But I was like, "[B]ut she's dead" and she wouldn't answer that question and so you have that moment of thinking, "[W]ell maybe she's not dead". It was really horrible, absolutely awful. (Mother, SIDS case)

### Joint home visit by specialist police and pediatrician

Joint home visits (JHV) by specialist police and a pediatrician (or specialist nurse) accompanied by the parents are strongly recommended by national statutory guidance (2) but these only took place in 15/19 SUDI cases that died at home. In the remaining four cases, specialist police conducted scene examinations without support from clinicians and, in two cases, in the absence of parents.

Most parents considered the JHV as a positive or neutral experience. Parents valued different aspects of JHVs: being provided with information, being given support when returning to the scene of death, coming to an understanding of possible reasons why their baby may have died, and being treated with compassion and non-judgemental attitudes by professionals. Poor communication was a problem for some parents, who felt uncomfortable with detailed questioning and having to retell their version of events again. A few parents did not understand why a JHV was required. For a few mothers the JHV was intensely difficult; they were so distraught that they could not bear to talk to professionals at all or face returning home to the scene of the death.

> I always felt I should go back and say thank you to the police who attended. (Mother, SIDS case)

I think the practicalities, as well of everything that comes after a death in the family, that them being able to do it so quickly afterwards is really good because then it was done, if I'm honest. (Mother, SIDS cases)

I couldn't understand why the doctors were here … [W]hy would they want to come and look at her bedroom? … The pediatrician was slightly ... not rude but to the point … "Did you have the heating on?" … "I don't know what day it is at the moment and no, the heating wasn't on". (Mother, medically explained death)

The professionals who took part in JHVs were overwhelmingly in favor of them, often stating that they were the most useful part of the JAA, in that they had a much greater understanding of the circumstances of the death and general home environment. The police valued the presence of the pediatrician as they felt this reduced parental anxiety about their involvement. Compared to JHVs, police visits alone to examine death scenes led to more parental distress and, at times, notable findings were not recognized.

… So I think that works well … I wanted it to look like it's a medical professional taking the lead here and we were there and supporting. I think the home visit is very good. Because you've got that … two different lenses really you know. (Police officer, medically explained case)

I felt it went quite well … I would say that the police handled it very sensitively … But Mum was able to sort of demonstrate to us on the double bed exactly where the baby was, what position Mum was in, what position Dad was in … I think they found it helpful to do that, although distressing, as it is for all parents. (Specialist nurse, SIDS case)

It felt like he was just checking everything in the house … [Y]ou're on pins by this stage anyway, your life is shit, it can't get any worse than this and then you've got someone peering about your house like you're a murderer. (Father, SIDS case — police visit without pediatrician)

I mean we have been out [to the home] since then, but yes probably we did [miss details], we did on the sort of precise sleeping arrangements. Yes I'm sure we did. (Specialist nurse, SIDS case without JHV)

### The role of uniformed police

In 10 families the actions of non-specialist uniformed police officers caused considerable additional distress; these events were all corroborated by police records. In contrast to the specialist police teams, uniformed officers have no prior training in managing SUDI cases, although often they are the first professionals to attend the home after parents contact emergency services. Uniformed police seemed to treat the home as a crime scene and prioritized investigation of "the crime" over supporting the parents. Frequently, uniformed police refused parents access to collect vital possessions such as keys or mobile telephones, demanding that families leave their homes immediately. In three cases, parents were not allowed to go to hospital with their infants, or had their baby removed from them while they waited for the ambulance to attend, and these actions were hugely distressing to parents. All these actions were contrary to local multi-agency SUDI protocols and they often caused difficulties for other professionals subsequently by traumatizing parents and even preventing analyses of death scenes. A few families, however, commented positively about uniformed police offering them emotional support and providing family members with transport to the hospital.

> The ambulance just took him ... and the next thing the police were everywhere ... We said can we go and see him and they said no, we had to wait ... but they just wouldn't let us go ... (Mother, SIDS case)

> ... So the police had gone in with great big size 10 boots and caused a lot of distress to the family, ahead of us getting there so ... we had to recoup all of that ... Then it [the JHV] went quite well but we clearly could not look properly at the place where the baby had been sleeping, because the police had removed all the bedding and so it was not how it had been. (Pediatrician, medically explained death)

## Contact with social care

Social workers only made direct contact with five families. Generally, they took part in the multi-agency discussions but only became more involved if child safeguarding concerns became apparent or if they felt they could provide families with support. Parents were typically very appreciative of support from social care. However, in two families safeguarding concerns arose after social care started working with them, and these parents felt misled, in that they thought they were being offered support and only later realized their parenting was being assessed. The social workers also found this issue difficult, particularly as the safeguarding concerns had not been apparent initially.

> To me that [the death] was just an excuse for the social workers to get involved, they wanted to be fully on me because there's been domestic violence between me and the Dad. (Mother, SIDS case)

> ... So I had kind of gone in and was genuinely trying to offer some support for Mum and the children, and I was talking about bereavement counseling and things like that ... [I]t was only when I picked up the case file ... that I thought, there are too many other risk factors here that are going on. (Social worker, SIDS case)

## Follow-up for bereaved families

Follow-up experiences were variable. Parents appreciated contact from pediatricians but were distressed by long waits for information; most families waited nearly six months to obtain the cause of death, with half the families having no contact with the pediatrician or specialist nurse in the interim. Many parents felt that they had to chase pediatricians to remain updated with the progress of investigations. Parents valued the chance to discuss the cause of death in detail with pediatricians.

> The pediatrician was really good at this, how she read it to me; she was very clear and thorough. That I liked ... Them coming to your home and speaking to you before coroner's court, I would absolutely agree with that ... (Mother, medically explained death)

> … [L]ike they were supposed to keep in touch with me … just even if they never had any news … I don't like the way it was done about that. I had to keep phoning and pestering them to know if there was anything ... (Mother, medically explained death)

Few families had follow-up contact with the police, usually by telephone; for some, this caused distress as they felt under ongoing suspicion despite no professionals raising child safeguarding concerns. However, many parents felt the police returned any property sensitively, following the end of investigations.

> My husband said the police officer was lovely. He took my husband in a room, and they'd even put her clothes in a gift box and tissue paper inside, and they had even put a nappy in. (Mother, SIDS case)

## Emotional support

Many families felt let down by the lack of emotional support provided by the JAA and struggled to access bereavement services themselves. Pediatricians and specialist nurses commented that they were unable to provide the level of support that some families needed. Parents often obtained support from family doctors; in the year after the death mothers had a mean of 5.6 (95%: CI 3.0-8.3) consultations for bereavement issues and fathers 3.3 (95% CI: 0.2-6.8). However, some parents did not attend their doctor at all, and in four cases the parental medical record summary made no reference to the death. Families also used other bereaved parents for support either informally or through organizations. Officially, health visitors only have a role in families with children of pre-school age; despite this, some mothers had continuing contact, which they valued highly, but others felt let down by the lack of contact. However, not all parents wanted emotional support from professionals; many were content with the support given to them from their families and friends.

> But then I got in touch with my friend's health visitor … She wasn't my health visitor and I hadn't got a baby anymore but she comes about every two weeks … But she's lovely. (Mother, SIDS case)

> I mean we went over it before … in hindsight, how pleased we were with the clinical side of things but disappointed with the mental health support. (Father, medically explained death)

## Strengths and limitations of study

In this study, I was able to obtain a very detailed understanding of cases due to the comparison of data within each case from interviews and case records. This enabled me to confirm parents' accounts that seemed questionable, such as some of the actions of uniformed police, and it was vital to the study of SIDS parents' understanding of risk factors. As with all qualitative research, limitations include that few people participate, and results may be highly subjective and therefore difficult to generalize. I did indeed struggle to recruit bereaved families and this was particularly apparent where there were long delays in the JAA process, in which families were lost to follow-up, preventing recruitment. I had previously audited JAA processes in part of the study area showing that only 64% of families were offered follow-up after SUDI (21); this could suggest that non-recruited families had significantly poorer experiences of the JAA than recruited ones. However, despite the limited recruitment, I captured a wide diversity of parental and professional experiences with recruited cases from socially diverse background. The results of this study concur with other research into bereaved parents' needs. Previously, I had conducted a systematic literature review of parents' needs following sudden child death; these included wanting to know why their child died, to have follow-up appointments with physicians to discuss the death, and to receive emotional support (6).

I would suggest that given the diversity of experiences, theoretical saturation of data, and rigorous approach to data analysis, the findings of this study are likely to be relevant to all professionals investigating unexpected child deaths with similar detailed child death review processes.

## Conclusions

### Helping parents by improving the investigation of SUDI

It is possible to thoroughly investigate sudden infant deaths while being supportive and compassionate to families. Bereaved families particularly want detailed information about why their child died; many can understand the role of modifiable risk factors in SIDS even when this relates to parental actions. Professionals may be reassured that sharing this detailed information with parents does not seem to relate to parental self-blame. Parents really struggle with long waits for information during the investigative process and this can increase their distress. Most parents found the JHV helpful but a small minority of mothers found it intensely distressing. There were issues with uniformed police who had little knowledge of SUDI, increasing parents' distress by starting criminal investigations and limiting parents' access to their home and possessions. These actions made subsequent investigation by specialist police and pediatricians more challenging.

Although the overall experience for most parents was positive, there are clearly ways in which SUDI investigations could be improved. The suggestions made here arise from this research study, some of which has been incorporated into the latest UK guidance for investigating unexpected infant and child deaths (22).

1. Healthcare professionals investigating SUDI should be adequately trained for this role.

Parents want detailed information about the complete causes of death, and this information will only be available if professionals are appropriately trained to identify relevant risk factors and confident in discussing these with parents. If these issues are not recognized and shared with parents, they cannot protect a child born subsequently, which parents will clearly wish to do. SUDI is a relatively rare event and one that most pediatricians encounter only occasionally. In the three years of this study, there were approximately 40 SUDI cases annually in the West Midlands region. Each local area has their own system of ensuring that pediatricians or specialist nurses are available for SUDI cases, leading to large numbers of healthcare professionals investigating deaths only occasionally. As a result, it may make it difficult for individuals to develop expertise in SUDI and particularly in death scene examination. This issue was also highlighted in my PhD research, analysing CDR data in the West Midlands, which revealed that the JAA frequently failed to identify deaths probably due to accidental asphyxia and did not always recognize modifiable risk factors (23).

## 2. Specialist police officers should investigate SUDI wherever possible.

Many parents spoke of the distress caused by uniformed non-specialist police officers commencing crime scene investigations, and professionals spoke of the difficulties this caused subsequently, both in their working relationships with families and death scene examination. Ideally, specialist non-uniformed police should be available at all times to manage cases of unexpected child death. If immediate SUDI response remains a uniformed police responsibility, police authorities should recognize the need for training and clear guidance for all officers on the immediate management of SUDI prior to the involvement of specialist officers.

## 3. Specialist police officers and pediatricians should conduct joint home visits routinely.

Parents expressed a clear preference for a JHV by police and pediatrician, and professionals felt strongly that this was a sensitive and effective approach. When police examined death scenes without pediatric support, important information was missed and parents found these visits much more distressing than joint visits. Given these findings, it would suggest that wherever possible police and pediatricians should work together investigating unexpected child deaths.

## 4. Professionals should create a flexible approach to enable full engagement with all parents.

Although most mothers were willing to talk to pediatricians and police, and participate in the JHV, a few were so distressed that they could not, so other relatives engaged with the professionals on their behalf. As most mothers are the primary caregivers, this situation risks losing important information, particularly concerning the final sleep. In cases where mothers are this distressed, it may be that a more flexible approach to investigation is needed. Forensic considerations may require that police conduct an initial scene examination without the mother but a JHV could be arranged some days later when the mother feels able and ready to give her account of events.

5. Parents should be kept up to date with the progress of investigations.

Parents spoke at length about the anxiety of waiting to hear why their child had died, and of feeling forgotten by professionals while they waited. Early in the investigation, a professional should be identified to keep in contact with the parents; even if only to tell them that the results are still awaited and to give an idea of timescales. Regular contact should enable parents to ask questions of professionals and help them feel supported. All professionals should be aware of the potential for increased distress caused by delayed information and should therefore seek to streamline processes where possible, keeping the parents' needs at the forefront of the investigation.

6. Parents should receive full information about the cause of death.

Parents made it clear in the study that they wanted to understand as fully as possible why their child died; many understood the role of modifiable risk factors even when these related to parental actions. Parents should be offered an opportunity to talk through all the information concerning the death, including the post-mortem examination report with an experienced healthcare professional.

7. Parents should be assisted to access bereavement services.

Many, but not all, parents will want help from bereavement services for themselves or their surviving children. Often these services are independent from healthcare services and they rely on clients referring themselves for support. Many parents have said how difficult they found this, feeling unable to even make a telephone call to explain their situation. Professionals could proactively assist parents who want support to make these initial contacts.

## Acknowledgements

I would like to thank the many families who shared their stories with me, enabling me to learn from them; without them the project would not have been possible. I also thank the Department of Pathology at Birmingham Women's Hospital for their help with identifying suitable cases, and my PhD supervisors, Dr Peter Sidebotham and Professor Frances Griffiths, both from Warwick Medical School, UK.

# References

1. Royal College of Pathologists, Royal College of Paediatrics and Child Health. Sudden unexpected death in infancy; a multi-agency protocol for care and investigation. Royal College of Pathologists, Royal College of Paediatrics and Child Health 2004.

2. HM Government. Working Together to Safeguard Children: A guide to inter-agency working to safeguard and promote the welfare of children. London: Department for Education,; 2015.

3. Vincent S. Child Death Review Processes: A Six-Country Comparison. Child Abuse Review. 2014;23(2):116-29. https://doi.org/10.1002/car.2276.

4. Fraser J, Sidebotham P, Frederick J, Covington T, Mitchell EA. Learning from child death review in the USA, England, Australia, and New Zealand. Lancet. 2014;384(9946):894-903. https://doi.org/10.1016/S0140-6736(13)61089-2.

5. Sidebotham P, Pearson G. Responding to and learning from childhood deaths. BMJ. 2009;338:b531. https://doi.org/10.1136/bmj.b531.

6. Garstang J, Griffiths F, Sidebotham P. What do bereaved parents want from professionals after the sudden death of their child: a systematic review of the literature. BMC pediatrics. 2014;14(1):269. https://doi.org/10.1186/1471-2431-14-269.

7. Limerick S. Family and health-professional interactions. Ann N Y Acad Sci. 1988;533:145-54. https://doi.org/10.1111/j.1749-6632.1988.tb37243.x.

8. Carlson JA. The psychologic effects of sudden infant death syndrome on parents. J Pediatr Health Care. 1993;7(2):77-81. https://doi.org/10.1016/0891-5245(93)90077-U.

9. Dyregrov A. Parental reactions to the loss of an infant child: a review. Scand J Psychol. 1990(4):266-80. https://doi.org/10.1111/j.1467-9450.1990.tb00839.x.

10. Ostfeld BM, Ryan T, Hiatt M, Hegyi T. Maternal grief after sudden infant death syndrome. J Develop Behav Ped. 1993;14(3):156-62. https://doi.org/10.1097/00 004703-199306010-00005.

11. Stroebe M, Stroebe W, Schoot Rv, Schut H, Abakoumkin G, Li J. Guilt in Bereavement: The Role of Self-Blame and Regret in Coping with Loss: e96606. PLoS One. 2014;9(5). https://doi.org/10.1371/journal.pone.0096606.

12. Kotsubo CZ. Helping families survive S.I.D.S. Nursing. 1983;13(5):94-6. https://doi.org/10.1097/00152193-198305000-00028.

13. McClain ME, Shaefer SJ. Supporting families after sudden infant death. J Psychosoc Nurs Ment Health Serv. 1996;34(4):30-4.

14. Garstang J. Why did my baby die? An evaluation of parental and professional experiences of joint agency investigations following sudden unexpected death in infancy Warwick; 2015.

15. Garstang J, Griffiths F, Sidebotham P. Parental understanding and self-blame following sudden infant death: A mixed-methods study of bereaved parents' and professionals' experiences. BMJ Open. 2016;6(5):e011323. https://doi.org/10.1136/bmjopen-2016-011323.

16. Garstang J, Griffiths F, Sidebotham P. Rigour and Rapport: a qualitative study of parents' and professionals' experiences of joint agency infant death investigation. BMC pediatrics. 2017. https://doi.org/10.1186/s12887-017-0803-2.

17. Fleming P, Blair P, Bacon CJ, Berry P. Sudden unexpected deaths in infancy: The CESDI SUDI Studies 1993-1996. London: The Stationery Office; 2000.

18. Zigmond AS, Snaith RP. The hospital anxiety and depression scale. Acta Psychiatr Scand. 1983;67(6):361-70. https://doi.org/10.1111/j.1600-0447.1983.tb09716.x.

19. Bryman A, Burgess RG, editors. Analyzing Qualitative Data. London: Routledge; 1994. https://doi.org/10.4324/9780203413081.

20. Holloway I. Qualitative Research in Nursing and Healthcare: Chichester: Wiley; 2013.

21. Garstang J, Debelle G, Aukett A. Investigating Unexpected Child Deaths: An Audit of the New Joint Agency Approach. Child Abuse Review. 2015;24(5):378-84. https://doi.org/10.1002/car.2271.

22. The Royal College of Pathologists, The Royal College of Paediatrics and Child Health. Sudden unexpected death in infancy and childhood. Multi-agency guidelines for care and investigation. London; 2016.

23. Garstang J, Ellis C, Griffiths F, Sidebotham P. Unintentional asphyxia, SIDS, and medically explained deaths: a descriptive study of outcomes of child death review (CDR) investigations following sudden unexpected death in infancy. Forensic Sci Med Pathol. 2016;12(4):407-15. https://doi.org/10.1007/s12024-016-9802-0.

# 8

# Parental Grief

Richard D Goldstein, MD

*Division of General Pediatrics, Department of Medicine,*
*Boston Children's Hospital and Harvard Medical School, Boston, USA*

## Introduction

A seemingly healthy infant dies suddenly and unexpectedly. A parent or someone the parent trusted with their infant was nearby, but the moment of death went unwitnessed. The forensic process ensues, including parent and guardian interviews, a death scene investigation, and autopsy. But another highly consequential process also begins: the process through which the infant's parents contend with their profound loss. As they seek an explanation, and the typically inconclusive results of the forensic process become known, they will experience intense emotions and a crisis of meaning. They will continue to face the complexities of coping with their loss for the rest of their lives. Medical relationships during involvement with sudden infant death syndrome (SIDS) begin and occur in a context of grief.

Medical and investigative interactions occur at the time of death, during the investigations, and as results are shared. Bereavement-related supportive services may be available; they may or may not meet the parents' needs (a situation which is explored in more detail in Chapter 7). There is rarely a plan or anticipatory guidance provided for the future once the death investigation is concluded. The family's usual medical care providers may not feel qualified to offer their assessment or advice, provided they even become aware of the challenges the family faces. All of these services and interactions will be influenced by the parents' grief, just as their grief will be influenced by the interactions. We can improve our care in this area with an awareness of the parents' emotional state and their needs. In the following, we present the state of knowledge about psychological coping following the loss of a young child and the process of grief that is seen.

## Important Concepts

Grief is the emotional adaptation to loss and the way it is expressed. Those who interact with parents around the time of unexpected infant death would agree that the emotional state of the parents is extremely raw and intense. First moments in dealing with significant losses are predictably overwhelming but, from the perspective of grief research, the quality of grief in this setting underscores important concepts at the heart of the current theoretical understanding of grief.

Conceptually, grief is an attachment reaction. Attachment can be thought of in a behavioral sense as a naturally occurring system that protects individuals by discouraging prolonged separation from their primary attachment figure (1). The attachment bond between a parent and a child is considered the strongest human attachment bond (2). In the case of a young, dependent child, this is self-evident. The survival of a young child depends on the protection and nurturing of his or her parent. But the strength of this bond is bi-directional: a parent's self-concept and self-worth are strongly tied to meeting their obligations to their child. This includes, at a baseline, protecting them from harm, but also providing for their future, a future they have imagined since becoming aware of their pregnancy. Their child's safety and future is an extension of their identity. Death brings an end to the infant and the reality of that future, but not to the bond or the meaning embedded in it (3). Grief can be understood as an effort to maintain these bonds in the face of loss. In addition to the empirically based evidence that will be reviewed later, the innate process that seeks to restore these bonds has been understood through two important ways of conceptualization: stage models of grief and process models of grief.

### Stage models of grief

Stage models of grief attempt to describe the changing emotional states and tasks that are commonly seen following death, as attempts are made to adapt and preserve the attachment bond. The work of Elizabeth Kübler-Ross (4) is a well-known example of a stage model, although her work's primary focus was on how a person reckoned with their personal impending death. She described five stages a person goes through, following a significant loss: [1] denial and isolation; [2] anger; [3] bargaining; [4] depression; and [5] acceptance. The first four stages are negative conditions that are ultimately passed once a person learns to accept the loss. These negative stages can be seen from the perspective of frustrated attachment ties and the feelings that occur during efforts to reactivate them. The presence of these stages has been empirically demonstrated, although the population in question was made up of elderly, surviving life partners without pathological levels of grief (5). The current status of the Kübler-Ross stages is that they are regarded as descriptive and informative, but should not be taken as a strict sequence to be accomplished in some fixed period of time. Experience has found that people move back and forth between stages, retaining and revisiting feelings from "earlier" stages long after grief has "resolved". The persistence of these stages has not been implicated as a key feature of pathological grief.

The inherent limitations to the stage conceptualization, particularly with its suggestion of a linear process, has been noted since stages of accommodation to loss were first proposed, as for example, can be found in Bowlby and Parkes' four stages of normal adaptation to loss: [1] numbness; [2] yearning and searching; [3] disorganization and despair; and [4] reorganization (6). Similar to Kübler-Ross's later proposal, this conceptualization remains relevant as another informative framework shedding light on the emotional states involved as a person strives to maintain a meaningful relationship (attachment) following loss, reconceiving their relationship with that person. While there may be a more typical sequence where certain feelings predominate, following a stereotypic sequence does not indicate healthier bereavement. It is also important to note that acceptance may not be the final, resolved state of a parents' grief. It may not be reasonable to recognize that a parent must strive to maintain their attachment bond to their deceased infant, yet also expect them to accept their infant's absence from the world or feel that other relationships can replace it. The idea of reorganization may better illuminate this stage of adaptation, where the loss is reconceived and incorporated into a satisfying but changed life.

## Process models of grief

Important insights into the process through which this reconceiving of attachment occurs can be found in the Dual Process Model of Coping with Bereavement (7). The Dual Model brings attention to the way in which people accommodate to the absence of a significant figure while maintaining bonds, illustrating the adjustments necessary to keep the process sustained and yet tolerable. It highlights an oscillation between two kinds of adjustments involved in the coping process. Loss orientation refers to thoughts and feelings which are directed toward important elements of the loss. For example, remembering the sensations that were experienced while embracing their infant when he or she was alive is loss-oriented and generally creates intense emotions of yearning and pain. The fact that such experiences are no longer possible as they once were must be dealt with in order to be reconceived as tolerable remembrances of special aspects of their relationship.

Alternatively, restoration orientation involves the times when attention is diverted from what has been lost. Time may be spent apathetically on mundane tasks or in settings where memories of the deceased are not intrusive. Life occurs without pain and time goes on. A parent may feel guilty or disloyal to their child when they discover they are enjoying themselves, or that they have gone for a long period of time without noticing their sorrow, yet it is in this way that reorganization may occur. The dynamic of oscillating from loss orientation to restorative orientation is found in normal grief. Hindrances or imbalances in the oscillation suggest a more problematic process.

## Normal Grief

Most grief is not pathological. Stage theories of adjustment describe an anticipated, acute experience of loss that is normal. It may be dramatic and can often involve negative emotions that are only considered normal in this context. Parents are stunned and dazed by their loss. There is a high level of emotional distress, especially intense sadness and yearning. Intrusive thoughts and dysphoria are to be expected. Acute grief involves affective, behavioral, and cognitive elements that are considered normal so long as they conform to cultural norms and do not persist (8). It may be interesting to note that in sudden infant death, the immediate expression of loss by parents has been found to be the same regardless of what the cause of death is ultimately determined to be (9).

Behavioral aspects of acute grief include social withdrawal, fatigue, irritability, sleep disturbance, and somatic complaints. These behavioral reactions may limit the ability of professionals to conduct an interpersonal assessment of the acutely bereaved. There are also cognitive consequences of significant loss that have an influence on our interactions with parents in the acute setting. An altered sense of reality and problems with memory and concentration are normal. Cognitive reaction time is significantly delayed (10) and there are diminished attention and lower scores in global cognitive performance (11). Normal grief involves preoccupation, lowered self-esteem, and self-reproach. Rumination — i.e. repetitive, self-focused thoughts and behaviors focused on negative emotions ("I'm so sad") and the bereaved person's difficult circumstances ("how can I live with this?") — has been shown to be prevalent in bereaved parents (12).

While not everyone ruminates, those who exhibit higher levels of rumination regard it as a way to help solve the dilemmas their loss has occasioned. However, research has shown that they are less able to make sense of their loss. This is important because meaning making predicts grief severity (13). Parents who are better able to make sense of their child's death have better post-loss adjustment. Tellingly, 45% of bereaved parents cannot make sense of their loss and 21% can find no benefits to their post-loss experiences (14, 15). Better grief outcomes rely on a parent's ability to find meaning in their child's life and their death (16).

In addition to behavioral and cognitive aspects, acute grief has affective dimensions. Depression, despair and dejection, anxiety, guilt, anhedonia, and isolation may be part of normal coping with regards to a loss (17). These are well-described and accepted parts of normal adjustment to significant loss, with an expectation that the intense presentation of these symptoms will resolve in a time-limited manner. Mourning is the culturally sanctioned manner that allows the symptoms to be experienced and not challenged, providing quarantine for the bereaved while they "recover".

Informally, the affective dimensions of grief are sometimes spoken about as a kind of depression; alternatively, they may be spoken of in terms of psychic trauma and thus considered a variant of post-traumatic stress disorder (PTSD). But once one considers diagnostic categories of psychological pathology, this lack of precision becomes inaccurate. Pathological bereavement is increasingly understood in terms of prolonged grief disorder (PGD), now set for inclusion in ICD-11 (18, 19). Certain aspects of pathological grief, presented below, distinguish it from other psychiatric diagnoses. The intensity of PGD is related to the strength of the attachment bond, and whereas in depression the intensity is related to a withdrawal from attachment figures, in PTSD it is related to the enormity of the stressor event. PGD involves abnormal preoccupation with the deceased, but the preoccupation in depression is with low self-esteem and in PTSD with a sense of personal safety. Intrusions in PGD are positive remembrances that provoke yearning or emotional pain, whereas the intrusive thoughts in depression are self-referential and negative and in PTSD are marked by helplessness and fear (20). PGD has been shown to be a distinguishable syndrome by confirmatory factor analysis (21), distinct from grief-related depression (22), anxiety (23), major depressive disorder (24), or PTSD (19). People with disordered grief may also be clinically depressed or have diagnostic levels of post-traumatic stress, but pathological grief is a separate affective category that entails a different therapeutic approach.

## Prolonged Grief Disorder

Although the dimensions of normal grief are significant, some bereaved persons experience more intense grief, which lasts longer than would be expected according to social norms and causes impairment in daily functioning. In these instances, the coping abilities of the bereaved leave them unable to adapt to their loss. The high levels of distress that are initially experienced do not abate, and the bereaved fail to achieve integrated grief. Prolonged grief disorder (PGD), also called complicated grief or persistent complex bereavement disorder, defines this pathological category of grief (19). Prolonged grief disorder affects 2-3% of the general population, with a pooled prevalence of 9.8% (25). Research establishing PGD initially focused on spousal loss later in life, which is the most common type of loss currently experienced, but now extends to many other populations and types of loss with consistent findings.

Prolonged grief disorder is a diagnosis used for bereaved persons who are abnormally affected (19). Its criteria require that the grief lasts for a period of greater than six months after a significant loss, along with clinically significant impairment in social, occupational, or other important areas of functioning. Separation distress must be present, manifest as yearning and physical or emotional suffering on daily basis or to a disabling degree. In addition, at least five cognitive, emotional, or behavioral symptoms must be present daily or to a disabling degree. These symptoms include role confusion or a diminished sense of self; difficulty accepting the loss; avoidance of reminders of the deceased; loss of trust; anger; difficulty "moving on"; emotional numbness; feeling that life is empty, meaningless, or unfulfilling; feeling stunned, dazed, or shocked by the loss.

Research to judge the significance of PGD in bereaved parents is plagued by inconsistent methodologies and varied indicators of grief outcomes. Among the populations studied, however, it would be fair to conclude that the risk for complex bereavement following the death of a child is greater than twice that reported in other forms of loss (26) and, in certain situations, may approach a sevenfold increase (27).

## Is Parental Grief Distinct?

Many aspects of the death of a young child predict greater difficulty in grief for parents of dependent children who have died. The loss of a child is considered among the worst experiences when rated in life event scales (28). The loss is against the normal order of things (29). As stated above, insofar as grief reflects attachment, parental grief is a special case. The loss is hostile to defining elements of the close attachment relationship: to the feelings, hopes, and meanings projected onto the child by the parents; to the protective obligations of a parent; and to the closeness and intensity of the parent-child relationship. The loss is hostile to the assumed and socially assigned responsibilities of a parents. The loss attacks the very premise of all that being a parent incorporates.

As well as the psychological aspects of the bereavement adjustment, the death of a young child is associated with worsened physical health and mortality in parents. Research indicates that bereavement following the death of a young child is accompanied by a significant increase in mortality, physical health problems, and mental health difficulties in bereaved parents. Mortality from both natural and unnatural causes remains elevated for up to 18 years in mothers, with a nearly fourfold increased risk of death by unnatural causes in the three months following the death (30, 31). Fathers have an increased rate of death by unnatural causes for three years, and unexpected death leads to further increased risk (31). Bereaved parents have more health problems (32), including increased cardiovascular-related disease (33), more diagnoses of chronic medical conditions, and a greater than 10-fold rate of health-related work absence (34).

Research has shown increased levels of unresolved, complicated, or prolonged grief in parents of children dying from virtually any cause. Poorer outcomes in bereaved parents, and features that are consistent with PGD, are seen in much of the parental grief literature. Parental grief after the loss of a child is well documented to be more intense, complicated, and long-lasting, with huge fluctuations over time in comparison to grief related to any other type of loss (35). This view is remarkably unchallenged. Loss-related risk factors that have been shown to complicate bereavement and adjustment include the nature of the death (13); the bereaved person's relationship with the deceased, with more grief intensity experienced by parents who have lost a child than by adults who have lost either spouses or parents; and the existence of unresolved issues or an inability to find meaning. Personal risk factors include pre-existing psychological morbidity and vulnerabilities (36), gender (37), social context, and role (38); including the role as a parent and the role as a competent adult. Research specific to parental loss points to more severe grief outcomes associated with the death of a younger child (39), parent-child kinship (40), a more dependent relationship (31), and being a mother (41). Sudden death in the home also carries increased risk (41), as does a lack of preparation for death (42). Parents whose only child has died experience greater symptoms (43). Parental grief may not be an entirely distinct experience but evidence is consistent that it is more severe. In bereaved parents with prolonged grief, 80% wished to die at some point following the loss (44).

## Considerations Particular to SIDS

Research on parental bereavement adjustment following SIDS has become much less common in the "Back to Sleep" era. Whether due to the decreased incidence of SIDS, a bias against the legitimacy of the SIDS diagnosis, or an accusatory environment in these cases, very few of the more commonly used grief indicator measures have been used to study grief following SIDS. The grief in these parents, however, is extremely severe in whatever population it has been studied. Research on parental grief following a SIDS death has shed light on the greater psychological burdens for parents after the sudden death of a child (45), when approximately two-thirds of parents whose children died from SIDS, suicide, or accidents have pathological levels of grief 18 months following the death. Parents whose infants died from SIDS experience higher levels of isolation (46), with feelings of self-blame and guilt increasing in the months following the infant's death (47). Research samples consistently show high levels of prolonged grief-related symptoms and extraordinary amounts of self-blame, especially in mothers (48).

## Next Steps

In many ways, insights gained through better understanding the severe form of grief observed in parents following their child's death from SIDS have great potential to increase the understanding of important areas of investigation in bereavement research. This population of parents has the power to inform important questions in PGD and its treatment. Their high levels of grief-related symptoms and pathology distinguish these parents as a "boundary population". Their experience may not be typical, or especially common, in comparison to the prevalence of bereavement after the death of a life partner, yet the severity of their symptoms provides important insights into the diagnostic categorization of pathological grief. Their symptom severity raises important questions about the specificity of criteria for prolonged grief disorder, namely whether a condition should be labeled as pathological when it is a highly prevalent outcome of an event with relatively high incidence. As the disorder becomes established, it is valid to consider whether parental grief requires a modified set of diagnostic criteria, in order to identify the subpopulation of bereaved parents with the most heightened risk for pathology.

Bereavement support is generally regarded as helpful in parental grief, but its outcomes are relatively unstudied. Some promising cognitive behavioral approaches to grief support rely on motivating the bereaved with activities and structure, based upon the view that quotidian tasks act as "hidden regulators" of behavior (49). The pervasive isolation and self-blame seen in these parents after SIDS contributes to their bereavement outcomes, in part, by removing many of those regulators from people's lives. Interventions aimed at invigorating daily structure and activities may demonstrate therapeutic efficacy.

## Conclusions

Mortality from SIDS/sudden and unexpected infant death remains significant at this unique time in human history, a time when the death of a child is an uncommon event, and, indeed, when a typical death is not the death of a child (50). As long as these deaths occur, there will be an important population of bereaved parents with significant needs affecting their own health and productivity, as well as the health of their young families. Their intense feelings of responsibility and failure in their role as parent to their infant, provoked by their loss, are rooted in the same attachment bonds that would strengthen their abilities as parents had the death not occurred.

A child's death from SIDS is a profound loss. Parental grief in its aftermath is severe, with physical, behavioral, cognitive, and emotional dimensions. This grief influences every medical encounter related to the death, from information gathering to the sharing of conclusions. Most parents' difficulties are under-recognized and unaddressed, as they struggle under the weight of adjusting to a loss from which they will not fully recover. There is an important role for research and support in this area.

## References

1. Bowlby J. Attachment. New York: Basic Books; 1969/1982.

2. Crowell JA, Treboux D, Gao Y, Fyffe C, Pan H, Waters E. Assessing secure base behavior in adulthood: Development of a measure, links to adult attachment representations, and relations to couples' communication and reports of relationships. Dev Psychol. 2002;38(5):679-93. https://doi.org/10.1037/0012-1649.38.5.679.

3. Bowlby J. Disruption of affectional bonds and its effects on behavior. Can Mental Hlth Suppl. 1969;59(12):1-12.

4. Kübler-Ross E. On death and dying. New York: Collier Book/Macmillan Publishing Co, 1970.

5. Maciejewski PK, Zhang B, Block SD, Prigerson HG. An empirical examination of the stage theory of grief. JAMA. 2007;297(7):716-23. https://doi.org/10.1001/jama.297.7.716.

6. Bowlby J, Parkes CM. Separation and loss within the family. In: The child in his family. Ed Anthony EJ. New York: Wiley, 1970. p. 197-216.

7. Stroebe M, Schut H. The dual process model of coping with bereavement: Rationale and description. Death Stud. 1999;23(3):197-224. https://doi.org/10.1080/074811899201046.

8. Bonanno GA, Moskowitz JT, Papa A, Folkman S. Resilience to loss in bereaved spouses, bereaved parents, and bereaved gay men. J Pers Soc Psychol. 2005;88(5):827-43. https://doi.org/10.1037/0022-3514.88.5.827.

9. Smialek Z. Observations on immediate reactions of families to sudden infant death. Pediatrics. 1978;62(2):160-5.

10. O'Connor MF, Arizmendi BJ. Neuropsychological correlates of complicated grief in older spousally bereaved adults. J Gerontol B Psychol Sci Soc Sci. 2014;69(1):12-18. https://doi.org/10.1093/geronb/gbt025.

11. Hall CA, Reynolds CF 3rd, Butters M, Zisook S, Simon N, Corey-Bloom J, et al. Cognitive functioning in complicated grief. J Psychiatr Res. 2014;58:20-5. https://doi.org/10.1016/j.jpsychires.2014.07.002.

12. Schwab R. Gender differences in parental grief. Death Stud. 1996;20(2):103-13. https://doi.org/10.1080/07481189608252744.

13. Keesee NJ, Currier JM, Neimeyer RA. Predictors of grief following the death of one's child: The contribution of finding meaning. J Clin Psychol. 2008;64(10):1145-63. https://doi.org/10.1002/jclp.20502.

14. Ronen R, Packman W, Field NP, Davies B, Kramer R, Long JK. The relationship between grief adjustment and continuing bonds for parents who have lost a child. Omega (Westport). 2009;60(1):1-31. https://doi.org/10.2190/OM.60.1.a.

15. Lichtenthal WG, Neimeyer RA, Currier JM, Roberts K, Jordan N. Cause of death and the quest for meaning after the loss of a child. Death Stud. 2013;37(4):311-42. https://doi.org/10.1080/07481187.2012.673533.

16. Rogers CH, Floyd FJ, Seltzer MM, Greenberg J, Hong J. Long-term effects of the death of a child on parents' adjustment in midlife. J Fam Psychol. 2008;22(2):203-11. https://doi.org/10.1037/0893-3200.22.2.203.

17. Zisook S, Shuchter SR. Uncomplicated bereavement. J Clin Psychiatry. 1993;54(10):365-72.

18. Prigerson HG, Maciejewski PK. Rebuilding consensus on valid criteria for disordered grief. JAMA Psychiatry. 2017;74(5):435-6. https://doi.org/10.1001/jamapsychiatry.2017.0293.

19. Prigerson HG, Horowitz MJ, Jacobs SC, Parkes CM, Aslan M, Goodkin K, et al. Prolonged grief disorder: Psychometric validation of criteria proposed for DSM-V and ICD-11. PLoS Med. 2009;6(8):e1000121. https://doi.org/10.1371/journal.pmed.1000121.

20. Shear MK. Clinical practice. Complicated grief. N Engl J Med. 2015;372(2):153-60. https://doi.org/10.1056/NEJMcp1315618.

21. Boelen PA, van de Schoot R, van den Hout MA, de Keijser J, van den Bout J. Prolonged Grief Disorder, depression, and posttraumatic stress disorder are distinguishable syndromes. J Affect Disord. 2010;125(1-3):374-8. https://doi.org/10.1016/j.jad.2010.01.076.

22. Prigerson HG, Frank E, Kasl SV, Reynolds CF 3rd, Anderson B, Zubenko GS, et al. Complicated grief and bereavement-related depression as distinct disorders: Preliminary empirical validation in elderly bereaved spouses. Am J Psychiatry. 1995;152(1):22-30. https://doi.org/10.1176/ajp.152.1.22.

23. Prigerson HG, Bierhals AJ, Kasl SV, Reynolds CF 3rd, Shear MK, Newsom JT, et al. Complicated grief as a disorder distinct from bereavement-related depression and anxiety: A replication study. Am J Psychiatry. 1996;153(11):1484-6. https://doi.org/10.1176/ajp.153.11.1484.

24. Prigerson HG, Maciejewski PK, Reynolds CF 3rd, Bierhals AJ, Newsom JT, Fasiczka A, et al. Inventory of Complicated Grief: A scale to measure maladaptive symptoms of loss. Psychiatry Res. 1995;59(1-2):65-79. https://doi.org/10.1016/0165-1781(95)02757-2.

25. Lundorff M, Holmgren H, Zachariae R, Farver-Vestergaard I, O'Connor M. Prevalence of prolonged grief disorder in adult bereavement: A systematic review and meta-analysis. J Affect Disord. 2017;212:138-49. https://doi.org/10.1016/j.jad.2017.01.030.

26. Kreicbergs UC, Lannen P, Onelov E, Wolfe J. Parental grief after losing a child to cancer: Impact of professional and social support on long-term outcomes. J Clin Oncol. 2007;25(22):3307-12. https://doi.org/10.1200/JCO.2006.10.0743.

27. Kristensen P, Dyregrov K, Dyregrov A, Heir T. Media exposure and prolonged grief: A study of bereaved parents and siblings after the 2011 Utoya Island terror attack. Psychol Trauma. 2016;8(6):661-7. https://doi.org/10.1037/tra0000131.

28. Holmes TH, Rahe RH. The Social Readjustment Rating Scale. J Psychosom Res. 1967;11(2):213-18. https://doi.org/10.1016/0022-3999(67)90010-4.

29. Neugarten BL. Time, age, and the life cycle. Am J Psychiatry. 1979;136(7):887-94. https://doi.org/10.1176/ajp.136.7.887.

30. Li J, Precht DH, Mortensen PB, Olsen J. Mortality in parents after death of a child in Denmark: A nationwide follow-up study. Lancet. 2003;361(9355):363-7. https://doi.org/10.1016/S0140-6736(03)12387-2.

31. Li J, Laursen TM, Precht DH, Olsen J, Mortensen PB. Hospitalization for mental illness among parents after the death of a child. N Engl J Med. 2005;352(12):1190-6. https://doi.org/10.1056/NEJMoa033160.

32. Lannen PK, Wolfe J, Prigerson HG, Onelov E, Kreicbergs UC. Unresolved grief in a national sample of bereaved parents: Impaired mental and physical health 4 to 9 years later. J Clin Oncol. 2008;26(36):5870-6. https://doi.org/10.1200/JCO.2007.14.6738.

33. Rogers CH, Floyd FJ, Seltzer MM, Greenberg J, Hong JK. Long-term effects of the death of a child on parents' adjustment in midlife. J Fam Psychol. 2008;22(2):203-11. https://doi.org/10.1037/0893-3200.22.2.203.

34. Wilcox HC, Mittendorfer-Rutz E, Kjeldgard L, Alexanderson K, Runeson B. Functional impairment due to bereavement after the death of adolescent or young adult offspring in a national population study of 1,051,515 parents. Soc Psychiatry Psychiatr Epidemiol. 2015;50(8):1249-56. https://doi.org/10.1007/s00127-014-0997-7.

35. Rando TA. Parental loss of a child. Champaign, Ill.: Research Press, 1986.

36. Bonanno GA, Wortman CB, Lehman DR, Tweed RG, Haring M, Sonnega J, et al. Resilience to loss and chronic grief: A prospective study from preloss to 18-months postloss. J Pers Soc Psychol. 2002;83(5):1150-64. https://doi.org/10.1037/0022-3514.83.5.1150.

37. Vance JC, Boyle FM, Najman JM, Thearle MJ. Gender differences in parental psychological distress following perinatal death or sudden infant death syndrome. Br J Psychiatry. 1995;167(6):806-11. https://doi.org/10.1192/bjp.167.6.806.

38. Malkinson R, Rubin SS, Witztum E. Therapeutic issues and the relationship to the deceased: Working clinically with the two-track model of bereavement. Death Stud. 2006;30(9):797-815. https://doi.org/10.1080/07481180600884723.

39. Wijngaards-de Meij L, Stroebe M, Stroebe W, Schut H, Van den Bout J, van der Heijden PG, et al. The impact of circumstances surrounding the death of a child on parents' grief. Death Stud. 2008;32(3):237-52. https://doi.org/10.1080/07481180701881263.

40. Middleton W, Raphael B, Burnett P, Martinek N. A longitudinal study comparing bereavement phenomena in recently bereaved spouses, adult children and parents. Aust N Z J Psychiatry. 1998;32(2):235-41. https://doi.org/10.3109/00048679809062734.

41. Michon B, Balkou S, Hivon R, Cyr C. Death of a child: Parental perception of grief intensity — End-of-life and bereavement care. Paediatr Child Health. 2003;8(6):363-6.

42. Meert KL, Shear K, Newth CJ, Harrison R, Berger J, Zimmerman J, et al. Follow-up study of complicated grief among parents eighteen months after a child's death in the pediatric intensive care unit. J Palliat Med. 2011;14(2):207-14. https://doi.org/10.1089/jpm.2010.0291.

43. Wijngaards-de Meij L, Stroebe M, Schut H, Stroebe W, van den Bout J, van der Heijden P, et al. Couples at risk following the death of their child: Predictors of grief versus depression. J Consult Clin Psychol. 2005;73(4):617-23. https://doi.org/10.1037/0022-006X.73.4.617.

44. Zisook S, Iglewicz A, Avanzino J, Maglione J, Glorioso D, Zetumer S, et al. Bereavement: Course, consequences, and care. Curr Psychiatry Rep. 2014;16(10):482. https://doi.org/10.1007/s11920-014-0482-8.

45. Dyregrov K, Nordanger D, Dyregrov A. Predictors of psychosocial distress after suicide, SIDS and accidents. Death Stud. 2003;27(2):143-65. https://doi.org/10.1080/07481180302892.

46. Lang A, Gottlieb LN, Amsel R. Predictors of husbands' and wives' grief reactions following infant death: The role of marital intimacy. Death Stud. 1996;20(1):33-57. https://doi.org/10.1080/07481189608253410.

47. Ostfeld BM, Ryan T, Hiatt M, Hegyi T. Maternal grief after sudden infant death syndrome. J Dev Behav Pediatr. 1993;14(3):156-62. https://doi.org/10.1097/00004703-199306010-00005.

48. Garstang J, Ellis C, Griffiths F, Sidebotham P. Unintentional asphyxia, SIDS, and medically explained deaths: A descriptive study of outcomes of child death review (CDR) investigations following sudden unexpected death in infancy. Forensic Sci Med Pathol. 2016;12(4):407-15. https://doi.org/10.1007/s12024-016-9802-0.

49. Hofer MA. Relationships as regulators: A psychobiologic perspective on bereavement. Psychosom Med. 1984;46(3):183-97. https://doi.org/10.1097/00006842-198405000-00001.

50. Walter T. A new model of grief: Bereavement and biography. Mortality. 1996;1:7-25. https://doi.org/10.1080/713685822.

# 9 Promoting Evidence-Based Public Health Recommendations to Support Reductions in Infant and Child Mortality: The Role of National Scientific Advisory Groups

Jeanine Young, BSc(Hons), PhD

*School of Nursing, Midwifery, and Paramedicine,*
*University of the Sunshine Coast, Queensland, Australia*

## Introduction

Public health programs are tasked with using the best available evidence to make informed decisions in supporting campaigns, guidelines, policies, and advice in order to improve the health and wellbeing of countries, communities, families, and individuals (1). Public health programs, which focus on reducing preventable infant and child mortality, target modifiable factors that parents, caregivers, and health professionals can influence the most in order to promote the optimal conditions in which infants and children may survive, grow, and thrive (2, 3). The "Reduce the Risk of Sudden Infant Death Syndrome (SIDS)" and subsequent "Safe Sleeping" campaigns (4, 5) are key components of successful public health programs, which promote evidence-based risk reduction strategies to reduce infant mortality (2, 6). Although national campaigns and programs may vary in style, number, and content of key messages, countries that have adopted similar risk reduction programs, and in particular the advice to sleep babies on their backs, have experienced marked reductions in sudden and unexpected infant deaths (2, 4, 5, 7).

## Essentials of an Evidence-Based Public Health Approach

Evidence underpinning public health recommendations comes from a systematic study of completed, peer reviewed, and publicly available research (1, 8). To ensure that public health practice is underpinned by evidence, it has been proposed that five key activities need to be undertaken (1). These activities include [1] evaluating needs for new or improved programs or practices; [2] identifying the best available evidence on programs and practices that potentially meet the needs; [3] collecting the best available information on appropriate programs and practices; [4] selecting programs that fit together with community and population needs and values; and [5] evaluating the impact on health and wellbeing of putting selected programs into practice (1, 9). In addition, high-quality programs are those which deliver public health initiatives that have been demonstrated to be population-centered, equitable, proactive, health promoting, risk-reducing, vigilant, transparent, effective, and efficient (9, 10).

## The Role of Scientific Advisory Groups

Governments and public health organizations have recognized the importance of expert advice in facilitating efficient access to the best available evidence to support sound public health practice and policy making (11, 12). Access to, and knowledge of, good clinical practice also requires an understanding of the needs of stakeholder groups and the systems they work within, in order to translate evidence into practice. Thus "scientific" or "expert" advisory groups, on a local and national scale, have an important role in assisting with both access to, and translation of, best available evidence to inform clinical practice, individual- and community-based strategies, and national public health campaigns (13). Specific functions of advisory groups may vary, depending on the topic or area with which they have been established to assist. However, generally scientific advisory groups perform three broad functions (13, 14). First, group members provide expertise, ranging from very specific tacit knowledge through to general advice on broad, scientific, or practice strategies. Second, participants lend their reputation to the organization they are representing, in effect signaling scientific quality and credibility to external bodies. Third, members share their academic and scientific networks with the organization to assist in providing critical resources to enable the organization in achieving its goals. For example, this may include access to expert consultants or opportunities for collaborative research.

Most countries around the world that have initiated national campaigns to reduce the risk of sudden unexpected death in infancy have established expert groups or forums to assist in a continual review of the dynamic and emerging evidence base relating to infant care. Continual review and critique of new research is essential in order to ensure that recommendations, and the strategies used in dissemination of those recommendations, are based on the most current, relevant, and best available evidence

(4, 5, 7). In this chapter, the Red Nose National Scientific Advisory Group, established to work collaboratively with the Australian national organization Red Nose Saving Little Lives (formerly SIDS and Kids), will be used as a case study to illustrate the role of a scientific advisory committee in supporting a nationally recognized, not-for-profit organization to achieve its vision in reducing infant and child deaths. A brief synopsis of the organization's history and current vision and mission will be provided. Both focal responsibilities, including priority setting undertaken by the scientific advisory group, and the advantages of having a national reference group will be discussed, together with common pitfalls to avoid. The sharing of experiences of one particular national advisory group in this chapter is not intended to represent the depth and breadth of the terms of reference that may be undertaken by similar groups established in the many nations which have instituted a safe sleeping public health campaign; however, it is likely that many commonalities will exist.

## Supporting Evidence-Based National Safe Sleeping Recommendations: The Australian Experience

In Australia, Red Nose Saving Little Lives is a high-profile and well-respected national not-for-profit organization with a successful history spanning 40 years. The history of both Red Nose and other SIDS support organizations is explored in more depth in Chapter 4; Red Nose itself is renowned for delivering a national safe infant sleeping health promotion program; bereavement support for families who have experienced an infant or child death; advocacy; and support for research into sudden infant deaths, perinatal deaths, and stillbirth (15). The organization has evolved markedly since it was founded in 1977 as the Sudden Infant Death Research Foundation Inc. under the stewardship of Kaarene Fitzgerald, following the sudden and unexpected death of her infant son, Glenn. By 1986, the creation of similar organizations in other states and territories to address the phenomenon of SIDS led to the formation of the National SIDS Council of Australia (16). This latter organization and its leaders, the majority of whom were bereaved parents in the organization's infancy, were instrumental in establishing the SIDS International and the Global Strategy Task Force (15). These transnational forums continue to facilitate and nurture collaboration between researchers, educators, and bereaved parents to achieve a shared vision of reducing infant and child mortality.

Public health campaigns led by the National SIDS Council of Australia in the 1990s have been credited with the 80% reduction in sudden infant deaths achieved in the two decades following the first "Reduce the Risks of SIDS" campaign in 1991 (3, 6). The organization's name changed to SIDS and Kids in 2002 in order to recognize the organization's history and its future, as the remit expanded from SIDS to include pregnancy loss, sudden unexpected death in infancy (SUDI), including SIDS and fatal sleeping accidents, and sudden childhood deaths (15). In October 2016, SIDS and Kids restructured and rebranded its organization and support service as Red Nose Saving

Little Lives, in order to improve efficiency in service delivery, increase opportunities to meet the needs of Australian families, and achieve the organization's vision of a future where no child dies suddenly or unexpectedly during pregnancy, infancy, or their pre-school years (15, 17). To accomplish this vision, Red Nose is committed to its mission of reducing preventable deaths of babies and children and supporting bereaved families through the delivery of evidence-based education, bereavement support, and advocacy (17).

## Red Nose National Scientific Advisory Group: A Case Study

### History

As Australia's lead organization in reducing sudden and unexpected infant and child deaths, and in its role of advocating on the behalf of bereaved parents, Red Nose has recognized that it has a key role in the translation of scientific evidence into practice; the provision of advice to health professionals, parents, and the broader community; and the maintenance of standards. The SIDS and Kids National Scientific Advisory Group (NSAG) was established in 2004, following a national pathology workshop held in Canberra in March 2004, sponsored by SIDS and Kids (18) as an idea proposed by Professor Roger Byard to the SIDS and Kids Chief Executive Officer. The SIDS and Kids NSAG was renamed the Red Nose National Scientific Advisory Group (herein referred to as NSAG) in October 2016 with the rebranding of the national organization mentioned above.

### Purpose, membership, and terms of reference

NSAG is a multidisciplinary group of health professionals and researchers who promote and support Red Nose's agenda in research, community and health professional education, and bereavement care. The leading responsibility of NSAG is to ensure that information provided to parents and health professionals is based upon the best available evidence and meets the needs of parents and carers living and working in contemporary Australian society (18, 19). The primary purpose of the group is to enable and support Red Nose to achieve its mission, through providing a forum that facilitates the translation of scientific evidence into evidence-based infant care advice which influences practice for health professionals, parents, and policy makers. In addition, NSAG actively engages with services and agencies for the maintenance of policy and standards that relate to optimal infant care.

NSAG membership is voluntary and made up of multidisciplinary, multistate representation. Members meet up to four times per year, by teleconference or face-to-face modes. Membership comprises up to 14 people who work in the areas of perinatal, infant, and early childhood health and mortality and have an active commitment to the work of Red Nose. Nomination to NSAG, including nomination of Chair, is by the group and approved by the Red Nose National Board. The terms of reference for NSAG also allow resource people to be co-opted to the group to source specific advice or achieve priority goals, as required (18). During the period 2004-17, this interprofessional team has included neonatal and child health nurses, midwives, neonatologists, obstetricians, forensic pathologists, perinatal pathologists, physiologists, neuroscientists, epidemiologists, maternal and child health educators, and academic researchers with experience in acute, community, and primary healthcare settings including Indigenous heath. The breadth of professional experience provided by members ensures a rich and valuable bank from which to draw the knowledge and expertise required for NSAG to achieve its goals. Membership includes the Red Nose Chief Executive Officer (CEO), a consumer advocate, and an Australian Indigenous academic/researcher representative. Since the establishment of NSAG, and until July 2017, each incumbent for the Red Nose CEO and national educator role (key support role to NSAG) has possessed a clinical/health professional background. The skills brought to these Red Nose positions have been invaluable in terms of understanding the needs of stakeholder groups, the systems they work within, and the influence required, and the understanding gained has formed an effective bridge for translating the work of the NSAG members into priority actions for Red Nose to disseminate to the wider community.

Like similar scientific advisory groups, NSAG is an independent group of advisors chartered by the Red Nose Board of Directors, and provides expert review and guidance to improve the rigor and credibility of Red Nose public health and bereavement support programs and activities. More specifically, terms of reference for NSAG include provision of advice to Red Nose on research development, research, and policy initiatives, as well as public and health professional education programs. NSAG's remit includes identification of gaps; liaison between Red Nose and other agencies working in the area of perinatal and infant mortality to promote a united, consistent, and cohesive approach to policy change and/or education; and facilitation of Australian and international collaborative research activities including establishing research priorities, identification of funding sources, and support of the scientific component of Red Nose conferences and meetings. NSAG members are also available as media spokespeople for Red Nose in their area of expertise, and contribute to review panels relating to research or education initiative funding submissions, where appropriate (18).

During the last decade, the outcomes of NSAG's activities, on behalf of Red Nose, have been considerable. These include, but are not limited to, the availability of the first Red Nose (SIDS and Kids) endorsed eLearning program for safe infant sleeping (2010) in collaboration with Queensland Health in 2010 (20); the launch of a revised public health campaign "Sleep Safe My Baby" in 2012 (3); participation in the GAPS workshop, an international research priority setting workshop for SUDI in 2015 (7); and the development of national guidelines for safe infant sleeping using the NHMRC guidelines framework (currently under development) (21).

Several activities of NSAG, some of which comprise core business, will now be described to highlight the contribution of a scientific advisory group to furthering the work of a public health organization committed to using, and expanding, the evidence base in order to reduce perinatal and infant mortality.

## Evidence-based recommendations and resources

One of the major activities of NSAG is informing the content of Red Nose's suite of parent and health professional education resources, which are made publicly available in a variety of written and electronic media, in order to ensure that these are based on quality evidence. Prior to 2004, resources were developed through expert working groups established by Red Nose (as SIDS and Kids) to review and revise public health campaign resources, and were primarily print-based. Since 2004, a comprehensive suite of evidence-based safe infant sleeping resources designed for use by parents and/or health professionals has been developed in collaboration with NSAG, together with a process to ensure both periodic critical review and revision to incorporate relevant and recent quality evidence, and the identification of priority areas for further resource development. The Red Nose education suite comprises safe sleeping information brochures and posters designed primarily for parents, health professionals, and childcare providers to support the Australian safe sleeping public health campaign (last revised in 2012 and launched as the "Sleep Safe My Baby Campaign"), a childcare education kit, mobile-technology-based applications, and more detailed Red Nose position statements on a variety of infant care topics suitable for health professionals, students, and parents, including sleep position, sleep location and environment, breastfeeding, oesophageal reflux and sleep position, and immunization. All resources are also made available electronically via the Red Nose website.[1] This enables more rapid dissemination of updated information as soon as it becomes available.

New position statements, or revisions of current resources, are drafted by an NSAG member and/or subcommittee and presented to the group for comment prior to finalization of content. Statements are then subsequently formatted and presented to the Red Nose Board, before being made publicly available. Red Nose directly supports this work through allocation of time and resources via the organization's national education and librarian roles. These Red Nose staff members attend NSAG meetings, support NSAG members, and provide important feedback, particularly regarding identification of priority areas for further resource or policy development based on frequently asked questions and enquiries made to Red Nose around a variety of infant care topics.

The process of review by an expert and volunteer multidisciplinary group has provided an efficient forum through which to consolidate expertise and identify gaps and/or inconsistencies in resources across states and territories, together with opportunities for improvements in the sharing of information and the facilitation

---

1   See https://rednose.com.au for more information.

of endorsement of resources by health professional organizations. For example, the development of a Safe Infant Sleeping eLearning resource arose from a research project led by an NSAG member in the state of Queensland in 2010, to support implementation of the Queensland statewide safe infant sleep policy and guidelines (22, 23).[2] This eLearning program provided the evidence base underpinning current public health recommendations and the safe sleeping policy and incorporated links to Red Nose information statements; in a reciprocal arrangement, new education materials developed for this eLearning program were shared with Red Nose. This partnership led to a formal agreement between Queensland's Department of Health and Red Nose to provide this free education program as an electronic internet platform supported by Queensland Health's Clinical Skills Development Service and shared through a link to Red Nose for access by health professionals and parents throughout Australia and internationally (20).[3] This Red Nose preferred safe sleeping eLearning program has been endorsed for continuing professional education points by several professional organizations; has been incorporated into maternal and child health education requirements in several states; and has recorded over 9,000 successful completions by health professionals and parents. A subsequent sister program, the Aboriginal and Torres Strait Islander safe infant sleeping eLearning program was developed in 2012 in consultation with Indigenous stakeholder groups (24).[4] Both eLearning programs undergo periodic review and revision.

Since Australia's first "Reduce the Risk of SIDS" campaign in 1991, Red Nose has supported three national public health campaigns to raise awareness of messages in order to promote safe sleeping and reduce risk of sudden and unexpected infant deaths — in 1997, 2002, and 2012 (3, 25). In preparation for the launch of the 2012 "Sleep Safe, My Baby" Campaign, NSAG members convened an expert forum following the ISA-ISPID international conference held in Sydney, Australia, in October 2010 to review contemporary evidence and establish consensus for messages to be included in the national safe sleeping campaign. Agreement for five messages was established and published in a consensus paper (4); however, a meta-analysis of the relationship between breastfeeding and the risk of sudden infant death, although prepared, had not been published at the time of the forum. NSAG members actively lobbied for inclusion of breastfeeding in the new campaign, and after much debate about appropriate wording to be supportive of all parents regardless of feeding mode, "Breastfeed baby" was included in the 2012 national safe sleeping campaign (3). NSAG's role during this public health campaign preparation included support of Red Nose personnel in the development of health promotion messages, resources, and campaign materials; assistance during the campaign launch; and taking on the role of spokespeople for the organization on scientific matters during interactions with the media (19).

---

2   This eLearning resource is available at https://www.sdc.qld.edu.au/courses/126.

3   The free education program can be accessed via Red Nose at https://rednose.com.au/page/e-learning-education-package.

4   This eLearning program can be accessed at https://www.sdc.qld.edu.au/courses/123.

## Development of safe sleeping policy, clinical guidelines, and product safety standards

NSAG also supports Red Nose by providing content knowledge and scientific advice in its role in actively engaging with other Australian organizations, services and stakeholders involved in the maintenance of policy, guidelines, and standards that relate to infant mortality and safe infant sleeping. NSAG has actively lobbied for consistency in safe infant sleeping messages by supporting and informing professional groups, state and territory health departments, and community interest groups. This support specifically includes contributions as a key stakeholder in the development of position statements by professional organizations and government consultation, and priority research setting initiatives that address infant mortality (26, 27).

Clinical practice guidelines are increasingly becoming a familiar part of health professional practice, with the principal benefit being to improve the safety, quality and consistency of care received by patients and their families (28, 29). Various Australian states and territories have undertaken projects to establish state-based safe sleeping guidelines relevant to their state policy frameworks during the period 2008-17 (22, 30-32). In reviewing these policies, however, it is evident that much variation exists in contemporary policies and guidelines, with regard to content, wording, and approaches (33, 34). Many policies are not consistent with the current public health recommendations supported by Red Nose, and only succeed in further confusing parents, health professionals, and the public. Such confusion serves to ultimately undermine important public health messages (33, 35). Key stakeholder and consumer consultation is integral to successful consensus upon consistent messaging, which will underpin clear practice guidelines based on the best available evidence for use by parents and health professionals.

For example, successful recent collaborative projects and stakeholder consultation led by members of NSAG have achieved consistency between Red Nose's risk minimization and informed decision-making approach to shared sleeping (36) and position statements released by leading professional organizations (26, 37). NSAG members have been instrumental in lobbying for, and embarking upon, the development of national safe sleeping guidelines using the NHMRC clinical guidelines framework (completion due in 2018). Effective implementation of any successful national guidelines will be reliant on the content expertise within the guidelines group; the effectiveness of stakeholder consultation, particularly with professional organizations; and the utility of the guidelines being translated into practice across acute and community settings to support parents to adopt safe sleep recommendations, particularly for our most vulnerable families.

NSAG liaison with Australian government and non-government organizations in the development, maintenance, and/or promotion of standards (including the Australian Competition and Consumer Commission [ACCC]; the Queensland Office of Fair Trading's Department of Product Safety; Standards Australia; INPAA [formerly the Infant and Nursery Products Association of Australia]; and the Australian coronial system), have informed and supported several standards, investigations, and recommendations that relate to safe infant sleeping environments and infant products to ensure consistent messaging to the public. This work includes the ACCC investigation of convertible prams and pushchairs, the development of a voluntary standard for firmness of cot mattresses (38), and safety investigations into infant slings, infant hammocks, infant bean bags, and sleep cocoons, in collaboration with the Office of Fair Trading (16). Collaborative relationships and partnerships developed by NSAG members with these organizations have in turn facilitated the progress of research trials in novel areas in which standards are being developed, such as portable sleep spaces for Australian and New Zealand community settings and postnatal environments (39). Such partnerships and consultation with key stakeholders at each stage of the research process, from conception of the idea to the dissemination of study findings, in such dynamic and evolving research areas, are integral to the translation of research findings into safe, practical applications for use by families and contemporary product safety standards.

## Public representation and collaborative partnerships

Scientific advisory group members act as media spokespeople in their area of expertise, which assists the organization in maintaining a credible public profile, highlighting the role of Red Nose as a trusted public health organization actively engaged in issues relating to infant safety, family support, and furthering relevant research to benefit Australian families and their babies. The role of NSAG also extends to partnership with other stakeholder organizations in order to actively promote issues of importance in reducing infant mortality and supporting families. Examples include responses to government changes in monitoring infant formula legislation, tissue testing to assist in diagnosis of inherited metabolic disease, and expansion of Medicare rebates for lactation consultants to promote improved availability of breastfeeding support in the community (15). NSAG also engages in community advocacy and provides responses for parents and family members who seek further information about systems, processes, and investigations, including responses to recommendations for improvements.

## Role in research

Underpinning high-quality evidence to support the safe sleeping public health agenda is the need to explore, evaluate, and prioritize emerging research areas. NSAG members play an active role in research development and provide content expertise to assist Red Nose in prioritizing areas for future research investment (7). Activities of the group have included participation in research priority setting, both for the organization and internationally; committee support for scientific conferences and meetings; and scientific review of research submissions for collaborative funding. Areas identified by NSAG for future investigation include improvements to infant death investigation and classification systems, evaluations of the effectiveness of current public health campaigns, genetic-environmental interactions that influence SUDI risk, and progressing the stillbirth research and community education agenda (7).

## Conclusions

The work of NSAG is broad and varied, and focus is concentrated on sustainable strategies to support public health messages. NSAG, for example, neither engages in product endorsement nor attempts to police and respond to all inappropriate products, advertising, and media using imagery or messaging that promotes unsafe or suboptimal infant care practices. Such work would require full-time monitoring. Instead, the group focuses on collaborating with key stakeholders to extend the reach of public health messages to the wider audience through positive engagement in policy, guidelines, and standards development and provision of resources that promote evidence-based public health recommendations.

In considering the work of Red Nose within Australia, a systems approach that recognizes key levels of engagement and influence is useful in examining the work of NSAG in the promotion of safe sleeping education and research that aims to reduce infant mortality (9, 10). These examples of NSAG activities were chosen to illustrate how the context in which scientific advisory bodies operate, and the nature of the partnerships developed over time, influence decision making at many different levels — from the micro- (professional) level through the meso- (institutional or organizational) level to the macro- (policy) level (40). Solid partnerships on a micro-level between researchers and healthcare professionals who form and/or collaborate with NSAG are essential in order to build credibility and trust and lay the groundwork for contextualized and relevant advice, with translation of evidence into practice and impact at institutional and policy levels.

During the 21st century, the development of safe infant sleeping programs has matured into a robust process where evidence-based methodologies and frameworks are increasingly adopted. Scientific advisory groups, such as NSAG, have a key role to play in organizations which are required to proactively respond to the dynamic and emerging evidence base upon which decisions are made at many levels. Furthermore, NSAG provides an organized forum in which to consider and evaluate emerging evidence for its quality and relevance to contemporary public health recommendations and parent advice, and to identify areas for future investigation. A scientific advisory group improves the way scientific advice is gathered and acted upon; it forms a conduit for knowledge translation into practical advice for families; and in so doing it improves public confidence in the quality of messages and the public profile of the public health organization. Organizational support in terms of funding meetings and resourcing specific projects with organizational personnel time is crucial. The dedication and commitment of NSAG volunteers is also considerable but is not without many benefits in terms of professional growth, strategic engagement and networking, personal satisfaction, and reciprocity.

Pivotal to future success in further reducing infant and child mortality are high-quality evidence and partnerships between public health organizations, health professionals, the scientific community, and consumer groups, in order to effectively translate evidence into action. Scientific advisory groups have an essential role to play in supporting public health organizations to deliver on quality, evidence-based education, bereavement support, and advocacy, so as to achieve the best possible outcomes for Australian families.

# References

1. Fink A. Evidence-based public health practice. Thousand Oaks: Sage Publications, 2013. https://doi.org/10.4135/9781506335100.

2. Moon RY, Hauck FR, Colson ER. Safe infant sleep interventions: What is the evidence for successful behavior change? Curr Pediatr Rev. 2016;12(1):67-75. https://doi.org/10.2174/1573396311666151026110148.

3. Young J, Watson K, Ellis L, Raven L. Responding to evidence: Breastfeed baby if you can — The sixth public health recommendation to reduce the risk of sudden and unexpected death in infancy. Breastfeed Rev. 2012;20(1):7-15.

4. Mitchell EA, Freemantle J, Young J, Byard RW. Scientific consensus forum to review the evidence underpinning the recommendations of the Australian SIDS and Kids safe sleeping health promotion programme — October 2010. J Paediatr Child Health. 2012;48(8):626-33. https://doi.org/10.1111/j.1440-1754.2011.02215.x.

5. Moon RY, & AAP Taskforce on Sudden Infant Death Syndrome. SIDS and other sleep-related infant deaths: Updated 2016 recommendations for a safe infant sleeping environment. Pediatrics. 2016;138(5):e20162940. https://doi.org/10.1542/peds.2016-2940.

6. Tursan d'Espaignet E, Bulsara M, Wolfenden L, Byard RW, Stanley FJ. Trends in sudden infant death syndrome in Australia from 1980 to 2002. Forensic Sci Med Pathol. 2008;4(2):83-90. https://doi.org/10.1007/s12024-007-9011-y.

7. Hauck FR, McEntire BL, Raven LK, Bates FL, Lyus LA, Willett AM, et al. Research priorities in sudden unexpected infant death: An international consensus. Pediatrics. 2017;140(2):e20163514. https://doi.org/10.1542/peds.2016-3514.

8. Reijneveld SA. Evidence on the effectiveness of public health practice: How should we proceed? Eur J Public Health. 2015;25(5):752-3. https://doi.org/10.1093/eurpub/ckv003.

9. Honoré PA, Scott W. Priority areas for improvement of quality in public health. Washington DC: Department of Health and Human Services, 2010.

10. Van Wave TW, Scutchfield FD, Honore PA. Recent advances in public health systems research in the United States. Annu Rev Public Health. 2010;31:283-95. https://doi.org/10.1146/annurev.publhealth.012809.103550.

11. Finch R. Current challenges in antimicrobial resistance and healthcare-associated infections: Role and organization of ARHAI. J Antimicrob Chemother. 2012;67 Suppl 1:i3-10. https://doi.org/10.1093/jac/dks204.

12. Green AC, Greenberg P, Fitzgerald G, Clutton C. Translating health research into clinical advice and health recommendations: The NHMRC experience 2000-2005. Intern Med J. 2006;36(6):335-7. https://doi.org/10.1111/j.1445-5994.2006.01089.x.

13. Ding WW, Murray F, Stuart TE. From bench to board: Gender differences in university scientists' participation in corporate scientific advisory boards. Acad Manage J. 2013;56(5):1443-64. https://doi.org/10.5465/amj.2011.0020.

14. Slade M, Bir, V, Chandler R, Fox J, Larsen J, Tew J, et al. The contribution of advisory committees and public involvement to large studies: Case study. BMC Health Serv Res. 2010;10:323. https://doi.org/10.1186/1472-6963-10-323.

15. SIDS and Kids Australia. SIDS and Kids Annual Report 2015. [Available from: https://rednose.com.au/downloads/Annual_Report_2015.pdf]. Accessed 29 September 2017.

16. SIDS and Kids Australia. SIDS and Kids Annual Report 13/14. [Available from: https://rednose.com.au/downloads/Annual_Report_2014.pdf]. Accessed 29 September 2017.

17. Red Nose Saving Little Lives. Our vision and purpose. [Available from: https://rednose.com.au/page/our-vision-and-purpose]. Accessed 29 September 2017.

18. Red Nose National Scientific Advisory Group. Red Nose National Scientific Advisory Group terms of reference. Melbourne: Red Nose National Scientific Advisory Group, 2017.

19. SIDS and Kids Australia. SIDS and Kids Annual Report 12/13. Melbourne: SIDS and Kids, 2013.

20. Young J, Higgins N, Raven L. Reach, effectiveness and sustainability of a safe infant sleeping e-Learning program. Women and Birth; 2013;26(Suppl 1):S21. https://doi.org/10.1016/j.wombi.2013.08.281.

21. Red Nose National Scientific Advisory Group. Minutes of March 2017 meeting. Melbourne: National Scientific Advisory Group, 2017.

22. Queensland Health. Safe infant care to reduce the risk of sudden unexpected deaths in infancy: Policy statement and minimum practice standards. Brisbane: Maternity, Child Health and Safety Branch, Queensland Health, 2008.

23. Queensland Health. Safe infant care to reduce the risk of sudden unexpected deaths in infancy. Policy statement and guidelines. Brisbane: Queensland Government, 2008.

24. Young J, Craigie L, Watson K, Cowan S, Barnes M. Safe sleep, every sleep: Reducing infant deaths in Indigenous communities. Women and Birth; 2015;28(Suppl 1):S31-2. https://doi.org/10.1016/j.wombi.2015.07.105.

25. Henderson-Smart DJ, Ponsonby AL, Murphy E. Reducing the risk of sudden infant death syndrome: A review of the scientific literature. J Paediatr Child Health. 1998;34(3):213-19. https://doi.org/10.1046/j.1440-1754.1998.00225.x.

26. Australian College of Midwives. Australian College of Midwives position statement on bed-sharing and co-sleeping. [Available from: https://www.midwives.org.au/resources/acm-position-statement-co-sleeping-and-bed-sharing]. Accessed 29 September 2017.

27. Commonwealth of Australia. National Aboriginal and Torres Strait Islander Health Plan 2013-2023. Canberra: Commonwealth of Australia, 2013.

28. Buchan HA, Currie KC, Lourey EJ, Duggan GR. Australian clinical practice guidelines — A national study. Med J Aust. 2010;192(9):490-4.

29. Sciarra E. The importance of practice guidelines in clinical care. Dimens Crit Care Nurs. 2012;31(2):84-5. https://doi.org/10.1097/DCC.0b013e3182445f62.

30. Queensland Health. Safe infant sleeping, co-sleeping and bed-sharing: Guideline. Version 1.0. QH-GDL-362:2013. Brisbane: Queensland Government, 2013.

31. Government of South Australia. Best practice indicators for Health, Families SA and Childcare staff: South Australian safe infant sleeping standards. Adelaide: SA Health, Government of South Australia, 2011.

32. Government of Western Australia. Operational directive: Statewide co-sleeping/bed-sharing policy for WA hospitals and health services. OD 0139/08. Perth: Department of Health, 2011.

33. Dodd J. Evaluation of the Department of Health Western Australian operational directive satewide co-sleeping/bed-sharing policy for WA Health hospitals and health services. Western Australia: Telethon Institute for Child Health Research under contract with the Department of Health, 2012.

34. Drever-Smith C, Bogossian F, New K. Co-sleeping and bed sharing in postnatal maternity units: A review of the literature and critique of clinical practice guidelines. Int J Childbirth. 2013;3(1):13-27. https://doi.org/10.1891/2156-5287.3.1.13.

35. Fetherston CM, Leach JS. Analysis of the ethical issues in the breastfeeding and bedsharing debate. Breastfeed Rev. 2012;20(3):7-17.

36. Red Nose National Scientific Advisory Group. Information statement: Sharing a sleep surface with a baby. Melbourne: National SIDS Council of Australia, 2006 (revised May 2015).

37. Young J, Watson K, Kearney L. ACM position statement on bed-sharing and co-sleeping — Literature review: Bed sharing and co-sleeping 2014. [Available from: https://www.midwives.org.au/resources/acm-position-statement-co-sleeping-and-bed-sharing]. Accessed 29 September 2017.

38. Joint Standards Australia/New Zealand Committee CS-003. Australia/New Zealand standard: Methods of testing infant products. Method 1: Sleep surfaces — Test for firmness. AS/NZS 88111.1:2013. New Zealand: Standards New Zealand Paerewa Aotearoa, 2013.

39. Young J, Kearney L, Watson K, Shipstone R, Cole R, Rutherford C, et al. Sustainable strategies to support parents and health professionals in providing evidence-based infant care: A multi-agency collaboration to reduce infant mortality. USC Research Showcase; 12 July; Innovation Centre, USC, Sippy Downs, University of the Sunshine Coast, Australia, 2017.

40. Blancquaert I. Managing partnerships and impact on decision-making: The example of health technology assessment in genetics. Community Genet. 2006;9(1):27-33. https://doi.org/10.1159/000090690.

# 10

# Risk Factors and Theories

Rachel Y Moon, MD[1] and
Fern R Hauck, MD, MS[2]

[1]*Department of Pediatrics, University of Virginia
School of Medicine, Charlottesville, Virginia, USA*
[2]*Department of Family Medicine, University of Virginia
School of Medicine, Charlottesville, Virginia, USA*

## Introduction

Identification of factors that increase risk of, or are protective against, sudden infant death syndrome (SIDS) has largely been accomplished through epidemiological case-control studies. Risk factors include side and prone positioning, prenatal and postnatal tobacco smoke exposure, sleeping on soft or cushioned surfaces (particularly sofas, couches, and armchairs), bed sharing, soft bedding, head covering and overheating, and prematurity. Protective factors include breastfeeding, pacifier use, and room sharing. In this chapter, we will discuss the evidence for these risk and protective factors. We will also review the leading theories for SIDS causation including the Triple Risk Hypothesis, rebreathing theory, and deficient arousal and autonomic regulation, and how these theories create a plausible explanation for the risk and protective factors for SIDS identified in case-control studies.

# Risk Factors

## Side and prone sleep position

The prone sleep position was noted in multiple case-control studies to be associated with SIDS (1-6), beginning in 1965 in the United Kingdom (UK) (7). Even before this, in 1944, Abramson reported that prone positioning was found in 68% of young infants who died of accidental mechanical suffocation in New York City (8). Public health campaigns, which first promoted non-prone positioning in the 1980s and then supine placement, only beginning in the 1990s in many Western countries, have all been associated with a decline in SIDS rates. Subsequent studies have confirmed the association of prone sleep positioning and an increased SIDS risk (adjusted odds ratio [aOR] 2.3-13.1) (9-11). Physiologic studies have demonstrated an association of prone positioning with an increased risk of hypercapnia and hypoxia (12-14), overheating (15), diminished cerebral oxygenation (16), altered autonomic control (17), and increased arousal thresholds (18).

Subsequent studies have identified that the risk of side sleep positioning is similar to that of prone positioning (aOR 2.0 and 2.6 respectively) (10). Side positioning also has a higher population-attributable risk than prone positioning (11), likely because many infants who are placed on their side are found prone (10). Placement in, or rolling to, the prone position, particularly when infants are unaccustomed to that position, places infants at extremely high risk of SIDS (aOR 8.7-45.4) (10, 19). Thus all caregivers, including childcare providers, family members, and friends, should place the infant in the supine position for every sleep.

## Prenatal and postnatal tobacco smoke, alcohol, and illicit drug exposure

Multiple studies have found that both in utero and environmental tobacco smoke exposure increase the risk of SIDS (20-24) in a dose-dependent manner (25-27). The strongest risk occurs with maternal smoking; there is a small independent risk when fathers smoke after the infant's birth (23, 28).

While it is difficult to separate out the effects of in utero and environmental smoke exposure, in utero exposure reduces lung compliance and volume, impairs arousal mechanisms, and decreases heart rate variability in response to stress (29, 30), all factors which may negatively impact an infant's ability to respond appropriately to the environment. Researchers have estimated that one-third of SIDS deaths could be prevented if in utero smoke exposure were eliminated (31, 32).

Substance abuse often involves more than one substance, and it is difficult to separate each effect from the others or to separate it from smoking. In addition, there are few studies that have examined the association between substance use and SIDS. In one study of Northern Plains American Indians, periconceptual maternal alcohol consumption was associated with a sixfold increased risk of SIDS, and binge drinking during the first trimester of pregnancy was associated with an eightfold increase (33). In another study, a maternal alcoholism diagnosis was associated with a sevenfold increased risk (34). Maternal drinking postnatally has also been found to be associated with increased SIDS risk (34, 35), especially when it occurs within the 24 hours prior to the infant's death. Additionally, although the data for maternal drug use and SIDS are conflicting, overall, maternal prenatal drug use, especially of opiates, is associated with a 2- to 15-fold increased risk of SIDS (36-38). Thus parents should not smoke during pregnancy, and there should be no smoking around the infant. In addition, alcohol and illicit drugs should not be consumed during pregnancy. There is also a substantial risk when smoking or consumption of alcohol or illicit drugs occurs in the context of infant-adult bed sharing (11, 39, 40).

## Soft or cushioned sleep surfaces (including sofas, couches, armchairs)

A firm sleep surface, such as a tight-fitting mattress in an infant cot (known in some countries as "cribs"), bassinet, play yard, or portable crib, is the safest sleep surface. Sofas, couches, and armchairs are particularly dangerous sleep surfaces; compared with a crib mattress, these surfaces confer up to 67 times higher risk of infant death (41-43). A recent study in the United States (US) found that deaths on sofas comprised 12.9% of all infant sleep-related deaths in 2004-12, including SIDS, accidental suffocation, and ill-defined deaths (44). Parents should be counseled about the risk of placing the infant for sleep, or falling asleep with an infant, on a sofa, couch, or similarly cushioned surface.

Infants are also often placed to sleep in car seats, strollers, swings, infant carriers, and slings, often because the infant will fall asleep more quickly or because of the belief that sleeping in a sitting position will alleviate gastroesophageal reflux. However, sitting in a car seat or similar sitting device exacerbates gastroesophageal reflux (45) and is thus not recommended for that purpose. Additionally, young infants may not have adequate head control to support their airway when sleeping in such sitting devices, and sleeping in these devices may lead to accidental death (46). Slings are of particular concern in this regard, and infants who are carried in slings should have their heads visible and outside of the sling to minimize the risk of suffocation (47).

## Bed sharing

Bed sharing is defined as the infant sleeping on the same surface as another person. The practice of bed sharing is common in many cultures and facilitates breastfeeding (48, 49), which is known to be a protective factor against SIDS (50). However, in case-control studies, bed sharing has been associated with an increased risk of SIDS (39, 41), and it is believed that soft mattresses, other soft bedding, the risk of overheating, and the risk of overlay contribute to this increased risk.

It is clear that there is increased risk of infant death when bed sharing occurs when one or both parents are smokers (even if they do not smoke in the bed), when there was maternal smoking during pregnancy, when the adult bed sharer has drunk alcohol or taken arousal-altering medications or drugs, when the bed sharing takes place on a couch or sofa, when there is soft bedding, when bed sharing lasts for the entire night, and when the infant is <11 weeks of age (11, 39, 40). Indeed, bed sharing was found in one US analysis of infant deaths to be the most important risk factor for death for infants <4 months of age (51).

However, there is controversy about bed sharing for infants who are breastfed and whose parents are non-smokers and have not consumed alcohol, medications, or illicit drugs. Case-control studies have had conflicting conclusions. An individual-level analysis of 19 studies from nine datasets in the UK, Europe, Australia, and New Zealand, with 1,472 SIDS cases and 4,679 controls, found that bed sharing for these low-risk infants was associated with a fivefold increased risk of SIDS in the first three months of life (aOR 5.1, 95% CI: 2.3-11.4) and an eightfold increased risk in the first two weeks of life (aOR 8.3, 95% CI: 3.7-18.6) (52). In this study, there was no increased risk of SIDS if the bed-sharing infant was >3 months old. However, this study has been criticized for the large amount of imputed missing data on parental alcohol and drug use (53). Another analysis of data from two English studies, with 400 SIDS infants and 1,386 controls, found that, although bed sharing with a smoker or an adult who had recently consumed >2 units of alcohol was associated with an increased risk of SIDS, infants younger than 98 days of age who bed shared with an adult who was a non-smoker and did not recently consume alcohol were not at increased risk for SIDS (OR 1.6, 95%: CI 0.96-2.7) (43). Both of these studies are limited by small sample size in the subanalyses (54).

Recommendations regarding bed sharing differ. In the Netherlands, parents are advised not to bed share if the infant is <3 months old. In the US, parents are advised to avoid bed sharing for the first year but instead to have the infant sleep on a separate sleep surface close to the parents' bed (55). Because there is no increased SIDS risk if bed sharing does not last the entire night (11), parents are encouraged to bring the infant to the bed for feeding and comforting, and then to return the infant to his/her own sleep space when the parent is ready to go to sleep. Other countries, including Australia and the UK, recommend against bed sharing, particularly when the parent is a smoker or has consumed alcohol, drugs, or arousal-altering medication (56, 57).

## Soft bedding

The presence of soft bedding, including pillows, blankets, sheepskins, bumper pads, and positioners, in the infant sleep environment has been shown to increase the risk for infant death fivefold, independent of the sleep position, and 21-fold when the infant is in the prone sleep position (9). In addition, the US Consumer Product Safety Commission has reported an increased risk of accidental suffocation and asphyxial deaths associated with soft bedding use (58). Soft bedding increases the risk of overheating and head covering, both of which have been associated with increased SIDS risk. Finally, in an analysis of US child deaths, the presence of soft bedding in the infant sleep environment was reported to be the most important risk factor for sudden and unexpected death in infants 4 months and older (51).

Infants are safest when they do not sleep with blankets (53, 59). If parents are concerned that their infant will become cold, an infant sleeping bag, sleeping sack, or wearable blanket is recommended as an alternative to blankets. A safe infant sleeping bag is one in which the infant cannot slip inside the bag and the head cannot become covered. One Dutch study found that the odds ratio for a sleeping bag was 0.30 (95% CI: 0.13-0.67); however, when adjusted for confounders, the odds ratio was no longer statistically significant (aOR 0.73 (95% CI: 0.29-6.43)) (60). Cot bumpers and similar products that attach to the cot sides are not recommended because of the risk of entrapment between the mattress or cot and the bumper, the risk of suffocation against the bumper, and the risk of strangulation with bumper pad ties (61, 62).

## Head covering and overheating

In one case-control study, 24.6% of SIDS victims had their heads covered by bedding, compared with 3.2% of control infants during last sleep (63). Duvets, blankets, and quilts should be avoided in the infant sleep environment, as they may cover the infant's head or face and obstruct breathing (11, 63).

## Prematurity

Infants who are born preterm or with low birth weight are at fourfold risk of SIDS, compared to full term, normal birth weight infants (64, 65). Despite overall declines in SIDS rates, the rates among infants born preterm or with low birth weight still remain higher (66). Much of this may be due to an immature autonomic system, with impaired arousal mechanisms and an increased risk for hypercarbia. The increased SIDS risk does not appear to be related to apnea of prematurity, as there is no evidence that these episodes of apnea precede SIDS deaths (67). The increased risk of SIDS, however, may also be related to prone sleep positioning. Preterm infants are at equal or increased SIDS risk when placed prone (68). Further, they are more likely to be placed prone after hospital discharge, presumably because they were placed prone in the neonatal intensive care unit as a means to improve ventilatory status while requiring mechanical ventilation (69). It is therefore recommended that preterm infants be placed supine as soon as they are clinically stable, so that they and their parents can become accustomed to the supine position before the infant is discharged to home. The American Academy of Pediatrics recommends that this transition to the supine position occur by 32 weeks post-menstrual age (70).

## Protective Factors

### Breastfeeding

Multiple studies have demonstrated that breastfeeding provides protection against SIDS (50). Studies do not distinguish between direct breastfeeding and feeding with expressed breast milk. A meta-analysis of 18 case-control studies found that any breastfeeding was protective, but that the protective effect increased with increased duration and exclusivity of breastfeeding (50). A recent individual-level analysis of eight case-control studies in the US, Europe, Australia, and New Zealand found that two months of breastfeeding was required before a protective effect against SIDS was seen, and that this protective effect is seen with any amount of breastfeeding, regardless of exclusivity (70). Parents are encouraged to feed the infant with breast milk as much and for as long as possible.

### Dummy (pacifier) use

Several case-control studies and meta-analyses have found a strong protective effect with dummy (also known as pacifier) use (71-73). Although the mechanism of protection is yet unclear, proposed mechanisms include increased arousability and improved autonomic control (74). Others note that non-nutritive sucking of the pacifier may alter the upper airway diameter (75). However, it should be noted that the protective effect of dummy use is seen if the dummy is used when the infant is falling asleep, even though the dummy often falls out of the mouth soon after the onset of sleep (76, 77). Because the mechanism by which dummy use confers protection is still unclear, some experts are reluctant to recommend dummy use as a SIDS risk reduction strategy. However, in some countries, such as the US, dummy use is promoted as a risk reduction strategy. Because there is some concern that dummy use may interfere with breastfeeding initiation, introduction of a dummy for infants who are directly breastfed should be delayed until breastfeeding has been well established. In infants who are fed with formula or expressed breast milk, a dummy can be introduced at any time. If the dummy is not accepted by the infant, it should not be forced.

### Room sharing

The safest place in which an infant can sleep is in the parental bedroom, on a separate sleep surface; this reduces the risk of SIDS by as much as 50% (39, 41, 42, 78, 79). Infants who have died of SIDS while sleeping in a separate room are more likely to have been found with their heads covered by bedding and to have rolled into the prone position if they had been placed on their sides for sleep (80). It is recommended that the infant sleep surface be placed close to the parents' bed, to allow for easy monitoring and feeding. Room sharing, without bed sharing, is recommended for the first 6-12 months of life (55, 56, 57, 81, 82).

## Theories

There have been multiple theories over the years regarding the etiology and mechanisms of SIDS. This may be partly because the successes in reducing the SIDS rates have come from epidemiological studies. Thus there has been considerable research into the underlying mechanisms that may underpin the risk factors identified in these epidemiological studies.

For many years, it was believed that apneic events, including apparent life-threatening events, were precursors to SIDS. Home apnea monitors were often prescribed for these infants as a means to prevent SIDS. However, subsequent research found that apparent life-threatening events and apnea did not predict SIDS. Indeed, the increase in the use of apnea monitors beginning in the 1970s did not correlate with a decline in the SIDS rate (67).

Because many deaths occurred in cribs, much attention has been paid to sleep surfaces. One theory has attributed SIDS to toxic gases and has proposed that gases such as antimony, arsenic, or phosphorus can be released from infant mattresses (in particular, old mattresses) and cause toxicity when inhaled. However, no data support this theory. In addition, case-control studies have found no benefit to wrapping mattresses in plastic to reduce toxic gas emission (83, 84).

Another theory that focuses on the infant sleep environment proposed that, in specific situations, infants may rebreathe exhaled carbon dioxide. Relevant situations include when the infant is prone and/or when the infant's face is close to bedding. It is theorized that, in these conditions, a "pocket" of exhaled carbon dioxide collects around the infant's face, and the infant, rather than inhaling oxygen, inhales the exhaled carbon dioxide. The infant thus becomes increasingly hypercarbic and eventually succumbs to death if there is no stimulus that interrupts the rebreathing (85, 86). It has been suggested that the rebreathing theory could explain some of the risk posed by soft bedding and prone sleeping. However, there are no physiologic data from infants who died for which evidence supporting rebreathing has been documented.

In recent years, there has been growing consensus among scientists that SIDS is multifactorial in origin. The Triple Risk Hypothesis (87) (Figure 10.1) proposes that when a vulnerable infant, such as one born preterm or one exposed to maternal smoking, is at a critical but unstable developmental period in homeostatic control and is exposed to an exogenous stressor, such as being placed prone to sleep, then SIDS may occur. The model proposes that infants will die of SIDS only if all three factors are present, and that the vulnerability lies dormant until they enter the critical developmental period

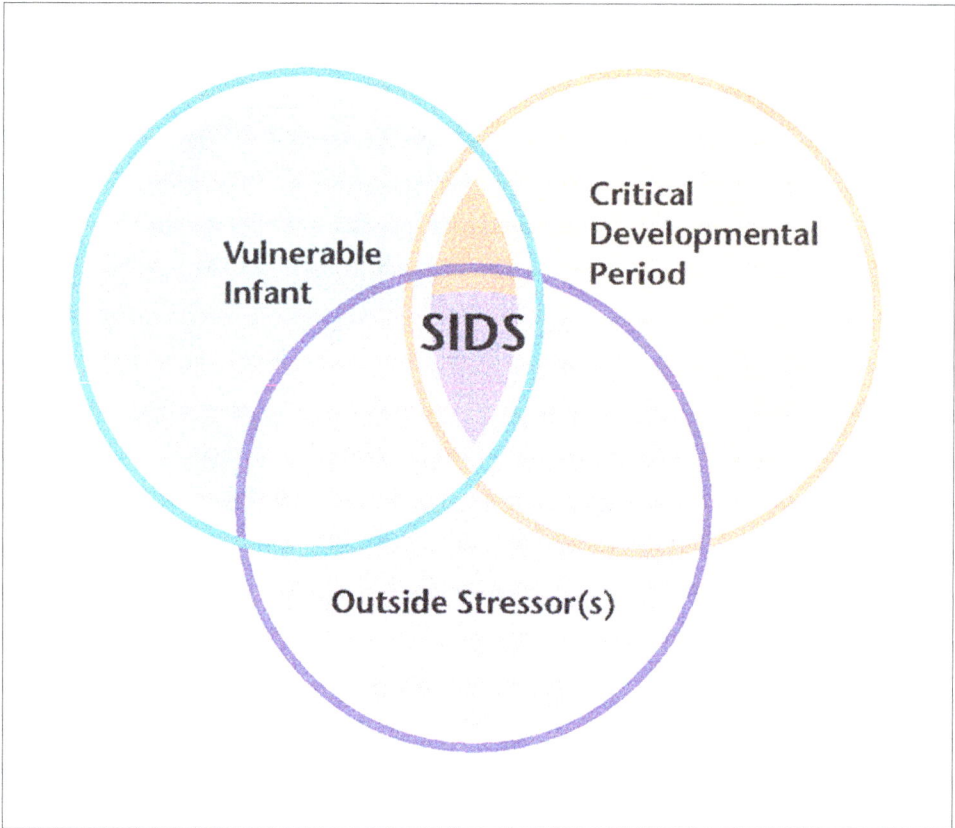

Figure 10.1: Triple Risk Hypothesis. (Adapted by the National Institutes of Health with permission from (87).)

and are exposed to an exogenous stressor. SIDS usually occurs during sleep, and the peak incidence is between 2-4 months of age, when sleep patterns are rapidly maturing. The final pathway to SIDS is widely believed to involve immature cardiorespiratory control, in conjunction with a failure of arousal from sleep (86, 88, 89). Support for this hypothesis comes from numerous physiological studies showing that the major risk factors for SIDS (prone sleeping, maternal smoking, prematurity, head covering) have significant effects on blood pressure, heart rate, and their control (90), and also impair arousal from sleep (91).

## Conclusions

Epidemiological case-control studies have been critical in identifying factors that are associated with an increased or decreased risk of SIDS. As such, great strides have been made in our understanding of the risk and protective factors for SIDS based on epidemiologic research, leading to educational interventions that have resulted in dramatic declines in SIDS rates. Theories regarding the pathophysiology of SIDS are myriad, but they all rely upon understanding the mechanisms by which these factors increase or decrease SIDS risk. However, further research — especially on the physiological mechanisms that contribute to or cause SIDS — is essential to achieving the reduction of SIDS rates to lowest levels possible.

## Acknowledgements

The authors thank their families for their continuous support.

## References

1. Mitchell EA, Scragg R, Stewart AW, Becroft DMO, Taylor BJ, Ford RPK, et al. Results from the first year of the New Zealand cot death study. NZ Med J. 1991;104:71-6.

2. Ponsonby A-L, Dwyer T, Gibbons LE, Cochrane JA, Wang Y-G. Factors potentiating the risk of sudden infant death syndrome associated with the prone position. N Engl J Med. 1993;329:377-82. https://doi.org/10.1056/NEJM199308053290601.

3. Dwyer T, Ponsonby A-L, Gibbons LE, Newman NM. Prone sleeping position and SIDS: Evidence from recent case-control and cohort studies in Tasmania. J Paediatr Child Health. 1991;27:340-3. https://doi.org/10.1111/j.1440-1754.1991.tb00415.x.

4. Irgens LM, Markestad T, Baste V, Schreuder P, Skjaerven R, Oyen N. Sleeping position and sudden infant death syndrome in Norway 1967-91. Arch Dis Child. 1995;72:478-82. https://doi.org/10.1136/adc.72.6.478.

5. Taylor JA, Krieger JW, Reay DT, Davis RL, Harruff R, Cheney LK. Prone sleep position and the sudden infant death syndrome in King County, Washington: A case-control study. J Pediatr. 1996;128:626-30. https://doi.org/10.1016/S0022-3476(96)80126-0.

6. Fleming P, Gilbert R, Azaz Y, Berry PJ, Rudd PT, Stewart A, et al. Interaction between bedding and sleeping position in the sudden infant death syndrome: A population based case-control study. BMJ. 1990;301:85-9. https://doi.org/10.1136/bmj.301.6743.85.

7.  Carpenter RG, Shaddick CW. Role of infection, suffocation, and bottle-feeding in cot death; An analysis of some factors in the histories of 110 cases and their controls. Br J Prev Soc Med. 1965;19:1-7. https://doi.org/10.1136/jech.19.1.1.

8.  Abramson H. Accidental mechanical suffocation in infants. J Pediatr. 1944;25:404-13. https://doi.org/10.1016/S0022-3476(44)80005-1.

9.  Hauck FR, Herman SM, Donovan M, Iyasu S, Merrick Moore C, Donoghue E, et al. Sleep environment and the risk of sudden infant death syndrome in an urban population: The Chicago Infant Mortality Study. Pediatrics. 2003;111(5 Pt 2):1207-14.

10. Li DK, Petitti DB, Willinger M, McMahon R, Odouli R, Vu H, et al. Infant sleeping position and the risk of sudden infant death syndrome in California, 1997-2000. Am J Epidemiol. 2003;157(5):446-55. https://doi.org/10.1093/aje/kwf226.

11. Fleming PJ, Blair PS, Bacon C, Bensley D, Smith I, Taylor E, et al. Environment of infants during sleep and risk of the sudden infant death syndrome: Results of 1993-5 case-control study for confidential inquiry into stillbirths and deaths in infancy. BMJ. 1996;313(7051):191-5. https://doi.org/10.1136/bmj.313.7051.191.

12. Kanetake J, Aoki Y, Funayama M. Evaluation of rebreathing potential on bedding for infant use. Pediatr Int. 2003;45(3):284-9. https://doi.org/10.1046/j.1442-200X.2003.01708.x.

13. Kemp JS, Livne M, White DK, Arfken CL. Softness and potential to cause rebreathing: Differences in bedding used by infants at high and low risk for sudden infant death syndrome. J Pediatr. 1998;132:234-9. https://doi.org/10.1016/S0022-3476(98)70437-8.

14. Patel AL, Harris K, Thach BT. Inspired $CO_2$ and $O_2$ in sleeping infants rebreathing from bedding: Relevance for sudden infant death syndrome. J Appl Physiol. 2001;91:2537-45.

15. Tuffnell CS, Petersen SA, Wailoo MP. Prone sleeping infants have a reduced ability to lose heat. Early Hum Dev. 1995;43(2):109-16. https://doi.org/10.1016/0378-3782(95)01659-7.

16. Wong FY, Witcombe NB, Yiallourou SR, Yorkston S, Dymowski AR, Krishnan L, et al. Cerebral oxygenation is depressed during sleep in healthy term infants when they sleep prone. Pediatrics. 2011;127(3):e558-65. https://doi.org/10.1542/peds.2010-2724.

17. Yiallourou SR, Walker AM, Horne RS. Prone sleeping impairs circulatory control during sleep in healthy term infants: Implications for SIDS. Sleep. 2008;31(8):1139-46.

18. Horne RS, Ferens D, Watts AM, Vitkovic J, Lacey B, Andrew S, et al. The prone sleeping position impairs arousability in term infants. J Pediatr. 2001;138(6):811-16. https://doi.org/10.1067/mpd.2001.114475.

19. Mitchell EA, Thach BT, Thompson JMD, Williams S. Changing infants' sleep position increases risk of sudden infant death syndrome. Arch Pediatr Adolesc Med. 1999;153:1136-41. https://doi.org/10.1001/archpedi.153.11.1136.

20. Anderson HR, Cook DG. Passive smoking and sudden infant death syndrome: Review of the epidemiological evidence. Thorax. 1997;52(11):1003-9. https://doi.org/10.1136/thx.52.11.1003.

21. Blair PS, Fleming PJ, Bensley D, Smith I, Bacon C, Taylor E, et al. Smoking and the sudden infant death syndrome: Results from 1993-5 case-control study for confidential inquiry into stillbirths and deaths in infancy. BMJ. 1996;313:195-8. https://doi.org/10.1136/bmj.313.7051.195.

22. Haglund B. Cigarette smoking and sudden infant death syndrome: Some salient points in the debate. Acta Paediatr Suppl. 1993;82 Suppl 389:37-9. https://doi.org/10.1111/j.1651-2227.1993.tb12872.x.

23. Mitchell EA, Ford RP, Stewart AW, Taylor BJ, Becroft DM, Thompson JM, et al. Smoking and the sudden infant death syndrome. Pediatrics. 1993;91(5):893-6.

24. Klonoff-Cohen HS, Edelstein SL, Lefkowitz ES, Srinivassan IP, Kaegi D, Chang JC, et al. The effect of passive smoking and tobacco exposure through breast milk on sudden infant death syndrome. JAMA. 1995;273(10):795-8. https://doi.org/10.1001/jama.1995.03520340051035.

25. MacDorman MF, Cnattingius S, Hoffman HJ, Kramer MS, Haglund B. Sudden infant death syndrome and smoking in the United States and Sweden. Am J Epidemiol. 1997;146(3):249-57. https://doi.org/10.1093/oxfordjournals.aje.a009260.

26. Schoendorf KC, Kiely JL. Relationship of sudden infant death syndrome to maternal smoking during and after pregnancy. Pediatrics. 1992;90(6):905-8.

27. Haglund B, Cnattingius S. Cigarette smoking as a risk factor for sudden infant death syndrome: A population-based study. Am J Public Health. 1990;80(1):29-32. https://doi.org/10.2105/AJPH.80.1.29.

28. Liebrechts-Akkerman G, Lao O, Liu F, van Sleuwen BE, Engelberts AC, L'Hoir MP, et al. Postnatal parental smoking: An important risk factor for SIDS. Eur J Pediatr. 2011;170(10):1281-91. https://doi.org/10.1007/s00431-011-1433-6.

29. Fifer WP, Fingers ST, Youngman M, Gomez-Gribben E, Myers MM. Effects of alcohol and smoking during pregnancy on infant autonomic control. Dev Psychobiol. 2009;51(3):234-42. https://doi.org/10.1002/dev.20366.

30. Richardson HL, Walker AM, Horne RS. Maternal smoking impairs arousal patterns in sleeping infants. Sleep. 2009;32(4):515-21. https://doi.org/10.1093/sleep/32.4.515.

31. Mitchell EA, Milerad J. Smoking and the sudden infant death syndrome. Rev Environ Health. 2006;21(2):81-103. https://doi.org/10.1515/REVEH.2006.21.2.81.

32. Dietz PM, England LJ, Shapiro-Mendoza CK, Tong VT, Farr SL, Callaghan WM. Infant morbidity and mortality attributable to prenatal smoking in the US. Am J Prev Med. 2010;39(1):45-52. https://doi.org/10.1016/j.amepre.2010.03.009.

33. Iyasu S, Randall LL, Welty TK, Hsia J, Kinney HC, Mandell F, et al. Risk factors for sudden infant death syndrome among northern plains Indians. JAMA. 2002;288(21):2717-23. https://doi.org/10.1001/jama.288.21.2717.

34. O'Leary CM, Jacoby PJ, Bartu A, D'Antoine H, Bower C. Maternal alcohol use and sudden infant death syndrome and infant mortality excluding SIDS. Pediatrics. 2013;131(3):e770-8. https://doi.org/10.1542/peds.2012-1907.

35. L'Hoir MP, Engelberts AC, van Well GTJ, Westers P, Mellenbergh GJ, Wolters WHG, et al. Case-control study of current validity of previously described risk factors for SIDS in the Netherlands. Arch Dis Child. 1998;79:386-93. https://doi.org/10.1136/adc.79.5.386.

36. Durand DJ, Espinoza AM, Nickerson BG. Association between prenatal cocaine exposure and sudden infant death syndrome. J Pediatr. 1990;117(6):909-11. https://doi.org/10.1016/S0022-3476(05)80133-7.

37. Kandall SR, Gaines J, Habel L, Davidson G, Jessop D. Relationship of maternal substance abuse to subsequent sudden infant death syndrome in offspring. J Pediatr. 1993;123(1):120-6. https://doi.org/10.1016/S0022-3476(05)81554-9.

38. Ward SL, Bautista D, Chan L, Derry M, Lisbin A, Durfee MJ, et al. Sudden infant death syndrome in infants of substance-abusing mothers. J Pediatr. 1990;117(6):876-81. https://doi.org/10.1016/S0022-3476(05)80125-8.

39. Carpenter RG, Irgens LM, Blair PS, England PD, Fleming PJ, Huber J, et al. Sudden unexplained infant death in 20 regions in Europe: Case control study. Lancet. 2004;363:185-91. https://doi.org/10.1016/S0140-6736(03)15323-8.

40. Vennemann MM, Hense HW, Bajanowski T, Blair PS, Complojer C, Moon RY, et al. Bed sharing and the risk of sudden infant death syndrome: Can we resolve the debate? J Pediatr. 2012;160(1):44-8 e2.

41. Tappin D, Ecob R, Brooke H. Bedsharing, roomsharing, and sudden infant death syndrome in Scotland: A case control study. J Pediatr. 2005;147(1):32-7. https://doi.org/10.1016/j.jpeds.2005.01.035.

42. Blair PS, Fleming PJ, Smith IJ, Platt MW, Young J, Nadin P, et al. Babies sleeping with parents: Case-control study of factors influencing the risk of the sudden infant death syndrome. CESDI SUDI research group. BMJ. 1999;319(7223):1457-62. https://doi.org/10.1136/bmj.319.7223.1457.

43. Blair PS, Sidebotham P, Pease A, Fleming PJ. Bed-sharing in the absence of hazardous circumstances: Is there a risk of sudden infant death syndrome? An analysis from two case-control studies conducted in the UK. PLoS One. 2014;9(9):e107799. https://doi.org/10.1371/journal.pone.0107799.

44. Rechtman LR, Colvin JD, Blair PS, Moon RY. Sofas and infant mortality. Pediatrics. 2014;134(5):e1293-300. https://doi.org/10.1542/peds.2014-1543.

45. Orenstein SR, Whitington PF, Orenstein DM. The infant seat as treatment for gastroesophageal reflux. N Engl J Med. 1983;309(13):760-3. https://doi.org/10.1056/NEJM198309293091304.

46. Batra EK, Midgett JD, Moon RY. Hazards associated with sitting and carrying devices for children two years and younger. J Pediatr. 2015;167(1):183-7. https://doi.org/10.1016/j.jpeds.2015.03.044.

47. Bergounioux J, Madre C, Crucis-Armengaud A, Briand-Huchet E, Michard-Lenoir AP, Patural H, et al. Sudden deaths in adult-worn baby carriers: 19 cases. Eur J Pediatr. 2015;174(12):1665-70. https://doi.org/10.1007/s00431-015-2593-6.

48. Blair PS, Heron J, Fleming PJ. Relationship between bed sharing and breastfeeding: Longitudinal, population-based analysis. Pediatrics. 2010;126(5):e1119-26. https://doi.org/10.1542/peds.2010-1277.

49. Huang Y, Hauck FR, Signore C, Yu A, Raju TN, Huang TT, et al. Influence of bedsharing activity on breastfeeding duration among US mothers. JAMA Pediatr. 2013;167(11):1038-44. https://doi.org/10.1001/jamapediatrics.2013.2632.

50. Hauck FR, Thompson J, Tanabe KO, Moon RY, Vennemann M. Breastfeeding and reduced risk of sudden infant death syndrome: A meta-analysis. Pediatrics. 2011;128(1):103-10. https://doi.org/10.1542/peds.2010-3000.

51. Colvin JD, Collie-Akers V, Schunn C, Moon RY. Sleep environment risks for younger and older infants. Pediatrics. 2014;134(2):e406-12. https://doi.org/10.1542/peds.2014-0401.

52. Carpenter R, McGarvey C, Mitchell EA, Tappin DM, Vennemann MM, Smuk M, et al. Bed sharing when parents do not smoke: is there a risk of SIDS? An individual level analysis of five major case-control studies. BMJ Open. 2013;3(5):e002299. https://doi.org/10.1136/bmjopen-2012-002299.

53. Blair PS, Sidebotham P, Evason-Coombe C, Edmonds M, Heckstall-Smith EM, Fleming P. Hazardous cosleeping environments and risk factors amenable to change: Case-control study of SIDS in south west England. BMJ. 2009;339:b3666. https://doi.org/10.1136/bmj.b3666.

54. Moon RY, & Task Force on Sudden Infant Death Syndrome. SIDS and other sleep-related infant deaths: Evidence base for 2016 updated recommendations for a safe infant sleeping environment. Pediatrics. 2016;138(5):e20162940. https://doi.org/10.1542/peds.2016-2940.

55. Moon RY, & Task Force on Sudden Infant Death Syndrome. SIDS and other sleep-related infant deaths: Updated 2016 recommendations for a safe infant sleeping environment. Pediatrics. 2016;138(5):e20162938. https://doi.org/10.1542/peds.2016-2940.

56. The Lullaby Trust. Sudden infant death syndrome: A guide for professionals. London, England: The Lullaby Trust, 2013.

57. Red Nose National Scientific Advisory Group (NSAG). Information statement: Sleeping with a baby. [Available from: https://rednose.com.au/article/sharing-a-sleepsurface-with-a-baby]. Accessed 5 October 2017.

58. Chowdhury RT. Nursery product-related injuries and deaths among children under age five. Washington, DC: U.S. Consumer Product Safety Commission, 2014.

59. Mitchell EA, Blair PS. SIDS prevention: 3000 lives saved but we can do better. NZ Med J. 2012;125(1359):50-7.

60. L'Hoir MP, Engelberts AC, van Well GTJ, McClelland S, Westers P, Dandachli T, et al. Risk and preventive factors for cot death in The Netherlands, a low-incidence country. Eur J Pediatr. 1998;157:681-8. https://doi.org/10.1007/s004310050911.

61. Thach BT, Rutherford GW, Harris K. Deaths and injuries attributed to infant crib bumper pads. J Pediatr. 2007;151:271-4. https://doi.org/10.1016/j.jpeds.2007.04.028.

62. Scheers NJ, Woodard DW, Thach BT. Crib bumpers continue to cause infant deaths: A need for a new preventive approach. J Pediatr. 2016;169:93-7 e1. https://doi.org/10.1016/j.jpeds.2015.10.050.

63. Blair PS, Mitchell EA, Heckstall-Smith EM, Fleming PJ. Head covering — A major modifiable risk factor for sudden infant death syndrome: A systematic review. Arch Dis Child. 2008;93(9):778-83. https://doi.org/10.1136/adc.2007.136366.

64. Malloy MH, Hoffman HJ. Prematurity, sudden infant death syndrome, and age of death. Pediatrics. 1995;96(3 Pt 1):464-71.

65. Sowter B, Doyle LW, Morley CJ, Altmann A, Halliday J. Is sudden infant death syndrome still more common in very low birthweight infants in the 1990s? Med J Aust. 1999;171(8):411-13.

66. Malloy MH. Prematurity and sudden infant death syndrome: United States 2005-2007. J Perinatol. 2013;33(6):470-5. https://doi.org/10.1038/jp.2012.158.

67. Ramanathan R, Corwin MJ, Hunt CE, Lister G, Tinsley LR, Baird T, et al. Cardiorespiratory events recorded on home monitors: Comparison of healthy infants with those at increased risk for SIDS. JAMA. 2001;285(17):2199-207. https://doi.org/10.1001/jama.285.17.2199.

68. Oyen N, Markestad T, Skjaerven R, Irgens LM, Helweg-Larsen K, Alm B, et al. Combined effects of sleeping position and prenatal risk factors in sudden infant death syndrome: The Nordic epidemiological SIDS study. Pediatrics. 1997;100(4):613-21. https://doi.org/10.1542/peds.100.4.613.

69. Gillies D, Wells D, Bhandari AP. Positioning for acute respiratory distress in hospitalised infants and children. Cochrane Database Syst Rev. 2012;7:CD003645. https://doi.org/10.1002/14651858.CD003645.pub3.

70. Thompson JMD, Tanabe K, Moon RY, Mitchell EA, McGarvey C, Carpenter R, et al. A pooled analysis of breastfeeding and sudden infant death syndrome: How much is enough to reduce the risk? Under review.

71. Alm B, Wennergren G, Mollborg P, Lagercrantz H. Breastfeeding and dummy use have a protective effect on sudden infant death syndrome. Acta Paediatr. 2016;105(1):31-8. https://doi.org/10.1111/apa.13124.

72. Hauck FR, Omojokun OO, Siadaty MS. Do pacifiers reduce the risk of sudden infant death syndrome? A meta-analysis. Pediatrics. 2005;116(5):e716-e23. https://doi.org/10.1542/peds.2004-2631.

73. Li DK, Willinger M, Petitti DB, Odouli R, Liu L, Hoffman HJ. Use of a dummy (pacifier) during sleep and risk of sudden infant death syndrome (SIDS): Population based case-control study. BMJ. 2006;332(7532):18-22. https://doi.org/10.1136/bmj.38671.640475.55.

74. Yiallourou SR, Poole H, Prathivadi P, Odoi A, Wong FY, Horne RS. The effects of dummy/pacifier use on infant blood pressure and autonomic activity during sleep. Sleep Med. 2014;15(12):1508-16. https://doi.org/10.1016/j.sleep.2014.07.011.

75. Tonkin SL, Vogel SA, Gunn AJ. Upper airway size while sucking on a pacifier in an infant with micrognathia. J Paediatr Child Health. 2008;44(1-2):78-9. https://doi.org/10.1111/j.1440-1754.2007.01259.x.

76. Franco P, Scaillet S, Wermenbol V, Valente F, Groswasser J, Kahn A. The influence of a pacifier on infants' arousals from sleep. J Pediatr. 2000;136(6):775-9.

77. Weiss P, Kerbl R. The relatively short duration that a child retains a pacifier in the mouth during sleep: Implications for sudden infant death syndrome. Eur J Pediatr. 2001;160:60-70. https://doi.org/10.1007/s004310000638.

78. Scragg RKR, Mitchell EA, Stewart AW, Ford RPK, Taylor BJ, Hassall IB, et al. Infant room-sharing and prone sleep position in sudden infant death syndrome. Lancet. 1996;347:7-12. https://doi.org/10.1016/S0140-6736(96)91554-8.

79. Mitchell EA, Thompson JMD. Co-sleeping increases the risk of SIDS, but sleeping in the parents' bedroom lowers it. In: Sudden infant death syndrome: New trends in the nineties. Ed Rognum TO. Oslo, Norway: Scandinavian University Press, 1995. p. 266-9.

80. Blair PS, Platt MW, Smith IJ, Fleming PJ. Sudden infant death syndrome and the time of death: Factors associated with night-time and day-time deaths. Int J Epidemiol. 2006;35(6):1563-9. https://doi.org/10.1093/ije/dyl212.

81. Mitchell EA. Risk factors for SIDS. BMJ. 2009;339:b3466. https://doi.org/10.1136/bmj.b3466.

82. Vennemann MM, Bajanowski T, Brinkmann B, Jorch G, Sauerland C, Mitchell EA. Sleep environment risk factors for sudden infant death syndrome: The German sudden infant death syndrome study. Pediatrics. 2009;123(4):1162-70. https://doi.org/10.1542/peds.2008-0505.

83. Blair P, Fleming P, Bensley D, Smith I, Bacon C, Taylor E. Plastic mattresses and sudden infant death syndrome. Lancet. 1995;345(8951):720. https://doi.org/10.1016/S0140-6736(95)90891-9.

84. Wilson CA, Taylor BJ, Laing RM, Williams SM, Mitchell EA. Clothing and bedding and its relevance to sudden infant death syndrome: Further results from the New Zealand Cot Death Study. J Paediatr Child Health. 1994;30(6):506-12. https://doi.org/10.1111/j.1440-1754.1994.tb00722.x.

85. Kemp Js, Thach BT. Sudden death in infants sleeping on polystyrene-filled cushions. N Engl J Med. 1991;324:1858-64. https://doi.org/10.1056/NEJM199106273242605.

86. Kinney HC, Thach BT. The sudden infant death syndrome. N Engl J Med. 2009;361(8):795-805. https://doi.org/10.1056/NEJMra0803836.

87. Filiano JJ, Kinney HC. A perspective on neuropathologic findings in victims of the sudden infant death syndrome: The triple-risk model. Biol Neonate. 1994;65:194-7. https://doi.org/10.1159/000244052.

88. Moon RY, Fu LY. Sudden infant death syndrome. Pediatr Rev. 2007;28(6):209-14. https://doi.org/10.1542/pir.28-6-209.

89. Harper RM, Kinney HC, Fleming PJ, Thach BT. Sleep influences on homeostatic functions: Implications for sudden infant death syndrome. Respir Physiol. 2000;119(2-3):123-32. https://doi.org/10.1016/S0034-5687(99)00107-3.

90. Horne RS, Witcombe NB, Yiallourou SR, Scaillet S, Thiriez G, Franco P. Cardiovascular control during sleep in infants: Implications for sudden infant death syndrome. Sleep Med. 2010;11(7):615-21. https://doi.org/10.1016/j.sleep.2009.10.008.

91. Franco P, Kato I, Richardson HL, Yang JS, Montemitro E, Horne RS. Arousal from sleep mechanisms in infants. Sleep Med. 2010;11(7):603-14. https://doi.org/10.1016/j.sleep.2009.12.014.

# 11 Shared Sleeping Surfaces and Dangerous Sleeping Environments

Jeanine Young, BSc(Hons), PhD and
Rebecca Shipstone, BSocSci

*School of Nursing, Midwifery, and Paramedicine,*
*University of the Sunshine Coast, Queensland, Australia*

## Introduction

Whether, and in what circumstances, the risk of sudden unexpected death in infancy (SUDI) is increased when an infant shares a sleep surface with another person has been the subject of extensive and vexed debate over the past two decades (1-6). This is largely because of opposing views as to the potential benefits and risks associated with this practice. Researchers remain divided on their stance towards shared sleeping and SUDI. While the United States American Academy of Pediatrics has strongly recommended against sharing a sleep surface with an infant for many years (7-9), a number of researchers in the United Kingdom and Australia question labeling a common sleeping practice a "risk factor" to be advised against. Instead the circumstances, rather than the shared sleeping itself, are recognized as the potential risk (3, 10-12). Whatever one's personal standpoint, from a clinical perspective, parents are entitled to clear information about the risks and benefits of shared sleeping to enable them to make a well-informed decision concerning the infant care practices they adopt. Health professionals, in both hospital and community settings, play a pivotal role in ensuring that parents are provided with this information, ideally in a non-judgemental manner that is relevant to their specific circumstances.

This chapter commences by defining the important terms used throughout. Second, it examines the prevalence of shared sleeping in both Western and non-Western countries and cultures. Third, it reviews the evidence base concerning the benefits and the risks of sharing a sleep surface with an infant. Fourth, the use of a risk-minimization, as opposed to a risk-elimination, approach in the provision of safe sleeping advice and education is discussed. Finally, the recent move towards devices designed to overcome the risk associated with "direct" shared sleeping, while still maintaining the close mother-infant proximity needed to facilitate breastfeeding, is discussed.

## Definitions

Various terms have been used in the literature to define environments in which an infant sleeps in close proximity to a caregiver, including co-sleeping, bed sharing, and room sharing.

**Co-sleeping** is most commonly defined as a mother and/or her partner (or any other person) being asleep on the same sleep surface as an infant (13-15). However, it was used originally and more broadly to include both room-sharing and bed-sharing practices (7, 9, 12, 16). Variation in definitions frequently creates confusion, particularly since there is evidence that room sharing decreases the risk of SUDI by as much as 50% (7, 17-20), and that it is safer than both sharing a sleep surface (17, 18, 21) and solitary sleeping (when an infant is in a separate room) (18, 20-23).

Bed sharing is frequently used synonymously with co-sleeping (1, 11, 24) to refer to an infant sleeping on the same surface as another person. It has also been defined as bringing an infant onto a surface where sleep is possible, whether intended or not (13, 15, 25). This definition of bed sharing includes instances where the caregiver is awake. The latter, more inclusive definition can be problematic. While there is evidence that sleeping on the same surface as an infant may increase the risk of SUDI under particular conditions (2, 26, 27), there is no evidence that bringing an infant into bed for a short time for feeding or comfort while the caregiver is awake poses any risk (28, 29). In fact, this practice (which would meet the broader definition of bed sharing) is encouraged in postnatal environments which promote skin-to-skin contact as part of Baby Friendly Health Initiatives to support breastfeeding initiation and duration (30, 31).

For clarity, in this chapter the terms *sharing a sleep surface* and *shared sleeping* will generally be used in preference to the terms bed sharing and co-sleeping, which will be taken to be synonymous.

**Room sharing** is defined as the practice of sleeping an infant in their own safe sleeping place in the same room as an adult caregiver. There is consensus among researchers that room sharing between committed caregivers and an infant is protective against SUDI (17, 18, 32) and should be encouraged.

The use of the above defined terminology allows for differentiation of the risks associated with solitary sleeping, room sharing, and environments in which baby and caregiver share the same sleep surface, without creating unnecessary terminological confusion.

## Prevalence of Shared Sleeping

Sharing a sleep surface with an infant is a normal and often valued part of infant care in many different cultures. Anthropologists consider it highly probable that infants slept near or on their mother's body to be fed and nurtured over the course of human evolution, in order to maximize the chances of infant survival and flourishing (33). Today, in most non-Western cultures, mother-infant contact during sleeping remains the norm (34, 35), and it is also commonly practiced in Western societies (36-38).

Shared sleep behavior has been surveyed in many Western countries, including the United States, the United Kingdom, New Zealand, and Australia (9, 36, 39-48), with some studies reporting that the prevalence of shared sleeping has increased over the past two decades (32, 49). In the United States, a large national infant care practice study found that the prevalence of shared sleeping nearly doubled between 1993 and 2010. For the 2001-10 period, 46% of parents reported sharing a sleep surface with their infant (aged less than 9 months) at some point in the previous fortnight, while 13.5% reported *usually* sleeping with their infant (39). In another national survey, 42% of mothers reported *any* shared sleeping at 2 weeks of age (40). A third recent study found that almost 60% of mothers reported sharing a sleep surface with their infant at least once (41).

In England, local and national studies show that almost half of all neonates shared a sleep surface with their parents at least once, for all or part of the night (local = 47%, national = 46%), and a fifth of babies slept in the parental bed on a regular basis over the first year of life (42). Similar or higher rates of surface sharing at 3 months of age have been previously reported in other European countries, including Ireland (21%), Germany (23%), Italy (24%), Scotland (25%), Austria (30%), Denmark (39%), and Sweden (65%) (37, 43).

Reports in Australia indicate a population prevalence of sharing a sleep surface of 40-80%, depending on infant age at the time of measurement (45-47, 50, 51). A small study conducted in South Australia demonstrated that 80% of young babies spent some time sharing a sleep surface for at least part of the night (47). A larger Queensland infant care practice study (n=2,534) demonstrated that shared sleeping was common, being the usual practice of 46% of parents when their infants were 3 months of age. Although most infants (51%) were brought into bed for short periods of between one and three hours, almost a third (31%) shared a sleep surface for six hours or more per night (45, 46). More recently a Victorian study surveying 1,126 respondent mothers attending the Maternal and Child Health Service for their infant's eight-week visit found that 44.7% of participants (n=503) had shared a sleep surface with their infant on at least one occasion since birth (52). Studies of shared sleeping incidence in Western countries, in which sharing a sleep surface is discouraged, may underrepresent the prevalence. Ball and colleagues (53) found that 40% of parents reported where they "intended" their infant to sleep (i.e. a cot), even if the infant had slept in a combination of cot and parental bed.

Recent studies in non-Western countries generally document a greater prevalence of shared sleep arrangements, including Brazil (48%) (54), Thailand (68%) (44), and Malaysia (74%) (55). There are also ethnic and cultural differences within the culturally diverse societies of Western countries, with shared sleeping common among specific subgroups (36). These include breastfeeding mother-infant dyads (36, 47, 56, 57), recent immigrant populations from non-Caucasian countries (36), and indigenous populations (9, 48, 50, 58-60). Shared sleeping is a well-documented characteristic of infant care culture among Māori families in New Zealand (48, 61), with 65% of Māori mothers sharing a sleep surface with their babies for part or all of the night (58). Sharing the same sleep surface is also the usual, often valued, and accepted way for Australian Aboriginal infants and their parents to sleep (62). Studies have found that 68-77% of Aboriginal babies share a sleep surface, with the incidence higher in regional than in metropolitan localities (50, 60). However, as researchers such as Ball and Volpe (36) and Blair (63) observe, since the advantages and risks of shared sleeping are perceived in accordance with the dominant values of any given society, the validity of these subpopulations' cultural and behavioral differences is rarely recognized in public health safe infant sleep information.

It is clear that shared sleeping prevalence differs according to country and culture, as well as by age at measurement, frequency, and duration. Also differing among countries, communities, and cultures are the demographics of mothers who share a sleep surface, as well as the impact of the shared-sleep environment on the infant. In the United States, shared sleeping is reported to occur more frequently among young, single, poorly educated mothers living in disadvantaged circumstances (36, 64, 65). Conversely, in England, shared sleeping straddles all social classes (37, 42), as it does in Sweden and numerous non-Western cultures, where it is simply perceived as a normal family activity (66). While both the prevalence of shared sleeping and the incidence of SUDI is high in certain cultures, including black (United States), Māori, and Aboriginal populations, other culturally distinct groups such as South Asian families in the United Kingdom (predominantly Bangladeshi and Pakistani) (36, 67-69), Pacific Islanders in New Zealand (70), and Southern Europeans (71), and Thais in Australia (72) have a similarly high incidence of shared sleeping, without a correspondingly higher rate of SUDI. This gives weight to the argument that it is not the shared-sleep environment per se that carries the risk, but the circumstances in which the surface sharing occurs, particularly the presence of other known risk factors for SUDI. These have been shown to be low in those populations with high shared-sleep prevalence but low SUDI incidence (37, 68).

# Benefits of Shared Sleeping

Anthropological studies of parent-infant shared sleeping have found sleeping with an infant to be associated with improved settling with reduced crying (73), improved maternal and infant sleep and increased arousals (25, 52, 73-75), increased duration of breastfeeding (38, 39, 76, 77), and reduced formula supplementation (78).

Support for the beneficial effects of shared-sleep environments is also provided in studies of the physiology of mother infant-contact (34, 37). Studies of skin-to-skin contact (kangaroo care) among preterm and newborn infants have documented the benefits of continuous infant-mother contact, including improved cardiorespiratory stability, oxygenation, and thermoregulation (79-81); longer periods of infant sleep and more restful sleep (80, 82, 83); reduced crying (81); and enhanced milk production along with more successful, frequent, and longer duration of breastfeeding (12, 84, 85).

Enhanced maternal-infant bonding, attachment, and maternal responsiveness, particularly when shared sleeping is combined with breastfeeding, have also been associated with shared sleeping in numerous studies (34, 38, 52, 53, 73, 79, 86-92). These studies predominantly measure maternal bonding by mothers' perceptions of and/or reasons for bed sharing, and by observations of mother-infant interaction during breastfeeding. Mitchell and colleagues' (93) recent study of shared sleeping and maternal bonding is the first study to attempt to directly test the association between maternal bonding and shared sleeping, using the Postpartum Bonding Questionnaire (PBQ) (94). An inverse relationship between bonding and shared sleeping was reported. However, this study did not control for either maternal depression or postpartum traumatic stress disorder. These conditions have repeatedly been shown to be associated with high scores on the PBQ, and this was acknowledged as a limitation of the research. Mitchell et al. (93) also did not differentiate between planned and reactive shared sleeping. Mileva-Seitz and colleagues (95) contend that the difference between reactive and intentional shared sleeping is crucial for the interpretation of findings. A recent Australian study found that mothers who planned to sleep with their baby viewed their shared sleeping as beneficial for baby, mother, and family, whereas mothers who did not plan to surface share (reactive bed sharers) reported that they did so predominantly out of a desperate need for sleep (52). Ramos and colleagues (96) have also previously shown that intentional shared-sleeping parents are more likely to endorse and be satisfied with shared sleep. Given the study's finding (93) that shared-sleeping mothers scored more highly on items relating to feelings of anger, irritation, and annoyance towards their infant, differentiating between these groups seems prima facie an important consideration.

Closely related, a study of child attachment security recently found a pattern of greater secure attachment in bed-sharing infants; it also found that infants who had never bed shared at 2 months had greater odds of developing resistant attachment at 14 months (colloquially, becoming a "clingy" child reluctant to separate from their mother) (87). Some caution in interpreting these results should be noted, however, due the absence of a dose response — the "some bed sharing" group demonstrated more secure attachment than the most frequently bed-sharing children. Again, the consideration for maternal and family rationales for bed sharing is important in the interpretation of results.

Another benefit of shared sleep is the long-term positive effect it has into adulthood. Longitudinal studies have suggested that those who shared the parental bed as infants and children become adults with higher self-esteem, and better social skills and emotional outcomes (38, 97, 98).

## Breastfeeding and shared sleeping

Breastfeeding is universally recognized as the optimal way to feed infants, due to the numerous health benefits for both infants and their mothers (99). In Australia, breastfeeding initiation rates are high (96%), although only 39% of infants exclusively breastfeed to 3 months of age, with the figure falling to 15% by around 6 months (100). Breastfeeding and sharing a sleep surface constitute an integrated care system which is mutually reinforcing; breastfeeding promotes shared sleep, which increases breastfeeding frequency and extends duration of breastfeeding by months (5, 38, 39, 77). Sustained skin-to-skin contact between mother and infant in the first 24 hours post-birth is critical to establishing optimal breastfeeding (35, 101, 102). There is also a strong association between breastfeeding and infant sleep patterns, with breastfed infants exhibiting night waking behavior that is necessary both for nourishment and for ongoing stimulation of breastmilk production in the mother (33, 103).

Population-based analysis has confirmed that shared sleeping patterns significantly affect breastfeeding up to, and beyond, the age of 12 months (39, 54, 57). In studies of infant sleep and feeding method, the most common reason given by mothers for sharing a sleep surface was convenience of night-time breastfeeding (34, 56, 59, 88-92, 104). Mothers who were committed to breastfeeding used shared sleeping to accommodate the fragmentary nature of infant sleep and ameliorate frequent night-time feeds (34, 90, 92, 104), often commenting that when bed sharing they barely needed to awaken in order to latch the infant on the breast (34, 56, 88, 89, 92, 104, 105).

Breastfeeding is also important to the way in which shared sleeping occurs. Several studies on mother-infant sleep behavior have documented that mothers and infants who routinely bed share and breastfeed sleep near to, and facing, each other, and experience a high degree of arousal overlap (waking at the same time) (12). Specifically, a video study of mothers in their home environment (106) showed that breastfeeding mothers sleep in a lateral position facing their infant and curled around them. The infant is flat on the mattress, below pillow height, level with their mother's breasts, and sleep in the space created by the mother's arm. The mother's arm is positioned above her infant's head and her knees are drawn up under her infant's feet. These results suggest that a breastfeeding, bed-sharing mother's characteristic sleep position "represents an instinctive behavior on the part of a breastfeeding mother to protect her infant during sleep" (107) (p. 25). This contrasts with formula-feeding mothers who did not adopt the "protective" position. Rather, formula-feeding mothers placed their infants high in the bed, either on or between pillows, and frequently turned their backs on their infants while sleeping (73, 106). Given the well-recognized importance of close contact in establishing breastfeeding, and the need for frequent sucking, anthropologists and infant physiologists consider that mother-infant sleep contact in the form of shared sleeping is a normal, species-typical parenting behavior for humans (12, 107, 108). A positive link has been identified between breastfeeding and both shared sleeping and room-sharing practices in early life to the appropriate early regulation of the hypothalamic-pituitary-adrenal axis (HPA-axis), or the ability to respond and adapt to stressors (109, 110). Regulation of this stress response is an important factor for psychological health (111).

Since breastfeeding is protective against SUDI (112-114) and confers significant health benefits for both infants and mothers (115, 116), while both not-breastfeeding (20, 117) and solitary sleep in a separate room (21, 23, 32, 118) are well-established, independent risk factors, it is desirable to encourage and support exclusive breastfeeding. Shared sleeping is an infant care practice significantly associated with breastfeeding longevity. Indeed, McKenna and Gettler (35) most recently proposed that in order to resolve the bed-sharing debate, the term "breastsleeping" be used to acknowledge that the breastfeeding shared-sleeping mother-infant dyad "exhibits such vastly different behavioral and physiological characteristics compared with the bottle/formula feeding bed-sharing dyad, it must be distinguished and given its own epidemiological category" (p. 21).

## Risks Associated with Shared Sleeping

Despite the above described benefits, under some circumstances sharing a sleep surface with an infant is strongly associated with SUDI.

Numerous studies have reported a very significantly increased risk of infant death when infants slept with parents who smoke, with odds ratios (OR) generally ranging between 3.9 and 17.7 (11, 18, 21, 24, 27, 28, 70, 119-122). Carpenter's (18) large case-control study in 20 European regions found the risk of surface sharing was 10-fold greater amongst mothers who smoked. For mothers who did not smoke during pregnancy, the risk associated with shared-sleep environments was very small (OR at 10 weeks 1.56 [95% CI: 0.91-2.68], and only significant during the first eight weeks of life (OR at 2 weeks 2.4 [95% CI: 1.2-4.6]). Vennemann and colleagues' (27) meta-analysis of 11 published studies on the relationship between shared sleeping and SUDI showed a significant risk for smoking mothers (OR 6.27 [95% CI: 3.94-9.99]). The three papers included in this analysis that reported the risk of shared sleeping among non-smoking parents found the risk to be only slightly, and not significantly, increased

(OR 1.66 [95% CI: 0.91-3.01]). More recently, Blair, Sidebotham, Pease, and Fleming's (24) pooled data from two previous case-control investigations in the United Kingdom found that for infants who slept next to a parent who smoked (but had not consumed alcohol), the risk was four times greater than for those who did not share a sleep surface. A dose-response effect has also been reported when bed sharing, related to whether only the partner smokes, only the mother smokes, or both parents smoke (119).

A more pronounced effect of smoking and shared sleep among younger age groups has been reported in at least two studies (18, 119). In 2004, Carpenter and colleagues (18) demonstrated an interaction with age such that if the mother smoked significant risks were associated with shared sleeping in the first weeks of life (OR at 2 weeks 27.0 [95% CI: 13.3-54.9]). More recently, Carpenter et al. (119) reported that infants who share a sleep surface at 2 weeks of age and whose parents both smoke are at a 65-fold risk of sudden infant death syndrome (SIDS), compared with infants who room shared with non-smoking parents.

There is also evidence of a highly significant interaction between sharing a sleep surface and parental use of alcohol, drugs, or other sedating medication, over and above the risk associated with smoking (11, 21, 119, 121-123). Blair and colleagues (11) report a multivariable odds ratio of 53.26 [95% CI: 4.07-696.96] among SIDS compared to random control infants. When SIDS infants were compared to high-risk controls with similar sociodemographic characteristics the risk, while remaining significant, lowered considerably (OR 11.76 [95% CI: 1.40-99.83]). Subsequent pooled data analyses by the authors have reported a multivariable risk that was 18 times greater when sharing a sleep surface with an adult who had consumed more than two units of alcohol. In Australia, a retrospective case series study examining sleep-related infant deaths from 2008 to 2010 found that alcohol or drug use was present in 70% of infant deaths involving surface sharing (124). As with smoking, the interaction between substances and shared sleep was found to be more pronounced in the younger age groups (aOR at 2 weeks 89.7 [95% CI: 25.3-317.7]) (119).

More generally, studies have documented a risk associated with shared sleeping with younger infants (18, 21, 29, 32, 125) and for infants who were preterm or low birth weight (18, 119, 121). The risk among young infants has been shown to persist even among non-smoking parents (18, 21, 27, 32). Vennemann and colleagues (27) found that the risk of SUDI while bed sharing was 10 times higher among infants aged less than 3 months. Blair et al. (24) and Carpenter et al. (119) both report a fivefold increased risk for infants aged less than 3 months.

Sharing a sofa is also associated with a very high risk of SUDI. A recent meta-analysis (123) found a 23-fold pooled risk for sofa sharing, which is almost eight times the pooled risk for bed sharing. Parental alcohol and drugs use were implicated, in addition to low birth weight, and mechanical suffocation by wedging. In the UK in the SWISS (South West Infant Sleep Scene Study), a sixth of all SUDI occurred when an infant slept on a sofa with a parent (126). For most sofa-sharing deaths, sofa sharing was not the usual practice, and often parents unintentionally fell asleep while settling and feeding their infant (41, 127). Of significant concern, at least a proportion of sofa-sleeping deaths appear to have been an unintended consequence of the advice never to bed share, as parents tried to avoid feeding their infants in the parental bed because they had been told this was a risk (127, 128). A 2010 survey of nearly 5,000 mothers in the United States found that to avoid bed sharing, 55% of mothers fed their infants at night on chairs, recliners, or sofas, and 40% of these admitted to falling asleep with their infants while doing so (41). Similar findings have been reported in the United Kingdom (11, 127).

Studies have reported the risk associated with shared sleeping when coupled with a soft sleep surface, and pillow use (26, 120, 129). Shared sleeping may also increase the risk of overheating rebreathing, airway obstructions, and head covering (7, 9, 130-132), all of which are risk factors for SUDI. Unintentional suffocation is becoming increasingly recognized as a significant contributor to SUDI (26, 133-138). Unsuitable bedding, temporary sleeping arrangements, and a shared sleeping partner have been attributes of accidental suffocation deaths of infants (26, 136, 138). The recognition of the contribution of suffocation at least partially explains findings that the risk of infant death is increased where there are multiple bed sharers (129), alcohol and other substance use (11, 21, 119),[1] and the surface sharer is unusually overtired (18, 122).

The strongest predictor of SUDI has been identified as the combination of recent maternal alcohol consumption and sleeping together with an infant on a soft shared surface (bed or sofa) (11, 119, 123, 127). Cumulatively, the above described findings lead researchers to concur that parents should be strongly advised against sharing a sleep surface when either parent smokes, or has consumed alcohol or drugs, or is sleeping on a couch, sofa, or other inappropriate sleep surface. They should also be made aware that the risks associated with shared sleeping are particularly high if their infant is very young, premature, or of low birth weight, even if they do not smoke (1, 24, 27, 119).

## Shared Sleeping Risks in the Absence of Known Hazards

Where researchers cannot reach a consensus is on whether there is a risk associated with shared sleeping in all circumstances. Recently, two individual-level analyses (24, 119) using data from large population-based case-control studies have aimed to quantify whether there is a risk of SUDI associated with shared sleeping in the absence of known hazards, particularly, smoking, alcohol, and other substance use. Both studies concurred that parental smoking, alcohol, and drug use increased the risk of SIDS significantly

---

1    Suffocation may not explain the interaction between SUDI and drug use in its entirety. Carpenter et al. (119) found that the use of any illegal drugs by the mother increased the risk of death 11-fold and the use of alcohol fivefold, even when room sharing. However, other studies have found no associated risk when the parents did not surface share (11). The precise nature of this interaction remains unexplained, although it is likely also related to social determinants of health that tend to be more prevalent amongst substance-using populations.

when shared sleeping was a factor, particularly among the younger age group of infants. However, in the absence of these factors, among older infants different conclusions were reached regarding the risk of bed sharing.

Carpenter and colleagues (119) reported a significantly increased risk of SIDS when shared sleeping occurred in the absence of parental smoking or alcohol consumption for infants aged 3 months or less (aOR = 5.1 [95% CI: 2.3-11.4]). No increased risk was reported among the older age group (aOR = 1.0 [95% CI: 0.3-3.1]). Blair and colleges (24) also found that the risk of bed sharing in the absence of known hazards was elevated among young infants (aged less than 98 days); however, it did not reach significance. However, for infants older than 3 months, bed sharing in the absence of other hazards was significantly protective, with the researchers reporting that the risk halved among this group of infants (OR 0.1 [95% CI: 0.01-0.5] p=0.009). Only one death (0.6%) occurred in an infant older than 3 months of age in the absence of alcohol, smoking, or sofa sharing, compared to 8.5% among controls. Preliminary data from a retrospective study of SUDI in Australia also indicate that the incidence of SUDI involving shared sleeping in the absence of known risk factors is low. Only three of 58 (5%) SUDI involving shared sleeping occurred among infants 3 months of age or older whose mothers neither smoked nor slept on a couch with the infant (139).

Importantly, it is in the conclusions drawn from these statistics, rather than in the findings themselves, that these two groups of researchers differ most significantly. Carpenter and colleagues (119) draw three distinct, yet related, conclusions. First, they conclude that bed-sharing infants aged over 3 months, whose parents do not smoke or consume alcohol or other substances and do not sleep on a sofa, are of very low risk. However, they consider this to be an inconsequentially small group. While it is mentioned both in this study and elsewhere (140), it should be noted that only one UK study (24) has reported on the prevalence of this low-risk bed sharing (8.5%). Noteworthy is that this is still a considerably larger group than some indigenous populations, such as Australian Aboriginals, who constitute 2.4% of the total population. Second, Carpenter et al. (119) conclude that their findings regarding shared-sleeping risk are sufficient to recommend that "professionals and the literature take a more definitive stand against bed-sharing" (p. 10). They further conclude that any negative effect of such a stance on breastfeeding promotion is justified, on the basis that the "costs of bed-sharing ... far outweigh any benefits from increased breast feeding rates" (p. 9).

In contrast, Blair and colleagues determine that despite the findings of these recent studies, the question of whether there is an increased risk of SUDI for an infant routinely sharing a bed with a breastfeeding mother who does not smoke, drink alcohol, or use other recreational or sedating drugs, and who is aware of how to maximize the safety of the sleep environment for the infant remains unclear (1). As such, acknowledging the low risk of this group reported by both studies, they consider that to give blanket advice to all parents never to bed share does not reflect the evidence, particularly given that it has been shown to influence parents to seek alternative, more dangerous sleep surfaces, such as a sofa (24). Third, they consider that, given the considerable evidence of an interdependent, positive relationship between shared sleeping and breastfeeding, the "inherent advantages to the infant need to be considered in addition to the possible risk of SIDS" (24) (p. 6).

The debate, it seems, has never been more polarized. As Ball and Volpe (36) and Cunningham (52) observe, the crux of the problem is that the question of infant sleep location is caught between two competing, and at times contradictory, public health agendas: safeguarding agendas (focused on reducing hazardous sleep environments known to increase infant mortality or adverse events) and wellbeing agendas (those centered around the promotion of breastfeeding, appropriate growth and development, and secure attachment relationships).

Of note, the most recent analysis of the evidence regarding shared-sleep environments (95) determines that conclusive evidence as to the risks of shared sleeping is lacking. However, the researchers assert that this is not due to negative findings, but rather because of a lack of focus on current gaps in knowledge. Consequently, Mileva-Seitz and colleagues (95) call for the end of the single-discipline, pediatrics-dominated approach, arguing that a cross-fertilization within the field is both imperative and long overdue. "It's time for pediatrics/epidemiology, anthropology/evolutionary psychology and psychiatry/developmental psychology to join forces in a new subfield that we label psychoanthropediatrics" (p. 16).

## Delivering the Best Possible Advice: Risk Minimization versus Risk Elimination

The translation of epidemiological findings regarding shared sleeping risk into recommendations and policy for families and health professionals has resulted in two divergent approaches: one focused on risk elimination and the other focused on risk minimization (52, 141).

Proponents of a risk elimination approach seek to reduce the incidence of SUDI by eliminating those risk factors that are considered to be within parents' control. Adopting a risk elimination standpoint, many public health bodies, most notably the American Academy of Pediatrics, advise parents never to share a sleep surface with their infant (7, 9, 119, 141). At the local level this recommendation has frequently been translated into aggressive anti-shared-sleeping campaigns that have served more to offend and anger than to dissuade parents from sharing a sleep surface with their infant (127). Examples include campaigns featuring bedheads as tombstones, infants sleeping with meat cleavers, and horror "fairy-tales" ending in death.

Irrespective of how aggressive, or otherwise simplistic, the message never to sleep with an infant is, an increasing number of researchers question whether a risk elimination approach is appropriate at all (4, 36, 127, 141-143). First, such recommendations imply that any SUDI that occurs in the context of shared sleeping may be directly attributable to the surface sharing rather than to other risk factors that may be present (127, 141). Moreover, simplistic rhetoric equating safe infant sleep with sleeping alone can obscure the importance of both room sharing and breastfeeding (which is associated with night-time mother-infant proximity) to SUDI reduction (4). As such, it does not accurately reflect the research evidence which, as discussed above, is nuanced and far from straightforward. Second, a risk elimination approach does not take account of research findings that the majority of parents who share a sleep surface do not intend to do so (52, 53). For these parents, surface sharing most frequently occurs under conditions of stress, as they try to sooth an unsettled infant in the context of sleep deprivation (144). Simple advice for parents never to sleep with their infants, a risk elimination approach, is therefore argued to be impractical for new parents. Third, blanket advice against shared-sleep environments has failed to emulate the previous success of infant sleep position advice. This is because the risk elimination approach does not account for the culturally embedded nature of shared sleeping, which results in the recommendations being largely rejected by their target populations (4, 36, 127).

It is increasingly acknowledged that risk minimization polices will be more effective in reducing preventable infant deaths, because risk minimization acknowledges that infants will be placed to sleep, intentionally or unintentionally, in their parent's bed at some stage, particularly if they are breastfed (12, 34, 52, 88, 141, 145). Advocates of a risk minimization approach contend that in providing safe infant sleep advice, recommendations and policies should consider the documented benefits of shared sleeping, the need to promote and support breastfeeding, the high prevalence and culturally embedded nature of shared sleeping, and the right of parents to make informed choices about their infant's care (4). Parents should be provided with information that includes benefits, risks, and strategies to reduce the risk and increase safety associated with shared sleep environments, should they decide to, or have no option but to, share a sleep surface with their infant (5, 12, 21, 36, 73, 113, 127, 146). This approach does not prevent providing information about the known dangers of some shared-sleeping practices, nor the circumstances in which it should be avoided altogether (4). Rather, a risk minimization approach simply recognizes that successful interventions to reduce the risk of sleep-related infant death need to address the unique needs and influences of the families they are targeting (4, 36, 85, 141). Parents can then be supported to ensure that they are aware of specific hazardous circumstances and can make informed decisions about sharing a sleep surface with their infant. This risk minimization approach is consistent with, and supported by, recommendations for health professional practice proposed by UNICEF (15, 25, 102, 147), the National Institute for Health and Care Excellence (145), the Australian College of Midwives (148), and Red Nose (formerly SIDS and Kids Australia) (149, 150).

# Future Directions

To overcome the risk associated with "direct" shared sleeping, while respecting its social value and importance for initiating and maintain breastfeeding, several devices have been designed to promote safer sleep in close proximity to a parent. These have been termed side-car cots, co-sleepers, safe sleep enablers, and infant safe sleep devices (ISSDs) in the literature (151). There are several sleep enablers available on the market for domestic use, such as the Finnish Baby Box or the Safe and Secure Sleeper, but there has been little formal research into the safety or acceptability of these devices. In addition, these devices may have sides too high to allow physical contact while the infant is contained in the device (e.g. the Baby Box), or they may have design features such as a flexible sleep surface that is reliant on being placed on a firm, flat surface for safe use (e.g. the Safe and Secure Sleeper). Devices to enable "safer" sleep in the context of close contact with a primary caregiver which have been, or are currently being, evaluated are side-car cots, the Change for our Children Pēpi-Pod® Program and First Days Pēpi-Pod® Sleep Space in New Zealand, and the Pēpi-Pod® Program in Australia.

## Side-car cots

Several studies have reported on the use of side-car cots in postnatal care. These three-sided bassinettes temporarily fix to the mother's hospital bed to facilitate a level, but separate, sleep surface for an infant which is easily accessed by the mother (152). Trials based in the United Kingdom of the NECOT side-car cot were positive in relation to frequency of mother-infant interaction, infant safety, and establishment of breastfeeding (153). Further trials within institutions have demonstrated it to be a positive alternative to free-standing cots for participants, and a safer option for infant handling (154). However, the side-car cot did not demonstrate improved breastfeeding outcomes, nor did it impact shared sleeping practice post-discharge (152).

## The Pēpi-Pod® and Wahakura programs: New Zealand

The Change for our Children Pēpi-Pod® Program was specifically developed to address high Māori infant mortality rates. Billed as the sister to the Māori Wahakura, a flax woven basket (155, 156), the Pēpi-Pod® is a rectangular polypropylene box with a fitted mattress and bed linen to be used on the parent bed. Additionally, the Pēpi-Pod® Program incorporates safe sleep education, and the families involved undertake to spread safe infant sleep messages amongst their social network (157, 158). Both the Pēpi-Pod® and the Wahakura provide a zone of physical protection while an infant sleeps, which reduces risk of suffocation, particularly when an infant is placed in a shared-sleep environment. The community-based Pēpi-Pod® and Wahakura programs have been supported by New Zealand's Ministry of Health, with over 15,000 pods and approximately 1,500 handwoven Wahakura distributed through the country

(151, 158). Findings to date have demonstrated a significant fall in infant mortality over the intervention period (2011-14), from 2.4 to 1.9 per 1,000 within the whole population and from 4.5 to 3.5 per 1,000 within the Māori population (151, 159).

A randomized controlled trial with 200 mainly Māori families comparing the Wahakura with a standard bassinet has been conducted to evaluate safety and potential effects on infant sleep position, head covering, breastfeeding, bed sharing, and maternal sleep and fatigue (160). No significant differences were found in risk behaviors for infants who slept in Wahakura compared with bassinets. However, there was a significant benefit relating to breastfeeding, with the Wahakura group reporting twice the level of exclusive breastfeeding at 6 months (22.5% vs 10.7%, p=0.04) (160). The authors concluded that Wahakura were relatively safe, and can be promoted as an alternative to direct infant-adult surface sharing (160).

Most recently, a smaller version of the Pēpi-pod® (the First Days Pod), developed for use in birthing facilities, is currently being trialed in New Zealand (161). A collaborative study will commence in mid-2017 in Queensland, Australia, as part of a randomized controlled trial of safe sleep enablers in postnatal environments (162).

## Pēpi-Pod® sleep space and the Pēpi-Pod® program: Australia

Many Aboriginal and Torres Strait Islander families surface share as a cultural norm and experience social determinants of health that increase the risk of SUDI fourfold, compared to non-Indigenous infants. In collaboration with the NZ Pēpi-Pod® Program, the pilot Pēpi-Pod® Program was launched in Queensland in 2013, facilitated by health services working with Aboriginal and Torres Strait Islander families (163). Responses relating to use, acceptability, convenience, and safety of the infant sleep space have been positive. A larger trial of this program (n=300) has also commenced in remote, regional, and urban Aboriginal communities in Queensland (163). No adverse events have been reported with the use of the Pēpi-Pod® in the Queensland study (164). Preliminary data suggest that the use of the Pēpi-Pod® reduces direct surface sharing with caregivers who are smokers (165).

Although as yet only preliminary, the findings of studies evaluating safe shared-sleep enablers are nevertheless encouraging. Importantly, those shared-sleep enablers trialed have been acceptable to culturally diverse groups in which risk factors for SUDI are associated with social determinants of health that are not easily amendable to change. Safe shared-sleep enablers may represent a way forward that diminishes the risk associated with certain forms of direct surface sharing, while simultaneously allowing for enhanced breastfeeding, close contact, and maternal responsiveness associated with shared-sleep environments.

## Conclusions

Sharing a sleep surface with an infant is a prevalent parenting practice associated with both positive and negative outcomes. Whether it is beneficial or dangerous depends on a range of factors, including the reasons for, and circumstances in which, shared sleeping occurs, as well as the social and biological connection between the infant and the caregiver. Indeed, so variable is the range of factors associated with shared sleeping and the impact it has on different families that it is inappropriate and possibly harmful to recommend against shared sleeping in any unqualified way, without awareness and consideration of the individual family circumstances, as well as the broader social and cultural context in which it occurs. The proliferation of mixed and oftentimes contradictory infant care messages that have resulted from the polarized debate between advocates and opponents of shared-sleep environments has served only to confuse and alienate families, rather than to educate, empower, and protect them. From a public health perspective, clinicians have a duty of care to provide families with unbiased, accurate, and up-to-date evidence that includes both the benefits and the risks associated with shared-sleep environments, to enable informed decision making. As such, a risk minimization approach is supported. Future research should involve multidisciplinary approaches, and should continue to investigate new and innovative approaches to improve the safety of infant sleep, while recognizing the social and cultural importance of shared-sleep environments to many families. In this regard, the findings of studies involving safe shared-sleep enablers are promising, and may bridge a hitherto longstanding divide.

## References

1.  Fleming PJ, Blair PS, Pease A. Sudden unexpected death in infancy: Aetiology, pathophysiology, epidemiology and prevention in 2015. Arch Dis Child. 2015;100(10):984-8. https://doi.org/10.1136/archdischild-2014-306424.

2.  Mitchell EA, Taylor BJ, Ford RP, Stewart AW, Becroft DM, Thompson JM, et al. Four modifiable and other major risk factors for cot death: The New Zealand study. J Paediatr Child Health. 1992;28(Suppl 1):S3-8. https://doi.org/10.1111/j.1440-1754.1992.tb02729.x.

3.  Mitchell EA, Freemantle J, Young J, Byard RW. Scientific consensus forum to review the evidence underpinning the recommendations of the Australian SIDS and Kids safe sleeping health promotion programme — October 2010. J Paediatr Child Health. 2012;48(8):626-33. https://doi.org/10.1111/j.1440-1754.2011.02215.x.

4.  Gettler LT, McKenna JJ. Never sleep with baby? Or keep me close but keep me safe: Elimininating inappropriate "safe infant sleep" rhetoric in the United States. Curr Pediatr Rev. 2010;6:71-7. https://doi.org/10.2174/157339610791317250.

5.  Ball HL. The latest on bed sharing and breastfeeding. Community Pract. 2012;85(11):29-31.

6.  Horsley T, Clifford T, Barrowman N, Bennett S, Yazdi F, Sampson M, et al. Benefits and harms associated with the practice of bed sharing: A systematic review. Arch Pediatr Adolesc Med. 2007;161(3):237-45. https://doi.org/10.1001/archpedi.161.3.237.

7.  Moon RY, & Taskforce on Sudden Infant Death Syndrome. SIDS and other sleep-related infant deaths: Expansion of recommendations for a safe infant sleeping environment. Pediatrics. 2011;128(5):e1341-67. https://doi.org/10.1542/peds.2011-2285.

8.  American Academy of Pediatrics (AAP) Task Force on Infant Sleep Position and Sudden Infant Death Syndrome. Changing concepts of sudden infant death syndrome: Implications for infant sleeping environment and sleep position. Pediatrics. 2000;105(3):650-6. https://doi.org/10.1542/peds.105.3.650.

9.  Moon RY, & Taskforce on Sudden Infant Death Syndrome. SIDS and other sleep-related infant deaths: Evidence base for 2016 updated recommendations for a safe infant sleeping environment. Pediatrics. 2016;138(5):e20162940. https://doi.org/10.1542/peds.2016-2940.

10. Blair PS, Fleming PJ. Epidemiological investigation of sudden infant death syndrome infants — Recommendations for future studies. Child Care Health Dev. 2002;28(Suppl 1):49-54. https://doi.org/10.1046/j.1365-2214.2002.00014.x.

11. Blair PS, Sidebotham P, Evason-Coombe C, Edmonds M, Heckstall-Smith EM, Fleming PJ. Hazardous cosleeping environments and risk factors amenable to change: Case-control study of SIDS in south west England. BMJ. 2009;339:b3666. https://doi.org/10.1136/bmj.b3666.

12. McKenna JJ, Ball HL, Gettler LT. Mother-infant cosleeping, breastfeeding and sudden infant death syndrome: What biological anthropology has discovered about normal infant sleep and pediatric sleep medicine. Am J Phys Anthropol. 2007;Suppl 45:133-61. https://doi.org/10.1002/ajpa.20736.

13. Queensland Health. Safe infant sleeping, co-sleeping and bed-sharing: Guideline. QH-GDL-362:2013. Brisbane: Queensland Government, 2013.

14. Queensland Health. Safe infant care to reduce the risk of sudden unexpected deaths in infancy: Policy statement and guidelines. Brisbane: Queensland Government, 2008.

15. Infant Sleep Information Source (ISIS). Information for parents and carers United Kingdom: Collaboration between Durham University Parent-Infant Sleep Lab and UNICEF United Kingdom, National Childbirth Trust, The Breastfeeding Network,

Lactation Consultants of Great Britain and Association of Breastfeeding Mothers. [Available from: https://www.isisonline.org.uk]. Accessed 9 October 2017.

16. McKenna JJ, Thoman EB, Anders TF, Sadeh A, Schechtman VL, Glotzbach SF. Infant-parent co-sleeping in an evolutionary perspective: Implications for understanding infant sleep development and the sudden infant death syndrome. Sleep. 1993;16(3):263-82. https://doi.org/10.1093/sleep/16.3.263.

17. Mitchell EA, Thompson JM. Co-sleeping increases the risk of SIDS, but sleeping in the parents' bedroom lowers it. In: Sudden infant death syndrome: New trends in the nineties. Ed Rognum T. Oslo: Scandinavian University Press, 1995. p. 266-9.

18. Carpenter RG, Irgens LM, Blair PS, England PD, Fleming PJ, Huber J, et al. Sudden unexplained infant death in 20 regions in Europe: Case control study. Lancet. 2004;363(9404):185-91. https://doi.org/10.1016/S0140-6736(03)15323-8.

19. Blair PS, Platt MW, Smith IJ, Fleming PJ. Sudden infant death syndrome and the time of death: Factors associated with night-time and day-time deaths. Int J Epidemiol. 2006;35(6):1563-9. https://doi.org/10.1093/ije/dyl212.

20. Vennemann MM, Bajanowski T, Brinkmann B, Jorch G, Sauerland C, Mitchell EA. Sleep environment risk factors for sudden infant death syndrome: The German sudden infant death syndrome study. Pediatrics. 2009;123(4):1162-70. https://doi.org/10.1542/peds.2008-0505.

21. Blair PS, Fleming PJ, Smith IJ, Platt MW, Young J, Nadin P, et al. Babies sleeping with parents: Case-control study of factors influencing the risk of the sudden infant death syndrome. BMJ (Clinical research ed). 1999;319:1457-61. https://doi.org/10.1136/bmj.319.7223.1457.

22. Horne RS, Hauck FR, Moon RY. Sudden infant death syndrome and advice for safe sleeping. BMJ. 2015;350:h1989. https://doi.org/10.1136/bmj.h1989.

23. Scragg RK, Mitchell EA, Stewart AW, Ford RP, Taylor BJ, Hassall IB, et al. Infant room-sharing and prone sleep position in sudden infant death syndrome. Lancet. 1996;347(8993):7-12. https://doi.org/10.1016/S0140-6736(96)91554-8.

24. Blair PS, Sidebotham P, Pease A, Fleming PJ. Bed-sharing in the absence of hazardous circumstances: Is there a risk of sudden infant death syndrome? An analysis from two case-control studies conducted in the UK. PLoS One. 2014;9(9):e107799. https://doi.org/10.1371/journal.pone.0107799.

25. UNICEF UK Baby Friendly Initiative. Babies sharing their mothers' bed while in hospital: A sample policy. London: UNICEF, 2004.

26. Kemp JS, Unger B, Wilkins D, Psara RM, Ledbetter TL, Graham A, et al. Unsafe sleep practices and an analysis of bedsharing among infants dying

suddenly and unexpectedly: Results of a four-year, population-based, death-scene investigation study of sudden infant death syndrome and related deaths. Pediatrics. 2000;106(3):e41-e.

27. Vennemann MM, Hense HW, Bajanowski T, Blair PS, Complojer C, Moon RY, et al. Bed sharing and the risk of sudden infant death syndrome: Can we resolve the debate? J Pediatr. 2012;160(1):44-8.e2. https://doi.org/10.1016/j.jpeds.2011.06.052.

28. Fleming PJ, Blair PS, Bacon C, Bensley D, Smith I, Taylor E, et al. Environment of infants during sleep and risk of the sudden infant death syndrome: Results of 1993-5 case-control study for confidential inquiry into stillbirths and deaths in infancy. BMJ. 1996;313(7051):191-5. https://doi.org/10.1136/bmj.313.7051.191.

29. McGarvey C, McDonnell M, Chong A, O'Regan M, Matthews T. Factors relating to the infant's last sleep environment in sudden infant death syndrome in the Republic of Ireland. Arch Dis Child. 2003;88(12):1058-64. https://doi.org/10.1136/adc.88.12.1058.

30. Baby Friendly Health Initiatives Australia. Standards for implementation of the ten steps to successful beastfeeding. The gobal criteria for baby friendly hospitals in Australia. Canberra: Australian College of Midwives, 2009.

31. World Health Organization (WHO), & UNICEF. Baby-friendly hospital initiative: Revised, updated and expanded for intergrated care. Geneva: World Health Organization, UNICEF, and Wellstart International, 2009.

32. Tappin D, Ecob R, Brooke H. Bedsharing, roomsharing, and sudden infant death syndrome in Scotland: A case-control study. J Pediatr. 2005;147(1):32-7. https://doi.org/10.1016/j.jpeds.2005.01.035.

33. Gettler LT, McKenna J. Evolutionary perspectives on mother-infant sleep proximity and breastfeeding in a laboratory setting. Am J Phys Anthropol. 2011;144(3):454-62. https://doi.org/10.1002/ajpa.21426.

34. Ball HL. Reasons to bed-share: Why parents sleep with their infants. J Reprod Infant Psychol. 2002;20(4):207-21. https://doi.org/10.1080/0264683021000033147.

35. McKenna JJ, Gettler LT. There is no such thing as infant sleep, there is no such thing as breastfeeding, there is only breastsleeping. Acta Paediatr. 2016;105(1):17-21. https://doi.org/10.1111/apa.13161.

36. Ball HL, Volpe LE. Sudden infant death syndrome (SIDS) risk reduction and infant sleep location — Moving the discussion forward. Soc Sci Med. 2013;79:84-91. https://doi.org/10.1016/j.socscimed.2012.03.025.

37. Blair PS. Perspectives on bed-sharing. Curr Pediatr Rev. [Available from: https://www.ispid.org/fileadmin/user_upload/textfiles/articles/CPR12_Blair_Bed_Sharing.pdf]. Accessed 9 October 2017.

38. McKenna JJ, McDade T. Why babies should never sleep alone: A review of the co-sleeping controversy in relation to SIDS, bedsharing and breast feeding. Paediatr Respir Rev. 2005;6(2):134-52. https://doi.org/10.1016/j.prrv.2005.03.006.

39. Colson ER, Willinger M, Rybin D, Heeren T, Smith LA, Lister G, et al. Trends and factors associated with infant bed sharing, 1993-2010: The national infant sleep position study. JAMA Pediatr. 2013;167(11):1032-7. https://doi.org/10.1001/jamapediatrics.2013.2560.

40. Hauck FR, Signore C, Fein SB, Raju T. Infant sleeping arrangements and practices during the first year of life. Pediatrics. 2008;122(Suppl 2):s113-20. https://doi.org/10.1542/peds.2008-1315o.

41. Kendall-Tackett K, Cong Z, Hale TW. Mother-infant sleep locations and nighttime feeding behavior: US data from the survey of mothers' sleep and fatigue. Clin Lact. 2010;1(1):27-31. https://doi.org/10.1891/215805310807011837.

42. Blair PS, Ball HL. The prevalence and characteristics associated with parent-infant bed-sharing in England. Arch Dis Child. 2004;89(12):1106-10. https://doi.org/10.1136/adc.2003.038067.

43. Nelson EA, Taylor BJ, & ICCPS Study Group. International child care practices study: Infant sleeping environment. Early Hum Dev. 2001;62(1):43-55. https://doi.org/10.1016/S0378-3782(01)00116-5.

44. Anuntaseree W, Mo-Suwan L, Vasiknanonte P, Kuasirikul S, Ma-a-lee A, Choprapawon C. Factors associated with bed sharing and sleep position in Thai neonates. Child Care Health Dev. 2008;34(4):482-90. https://doi.org/10.1111/j.1365-2214.2008.00832.x.

45. Young J, Battistutta D, O'Rouke P, Thompson JM. Infant care practices related to sudden infant death syndrome in Queensland 2002. Brisbane: Queensland Health, 2008.

46. Young J, Thompson JM. Recommendations for real life: The nature of shared sleep environments in Queensland and implication for effective safe infant sleeping messages. Forensic Sci Med Pathol. 2009;5(2):115.

47. Rigda RS, McMillen IC, Buckley P. Bed sharing patterns in a cohort of Australian infants during the first six months after birth. J Paediatr Child Health. 2000;36(2):117-21. https://doi.org/10.1046/j.1440-1754.2000.00468.x.

48. Tuohy PG, Smale P, Clements M. Ethnic differences in parent/infant co-sleeping practices in New Zealand. N Z Med J. 1998;111(1074):364-6.

49. Blair PS, Sidebotham P, Berry P, Evans M, Fleming PJ. Major epidemiological changes in sudden infant death syndrome: A 20-year population-based study in the UK. Lancet. 2006;367(9507):314-19. https://doi.org/10.1016/S0140-6736(06)67968-3.

50. Panaretto KS, Smallwood VE, Cole P, Elston J, Whitehall J. Sudden infant death syndrome risk factors in north Queensland: A survey of infant-care practices in Indigenous and non-Indigenous women. J Paediatr Child Health. 2002;38(2):129-34. https://doi.org/10.1046/j.1440-1754.2002.00759.x.

51. Schluter PJ, Young J. Reducing the risk of sudden infant death syndrome: What infant care practices are being used by primary care-givers in Queensland? Neontal, Paediatric and Child Health Nursing. 2002;5(2):27-35.

52. Cunningham H. Infant sleep practices: Exploring the prevalence and circumstances of bed-sharing in the first eight weeks of life [MPH]. Victoria: La Trobe University, 2015.

53. Ball HL, Hooker E, Kelly PJ. Where will the baby sleep? Attitudes and practices of new and experienced parents regarding cosleeping with their newborn infants. Amer Anthrop. 1999;101(1):143-51. https://doi.org/10.1525/aa.1999.101.1.143.

54. Santos IS, Mota DM, Matijasevich A, Barros AJD, Barros FC. Bed-sharing at 3 months and breast-feeding at 1 year in southern Brazil. J Pediatr. 2009;155(4-4):505-9.

55. Tan KL, Ghani SN, Moy FM. The prevalence and characteristics associated with mother-infant bed-sharing in Klang district, Malaysia. Med J Malaysia. 2009;64(4):311-15.

56. Ball HL. Breastfeeding, bed-sharing, and infant sleep. Birth. 2003;30(3):181-8. https://doi.org/10.1046/j.1523-536X.2003.00243.x.

57. Blair PS, Heron J, Fleming PJ. Relationship between bed sharing and breastfeeding: Longitudinal, population-based analysis. Pediatrics. 2010;126(5):e119-e1126. https://doi.org/10.1542/peds.2010-1277.

58. Tipene-Leach D, Hutchison L, Tangiora A, Rea C, White R, Stewart A, et al. SIDS-related knowledge and infant care practices among Māori mothers. N Z Med J. 2010;123(1326):88-96.

59. Abel S, Park J, Tipene-Leach D, Finau S, Lennan M. Infant care practices in New Zealand: A cross-cultural qualitative study. Soc Sci Med. 2001;53:1135-48. https://doi.org/10.1016/S0277-9536(00)00408-1.

60. Eades SJ, Read AW, & Bibbulung Gnarneep Team. Infant care practices in a metropolitan aboriginal population. J Paediatr Child Health. 1999;35(6):541-4. https://doi.org/10.1046/j.1440-1754.1999.00425.x.

61. Tipene-Leach D, Baddock SA, Williams S, Jones R, Tangiora A, Abel S, et al. Methodology and recruitment for a randomised controlled trial to evaluate the safety of wahakura for infant bedsharing. BMC Pediatr. 2014;14(1):1-10. https://doi.org/10.1186/1471-2431-14-240.

62. Desmosthesous C, Desmosthesous T. The Indigenous safe sleep project: Closing the gap on knowledge, resources and access in Queensland. Brisbane: Sids and Kids Queensland, 2011.

63. Blair PS. Putting co-sleeping into perspective. Jornal de Pediatria (Rio J). 2008;84(2):99-101. https://doi.org/10.2223/JPED.1775.

64. Willinger M, Ko C, Hoffman HJ, Kessler RC, Corwin MJ. Trends in infant bed sharing in the United States, 1993-2000: The national infant sleep position study. Arch Pediatr Adolesc Med. 2003;157(1):43-9. https://doi.org/10.1001/archpedi.157.1.43.

65. Lahr MB, Rosenberg KD, Lapidus JA. Maternal-infant bedsharing: Risk factors for bedsharing in a population-based survey of new mothers and implications for SIDS risk reduction. Matern Child Health J. 2007;11(3):277-86. https://doi.org/10.1007/s10995-006-0166-z.

66. Welles-Nystrom B. Co-sleeping as a window into Swedish culture: Considerations of gender and health care. Scand J Caring Sci. 2005;19(4):354-60. https://doi.org/10.1111/j.1471-6712.2005.00358.x.

67. Ball HL, Moya E, Fairley L, Westman J, Oddie S, Wright J. Bed- and sofa-sharing practices in a UK biethnic population. Pediatrics. 2012;129(3):e673-81. https://doi.org/10.1542/peds.2011-1964.

68. Ball HL, Moya E, Fairley L, Westman J, Oddie S, Wright J. Infant care practices related to sudden infant death syndrome in South Asian and white British families in the UK. Paediatr Perinat Epidemiol. 2012;26(1):3-12. https://doi.org/10.1111/j.1365-3016.2011.01217.x.

69. Gantley M, Davies DP, Murcott A. Sudden infant death syndrome: Links with infant care practices. BMJ. 1993;306(6869):16-20. https://doi.org/10.1136/bmj.306.6869.16.

70. Mitchell EA, Tuohy PG, Brunt JM, Thompson JM, Clements MS, Stewart AW, et al. Risk factors for sudden infant death syndrome following the prevention campaign in New Zealand: A prospective study. Pediatrics. 1997;100(5):835-40. https://doi.org/10.1542/peds.100.5.835.

71. Kilkenny M, Lumley J. Ethnic differences in the incidence of the sudden infant death syndrome (SIDS) in Victoria, Australia 1985-1989. Paediatr Perinat Epidemiol. 1994;8(1):27-40. https://doi.org/10.1111/j.1365-3016.1994.tb00433.x.

72. Rice PL, Naksook C. Child rearing and cultural beliefs and practices amongst Thai mothers in Victoria, Australia: Implications for the sudden infant death syndrome. J Paediatr Child Health. 1998;34(4):320-4. https://doi.org/10.1046/j.1440-1754.1998.00234.x.

73. Young J. Night-time behavior and interactions between mothers and their infants of low risk for SIDS: A longtitudinal study of room sharing and bed-sharing [PhD]. Bristol: University of Bristol (United Kingdom), 1999.

74. Mosko SS, Richard CA, McKenna J. Infant arousals during mother-infant bed sharing: Implications for infant sleep and sudden infant death syndrome research. Pediatrics. 1997;100(5):841-9. https://doi.org/10.1542/peds.100.5.841.

75. Mosko SS, Richard CA, McKenna JJ. Maternal sleep and arousals during bedsharing with infants. Sleep. 1997;20(2):142-50. https://doi.org/10.1093/sleep/20.2.142.

76. McKenna J, Mosko S, Richard C. Bedsharing promotes breastfeeding. Pediatrics. 1997;100(2):214-19. https://doi.org/10.1542/peds.100.2.214.

77. Huang Y, Hauck FR, Signore C, Yu A, Raju TN, Huang TT, et al. Influence of bedsharing activity on breastfeeding duration among US mothers. JAMA Pediatr. 2013;167(11):1038-44. https://doi.org/10.1001/jamapediatrics.2013.2632.

78. Pemberton D. Breastfeeding, co-sleeping and the prevention of SIDS. Br J Midwifery. 2005;13(1):12-18. https://doi.org/10.12968/bjom.2005.13.1.17315.

79. Hunt F. The importance of kangaroo care on infant oxygen saturation levels and bonding. J Neonatal Nurs. 2008;14(2):47-51. https://doi.org/10.1016/j.jnn.2007.12.003.

80. Ferber SG, Makhoul IR. The effect of skin-to-skin contact (kangaroo care) shortly after birth on the neurobehavioral responses of the term newborn: A randomized, controlled trial. Pediatrics. 2004;113(4):858-65. https://doi.org/10.1542/peds.113.4.858.

81. Christensson K, Cabrera T, Christensson E, Uvnas-Moberg KW. Separation distress call in the human neonate in the absence of maternal body contact. Acta Paediatr Scand. 1995;84(5):468-73. https://doi.org/10.1111/j.1651-2227.1995.tb13676.x.

82. Ludington SM. Energy conservation during skin-to-skin contact between premature infants and their mothers. Heart Lung. 1990;19(5 Pt 1):445-51.

83. Ludington-Hoe SM, Johnson MW, Morgan K, Lewis T, Gutman J, Wilson PD, et al. Neurophysiologic assessment of neonatal sleep organization: Preliminary results of a randomized, controlled trial of skin contact with preterm infants. Pediatrics. 2006;117(5):e909-23. https://doi.org/10.1542/peds.2004-1422.

84. Moore ER, Anderson GC, Bergman N, Dowswell T. Early skin-to-skin contact for mothers and their healthy newborn infants. Cochrane Database Syst Rev. 2012;5:CD003519-CD. https://doi.org/10.1002/14651858.CD003519.pub3.

85. Baddock SA, Galland BC, Bolton DP, Williams SM, Taylor BJ. Differences in infant and parent behaviors during routine bed sharing compared with cot sleeping in the home setting. Pediatrics. 2006;117(5):1599-607. https://doi.org/10.1542/peds.2005-1636.

86. Young J. Bedsharing with babies: The facts. RCM Midwives Journal. 1998;1(11):338-41.

87. Mileva-Seitz VR, Luijk MP, van Ijzendoorn MH, Bakermans-Kranenburg MJ, Jaddoe VW, Hofman A, et al. Association between infant nighttime-sleep location and attachment security: No easy verdict. Infant Ment Health J. 2016;37(1):5-16. https://doi.org/10.1002/imhj.21547.

88. McKenna JJ, Volpe LE. Sleeping with baby: An internet-based sampling of parental experiences, choices, perceptions, and interpretations in a western industrialized context. Infant Child Dev. 2007;16(4):359-85. https://doi.org/10.1002/icd.525.

89. Rowe J. A room of their own: The social landscape of infant sleep. Nurs Inq. 2003;10(3):184-92. https://doi.org/10.1046/j.1440-1800.2003.00167.x.

90. Ateah CA, Hamelin KJ. Maternal bedsharing practices, experiences, and awareness of risks. J Obstet Gynecol Neonatal Nurs. 2008;37(3):274-81. https://doi.org/10.1111/j.1552-6909.2008.00242.x.

91. Baddock SA, Galland BC, Taylor BJ, Bolton DP. Sleep arrangements and behavior of bed-sharing families in the home setting. Pediatrics. 2007;119(1):e200-7. https://doi.org/10.1542/peds.2006-0744.

92. Chianese J, Ploof D, Trovato C, Chang JC. Inner-city caregivers' perspectives on bed sharing with their infants. Acad Pediatr. 2009;9(1):26-32. https://doi.org/10.1016/j.acap.2008.11.005.

93. Mitchell EA, Hutchison BL, Thompson J, Wouldes T. Exploratory study of bed-sharing and maternal-infant bonding. J Paediatr Child Health. 2015;51(8):820-5. https://doi.org/10.1111/jpc.12833.

94. Brockington IF, Oates J, George S, Turner D, Vostanis P, Sullivan M, et al. A screening questionnaire for mother-infant bonding disorders. Arch Womens Ment Health. 2001;3(4):133-40. https://doi.org/10.1007/s007370170010.

95. Mileva-Seitz VR, Bakermans-Kranenburg MJ, Battaini C, Luijk MP. Parent-child bed-sharing: The good, the bad, and the burden of evidence. Sleep Med Rev. 2017;32:4-27. https://doi.org/10.1016/j.smrv.2016.03.003.

96. Ramos KD, Youngclarke D, Anderson JE. Parental perceptions of sleep problems among co-sleeping and solitary sleeping children. Infant Child Dev. 2007;16(4):417-31. https://doi.org/10.1002/icd.526.

97. Mosenkis J. The effects of childhood co-sleeping on later life development [MSc]. Chicago: The University of Chicago, 1998.

98. Okami P, Weisner T, Olmstead R. Outcome correlates of parent-child bedsharing: An eighteen-year longitudinal study. J Dev Behav Pediatr. 2002;23(4):244-53. https://doi.org/10.1097/00004703-200208000-00009.

99. World Health Organisation (WHO). Infant and young child feeding: Model chapter for text books for medical students and allied health professionals. Geneva: World Health Organisation, 2009.

100. Australian Institute of Health and Welfare. A picture of Australia's children 2012. Canberra: Australian Institute of Health and Welfare, 2012.

101. Nyqvist KH, Anderson GC, Bergman N, Cattaneo A, Charpak N, Davanzo R, et al. State of the art and recommendations. Kangaroo mother care: Application in a high-tech environment. Acta Paediatr. 2010;99(6):812-19. https://doi.org/10.1111/j.1651-2227.2010.01794.x.

102. UNICEF UK Baby Friendly Initiative. Caring for your baby at night: A guide for parents. London: UNICEF, 2012.

103. Galbally M, Lewis A, McEgan K, Scalzo K, Islam FA. Breastfeeding and infant sleep patterns: An Australian population study. J Paediatr Child Health. 2013;49(2):e147-52. https://doi.org/10.1111/jpc.12089.

104. Hooker E, Ball HL, Kelly PJ. Sleeping like a baby: Attitudes and experiences of bedsharing in northeast England. Med Anthropol. 2001;19(3):203-22. https://doi.org/10.1080/01459740.2001.9966176.

105. Rudzik AE, Ball HL. Exploring maternal perceptions of infant sleep and feeding method among mothers in the United Kingdom: A qualitative focus group study. Matern Child Health J. 2016;20(1):33-40. https://doi.org/10.1007/s10995-015-1798-7.

106. Ball HL. Parent-infant bed-sharing behavior: Effects of feeding type and presence of father. Hum Nat. 2006;17(3):301-18. https://doi.org/10.1007/s12110-006-1011-1.

107. Ball HL. Research overview: Bed-sharing and co-sleeping. New Digest. 2009;48:22-7.

108. Fleming PJ, Blair PS. New knowledge, new insights, and new recommendations. Arch Dis Child. 2006;91(10):799-801. https://doi.org/10.1136/adc.2005.092304.

109. Beijers R, Riksen-Walraven JM, de Weerth C. Cortisol regulation in 12-month-old human infants: Associations with the infants' early history of breastfeeding and co-sleeping. Stress. 2013;16(3):267-77. https://doi.org/10.3109/10253890.2012.742057.

110. Tollenaar MS, Beijers R, Jansen J, Riksen-Walraven JM, de Weerth C. Solitary sleeping in young infants is associated with heightened cortisol reactivity to a bathing session but not to a vaccination. Psychoneuroendocrinology. 2012;37(2):167-77. https://doi.org/10.1016/j.psyneuen.2011.03.017.

111. Lupien SJ, McEwen BS, Gunnar MR, Heim C. Effects of stress throughout the lifespan on the brain, behavior and cognition. Nat Rev Neurosci. 2009;10(6):434-45. https://doi.org/10.1038/nrn2639.

112. Hauck FR, Thompson JM, Tanabe KO, Moon RY, Vennemann MM. Breastfeeding and reduced risk of sudden infant death syndrome: A meta-analysis. Pediatrics. 2011;128(1):103-10. https://doi.org/10.1542/peds.2010-3000.

113. Young J, Watson K, Ellis L, Raven L. Responding to evidence: Breastfeed baby if you can — The sixth public health recommendation to reduce the risk of sudden and unexpected death in infancy. Breastfeed Rev. 2012;20(1):7-15.

114. Vennemann MM, Bajanowski T, Brinkmann B, Jorch G, Yucesan K, Sauerland C, et al. Does breastfeeding reduce the risk of sudden infant death syndrome? Pediatrics. 2009;123(3):e406-10. https://doi.org/10.1542/peds.2008-2145.

115. Bartick MC, Stuebe AM, Schwarz EB, Luongo C, Reinhold AG, Foster EM. Cost analysis of maternal disease associated with suboptimal breastfeeding. Obstet Gynecol. 2013;122(1):111-19. https://doi.org/10.1097/AOG.0b013e318297a047.

116. Duijts L, Jaddoe VW, Hofman A, Moll HA. Prolonged and exclusive breastfeeding reduces the risk of infectious diseases in infancy. Pediatrics. 2010;126(1):e18-25. https://doi.org/10.1542/peds.2008-3256.

117. Chen A, Rogan WJ. Breastfeeding and the risk of postneonatal death in the United States. Pediatrics. 2004;113(5):e435-9. https://doi.org/10.1542/peds.113.5.e435.

118. Where should babies sleep — Alone or with parents? BMJ. 1999;319(7223).

119. Carpenter R, McGarvey C, Mitchell EA, Tappin DM, Vennemann MM, Smuk M, et al. Bed sharing when parents do not smoke: Is there a risk of SIDS? An individual level analysis of five major case-control studies. BMJ Open. 2013;3(5):e002299. https://doi.org/10.1136/bmjopen-2012-002299.

120. Fu LY, Moon RY, Hauck FR. Bed sharing among black infants and sudden infant death syndrome: Interactions with other known risk factors. Acad Pediatr. 2010;10(6):376-82. https://doi.org/10.1016/j.acap.2010.09.001.

121. McGarvey C, McDonnell M, Hamilton K, O'Regan M, Matthews T. An 8-year study of risk factors for SIDS: Bed-sharing versus non-bed-sharing. Arch Dis Child. 2006;91(4):318-23. https://doi.org/10.1136/adc.2005.074674.

122. Scragg RK, Mitchell EA, Taylor BJ, Stewart AW, Ford RP, Thompson J, et al. Bed sharing, smoking, and alcohol in the sudden infant death syndrome. BMJ. 1993;307(6915):1312-18. https://doi.org/10.1136/bmj.307.6915.1312.

123. Fleming PJ, Vennemann MM, Moon RY, Kiechl-Kohlendorfer U, Hauck FR, Byard RW, et al. Sofa-sharing: A meta-analysis. International Conference on Stillbirth, SIDS and Infant Survival; 4-7 October; Baltimore, Maryland, 2012.

124. Bugeja L, Dwyer J, McIntyre SJ, Young J, Stephan KL, McClure RJ. Sleep-related infant deaths in Victoria: A retrospective case series study. Matern Child Health J. 2016;20(5):1032-40. https://doi.org/10.1007/s10995-015-1888-6.

125. Ruys JH, de Jonge GA, Brand R, Engelberts AC, Semmekrot BA. Bed-sharing in the first four months of life: A risk factor for sudden infant death. Acta Paediatr. 2007;96(10):1399-403. https://doi.org/10.1111/j.1651-2227.2007.00413.x.

126. Blair PS, Sidebotham P, Evason-Coombe C, Edmonds M, Heckstall-Smith EMA, Fleming PJ. Hazardous cosleeping environments and risk factors amenable to change: Case-control study of SIDS in south west England. BMJ. 2009;339:b3666. https://doi.org/10.1136/bmj.b3666.

127. Blair PS, Fleming PJ. Bed-sharing advice — An alternative strategy? International Conference on Stillbirth, SIDS and Infant Survival; 4-7 October; Baltimore, Maryland, 2012.

128. Bartick MC, Smith LJ. Speaking out on safe sleep: Evidence-based infant sleep recommendations. Breastfeed Med. 2014;9(9):417-22. https://doi.org/10.1089/bfm.2014.0113.

129. Hauck FR, Herman SM, Donovan M, Iyasu S, Merrick Moore C, Donoghue E, et al. Sleep environment and the risk of sudden infant death syndrome in an urban population: The Chicago infant mortality study. Pediatrics. 2003;111(5 Pt 2):1207-14.

130. Blair PS, Mitchell EA, Heckstall-Smith EM, Fleming PJ. Head covering — A major modifiable risk factor for sudden infant death syndrome: A systematic review. Arch Dis Child. 2008;93(9):778-83. https://doi.org/10.1136/adc.2007.136366.

131. Ball HL. Airway covering during bed-sharing. Child Care Health Dev. 2009;35(5):728-37. https://doi.org/10.1111/j.1365-2214.2009.00979.x.

132. Baddock SA, Galland BC, Beckers MGS, Taylor BJ, Bolton DGP. Bed-sharing and the infant's thermal environment in the home setting. Arch Dis Child. 2004;89(12):1111-6. https://doi.org/10.1136/adc.2003.048082.

133. Drago DA, Dannenberg AL. Infant mechanical suffocation deaths in the United States, 1980-1997. Pediatrics. 1999;103(5):e59. https://doi.org/10.1542/peds.103.5.e59.

134. Hayman R, Dalziel S, Baker N. The context and circumstances of unintentional suffocation in place of sleep in New Zealand. International Conference on Stillbirth, SIDS and Infant Survival; 4-7 October; Baltimore, Maryland, 2012.

135. Byard RW. Overlaying, co-sleeping, suffocation, and sudden infant death syndrome: The elephant in the room. Forensic Sci Med Pathol. 2015;11(2):273-4. https://doi.org/10.1007/s12024-014-9600-5.

136. Li L, Zhang Y, Zielke RH, Ping Y, Fowler DR. Observations on increased accidental asphyxia deaths in infancy while cosleeping in the State of Maryland. Am J Forensic Med Pathol. 2009;30(4):318-21. https://doi.org/10.1097/PAF.0b013e31819df760.

137. Byard RW, Elliott J, Vink R. Infant gender, shared sleeping and sudden death. J Paediatr Child Health. 2012;48(6):517-19. https://doi.org/10.1111/j.1440-1754.2011.02226.x.

138. Combrinck M, Byard RW. Infant asphyxia, soft mattresses, and the "trough" effect. Am J Forensic Med Pathol. 2011;32(3):213-14. https://doi.org/10.1097/PAF.0b013e31822abf68.

139. Hamill K, Young J, Shipstone R. Co-sleeping: Is there an increased risk of sudden unexpected death in infancy (SUDI) if no other risk factors are present? ISA-ISPID Congress: The 2016 International Conference on Stillbirth, SIDS and Baby Survival; 7-10 September; Montevideo, Uruguay, 2016.

140. Mitchell EA. Bed sharing and the risk of sudden infant death: Parents need clear information. Curr Pediatr Rev. 2010;6:63-6. https://doi.org/10.2174/157339610791317133.

141. Fetherston CM, Leach JS. Analysis of the ethical issues in the breastfeeding and bedsharing debate. Breastfeed Rev. 2012;20(3):7-17.

142. Wennergren G. No bed sharing or safer bed sharing? Acta Paediatr. 2016;105(11):1321. https://doi.org/10.1111/apa.13517.

143. Blanchard DS, Vermilya HL. Bedsharing: Toward a more holistic approach in research and practice. Holist Nurs Pract. 2007;21(1):19-25. https://doi.org/10.1097/00004650-200701000-00005.

144. Pease A. Just this once: The role of disrupted routines on decision-making for infant care among mothers with babies at higher risk of SIDS. ISA-ISPID Congress: The 2016 International Conference on Stillbirth, SIDS and Baby Survival; 7-10 September; Montevideo, Uruguay, 2016.

145. National Institute for Health and Care Excellence (NICE). Postnatal care up to 8 weeks after birth. [Available from: https://www.nice.org.uk/guidance/cg37/chapter/1-Recommendations#maintaining-infant-health]. Accessed 9 October 2017.

146. Baddock SA. Co-sleeping: An ecological parenting practice. In: Sustainability, midwifery and birth. Eds Davies L, Daellenbach R, Kensington M. London: Routledge, 2011. p. 207-17.

147. Ball H, Blair PS. The health professional's guide to "caring for your baby at night". [Available from: https://www.unicef.org.uk/babyfriendly/wp-content/uploads/sites/2/2011/11/Caring-for-your-Baby-at-Night-A-Health-Professionals-Guide.pdf]. Accessed 10 January 2018.

148. Australian College of Midwives. Position statement on bed-sharing and co-sleeping. Canberra: Australian College of Midwives, 2014.

149. Red Nose Australia. Information statement: Sharing a sleep surface with a baby. [Available from: https://rednose.com.au/article/sharing-a-sleep-surface-with-a-baby]. Accessed 9 October 2017.

150. Red Nose Australia. Safe sleeping: A guide to assist sleeping your baby safely. Melbourne: Red Nose Australia, 2016.

151. Mitchell ES, Cowan S, Tipene-Leach D. The recent fall in postperinatal mortality in New Zealand and the safe sleep programme. Acta Paediatr. 2016;105(11):1312-20. https://doi.org/10.1111/apa.13494.

152. Ball HL, Ward-Platt MP, Howel D, Russell C. Randomised trial of sidecar crib use on breastfeeding duration (NECOT). Arch Dis Child. 2011;96(7):630-4. https://doi.org/10.1136/adc.2010.205344.

153. Ball HL, Ward-Platt MP, Heslop E, Leech SJ, Brown K. Randomised trial of infant sleep location on the postnatal ward. Arch Dis Child. 2006;91(12):1005-10. https://doi.org/10.1136/adc.2006.099416.

154. Tully KP, Ball HL. Postnatal unit bassinet types when rooming-in after cesarean birth: Implications for breastfeeding and infant safety. J Hum Lact. 2012;28(4):495-505. https://doi.org/10.1177/0890334412452932.

155. Abel S, Tipene-Leach D. SUDI prevention: A review of Māori safe sleep innovations for infants. N Z Med J. 2013;126(1379):86-94.

156. Abel S, Stockdale-Frost A, Rolls R, Tipene-Leach D. The wahakura: A qualitative study of the flax bassinet as a sleep location for New Zealand Māori infants. N Z Med J. 2015;128(1413):12-19.

157. Cowan S. Using Pēpi-Pods: Report on feedback from families who used protected sleeping spaces for babies following the Christchurch earthquake of February 2011. Christchurch: Change for our Children Ltd, 2012.

158. Cowan S, Bennett S, Clarke J, Pease A. An evaluation of portable sleeping spaces for babies following the Christchurch earthquake of February 2011. J Paediatr Child Health. 2013;49(5):364-8. https://doi.org/10.1111/jpc.12196.

159. Cowan S. Their first 500 sleeps: Pēpi-Pod report 2012-2014. Christchurch: Change for our Children Ltd, 2015.

160. Baddock SA, Tipene-Leach D, Williams SM, Tangiora A, Jones R, Iosua E, et al. Wahakura versus bassinet for safe infant sleep: A randomized trial. Pediatrics. 2017;139(2):e20160162. https://doi.org/10.1542/peds.2016-0162.

161. Cowan S. First days: Report on a trial run of a small-sized infant sleep space for safer co-sleeping in postnatal facilities. Christchurch: Change for our Children Ltd, 2016.

162. Young J. Safe sleep advice to safe sleep action: Practical infant care recommendations for parents and culturally appropriate approaches to reducing infant deaths in Indigenous communities. Possums Conference 2017: New clinical tools for early life care — Mood, breastfeeds, sleep and crying; 2-4 February; Brisbane, Australia, 2017.

163. Young J, Craigie L, Watson K, Kearney L, Cowan S, Barnes M. Safe sleep, every sleep: Reducing infant deaths in Indigenous communities. Women and Birth. 2015;28(Suppl 1):S31-2. https://doi.org/10.1016/j.wombi.2015.07.105.

164. Salm Ward TC. Reasons for mother-infant bed-sharing: A systematic narrative synthesis of the literature and implications for future research. Matern Child Health J. 2015;19(3):675-90. https://doi.org/10.1007/s10995-014-1557-1.

165. Young J, Watson K, Craigie L, Cowan S, Kearney L. Advice to action: Uniting cultural practices and safe sleep environments for vulnerable Indigenous Australian infants. ISA-ISPID Congress: The 2016 International Conference on Stillbirth, SIDS and Baby Survival; 7-10 September; Montevideo, Uruguay, 2016.

# 12 Preventive Strategies for Sudden Infant Death Syndrome

Peter Sidebotham, MBChB, PhD[1],
Francine Bates, BA(Hons)[2],
Catherine Ellis, MSc[3] and
Lucy Lyus, MA(Hons)[2]

[1] *Warwick Medical School, University of Warwick, Coventry, UK*
[2] *The Lullaby Trust, London, UK*
[3] *Faculty of Health and Life Sciences, University of Coventry, Coventry, UK*

## Introduction

The impact on sudden infant death rates of the "Back to Sleep" or "Reduce the Risk" campaigns introduced across many countries in the late 1980s and early 1990s has been hailed as one of the great public health success stories of the 20th century (1, 2). Many countries around the world saw substantial reductions in their sudden infant death syndrome (SIDS) rates around the time of introduction of the campaigns (Figure 12.1), with falls of between 42% and 92% (Figure 12.2). The rate of SIDS was halved in the United Kingdom (UK) in just one year, and in New Zealand in two years (1, 3). Instituting a "Back to Sleep" campaign has been estimated to have saved 3,000 lives in New Zealand, 17,000 lives in the UK, and 40,000 lives in the United States (3).

Since the initial drop-off immediately after the "Back to Sleep" campaigns, the rate of SIDS has continued to decline in line with overall post-neonatal mortality (4). For example, in England and Wales, SIDS rates fell from an average of 2.27 per 1,000 live births in 1986-88 to 0.66 per 1,000 live births in 1993-95 and 0.32 per 1,000 live births in 2012-14 (5). These reductions have been accompanied by a shift in the demographics

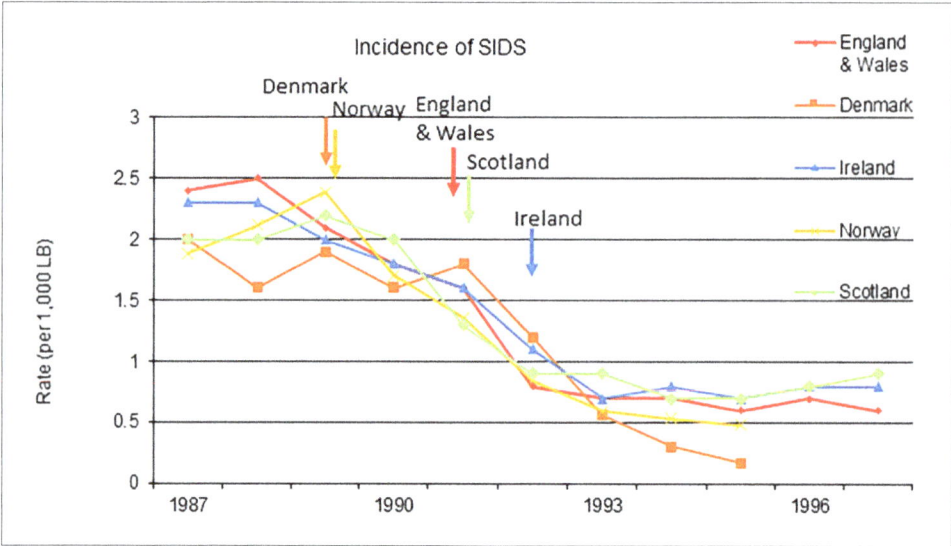

Figure 12.1: Epidemiology of SIDS in selected European countries in relation to "Back to Sleep" campaigns. (Based on (1).) X-axis represents year.

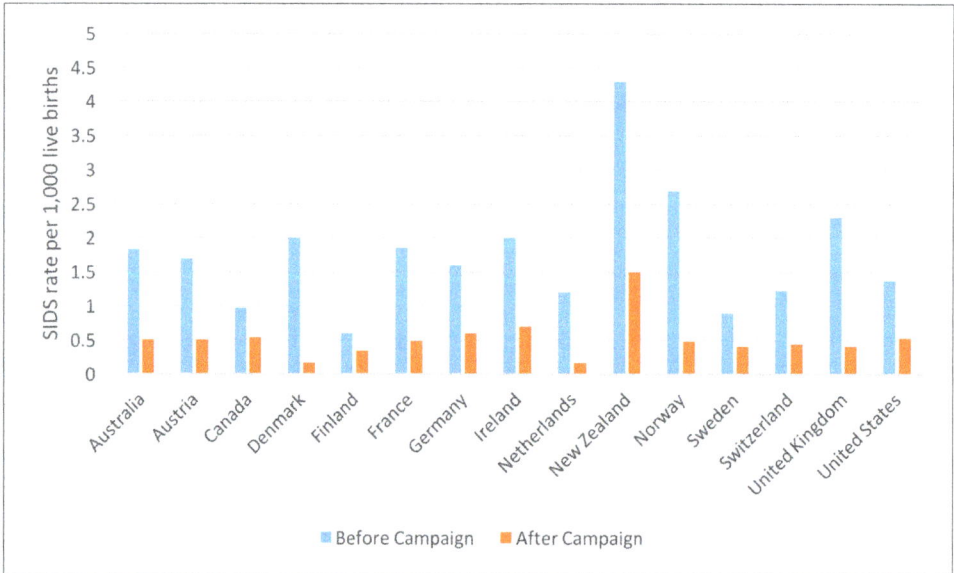

Figure 12.2: Changes in SIDS rates in different countries following "Back to Sleep" campaigns. (Based on (34).)

of SIDS cases, such that most cases now occur in high-risk families with multiple recognized risk factors (6). As a result, SIDS rates are much higher in families from deprived socioeconomic backgrounds and particular population groups, such as the Māori population in New Zealand (7) or the Indigenous and black populations in the United States (8). While these campaigns appear to have effectively reached some segments of our population and resulted in behavioral change, this is not universal.

In order to better understand how we can reach those higher-risk groups and achieve further reductions in SIDS rates, we need a better understanding of the nature and impact of preventive strategies. In this chapter we will outline the principles of public health approaches to prevention and the evidence base for different strategies; in light of this, we will consider the evidence for current approaches to further reduce the risk of SIDS.

## Principles of Effective Preventive Strategies

Like many causes of mortality and morbidity, SIDS is a complex phenomenon with multiple, interacting risk factors. As such, it is unlikely that any single preventive approach will achieve universal success. Rather, more complex, multifaceted community-based approaches may contribute to further reductions in SIDS mortality. Much can be learned in this regard from public health approaches to injury prevention (2, 9, 10). Approaches to injury prevention are often conceptualized in terms of three domains of Education, Environmental Modification, and Enforcement of legislation or regulations (9). To this can be added a fourth aspect of Empowerment (Figure 12.3, Table 12.1).

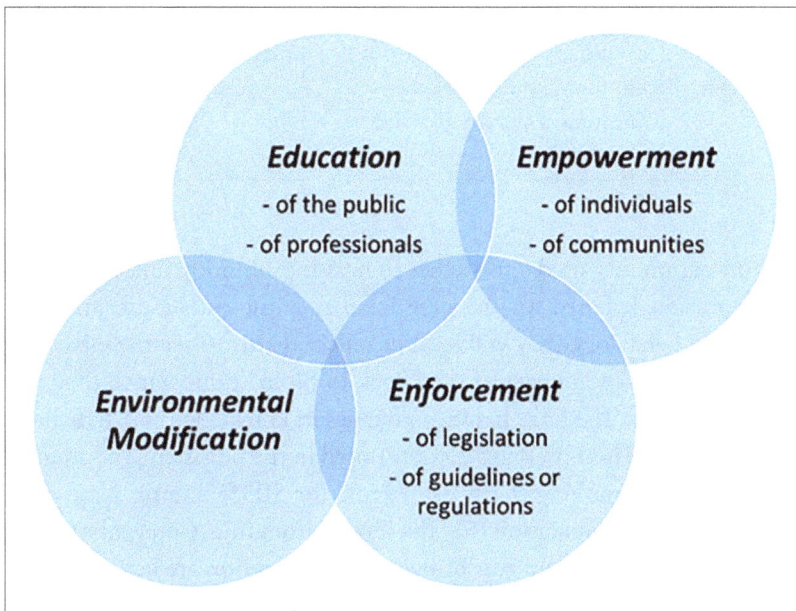

**Education**
- of the public
- of professionals

**Empowerment**
- of individuals
- of communities

**Environmental Modification**

**Enforcement**
- of legislation
- of guidelines or regulations

Figure 12.3: Public health approaches to injury prevention. (Authors' own work.)

Table 12.1: Public health approaches to injury prevention and their application to SIDS prevention.

| Domain | Examples from injury prevention | Examples of (potential) application to SIDS prevention |
|---|---|---|
| **Education** | | |
| • of the public | Teaching children road safety skills | "Back to Sleep" campaigns |
| • of professionals | Training health visitors in recognizing home safety hazards | Training midwives to model safe sleeping in maternity wards |
| **Environmental modification** | | |
| | Road speed restrictors in residential areas | Provision of safe sleeping cribs (Wahakura, Pēpi-Pods®) |
| | Child-resistant packaging of medication | Baby sleeping bags |
| **Enforcement** | | |
| • of legislation | Legislation on motorcycle helmets and seat belts | Legislation to reduce parental cigarette smoking |
| • of guidelines or regulations | Audit of home safety advice given by pediatricians | Inclusion of safe sleeping advice in parent-held child health records |
| **Empowerment** | | |
| | Multifaceted project empowering local groups within a high-risk community: the Waitakere community injury prevention project (11) | Little Lullaby (www.littlelullaby.org.uk): online support network for young parents |

The most commonly used approaches to health promotion and injury prevention have been educational, based on the premise that if the public are informed about health-promoting behaviors, they will tend to follow them. While these have had some effect (as evidenced by the impact of the "Back to Sleep" campaigns), they tend to be limited in their impact. The links between changes in knowledge and actual changes in behavior are weak (9). This is perhaps demonstrated in the persistence of unsafe sleeping practices and parental smoking (both risk factors for SIDS) among some of the most vulnerable groups in the population (6). The lessons from injury prevention suggest that educational approaches based on fear or negative information are less likely to result in sustained behavioral change than more positive approaches— for example, motivational interviewing (9).

In the field of injury prevention, approaches based on environmental or product modification and on enforcing legislation have typically been shown to have a greater impact on outcomes (9). Many examples exist within the published literature of successful interventions which have contributed to reductions in mortality and morbidity. These include child-resistant containers for medication, flame-retardant sleepwear for children, and traffic-calming measures in residential areas. Often these environmental measures are most successful when combined with legislation, as has been seen in the impact of seatbelt and motorcycle helmet legislation in many countries, and in the legislation requiring secure fencing around domestic swimming pools in countries such as Australia and New Zealand.

One of the key differences between educational approaches and those relying on environmental modification or legislation is that the latter are more passive approaches: once implemented, they do not require repeated behavioral changes by individuals (9). In contrast, educational approaches rely on individuals learning the lessons and then consistently implementing them on every occasion of potential risk. This may be particularly pertinent in relation to safe sleep messages for SIDS prevention. Often SIDS deaths occur in circumstances that are out of the ordinary: when a parent gets out of bed to feed their infant and then falls asleep with the infant on a sofa; following a party where parents have been drinking and then without thinking take the infant into their bed; when a family is staying in temporary accommodation or visiting relatives and they do not follow their usual routine.

While there is a growing evidence base in relation to injury prevention efforts, there are still major limitations in our knowledge of what works. There is a paucity of well-designed outcome studies, and the (fortunately) low mortality rates mean that randomized-controlled trials of single, simple interventions with mortality as the primary outcome are unlikely to be helpful in measuring effectiveness. This may be particularly true for SIDS prevention approaches. Nevertheless, it is important both that we learn from the evidence that is available and that our ongoing approaches to prevention are based on the best available evidence (bearing in mind that an absence of evidence of effectiveness does not necessarily equate to evidence of a lack of effectiveness).

A number of key components for successful campaigns can be identified (Table 12.2) (2, 10, 12).

Table 12.2: Key components for successful prevention campaigns.

| | Component | Key elements |
|---|---|---|
| 1. | Establish, as far as possible, a strong scientific basis for intervention. | This should include understanding of the nature, prevalence, and impact of the issue being considered; the evidence for the effectiveness and cost-effectiveness of any proposed interventions and any gaps in current evidence; and clarity over how any impact will be measured. It is important, also, that interventions are grounded in a strong understanding of theories of behavioral change. |
| 2. | Focus on a limited number of simple, achievable interventions. | Trying to incorporate too wide a spread of interventions may make a program unachievable and may limit the value of any individual component; nevertheless, there is evidence that programs that combine different elements (e.g. public education around safe sleep combined with provision of low-cost safe bassinettes) may be more effective than those that focus solely on one element. |
| 3. | Involve the community in planning, promoting and delivering the intervention. | This is a key element of empowerment, and there is evidence that interventions that come from the community and involve key players in the community are likely to be more effective and sustainable in the long term. This includes identifying key stakeholders and getting them on board. Careful consideration needs to be given as to whether an intervention is to be universal or targeted at particular groups; if targeted, it is essential that the relevant groups are involved in designing and delivering the intervention. Effective interventions need to be tailored to the community they are targeted to. |
| 4. | Promote strong, focused leadership that is inclusive in its approach. | Ensure that key players in different agencies and sectors are on board; have a clear vision and goal that can be well articulated. High-profile or charismatic leaders can lend significant support to a program, as was seen with the engagement of Anne Diamond, a high-profile broadcaster, in the UK "Reduce the Risks" campaign. |
| 5. | Develop a long-term strategy. | Short-term interventions are unlikely to lead to sustained change. Perseverance is essential so that the impact of any intervention is not lost as the next generation or cohort of parents comes through. |

| 6. | Ensure that the intervention is affordable. | Seeking out appropriate funding, for example through industry partnerships; making any individual intervention low-cost and affordable. |
|---|---|---|
| 7. | Monitor the results using sound evaluation methods. | This should include robust local and national surveillance, and may require measurement of proxy outcomes (such as uptake of safe sleeping advice) as well as the primary outcome (reduction in SIDS deaths). |

## Understanding Behavioral Change

Human behaviors are complex phenomena and understanding what underlies particular behaviors, and what influences any changes in behavior, is essential to the development and implementation of effective interventions that aim to change behavior. The field of behavioral change theory has sought to bring clarity to these issues. There are two components to behavioral change theory: first, the process of describing and understanding the behavior; and second, the process of understanding how that behavior might be changed and which elements are important in achieving and sustaining a change in behavior.

There are many behavioral change theories described in the literature, and many more theorists. These theories recognize the "work" required, or the significance of "personal investment" by the individual and their ability to make a change to their behavior; and the personal resources (knowledge, skills, and attitudes) required for behavioral change. They also acknowledge the influence of external factors, recognizing that having the personal resources (knowledge, skills, or behaviors) required for behavioral change does not always translate into a change in behavior: many smokers are well aware of the risks of smoking and yet continue to smoke. Later theories attempt to build on this, situating behavioral change within the wider environmental context, acknowledging the latter as an important factor in the individual's ability to change. Table 12.3 describes some of the most prominent theories applicable to health interventions.

Table 12.3: Behavioral change theories relevant to health interventions.

| Theory | Description |
|---|---|
| Learning theory | Learning theory is more commonly applied to child development and education; however, it is equally applicable to lifelong learning and to facilitating behavioral change in adulthood. Learning theory states that skills and behavior are learned gradually through experience, observation, and replication of that behavior or skill which builds competence over time. |

| Social learning theory | Social learning theory states that behavior is determined by the interaction between personal, environmental, and behavioral elements; therefore an individual's knowledge acquisition is based on the observation of others within social interactions and experiences, and on exposure through the media — for example, watching violence on television can incite violent behavior in individuals (13). |
|---|---|
| Social cognitive theory | Bandura further developed the social learning theory to identify self-efficacy (the extent to which the individual believes they can master a skill or have control over a situation) as a central factor in an individual's ability to change their behavior; he called this "social cognitive theory" in order to emphasize the role of cognition (understanding) in behavior development (14). |
| The theory of reasoned action | The theory of reasoned action aims to explain the relationship between attitude and behavior, by predicting behavior based on the attitudes and intentions of the individual, including instances where the individual considers the consequences of engaging in the behavior prior to doing so. This theory identifies that the strength of intention expressed by the individual influences the likelihood of them engaging in the behavior, but it also acknowledges that both personal attitudes and social or other external pressures influence intention (15). |
| The theory of planned behavior | The theory of planned behavior, which builds on the theory of reasoned action, states that an individual's attitude, the subjective norms (social acceptability of a behavior in a given community), and perceived behavioral control (self-efficacy) towards the behavior all influence behavioral intention and actual performance of the behavior. This theory acknowledges that the individual is not always in control of all the factors that affect behavior performance. This means that actual behavior performance is proportional to the amount of control the individual has and the strength of their intention to perform the behavior (16). This theory incorporates self-efficacy as an important element, recognizing that behavior is strongly influenced by an individual's confidence in their ability to perform a task, whether that be stopping smoking or believing they are able to breastfeed. This theory offers a more comprehensive explanation of behavioral change and acknowledges that both personal (internal) and external factors influence the success or failure in changing behavior. This theory is often used to underpin behavior change programs in health. |

| Transtheoretical or stages of change model | This is a combination of various behavioral change theories and offers a five-step process model for behavioral change. The process involves pre-contemplation, contemplation, preparation for action, action, and maintenance. An individual will move between these stages, ideally progressively; however, individuals may regress to an earlier stage depending on internal (self-efficacy) or external factors that may influence this trajectory. Once the desired behavioral change has been achieved, maintenance is the goal but relapse to a previous stage can occur (17). However, Lumley et al. (18) noted that data from one research study (19) and a systematic review (20) suggest that the stages of change model may not apply in pregnancy, and that stage changes in early pregnancy are not sustained (18). |
| --- | --- |

To summarize, individuals learn and acquire knowledge through observation of others, personal experience, and social interaction. Replication of that skill or behavior, and the feedback — either positive or negative — that the individual receives for performing a skill or engaging in a particular behavior, reinforce the experience of learning for that individual. In addition, internal resources such as self-belief — based on previous experience and learning, perceived control over a situation, and desire (intention and motivation) to change — and external factors such as social norms (peer pressure and community norms) and environmental factors will influence how the individual approaches, and is able to engage in, changing their behavior and maintaining that change in the long term.

## Challenges with motivating behavioral change

Having an understanding of the complexity of human behavior and the challenges of achieving behavioral change should be the foundation for behavioral change interventions. However, the theoretical basis of an intervention is not always explicit. In a systematic review of interventions (18), those with explicit theoretical foundations were reported to be more successful than those that did not report a specific theoretical approach.

Interventions need to be "relatable" to the "target" group. Interventions that are not perceived as relevant to the individual, do not meet the immediate needs of the participant, or fail to identify competing priorities for the individual are unlikely to be successful or to result in a sustained behavioral change (21, 22). Interventions that meet the perceived need of, or are perceived to be beneficial to, the individual, or that occur where individuals are motivated to change are more likely to be successful (23, 24).

The method of participation can also be significant. Participants who are "compelled" to attend a program may feel stigmatized and marginalized further by being identified as a "target" or "at risk" population. Where a participant's financial support or housing provision are dependent on attendance, the motivation or pressure to attend and engage is external and therefore not likely to be sustained or considered relevant by the participant (25). Some programs may experience high rates of attrition where the nature of an intervention is intensive, or where it is viewed as intrusive or authoritarian; or they may experience non-compliance when the intervention is perceived as ineffective.

The relationship between the provider and the recipient has also been identified as a significant factor that can impact on the success of an intervention. A systematic review by Petosa and Smith (26) found that peer mentoring was successful and cost-effective in a wide range of behavioral change programs in health settings, as well as being effective with diverse, disadvantaged, and hard-to-reach populations. Similarly, Anderson et al. (27) found that using peer counsellors to support low-income Latina mothers to breastfeed increased initiation and duration of breastfeeding compared to the control group receiving usual breastfeeding support offered by maternity professionals. Olds et al. (28) stated that the success of the Family Nurse intervention in the US was dependent upon the knowledge and skills of the trained provider. Based on this evidence, it seems likely that different types of interventions will require different approaches and will need to be delivered by suitably prepared providers; the "qualification" of the provider will be determined by the intervention, as well as by the acceptability to the participants.

Behavioral change interventions vary in nature, from mass public health campaigns to targeted population and individually tailored single or complex multimodal interventions. Mass campaigns aimed to change behavior, such as the "Back to Sleep" campaigns in the early 1990s, were successful due to the clear and simple message being delivered. However, little personal sacrifice was required of parents to change the sleep position of the infant. It is far more challenging to change the smoking behavior of pregnant women who enjoy smoking, especially when smoking is intertwined with their identity and with peer group social activity, and when it is accepted as the norm within their local community (29). Despite awareness of the harm of smoking during pregnancy and after birth, translating knowledge of harm into stopping smoking is much more complicated and requires personal motivation and sacrifice.

## Current Approaches and Evidence of Effectiveness

In a systematic review of infant safe sleep interventions, Salm Ward and Balfour identified 29 papers that reported on intervention results for an intervention or educational program to increase the safety of the infant sleep environment (30). The majority of studies identified by Salm Ward and Balfour were based on education of families and carers of newborn infants; there were seven studies that reported on a direct intervention, such as the provision of cribs or infant blankets. One of the challenges in evaluating the effectiveness of any prevention effort is that the low overall rates of SIDS mean that it is unlikely that any but the largest national interventions will be able to demonstrate any impact on the primary outcome of reducing SIDS. Most intervention studies therefore rely on demonstrating impacts on proxy measures such as knowledge of safe sleep messages. The majority of the studies in the systematic review mentioned above measured outcomes by self-report questionnaires, with only a small number carrying out direct observation of safe sleep practices.

The systematic review by Salm Ward and Balfour was able to demonstrate improvements in knowledge of safe sleep messages in 9 out of 11 studies (30). However, lower rates of change in actual safe sleep practices were observed, with only 12 out of 20 studies demonstrating improvements in intention to practice, or actual use of, supine sleeping; 5 out of 12 studies showing improvements in planned or reported sleep location; 4 out of 10 reported improvements in relation to unsafe items in the crib; and only 1 out of 7 studies reporting an improvement in smoking-related behavior, with a reported decrease in bed sharing among smoking mothers post-intervention.

These findings are important in highlighting the current paucity of evidence around the effectiveness of preventive interventions. It is pertinent that the majority of intervention studies have been based on education of parents, with very few incorporating more direct interventions designed to modify the environment. As highlighted in the sections above, education-based strategies may be the least effective public health tools in comparison to those based on empowerment, environmental modification, or enforcement. This may be particularly important in relation to the population groups most at risk of SIDS. In a commentary on the high levels of bed sharing among smoking mothers in the Māori population in New Zealand, Abel and Tipene-Leach (31) highlighted that "[t]he classic approach to preventing SIDS deaths has been to define the risk factors, devise the appropriate messages and then design and implement an information-sharing health promotion campaign. Indeed, this has worked very well in mainly middle class, white communities in which advice to change from the prone to the back sleeping position was associated with a huge decrease in post-neonatal death in the 1990s. However, it has not been as effective amongst Māori, whose infants are now significantly over-represented" (p. 87).

In the following sections, we will examine some of the evidence around different preventive approaches for SIDS based on education or empowerment, and those based on engineering, environmental modification, and enforcement. We finish the chapter with a consideration of combined strategies to influence behavioral change in relation to smoking in pregnancy.

## Approaches Based on Education or Empowerment

### Public health campaigns

The first mass public health campaigns to promote supine sleeping appeared in the late 1980s and early 1990s, after two decades of high sudden infant death rates in industrialized countries, a period that has been described as a "SIDS pandemic" (32). During this time it was common practice for infants to be slept in the prone position, ostensibly to avoid aspiration of vomit; indeed, this practice was recommended. By the mid-1980s, however, a growing evidence base from observational studies linked prone sleeping to SIDS, and by 1991 the UK, Australia, and New Zealand all introduced campaigns to encourage parents to sleep infants supine, following earlier examples in countries such as the Netherlands and Norway (1).

## "Back to Sleep"

The UK's campaign became known as "Back to Sleep" and was led by the Department of Health in conjunction with the Foundation of the Study for Infant Deaths (FSID, now known as The Lullaby Trust). The primary message was initially not to sleep infants prone; this was later revised to recommend the supine position exclusively, after research showed side positioning to be unstable, leading some infants to roll prone (6). Other recommendations included avoidance of smoking and not allowing infants to overheat, and Australia and New Zealand also recommended breastfeeding in their initial campaigns (1). The US launched their "Back to Sleep" (now known as "Safe to Sleep") campaign in 1994, one of the last countries with high SIDS rates to do so. Campaign activities consisted of mass mail-outs of information to professionals, as well as public service announcements on the radio and television (33).

The various "Back to Sleep" campaigns were undeniably successful in bringing about a rapid and marked decline in rate of SIDS, but what made them so successful? Primarily, it is in the strength of the intervention itself, of sleeping infants supine. The number of parents sleeping their infant prone declined dramatically in line with the fall in SIDS rates, suggesting the intervention was responsible for the drop rather than random cyclic fluctuations among SIDS deaths (34). Second, the campaigns revolved around one central message that was relatively easy to understand and simple to implement: avoid sleeping your infant on his or her front. Further recommendations were added later — for example, the use of a firm, flat surface and avoiding the use of soft bedding in the US in 1996 (33) — but the simplicity and clarity of "Back to Sleep" as a slogan might have helped parents to understand the conveyed action. Third, the involvement of the media and influential spokespeople such as Anne Diamond (in the UK) and Tipper Gore (wife of then-Vice President Al Gore in the US) heightened public awareness and highlighted emotive case studies, which helped to increase the effectiveness of a campaign by conveying that no infants are "immune" and all are at risk (35). Last, Van Wouwe and Hirasing (32) conclude that universal child healthcare is an important component of the success of the campaigns, attributing the Netherlands' rapid and steep decline following their campaign to a nationwide healthcare system that allows for close surveillance and timely intervention by professionals. This may be seen in contrast to countries like the US, which lacks universal healthcare and continues to have one of the highest rates of sudden infant death worldwide (36).

Most countries have since moved away from "Back to Sleep" as a primary campaign message, as other risk factors have taken over from prone sleeping in terms of prevalence and impact on SIDS rates. SIDS is now most likely to occur in deprived families, with infants often found supine and in bed-sharing situations, particularly in hazardous circumstances (6). However, non-recommended infant sleep practices do occur on a wider level: one recent study that video-recorded infant sleep environments at 1, 3 and 6 months found that 10-21% of infants were slept on a non-recommended surface, 14-33% were placed non-supine, and 87-93% had loose or soft bedding or other items nearby (37). This indicates a continuing need for safer sleep education and guidance. In their most recent recommendations, the American Academy of Pediatrics noted the incidence of "sleep-related deaths" and expanded their guidelines to move away from focusing only on SIDS to focus on a safe sleep environment that can reduce the risk of all sleep-related infant deaths, including SIDS (38).

## Baby Essentials Online

In an attempt to extend the reach of educational interventions, the internet offers a convenient and cost-effective platform. One such intervention, "Baby Essentials Online" (39), was launched as a national campaign in New Zealand. This e-learning tool, originally prepared for professionals, aimed to increase parental awareness of a safe sleep environment for all infants. The tool was culturally inclusive, infant-focused, and aimed to encourage vulnerable parents to gain knowledge and confidence, and to engage in conversations with others about safe sleeping conditions for infants. The intervention was promoted and supported by an existing network of Safe Sleep Champions from the District Health Boards; a monitoring template gathered data about internet usage of the tool; and a pre- & post-activity test gauged individuals' reported learning outcomes. Increased confidence was noted for participants who engaged with the material for longer and for populations identified as having increased risk for SIDS. The intervention cost was NZ$1.11 per completed session. This demonstrates that a national online education intervention can be successful and cost-effective in delivering a consistent safe sleep message, with broad reach and large-scale participation. Focused educational interventions that engage adolescents might yield benefits for their health, potentially preventing engagement with unhealthy behaviors and in reducing SIDS risks for young parents. An interactive, culturally sensitive health education program that aimed to raise awareness of the health risks related to SIDS with adolescent students was delivered across inner-city schools in New Jersey, USA (40). Evaluation found that students who participated in the program demonstrated increased awareness of health risks related to SIDS compared with same-grade students and a convenience sample of parents who were tested prior to the commencement of the school-based program.

"Back to Sleep" was the last major safer sleeping campaign to run in the UK. In 2015 The Lullaby Trust renewed campaigning efforts with the development of Safer Sleep Week: an annual week-long campaign held every March. The aim was to increase the reach and impact of safer sleep advice for parents, professionals, and anyone involved in the care of an infant. Activities during Safer Sleep Week include national and locally targeted press releases, dissemination of toolkits for displays at health and children's centers, fundraising events, and educational talks for professionals. Moon, Hauck, and Colson highlight the need for such multistranded activity, which supports parents and professionals to form their own rationale for safer sleep, rather than reliance on a catchy "soundbite" that may not convey enough information to encourage behavioral change (35).

Awareness weeks (as well as days and months) are a relatively cost-effective and easy way to educate the public on a specific issue compared to larger mainstream campaigns (41). They are a widely used tactic: the National Health Service (NHS) in England notes more than 50 awareness campaigns for 2016-17 (42), but there are dozens more that take place every year, from Dementia Awareness Week to World Asthma Day. Safer Sleep Week is one of several related to SIDS and infant mortality, including Pregnancy and Infant Loss Awareness Day (15 October), Baby Loss Awareness Week (9-15 October), and, in the USA, SIDS Awareness Month (October).

Despite the widespread use of such campaigns, there are few data on their effectiveness, as only a minority of published papers on awareness campaigns include an impact evaluation (43). Evaluation of an awareness campaign can be costly, which negates the cost-saving benefits of shorter-term campaigns, and traditional methods such as pre-post surveys are not always possible (41). Where awareness campaigns have been evaluated, analysis of webpage visits, internet searches on the issue, and engagement through social media platforms such as Twitter have found that they have been successful in raising awareness through increased traffic (41, 43). However, Purtle and Roman point out that despite achieving their aim of increased awareness, it is not clear whether these measures translate into longer-term, meaningful behavioral change (43). To try to achieve this, it is recommended that successful awareness-raising campaigns include specific and clearly constructed aims and methods; seek to bring about impact on multiple levels and domains, including media coverage and political advocacy; and conduct a transparent evaluation of cost-effectiveness of the campaign (43).

Safer Sleep Week appears to be successfully raising awareness of ways to reduce the risk of SIDS. In 2017 it reached 3.6 million Twitter users, which was three times the number reached in the inaugural 2015 campaign of 1.2 million.[1] There was five times the amount of media coverage in 2017 compared to 2015, including broadcast and print, and a number of high-profile MPs were engaged through their websites and

---

1   These figures come from unpublished data produced by The Lullaby Trust, 2017.

Twitter, including the English Health Minister, who retweeted the campaign messaging. The 2017 campaign also saw targeted use of posters in infant-changing facilities as well as an animation in doctors' surgeries. This increasing engagement would suggest that Safer Sleep Week has been effective in raising awareness thus far, but further evaluation is required to assess its long-term impact and conversion to behavioral change.

## Targeted support for high-risk families

The debate of universal provision versus targeted services is contentious. Significant differences exist in maternal and child health service provision between high-income countries, with models ranging from universal services free at the point of access to insurance-based provision requiring a financial contribution. The identification of specific populations labeled "at risk" or "in need" of service interventions is problematic. At best, targeted service provision critically focuses resources and supports on the more vulnerable sections of society; at worst these populations are labeled, marginalized, and stigmatized.

Young and disadvantaged mothers are commonly grouped together and viewed as a potential high-risk group, lacking in parenting skills and requiring targeted intervention and monitoring. Mothers in these groups are often perceived as being resistant to changing their behavior or infant care practices. There are challenges for professionals in understanding and identifying what motivates individuals in different groups; what influences behavioral change in different populations; and which interventions work and are relevant and acceptable to different population groups. The next section presents several interventions that demonstrate varying degrees of success in improving outcomes for groups identified as being at increased risk for experiencing sudden unexpected death in infancy.

### Parenting support interventions

Educational interventions that have been evaluated as successful in modifying parental behavior include the Family-Nurse Partnership (FNP) model that originates from the USA (28). This is a targeted, intensive home visiting program for vulnerable, young, first-time parents, delivered between early pregnancy and the child's second birthday. The model has been hailed as a success in the USA and was piloted in the UK. A recent randomized controlled trial to evaluate the impact of the pilot identified some minor benefits such as improvements in early child development and increased self-efficacy of the mothers (44). However, there was no impact on the primary outcome measures, including rates of smoking, reduction in preterm births or low birth weight infants, pregnancy intervals, or rates of emergency attendances or admissions to hospital. The relative success of the FNP in the USA compared to the UK may be due to the absence of universally available services that support parents. In the UK, health and parenting services are universally available and therefore parents may feel marginalized by being referred to a more intensive service. Ethically, there is little justification for providing an expensive, targeted service when no discernible benefit is identified; however, there may be hidden benefits that are not well captured in the pre-defined outcome measures of a randomized controlled trial.

A study evaluating a parent support program, using home visits and supported parent groups with young disadvantaged parents in an area of Sydney, Australia, describes the experiences of staff and identifies important components that contributed to program success (23). The program aimed to enhance parenting skills and link families to additional services. Focus groups with staff identified two key themes that contributed to the success of the program; "connecting" and "facilitating learning". "Connecting" with the young mothers reflected the development of a relationship as a key component, building trust between the worker and young women in order to move to "facilitating learning". Learning was facilitated through using behavior role modeling through interactions with children, other mothers, and workers; such modeling was reported as the most effective way to facilitate social and parenting skill development and formal and informal education sessions. Formal education sessions were offered but the most effective sessions were informal and led by issues raised by the mothers themselves, allowing the focus for education to be centered on their perceived needs and priorities, which encouraged continued engagement with the program. This participant-centered intervention achieved its objectives of encouraging self-reliant mothers confident to parent their children. Staff reported that the mothers left the program when they felt ready, but there was an open-door policy for the mothers should they require support in the future. This intervention acknowledges that parenting happens within the context of other priorities for parents living in poverty, with low income and poor resources. Dealing with these issues, as part of a parenting program, promotes resilience and supports parents to provide a safe and nurturing environment for their children.

### Support for families who have experienced a previous unexpected infant death

Siblings born subsequently to an infant who died of SIDS carry an increased risk of sudden infant death, from both explained and unexplained causes (45). Families in which an infant dies of SIDS are more likely to have significant risk factors, including smoking, being a younger mother of higher parity, and a lack of income, which are likely to remain present for subsequent children (46). These factors, combined with strong feelings of anxiety at the prospect of a new infant (47), mean that families bereaved by SIDS constitute a vulnerable group who are in need of support and could benefit from targeted preventative interventions.

The Care of the Next Infant (CONI) program was developed in the late 1980s with financial support from the Foundation for the Study of Infant Deaths. The aim was to provide multidisciplinary care to families expecting a new infant following

SIDS. Co-ordinated on a local level, usually by health visitors, the scheme is available to approximately 90% of England and Wales and 100% of Northern Ireland and is now incorporated into The Lullaby Trust's wider services for bereaved parents (48). Core elements of the scheme are frequent home visits from a specialist health visitor; weekly weigh-ins to plot development on a growth chart; provision of an apnea monitor, room thermometer, symptom diary, and a Baby Check guide (see below); and, where available, fast-track access to acute pediatric care. The program is available for families for up to six months after their infant is born, or until two months after the age at which their previous infant died, whichever is longer. The extended families of SIDS infants are eligible for support under the CONI Plus scheme, which also covers families whose infant died suddenly of causes other than SIDS or whose infant has suffered an apparent life-threatening event (ALTE). CONI has been recommended by the Department of Health as part of their strategy to prevent sudden unexpected death in infancy (49).

A 2011 analysis of data from families enrolled in the CONI scheme confirmed that they were a group faced with an over-representation of risk factors: parents were twice as likely to smoke and five times more likely to be unemployed than national averages, and had a higher number of births (48). Compared to national averages, infants supported through CONI were twice as likely to be of low birth weight, were 50% more likely to be born prematurely, and were only half as likely to be breastfed.

The CONI program is not so much an intervention as a package of care to support vulnerable families at a most difficult time, but each component of the CONI scheme can also be evaluated for effectiveness. Intensive home visiting by healthcare professionals has been associated with a reduced prevalence of sudden infant death in high-risk families (50). Health visitors are well placed to carry out these visits, as they can provide continuity of care and have the skills to be able to "befriend" the bereaved family, listen to their worries, develop strategies to help them, and identify causes for concern (51). Frequent home support can also aid parental bonding with the new infant during a time of high anxiety and stress, helping them to develop their relationship and create a stable long-term attachment. Poor postnatal weight gain is associated with an increased risk of SIDS (52); regular weigh-ins help to track growth and provide reassurance for parents. Room thermometers are provided as part of the CONI program, as overheating has long been known to be a risk factor for SIDS (53). The evidence base behind Baby Check can be found later in this chapter, and symptom diaries play a similar role of encouraging parents to identify changes in their infant and empowering them to contact help if they appear unwell.[2] It is only the movement or apnea monitors that are not well supported by an evidence base, as they have been shown in many studies not to have any impact on prevention of SIDS (54). Apnea monitors in the CONI program are distributed only

---

2   This information is sourced from unpublished data provided by The Lullaby Trust, 2017.

as a short-term tool to assuage parental anxiety while their infant sleeps, and parents are told that the monitor will not prevent death (48).

Deaths of infants enrolled in the CONI scheme have occurred. In one sample of 6,373 infants, 41 died unexpectedly, of which 18 were repeat SIDS (6.43 per 1,000) (55), and in a later study there were 6 unexpected deaths in CONI Plus, out of a sample of 6,487 (2.15 per 1,000) (56). These rates are much higher than national averages; however, as families who have already suffered a SIDS death have an elevated risk compared to that of the general population (46), this measure cannot accurately be used as an evaluation of the effectiveness of the CONI program, and at present there is limited direct evidence to support such targeted campaigns.

## Peer support programs

### Little Lullaby

As mentioned earlier in the chapter, interventions that are tailored for a specific community are more likely to be effective and sustainable, particularly if the community is engaged in design and implementation. However, there is currently very little research published on community involvement using peer educators in SIDS risk-reduction strategies. One community of particular interest is young parents — that is, those aged under 20. Young parents, particularly young mothers, have been consistently associated with an increased risk of SIDS in their children (57).

Little Lullaby is a Big Lottery-funded project aimed at empowering young parents to reduce their risk of SIDS through peer support and education.[3] Originally known as Bubbalicious, Little Lullaby was developed by The Lullaby Trust and launched in 2009. The program deploys the skills of specially trained young parents known as Little Lullaby Ambassadors, who have completed a nationally accredited training course, in order to raise awareness of SIDS and deliver safer sleep advice. Ambassadors create content such as blogs and videos for the Little Lullaby website and linked social media accounts, and also deliver peer-to-peer educational workshops. Young parents can also receive peer support by registering as a member of the website's forum to chat to other young parents about parenting, as well as other issues pertinent to young parents, such as education and housing.

Between 2013 and 2016, Little Lullaby exceeded its targets to reach over 80,000 young parents. Most of these were unique online users, including 900 registered members of the website. The length of time users stayed on the website increased by over 50% over that period, indicating that users were engaging with the materials. Outreach activities engaged with 934 young parents, of which 18 young parents completed Ambassador training (of 27 who enrolled) and led educational workshops reaching 281 young parents and 190 professionals. A further 184 professionals attended

---

3   See www.littlelullaby.org.uk for more information.

workshops led by Little Lullaby staff and more than 12,000 young parents were reached by professionals who had attended safer sleep training.[4]

An independent evaluation of Little Lullaby was conducted in 2016 (58). The evaluation highlighted raised awareness of SIDS among young parents, with 97% stating they had learnt something new about safer sleep, and 60% stating they would change their behavior. The majority of the remaining 40% said they already followed the advice. In young mothers, knowledge does not necessarily translate into safer sleep practice. Nevertheless, young parents interviewed as part of the evaluation indicated that they would change their infant sleep routine, including positioning and use of blankets and cot bumpers, and importantly were highly motivated to encourage others to do the same. Caraballo and colleagues raise the issue of grandmothers as a potential source of conflicting safer sleep advice that can influence young parents' decision making (57). The Little Lullaby evaluation found young parents challenging older generations, feeling reassured by the evidence-based information they received, and sharing materials with family members (58). This feeling of empowerment was directly attributed to the model of peer education, with respondents praising Little Lullaby for presenting information in a non-judgemental and supportive way. In addition, over 99% of professionals attending Little Lullaby training felt better equipped to talk to young parents about SIDS, and 91% said they would change their practice. Respondents indicated that Little Lullaby equipped them to have difficult conversations with young parents and to recognize that they may have underestimated young parents' capacity for engaging with SIDS research.

A key part of Little Lullaby's success in engaging with young parents has been its digital communication strategy. Involving young parents in the design of the website and the creation of their own content, such as blogs and videos, has created an informative environment that validates young parents as experts in their own right. As with other interventions targeting young people, social media platforms are becoming increasingly important: videos and quotes from young parents feature heavily on Facebook and Twitter feeds, and weekly Instagram "takeovers" are staged, where young parents post content about their lives and their own personal parenting tips.

## Approaches based on Engineering, Environmental Modification, and Enforcement

A wide range of approaches incorporating engineering and environmental modification have been developed to facilitate the provision of safe sleep environments for infants. These include the provision of equipment such as sleeping bags and safe cribs/bassinettes for infants, and also tools to support parents in the early recognition of illness. The evidence base for some of these will be examined below.

---

4   This information comes from an internal report from Little Lullaby, 2017.

There is some limited evidence of the effectiveness of enforcement of guidelines among professionals (for example, through audit/clinical governance). While it may be relatively easy to show through audits that professionals are giving out safe sleep messages, the actual impact of these on parenting behavior is less clearly established. So, for example, while the safe sleep messages in the UK are universally given out to new parents by midwives and health visitors, and are included in each child's personal child health record, evidence suggests that this does not always translate to retention and implementation of safe sleep practices among high-risk groups (59).

While many countries have adopted legislation and taxation measures to reduce cigarette uptake and use, to date, there have been no legislative measures of which we are aware that targets any parental behaviors in relation to their infants' safety. Individual parents may face criminal prosecution when there is evidence of sustained or severe neglect or abuse contributing to their child's death. Specifically, in the UK under the *Children and Young Persons Act 1933*, a person may be convicted of neglect if an infant dies of suffocation while co-sleeping with an adult deemed to be under the influence of alcohol (60). While such provisions exist in many countries where there is clear evidence of abuse or neglect contributing to a child's death, it is questionable whether wider criminalization of common parental practices, such as smoking or consuming alcohol or drugs, is currently appropriate or in the public interest. These are areas which should prompt ongoing public and political debate.

## Providing safe sleep environments

### Sleeping bags

Thick bedding and bedding that can cover an infant's head have been shown to be risk factors for SIDS (61). In a German study, the use of a duvet doubled the risk of SIDS compared to infants sleeping with a sleeping bag or light cotton blanket (62). However, the evidence for using sleeping bags as a preventive measure is limited. One study from the Netherlands showed a protective effect of using cotton sleeping sacks (63). Another study from the UK showed that infant sleeping bags were used more commonly in control infants than in those who died of SIDS, but this was not significant on multivariate analysis (64).

If infant sleeping bags are to be promoted as a preventive measure for SIDS, it is important that any potential risks associated with them are identified. In a study of safety reports to the Consumer Product Safety Commission in the USA, McDonnell and Moon identified 10 deaths in infants using infant sleeping bags ("wearable blankets" or "swaddle wraps") over an eight-year period (65). The authors reported that during that time, over 5 million swaddle wraps had been sold in the USA, and they pointed out that in nearly all of the deaths, other hazards were identified in the sleep environment.

The risks associated with prone sleeping and thick or loose bedding are such that, intuitively at least, infant sleeping bags carry great potential for prevention. As highlighted by Carpenter et al. (61), "risk of SIDS might be substantially reduced by putting infants to sleep supine with no bedding other than a jumper suit ... or in a well fitting cotton or acrylic sleeping bag of no more than 2-tog" (p. 189-90). However, we are not aware of any studies to date that have prospectively assessed the value of providing, or using, infant sleeping bags as a SIDS prevention measure.

## Wahakura/Pēpi-Pods®

The Pēpi-Pod® program in New Zealand had its origins in developing the use of a hand-woven Wahakura, which was being promoted in Māori communities to provide a safe infant sleep space for vulnerable infants to reduce the risk of SIDS. The Wahakura could be taken into the parents' bed, but offered a discrete safe space for the infant to sleep which reduced the risks associated with parent-infant bed sharing (66). The motivation for developing these Wahakura was a recognition of continuing high SIDS rates among the Māori population, among whom it was recognized that bed sharing was a culturally valued behavior and common practice. This left health workers with the challenge of finding a safer sleep environment that was both culturally acceptable and practical (31). The Wahakura provided this, but the high costs of production meant that it was not sustainable as a large-scale preventive effort. The Pēpi-Pod®, made from the bottom section of a plastic clothes container and provided along with a simple mattress, a sheet/merino blanket set, and safer sleep instructions, proved a cheap and sustainable alternative (31).

The Christchurch earthquakes expedited the introduction of the Pēpi-Pod® to provide portable sleep spaces (PSS) for infants in order to prevent the escalation of infants sleeping in potentially hazardous environments. This initial PSS intervention was evaluated well, and the program was extended to vulnerable families. PSS were distributed to vulnerable families accompanied by safe sleep education. Distributors were trained to deliver safe sleep messages and to show parents how to set up and use the PSS. PSS were distributed to infants less than 4 weeks old who had identified risk factors; the majority of PSS were distributed to Māori families. The PSS were acceptable to parents and were often used when the infant was in the parental bed. Parents reported valuing the safety aspect, convenience, and facilitation of breastfeeding and settling, as infants were in close proximity to their mother. Use of the PSS continued, in most cases, until the infant got too big to fit into the PSS, usually around 4 to 5 months of age. Adherence to safe sleep practices was high. During the period of the intervention, infant mortality (all causes) fell significantly from 2.4 per 1,000 live births in 2011 to 1.9 in 2014, and from 4.5 to 3.5 per 1,000 live birth for Māori (67).

The New Zealand portable sleep space program proved a very successful and popular intervention, accepted and used by mothers and communities; safe sleep messages are translating into behavioral change and there is effective "word of mouth" sharing of safe sleep messages. Similarly, there are a number of crib distribution programs in the USA. Hauck and colleagues evaluated Bedtime Basics for Babies (BBB) (68). Safe sleep knowledge and practice in vulnerable families were examined before and after the distribution of a Safe Sleep Kit. The kit included educational materials about reducing the risk of SIDS and encouraging breastfeeding; a free crib, plus crib sheet; a wearable blanket; and a pacifier. Findings revealed that if families had not received a crib, 38% of infants would be sharing a bed with either the parent or another person, and 4% would use a car seat for sleep. Pre- and post-intervention tests revealed improved parental knowledge of recommended sleep position from 76% to 94%; intended use of supine position increased from 84% to 87%; 38% of parents reported that they had bed shared the night before receipt of the crib, reducing to 16% after the intervention. Additionally, 90% reported that the infant slept in a crib after the intervention, compared with 51% pre-intervention. The evaluation noted minimal effects for breastfeeding or pacifier use, however.

The Bedtime Basics for Babies intervention was effective in improving parental knowledge and behavior in a large, vulnerable population and provided a safe sleep environment for the infants. Both the Pēpi-Pod® and crib distribution programs have been running for a number of years, possibly contributing to their success, as embedded and familiar interventions. Both report positive impact in reducing the risks for infants living in disadvantaged families. These interventions have evaluated well, and offer a real solution to the ongoing issues in reaching vulnerable families with an acceptable solution to resolve continued exposure to hazardous sleep environments for their infants.

### Baby boxes

Effective interventions can incorporate culture and tradition as a way of encouraging parental behavioral change, such as the distribution of "baby boxes", a longstanding tradition in Finland since 1938 (69). A cardboard box, intended to be repurposed as a bed, contains a mattress and fitted sheet, as well as supplies and clothing, and is given to every woman during her first pregnancy. Although these boxes were introduced prior to the SIDS "pandemic" of the 1970s and 1980s, and were not related in any way to SIDS prevention, the low infant mortality rate seen in Finland (70) has prompted other countries to take note.

In recent years a number of copy-cat cardboard baby box schemes have been set up in other countries, including the USA, Scotland, and England. Some are free interventions distributed by the healthcare system, as in Finland, such as pilot schemes in two regions of Scotland (71), in London (72), and in Alaska (73). The Scottish baby box is supported by the Scottish Government and is designed to reduce health inequality. These pilots have not focused on the box as a safe sleep tool but rather as part of wider strategies to reduce health inequalities. In contrast, some NHS trusts and local authorities are now offering free boxes and products to all newly delivered mothers as a safe sleep intervention. Mothers can only receive the box if they have participated in a video-based safer sleep training program. It is not clear how these schemes are being evaluated and whether data on the use of the box as a sleeping space are being systematically collected across the agencies which are participating. The industry in cardboard boxes has boomed in recent years and there are many other companies selling baby boxes either directly to the public or through specific retailers.

Despite their popularity, and in contrast to the Pēpi-Pod® and Wahakura used in New Zealand, the evidence base for these baby boxes is not straightforward. The box itself, as a separate sleep space with a firm and flat base, could be considered a safer space for infants to sleep, particularly if the alternative is the parental bed. While Finland's infant mortality rate reduced dramatically following the introduction of these boxes in the late 1930s, there is no evidence that the baby boxes themselves were instrumental in this reduction. Instead, it has been suggested that the introduction of free universal maternity care in the 1940s; improvements in healthcare, nutrition, and hygiene; and the requirement for mothers to attend antenatal care in order to receive a baby box are the real reasons for the observed decline in infant mortality (74, 75). There is an urgent need for further research on the value of the cardboard baby box as a SIDS risk-reduction strategy.

## Tools to facilitate recognition of illness

### Baby Check

A significant number of infants who die suddenly and unexpectedly, for either explained or unexplained reasons, show signs and symptoms of illness in the immediate 24 hours before death (76). They are also more likely to present at doctors' surgeries or to be admitted to hospital in the weeks leading to death (77). Both parents and professionals are liable to miss signs of serious illness, despite the high anxiety that symptoms such as fever can invoke in parents (78). A system that accurately assesses seriousness of illness can support concerned parents and enable professionals to administer appropriate treatment, and may help to prevent sudden infant death.

Baby Check is a scoring system that grades the severity of 19 signs and symptoms of illness (Table 12.4). The higher the score, the more serious the illness is (79). Early versions included a professional and a parent tool, but Baby Check is now designed primarily to be used at home to help parents understand whether they need to seek medical attention or not, and is not intended to replace parental judgement or diagnose specific conditions or diseases (80, 81).[5]

---

5   Baby Check exists as a simple illustrated booklet and is available as a downloadable app: (https://play.google.com/store/apps/details?id=com.sgs_lab.babycheck&hl=en_GB).

Table 12.4: Baby Check symptoms and scoring. (Authors' own work.)

| Symptom | Score |
|---|---|
| If your baby has an unusual cry | 2 |
| In the last 24 hours:<br>• If your baby has taken a little less fluid than usual; or<br>• If your baby has taken about half as much fluid as usual; or<br>• If your baby has taken very little fluid | 3<br>4<br>9 |
| If your baby has vomited at least half the feed after every one of the last three feeds | 4 |
| If your baby has had green vomit | 13 |
| If your baby has passed less urine than usual | 3 |
| If there has been a large amount of obvious blood in your baby's nappy (not just a streak on the stool) | 11 |
| If your baby has been drowsy and less alert than usual when awake score as follows:<br>• Occasionally drowsy; or<br>• Drowsy most of the time | 3<br>5 |
| If your baby seems more floppy than usual | 4 |
| If your baby is watching you less than usual | 4 |
| If your baby is responding less than usual to what is going on around | 5 |
| If a baby has breathing difficulty the lower chest and upper tummy will dip in with each breath. This is called "indrawing".<br>• If there is indrawing just visible with each breath; or<br>• If there is obvious or deep indrawing with each breath | 4<br>15 |
| • If your baby's body is much paler than usual; or<br>• If your baby has had an episode of going very pale at any time during the last 24 hours | 3<br>3 |
| If your baby is wheezing when breathing out | 3 |
| If your baby's nails are blue | 3 |
| Gently squeeze his or her big toe to make it white:<br>• If your baby's toe was completely white before the squeeze<br>• If your baby's toe color does not return within three seconds | 3<br>3 |
| • If your baby has a rash which covers a large part of the body; or<br>• If your baby has a rash which is raw or weeping and is bigger than the shaded area shown | 4<br>4 |

| If there is a bulge in the groin or scrotum which gets bigger with crying | 13 |
|---|---|
| • In a baby below 3 months, if the temperature is 38.0 °C or more<br>• In a baby above 3 months, if the temperature is 39.0 °C or more | 4<br>4 |
| If your baby has cried during the checks (more than a little grizzle) | 3 |

| What the total score means | |
|---|---|
| 0 to 7 | Your baby is only a little unwell, and medical attention should not be necessary. |
| 8 to 12 | Your baby is unwell, but is unlikely to be seriously ill. You may want advice from your doctor, health visitor or midwife. |
| 13 to 19 | Your baby is ill. Contact your doctor and arrange for your baby to be seen. |
| 20+ | Your baby may be seriously ill and should be seen by a doctor straight away. |

The signs and symptoms chosen for Baby Check were based on a study of 1,007 infants which, when scored in combination, were found to most accurately assess severity of illness in terms of specificity and sensitivity (79). They include fluid intake, circulation, level of alertness, temperature, and degree of intercostal recession, which are described in Baby Check in everyday language to make it easier for parental use. In early field trials mothers found the Baby Check scoring system to be both easy to use and useful. Comparing mothers' scores to those of nurses, 70% were able to use the system relatively competently to assess the severity of their infant's illness (81). Acceptability of Baby Check among professionals was also found to be high: 92% of GPs found that Baby Check gave an accurate assessment of infants' health, 84% found it useful, and 94% thought it would be useful for mothers (80).

In a retrospective application of Baby Check to a large UK dataset, Ward Platt and colleagues found that over a fifth of infants who died of SIDS were identifiably unwell in the 24 hours before death (76). A small proportion of these infants exhibited signs of severe illness, which might have been prevented with recognition and appropriate action by parents or by professionals. There are many reasons this may occur: parents are good at recognizing when their infants are not well, but they are not as good at recognizing illness that may require medical help (76), and parenting books can be vague on when to seek help (81). Should parents decide to seek help, they may then lack confidence to challenge a healthcare professional who decides their infant's symptoms are not severe, particularly if they are a younger or disadvantaged parent who may have previously faced stigma from professionals. On the professionals' part, signs and symptoms common in serious illness also occur in milder illness (79), making it difficult for less experienced or less confident doctors or nurses to distinguish between infants in need of treatment and infants who can be sent home (76).

Baby Check can help to overcome these barriers, by either providing reassurance to parents that their infant is not seriously ill, as is most commonly the case, or by bolstering their decision to seek medical opinion. A qualitative study on parents from disadvantaged backgrounds found that they used Baby Check spontaneously and felt it was helpful. It reduced anxiety, and increased confidence in coping with illness, seeking medical advice, and communicating with doctors (82).

While there is evidence that Baby Check can improve parents' confidence in recognizing and responding to signs of illness in their infant, there is, to date, no robust evidence of its effectiveness as a strategy for reducing SIDS rates. However, compared to other interventions for modifiable risk factors, which rely on significant behavioral change, the use of Baby Check as a tool may be more amenable to sustained change.

## Combined strategies to influence behavioral change: Smoking cessation in pregnancy

Following the reductions in prone sleeping, maternal smoking is recognized as the next most important modifiable risk factor for SIDS (83). While smoking rates in the general populations of high-income countries have decreased steadily over the last 40 years, Lumley et al. identified that those in lower socioeconomic groups, those of lower educational achievement, those living in poverty or receiving state financial support, younger women, and those who are less psychologically resilient or more marginalized and unsupported were more likely to continue to smoke (18). These population groups are also those who are most at risk of SIDS (6). Fleming and Blair also found that as the prevalence of smoking during pregnancy decreased in the general population between 1984 and 2003 from 30% to 20%, the proportion of SIDS mothers who smoked during pregnancy increased from 50% to 80% (84). Thus strategies to reduce maternal smoking among these most vulnerable groups should be a priority for SIDS prevention.

While pregnancy is a potential motivator to stop smoking, a recent systematic review of smoking cessation interventions identified that only around 6% of pregnant women stop smoking and many of these are in the latter stages of pregnancy (18). Following the birth, up to 50% of mothers return to smoking within the first postnatal month, and by 12 months this is reported to be up to 80% (29, 85). A number of public health strategies have supported the reduction in smoking rates, such as legislation on smoke-free public places, increased taxation on tobacco, and the recent introduction of standardized plain packaging with larger health warnings for tobacco products. Strategies aimed at the individual to support smoking cessation include health education, counseling, home visits, telephone and internet help, nicotine replacement therapy (NRT), fetal growth feedback offered at the antenatal scan appointment, exercise interventions, financial incentives, and the use of e-cigarettes. These interventions can be used alone or in combination. Evaluating what works in these strategies, or isolating the most effective component in combination approaches, remains a challenge, and for many the evidence base for their effectiveness is weak.

Pregnancy offers an opportunity for making changes to unhealthy behaviors. Individuals may be motivated to seek help, and professional support is often available. The antenatal booking appointment is often the first opportunity for the clinician to identify behaviors that have an adverse effect on the health of the mother and fetus. Information on the impact on the health of the fetus, support for stopping or reducing smoking, referral to smoking cessation services, or prescription of pharmacotherapy may be offered. However, the motivation of the individual to change their behavior is a significant factor in their engagement with services and in any subsequent behavioral change. Smoking cessation during pregnancy is often motivated by external influences — nausea, concern for fetal health, and social pressure, for example. Women who have a strong desire (self-efficacy) to stop smoking in the long term, for the benefit of their infant and their own health, are likely to be more successful than those women who "suspend" smoking during pregnancy and either intend to smoke after pregnancy or unintentionally relapse due to low motivation to remain abstinent (13, 85).

A systematic review by Chamberlain et al. included 102 studies examining counseling, health education, feedback of fetal health status, social support, and exercise interventions to support smoking cessation during pregnancy (86). The authors reported that there was good evidence to support the use of counseling interventions compared with less intensive interventions or usual care for smoking cessation in pregnancy, with a clear effect of smoking abstinence between birth and five months postpartum. Evidence was inconclusive for educational material, health education groups, peer support, and feedback interventions, or where these were provided as a component of a multimodal intervention. Only one study reviewed an exercise intervention, but the effect was unclear.

In another systematic review, Baxter and colleagues reviewed 12 studies that included counseling, counseling plus educational information, smoke-free home programs, and motivational interviewing interventions (87). Only the motivational interview intervention demonstrated a significant reduction in smoke exposure within the home at three months post-birth, although the smoking rate had not decreased in either intervention or control group, and smoking rates increased in both groups at 6 months of age. The systematic review by Lumley and colleagues reviewed 72 trials investigating the outcomes of smoking cessation interventions on smoking rates and perinatal health outcomes (18). Interventions included cognitive behavior therapy, educational and motivational interviewing, and feedback of fetal health or measurement. The evidence was presented for the primary intervention in multimodal strategies and the authors concluded overall that smoking cessation interventions reduce the proportion of women who continue to smoke in late pregnancy and improve outcomes for infants, reducing the number of low birth weight and preterm births (18).

## Telephone and internet support

There is conflicting evidence on whether or not telephone and internet-based support is successful for antenatal smoking cessation. A systematic review by Lavender et al. concluded that although telephone support may be a promising intervention for some pregnancy outcomes, there was no evidence that women were more likely to have reduced, or stopped, smoking at the end of pregnancy, or during the postnatal period, or that telephone support reduced the likelihood of smoking relapse (88). Another systematic review evaluated proactive and reactive telephone helplines supporting smoking cessation and found that telephone helplines can support people to stop; however, these calls are initiated by the individual, which increases the likelihood that they are ready and intend to stop, or want to resist relapse, and therefore are more motivated than others who do not contact helplines (89). This review also found a "dose-response" effect in number of contacts; three or more calls increased the chances of stopping, compared to a minimal intervention such as providing standard self-help materials, brief advice, or NRT. Telephone counseling and helplines provide accessible support to those who are motivated to seek help, and therefore such interventions may be useful and demonstrate measurable benefit compared to brief and self-help interventions.

## Real time feedback

Ultrasound monitoring of fetal development is commonplace in antenatal care and presents an opportunity to discuss maternal behavior related to the health and development of the fetus, supported by visual evidence and measurement. In a study of 129 participants, Reading et al. found that women who received detailed feedback about the growth and development of the fetus during their scan appointment were more likely to stop smoking and avoid alcohol during pregnancy (90). However, a systematic review by Nabhan and Faris concluded that there was insufficient evidence to suggest that either low or high detailed feedback during the scan appointment promoted behavioral change (91).

## Nicotine replacement therapy

While nicotine is known to have significant deleterious effects on the developing fetus, it is also known to metabolize much more quickly during pregnancy, which may act to protect the fetus from extended exposure to toxic levels of circulating nicotine. Therefore, NRT may be a viable option to support smoking cessation during pregnancy (92). Nicotine replacement products may be considered safer than smoking during pregnancy due to the reduction of exposure to the toxic products of combustion (93). A systematic review of five randomized controlled trials (RCTs) to determine the efficacy and safety of NRT to support smoking cessation in pregnancy, with or without behavioral support, found insufficient evidence of both efficacy and safety of use to recommend its use in pregnancy (94). However, adherence to treatment was low across all studies and the majority of participants did not complete the recommended course of NRT. A subsequent meta-analysis by Myung et al. revealed that pregnant smokers using NRT demonstrated an abstinence rate 1.8 times higher in late pregnancy than the control group; however, pregnant smokers using NRT had lower cessation rates compared to the non-pregnant smoking population (95). The pooled data revealed no significant impact on the birth outcomes for the infants between the subject and control groups. Myung concluded that there may be clinical evidence to support the use of NRT, and that NRT was generally safe for use with pregnant women.

### Electronic cigarettes

Electronic cigarettes (EC) have been available since 2007 and have been used by smokers as a cessation device, as a more socially acceptable habit than cigarette smoking to non-smokers, or as a substitute for cigarettes in areas that ban smoking in public places (96). Early studies have identified some physiological benefits of using ECs over conventional tobacco products, as they contain fewer of the harmful compounds of normal cigarettes and less carbon monoxide (97). Pregnant women may opt to use ECs, and indeed, they may be advised by healthcare practitioners to move to them as a safer and more socially acceptable alternative, or they may be encouraged to use them to support smoking cessation (98).

The evidence for ECs to support smoking cessation is inconclusive. A randomized trial by Bullen and colleagues found that smokers who planned to stop using ECs instead switched to long-term use of ECs, thereby undermining complete cessation, and that ECs were no more effective than NRT (99). A subsequent meta-analysis found that EC users were significantly less likely to have stopped smoking than non-users (100). Mark et al. conducted a survey with pregnant women on their use and attitudes toward ECs (101). Three-quarters of respondents viewed ECs as a smoking cessation device, 43% of women believed that ECs were less harmful to themselves and their fetus than conventional cigarettes, and 66% of those who had used ECs stated that they were unaware that ECs contained nicotine. Little longitudinal research evidence is available yet regarding the safety or consequences of long-term use of these devices, particularly for pregnant women and the infant; therefore, these devices are not recommended for use during pregnancy. However, there is a need for healthcare practitioners to provide accurate and comprehensive information to women who are considering the use of ECs as a safer alternative to cigarettes, or to support smoking cessation.

### Financial incentives

A meta-analysis in 2009 found that financial incentives were associated with a 24% increase of smoking abstinence in late pregnancy (18); however, this meta-analysis reviewed combined approach treatments and therefore it is difficult to identify specific efficacy of individual elements. A literature review by Higgins et al. specifically looked at the use of financial incentives for smoking cessation in economically disadvantaged pregnant smokers (102). The interventions consisted of vouchers (with differing monetary values per study) given to the women following biochemical verification of abstinence from smoking. Higgins found that the use of financial incentives improved mean birth weight and increased breastfeeding duration. A randomized controlled trial conducted in Glasgow, UK, for which 612 pregnant women were recruited, compared the use of usual smoking cessation services with those enhanced with a financial incentive (£400 worth of food vouchers). Results from the trial support that the use of financial incentives was successful in helping women to stop smoking during pregnancy, with 22.5% of the intervention group stopping by 34-38 weeks' gestation compared to just 8.6% in the control group. No differences in perinatal outcomes were noted between the control and incentive groups, however (103). Overall, there seems to be good evidence for the use of financial incentives to support smoking cessation in economically disadvantaged pregnant smokers, demonstrating a significant effect for both cessation rate and improved perinatal outcomes for the infant (86, 102-104).

In summary, a wide range of interventions are used in order to support smoking cessation. These interventions have generally been evaluated as combination interventions, and therefore the efficacy of individual components are difficult to identify. Some benefits can be shown from most interventions. Interventions with an identified theoretical foundation were evaluated as more successful than interventions with no explicit theoretical basis and a "dose-response" was noted in most interventions; those offering more intensive or more frequent contact and support were generally more successful. The most effective interventions in terms of smoking abstinence, perinatal health improvement, and extended duration of breastfeeding were those offering financial incentives. Moderate effects were reported in behavioral and counseling interventions, although the effective component was often difficult to identify. The least effective intervention appears to be NRT, and significant questions remain over the safety and efficacy of electronic cigarettes.

## Conclusions

In this chapter, we have reviewed the evidence for strategies designed to support the prevention of SIDS. The huge successes of the initial public health strategies of the 1990s are a testament to what can be achieved through concerted national efforts. The key to these has been the simplicity of the messages and the support of high-profile campaigns. However, the initial rapid declines in SIDS mortality have plateaued, and it seems clear that simply continuing with the same approaches will now only have marginal effects, particularly among those families most at risk of SIDS.

The current evidence suggests that education-based strategies on their own have only minimal benefits in terms of short-term improvements in knowledge and behavior, particularly among those at highest risk. Where education is combined with more direct interventions aimed at modifying the sleep environment, such as portable sleep spaces, there may be more scope for change. There is some emerging evidence of the effectiveness of these combined strategies, although the complexity of the interventions and the low incidence of the primary outcome (SIDS mortality) mean that robust intervention studies are hard to develop. This may be particularly so for more entrenched behaviors, such as parental smoking. If we are to engage with those most at risk, we need to have a deeper understanding of behavioral change, and to ensure that our interventions are more geared towards empowerment of individuals. This in turn may require high levels of professional support over prolonged time frames.

As we move forward in our efforts to reduce the risks of SIDS, it is more important than ever that our risk-reduction strategies are based on sound public health principles. The key elements of successful strategies outlined earlier (see Table 12.2) should facilitate more creative thinking around how we can engage with, and empower, those most at risk. We need to ensure that the strategies we use are based on the best current evidence, including a strong scientific basis rooted in behavioral change theories. Our interventions need to focus on a limited number of simple achievable interventions, delivered through combined programs that are appropriately resourced, long-term in nature, and recruit strong leadership that engages and empowers the target communities. Finally, we need to ensure that these programs have built-in robust monitoring and evaluation.

# References

1. Ponsonby AL, Dwyer T, Cochrane J. Population trends in sudden infant death syndrome. Semin Perinatol. 2002;26(4):296-305. https://doi.org/10.1053/sper.2002.34774.

2. Rivara FP, Johnston B. Effective primary prevention programs in public health and their applicability to the prevention of child maltreatment. Child Welfare. 2013;92(2):119-39.

3. Mitchell EA, Blair PS. SIDS prevention: 3000 lives saved but we can do better. N Z J Med. 2012;125(1359):50-7.

4. Goldstein RD, Trachtenberg FL, Sens MA, Harty BJ, Kinney HC. Overall postneonatal mortality and rates of SIDS. Pediatrics. 2016;137(1):e20152298. https://doi.org/10.1542/peds.2015-2298.

5. Office for National Statistics. Unexplained deaths in infancy, England and Wales: 2014. London: Office for National Statistics, 2016.

6. Blair PS, Sidebotham P, Berry PJ, Evans M, Fleming PJ. Major epidemiological changes in sudden infant death syndrome: A 20-year population-based

study in the UK. Lancet. 2006;367(9507):314-19. https://doi.org/10.1016/S0140-6736(06)67968-3.

7.  NZ Mortality Review Data Group. NZ Child and Youth Mortality Review Committee: 9th data report 2008-2012. DunedIn: University of Otago, 2013.

8.  Maternal and Child Health Bureau. Child health USA 2014. Rockville, Maryland: US Department of Health and Human Services, 2015.

9.  Deal LW, Gomby DS, Zippiroli L, Behrman RE. Unintentional injuries in childhood: Analysis and recommendations. Future Child. 2000;10(1):4-22. https://doi.org/10.2307/1602823.

10. Towner E, Dowswell T. Community-based childhood injury prevention interventions: What works? Health Promot Int. 2002;17(3):273-84. https://doi.org/10.1093/heapro/17.3.273.

11. Coggan C, Patterson P, Brewin M, Hooper R, Robinson E. Evaluation of the Waitakere Community Injury Prevention Project. Inj Prev. 2000;6(2):130-4. https://doi.org/10.1136/ip.6.2.130.

12. Klassen TP, MacKay JM, Moher D, Walker A, Jones AL. Community-based injury prevention interventions. Future Child. 2000;10(1):83-110. https://doi.org/10.2307/1602826.

13. Bandura A. Self-efficacy: Toward a unifying theory of behavioral change. Psychological Rev. 1977;84(2):191-215. https://doi.org/10.1037/0033-295X.84.2.191.

14. Bandura A. Social foundations of thought and action: A social cognitive theory. Englewood Cliffs; London: Prentice-Hall, 1986.

15. Fishbein M, Ajzen I. Belief, attitude, intention and behavior: An introduction to theory and research. Reading, Mass; London: Addison-Wesley, 1975.

16. Ajzan I. The theory of planned behavior. In: Handbook of social psychological theories. Eds Lange PAMV, Kruglanski AW, Higgins ET. London: SAGE, 2012. p. 438-60. https://doi.org/10.4135/9781446249215.n22.

17. Prochaska JO, Velicer WF. The transtheoretical model of health behavior change. AJHP. 1997;12(1):38-48. https://doi.org/10.4278/0890-1171-12.1.38.

18. Lumley J, Chamberlain C, Dowswell T, Oliver S, Oakley L, Watson L. Interventions for promoting smoking cessation during pregnancy. Cochrane Database Syst Rev. 2009. Jul 8(3):CD001055. https://doi.org/10.1002/14651858.CD001055.pub3.

19. Solomon LJ, Secker-Walker RH, Skelly JM, Flynn BS. Stages of change in smoking during pregnancy in low-income women. J Behav Med. 1996;19(4):333-44. https://doi.org/10.1007/BF01904760.

20. Riemsma RP, Pattenden J, Bridle C, Sowden AJ, Mather L, Watt IS, et al. Systematic review of the effectiveness of stage based interventions to promote smoking cessation. BMJ. 2003;326(7400):1175-7. https://doi.org/10.1136/bmj.326.7400.1175.

21. Jones LL, Atkinson O, Longman J, Coleman T, McNeill A, Lewis SA. The motivators and barriers to a smoke-free home among disadvantaged caregivers: Identifying the positive levers for change. Nicotine Tobacco Res. 2011;13(6):479-86. https://doi.org/10.1093/ntr/ntr030.

22. Ogden J, Karim L, Choudry A, Brown K. Understanding successful behavior change: The role of intentions, attitudes to the target and motivations and the example of diet. Health Educ Res. 2007;22(3):397-405. https://doi.org/10.1093/her/cyl090.

23. Mills A, Schmied V, Taylor C, Dahlen H, Schuiringa W, Hudson ME. Connecting, learning, leaving: Supporting young parents in the community. Health Soc Care Community. 2012;20(6):663-72. https://doi.org/10.1111/j.1365-2524.2012.01084.x.

24. Cowan S. Their first 500 sleeps: Pēpi-Pod Report 2012-2014. Christ Church, New Zealand: Change for our Children Limited, 2015.

25. Romagnoli A, Wall G. "I know I'm a good mom": Young, low-income mothers' experiences with risk perception, intensive parenting ideology and parenting education programmes. Health Risk & Society. 2012;14(3):273-89. https://doi.org/10.1080/13698575.2012.662634.

26. Petosa RL, Smith LH. Peer mentoring for health behavior change: A systematic review. Am J Health Educ. 2014;45(6):351-7. https://doi.org/10.1080/19325037.2014.945670.

27. Anderson AK, Damio G, Young S, Chapman DJ, Perez-Escamilla R. A randomized trial assessing the efficacy of peer counseling on exclusive breastfeeding in a predominantly Latina low-income community. Arch Pediatr Adolesc Med. 2005;159(9):836-41. https://doi.org/10.1001/archpedi.159.9.836.

28. Olds DL, Henderson CR Jr, Tatelbaum R, Chamberlin R. Improving the delivery of prenatal care and outcomes of pregnancy: A randomized trial of nurse home visitation. Pediatrics. 1986;77(1):16-28.

29. Nichter M, Nichter M, Adrian S, Goldade K, Tesler L, Muramoto M. Smoking and harm-reduction efforts among postpartum women. Qualitative Health Res. 2008;18(9):1184-94. https://doi.org/10.1177/1049732308321738.

30. Salm Ward TC, Balfour GM. Infant safe sleep interventions, 1990-2015: A review. J Community Health. 2016;41(1):180-96. https://doi.org/10.1007/s10900-015-0060-y.

31. Abel S, Tipene-Leach D. SUDI prevention: A review of Māori safe sleep innovations for infants. The New Zealand medical journal. 2013;126(1379):86-94.

32. Van Wouwe JP, Hirasing RA. Prevention of sudden unexpected infant death. Lancet. 2006;367(9507):277-8. https://doi.org/10.1016/S0140-6736(06)67969-5.

33. NIH. Safe to Sleep public education campaign. [Available from: https://www.nichd.nih.gov/sts/Pages/default.aspx]. Accessed 5 May 2017.

34. Blair P. Sudden infant death syndrome. In: Unexpected death in childhood: A handbook for practitioners. Eds Sidebotham P, Fleming P. Chichester, UK: Wiley, 2007. p. 41-60. https://doi.org/10.1002/9780470988176.ch4.

35. Moon RY, Hauck FR, Colson ER. Safe infant sleep interventions: What is the evidence for successful behavior change? Curr Pediatr Rev. 2016;12(1):67-75. https://doi.org/10.2174/1573396311666151026110148.

36. Taylor BJ, Garstang J, Engelberts A, Obonai T, Cote A, Freemantle J, et al. International comparison of sudden unexpected death in infancy rates using a newly proposed set of cause-of-death codes. Arch Dis Child. 2015;100(11):1018-23. https://doi.org/10.1136/archdischild-2015-308239.

37. Batra EK, Teti DM, Schaefer EW, Neumann BA, Meek EA, Paul IM. Nocturnal video assessment of infant sleep environments. Pediatrics. 2016;138(3):e20161533. https://doi.org/10.1542/peds.2016-1533.

38. Task Force On Sudden Infant Death Syndrome. SIDS and other sleep-related infant deaths: Updated 2016 recommendations for a safe infant sleeping environment. Pediatrics. 2016;138(5).

39. Cowan S, Pease A, Bennett S. Usage and impact of an online education tool for preventing sudden unexpected death in infancy. J Paediatr Child Health. 2013;49(3):228-32. https://doi.org/10.1111/jpc.12128.

40. Ostfeld BM, Esposito L, Straw D, Burgos J, Hegyi T. An inner-city school-based program to promote early awareness of risk factors for sudden infant death syndrome. J Adolescent Health. 2005;37(4):339-41. https://doi.org/10.1016/j.jadohealth.2004.12.002.

41. Ayers JW, Westmaas JL, Leas EC, Benton A, Chen Y, Dredze M, et al. Leveraging big data to improve health awareness campaigns: A novel evaluation of the great American smokeout. JMIR Public Health Surveillance. 2016;2(1):e16. https://doi.org/10.2196/publichealth.5304.

42. NHS Employers. Calendar of national campaigns 2017. [Available from: http://www.nhsemployers.org/your-workforce/retain-and-improve/staff-experience/health-work-and-wellbeing/sustaining-the-momentum/calendar-of-national-campaigns-2016%]. Accessed 11 October 2017.

43. Purtle J, Roman LA. Health awareness days: Sufficient evidence to support the craze? Am J Public Health. 2015;105(6):1061-5. https://doi.org/10.2105/AJPH.2015.302621.

44. Robling M, Bekkers MJ, Bell K, Butler CC, Cannings-John R, Channon S, et al. Effectiveness of a nurse-led intensive home-visitation programme for first-time teenage mothers (Building Blocks): A pragmatic randomised controlled trial. Lancet. 2016;387(10014):146-55. https://doi.org/10.1016/S0140-6736(15)00392-X.

45. Hunt CE. Sudden infant death syndrome and other causes of infant mortality: Diagnosis, mechanisms, and risk for recurrence in siblings. American journal of respiratory and critical care medicine. 2001;164(3):346-57. https://doi.org/10.1164/ajrccm.164.3.9910045.

46. Campbell MJ, Hall D, Stephenson T, Bacon C, Madan J. Recurrence rates for sudden infant death syndrome (SIDS): The importance of risk stratification. Arch Dis Child. 2008;93(11):936-9. https://doi.org/10.1136/adc.2007.121350.

47. Brooten D, Youngblut JM, Hannan J, Caicedo C, Roche R, Malkawi F. Infant and child deaths: Parent concerns about subsequent pregnancies. J Am Ass Nurse Practitioners. 2015;27(12):690-7. https://doi.org/10.1002/2327-6924.12243.

48. Waite A, McKenzie A, Daman-Willems C. CONI: Confirmation of continuing relevance after 20 years. Community Pract. 2011;84(1):25-9.

49. Health Inequalities Unit. Implementation plan for reducing health inequalities in infant mortality: A good practice guide. London: Department of Health, 2007.

50. Taylor EM, Spencer NJ, Carpenter RG. Evaluation of attempted prevention of unexpected infant death in very high-risk infants by planned health care. Acta Paediatr. 1993;82(1):83-6. https://doi.org/10.1111/j.1651-2227.1993.tb12522.x.

51. The Lullaby Trust. CONI protocol. London: The Lullaby Trust, 2017.

52. Blair PS, Nadin P, Cole TJ, Fleming PJ, Smith IJ, Platt MW, et al. Weight gain and sudden infant death syndrome: Changes in weight z scores may identify infants at increased risk. Arch Dis Child. 2000;82(6):462-9. https://doi.org/10.1136/adc.82.6.462.

53. Fleming P, Blair P, Bacon C, Berry P. Sudden unexpected deaths in infancy. The CESDI SUDI studies 1993-1996. London: The Stationery Office, 2000.

54. Committee on Fetus and Newborn AAoP. Apnea, sudden infant death syndrome, and home monitoring. Pediatrics. 2003;111(4 Pt 1):914-17.

55. Carpenter RG, Waite A, Coombs RC, Daman-Willems C, McKenzie A, Huber J, et al. Repeat sudden unexpected and unexplained infant deaths: Natural or unnatural? Lancet. 2005;365(9453):29-35. https://doi.org/10.1016/S0140-6736(04)17662-9.

56. Waite AJ, Coombs RC, McKenzie A, Daman-Willems C, Cohen MC, Campbell MJ, et al. Mortality of babies enrolled in a community-based support programme: CONI PLUS (Care of Next Infant Plus). Arch Dis Child. 2015;100(7):637-42. https://doi.org/10.1136/archdischild-2014-307232.

57. Caraballo M, Shimasaki S, Johnston K, Tung G, Albright K, Halbower AC. Knowledge, attitudes, and risk for sudden unexpected infant death in children of adolescent mothers: A qualitative study. J Pediatr. 2016;174:78-83 e2.

58. Gilchrist A. Little Lullaby evaluation 2014-2016. London: The Lullaby Trust, 2016.

59. Pease A. Factors influencing infant care practices in the sleep environment among families at high risk of sudden infant death syndrome. Bristol: University of Bristol, 2015.

60. *Children and Young Persons Act 1933* (UK) c 12.

61. Carpenter RG, Irgens LM, Blair PS, England PD, Fleming P, Huber J, et al. Sudden unexplained infant death in 20 regions in Europe: Case control study. Lancet. 2004;363(9404):185-91. https://doi.org/10.1016/S0140-6736(03)15323-8.

62. Vennemann MM, Bajanowski T, Brinkmann B, Jorch G, Sauerland C, Mitchell EA, et al. Sleep environment risk factors for sudden infant death syndrome: The German Sudden Infant Death Syndrome Study. Pediatrics. 2009;123(4):1162-70. https://doi.org/10.1542/peds.2008-0505.

63. L'Hoir MP, Engelberts AC, van Well GT, McClelland S, Westers P, Dandachli T, et al. Risk and preventive factors for cot death in The Netherlands, a low-incidence country. Eur J Pediatr. 1998;157(8):681-8. https://doi.org/10.1007/s004310050911.

64. Blair PS, Sidebotham P, Evason-Coombe C, Edmonds M, Heckstall-Smith EM, Fleming P. Hazardous cosleeping environments and risk factors amenable to change: Case-control study of SIDS in south west England. BMJ. 2009;339:b3666. https://doi.org/10.1136/bmj.b3666.

65. McDonnell E, Moon RY. Infant deaths and injuries associated with wearable blankets, swaddle wraps, and swaddling. J Pediatr. 2014;164(5):1152-6. https://doi.org/10.1016/j.jpeds.2013.12.045.

66. Tipene-Leach D, Abel S. The Wahakura and the safe sleeping environment. J Primary Health Care. 2010;2(1):81.

67. Cowan S, Bennett S, Clarke J, Pease A. An evaluation of portable sleeping spaces for babies following the Christchurch earthquake of February 2011. J Paediatr Child Health. 2013;49(5):364-8. https://doi.org/10.1111/jpc.12196.

68. Hauck FR, Tanabe KO, McMurry T, Moon RY. Evaluation of Bedtime Basics for Babies: A national crib distribution program to reduce the risk of sleep-related sudden infant deaths. J Community Health. 2015;40(3):457-63. https://doi.org/10.1007/s10900-014-9957-0.

69. Moon RY, & Task Force On Sudden Infant Deaths. SIDS and other sleep-related infant deaths: Evidence base for 2016 updated recommendations for a safe infant sleeping environment. Pediatrics. 2016;138(5). https://doi.org/10.1542/peds.2016-2940.

70. Statistics Finland. Causes of death: Appendix table 3. Mortality during infant and perinatal period 1987-2015. [Available from: http://www.stat.fi/til/ksyyt/2015/ksyyt_2015_2016-12-30_tau_005_en.html]. Accessed 11 October 2017.

71. Ross L. Baby boxes: Improving wellbeing outcomes in Scotland. J Health Visiting. 2017;5(4):172-5. https://doi.org/10.12968/johv.2017.5.4.172.

72. Murphy M. UK's first Baby Box programme launched at London NHS Trust. British J Midwifery. 2016;24(7):521-2. https://doi.org/10.12968/bjom.2016.24.7.521.

73. Demer L. Rash of sleep-related infant deaths troubles health officials. Alaska Dispatch News [internet]; 14 February 2015. [Available from: https://www.adn.com/health/article/rash-infant-deaths-related-sleeping-alarms-health-officials/2015/02/15/]. Accessed 1 June 2017.

74. Lee H. Why Finnish babies sleep in cardboard boxes. BBC News [internet]; 4 June 2013. [Available from: http://www.bbc.co.uk/news/magazine-22751415]. Accessed 1 June 2017.

75. Cassain E. Do baby boxes really save lives? BBC News [internet]; 25 March 2017. [Available from: http://www.bbc.co.uk/news/magazine-39366596]. Accessed 1 June 2017.

76. Ward Platt M, Blair PS, Fleming PJ, Smith IJ, Cole TJ, Leach CE, et al. A clinical comparison of SIDS and explained sudden infant deaths: How healthy and how normal? CESDI SUDI Research Group. Confidential Inquiry into Stillbirths and Deaths in Infancy study. Arch Dis Child. 2000;82(2):98-106. https://doi.org/10.1136/adc.82.2.98.

77. Ford RP, Mitchell EA, Stewart AW, Scragg R, Taylor BJ. SIDS, illness, and acute medical care. New Zealand Cot Death Study Group. Arch Dis Child. 1997;77(1):54-5. https://doi.org/10.1136/adc.77.1.54.

78. Wilkinson A. Pre-hospital assessment of a child under one year old with fever. Emergency Nurse. 2017;24(10):28-33. https://doi.org/10.7748/en.2017.e1663.

79. Morley CJ, Thornton AJ, Cole TJ, Fowler MA, Hewson PH. Symptoms and signs in infants younger than 6 months of age correlated with the severity of their illness. Pediatrics. 1991;88(6):1119-24.

80. Morley CJ, Thornton AJ, Green SJ, Cole TJ. Field trials of the Baby Check score card in general practice. Arch Dis Child. 1991;66(1):111-14. https://doi.org/10.1136/adc.66.1.111.

81. Thornton AJ, Morley CJ, Green SJ, Cole TJ, Walker KA, Bonnett JM. Field trials of the Baby Check score card: Mothers scoring their babies at home. Arch Dis Child. 1991;66(1):106-10. https://doi.org/10.1136/adc.66.1.106.

82. Kai J. "Baby Check" in the inner city — Use and value to parents. Family Practice. 1994;11(3):245-50. https://doi.org/10.1093/fampra/11.3.245.

83. Mitchell EA, Milerad J. Smoking and the sudden infant death syndrome. Rev Environmental Health. 2006;21(2):81-103. https://doi.org/10.1515/REVEH.2006.21.2.81.

84. Fleming P, Blair PS. Sudden infant death syndrome and parental smoking. Early Hum Dev. 2007;83(11):721-5. https://doi.org/10.1016/j.earlhumdev.2007.07.011.

85. Mullen PD. How can more smoking suspension during pregnancy become lifelong abstinence? Lessons learned about predictors, interventions, and gaps in our accumulated knowledge. Nicotine Tobacco Res. 2004;6(Suppl 2):S217-38. https://doi.org/10.1080/14622200410001669150.

86. Chamberlain C, O'Mara-Eves A, Oliver S, Caird JR, Perlen SM, Eades SJ, et al. Psychosocial interventions for supporting women to stop smoking in pregnancy. Cochrane Database Syst Rev. 2013. 10:CD001055. https://doi.org/10.1002/14651858.CD001055.pub4.

87. Baxter S, Blank L, Everson-Hock ES, Burrows J, Messina J, Guillaume L, et al. The effectiveness of interventions to establish smoke-free homes in pregnancy and in the neonatal period: A systematic review. Health Educ Res. 2011;26(2):265-82. https://doi.org/10.1093/her/cyq092.

88. Lavender T, Richens Y, Milan SJ, Smyth RM, Dowswell T. Telephone support for women during pregnancy and the first six weeks postpartum. Cochrane Database Syst Rev. 2013. 7:CD009338. https://doi.org/10.1002/14651858.CD009338.pub2.

89. Stead LF, Hartmann-Boyce J, Perera R, Lancaster T. Telephone counselling for smoking cessation. Cochrane Database Syst Rev. 2013. 8:CD002850. https://doi.org/10.1002/14651858.CD002850.pub3.

90. Reading AE, Campbell S, Cox DN, Sledmere CM. Health beliefs and health care behavior in pregnancy. Psychological Med. 1982;12(2):379-83. https://doi.org/10.1017/S0033291700046717.

91. Nabhan AF, Faris MA. High feedback versus low feedback of prenatal ultrasound for reducing maternal anxiety and improving maternal health behavior in pregnancy. Cochrane Database Syst Rev. 2010. 4:CD007208.

92. Dempsey D, Jacob P 3rd, Benowitz NL. Accelerated metabolism of nicotine and cotinine in pregnant smokers. Journal Pharm Exp Theraputics. 2002;301(2):594-8. https://doi.org/10.1124/jpet.301.2.594.

93. Benowitz N, Dempsey D. Pharmacotherapy for smoking cessation during pregnancy. Nicotine Tobacco Res. 2004;6(Suppl 2):S189-202. https://doi.org/10.1080/14622200410001669169.

94. Coleman T, Chamberlain C, Cooper S, Leonardi-Bee J. Efficacy and safety of nicotine replacement therapy for smoking cessation in pregnancy: Systematic review and meta-analysis. Addiction. 2011;106(1):52-61. https://doi.org/10.1111/j.1360-0443.2010.03179.x.

95. Myung SK, Ju W, Jung HS, Park CH, Oh SW, Seo H, et al. Efficacy and safety of pharmacotherapy for smoking cessation among pregnant smokers: A meta-analysis. BJOG. 2012;119(9):1029-39. https://doi.org/10.1111/j.1471-0528.2012.03408.x.

96. Etter JF. Electronic cigarettes: A survey of users. BMC Public Health. 2010;10:231. https://doi.org/10.1186/1471-2458-10-231.

97. Breland A, Soule E, Lopez A, Ramoa C, El-Hellani A, Eissenberg T. Electronic cigarettes: What are they and what do they do? Ann NY Acad Sci. 2017;1394(1):5-30. https://doi.org/10.1111/nyas.12977.

98. England LJ, Anderson BL, Tong VT, Mahoney J, Coleman-Cowger VH, Melstrom P, et al. Screening practices and attitudes of obstetricians-gynecologists toward new and emerging tobacco products. Am J Obstet Gynecol. 2014;211(6):695 e1-7.

99. Bullen C, Howe C, Laugesen M, McRobbie H, Parag V, Williman J, et al. Electronic cigarettes for smoking cessation: A randomised controlled trial. Lancet. 2013;382(9905):1629-37. https://doi.org/10.1016/S0140-6736(13)61842-5.

100. Grana R, Benowitz N, Glantz SA. E-cigarettes: A scientific review. Circulation. 2014;129(19):1972-86. https://doi.org/10.1161/CIRCULATIONAHA.114.007667.

101. Mark KS, Farquhar B, Chisolm MS, Coleman-Cowger VH, Terplan M. Knowledge, attitudes, and practice of electronic cigarette use among pregnant women. J Addiction Med. 2015;9(4):266-72. https://doi.org/10.1097/ADM.0000000000000128.

102. Higgins ST, Washio Y, Heil SH, Solomon LJ, Gaalema DE, Higgins TM, et al. Financial incentives for smoking cessation among pregnant and newly postpartum women. Preventive Med. 2012;55(Suppl):S33-40. https://doi.org/10.1016/j.ypmed.2011.12.016.

103. Tappin D, Bauld L, Purves D, Boyd K, Sinclair L, MacAskill S, et al. Financial incentives for smoking cessation in pregnancy: Randomised controlled trial. BMJ. 2015;350:h134. https://doi.org/10.1136/bmj.h134.

104. Lussier JP, Heil SH, Mongeon JA, Badger GJ, Higgins ST. A meta-analysis of voucher-based reinforcement therapy for substance use disorders. Addiction. 2006;101(2):192-203. https://doi.org/10.1111/j.1360-0443.2006.01311.x.

# 13

# The Epidemiology of Sudden Infant Death Syndrome and Sudden Unexpected Infant Deaths: Diagnostic Shift and other Temporal Changes

Carrie K Shapiro-Mendoza, PhD, MPH[1],
Sharyn Parks, PhD, MPH[1],
Alexa Erck Lambert, MPH[2],
Lena Camperlengo, DrPH[1],
Carri Cottengim, MA[1] and
Christine Olson, MD[1]

[1]*Division of Reproductive Health, Centers for Disease Control and Prevention, Atlanta, Georgia, USA*
[2]*DB Consulting Group, Inc, Silver, Spring, Maryland, USA*

## Introduction

To provide a detailed review of the changing epidemiology related to sudden infant death syndrome (SIDS) and sudden unexpected infant deaths (SUID), this chapter begins with an overview of the international system used to code and monitor SIDS trends around the world. Next, we describe the diagnostic shift in reporting and provide possible explanations as to why it occurred. We include a discussion of why using a single code to monitor sudden unexpected and unexplained infant deaths is no longer informative and discuss how new efforts to group codes for surveillance may allow for more consistent monitoring and comparison across jurisdictions and countries. Finally, we provide a description of the epidemiologic profile of SIDS and SUID, including information about current rates and historical trends, and sudden unexpected death in children 1 year old and over.

## Current Practice for Coding Cause of Sudden Infant Deaths

Vital statistics data, specifically records from live birth and infant death registration, are the typical source of information on population trends in SIDS and SUID. Causes of death are reported on infant death certificates by a death certifier, who, for unexpected infant deaths without an immediately obvious cause, can be a medical examiner, coroner, or forensic pathologist. To facilitate comparisons across jurisdictions and countries, underlying causes of death reported on death certificates are assigned an International Classification of Diseases or ICD code (1).

The International Classification of Diseases (ICD) coding system was developed by the World Health Organization to catalogue diseases, health conditions, and mortality causes. The coding system is used to monitor death trends and statistics within, and across, jurisdictions and countries (2). The ICD is currently in its 10th Revision (ICD-10). SIDS, first defined in 1969 (3), did not have a unique ICD code assigned until the ICD-9 in 1979. However, in 1973, the US National Center for Health Statistics (NCHS) created a distinct ICD-8 code for SIDS (795.0) for use in the United States (4). SIDS was introduced worldwide in ICD-9 as 798.0. In ICD-10, R95 is the code for SIDS. The SIDS code is indexed in the ICD chapter of nonspecific causes of death.

The underlying cause of death reported on the death certificate is assigned an ICD code by a computer (using a complex classification algorithm) or by a person called a nosologist (5). In the US, several terms can result in an infant death being assigned the SIDS code R95 (6). Some of these terms are SIDS, cot death, crib death, sudden unexplained (or unexpected) death in infancy, and sudden unexplained (or unexpected) infant death. Once coded, researchers can use data to make consistent comparisons of trends across jurisdictions and countries, evaluate programs, and monitor progress in reaching objectives toward reducing associated risk factors and mortality. For example, linking consistently coded infant death certificates to birth registration records facilitates more in-depth description of SIDS and other SUID epidemiology.

### Grouping ICD Codes to examine trends in SUID

Diagnostic preferences, and the resulting ICD coding differences, have led to wide variation in how deaths are represented in vital statistics. Depending upon the individual death certifier, nosologist, and the organizational and political culture within which each of those operates, two essentially identical infant deaths can be assigned different codes.

As such, relying on a single ICD code (e.g. R95) to monitor unexplained infant deaths across jurisdictions and countries has become uninformative and insufficient (7, 8). Consequently, researchers began grouping ICD codes for SIDS, accidental suffocation, and other nonspecific conditions together to comprise a more meaningful entity for surveillance and research purposes (7, 9-11). Together, these deaths are conceptualized as SUID or sudden unexpected (or unexplained) death in infancy (SUDI). SUDI is the preferred term in Europe and Australia (12, 13), whereas SUID is more commonly used in the United States (14, 15). We will use the term SUID throughout this chapter.

In 2006, Shapiro-Mendoza et al. (10) used ICD-9 codes and ICD-10 codes to define SUID as any infant death (0-364 days) with the following ICD-9/10 codes: SIDS (795.0/R95), unknown cause (799.9/R99), accidental suffocation or strangulation in bed (E913/W75), other accidental suffocation and strangulation (E913.1-913.9/W76-W77, W81-W84), and neglect, abandonment, and other maltreatment syndromes (E967, E968.4/Y06-Y07). From this larger group, the authors identified causes of death, which constituted most United States SUID cases (ICD-9/10 codes: SIDS (795.0/R95), unknown cause (799.9/R99), and accidental suffocation or strangulation in bed (E913/W75). In 2015, the NCHS recognized the value of grouping the codes and began using these three codes to more consistently track trends in SUID by grouping causes of death (11). This same group of codes is used to define SUID for the United States Healthy People 2020 initiative, where SUID is among the health indicators measured (16).

In 2015, an international group of researchers compared SUID rates across eight high-income countries (Australia, Canada, Germany, Japan, the Netherlands, New Zealand, England and Wales, and the United States) (7). To aid international comparisons they grouped seven ICD-10 codes (R95, R96, R98 and R99, W75, W78, and W79). These codes represented potential SUID or deaths where an unsafe sleep environment (e.g. bed sharing), or ill-defined agonal events (choking or aspiration of food contents) could have been associated with the death. The authors excluded deaths with distinct clinical causes such as head injuries, infections, and metabolic disorders. Using the seven selected ICD codes, the authors compared frequencies both by individual code and in aggregate and found that no code or groups of codes were used consistently across countries (Table 13.1). Even with the consistent seven-code grouping, the range of SUID rates observed across countries could be explained by additional, country-specific, ICD-10 codes. Additional codes used in the United States are listed in Table 13.1 (17, 18).

Table 13.1: ICD-10 codes commonly used to classify unexplained infant deaths in selected countries

| ICD-10 Code | ICD-10 Label (1) | Countries Where Used | Comments |
|---|---|---|---|
| **Chapter R: Symptoms, signs, and abnormal findings, not elsewhere classified** | | | |
| R95 | Sudden infant death syndrome (SIDS) | Most commonly used SUID code in all countries except Japan (7) | SIDS was not defined until 1969 (3). |
| R96 | Other sudden death, cause unknown | Japan (7) | More than 80% of Japan's SUID cases do not have autopsies, suggesting that this may be a reason why Japan uses R96 more often than R95 (7). |
| R98 | Unattended death | Australia, Germany, Japan, Netherlands (7) | An ill-defined and unknown cause of mortality. |
| R99 | Other ill-defined and unspecified causes of mortality | Netherlands, England & Wales, Canada, United States, Australia (7) | Remains an "ill-defined" cause of death (2). In the United States, death certificates that list "pending investigation" with no tentative cause of death and that do not update the cause of death by the time the national file is finalized are coded as R99 (9, 10). |
| **Chapter V-Y: External causes of morbidity and mortality** | | | |
| W75 | Accidental suffocation and strangulation in bed | New Zealand, United States, Japan, Netherlands (7, 9, 10, 18) | Leading cause of unintentional injury-related infant death in the US (18). |
| W78 & W79 | Inhalation of gastric contents (W78); Inhalation and ingestion of food, causing obstruction of respiratory tract (W79) | Japan, Netherlands, Germany (7) | Grouped by Taylor and colleagues to describe agonal or secondary events related to SUID (7). |
| W84 | Unspecified threat to breathing | Not monitored in Taylor study; (7)monitored in some US jurisdictions (17, 18) | Infrequently used in the United States (59). |
| Y10-Y34 | Deaths of undetermined intent | United States (17) | Used by death certifiers in New York City, US. |

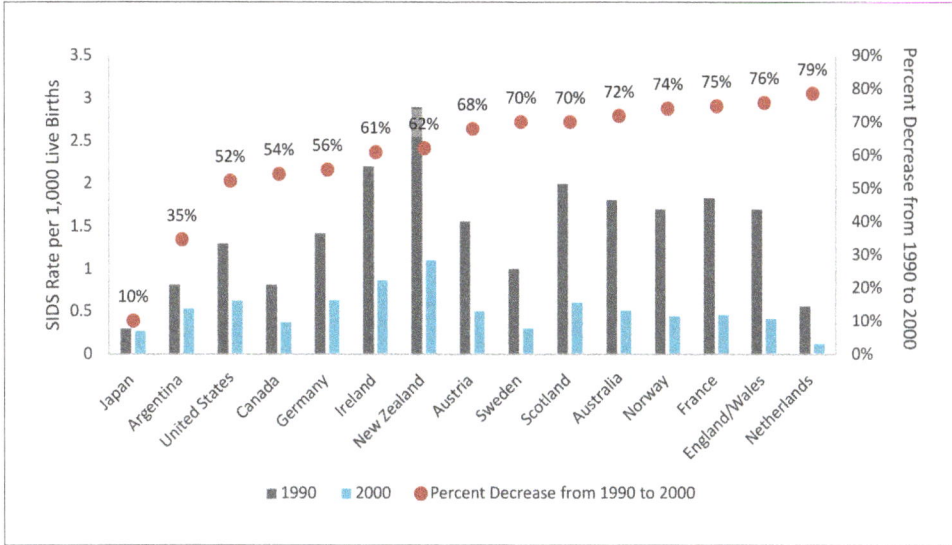

Figure 13.1: International SIDS rates 1990 and 2000 and per cent decrease from 1990-2000. (Adapted from (19).) Note: SIDS is defined by ICD-10 code R95.

## Historical Trends in SIDS and SUID

### SIDS rates before and after the promotion of back sleeping

Internationally, the implementation of risk reduction campaigns emphasizing back sleeping in the late 1980s and early 1990s resulted in a decline in SIDS rates in several countries (19-32). SIDS rates in 1990 and 2000 are shown in Figure 13.1. In 1990, before the campaigns, SIDS rates ranged from 0.30 deaths per 1,000 live births in Japan to 2.90 deaths per 1,000 live births in New Zealand, with most countries reporting rates between 1.00-2.00 deaths per 1,000 live births (19). In 2000, SIDS rates ranged from 0.12 deaths per 1,000 live births in the Netherlands to 1.10 deaths per 1,000 live births in New Zealand. The per cent decrease also varied by country; ranging from a 10% decrease in Japan to a 79% decrease in the Netherlands.

The greatest declines in SIDS rates occurred mainly in the first few years following these risk reduction campaigns (19). For example, from 1987-94 in Quebec, Canada, there had been little variability in the SIDS rate (0.50-0.57 deaths per 1,000 live births), but in the first couple of years following the 1993-94 "Back to Sleep" campaign, a 37% decrease in the SIDS rate (0.41 in 1995 and 0.32 in 1996) was observed (33). Similarly, in the United States, the steepest decline in SIDS rates occurred shortly after the American Academy of Pediatrics (AAP) non-prone sleep recommendation in 1992 and the national "Back to Sleep" campaign implemented in 1994 (Figure 13.2) (34, 35). There was a 41% decrease from 1.30 deaths per 1,000 live births in 1989-91 to 0.77 per

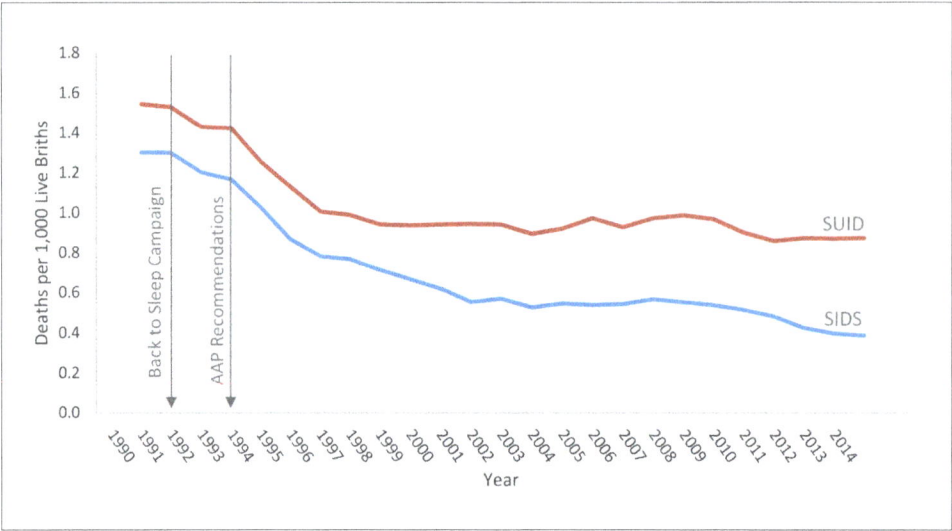

Figure 13.2: Trends in SUID and SIDS, United States, 1990-2014. SUID: ICD-10 codes R95, R99, W75; SIDS: ICD-10 code R95. (Based on data obtained from the online query system for the CDC/NCHS's National Vital Statistics System (58, 59).)

1,000 live births in 1995-98 (10). In late 1996, the AAP revised its sleep position statement and emphasized supine over both lateral and prone sleep position and this modification was integrated into the "Back to Sleep" campaign materials (34). However, when comparing the SUID rate from 1995-98 to 1999-2001 (0.77 to 0.61 deaths per 1,000 live births), the 22% decline was not as dramatic compared to earlier years (10).

## Diagnostic Shift

Studies in Australia (36, 37), England and Wales (38), and the United States (9, 10) showed that some of the decline in SIDS rates in the late 1990s was likely due to a diagnostic shift (Table 13.2). Data on trends in SIDS rates over the last 20 years reflect this diagnostic shift or change in reporting. As SIDS rates declined, rates of death attributed to other causes like unintentional injuries (e.g. accidental suffocation), and ill-defined conditions (e.g. undetermined, unknown, and unascertained causes) increased. For example, in South Australia, the decline in SIDS rates from 1994-98 was offset by increased deaths classified as undetermined (36). In England and Wales, the decline in SIDS in 1997-98 was accompanied by an increase in deaths attributed to non-SIDS causes including infectious diseases, metabolic disorders, and ill-defined conditions. According to the UK vital statistics office, many of the post-neonatal deaths that would have been classified as SIDS in 1997 were classified as unknown, unascertained, or ill-defined conditions in 1998 (38). In the United States, the diagnostic shift occurred from 1999-2001 and was evidenced by a decline in SIDS (R95) rates offset by increasing rates of unknown causes (R99) and accidental suffocation and strangulation in bed (W75) (9, 10).

Table 13.2: Diagnostic shift: Changes in reporting of causes of sudden death in infants.

| Country or Jurisdiction | Years when diagnostic shift occurred | Shift from SIDS to what other cause(s) | Explanations — change in definition for SIDS and other SUID |
|---|---|---|---|
| United States (9, 10) | 1999-2001 | • Unknown/ unspecified<br>• Accidental suffocation and strangulation in bed | • Reluctance of death certifiers to assign SIDS as the cause of death unless a thorough investigation had been conducted<br>• Improved death scene investigations |
| South Australia (36) | 1994-98 | • Undetermined cause | • Improved death scene investigations including scene reconstructions |
| England and Wales (38, 43) | 1997-98 | • Unknown, unascertained, or ill-defined conditions | • Change to the definition of SIDS and improved diagnosis from post-mortem investigation of deaths |

## Explanations for the diagnostic shift

There are multiple explanations for the diagnostic shift, including diagnostic preferences and policies about cause-of-death determinations and improved case investigations (36, 38, 39).

### Diagnostic preferences and policies about cause-of-death determinations

Although historical accounts of SIDS have existed since biblical times (40), it was not until 1969 that the pediatric pathologist Bruce Beckwith coined and defined the term SIDS at an international conference about the causes of sudden deaths in infants (3). Beckwith defined SIDS as "the sudden death of any infant or young child which is unexpected by history, and in which a thorough post-mortem examination fails to demonstrate an adequate cause of death". Formal recognition of SIDS as a cause of death encouraged etiologic research. A subsequent definition, characterized in 1989 by an international panel of experts (41), limited SIDS to infants less than 1 year old and added a death scene investigation as a requisite. This expert panel also declared that cases that remain unresolved following a thorough case investigation, such as suspected cases of abuse, neglect, and accidental asphyxiation, could be classified as undetermined or unexplained. Because forensic pathologists and scientific researchers have been unable to agree on specific criteria for defining SIDS, other attempts to refine the definition have been largely unsuccessful (41, 42). Consequently, SIDS remains a diagnosis of exclusion.

Some pathologists choose to follow the 1989 definition (41) strictly and are hesitant to assign SIDS as a cause of death in the absence of a scene investigation or a complete post-mortem examination including histology, microbiology, toxicology, and multidisciplinary review (43-45). Instead, these unexplained deaths are classified with terms which reflect the uncertainty about the cause of death: they are classified as unascertained in the United Kingdom (UK), and undetermined in the United States (US) (43, 46). Other death certifiers prefer to classify unexplained infant deaths as sudden unexpected (or unexplained) infant death or SUID to denote uncertainty about the possibility that unintentional injury could have contributed to the death. The level of evidence used to classify a death as suffocation or asphyxia varies among death certifiers (47). The determination of suffocation or asphyxia as the cause of death is complicated because these deaths are often unwitnessed events and lack biological evidence to distinguish SIDS from suffocation (36, 43, 48-50).

In 2003, a UK survey asked pathologists about the circumstances in which they would need to classify an infant death as unascertained as opposed to SIDS. More than two-thirds stated that sharing a sleep surface with an adult, or other uncertain situations, were reasons to classify a death as unascertained (43). More than one-third (38%) stated that they did not deem SIDS as serving a useful purpose as a cause of death. In 2004, the Kennedy Report was published in the UK (45), which standardized procedures for death scene investigation, autopsy, and cause-of-death determination. The report recognized that inconsistent certification practices existed and instructed coroners to avoid the term unascertained and instead to use SIDS to classify unexplained infant deaths (45). Despite the dissemination of these standardized practices, a 2010 UK study (51) found that pathologists still did not agree on definitions for the terms SIDS, SUID, and unascertained, and also could not agree on the components of a complete autopsy.

In the US, lack of consensus among medical examiners and coroners also exists. In 2004, about 5% of US medical examiner and coroner offices reported not using the term SIDS for death certification (8). Ten years later, 50% of medical examiners and coroners surveyed stated they did not use SIDS for death certification (47). Moreover, even with a complete autopsy reporting no specific pathology or autopsy findings to explain the death, only 38% of medical examiners and coroners assigned SIDS as the cause of death when given a scenario of an infant who died unexpectedly in a safe sleep environment (i.e. alone, on their back, in a crib, without soft objects or bedding). The terms SUID or undetermined were the classifications the medical examiners and coroners preferred to choose when classifying this death.

In addition to diagnostic preferences, in some jurisdictions, death certifiers are bound by office policies to apply jurisdictional definitions of SIDS and other SUID terms. For example, the New York City Medical Examiner Office has a policy stating that a sudden death cannot be classified as SIDS if an infant is found in an unsafe sleep environment (e.g. prone sleeping, soft bedding, shared sleep surface) (17). Some prominent US medical examiners have published statements proposing that their colleagues stop using SIDS in favor of undetermined cause and that international classification systems should exclude SIDS as a cause of death altogether (8, 52).

## Improved infant death investigations

In the 1980s, Bass and colleagues (53) conducted a case series investigation of presumed SIDS cases and documented the importance of death scene investigation in differentiating unexplained causes (e.g. SIDS) from other accidental and environmental mechanisms of the death (e.g. accidental asphyxiation in an unsafe sleep environment). In 1989, an international panel of experts promoted the value of the death scene investigation by incorporating it as part of the SIDS definition (41). Nonetheless, standardized scene investigation guidelines were not available until 1996 when the US Centers for Disease Control and Prevention (CDC) and multiple stakeholders recommended national guidelines for conducting SUID investigations (54). The CDC distributed these guidelines to medical examiner and coroner offices throughout the US. In 2004, the UK developed and recommended its own case investigation protocol, the Kennedy Report (45), described earlier. In drafting the Kennedy Report, the authors engaged many stakeholders and gained approval from the Royal College of Pathologists and the Royal College of Paediatrics and Child Health. In 2006, CDC and numerous stakeholders revised the 1996 recommendations and received endorsement from key professional organizations (14). The recommendations were widely disseminated to medical examiners, coroners, law enforcement investigators, and child advocates across the US, as well as an international team from the UK, via a comprehensive train-the-trainer program.

With more inclusive death scene investigations came a reduction in the use of the term SIDS. Per the 1989 definition (41), SIDS should only be designated as a cause of death in cases where a death scene investigation and autopsy were conducted and were unable to establish a precise cause of death. Improved death scene investigations with scene reconstructions and timely witness interviews assist the death certifier in understanding the role of potentially hazardous conditions in the immediate sleep environment that may have contributed to an infant death. For example, seeing a scene photo of an infant's airway in relation to soft objects like pillows and blankets or reading a witnessed account of a caregiver overlaying an infant on a shared sleep surface provides invaluable knowledge about the circumstances and factors contributing to an infant death, especially when the autopsy findings cannot explain the death. This improved knowledge likely contributed to the increase in classifying deaths as unknown and undetermined causes or accidental suffocation (48, 55, 56). For example, in Detroit, Michigan, increasing understanding of sleep position and other sleep environment hazards led to a decline in the use of SIDS and a marked increase in accidental asphyxia diagnoses (57).

## Recent SIDS and SUID Trends

### Variation across countries

Recent SIDS rates vary across high-income countries (2012-14), ranging from 0.05 deaths per 1,000 live births in Sweden to 0.39 deaths per 1,000 live births in the US (Figure 13.3). This variation is likely due to the differential coding patterns ascribed to unexplained infant deaths across countries (7). In a cross-country analysis using 2002-10 data, Taylor et al. showed a significant decline in rates of SUID in all countries, except the US and New Zealand. There was no significant change in SUID rates for the US and only a non-significant decline in New Zealand. Figure 13.4 shows SUID rates from eight countries including the US and New Zealand in 2002-04, 2005-07, and 2008-10 and the percentage changes from 2002-04 to 2008-10. Despite declining rates in all countries except the US, SUID remained the primary contributor to overall post-neonatal mortality, constituting one-third to half of all post-neonatal deaths in Australia, Canada, Germany, Japan, New Zealand, England and Wales, and the US. In the Netherlands, where SUID rates are typically among the lowest in the world, SUID accounted for 18% of post-neonatal deaths.

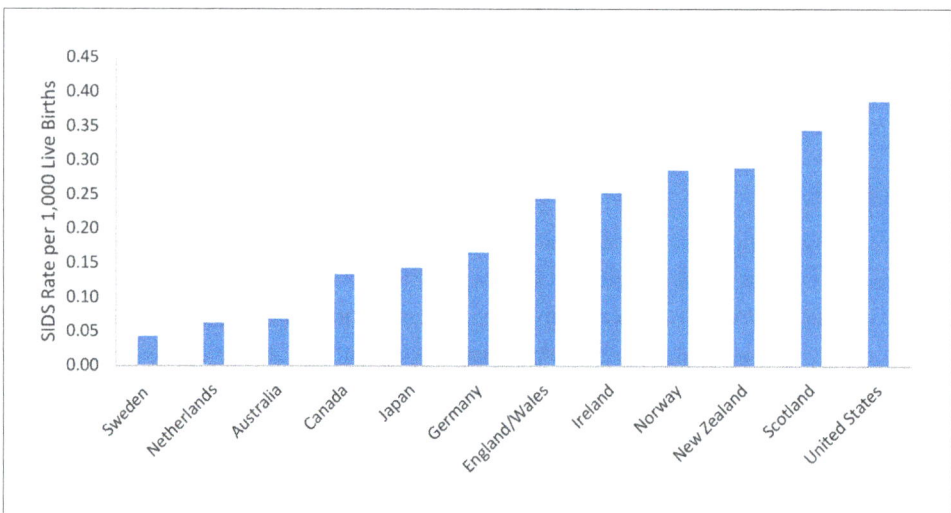

Figure 13.3: International SIDS rates, most recent data available. Note: SIDS is defined by ICD-10 code R95. (Source details for these rates are provided in the following table.)

| Country | Year | Source |
|---|---|---|
| Sweden (103) | 2014 | Health and Welfare Statistical Databases |
| Netherlands (104, 105) | 2014 | Dutch Central Bureau of Statistics |
| Australia (4) | 2015 | Australian Bureau of Statistics |
| Canada (106) | 2012 | Statistics Canada |
| Japan (106) | 2015 | Ministry of Health, Labor and Welfare: Handbook of Health and Welfare Statistics |
| Germany (107, 108) | 2014 | Federal Office of Statistics |
| England/Wales (108, 109) | 2013 | Office for National Statistics |
| Ireland (104) | 2014 | Central Statistics Office |
| Norway (104, 110) | 2012 | Statistics Norway |
| New Zealand (111) | 2012 | New Zealand Ministry of Health |
| Scotland (105) | 2015 | National Records of Scotland |
| United States (112) | 2014 | National Center for Health Statistics |

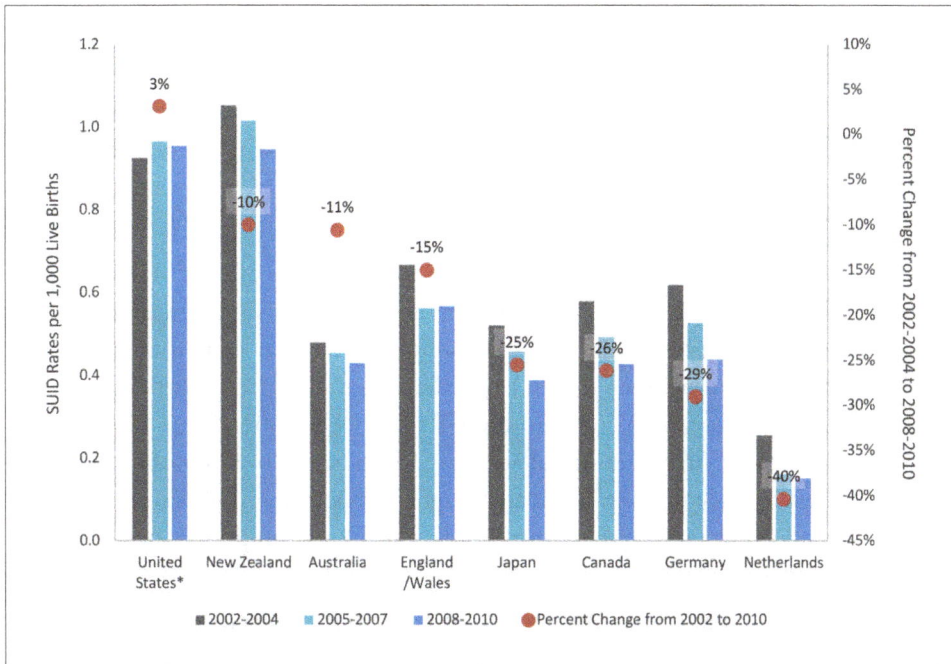

Figure 13.4: International SUID rates 2002-04, 2005-07 and 2008-10 and per cent decrease from 2002-10. SUID: ICD-10 codes R95, R96, R98, R99, W75, W78, and W79. (Source: Rachel Moon, unpublished data, November 2016; and Taylor et al. 2015 (7).)

With approximately 4 million births per year, the US is unique because of its large number of births (and infant deaths) and has the ability to show SIDS and SUID rates using 25 years of data, 1990-2014 (Figure 13.2). The SIDS rate in the US declined dramatically, from 1.30 deaths per 1,000 live births in 1990 to 0.39 deaths per 1,000 live births in 2014, a 70% decrease (58, 59). Since about 2000, the decline in the SIDS rate has slowed substantially, resulting in a 30.2% decrease in SIDS rate from 2001-14 compared with a 52.3% decrease the decade before (1990-2000).

The US SUID rate followed a trend similar to SIDS from 1990 until 1997 (Figure 13.2), at which point the declines in SUID were less pronounced than the declines in SIDS. This is likely due to the diagnostic shift, which began in the late 1990s, as mentioned above. As fewer deaths were classified as SIDS, increasing numbers of deaths were classified as undetermined causes or accidental suffocation and strangulation in bed. From 1990-98, the SUID rate declined rapidly from 1.55 to 0.95 deaths per 1,000 live births, a 39.3% decrease, and remained at 0.95 deaths per 1,000 live births from 1998-2002 (10, 59). In 2003, the rate declined to 0.90 deaths per 1,000 and then increased to a peak of 0.99 deaths per 1,000 live births in 2008. Since 2008, SUID rate declined to 0.88 deaths per 1,000 live births in 2014 (59).

## Selected demographic characteristics

Historically, SIDS has been described in terms of its distinct set of characteristics, including age at death, season of death, and sex. Variations in SIDS rates by race/ethnicity and gestational age have also been clearly established. In this section, we describe these characteristics of SIDS and include discussion of SUID where data are available.

### Age at death

SIDS has a unique age-at-death distribution with approximately 80% of SIDS occurring in the first four months after birth and a peak in SIDS typically observed at 2-3 months of age (9, 10, 21, 23, 24, 26, 60, 61). For example, in Ireland, more than half (59%) of SIDS cases occurred between 2 and 4 months of age and 83% occurred in the first 6 months of age from 1993-97 (26). In the US from 1999-2001, about 80% of SIDS deaths occurred in the first 4 months of age and 90% occurred by 6 months of age (10). Following the US "Back to Sleep" campaign, higher proportions of SIDS cases occurred in the neonatal period and after 6 months of age, and a lower proportion occurred from 1-3 months of age (10, 62).

Given the diagnostic shift, however, it is important to describe the age-of-death distribution for SUID as well. Like SIDS, most SUID occurs in younger rather than older infants. US data from 2011-13 examining racial and ethnic differences in SUID rates showed that 76-86% of SUID occur between 0-4 months of age, with a peak at 1-2 months across all racial and ethnic groups (63). Comparing 1995-97 to 2011-13, small increases were observed in the proportion of SUID cases occurring in the neonatal period and after 6 months of age. Like SIDS, this was accompanied by a decline in the proportion of deaths from 1-3 months of age.

## Seasonality

In early studies of SIDS, before implementation of risk reduction campaigns, a higher incidence of SIDS was reported during the fall and winter than in the spring and summer across several high-income countries (10, 60, 64-68). However, this seasonal difference appears to have attenuated over the years (24, 39, 69-73). In a recent SUID study comparing US data from 1995-97 and 2011-13, a decreasing proportion of winter deaths and increasing proportion of summer deaths occurred among non-Hispanic whites, non-Hispanic blacks and Hispanics (63). The net result is an equal distribution of SUID throughout the year for all racial and ethnic groups.

## Race/ethnicity

Rates of SIDS and SUID vary among racial and ethnic groups in several countries. In a 2007 German case-control study of SIDS risk factors, the odds of SIDS were slightly, but not statistically significantly, higher among infants with at least one non-European parent [odds ratio (OR) (95% CI): 1.22 (0.45 to 3.33)] (74). Studies of SUID in New Zealand have revealed significant racial/ethnic disparities. Maori or Pacific Islander infants comprise 83% of all SUID, but only 15% of the New Zealand population (75, 76). Aboriginal populations in Australia have also been shown to have significantly higher rates of SIDS than non-Aboriginals (0.61 versus 0.17 deaths per 1,000 live births) (77). A similar disparity has been observed among the Indigenous population in Canada (78). US data from 2013 show that SUID rates (deaths per 1,000 live births) are highest in American Indian/Alaska Native (1.70) and non-Hispanic black (1.73) populations compared to non-Hispanic whites (0.85). Rates are lowest in Asian/Pacific Islander (0.29) and Hispanic (0.49) populations (11). There is also variation in SUID rates among Hispanic subgroups: 0.48 for Hispanics of Mexican origin, 0.67 for Puerto Rican origin, and 0.18 for Central and South American origin (11).

Following the "US Back to Sleep" campaign, from 1995-2013, the SUID for non-Hispanic whites has remained close to 1.00 deaths per 1,000 live births. However, across other racial and ethnic groups, SUID rates have declined differentially (Figure 13.5). Declines were most marked for the groups with the highest rates (American Indian/ Alaska Natives and non-Hispanic blacks), but modest declines were observed for all racial/ethnic groups. From 1995-2013, rates were highest for American Indian/Alaska Natives (2.15) and non-Hispanic blacks (1.89), followed by non-Hispanic whites (0.88); rates were lowest for Asian/Pacific Islanders (0.42) and Hispanics (0.54) (63).

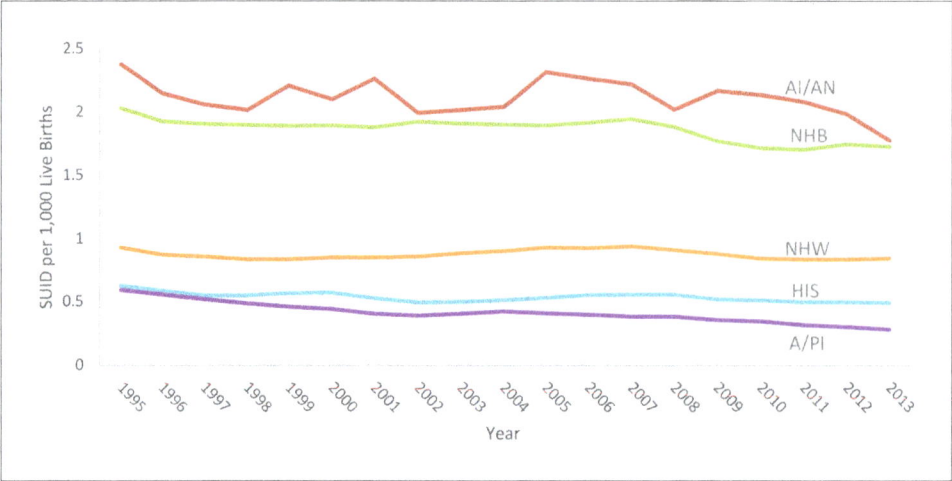

Figure 13.5: Trends in SUID-rates per 100,000 live births by race/ethnicity, United States, 1995-2013. Key: **AI/AN**: American Indian/Alaska Native, **NHB**: non-Hispanic black, **NHW**: non-Hispanic white, **HIS**: Hispanic, **A/PI**: Asian/Pacific Islander. **SUID**: Underlying ICD-10 Codes R95, R99, and W75. (Based on data obtained from the online query system for the CDC/NCHS's National Vital Statistics System (58, 59).)

## Sex

The SIDS literature over the past several decades clearly establishes a higher risk of SIDS in males than females (21, 24, 26, 61, 64, 71, 79-82). In 2014, the US reported SIDS rates of 0.45 deaths per 1,000 live births for males and 0.38 for females (83). One hypothesis is that a single recessive x-linked gene may be related to an infant's likelihood of suffering fatal, acute anoxic events (84). Another hypothesis is that these differences may be due to inherent sex differences in brain structure and function, which influence arousal during sleep (85-87). These hypotheses may explain why the relative sex distribution of cases has remained consistent despite declining overall incidence.

## Gestational age at birth

Preterm birth (<37 weeks' gestation) is a well-documented risk factor for SIDS (11, 12, 21, 70, 88-92). In the US, the risk of SIDS declines as gestational age at birth increases. For example, Malloy (91) found that the postneonatal SIDS rate varied by weeks of gestational age at the time of birth: 24-28 (1.23 deaths per 1,000 live births), 29-32 (1.23 deaths per 1,000 live births), 33-36 (0.78 deaths per 1,000 live births) and 37-42 (0.37 deaths per 1,000 live births) weeks' gestation among post-neonatal infants during 2005-07. SIDS was 2.6, 2.7 and 1.9 times more likely when the infant was born at 24-28, 29-32 and 33-36 weeks' gestation compared to full term (37-42 weeks gestation).

Following a peak in 2006, preterm birth rates declined from 2007-14 (93, 94). In examining the relationship between SUID and preterm births, using US vital statistics data from 1995-2013, it was found that declines in preterm SUID rates have been greater than declines in term SUID rates (63). The SUID rate among preterm infants was 2.25 deaths per 1,000 live births in 1995-97 and 1.72 deaths per 1,000 live births in 2011-13, a 23% decrease. The SUID rate among term infants was 0.89 deaths per 1,000 live births in 1995-97 and 0.76 deaths per 1,000 live births in 2011-13, a 15% decrease.

## Epidemiology of Unexplained Child Deaths

While epidemiologic data on SIDS and SUID demonstrate declining rates throughout a child's first year of life, less is known about sudden death beyond infancy. Sudden unexplained death in childhood (SUDC) is the sudden and unexpected death of a child 1 year old and older that remains unexplained after a thorough review of the child's death, including clinical history, death scene investigation, autopsy, and ancillary testing (95). Like SIDS, the etiology of SUDC eludes scientists and explanations for these events are likely multifactorial. Although there is an ICD code for SIDS, there is not one for SUDC, thereby making comparable incidence estimates challenging (96).

In the literature, rates of SUDC vary from 0.1-1.4 per 100,000 children aged 1-4 years for SUDC (96). SUDC occurs most commonly between 1 and 4 years of age and accounts for approximately 10% of unexpected childhood deaths (96, 97). More males than females are affected, at a ratio of approximately 2:1 (95, 97). Like SIDS, SUDC most often occurs during sleep, making most of these deaths unwitnessed. Furthermore, children are most often found in a prone position with about half found facedown on the sleep surface (95, 98). The general prevalence of febrile seizures among US and European living children is 2-5% prevalence (96); two small case series investigations (95, 96) reported a higher frequency (24%-32%) of febrile seizure history among SUDC cases indicating one possible common pathway to SUDC. Our understanding of SUDC is limited and more studies are need to improve scientific knowledge (96). The US Sudden Death in the Young Case Registry is a potential data source to study SUDC incidence and etiology (99). If cardiac, neurologic, or genetic contributing factors can be clearly identified and characterized, there may be prevention measures that can be implemented to prevent some of these tragic events.

## Conclusions

The diagnostic shift has made surveillance of SIDS challenging, as we can no longer rely on a single ICD code to monitor and compare trends, especially across jurisdictions and countries. Until researchers and forensic experts can agree on standardized definitions and criteria to define and classify SIDS and SUID, grouping ICD codes to reflect SUID is an important option for surveillance and research purposes (7, 100, 101).

Although a dramatic decline in SIDS and SUID occurred in the 1990s following risk reduction campaigns like "Back to Sleep", progress in reducing SIDS and SUID rates has slowed. High rates of SIDS and SUID still exist among some racial and ethnic groups, especially among Indigenous populations in high-income countries and among US non-Hispanic black populations. These high-risk populations need targeted, evidence-based interventions implemented to lower their rates of SUID. Surveillance using information collected from comprehensive multidisciplinary review structures like child death review teams may also improve our knowledge about the circumstances and events contributing to unexplained infant and child deaths (15, 99, 102). This knowledge may contribute to an understanding of factors that can be modified and inform the development and implementation of effective prevention programs.

## References

1.  International statistical classification of diseases and related health problems. ICD-10 Version:2010. [Available from: http://apps.who.int/classifications/apps/icd/icd10online/]. Accessed 12 October 2016.

2.  World Health Organization. History of the development of the ICD. [Available from: http://www.who.int/classifications/icd/en/HistoryOfICD.pdf]. Accessed 22 October 2017.

3.  Beckwith JB. The sudden infant death syndrome. Curr Probl Pediatr. 1973;3(8):1-36. https://doi.org/10.1016/S0045-9380(73)80020-9.

4.  MacDorman MF, Rosenberg HM. Trends in infant mortality by cause of death and other characteristics, 1960-88. Data from the National Vital Statistics System. Vital and Health Statistics Series 20. 1993;20(20):1-57.

5.  Kim SY, Shapiro-Mendoza CK, Chu SY, Camperlengo LT, Anderson RN. Differentiating cause-of-death terminology for deaths coded as sudden infant death syndrome, accidental suffocation, and unknown cause: An investigation using US death certificates, 2003-2004. J Forensic Sci. 2012;57(2):364-9. https://doi.org/10.1111/j.1556-4029.2011.01937.x.

6.  Shapiro-Mendoza CK, Kim SY, Chu SY, Kahn E, Anderson RN. Using death certificates to characterize sudden infant death syndrome (SIDS): Opportunities and limitations. J Pediatr. 2010;156(1):38-43. https://doi.org/10.1016/j.jpeds.2009.07.017.

7.  Taylor BJ, Garstang J, Engelberts A, Obonai T, Cote A, Freemantle J, et al. International comparison of sudden unexpected death in infancy rates using a newly

proposed set of cause-of-death codes. Arch Dis Child. 2015;100(11):1018-23. https://doi.org/10.1136/archdischild-2015-308239.

8.  Camperlengo LT, Shapiro-Mendoza CK, Kim SY. Sudden infant death syndrome: Diagnostic practices and investigative policies, 2004. Am J Forensic Med Pathol. 2012;33(3):197-201. https://doi.org/10.1097/PAF.0b013e3181fe33bd.

9.  Malloy MH, MacDorman M. Changes in the classification of sudden unexpected infant deaths: United States, 1992-2001. Pediatrics. 2005;115(5):1247-53. https://doi.org/10.1542/peds.2004-2188.

10. Shapiro-Mendoza CK, Tomashek KM, Anderson RN, Wingo J. Recent national trends in sudden, unexpected infant deaths: More evidence supporting a change in classification or reporting. Am J Epidemiol. 2006;163(8):762-9. https://doi.org/10.1093/aje/kwj117.

11. Mathews TJ, MacDorman MF, Thoma ME. Infant mortality statistics from the 2013 period linked birth/infant death data set. National Vital Statistics Reports. 2015;64(9):1-30.

12. Leach CE, Blair PS, Fleming PJ, Smith IJ, Platt MW, Berry PJ, et al. Epidemiology of SIDS and explained sudden infant deaths. CESDI SUDI Research Group. Pediatrics. 1999;104(4):e43. https://doi.org/10.1542/peds.104.4.e43.

13. Platt MW, Blair PS, Fleming PJ, Smith IJ, Cole TJ, Leach CE, et al. A clinical comparison of SIDS and explained sudden infant deaths: How healthy and how normal? CESDI SUDI research group confidential inquiry into stillbirths and deaths in infancy study. Arch Dis Child. 2000;82(2):98-106. https://doi.org/10.1136/adc.82.2.98.

14. Camperlengo L, Shapiro-Mendoza CK, Gibbs F. Improving sudden unexplained infant death investigation practices: An evaluation of the centers for disease control and prevention's SUID investigation training academies. Am J Forensic Med Pathol. 2014;35(4):278-82. https://doi.org/10.1097/PAF.0000000000000123.

15. Shapiro-Mendoza CK, Camperlengo LT, Kim SY, Covington T. The sudden unexpected infant death case registry: A method to improve surveillance. Pediatrics. 2012;129(2):e486-93. https://doi.org/10.1542/peds.2011-0854.

16. US Department of Health and Human Services. MICH-1.9 Reduce the rate of infant deaths from sudden unexpected infant deaths (includes SIDS, unknown cause, accidental suffocation, and strangulation in bed). [Available from: https://www.healthypeople.gov/2020/topics-objectives/objective/mich-19-0]. Accessed 22 October 2017.

17. Senter L, Sackoff J, Landi K, Boyd L. Studying sudden and unexpected infant deaths in a time of changing death certification and investigation practices:

Evaluating sleep-related risk factors for infant death in New York City. Matern Child Health J. 2011;15(2):242-8. https://doi.org/10.1007/s10995-010-0577-8.

18. Borse NN, Gilchrist J, Dellinger AM, Rudd RA, Ballesteros MF, Sleet DA. CDC childhood injury report: Patterns of unintentional injuries among 0-19 year olds in the United States, 2000-2006. Atlanta, GA: US Department of Health and Human Services, Centers for Disease Control and Prevention, National Center for Injury Prevention and Control, 2008.

19. Hauck FR, Tanabe KO. International trends in sudden infant death syndrome: Stabilization of rates requires further action. Pediatrics. 2008;122(3):660-6. https://doi.org/10.1542/peds.2007-0135.

20. Bergman NJ. Hypothesis on supine sleep, sudden infant death syndrome reduction and association with increasing autism incidence. World J Clin Pediatr. 2016;5(3):330-42. https://doi.org/10.5409/wjcp.v5.i3.330.

21. Fleming PJ, Blair PS, Pease A. Sudden unexpected death in infancy: Aetiology, pathophysiology, epidemiology and prevention in 2015. Arch Dis Child. 2015;100(10):984-8. https://doi.org/10.1136/archdischild-2014-306424.

22. Mitchell EA, Cowan S, Tipene-Leach D. The recent fall in postperinatal mortality in New Zealand and the Safe Sleep programme. Acta Paediatr. 2016;105(11):1312-20. https://doi.org/10.1111/apa.13494.

23. Arnestad M, Andersen M, Vege A, Rognum TO. Changes in the epidemiological pattern of sudden infant death syndrome in southeast Norway, 1984-1998: Implications for future prevention and research. Arch Dis Child. 2001;85(2):108-15. https://doi.org/10.1136/adc.85.2.108.

24. Blair PS, Sidebotham P, Berry PJ, Evans M, Fleming PJ. Major epidemiological changes in sudden infant death syndrome: A 20-year population-based study in the UK. Lancet. 2006;367(9507):314-19. https://doi.org/10.1016/S0140-6736(06)67968-3.

25. McGarvey C, McDonnell M, Chong A, O'Regan M, Matthews T. Factors relating to the infant's last sleep environment in sudden infant death syndrome in the Republic of Ireland. Arch Dis Child. 2003;88(12):1058-64. https://doi.org/10.1136/adc.88.12.1058.

26. Mehanni M, Cullen A, Kiberd B, McDonnell M, O'Regan M, Matthews T. The current epidemiology of SIDS in Ireland. Ir Med J. 2000;93(9):264-8.

27. Office for National Statistics. Health Statistics Quarterly, No. 24, Winter 2004. [Available from: http://webarchive.nationalarchives.gov.uk/20160105160709/http://ons.gov.uk/ons/rel/hsq/health-statistics-quarterly/no--24--winter-2004/index.html]. Accessed 22 October 2017.

28. Willinger M, Ko CW, Hoffman HJ, Kessler RC, Corwin MJ. Factors associated with caregivers' choice of infant sleep position, 1994-1998: The National Infant Sleep Position Study. JAMA. 2000;283(16):2135-42. https://doi.org/10.1001/jama.283.16.2135.

29. Wennergren G, Alm B, Oyen N, Helweg-Larsen K, Milerad J, Skjaerven R, et al. The decline in the incidence of SIDS in Scandinavia and its relation to risk-intervention campaigns. Nordic epidemiological SIDS study. Acta Paediatr. 1997;86(9):963-8. https://doi.org/10.1111/j.1651-2227.1997.tb15180.x.

30. Mitchell EA, Brunt JM, Everard C. Reduction in mortality from sudden infant death syndrome in New Zealand: 1986-92. Arch Dis Child. 1994;70(4):291-4. https://doi.org/10.1136/adc.70.4.291.

31. Markestad T, Skadberg B, Hordvik E, Morild I, Irgens LM. Sleeping position and sudden infant death syndrome (SIDS): Effect of an intervention programme to avoid prone sleeping. Acta Paediatr. 1995;84(4):375-8. https://doi.org/10.1111/j.1651-2227.1995.tb13653.x.

32. Hiley CM, Morley CJ. Evaluation of government's campaign to reduce risk of cot death. BMJ (Clinical research ed). 1994;309(6956):703-4. https://doi.org/10.1136/bmj.309.6956.703.

33. Cote A, Russo P, Michaud J. Sudden unexpected deaths in infancy: What are the causes? J Pediatr. 1999;135(4):437-43. https://doi.org/10.1016/S0022-3476(99)70165-4.

34. Willinger M, Hoffman HJ, Wu KT, Hou JR, Kessler RC, Ward SL, et al. Factors associated with the transition to nonprone sleep positions of infants in the United States: The National Infant Sleep Position Study. JAMA. 1998;280(4):329-35. https://doi.org/10.1001/jama.280.4.329.

35. National Institute of Child Health and Human Development. Safe to Sleep® Public Education Campaign. [Available from: http://www.nichd.nih.gov/sts/Pages/default.aspx]. Accessed 22 October 2017.

36. Mitchell E, Krous HF, Donald T, Byard RW. Changing trends in the diagnosis of sudden infant death. Am J Forensic Med Pathol. 2000;21(4):311-14. https://doi.org/10.1097/00000433-200012000-00002.

37. Byard RW, Beal SM. Has changing diagnostic preference been responsible for the recent fall in incidence of sudden infant death syndrome in South Australia? J Paediatr Child Health. 1995;31(3):197-9. https://doi.org/10.1111/j.1440-1754.1995.tb00785.x.

38. Office for National Statistics. Trends in cot death. Health Statistics Quarterly, No. 5, Spring 2000. [Available from: http://webarchive.nationalarchives.gov.

uk/20160105160709/http://ons.gov.uk/ons/rel/hsq/health-statistics-quarterly/
no--5--spring-2000/index.html]. Accessed 22 October 2017.

39. Shapiro-Mendoza CK, Kimball M, Tomashek KM, Anderson RN, Blanding S. US infant mortality trends attributable to accidental suffocation and strangulation in bed from 1984 through 2004: Are rates increasing? Pediatrics. 2009;123(2):533-9. https://doi.org/10.1542/peds.2007-3746.

40. The Official King James Bible Online. I Kings 3:19. [Available from: http://wwwkingjamesbibleonlineorg]. Accessed 22 October 2017.

41. Willinger M, James LS, Catz C. Defining the sudden infant death syndrome (SIDS): Deliberations of an expert panel convened by the National Institute of Child Health and Human Development. Pediatr Pathol. 1991;11(5):677-84. https://doi.org/10.3109/15513819109065465.

42. Krous HF, Beckwith JB, Byard RW, Rognum TO, Bajanowski T, Corey T, et al. Sudden infant death syndrome and unclassified sudden infant deaths: A definitional and diagnostic approach. Pediatrics. 2004;114(1):234-8. https://doi.org/10.1542/peds.114.1.234.

43. Limerick SR, Bacon CJ. Terminology used by pathologists in reporting on sudden infant deaths. J Clin Pathol. 2004;57(3):309-11. https://doi.org/10.1136/jcp.2003.013052.

44. Corey TS, Hanzlick R, Howard J, Nelson C, Krous H, & NAME Ad Hoc Committee on Sudden Unexplained Infant Death. A functional approach to sudden unexplained infant deaths. Am J Forensic Med Pathol. 2007;28(3):271-7. https://doi.org/10.1097/01.paf.0000257385.25803.cf.

45. Kennedy H, Royal College of Pathologists, Royal College of Paediatrics and Child Health. Sudden unexpected death in infancy: A multi-agency protocol for care and investigation. [Available from: http://www.rcpch.ac.uk/sites/default/files/page/SUDI_report_for_web.pdf]. Accessed 22 October 2017.

46. Byard RW. SUDI or "undetermined": Does it matter? Forensic Sci Med Pathol. 2009;5(4):252. https://doi.org/10.1007/s12024-009-9129-1.

47. Shapiro-Mendoza CK, Parks SE, Brustrom J, Andrew T, Camperlengo L, Fudenberg J, et al. Variations in cause-of-death determination for sudden unexpected infant deaths. Pediatrics. 2017; 140(1): e20170087. https://doi.org/10.1542/peds.2017-0087.

48. Garstang J, Ellis C, Sidebotham P. An evidence-based guide to the investigation of sudden unexpected death in infancy. Forensic Sci Med Pathol. 2015;11(3):345-57. https://doi.org/10.1007/s12024-015-9680-x.

49. Goldstein RD, Trachtenberg FL, Sens MA, Harty BJ, Kinney HC. Overall postneonatal mortality and rates of SIDS. Pediatrics. 2016;137(1): e20152298. https://doi.org/10.1542/peds.2015-2298.

50. Hauck FR, Signore C, Fein SB, Raju TN. Infant sleeping arrangements and practices during the first year of life. Pediatrics. 2008;122 Suppl 2:S113-20. https://doi.org/10.1542/peds.2008-1315o.

51. Gould SJ, Weber MA, Sebire NJ. Variation and uncertainties in the classification of sudden unexpected infant deaths among paediatric pathologists in the UK: Findings of a National Delphi Study. J Clin Pathol. 2010;63(9):796-9. https://doi.org/10.1136/jcp.2010.079715.

52. Nashelsky MB, Pinckard JK. The death of SIDS. Academic Forensic Pathology. 2011;1(1):92-8.

53. Bass M, Kravath RE, Glass L. Death-scene investigation in sudden infant death. N Engl J Med. 1986;315(2):100-5. https://doi.org/10.1056/NEJM198607103150206.

54. Centers for Disease Control and Prevention. Guidelines for death scene investigation of sudden, unexplained infant deaths: Recommendations of the interagency panel on sudden infant death syndrome. Morb Mortal Wkly Rep. 1996;45(RR-10):1-6.

55. Gornall J. Does cot death still exist? BMJ (Clinical research ed). 2008;336(7639):302-4. https://doi.org/10.1136/bmj.39455.496146.AD.

56. Hanzlick R. A perspective on medicolegal death investigation in the United States: 2013. Acad Forensic Pathol. 2014;4:2-9. https://doi.org/10.23907/2014.001.

57. Pasquale-Styles MA, Tackitt PL, Schmidt CJ. Infant death scene investigation and the assessment of potential risk factors for asphyxia: A review of 209 sudden unexpected infant deaths. J Forensic Sci. 2007;52(4):924-9. https://doi.org/10.1111/j.1556-4029.2007.00477.x.

58. CDC WONDER On-line Database. Centers for Disease Control and Prevention, National Center for Health Statistics. Compressed Mortality File 1979-1998, as compiled from Compressed Mortality File CMF 1968-1988, Series 20, No. 2A, 2000 and CMF 1989-1998, Series 20, No. 2E, 2003. [Available from: https://wonder.cdc.gov/cmf-icd9.html]. Accessed 22 October 2017.

59. CDC WONDER On-line Database. Centers for Disease Control and Prevention, National Center for Health Statistics. Compressed Mortality File 1999-2014, released December 2016, from the Compressed Mortality File 1999-2015, Series 20, No. 2U, 2016. [Available from: http://wonder.cdc.gov/cmf-icd10.html]. Accessed 22 October 2017.

60. Beal SM, Baghurst P, Antoniou G. Sudden infant death syndrome (SIDS) in South Australia 1968-97. Part 2: The epidemiology of non-prone and non-covered SIDS infants. J Paediatr Child Health. 2000;36(6):548-51. https://doi.org/10.1046/j.1440-1754.2000.00576.x.

61. Office for National Statistics. Unexplained deaths in infancy, 2006. Health Statistics Quarterly, No. 39, Autumn 2008. [Available from: http://webarchive.nationalarchives.gov.uk/20160105160709/http://ons.gov.uk/ons/rel/hsq/health-statistics-quarterly/no--39--autumn-2008/index.html]. Accessed 22 October 2017.

62. Malloy MH, Freeman DH. Age at death, season, and day of death as indicators of the effect of the back to sleep program on sudden infant death syndrome in the United States, 1992-1999. Arch Pediatr Adolesc Med. 2004;158(4):359-65. https://doi.org/10.1001/archpedi.158.4.359.

63. Parks SE, Shapiro-Mendoza CK, Lambert AE. Racial/ethnic trends in sudden unexpected infant deaths — United States 1995-2013. Paediatrics. 2017; 139(6):e20163844. https://doi.org/10.1542/peds.2016-3844.

64. Vege A, Rognum TO, Opdal SH. SIDS — Changes in the epidemiological pattern in eastern Norway 1984-1996. Forensic Sci Int. 1998;93(2-3):155-66. https://doi.org/10.1016/S0379-0738(98)00048-6.

65. Peterson DR, Sabotta EE, Strickland D. Sudden infant death syndrome in epidemiologic perspective: Etiologic implications of variation with season of the year. Ann NY Acad Sci. 1988;533:6-12. https://doi.org/10.1111/j.1749-6632.1988.tb37229.x.

66. Centers for Disease Control and Prevention. Seasonality in sudden infant death syndrome — United States, 1980-1987. MMWR Morb Mortal Wkly Rep. 1990;39(49):891-5.

67. Gupta R, Helms PJ, Jolliffe IT, Douglas AS. Seasonal variation in sudden infant death syndrome and bronchiolitis — A common mechanism? Am J Respir Crit Care Med. 1996;154(2 Pt 1):431-5. https://doi.org/10.1164/ajrccm.154.2.8756818.

68. Douglas AS, Helms PJ, Jolliffe IT. Seasonality of sudden infant death syndrome in mainland Britain and Ireland 1985-95. Arch Dis Child. 1998;79(3):269-70. https://doi.org/10.1136/adc.79.3.269.

69. Blair PS, Platt MW, Smith IJ, Fleming PJ, Group CSR. Sudden infant death syndrome and sleeping position in pre-term and low birth weight infants: An opportunity for targeted intervention. Arch Dis Child. 2006;91(2):101-6. https://doi.org/10.1136/adc.2004.070391.

70. Fleming PJ, Blair, PS, Bacon, C., Berrty PJ, editors. Sudden unexpected death in infancy. The CESDI SUDI studies 1993-1996. London; The Stationary Office: 2000 ISBN 0 11 322299 8.

71. Adams EJ, Chavez GF, Steen D, Shah R, Iyasu S, Krous HF. Changes in the epidemiologic profile of sudden infant death syndrome as rates decline among California infants: 1990-1995. Pediatrics. 1998;102(6):1445-51. https://doi.org/10.1542/peds.102.6.1445.

72. Mitchell EA. What is the mechanism of SIDS? Clues from epidemiology. Dev Psychobiol. 2009;51(3):215-22. https://doi.org/10.1002/dev.20369.

73. Sloan CD, Gebretsadik T, Rosas-Salazar C, Wu P, Carroll KN, Mitchel E, et al. Seasonal timing of infant bronchiolitis, apnea and sudden unexplained infant death. PLoS One. 2016;11(7):e0158521. https://doi.org/10.1371/journal.pone.0158521.

74. Vennemann M, Bajanowski T, Butterfass-Bahloul T, Sauerland C, Jorch G, Brinkmann B, et al. Do risk factors differ between explained sudden unexpected death in infancy and sudden infant death syndrome? Arch Dis Child. 2007;92(2):133-6. https://doi.org/10.1136/adc.2006.101337.

75. Hutchison BL, Rea C, Stewart AW, Koelmeyer TD, Tipene-Leach DC, Mitchell EA. Sudden unexpected infant death in Auckland: A retrospective case review. Acta Paediatr. 2011;100(8):1108-12. https://doi.org/10.1111/j.1651-2227.2011.02221.x.

76. Mitchell EA, Stewart AW, Scragg R, Ford RP, Taylor BJ, Becroft DM, et al. Ethnic differences in mortality from sudden infant death syndrome in New Zealand. BMJ (Clinical research ed). 1993;306(6869):13-16. https://doi.org/10.1136/bmj.306.6869.13.

77. Alessandri LM, Read AW, Stanley FJ, Burton PR, Dawes VP. Sudden infant death syndrome and infant mortality in aboriginal and non-aboriginal infants. J Paediatr Child Health. 1994;30(3):242-7. https://doi.org/10.1111/j.1440-1754.1994.tb00626.x.

78. Wilson CE. Sudden infant death syndrome and Canadian Aboriginals: Bacteria and infections. FEMS Immunol Med Microbiol. 1999;25(1-2):221-6. https://doi.org/10.1111/j.1574-695X.1999.tb01346.x.

79. Willinger M, Hoffman HJ, Hartford RB. Infant sleep position and risk for sudden infant death syndrome: Report of meeting held January 13 and 14, 1994, National Institutes of Health, Bethesda, MD. Pediatrics. 1994;93(5):814-19. https://doi.org/10.1097/00006205-199407000-00006.

80. Moscovis SM, Hall ST, Burns CJ, Scott RJ, Blackwell CC. The male excess in sudden infant deaths. Innate Immun. 2014;20(1):24-9. https://doi.org/10.1177/1753425913481071.

81. Freemantle CJ, Read AW, de Klerk NH, McAullay D, Anderson IP, Stanley FJ. Sudden infant death syndrome and unascertainable deaths: Trends and disparities among Aboriginal and non-Aboriginal infants born in Western Australia from 1980 to 2001 inclusive. J Paediatr Child Health. 2006;42(7-8):445-51. https://doi.org/10.1111/j.1440-1754.2006.00895.x.

82. Richardson HL, Walker AM, Horne RS. Sleeping like a baby — Does gender influence infant arousability? Sleep. 2010;33(8):1055-60. https://doi.org/10.1093/sleep/33.8.1055.

83. Heron M. Deaths: Leading causes for 2014. National vital statistics reports from the Centers for Disease Control and Prevention, National Center for Health Statistics, National Vital Statistics System. 2016;65(5):1-96.

84. Mage DT, Donner EM. Is excess male infant mortality from sudden infant death syndrome and other respiratory diseases X-linked? Acta Paediatr. 2014;103(2):188-93. https://doi.org/10.1111/apa.12482.

85. Machaalani R, Waters KA. Neuronal cell death in the sudden infant death syndrome brainstem and associations with risk factors. Brain. 2008;131(Pt 1):218-28.

86. Paterson DS, Trachtenberg FL, Thompson EG, Belliveau RA, Beggs AH, Darnall R, et al. Multiple serotonergic brainstem abnormalities in sudden infant death syndrome. JAMA. 2006;296(17):2124-32. https://doi.org/10.1001/jama.296.17.2124.

87. Thordstein M, Lofgren N, Flisberg A, Lindecrantz K, Kjellmer I. Sex differences in electrocortical activity in human neonates. Neuroreport. 2006;17(11):1165-8. https://doi.org/10.1097/01.wnr.0000227978.98389.43.

88. MacDorman MF. Race and ethnic disparities in fetal mortality, preterm birth, and infant mortality in the United States: An overview. Semin Perinatol. 2011;35(4):200-8. https://doi.org/10.1053/j.semperi.2011.02.017.

89. Hauck FR, Tanabe, KO, Moon, RY. Racial and ethnic disparities in infant mortality. Semin Perinatol. 2011;35(4):209-20. https://doi.org/10.1053/j.semperi.2011.02.018.

90. Carlberg MM, Shapiro-Mendoza CK, Goodman M. Maternal and infant characteristics associated with accidental suffocation and strangulation in bed in US infants. Matern Child Health J. 2012;16(8):1594-601. https://doi.org/10.1007/s10995-011-0855-0.

91. Malloy MH. Prematurity and sudden infant death syndrome: United States 2005-2007. J Perinatol. 2013;33(6):470-5. https://doi.org/10.1038/jp.2012.158.

92. Malloy MH, Hoffman HJ. Prematurity, sudden infant death syndrome, and age of death. Pediatrics. 1995;96(3 Pt 1):464-71.

93. Martin JA, Osterman MJ, Kirmeyer SE, Gregory EC. Measuring gestational age in vital statistics data: Transitioning to the obstetric estimate. National Vital Statistics Reports: From the Centers for Disease Control and Prevention, National Center for Health Statistics, National Vital Statistics System. 2015;64(5):1-20.

94. Shapiro-Mendoza CK, Barfield WD, Henderson Z, James A, Howse JL, Iskander J, et al. CDC grand rounds: Public health strategies to prevent preterm birth. Morb Mortal Wkly Rep. 2016;65(32):826-30. https://doi.org/10.15585/mmwr.mm6532a4.

95. Krous HF, Chadwick AE, Crandall L, Nadeau-Manning JM. Sudden unexpected death in childhood: A report of 50 cases. Pediatr Dev Pathol. 2005;8(3):307-19. https://doi.org/10.1007/s10024-005-1155-8.

96. Hesdorffer DC, Crandall LA, Friedman D, Devinsky O. Sudden unexplained death in childhood: A comparison of cases with and without a febrile seizure history. Epilepsia. 2015;56(8):1294-300. https://doi.org/10.1111/epi.13066.

97. Hefti MM, Kinney HC, Cryan JB, Haas EA, Chadwick AE, Crandall LA, et al. Sudden unexpected death in early childhood: General observations in a series of 151 cases: Part 1 of the investigations of the San Diego SUDC Research Project. Forensic Sci Med Pathol. 2016;12(1):4-13. https://doi.org/10.1007/s12024-015-9724-2.

98. Kinney HC, Chadwick AE, Crandall LA, Grafe M, Armstrong DL, Kupsky WJ, et al. Sudden death, febrile seizures, and hippocampal and temporal lobe maldevelopment in toddlers: A new entity. Pediatr Dev Pathol. 2009;12(6):455-63. https://doi.org/10.2350/08-09-0542.1.

99. Burns KM, Bienemann L, Camperlengo L, Cottengim C, Covington TM, Dykstra H, et al. The Sudden Death in the Young Case Registry: Collaborating to understand and reduce mortality. Pediatrics. 2017;139(3): e20162757. https://doi.org/10.1542/peds.2016-2757.

100. Hunt CE, Darnall RA, McEntire BL, Hyma BA. Assigning cause for sudden unexpected infant death. Forensic Sci Med Pathol. 2015;11(2):283-8. https://doi.org/10.1007/s12024-014-9650-8.

101. Shapiro-Mendoza CK, Camperlengo L, Ludvigsen R, Cottengim C, Anderson RN, Andrew T, et al. Classification system for the sudden unexpected infant death case registry and its application. Pediatrics. 2014;134(1):e210-19. https://doi.org/10.1542/peds.2014-0180.

102. Fraser J, Sidebotham P, Frederick J, Covington T, Mitchell EA. Learning from child death review in the USA, England, Australia, and New Zealand. Lancet (London, England). 2014;384(9946):894-903. https://doi.org/10.1016/S0140-6736(13)61089-2.

103. Socialstyrelsen. Sweden Health and Welfare Statistical Databases. [Available from: http://www.socialstyrelsen.se/statistics/statisticaldatabase/causeofdeath]. Accessed 22 October 2017.

104. Statistics Netherlands. Birth; key figures 2014. [Available from: http://statline.cbs.nl/Statweb/publication/?DM=SLEN&PA=37422ENG&D1]. Accessed 22 October 2017.

105. Statistics Norway. Causes of death. [Available from: https://www.ssb.no/statistikkbanken/selectvarval/Define]. Accessed 22 October 2017.

106. Office for National Statistics. Births and infant deaths, England 2012 to 2014. [Available from: https://www.ons.gov.uk/peoplepopulationandcommunity/birthsdeathsandmarriages/deaths/adhocs/005621birthsandinfantdeathsengland2012to2014]. Accessed 22 October 2017.

107. Central Statistics Office. Infant mortality and stillbirths. [Available from: http://www.cso.ie/px/pxeirestat/Statire/SelectVarVal/Define.asp?maintable=VSA97&PLanguage=0]. Accessed 22 October 2017.

108. Statistiches Bundesamt (Federal Statistical Office). Live births. [Available from: https://www.destatis.de/EN/FactsFigures/SocietyState/Population/Births/Tables/LiveBirthDifference.html]. Accessed 22 October 2017.

109. Office for National Statistics. Births and infant deaths, England 2012 to 2014. [Available from: https://www.ons.gov.uk/peoplepopulationandcommunity/birthsdeathsandmarriages/deaths/adhocs/005621birthsandinfantdeathsengland2012to2014]. Accessed 22 October 2017.

110. National Records of Scotland. Vital events reference tables 2015: Section 4 — Stillbirths and infant deaths. [Available from: https://www.nrscotland.gov.uk/statistics-and-data/statistics/statistics-by-theme/vital-events/general-publications/vital-events-reference-tables/2015/section-4-stillbirths-and-infant-deaths]. Accessed 22 October 2017.

111. Ministry of Health. Fetal and infant deaths 2012. [Available from: http://www.health.govt.nz/publication/fetal-and-infant-deaths-2012]. Accessed 22 October 2017.

112. CDC WONDER Online Database. Centers for Disease Control and Prevention. Compressed Mortality File: Underlying cause of Death. [Available from: http://wonder.cdc.gov/]. Accessed 22 October 2017.

# 14 Future Directions in Sudden Unexpected Death in Infancy Research

Heather E Jeffery, MBBS, MPH, PhD

*Sydney School Public Health, University of Sydney, NSW, Australia*

## Introduction

This chapter on sudden unexpected death in infancy (SUDI) (both explained and unexplained) outlines the background to gaps in practice, advances in our understanding of SUDI, non-compliant aspects of prevention, and needs and education of parents and health providers. From this outline the fourth section on future directions is developed.

SUDI is defined as the death of an infant aged less than 12 months that is sudden and unexpected "in which there is death (or collapse leading to death), which would not have been reasonably expected to occur 24 hours previously and in whom no pre-existing medical cause of death is apparent. It includes those deaths for which a cause is ultimately found (explained SUDI) and those that remain unexplained following investigation" (1).

## I. Gaps in Practice

The future of SUDI research remains dependent on accurate investigation and classification of death. This is frequently suboptimal. This section will discuss models of best practice, delineation of a standardized process of investigation, application of standardized percentile charts to SUDI from birth to 1 year, and a proposed simple classification that addresses potential asphyxia.

## Models of best practice

Various models of SUDI investigation with clear objectives and best practice standards have been defined. Garstang et al. (2015) have categorized the different models of SUDI investigation as coroner- or medical-examiner-led investigation, healthcare-led investigation, police-led investigation, and the joint-agency approach (2). All but police-led investigations have the potential to meet international minimum standards of SUDI investigation. The objectives outlined by Garstang et al. include:

- to identify, as far as is possible, any recognizable cause of death including accidental asphyxia, suspicious deaths, medical deaths, and sudden infant death syndrome (SIDS) where diagnostic criteria have been met

- to identify any factors contributing to the death, including factors in the physical or social environment, parental care, and service provision or need

- to support the family through a sensitive, respectful approach that allows them to grieve and recognizes their need for information

- to learn lessons for the prevention of future child deaths

- to ensure that all statutory requirements in relation to the death are fulfilled and that the public interest is served through the appropriate administration of justice and protection of children.

It is apparent that some models cannot fulfil these objectives because some individuals — for example, police — undertaking one or more of the three most important components of SUDI investigation (namely medical/developmental/social history, death scene investigation, or autopsy) have not been specifically trained to do so. While multi-agency and multidisciplinary engagement is intrinsic to the SUDI process and adds complexity, it is a necessity for accurate classification of death, for parental need and expectation, for research, and for prevention. The failure to reach an optimal investigatory process is hampering progress and needs correction for future improvement. The objectives and the process (Figure 14.1) required for an adequate standard can be used to assess the quality of each and every team providing SUDI investigation.

Rates of SUDI differ between, and within, countries, as do the ratio of explained to unexplained SUDI (3). Standards for the process of unraveling SUDI and SIDS have had sluggish uptake and been patchy in many countries. In response to this, several national bodies have developed models of care and guidelines and provided educational interventions to improve the process (1, 7). Arguably, while there is no global consensus on an international standard the most stringent of those published (4-6) is the Kennedy Report (1), recently updated together with the explicit protocols of the Centers for Disease Control (CDC) (7).

The development of a new classification system (4), if used correctly, enabled multidisciplinary practitioners to see the deficits when key pieces of investigation and/or information were missing — for example, competent history, death scene investigation,

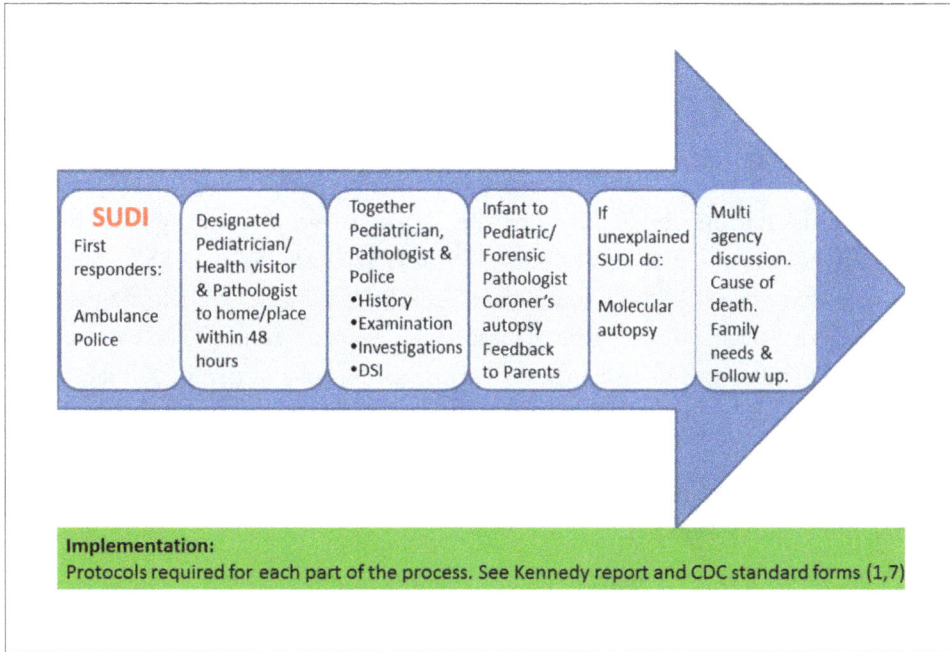

Figure 14.1: Process of SUDI investigation. (Adapted from (1, 7).)

or autopsy. Additional difficulties have seen diagnostic shifts (8, 9), not dissimilar to the very early approach of diagnosing SIDS as a respiratory illness causing the sudden infant death. Thus unascertained, undetermined, accidental suffocation, and strangulation have largely replaced SIDS. Furthermore, there are well-known causes of SUDI that are not necessarily included in investigations, to the detriment of parents in particular, but also researchers (see below).

The future of SUDI research depends on a reliable process that sorts unexplained from explained SUDI by employing a standardized process. The process may differ by country but a standardized process is essential, including the elements outlined in Figure 14.1. Autopsy protocols will require constant updating as new approaches such as molecular autopsy (10) and post-mortem magnetic resonance imaging improve diagnostic yield (11).

The Kennedy Report in 2004 and 2016 (1) defined the parts of this process, which became mandatory in the United Kingdom (UK) in 2008. The CDC (7) enabled an educational process to be implemented in the United States (US) using a hub and spoke model in a structured multi-agency, multiprofessional approach. Sustainability was incorporated by using a train-the-trainer-model for each state and each part of the process was clearly defined — for example, comprehensive forms for medical history and death scene investigation. The evaluation of the UK process indicated successful implementation of a multi-agency approach in the South West and the West Midlands regions of England (2, 12, 13). In the US the education surpassed expectations of numbers trained and positive self-reported responses to skills-based questions (14).

## SUDI from birth to 12 months, inclusive of neonatal SUDI

Analysis of risk factors for SUDI after the "Back to Sleep" campaign in the UK indicated a move to younger age at death (15). In New South Wales (NSW), Australia, a retrospective population study found that 23/828 (15%) of all SUDIs for the years 1996-2008 were neonatal and 66% of these were unexplained; in the first seven days, 42% of SUDIs remained unexplained (16). For each but one of the first 28 days there were deaths explained and unexplained (Figure 14.2). There was little difference in the modifiable and non-modifiable risk factors between the neonatal and post-neonatal groups, with an opportunity for prevention from the day of birth for mothers and staff working in maternity facilities.

A recent prospective population study of acute life-threatening events and SUDI during the first seven postnatal days in Australia revealed an annual incidence of 0.1 per 1,000 live births in NSW, where reporting by state and territory was optimal, most occurring on the day of birth (17). The incidence for Australia was half this and suggests the reticence of clinicians to report and/or investigate early neonatal SUDI. An awareness that SUDI does occur during the neonatal period and during the first week

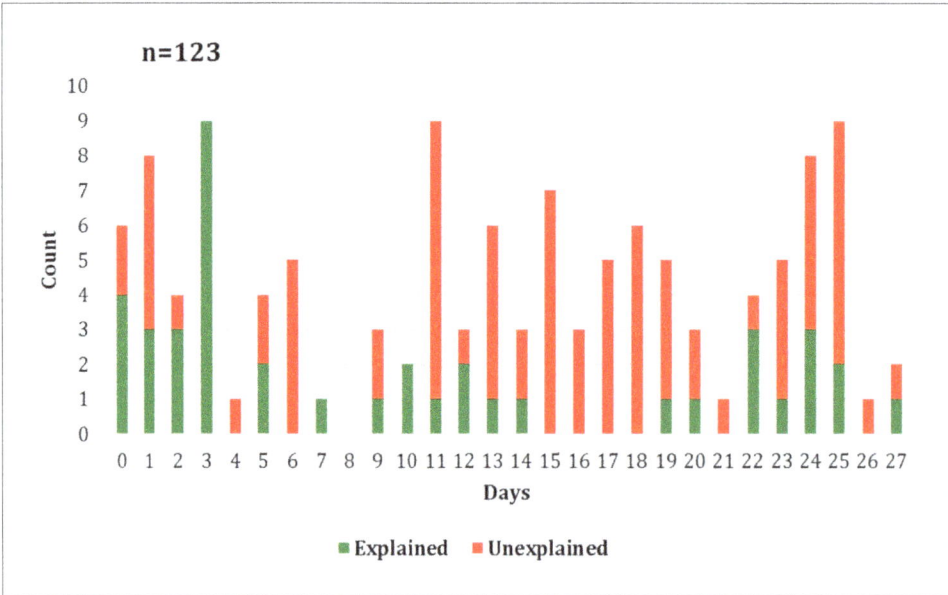

Figure 14.2: Explained and unexplained neonatal SUDI, NSW 1996-2008 (16).

of life justifies their inclusion in SUDI investigations. Excluding such infants introduces risk that a thorough investigation, including autopsy, is bypassed and explanation of "death" presumed by the neonatologist/doctor. Four of the 27 neonates who died in the prospective surveillance study (17) had either no or limited autopsy and their cause of death remained unexplained.

## Accurate measurements on standardized percentile charts

The availability of charts which provide percentiles on how a newborn and child should grow, rather than how they grow, are readily available at various websites — for example, INTERGROWTH-21st for term (18) and preterm infants (19), and World Health Organization (WHO) 0 to 5 years charts (20) — along with relevant publications (21-23).

The standards were developed in eight low-, middle- and high-income countries where the mother, newborn and child grew under selected optimal conditions for socioeconomic, health, and environmental circumstances. These charts provide standards and immediate and important information to the pathologist, pediatrician, and other health providers. These should form part of the pathologist's report. The medical history enables access to previous details on weight, length, and head circumference. These are valuable in defining expected normal growth or not. These charts are especially valuable for the increased preterm population amongst SUDI deaths, where growth differs until 64 weeks postmenstrual age (21), after which the WHO standards apply (23). Whether the infant was preterm or term, identification of growth <10th percentile for weight and weight-for-height, length, and head circumference must lead to a search for causes of possible growth reduction at birth or growth faltering after birth. Examinations of percentiles at birth and at death as well as inter-current measurements are relevant. Thus maternal and infant histories and percentiles are part of the complete medical history and examination of the SUDI infant and uncover unrecognized intrinsic factors.

## Simple classification system to address the potential contribution of asphyxia

There have been a number of proposals for a classification system for SIDS/SUDI that builds on that of Krous et al. 2004 (4). This has been provoked by the evidence for a diagnostic shift (8, 9) and for differences in International Classification of Disease (ICD)-10 coding (3). There is some confusion around the presence of risk factors and causality, the former being an association but not causal. There are differences in how pathologists interpret the definition of SIDS (24, 25). To overcome this and to provide better information for parents, prevention, research, and recognition of key missing components of the investigations, three simple systems have been published (26-29). Two of these classifications have also been tested (27, 28).

One suggestion to further simplify and "visualize" the definitions of SUDI is to unite these into one grid, as proposed in the UK (26), which provides evidence of adequacy, or not, of investigations and lists risk factors (see Table 14.1). Therefore

- if investigations were *inadequate*, cases would be classified as SUDI 0
- if investigations were *adequate*, if there were no intrinsic risk factors, and if there was a safe sleep environment, cases would be classified as SUDI 1
- if investigations were *adequate*, if there were intrinsic factors present, and if there was a safe sleep environment, classify as SUDI 2
- if investigations were *adequate*, if there were no or some intrinsic risk factors, and if there was an unsafe sleep environment, classify as SUDI 3
- if investigations were *adequate* and none of the above applies, cases would be classified as undetermined.

The grid provides a readily "digestible" classification that can be used by pathologists at the time of final autopsy report and at the multi-agency meeting This classification allows for inclusion of risk factors that may or may not have led to asphyxia, reducing the use of the terms undetermined or unascertained. Similarly, risk factors such as the infant found lying on soft pillows or bedding that may or may not have led to suffocation are not classified as causal. If suffocation (obstruction of the mouth and nose), airway obstruction, hanging, or wedging is unequivocally certain from the death scene investigation and/or post-mortem, then these deaths require descriptive evidence based on a standard definition and are explained. SUDI 0, 1, 2, 3 remain unexplained and all require a molecular autopsy as clarified in the next section.

Apart from classification, these categories have immediate value for quality assurance of the SUDI process. The use of intrinsic/extrinsic risk factors allows for application of current and future research findings with the potential to link risk factors to age at death, neuropathological, genetic, and metabolic findings.

## II. Advances in the Etiology of SUDI

Understanding of how SUDI occurs has been advanced by hypotheses that incorporate the known risk factors and are testable. These concepts have been elaborated in different ways over time (30, 31). The Triple Risk Hypothesis is a useful way to apply current and evolving research (32), incorporating a vulnerable infant (intrinsic factors — for example, preterm infant) in an age-dependent period (developmental) whose death is precipitated by an external agent or trigger (extrinsic factors — for example, prone sleep position).

Table 14.1 (right): Classification system for determining SUDI deaths. Refer to Appendix 14.1 for definitions. (Framework adapted from (26).)

**Unexplained: SUDI Classification**

Explained: Cause of death

| | History | Death scene | Abuse/neglect | Pathology | Intrinsic risk factors | Sleep environment | Classification |
|---|---|---|---|---|---|---|---|
| **Information not collected or incomplete to determine cause. (Circle all that apply: if ANY apply, classify SUDI 0.)** | History incomplete[1] | Death scene examination incomplete[2] | Abuse or neglect cannot be excluded with certainty | Incomplete pathology[3] | Intrinsic risk factors unknown | Details of sleep environment lacking | SUDI 0 |
| **All causes excluded. Infant in safe sleep environment*. Information complete, full investigation. ALL must apply to classify SUDI 1.** | History complete | Death scene examination complete | No evidence of abuse or neglect | Pathology complete | No intrinsic risk factors: • Term birth • Normal birth weight • Normal weight (≥10th P) • No preceding infectious disease last 2 weeks • No prenatal smoking | Safe sleep environment: • Placed to sleep on back • Placed in infant-specific bed • No pillows, heavy bedding, object in sleep environment • Face not covered • Not bed sharing <3 mo • Bed sharing — no other risks • Not exposed to smoking | SUDI 1 |
| **Safe sleep*, full investigation. With non-modifiable (intrinsic) risk factors#. ALL must apply to classify SUDI 2.** | History complete | Death scene examination complete | No evidence of abuse or neglect | Pathology complete | Presence of intrinsic risk factors: (circle all that apply) • Preterm birth • Low birth weight • Small for gestational age (<10th percentile) • Preceding infectious disease • Prenatal smoking | Safe sleep environment: • Placed to sleep on back • Placed in infant-specific bed • No pillows, heavy bedding, object in sleep environment • Face not covered • Not bed sharing <3 mo • Bed sharing — no other risks | SUDI 2 |
| **Unsafe sleep, full investigation. With modifiable risk (extrinsic) factors^, uncertain of contribution to death. Unsafe sleep environment MUST apply to classify SUDI 3.** | History complete | Death scene examination complete | No evidence of abuse or neglect, OR cannot be excluded with certainty | Pathology complete | Presence of intrinsic risk factors: (circle all that apply) • NIL • Preterm birth • Low birth weight • Small for gestational age • Preceding infectious disease • Prenatal smoking | Unsafe sleep environment (circle all that apply) • Placed to sleep prone/on side any age • Found prone or on side <6 mo • Soft pillows/heavy bedding • Face covered • Non-infant bedding e.g. sofa • Bed sharing <3 mo • Bed sharing (drugs/alcohol) any age • Exposed to smoking | SUDI 3 |
| Only if SUDI 0, 1, 2, 3 do not apply | | | | | | | Undetermined |
| If cause of death able to be determined | | | | | | | Explained |

[1] Complete history includes detailed history of events leading up to the death, together with medical, pregnancy and perinatal, social, and family history, plus an explicit review of any evidence suggesting past neglect or abuse of this child or other children in the family.

[2] Complete death scene investigation — detailed review of the scene of death by the pathologist/pediatrician and police in the light of the history given by the parents or carers.

[3] Complete pathological investigations to a standardized protocol, including gross pathology, histology, microbiology, toxicology, radiology, clinical chemistry, and any relevant metabolic investigations, including frozen section of liver stained for fat and genetic testing where appropriate.

* # ^ See definitions attached in Appendix 14.1.

The greatest advances have been in genetics and neuropathology of SUDI. These have established an increasing number of inherited or sporadic gene mutations, which can cause either sudden unexpected death (e.g. cardiac arrhythmias) or polymorphisms, which likely contribute to death but require additional factors. Conceptually, the discovery of specific brain pathology in up to 70% of unexplained SUDI (25) is in general similar to genetic advances, in that some pathology will be causative and other pathology contributory. This has significantly moved many SUDI cases from the unexplained to the explained causes of death with whole exome sequencing (WES) now available and affordable. These advances have clearly established that SUDI is multifactorial. Some elaboration of genetics and neuropathology is necessary to provide the background to future directions in research.

## Molecular autopsy

There have been advances in the genetic diagnosis of SUDI, with identification of genes associated with a direct (long QT syndrome (LQTS)) or indirect relationship (possibly subclinical until the infant is challenged by an extrinsic factor — for example, bed sharing) with sudden death, including cardiac, metabolic, infectious, and serotonergic functions. Hence there is a need for molecular autopsy or post-mortem genetic analysis. For example, in sudden and unexpected death in a cohort younger than 45 years, molecular autopsy of cardiac and epilepsy genes uncovered a likely or plausible cause of death in 40% of sequentially referred cases (10/25) (33). Earlier studies found similar results, with identification of 8.9 pre-symptomatic carriers per family (34).

The development of whole exome sequencing for rare diseases is accelerating. Most recently this rapid technique for examining the whole genome has uncovered potentially pathogenic genes in 20% of cases in a SIDS cohort in Switzerland, most commonly channelopathies (9%) and cardiomyopathies (7%) (35). Undoubtedly, as gene variants are tested for pathogenetic function, genetic diagnosis in SIDS will expand (36-38).

The recognition of a cardiac cause for SUDI from long QT interval and arrhythmia, LQTS, was proposed separately by Schwartz (39) and Maron (40) in 1976. The LQTS affects 1 in 2,500 individuals and presents clinically as syncope, seizures, or sudden death due to arrhythmia (41) or as an acute life-threatening event with ventricular fibrillation and brain death (42). In Italy, Schwartz et al. (1998) undertook a neonatal ECG screening of 33,034 newborns at 2-4 days with follow-up to 1 year (43). Subsequently 24 SIDS deaths occurred. Half of these infants had prolonged QT interval as newborns exceeding 440 milliseconds (ms) (95th percentile). Infants with a corrected QTc >440 ms had an odds ratio for SIDS of 41.3 (43). Maron argued that if SIDS was associated with inheritable LQTS then some parents would reveal the mutation, and 11/41 (26%) did so (40).

Acceptance of the extent of SUDI deaths due to cardiac arrhythmias from ECG and genetic evidence was slow, and implementation of ECG monitoring and/or genetic investigation of families of SUDI children variable. Subsequently, mutations in the genes encoding cardiac ion channels for sodium, potassium, and calcium involved in generating the cardiac action potential were recognized. These included Brugada syndrome and catecholaminergic polymorphic ventricular tachycardia (CPVT), which have been implicated in a sudden cardiac arrhythmic death due to ventricular tachycardia or fibrillation (44, 45). Similarly, cardiomyopathies with minimal histological or no gross pathological findings have been associated with SUDI (35, 46).

Estimates vary as to how many SIDS infants may be affected by cardiac arrthymias: 10-20% or higher. Klaver et al. in 2011 (44) estimated from population-based cohort studies that cardiac ion channelopathies are present in at least 20% of SIDS cases. In 2016, using next-generation sequencing of 100 genes associated with cardiac diseases, Hertz et al. found that 34% of 47 unexplained, fully investigated SUDI cases had variants with likely functional effects (47). Family and functional studies were not performed. The authors suggested the higher yield was due to the new next-generation sequencing method enabling analysis of a larger number of genes than previously possible.

As more than 95% of cardiac genetic deaths are autosomal dominant, there are important implications for first-degree relatives in particular, with sudden unexpected death a possible outcome (45, 48). As treatment is available, testing of all SIDS deaths or unexplained SUDI with molecular autopsy should be part of their investigation.

A focus on other genes such as PHOX2B — the disease-defining gene in congenital central hypoventilation syndrome (CCHS), which could mimic SIDS — has been suggested (49). In the Dutch population, Liebrects-Akkerman found that the POHX2B exon 3 polyalanine repeat was statistically associated with SIDS and serves as a genetic risk factor (50). Similarly, arguments have been made for the human connexion 43E42K gene mutation, the major gap junction protein in ventricular cardiomyocytes, identified recently in a 2-month-old SIDS infant (51). In addition to ion channels, cardiac gap channels are important for conduction of cardiac electrical activation and prevention of ventricular arrhythmia.

More recently SUDI in a 15-day-old infant remained unexplained after incomplete investigations. However, a molecular autopsy with WES revealed a CLCNKB variant, which encodes for the autosomal recessive renal disorder, Bartter's syndrome. Both parents were carriers and sudden death was proposed due to hypokalemia and/or volume depletion (52). Typical renal pathology was not confirmed as no traditional autopsy was performed.

The widening recognition that genetic causes underlie many SIDS deaths makes molecular autopsy mandatory for diagnosis, prevention, and future SIDS research. All unexplained SUDI require a molecular autopsy. Of most benefit would be WES, in order to identify those cardiac genes (LQTS, RDCC, cardiomyopathies) and others that have implication for family members and future children. There are clinical, ethical and cost considerations to implementing WES in all SUDI. These issues have been clearly outlined in the guidelines for cardiac genetic conditions known to cause SUDI (45, 53, 54). The clinical implications of the increasing number of genetic abnormalities underlying SIDS/unexplained SUDI highlight the need for pathologists, pediatricians, and the multidisciplinary team to support the family through future investigations and prevention of further sudden unexpected deaths.

The key points for best practice guidelines have been outlined (53, 54). The infrastructure required (laboratory genetic analysis, toxicology, and in the future proteomic and metabolomic investigations) and the necessary specialist expertise depending on genetic/metabolic findings will require a core team of pathologists, pediatricians, counselors, primary care physicians/nurses, psychologists, patient support groups assisted by experts in cardiac pathology, pediatric cardiologists and/or molecular genetic cardiologists, geneticists, neurologists, and/or pediatric respiratory/sleep specialists. Such a multidisciplinary model has already been developed for sudden cardiac death in the young (45).

The future of neonatal screening, universal or focused, for ECG changes to detect LQTS, and the place of screening for key cardiac arrhythmia/other genes in stillbirth, unexplained SUDI, and sudden unexplained child deaths require urgent international debate for consensus on best practice and the ability to update published new findings regularly via a web-based portal.

## Seizures

The role of seizures as a potential cause of SIDS/unexplained SUDI was observed when some infants presenting with an acute life-threatening event with demonstrable hypoxemia went on to a SIDS death (55, 56). These infants had documented apnea, hypoxemia, and autonomic behaviors during apparent sleep with evidence of seizure activity on EEG recordings, but normal interictal EEGs. Reflux during the seizure was also recorded, suggesting that reflux may be an integral part of the autonomic dysfunction accompanying temporal lobe seizures. The potential for high reflux to cause laryngeal-provoked apnea, with failure to respond to obstruction, makes such seizures particularly dangerous. Notable was a history of SIDS in siblings and seizures (55). In an 8-month-old infant with the rare observation of a witnessed seizure during sleep, a SIDS death ensued. The autopsy did not reveal a primary cause of death (57).

The entity sudden unexpected death in epilepsy (SUDEP) usually occurs during sleep as an unwitnessed event and young individuals are mostly found in the prone position (58). This observation was also noted in toddlers who died a sudden unexpected death in childhood during the night and during apparent sleep. Developmental hippocampal abnormalities were found at post-mortem and the authors proposed an unwitnessed seizure during sleep leading to cardiopulmonary arrest (59).

Recent investigation of documented unexplained SUDI found hippocampal abnormalities with focal granule cell bi-lamination in microscopic sections prepared in current forensic practice. This abnormal histology, a marker in temporal lobe epilepsy, occurred in 47/114 (47%) of unexplained SUDI compared with 3/39 (8%) explained SUDI. The authors concluded that seizures or cardiopulmonary dysfunction may underlie this abnormality (60). Bilateral hippocampal histology should now be part of the routine SUDI autopsy.

The possibility that seizures underlie some SUDI cases emphasizes the importance of a thorough medical and family history. Recent genetic analysis of SUDEP has uncovered pathological mutations in 46% (28/61) of common genes responsible for cardiac arrhythmias (such as LQTS) and dominant cardiac arrhythmia and epilepsy genes or possible pathological variants (61). Thus a molecular autopsy is indicated if the history is suggestive of seizures or the SUDI unexplained.

## Pulmonary hypertension

The very young neonate who dies a sudden unexpected death, often in a facility setting and often in the prone position and/or unsafe sleeping position, is frequently labeled an unexplained SUDI (17). However, the proximity of neonatal ultrasonography to delivery suites has identified pulmonary hypertension as one cause for hypoxemia in these cases, and either successful resuscitation or death has followed (17). Currently, such a severe functional abnormality is not usually pursued at post-mortem as the pathophysiology is considered a reversion to a fetal circulation or a failure in extrauterine adaptation.

Recent case reports in the neonatal period suggest that intra-acinar pulmonary artery architecture should be evaluated for abnormal thickening as seen in persistent pulmonary hypertension of the newborn (PPHN) (62). In this study two infants, who had been apparently well, presented with a short history of respiratory distress and rapid death at 12 and 28 postnatal days. The authors reviewed the literature with previous pathological pulmonary findings in SIDS infants and controls. However, the striking difference in these two infants is the later presentation of apparently well infants and the rapid progression to sudden death.

## Metabolic disorders

Metabolic dysfunction attributable to metabolic disorders underlies 1% to 2% of SIDS, mainly defects in hepatic fatty acid oxidation, the commonest being medium chain acyl-CoA dehydrogenase (MCAD) deficiency (63). A recent case-control study of SUDI in California found no difference after adjustment between cases and controls for inborn errors of metabolism. This confirmed that undiagnosed inborn errors of metabolism identified using tandem mass spectrometry testing are not associated with increased risk of SIDS, but did not include testing of broader SUDI classifications (63).

The contribution of mutant genes to infection is unclear, although mild infection is a common finding in the two weeks prior to SIDS deaths. The extent of bacterial and viral infection remains uncertain, as this depends on how diligently history of infection is sought and then how it is interpreted (64). Polymorphisms for certain cytokines such as interlukin-10 in Asian and Aboriginal populations may provide one hypothesis as to why overwhelming pro-inflammatory responses to bacterial toxins produce pathophysiology leading to SIDS. However, the mediator for altered responses was found to be cigarette smoke, which significantly reduced the anti-inflammatory responses implicated in SIDS (65).

## Intrinsic brainstem abnormality in SIDS and potential mechanisms leading to SIDS

The pathology found in the brainstem nuclei that are involved in cardiorespiratory, arousal, and laryngeal chemoreceptor function (LCR) is relatively common — up to 70% of infants classified as SIDS and confirmed in different research groups (66-69). The deficiency in serotonin receptors, especially in the raphe brainstem nuclei, and the association of SIDS with a promoter polymorphism of the serotonin transporter gene, suggest the potential for failure of this neurotransmitter network (66, 70, 71). The physiological determinants of these findings (72) and the normal infant cardiorespiratory physiology (73) provide insight as to how sudden death might occur.

Animal research has further illuminated potential mechanisms. In 2-3-day-old rat pups, medullary raphe 5 hydroxy tryptamine (5-HT, serotoninergic) neurons were eliminated by intra-cisterna magna injections of 5DHT. Compared with controls, minute ventilation decreased and arousal was delayed when challenged with repeated episodes of hypoxia during sleep at three ages. The authors suggested that altered medullary 5-HT neurons might contribute to deficient arousal and a SIDS death. Knockout mice deficient in serotonin die suddenly following hypoxic exposure (74).

Rat pups with a milder form of 5HT deficiency produced by exposure to maternal tryptophan deficiency, the essential amino acid precursor of serotonin, exhibited abnormal respiratory control at different postnatal ages compared with controls and had significantly less medullary 5HT but no difference in the number of 5-HT neurons (75). Tryptophan sufficiency may be one mechanism for the protective action of breastfeeding on SUDI. Infant formula has either no or limited added tryptophan. This may also explain the difference in sleep states in breast- compared with formula-fed infants, the former having more quiet than active sleep as neonates (76). The medullary raphe nuclei are involved in both sleep state and 5-HT transmission. More quiet sleep is potentially protective from brainstem 5-HT disturbed respiratory reflexes (66), such as the laryngeal chemoreflex (77), provoked by high reflux in active sleep (78).

Further elaboration of brainstem abnormality was defined in six SIDS and six control infants by proteomic examination. Hunt et al. 2016 (79) found abnormal expression patterns of 41 peptides from 9 proteins, confirmed by immunohistochemistry. The authors conclude that SIDS infants have abnormal neurodevelopment in the raphe and hypoglossal nuclei and pyramids in the brainstem, which may represent delayed neurological maturation and contribute to the pathogenesis of SIDS. The neurochemical abnormalities in the brainstem of SIDS have been carefully summarized (68).

Future opportunities lie in relating further proteomic and metabolomic studies with clinical data. New technologies enable acquisition of a whole organism's metabolic profile referred to as metabolic profiling or metabolomics. This approach revealed that in healthy normoglycemic individuals branched chain and aromatic amino acids were predictors of future diabetes up to 12 years before onset of clinical diabetes (80), thus potentially enabling prediction and prevention. Aligning risk factors, both intrinsic and extrinsic, with a targeted array of metabolites could reveal not only pathogenetic pathways and biomarkers, but also therapeutic possibilities. Serotonin metabolites would be of particular interest, given the current pathological, genetic, and physiological research implicating this pathway.

## III. Prevention of SUDI

### Non-supine sleep remains a significant problem with some parents and health providers

The success of the "Back to Sleep" public health prevention programs is considered largely responsible for the initial worldwide success in reduction of SIDS, with reductions of between 52% and 87%. However, rates have plateaued since 2005 in the US (81) and national trends in SUDI may be explained by diagnostic shift (8). This plateau in SUDI is also apparent in the annual child death review reports in NSW, Australia (82). As supine infant positioning has also plateaued for all races/ethnicities in the US, understanding parental concerns and targeting behavior change in a culturally appropriate manner is crucial (90). Mothers still identified that choking and infant comfort were reasons for choosing the non-supine position, whereas physician advice positively enhanced supine position. Of concern is that there was a statistically significant reduction in supine positioning comparing 2003 with 2007 (83).

Linneman (2016) has summarized the literature on health providers' knowledge, attitudes, and practices, specifically nurses who care for infants and provide preventive information for parents during hospitalization and in community settings (84). She undertook a systematic review around SUDI using the preferred reporting items for systematic reviews and meta-analyses (PRISMA) framework, and evaluated 18 articles, the majority questionnaires, dating from 1999 to 2016, from five countries (UK, Australia, Netherlands, Turkey, and most from the US). She found a gap between awareness of safe sleep recommendations and practice (83, 81). In particular, side sleeping was considered acceptable and frequently observed in most studies. The biggest barrier to following supine safe sleep by nurses was risk of aspiration cited in 12 of 15 studies, despite research evidence to the contrary (77, 81).

A similar conclusion was reached by Patton et al. (2015) in reviewing hospital research of nurses' knowledge and behaviors over a similar time span (85). In the research, 11 of 16 studies found that nurses were recommending incorrect sleep positions to mothers and, in five of these, nurses and mothers gave fear of aspiration as the reason for choosing a non-supine position. Moon et al. (2002) found by examining the results of 436 questionnaires to pediatricians that 67% of pediatricians recognized supine as the safest position (86). In a similar questionnaire, this figure for 552 pediatricians in Spain was 58% (87). These gaps in knowledge and behavior are in contrast to parents, who in a predominantly African-American population received a verbal supine recommendation from a healthcare professional and were nearly six times more likely to place their infant supine (85).

As preterm infants form an increasing number of total SUDIs, their intrinsic risk (88) is magnified by non-supine positioning for sleep (15). A large, nationally representative, population-based pregnancy risk assessment monitoring system of the CDC from 2000-08 found that late preterm infants were at risk for non-supine sleeping. Both late preterm and early term infants were significantly less likely than term infants to be placed in the supine sleep position, less likely to initiate and continue breastfeeding, and more likely to have second-hand smoke exposure at the time of the survey (89). Furthermore, only 66% of term infants were placed supine to sleep.

Individual and public education, together with policy expectations of 100% compliance, are suggested interventions to support behavior change. Several of these educational interventions are suitable for cluster-randomized trials. Clarifying and defining the exact intervention is crucial.

## Disparities in rates of SIDS/SUDI

There is remarkable similarity in recently published SIDS rates (2016) using ICD-10 coding R95 for SIDS in Canada, Australia, Germany, Japan, and England and Wales (range 0.3-0.5/1,000 live births). Netherlands is lowest at <0.2 and the US and New Zealand highest at 0.9 (3). However, there remain striking differences within countries and within Indigenous populations.

In the USA, the racial/ethnic differences over time from 1995 to 2013 were examined from linked birth and infant death data and SUDI rates determined per 100,000 live births. The consistently highest rates were for American Indian/Alaska Natives and non-Hispanic blacks, at 177 and 172 per 100,000 live births in 2013 respectively (90). Non-Hispanic whites were 84.5 per 100,000 live births, and the lowest rates per 100,000 live births were for Hispanic (49.3) and Asian/Pacific Islanders (28.3).

In Australia also a diagnostic shift has occurred and disparity exists when Indigenous SUDIs are compared with non-Indigenous SUDIs (91). The rates were 4.7 and 0.6 per 1,000 live births respectively. In New Zealand, Māori Indigenous SUDI rates were five times higher than non-Māori (92). Importantly, use of the traditional bedding for infants, a traditional flax bassinet (Wahakura) and the more recent version, Pēpi-Pods®, in an environment where bed sharing is common, seems to be successful (93). The post-neonatal mortality has fallen by 29% from 2009-15 (2.8 to 2.0 per 1,000 live births) especially in Māori infants. While 16,500 of these safe sleep devices were distributed to vulnerable families, prevention also included health promotion and education (93). The results of the randomized control trial of Wahakura compared with traditional bassinet demonstrate the safety of the Wahakura, with no difference in risk behaviors between the two groups. A significant benefit was the increase in full breastfeeding at 6 months in the Wahakura group: 22.5% versus 10.7% (94, 95).

Some of the disparities in rates of SUDI in Indigenous peoples and in non-Hispanic blacks in the US are related to known high risk factors — particularly non-supine positioning, but also bed sharing and smoking (83). The SUDI rates are four times lower for US Hispanics than African-Americans, and the former population are more likely to adhere to the recommendations of the American Academy of Pediatrics (AAP) for supine sleep positioning, breastfeeding, not bed sharing, and no smoke exposure. Interestingly, African-American families were more likely to be knowledgeable about SIDS (96). Knowledge does not equate to understanding. Changing behaviors will require more than knowledge.

The Institute of Medicine in the US found the sources of disparities in quality healthcare complex and systemic. A multilevel strategy is thus required and comprehensively outlined in a series of recommendations by Smedley et al. (2003) (97). The importance of unconscious bias in relation to safe sleep messages concerning the Māori population in New Zealand and the methods of overcoming such bias in health providers were reviewed by Houkamau et al. (2016) (98). The use of a diagnostic tool to assess bias and the importance of cross-cultural education for health providers were outlined. However, there may also be differences in intrinsic factors that contribute to disparity, and continued research for possible biological vulnerabilities is needed (99, 100).

Involving vulnerable communities in critically evaluating how and what targeted messages and interventions are introduced is essential if progress in SUDI reduction is to occur and disparities progressively eliminated. Policies are central to the underlying social determinants of health. While the WHO framework outlined by Solar and Irwin is complex, policies to reduce inequities are broadly framed around reducing health disadvantage, health gaps, and gradients, and are central to eliminating the disparities in preventable SUDI deaths (101).

## Changing behaviors of health providers and parents — Failure of evidence of risk into practice

Using Grol's 2004 (102) conceptual framework, which outlines barriers, incentives, and levels of influence when attempting to change behavior, Moon et al. (2016) have defined five categories of safe sleep interventions (103). These are health-messaging (the innovation), education of professionals (individual professionals), breaking down barriers (infant caregivers), culture and tradition (social context), and legislation (organizational, economic, and political context). Two barriers that have resisted change to infant safe sleep practices and operate at all five levels in Grol's framework are side sleeping and bed sharing with a young infant <12 weeks postnatal age due to fear of choking if the infant sleeps supine (82, 84, 103). The result of both behaviors is risk of prone and side positioning and thus SIDS. These behaviors exist particularly amongst disadvantaged families but also amongst some health providers.

To avoid "choking", infants have been placed on their side, which increases the risk of rolling to the prone position. Post-mortem anterior/lateral lividity has identified that at least 65 of 104 (63%) neonatal SUDIs were in the prone/side position at death, often with a history to the contrary (supine when placed and found), and many were co-sleeping (16). This suggests that non-intentional prone positioning is a risk if co-sleeping with a young infant. The figure of 63% is likely to be an underestimate, as fixed lividity is defined only several hours after death and thus position at death cannot be defined if death is more recent. The disparity in history of supine position when found and autopsy evidence of non-supine position at death has been noted previously (104, 105).

The concerns of health providers and parents need abating through direct evidence of safety of the supine position and risk of prone sleep positioning in infants. One educational approach is to provide an explanation of why prone sleep is risky. One mechanism for death in the prone position is activation and prolongation of the laryngeal chemoreceptor reflex (LCR) in active sleep (77). The reflex is vigorous in the young infant and diminishes with age. The LCR is activated by direct fluid stimulation/micro -stimulation of the laryngeal inlet and mucosa. The response is complex, with apnea, bradycardia, swallowing, startle, hypertension, and redistribution of blood flow.

Both the anatomy and physiology predispose the infant to activation of the LCR when prone. The anatomy when prone facilitates the LCR, as the esophagus is above the trachea or windpipe. The physiology is also facilitatory, as the LCR is active in the young infant and, when prone, stimulation results in reduced breathing. In addition, both swallowing and arousal, which are protective by preventing LCR stimulation, are decreased (77). Activation in active sleep can be due to postnasal secretions or the unusual high reflux event in active sleep (78, 106). Intrinsic and extrinsic factors prolong the LCR, including over-the-counter cold medications such as antihistamines (phenothiazine) (107), viral infection, and hyperthermia (reviewed by Reix 2007 (108)). Conversely,

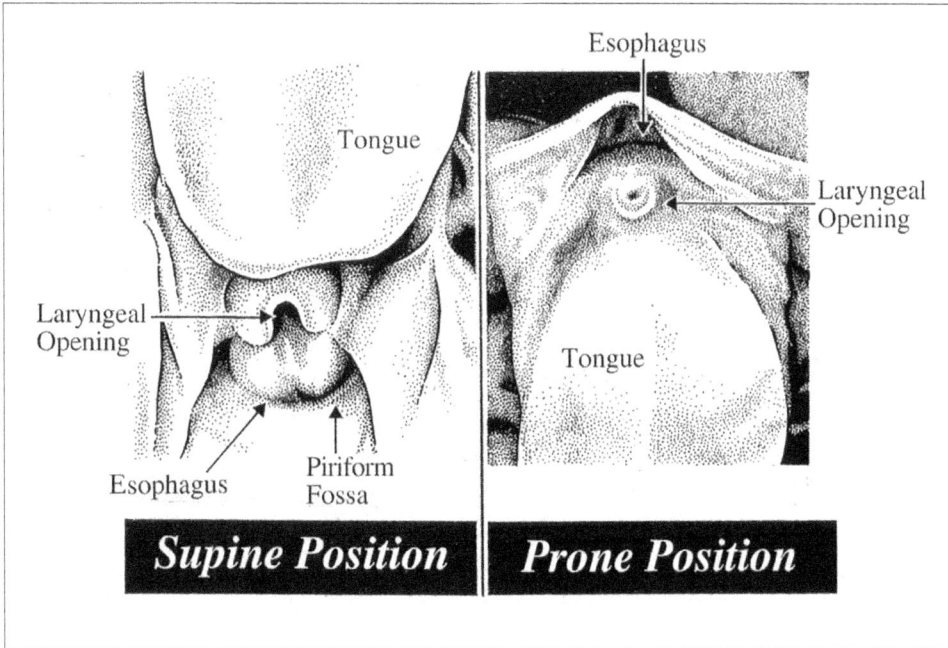

Figure 14.3: Anatomy of infant larynx in the prone and supine position. When prone, the esophagus (food pipe) is above the laryngeal opening, thus high reflux or postnasal secretions have direct access to stimulation of receptors around the laryngeal opening, leading to laryngeal chemoreceptor reflex apnea. When supine, the food pipe is below the laryngeal opening and the piriform fossae provide a temporary reservoir with protection from laryngeal chemoreflex stimulation. (Based on (77).)

serotonin micro-injected into the nucleus of the solitary tract in anesthetized newborn rats shortened the apnea and respiratory inhibition associated with the LCR (109), highlighting the potential physiological relevance of brainstem serotonin deficiency in SIDS (66, 67, 69, 70). The increase in quiet sleep in breastfed infants (76), reduction in respiratory infection from breastfeeding (110), and presence of tryptophan in breastmilk as a precursor of serotonin, with maximum circadian concentration in breastmilk at 0300 hours (111), are all potentially protective to LCR stimulation during sleep.

It is important for parents and health providers to have this information so that the rationale and safety for back sleeping is understood and fear of choking positively excluded. An easy way to translate this information, especially to health providers, is through a simple visual diagram (Figure 14.3) that depicts the anatomy and is derived from the actual macroscopic dissection. Such educational methods are amenable to clinical trials to measure change behavior and increase safe supine sleeping for infants.

## Modifiable risk and causative factors associated with preterm birth and SUDI

Preterm birth and low birth weight now constitute an increasing percentage of SIDS/SUDI and increased risk for SIDS compared with term infants (88). In the UK over 20 years the proportion of SIDS/SUDI with a history of preterm birth increased from 12% to 34% (15). In the state of NSW, Australia, the proportion doubled from 13% to 26% over five years (2011 to 2015).[1] Both intrinsic and extrinsic factors are contributory. The earlier the preterm birth, the more likely pathological factors are operating rather than physiological, and the more likely the newborn is to suffer neurodevelopmental impairment; up to 60% of very early preterm births are associated with maternal clinical or histological infection/ inflammation (112). The later preterm births are more often physiological, medically indicated, or iatrogenic (113).

Future prevention of SUDI could combine opportunities for prevention of preterm birth with prevention of SUDI and also stillbirth at the public health level, in school education, and during preconception, interbirth, and early pregnancy periods. Some of the principal social determinants, causes, and associations are common to stillbirth, preterm birth, and SUDI — including smoking, infection, substance and alcohol abuse, teen pregnancy, and unintended pregnancy (114).

The AAP recommendations for prevention of SIDS and SUDI include that pregnant women should receive regular prenatal care (115). Early care offers the best opportunity for prevention and early treatment, where pregnant women can then be triaged into preterm prevention clinics if at risk (113). In preterm labor, optimizing management with appropriate triage to a tertiary unit before delivery, tocolysis to ensure antenatal steroid cover, prophylactic antibiotics for preterm prelabor rupture of membranes, and magnesium sulphate for neuroprotection are highly relevant to improved neurodevelopmental outcomes (114, 116).

Behavioral modification addressing smoking and substance abuse, as well as early screening and effective treatment of bacterial vaginosis and other infections, are likely to prevent the potential for fetal neurological damage and postnatal neurodevelopmental impairment (113, 116). For example, smoking, a key risk factor for SUDI, preterm birth, and stillbirth, is amenable to reduction in pregnancy through interventions that target mental, emotional, and social (psychosocial) factors. Psychosocial interventions increased the proportion of women who had stopped smoking in late pregnancy by 35% and reduced the number of low birth weight infants by 17% and the number admitted to neonatal intensive care immediately after birth by 22% (117). Counseling, feedback, and incentives were effective. Further evidence is needed for the place of pharmacological interventions to reduce smoking during pregnancy.

---

1   This information is sourced from NSW Child Death Review Team (CDRT) data.

## IV. Parents and Health Providers

### What do parents want when their child is a SUDI?

This central question to SUDI discussion was investigated by Garstang et al. in a mixed studies systematic review (2014) (118). The clear answers were that parents wanted

- to be able to say goodbye
- to understand how and why their child died
- to feel supported by professionals.

The summary of recommendations for professionals from this study included (118):

*At the time of death*

- Offer all parents the chance to see and hold their child's body, even following a traumatic death.
- Allow families time and space to say goodbye to their child.

*Days after the death*

- Parents need to know how and why their child died; if this information is not available immediately, doctors should ensure that it is shared with parents at a later date.

*Weeks after the death*

- Parents should be offered follow-up appointments with pediatricians, bereavement teams, or family doctors, providing further opportunity to discuss their child's death and to provide emotional support.

To fulfil these responsibilities to parents, standard protocols are needed for medical history, death scene investigation, and pediatric or pediatric/forensic autopsy. These can be found on the CDC web site at (7, 119).[2] An updated pediatric/forensic autopsy protocol for SUDI is due by the end of 2017 on the Royal College of Pathologists, UK, website.[3]

However, advances in research on SUDI mean that these protocols/procedures are not static. For example, it is now possible to provide whole genome sequencing and to examine for genetic vulnerability to arrhythmias and other genetic diseases. This means that the medical history should incorporate a relevant "cardiac and genetic history". The death scene examination needs to thoroughly exclude other causes and to define any possible accidental asphyxia using doll re-enactment (120). Blood and tissue at autopsy need to be appropriately taken for genetic analysis. If gene positive, a multidisciplinary team needs to discuss findings together and the family needs to be expertly informed, supported, and followed over time.

---

2   See https://www.cdc.gov/sids/SUIDRF.htm and https://www.cdc.gov/sids/TrainingMaterial.htm).

3   See https://www.rcpath.org/profession/clinical-effectiveness/clinical-guidelines/autopsy-guidelines.html.

# V. Summary and Future Directions

Several recent publications have addressed the issue of future directions to understand and prevent SUDI (99, 121, 122). The drivers for this include a plateau in incidence of SUDI in most countries where data are available; the fact that SUDI remains a leading cause of post-neonatal death in most developed countries; and the constriction in funding for research into the causes of SUDI as the death rate has decreased since the first "Back to Sleep" public health campaigns.

The approaches to research have included individual author statements (121), review articles from selected SUDI/SUD researchers (122), and a research workshop summary held by the National Institute of Child Health and Human Development (NICHD) (99). The latter covered sudden unexpected death from fetal life to early childhood. Research priorities from the workshop were specific and addressed basic research, translation, public health, and training.

In contrast, the recent Global Action and Prioritization of Sudden infant death (GAPS) project was unique in that it included a broader range of stakeholders, including researchers and lay people. The aim was to use an international consensus process to define and direct future SUDI research, specifically by investigating the priorities of both expert and lay members of the SUDI community across countries (123). The methodology for the GAPS project was based on the priority-setting partnership model of the James Lind Alliance. Of the 19 participating countries, the top four participant responses were from the US (28%), UK (15%), Netherlands (14%), and Australia (10%). Following two surveys and three workshops, a consensus on the top 10 priorities for SUDI research were established with three broad themes:

- ensuring best practice data collection, management, and sharing (1 of 10 priorities)

- gaining a better understanding of the mechanisms underlying SUDI (6 of the 10)

- gaining a better understanding of the target populations and more effective communication of risk (3 of 10).

The top 10 priorities are yet to be released in a publication in the journal *Pediatrics* in 2017.[4]

Together, the researcher articles (99, 121, 122) and the stakeholder article (123) provide a set of objectives — setting standards for best practice, setting specific research priorities, and seeking to understand public health needs — in order to actively understand and reduce SUDI deaths. The way forward is to consider opportunities

---

4    The priorities were released in July 2017. See Hauck FR, McEntire BL, Raven LK, Bates FL, Lyus LA, Willett AM, et al. Research priorities in sudden unexpected infant death: An international consensus. Pediatrics. 2017 July;pii:e20150514 [Epub ahead of print]. https://doi.org./10.1542/peds.20163-3514.

under each of the GAPS headings, in addition to those specifically advanced at the NICHD workshop (99).

## Ensuring best practice data collection, management, and sharing

In addition to ensuring that key aspects of the SUDI investigatory process are complete (Figure 14.1) and that investigations into SUDI are standardized with published protocols, other standards are suggested and/or emphasized in this chapter. These include

- age of inclusion for SUDI: all neonatal sudden and unexpected deaths and infants up to 1 year

- autopsy by either a pediatric pathologist or conjoint pediatric/forensic pathologist

- use of standard WHO and INTERGROWTH-21st charts for assessment of growth

- use of a simple classification grid to sort minimum standards of investigation and separate risk factors from causality (Table 14.1; definitions in Appendix 14.1)

- molecular autopsy for all unexplained SUDI and SUDI with a history of seizures

- a multidisciplinary team to discuss issues arising and to ensure appropriate follow-up of the parents and family

- a process of yearly feedback to all stakeholders at state or country level on the audit of SUDI cases, with the opportunity to provide an update on new and applied research.

## Better understanding of the mechanisms underlying SUDI

1.  Goldstein et al. (99) highlight an important advance in the investigation and research into sudden unexpected deaths in pediatrics, namely Robert's Program at Boston Children's Hospital (37). This comprehensive program employs a multidisciplinary forensic/academic approach supported by grief counselors. Such programs, if established on a country/state/province basis, would provide up-to-date specialty investigations and provide answers for parents and future children on a statewide referral basis. Robert's Program provides a potentially rapid way forward for thorough investigation, including molecular autopsy and neuropathology, and a means to rapidly translate basic research into applied additional investigations. This is essential now that intrinsic brain abnormalities have been identified in unexplained SUDI and potential mechanisms uncovered. Similarly, as new gene mutations are discovered, these can be included in the genome search.

2. It is also important to develop a conjoint research approach with brain institutes and academic neuropathological departments, namely by

- engaging investigators skilled in proteomics and metabolomics to understand, predict (biomarkers), and prevent SUDI

- proposing conjoint research with brain institutes — for example, the Brain Research through Advancing Innovative Neurotechnologies® (BRAIN) funded by NIH; the Harvard brain science institute; brain and mind centers in major capitals in Australia; Brain Research Trust UK; and Oxford Neuroscience.

3. Finally, we must ensure that

- opportunities for genetic investigation of SUDI are utilized through cardiac, respiratory, neurological, and infection collaboration

- SUDI is listed as part of the investigation of rare diseases, as in the 100,000 genome project (38).

## Better understanding target populations and more effective communication of risk

1. The future of SUDI prevention must see an end to the very evident disparities within countries and between ethnic groups. Solutions need to be multipronged at policy level; to involve public health communication at community level, with the involvement of vulnerable communities; and to be specific to cultural needs (such as the Wahakura for safe sleep in the New Zealand Māori population (94, 95) and now the Australian Aboriginal population (124)). Valuable ways of approaching disparities (97, 98) should inform governments and non-government organizations, and these approaches should prioritize resources to the most disadvantaged communities with elevated rates of SUDI. Consideration and application of evidenced-based educational methods is recommended, using a mix of short didactic and focused skills-based teaching in a train-the-trainer application to such communities and to Indigenous health workers (125, 126). This approach has been successful in reducing early neonatal mortality (127).

2. In order to eradicate persistent erroneous messages from health providers concerning the safety of infant supine sleep (83, 84, 85,103), with a message that side sleeping is safer because of fear of aspiration, "convincing" communication is required. One method is using visual anatomy and physiology to explain why supine sleep is safe (Figure 14.3). Indeed, pediatricians, nurses, and all clinicians who encounter mothers and infants should be clear about the importance of safe infant sleep environments. A proactive preventive approach will save lives and is especially needed in disadvantaged communities identified in each country.

Most women in high-income countries access maternity services and some preconception clinics. This is an ideal time to implement prevention of both preterm birth and SUDI. As smoking is a very significant risk factor and affects both outcomes, special care is needed to effect a change in behavior through proven psychosocial interventions (117).

3. Parents are central in both prevention and investigation of SUDI. The importance of applying theories of behavior change to prevention is illustrated by the dual needs of infants for breastfeeding and safe sleeping in a visual outline by Brobheim at Georgetown University.[5] Garstang et al. (2014) have listed the three requests from parents after a SUDI and recommendations for professionals at the time of death, days after, and weeks after a SUDI (118).

## Conclusions

In conclusion, arriving at future directions for research has necessarily meant examining gaps in the process of investigation; the changing epidemiology, with an increasing number of SUDIs being preterm/low birth weight with elevated prevalence in disadvantaged communities; and advances in understanding of the genetic and neuropathophysiology of SUDI. This brief background underpins the reason that three elements of the GAPS project highlight that future attention needs to be paid to best practice and standards, understanding the mechanisms underlying SUDI, and communication with target populations in order to successfully reduce and prevent the number of SUDI cases.

## Acknowledgements

Thanks to Ms Monica Wolf, Director of Reviews, Child Death Review Team, NSW Ombudsman's Office, Sydney, for her major contribution to the development of Table 14.1 and the definitions in Appendix 14.1. Thanks also to Ms Emily Bek, advanced science and medical student, Sydney Medical School, for assistance with references, and to Dr Geoff Watson, Pathologist, at Royal Prince Alfred Hospital, Sydney, for the exacting dissection of infant anatomy that was used for the illustrative diagram in Figure 14.3.

---

5   See https://www.nappss.org/conceptual-model.php.

# References

1.  The Royal College of Pathologists. Sudden unexpected death in infancy and childhood: Multi-agency guidelines for care and investigation. 2nd ed. London, UK: The Royal College of Pathologists, 2016.

2.  Garstang J, Ellis C, Sidebotham P. An evidence-based guide to the investigation of sudden unexpected death in infancy. Forensic Sci Med Pathol. 2015;11:345-57. https://doi.org/10.1007/s12024-015-9680-x.

3.  Taylor BJ, Garstang J, Engelberts A, Obonai T, Cote A, Freemantle J, et al. International comparison of sudden unexpected death in infancy rates using a newly proposed set of cause-of-death codes. Arch Dis Child. 2015;100:1018-23. https://doi.org/10.1136/archdischild-2015-308239.

4.  Krous HF, Beckwith JB, Byard RW, Rognum TO, Bajanowski T, Corey T, et al. Sudden infant death syndrome and unclassified sudden infant deaths: A definitional and diagnostic approach. Pediatrics. 2004;114(1):234-8. https://doi.org/10.1542/peds.114.1.234.

5.  Bajanowski T, Vege A, Byard RW, Krous HF, Arnestad M, Bachs L, et al. Sudden infant death syndrome (SIDS) — Standardised investigations and classification: Recommendations. Forensic Sci Int. 2007;165:129-43. https://doi.org/10.1016/j.forsciint.2006.05.028.

6.  Sidebotham P, Fleming P. Unexpected death in childhood: A handbook for professionals. Chichester, UK: Wiley, 2007. https://doi.org/10.1002/9780470988176.

7.  Centers for Disease Control and Prevention. SUIDI Training Resources. [Available from: https://www.cdc.gov/sids/trainingmaterial.htm]. Accessed 23 October 2017.

8.  Shapiro-Mendoza CK, Tomashek KM, Anderson RN, Wingo J. Recent national trends in sudden, unexpected infant deaths: More evidence supporting a change in classification or reporting. Am J Epidemiol. 2006;163:762-9. https://doi.org/10.1093/aje/kwj117.

9.  Shapiro-Mendoza CK, Parks SE, Brustrom J, Andrew T, Camperlengo L, Fudenberg J, et al. Variations in cause-of-death determination for sudden unexpected infant deaths. Pediatrics. 2017:140(1):e20170087. https://doi.org/10.1542/peds.2017-0087.

10. Santori M, Blanco-Verea A, Gil R, Cortis J, Becker K, Schneider PM, et al. Broad-based molecular autopsy: A potential tool to investigate the involvement of subtle cardiac conditions in sudden unexpected death in infancy and early childhood. Archi Dis Child. 2015;100:952-6. https://doi.org/10.1136/archdischild-2015-308200.

11. Arthurs OJ, Hutchinson JC, Sebire NJ. Current issues in postmortem imaging of perinatal and forensic childhood deaths. Forensic Sci Med Pathol. 2017;13:58-66. https://doi.org/10.1007/s12024-016-9821-x.

12. Garstang J, Ellis C, Griffiths F, Sidebotham P. Unintentional asphyxia, SIDS, and medically explained deaths: A descriptive study of outcomes of child death review (CDR) investigations following sudden unexpected death in infancy. Forensic Sci Med Pathol. 2016;12:407-15. https://doi.org/10.1007/s12024-016-9802-0.

13. Sidebotham P, Blair PS, Evason-Coombe C, Edmond M, Heckstall-Smith E, Fleming P. Responding to unexpected infant deaths: Experience in one English region. Arch Dis Child. 2010;95(4):291-5.

14. Camperlengo L, Shapiro-Mendoza CK, Gibbs F. Improving sudden unexplained infant death investigation practices: An evaluation of the Centers for Disease Control and Prevention's SUID Investigation Training Academies. Am J Forensic Med Pathol. 2014;35:278-82. https://doi.org/10.1097/PAF.0000000000000123.

15. Blair PS, Sidebotham P, Berry PJ, Evans M, Fleming PJ. Major epidemiological changes in sudden infant death syndrome: A 20-year population-based study in the UK. Lancet (London, England). 2006;367:314-19. https://doi.org/10.1016/S0140-6736(06)67968-3.

16. Jeffery HE, Wang L, Carberry A. A preliminary investigation of neonatal SUDI in NSW 1996-2008: Opportunities for prevention. Sydney: NSW Commission for Children and Young People, 2010. [Available from: http://www.ombo.nsw.gov.au/news-and-publications/publications/reports/child-death-review-team/a-preliminary-investigation-of-neonatal-sudi-in-nsw-1996-2008-opportunities-for-prevention]. Accessed 23 October 2017.

17. Lutz T, Elliott E, Jeffery H. Sudden unexplained early neonatal death or collapse: A national surveillance study. Pediatr Res. 2016;80:493-8. https://doi.org/10.1038/pr.2016.110.

18. INTERGROWTH-21st. INTERGROWTH-21st Newborn Size at Birth Chart. [Available from: https://intergrowth21.tghn.org/articles/intergrowth-21st-newborn-size-birth-chart]. Accessed 23 October 2017.

19. INTERGROWTH-21st. INTERGROWTH-21st Very Preterm Size at Birth References and Z Scores (Standard Deviations). [Available from: https://intergrowth21.tghn.org/articles/intergrowth-21st-very-preterm-size-birth-references-and-z-scores-standard-deviations/]. Accessed 23 October 2071.

20. WHO Multicentre Growth Reference Study Group. WHO Child Growth Standards: Length/height-for-age, weight-for age, weight-for-length, weight-for-height and

body mass index-for-age: Methods and development. Geneva: World Health Organization, 2006.

21. Villar J, Giuliani F, Bhutta ZA, Bertino E, Ohuma EO, Ismail LC, et al. Postnatal growth standards for preterm infants: The Preterm Postnatal Follow-up Study of the INTERGROWTH-21(st) Project. Lancet Glob Health. 2015;3:e681-91. https://doi.org/10.1016/S2214-109X(15)00163-1.

22. Villar J, Ismail LC, Victora CG, Ohuma EO, Bertino E, Altman DG, et al. International standards for newborn weight, length, and head circumference by gestational age and sex: The Newborn Cross-Sectional Study of the INTERGROWTH-21st Project. Lancet. 2014;384(9946):857-68. https://doi.org/10.1016/S0140-6736(14)60932-6.

23. WHO Multicentre Growth Reference Study Group, & de Onis M. WHO Child Growth Standards based on length/height, weight and age. Acta Pædiatrica. 2006;95:76-85. https://doi.org/10.1111/j1651-2227.2006.tb02378.x.

24. Byard RW, Lee V. A re-audit of the use of definitions of sudden infant death syndrome (SIDS) in peer-reviewed literature. J Forensic Leg Med. 2012;19(8):455-6. https://doi.org/10.1016/j.jflm.2012.04.004.

25. Hunt CE, Darnall RA, McEntire BL, Hyma BA. Assigning cause for sudden unexpected infant death. Forensic Sci Med Pathol. 2015;11(2):283-8. https://doi.org/10.1007/s12024-014-9650-8.

26. Fleming PJ, Blair PS, Sidebotham PD, Hayler T. Investigating sudden unexpected deaths in infancy and childhood and caring for bereaved families: An integrated multiagency approach. BMJ. 2004;328:331-4. https://doi.org/10.1136/bmj.328.7435.331.

27. Randall BB, Wadee SA, Sens MA, Kinney HC, Folkerth RD, Odendaal HJ, et al. A practical classification schema incorporating consideration of possible asphyxia in cases of sudden unexpected infant death. Forensic Sci Med Pathol. 2009;5:254-60. https://doi.org/10.1007/s12024-009-9083-y.

28. Shapiro-Mendoza CK, Camperlengo L, Ludvigsen R, Cottengim C, Anderson RN, Andrew T, et al. Classification system for the sudden unexpected infant death case registry and its application. Pediatrics. 2014;134(1):e210-19. https://doi.org/10.1542/peds.2014-0180.

29. Blair PS, Byard RW, Fleming PJ. Sudden unexpected death in infancy (SUDI): Suggested classification and applications to facilitate research activity. Forensic Sci Med Pathol. 2012;8(3):312-15. https://doi.org/10.1007/s12024-011-9294-x.

30. Spinelli J, Collins-Praino L, Van Den Heuvel C, Byard RW. Evolution and significance of the triple risk model in sudden infant death syndrome. J Paediatri Child Health. 2017;53:112-15. https://doi.org/10.1111/jpc.13429.

31. Read DJC, Jeffery HE, Rahilly P. Sudden infant death syndrome and suspected "near miss": An overview for clinicians. Med J Aust. 1982;1(2):82-6.

32. Filiano JJ, Kinney HC. A perspective on neuropathologic findings in victims of the sudden infant death syndrome: The Triple-Risk Model. Neonatology. 1994;65:194-7. https://doi.org/10.1159/000244052.

33. Torkamani A, Muse ED, Spencer EG, Rueder M, Wagner GN, Lucas JR, et al. Molecular autopsy for sudden unexpected death. JAMA. 2016;316(14):1492-4. https://doi.org/10.1001/jama.2016.11445.

34. Tan HL, Hofman N, van Langen IM, van der Wal AC, Wilde AAM. Sudden unexplained death: Heritability and diagnostic yield of cardiological and genetic examination in surviving relatives. Circulation. 2005;112:207-13. https://doi.org/10.1161/CIRCULATIONAHA.104.522581.

35. Neubauer J, Lecca MR, Russo G, Bartsch C, Medeiros-Domingo A, Berger W, et al. Post-mortem whole-exome analysis in a large sudden infant death syndrome cohort with a focus on cardiovascular and metabolic genetic diseases. Eur J Hum Genetics. 2017;25:404-9. https://doi.org/10.1038/ejhg.2016.199.

36. Gando I, Morganstein J, Jana K, McDonald TV, Tang Y, Coetzee WA. Infant sudden death: Mutations responsible for impaired Nav1.5 channel trafficking and function. Pacing Clin Electrophysiol. 2017;40:703-12. https://doi.org/10.1111/pace.13087.

37. Boston Children's Hospital. Robert's Program: Overview. [Available from: robertsprogram@childrens.harvard.edu]. Accessed 23 October 2017.

38. Genomics England. The 100,00 Genomes Project. [Available from: https://www.genomicsengland.co.uk/the-100000-genomes-project]. Accessed 23 October 2017.

39. Schwartz PJ. Cardiac sympathetic innervation and the sudden infant death syndrome: A possible pathogenetic link. Am J Med. 1976;60:167-72. https://doi.org/10.1016/0002-9343(76)90425-3.

40. Maron BJ, Clark CE, Goldstein RE, Epstein SE. Potential role of QT interval prolongation in sudden infant death syndrome. Circulation. 1976;54:423-30. https://doi.org/10.1161/01.CIR.54.3.423.

41. van Norstrand DW, Ackerman MJ. Sudden infant death syndrome: Do ion channels play a role? Heart Rhythm. 2009;6(2):272-8. https://doi.org/10.1016/j.hrthm.2008.07.028.

42. Sauer CW, Marc-Aurele KL. A neonate with susceptibility to Long QT Syndrome type 6 who presented with ventricular fibrillation and sudden unexpected infant death. Am J Case Rep. 2016;17:544-8. https://doi.org/10.12659/AJCR.898327.

43. Schwartz PJ, Stramba-Badiale M, Segantini A, Austoni P, Bosi G, Giorgetti R, et al. Prolongation of the QT interval and the sudden infant death syndrome. NEJM. 1998;338:1709-14. https://doi.org/10.1056/NEJM199806113382401.

44. Klaver EC, Versluijs GM, Wilders R. Cardiac ion channel mutations in the sudden infant death syndrome. Int J Cardiol. 2011;152(2):162-70. https://doi.org/10.1016/j.ijcard.2010.12.051.

45. Semsarian C, Ingles J, Wilde AAM. Sudden cardiac death in the young: The molecular autopsy and a practical approach to surviving relatives. Eur Heart Journal. 2015;36:1290-6. https://doi.org/10.1093/eurheartj/ehv063.

46. Sweeting J, Semsarian C. Cardiac abnormalities and sudden infant death syndrome. Paediatr Resp Rev. 2014;15(4):301-6. https://doi.org/10.1016/j.prrv.2014.09.006.

47. Hertz CL, Christiansen SL, Larsen MK, Dahl M, Ferrero-Miliani L, Weeke PE, et al. Genetic investigations of sudden unexpected deaths in infancy using next-generation sequencing of 100 genes associated with cardiac diseases. Eur J Hum Genetics. 2016;24:817-22. https://doi.org/10.1038/ejhg.2015.198.

48. Semsarian C, Hamilton RM. Key role of the molecular autopsy in sudden unexpected death. Heart Rhythm. 2012;9:145-50. https://doi.org/10.1016/j.hrthm.2011.07.034.

49. Rand CM, Patwari PP, Carroll MS, Weese-Mayer DE. Congenital central hypoventilation syndrome and sudden infant death syndrome: Disorders of autonomic regulation. Sem Pediatr Neurol. 2013;20:44-55. https://doi.org/10.1016/j.spen.2013.01.005.

50. Liebrechts-Akkerman G, Liu F, Lao O, Ooms AHAG, van Duijn K, Vermeulen M, et al. PHOX2B polyalanine repeat length is associated with sudden infant death syndrome and unclassified sudden infant death in the Dutch population. Int J Legal Med. 2014;128:621-9. https://doi.org/10.1007/s00414-013-0962-0.

51. van Norstrand DW, Asimaki A, Rubinos C, Dolmatova E, Srinivas M, Tester DJ, et al. Connexin43 mutation causes heterogeneous gap junction loss and sudden infant death. Circulation. 2012;125:474-81. https://doi.org/10.1161/CIRCULATIONAHA.111.057224.

52. Lopez HU, Haverfield E, Chung WK. Whole-exome sequencing reveals CLCNKB mutations in a case of sudden unexpected infant death. Pediatr Dev Pathol. 2015;18(4):324-6. https://doi.org/10.2350/14-08-1543-CR.1.

53. Skinner JR, Duflou JA, Semsarian C. Reducing sudden death in young people in Australia and New Zealand: The TRAGADY initiative. Med J Aust. 2008;189:539-40.

54. Priori SG, Wilde AA, Horie M, Cho Y, Behr ER, Berul C, et al. HRS/EHRA/APHRS expert consensus statement on the diagnosis and management of patients with inherited primary arrhythmia syndromes. Heart Rhythm. 2013;10(12):1932-63. https://doi.org/10.1016/j.hrthm.2013.05.014.

55. Jeffery HE, Rahilly P, Read DJ. Multiple causes of asphyxia in infants at high risk for sudden infant death. Arch Dis Child. 1983;58:92-100. https://doi.org/10.1136/adc.58.2.92.

56. Hewertson J, Poets CF, Samuels MP, Boyd SG, Neville BG, Southall DP. Epileptic seizure-induced hypoxemia in infants with apparent life-threatening events. Pediatrics. 1994;94:148-56.

57. Kinney HC, McDonald AG, Minter ME, Berry GT, Poduri A, Goldstein RD. Witnessed sleep-related seizure and sudden unexpected death in infancy: A case report. Forensic Sci Med Pathol. 2013;9:418-21. https://doi.org/10.1007/s12024-013-9448-0.

58. Liebenthal JA, Wu S, Rose S, Ebersole JS, Tao JX. Association of prone position with sudden unexpected death in epilepsy. Neurol. 2015;84:703-9. https://doi.org/10.1212/WNL.0000000000001260.

59. Kinney HC, Armstrong DL, Chadwick AE, Crandall LA, Hilbert C, Belliveau RA, et al. Sudden death in toddlers associated with developmental abnormalities of the hippocampus: A report of five cases. Pediatr Dev Pathol. 2007;10(3):208-23. https://doi.org/10.2350/06-08-0144.1.

60. Kinney HC, Cryan JB, Haynes RL, Paterson DS, Haas EA, Mena OJ, et al. Dentate gyrus abnormalities in sudden unexplained death in infants: Morphological marker of underlying brain vulnerability. Acta Neuropathol. 2015;129:65-80. https://doi.org/10.1007/s00401-014-1357-0.

61. Bagnall RD, Crompton DE, Petrovski S, Lam L, Cutmore C, Garry SI, et al. Exome-based analysis of cardiac arrhythmia, respiratory control, and epilepsy genes in sudden unexpected death in epilepsy. Ann Neurol. 2016;79(4):522-34. https://doi.org/10.1002/ana.24596.

62. Zainun K, Hope K, Nicholson AG, Cohen MC. Abnormal muscularization of intra-acinar pulmonary arteries in two cases presenting as sudden infant death. Pediatr Dev Pathol. 2017;20:49-53. https://doi.org/10.1177/1093526616689311.

63. Rosenthal NA, Currier RJ, Baer RJ, Feuchtbaum L, Jelliffe-Pawlowski LL. Undiagnosed metabolic dysfunction and sudden infant death syndrome — A

case-control study. Paediatr Perinat Epidemiol. 2015;29(2):151-5. https://doi.org/10.1111/ppe.12175.

64. Pryce JW, Weber MA, Hartley JC, Ashworth MT, Malone M, Sebire NJ. Difficulties in interpretation of post-mortem microbiology results in unexpected infant death: Evidence from a multidisciplinary survey. J Clin Pathol. 2011;64(8):706-10. https://doi.org/10.1136/jclinpath-2011-200056.

65. Blackwell CC, Moscovis SM, Gordon AE, Al Madani OM, Hall ST, Gleeson M, et al. Ethnicity, infection and sudden infant death syndrome. FEMS Immunol Med Microbiol. 2004;42(1):53-65. https://doi.org/10.1016/j.femsim.2004.06.007.

66. Kinney HC, Richerson GB, Dymecki SM, Darnall RA, Nattie EE. The brainstem and serotonin in the sudden infant death syndrome. Annu Rev Pathol. 2009;4:517-50. https://doi.org/10.1146/annurev.pathol.4.110807.092322.

67. Duncan JR, Paterson DS, Hoffman JM, Mokler DJ, Borenstein NS, Belliveau RA, et al. Brainstem serotonergic deficiency in sudden infant death syndrome. JAMA. 2010;303:430-7. https://doi.org/10.1001/jama.2010.45.

68. Machaalani R, Waters KA. Neurochemical abnormalities in the brainstem of the sudden infant death syndrome (SIDS). Paediatr Respir Rev. 2014;15:293-300. https://doi.org/10.1016/j.prrv.2014.09.008.

69. Ozawa Y, Okado N. Alteration of serotonergic receptors in the brain stems of human patients with respiratory disorders. Neuropediatrics. 2002;33(3):142-9. https://doi.org/10.1055/s-2002-33678.

70. Narita N, Narita M, Takashima S, Nakayama M, Nagai T, Okado N. Serotonin transporter gene variation is a risk factor for sudden infant death syndrome in the Japanese population. Pediatrics. 2001;107:690-2. https://doi.org/10.1542/peds.107.4.690.

71. Lavezzi AM, Casale V, Oneda R, Weese-Mayer DE, Matturri L. Sudden infant death syndrome and sudden intrauterine unexplained death: correlation between hypoplasia of raphé nuclei and serotonin transporter gene promoter polymorphism. Pediatr Res. 2009;66:22-7. https://doi.org/10.1203/PDR.0b013e3181a7bb73.

72. Garcia AJ, Koschnitzky JE, Ramirez J-M. The physiological determinants of sudden infant death syndrome. Respir Physiol Neurobiol. 2013;189:288-300. https://doi.org/10.1016/j.resp.2013.05.032.

73. Horne RSC, Nixon GM. The role of physiological studies and apnoea monitoring in infants. Paediatr Respir Rev. 2014;15:312-18. https://doi.org/10.1016/j.prrv.2014.09.007.

74. Barrett KT, Dosumu-Johnson RT, Daubenspeck JA, Brust RD, Kreouzis V, Kim JC, et al. Partial raphe dysfunction in neurotransmission is sufficient to increase mortality after anoxic exposures in mice at a critical period in postnatal development. J Neurosci. 2016;36:3943-53. https://doi.org/10.1523/JNEUROSCI.1796-15.2016.

75. Penatti EM, Barina AE, Raju S, Li A, Kinney HC, Commons KG, et al. Maternal dietary tryptophan deficiency alters cardiorespiratory control in rat pups. J Appl Physiol. 2011;110:318-28. https://doi.org/10.1152/japplphysiol.00788.2010.

76. Heacock HJ, Jeffery HE, Baker JL, Page M. Influence of breast versus formula milk on physiological gastroesophageal reflux in healthy, newborn infants. J Pediatr Gastroenterol Nutr. 1992;14:41-6. https://doi.org/10.1097/00005176-1992010 00-00009.

77. Jeffery HE, Megevand A, Page M. Why the prone position is a risk factor for sudden infant death syndrome. Pediatrics. 1999;104:263-9. https://doi.org/10.1542/peds.104.2.263.

78. Jeffery HE, Heacock HJ. Impact of sleep and movement on gastro-oesophageal reflux in healthy, newborn infants. Archi Dis Child. 1991;66(10 Spec No):1136-9.

79. Hunt NJ, Phillips L, Waters KA, Machaalani R. Proteomic MALDI-TOF/TOF-IMS examination of peptide expression in the formalin fixed brainstem and changes in sudden infant death syndrome infants. J Proteomics. 2016;138:48-60. https://doi.org/10.1016/j.jprot.2016.02.022.

80. Wang TJ, Larson MG, Vasan RS, Cheng S, Rhee EP, McCabe E, et al. Metabolite profiles and the risk of developing diabetes. Nature Med. 2011;17(4):448-53. https://doi.org/10.1038/nm.2307.

81. American Academy of Pediatrics Task Force on Sudden Infant Death Syndrome. SIDS and other sleep-related infant deaths: Expansion of recommendations for a safe infant sleeping environment. Pediatrics. 2011;128(5):1030-9. https://doi.org/10.1542/peds.2011-2284.

82. NSW Child Death Review Team. Child death review report 2015. Sydney: NSW Ombudsman, 2015. [Available from: https://www.ombo.nsw.gov.au/__data/assets/pdf_file/0009/39474/CDRT_review_report_2015_final.pdf]. Accessed 23 October 2017.

83. Colson ER, Rybin D, Smith LA, Colton T, Lister G, Corwin MJ. Trends and factors associated with infant sleeping position: The national infant sleep position study, 1993-2007. Arch Pediatr Adolesc Med. 2009;163:1122-8. https://doi.org/10.1001/archpediatrics.2009.234.

84. Linneman JB. Nurses' knowledge, attitudes and practice of sudden unexpected infant death recommendations and safe sleep education: A systematic review. Farog, North Dakota: North Dakota State University, 2016.

85. Patton C, Stiltner D, Wright KB, Kautz DD. Do nurses provide a safe sleep environment for infants in the hospital setting? An integrative review. Adv Neonatal Care. 2015;15(1):8-22. https://doi.org/10.1097/ANC.0000000000000145.

86. Moon RY, Gingras JL, Erwin R. Physician beliefs and practices regarding SIDS and SIDS risk reduction. Clin Pediatr. 2002;41:391-5. https://doi.org/10.1177/000992280204100603.

87. de Luca F, Gómez-Durán EL, Arimany-Manso J. Paediatricians' practice about sudden infant death syndrome in Catalonia, Spain. Matern Child Health J. 2017;21:1267-76. https://doi.org/10.1007/s10995-016-2225-4.

88. Malloy MH. Prematurity and sudden infant death syndrome: United States 2005-2007. J Perinatol. 2013;33:470-5. https://doi.org/10.1038/jp.2012.158.

89. Hwang SS, Barfield WD, Smith RA, Morrow B, Shapiro-Mendoza CK, Prince CB, et al. Discharge timing, outpatient follow-up, and home care of late-preterm and early-term infants. Pediatrics. 2013;132:101-8. https://doi.org/10.1542/peds.2012-3892.

90. Parks SE, Erck Lambert AB, Shapiro-Mendoza CK. Racial and ethnic trends in sudden unexpected infant deaths: United States, 1995-2013. Pediatrics. 2017;139(6):e20168344. https://doi.org./10.1542/peds.2016-3844.

91. Freemantle CJ, Read AW, de Klerk NH, Charles AK, McAullay D, Stanley FJ. Interpretation of recent sudden infant death syndrome rates in Western Australia. J Paediatr Child Health. 2005;41(12):669-70. https://doi.org/10.1111/j.1440-1754.2005.00756.x.

92. Child and Youth Mortality Review Committee, Te Ròpù Arotake Auau Mate o te Hunga Tamariki, Taiohi. Fifth Report to the Minister of Health: Reporting mortality 2002-2008. Wellington, New Zealand: Child and Youth Mortality Review Committee, 2009.

93. Mitchell EA, Cowan S, Tipene-Leach D. The recent fall in postperinatal mortality in New Zealand and the Safe Sleep programme. Acta Paediatrica. 2016;105:1312-20. https://doi.org/10.1111/apa.13494.

94. Tipene-Leach D, Baddock S, Williams S, Jones R, Tangiora A, Abel S, et al. Methodology and recruitment for a randomised controlled trial to evaluate the safety of wahakura for infant bedsharing. BMC Pediatr. 2014;14:240. https://doi.org/10.1186/1471-2431-14-240.

95. Baddock SA, Tipene-Leach D, Williams SM, Tangiora A, Jones R, Iosua E, et al. Wahakura versus bassinet for safe infant sleep: A randomized trial. Pediatrics. 2017;139(2): pii: e20160162. https://doi.org/10.1542/peds.2016-0162.

96. Mathews AA, Joyner BL, Oden RP, Alamo I, Moon RY. Comparison of infant sleep practices in African-American and US Hispanic families: Implications for sleep-related infant death. J Immigr Minor Health. 2015;17(3):834-42. https://doi.org/10.1007/s10903-014-0016-9.

97. Smedley BD, Stith AY, Nelson AR, editors. Unequal Treatment: Confronting racial and ethnic disparities in health care. Washington (DC): National Academies Press (US), 2003.

98. Houkamau CA, Clarke K. Why are those most in need of sudden unexplained infant death (SUDI) prevention information the least likely to receive it? A comment on unconscious bias and Maori health. NZ Med J. 2016;129(1440):114-19.

99. Goldstein RD, Kinney HC, Willinger M. Sudden unexpected death in fetal life through early childhood. Pediatrics. 2016;137(6):e20154661 https://doi.org/10.1542/peds.2015-4661.

100. Goldstein RD, Trachtenberg FL, Sens MA, Harty BJ, Kinney HC. Overall postneonatal mortality and rates of SIDS. Pediatrics. 2016;137(1):e20152298. https://doi.org/10.1542/peds.2015-2298.

101. Solar O, Irwin A. A conceptual framework for action on the social determinants of health. Social Determinants of Health Discussion Paper 2 (Policy and Practice). Geneva: World Health Organization, 2010.

102. Grol R, Wensing M. What drives change? Barriers to and incentives for achieving evidence-based practice. Med J Aust. 2004;180(6 Suppl):S57-60.

103. Moon RY, Hauck FR, Colson ER. Safe Infant Sleep Interventions: What is the evidence for successful behavior change? 2016;12(1):67-75.

104. Pasquale-Styles MA, Tackitt PL, Schmidt CJ. Infant death scene investigation and the assessment of potential risk factors for asphyxia: A review of 209 sudden unexpected infant deaths. J Forensic Sci. 2007;52:924-9. https://doi.org/10.1111/j.1556-4029.2007.00477.x.

105. Byard RW, Jensen LL. How reliable is reported sleeping position in cases of unexpected infant death? J Forensic Sci. 2008;53(5):1169-71. https://doi.org/10.1111/j.1556-4029.2008.00813.x.

106. Page M, Jeffery HE, Marks V, Post EJ, Wood AK. Mechanisms of airway protection after pharyngeal fluid infusion in healthy sleeping piglets. J Appl Physiol. 1995;78:1942-9.

107. McKelvey GM, Post EJ, Wood AK, Jeffery HE. Airway protection following simulated gastro-oesophageal reflux in sedated and sleeping neonatal piglets during active sleep. Clin Exp Pharmacol Physiol. 2001;28:533-9. https://doi.org/10.1046/j.1440-1681.2001.03483.x.

108. Reix P, St-Hilaire M, Praud JP. Laryngeal sensitivity in the neonatal period: From bench to bedside. Pediatr Pulmonol. 2007;42(8):674-82. https://doi.org/10.1002/ppul.20645.

109. Donnelly WT, Bartlett D Jr, Leiter JC. Serotonin in the solitary tract nucleus shortens thelaryngeal chemoreflex in anaesthesized neonatal rats. Exp Physiol. 2016;101(7):946-61. https://doi.org/10.1113/EP085716.

110. Duijts L, Jaddoe VWV, Hofman A, Moll HA. Prolonged and exclusive breastfeeding reduces the risk ofiInfectious diseases in infancy. Pediatrics. 2010;126(1):e18-25 https://doi.org/10.1542/peds.2008-3256.

111. Cubero J, Valero V, Sanchez J, Rivero M, Parvez H, Rodriguez AB. The circadian rhythm of tryptophan in breast milk affects the rhythms of 6-sulfatoxymelatonin and sleep in newborn. Neuroendocrinology Letters. 2005;26(6):657-61.

112. Lahra MM, Jeffery HE. A fetal response to chorioamnionitis is associated with early survival after preterm birth. AJOG. 2004;190:147-51. https://doi.org/10.1016/j.ajog.2003.07.012.

113. Lamont RF. Setting up a preterm prevention clinic: A practical guide. BJOG. 2006;113 Suppl 3:86-92. https://doi.org/10.1111/j.1471-0528.2006.01130.x.

114. Shapiro-Mendoza CK. CDC Grand Rounds: Public health strategies to prevent preterm birth. MMWR. 2016;65(32): 826-30. https://doi.org/10.15585/mmwr.mm6532a4.

115. Task Force on Sudden Infant Death Syndrome. SIDS and other sleep-related infant deaths: Updated 2016 recommendations for a safe infant sleeping environment. Pediatrics. 2016;138:e20162938. https://doi.org/10.1542/peds.2016-2938.

116. Joergensen JS, Weile LKK, Lamont RF. The early use of appropriate prophylactic antibiotics in susceptible women for the prevention of preterm birth of infectious etiology. Expert Opin Pharmacother. 2014;15:2173-91. https://doi.org/10.1517/14656566.2014.950225.

117. Chamberlain C, O'Mara-Eves A, Porter J, Coleman T, Perlen SM, Thomas J, et al. Psychosocial interventions for supporting women to stop smoking in pregnancy. Cochrane Database Syst Rev. 2017;2:CD001055. https://doi.org/10.1002/14651858.CD001055.pub5.

118. Garstang J, Griffiths F, Sidebotham P. What do bereaved parents want from professionals after the sudden death of their child: A systematic review of the literature. BMC Pediatr. 2014;14:269. https://doi.org/10.1186/1471-2431-14-269.

119. CDC — Sudden infant death syndrome (SIDS) and sudden, unexpected infant death (SUID) — Reproductive health. [Available from: https://www.cdc.gov/sids/index.htm]. Accessed 23 October 2017.

120. Tabor PD, Ragan K. Infant death scene investigation. J Forensic Nurs. 2015;11:22-7; quiz E1.

121. Cutz E. The disappearance of sudden infant death syndrome — Reply. JAMA Pediatr. 2016;170:1026-7. https://doi.org/10.1001/jamapediatrics.2016.1782.

122. Waters KA. SIDS symposium — A perspective for future research. Paediatr Respir Rev. 2014;15:285-6. https://doi.org/10.1016/j.prrv.2014.09.005.

123. Lyus LH, Hauck F, McEntire B, Blair P, Raven LB, Bates F. International research priorities in SUDI: Findings of the GAPS project. 2016 Conference on Stillbirth, SIDS and Baby Survival; 8-10 September; Montevideo, Uruguay, 2016.

124. Young J, Watson K, Craigie L, Cowan S, Kearney L. Uniting cultural practices and safe sleep environments for vulnerable Indigenous Australian infants. Aust Nurs Midwifery J. 2017;24(9):37.

125. Forsetlund L, Bjørndal A, Rashidian A, Jamtvedt G, O'Brien MA, Wolf F, et al. Continuing education meetings and workshops: Effects on professional practice and health care outcomes. Cochrane Database Syst Rev. 2009:CD003030. https://doi.org/10.1002/14651858.CD003030.pub2.

126. Hill DA. SCORPIO: A system of medical teaching. Med Teach. 1992;14:37-41. https://doi.org/10.3109/01421599209044013.

127. Jeffery HE, Kocova M, Tozija F, Gjorgiev D, Pop-Lazarova M, Foster K, et al. The impact of evidence-based education on a perinatal capacity-building initiative in Macedonia. Med Educ. 2004;38:435-47. https://doi.org/10.1046/j.1365-2923.2004.01785.x.

# Appendix 14.1

## Sudden unexpected death in infancy: Proposed working definition and classifications

### Background

Sudden unexpected death in infancy (SUDI) is the death of an infant aged less than 12 months that is sudden and unexpected, where the cause was not immediately apparent at the time of death. Around 15% of all infant deaths in NSW (Australia) are SUDI (1).

SUDI are either

- **Explained SUDI** — deaths where a cause is found after investigation
- **Unexplained SUDI** — deaths where the cause remains unidentified after all investigations are completed. This includes deaths that are classified as sudden infant death syndrome (SIDS).

In NSW, the majority of SUDI — almost 75% — remain unexplained.

In NSW, there is no consistent classification of SUDI where a cause of death remains unexplained after investigation. Consistent classification can help to identify factors that may contribute to infant deaths, which is a key first step toward preventing future infant deaths.

The most commonly accepted framework for classifying SUDI is that proposed by Krous et al. in 2004 ("the San Diego definition"), which was broadly adopted at the SIDS and Kids Pathology Workshop in 2004 (2). There has been a major shift in SIDS diagnosis over the last decade and a major advance has been the identification of "modifiable risk factors" (3).

The following proposed classification framework takes into account key modifiable (extrinsic) and non-modifiable (intrinsic) SUDI risk factors, and draws from the earlier framework. The aim is to provide for a consistent approach to SUDI by coroners, pathologists, and Child Death Review Teams.

## Classification

Table 14.2: Unexplained SUDI.

| Classification | Definition |
| --- | --- |
| SUDI 0 | Post-death investigation is not sufficient, and a cause of death cannot be determined or excluded with certainty because of lack of information:<br>• Death scene examination is undocumented or insufficient.<br>• No or incomplete review of medical history of the child/family, including family interview (protocol) and review of clinical records.<br>• Autopsy not in compliance with the SIDS protocol, or missing tests or screens necessary to confirm or exclude a cause. |
| SUDI 1 | The infant was found in a safe sleeping environment with no evidence of accidental death, unexplained trauma, or abnormal presentation (1) prior to death. Following thorough investigation, all other possible causes have been excluded.<br>Safe sleep environment means:<br>• The infant was placed to sleep and found on their back (not prone, not on side).<br>• The infant was placed to sleep in their own infant-specific bedding (not in adult bedding or on a surface not designed for sleep).<br>• The infant was not exposed to tobacco smoke.<br>• The infant was not overdressed for the conditions or covered with heavy/adult/overly warm bedding.<br>• There were no soft pillows or other objects in sleep environment.<br>• The infant's face was not covered.<br>• There was no bed sharing <3 months of age.<br>Thorough investigation includes a minimum of<br>• Full and documented death scene examination<br>• Review of medical history of the child/family, including family interview with protocol and review of clinical records<br>• Autopsy in compliance with the SIDS protocol. |
| SUDI 2 | As above (SIDS), with the exception that non-modifiable (intrinsic) risk factors are identified:<br>• Low birth weight (less than 2,500 g)<br>• Preterm birth (less than 37 weeks)<br>• Small for gestational age (less than 10th percentile weight for age on relevant INTERGROWTH newborn charts for term and preterm infants).<br>• Preceding infectious illness (within the last two weeks)<br>• Prenatal smoking |

| SUDI 3 | The infant was found in an unsafe sleeping environment with modifiable (extrinsic) risk factors present, and following thorough investigation, mechanical asphyxia or suffocation cannot be determined or excluded with certainty.<br>Unsafe sleeping environment means:<br>• The infant was placed to sleep prone or on their side (and for infants less than 6 months, located prone or on their side).<br>• The infant was placed on a sleep surface with heavy or excess bedding.<br>• The infant was placed with soft pillows or other objects in sleep environment.<br>• The infant's face was covered.<br>• The infant slept in bedding not specifically designed for infant sleep (e.g. pram, sofa).<br>• An infant under 3 months of age was sharing a sleep surface with others (any circumstances), or an infant over 6 months was sharing a sleep surface with others, where evidence suggests that the other person/s were likely impaired by drugs or alcohol.<br>• The infant was exposed to smoking. |
|---|---|
| Undetermined | A finding of undetermined should only be applied in a SUDI context where the above classifications are insufficient.<br>This would include the sudden unexpected death of an infant not in a sleep environment and no cause found |

Table 14.3: Explained SUDI.

| SUDI Explained | The infant dies suddenly and unexpectedly and following investigation, a cause of death can be determined with certainty. | ICD 10 classification |
|---|---|---|

## Modifiable and non-modifiable risk factors for sudden unexpected death in infancy

Non-modifiable risk factors

Mitchell and Krous note that the "epidemiology of SIDS has been well described and has been largely consistent over time and place" with non-modifiable or intrinsic risk factors including certain social and personal characteristics (e.g. male preponderance), and (4):

- low birth weight (less than 2,500 g)

- preterm birth (less than 37 weeks' gestation)

- small for gestational age (less than 10th percentile on relevant WHO charts or INTERGROWTH newborn charts for term and preterm infants)
  - http://www.who.int/childgrowth/standards/en/
  - https://intergrowth21.tghn.org/articles/intergrowth-21st-newborn-size-birth-chart
  - http://www.who.int/childgrowth/standards/en/
  - https://intergrowth21.tghn.org/articles/intergrowth-21st-postnatal-growth-standards-and-z-scores-preterm-infants/
- preceding infectious illness

## Modifiable risk factors

There are also well-evidenced *modifiable* or extrinsic risk factors for SUDI, including placing infants to sleep prone (on their front); sharing a bed with an infant, particularly where other risks are present; placing infants in bedding not designed for them; exposing infants to tobacco smoke; excess thermal insulation and overheating; and placing loose bedding or other items in an infant's sleep environment (3, 4, 5, 6).

- **Prone sleeping**: Placing an infant to sleep in a prone position (on their front) is a significant risk factor for SUDI. The prone position increases the risk of rebreathing expired gases, overheating, and accidental suffocation — particularly for very young infants with limited head control and/or infants placed on soft bedding. Placing an infant to sleep on their side is also not recommended, as it may promote the infant rolling into a prone position.

- **Bed sharing**: Sleeping in the same bed as a baby can be unsafe if the infant gets caught under adult bedding or pillows; becomes wedged in gaps between the mattress and wall; or is rolled on or covered by an adult who sleeps very deeply, is affected by drugs or alcohol, and/or is extremely tired. Infants under 12 weeks have an increased risk of SUDI even if the parents do not smoke or drink alcohol, and the infant is breastfed.

- **Exposure to smoking**: Maternal smoking during pregnancy and in the infant's environment is a major risk factor for SUDI. Exposure to tobacco smoke has been shown to adversely affect infant arousal, and to increase the risk of premature birth and low birth weight, both of which are risk factors for SIDS. Tobacco smoke exposure is also linked to decreased lung growth and increased rates of respiratory tract infections, otitis media (ear infection), and childhood asthma, with the severity of these problems increasing with increased exposure. Research indicates that bed sharing with an infant greatly increases the risk for SIDS if either or both of the parents smoke. Strategies to minimize a baby's exposure to tobacco smoke, such as keeping windows open, avoiding smoking near the baby, or smoking outside, are not completely effective in reducing an infant's exposure to tobacco smoke (7, 8).

- **Excess bedding and clothing**: The risk of dying suddenly and unexpectedly is increased if an infant is placed prone, and that risk is even further increased if the infant is placed prone under heavy bedding or if their head becomes covered by bedding in any position. Excessive clothing and/or bedding can contribute to the risk of thermal stress by providing insulation which prevents infants from regulating their temperature. This can occur when a baby's head or face becomes covered by bedding, or when an infant is wrapped or dressed in overly warm clothing, and is unable to cool down by evaporation of sweat.

- **Bedding that is not designed for infants and/or for sleeping**: Placing a baby to sleep on a surface not specifically designed for infants to sleep increases the risk of SUDI. Examples of inappropriate surfaces include sofas, chairs, adult bedding, car seats, strollers, and slings. Risks to infants placed to sleep on these surfaces include suffocation, entrapment, strangulation, and assuming positions that can cause airway obstruction.

- **Soft pillows or other objects in sleep environment**: Loose soft items in an infant's sleep environment pose a potential risk of suffocation or overheating. Pillows, quilts, sheepskins, and other soft surfaces have been noted to increase the risk of SIDS fivefold, independent of sleep position.

## Safe sleeping

**Safe sleep environment** means:
- The infant was placed to sleep and found on their back (not prone or on side).
- The infant was placed to sleep in their own infant-specific bedding (not in adult bedding, and not on a sofa or any other surface not designed for infant sleep).
- The infant was not exposed to tobacco smoke.
- The infant was not overdressed for the conditions or covered with heavy/adult/overly warm bedding.
- The infant's face was not covered.
- There were no soft pillows or other objects in sleep environment.
- The infant was not bed sharing at the age of <3 months.

# References to Appendix 14.1

1. NSW Child Death Review Team 2016 Child Death Review Report 2015. NSW Ombudsman, Sydney. [Available from: https://www.ombo.nsw.gov.au/data/assets/ pdf_file/0009/39474/CDRT_review_report_2015_final.pdf].

2. Byard RW, Ranson D, Krous HF. National Australian Workshop Consensus on the definition of SIDS and initiation of a uniform autopsy approach to unexpected infant and early childhood death. For Sci Med Pathol. 2005;1(4):289-92. https:// doi.org/10.1385/FSMP:1:4:289.

3. American Academy of Pediatrics Task Force on Sudden Infant Death Syndrome. The changing concept of sudden infant death syndrome: Diagnostic coding shifts, controversies regarding the sleeping environment, and new variables to consider in reducing risk. Pediatrics. 2005;116:1245-55. https://doi.org/10.1542/ peds.2005-1499.

4. Mitchell EA, Krous HF. Sudden unexpected death in infancy: A historical perspective. J Paediatr Child Health. 2015;51:108-12. https://doi.org/10.1111/ jpc.12818.

5. American Academy of Pediatrics Task Force on Sudden Infant death Syndrome. SIDS and other sleep-related infant deaths: Expansion of recommendations for a safe infant sleeping environment. Pediatrics. 2011;128(5):1030-9. https://doi. org/10.1542/peds.2011-2284.

6. American Academy of Pediatrics Task Force on Sudden Infant Death Syndrome. SIDS and other sleep-related infant deaths: Updated 2016 recommendations for a safe infant sleeping environment. Pediatrics. 2016;138:e20162938. https://doi. org/10.1542/peds.2016-2938.

7. DiFranza JR, Aligne CA, Weitzman M. Prenatal and postnatal environmental tobacco smoke exposure and children's health. Pediatrics. 2004;113(Suppl 3):1007-15.

8. Moon RY, Fu L. Sudden infant death syndrome: An update. Pediatrics in Review. 2012;33:314. https://doi.org./10.1542/pir.33-7-314.

# 15 Observational Investigations from England: The CESDI and SWISS Studies

Peter S Blair, BSc, MSc, PhD,
Anna S Pease, MA, MSc, PhD and
Peter J Fleming, MD, PhD

*The University of Bristol, Bristol, UK*

## Introduction

Emerging evidence in the 1980s of a link between infants positioned to sleep on their front (prone) and sudden infant death syndrome (SIDS) eventually led to a national "Back to Sleep" campaign in England and Wales in November 1991 (1-6). The SIDS rate dramatically fell by two-thirds (67%) in just four years, from a peak of 1,597 SIDS deaths in 1988 to 531 deaths by 1992 (7). To monitor the characteristic profile of this reduced number of deaths, and identify further potential risk factors associated with SIDS, a case-control study was commissioned as part of a Confidential Enquiry into Stillbirths and Deaths in Infancy (CESDI) and conducted via the University of Bristol between 1993 and 1996 across a third of England (8, 9). A similar study in a smaller geographical area, the South West Infant Sleep Scene Study (SWISS), collecting additional details surrounding the infant sleeping environment, was conducted 10 years later between 2003 and 2006 by the same team (10). Both studies have been instrumental in providing the evidence base for SIDS risk reduction campaigns worldwide and reducing these deaths nationally by a further 60% to 212 SIDS deaths in 2014. This is a review of the main findings, the changes in risk profile over time, and what can be learnt from combining the data from these two studies.

## The Optimal Study Design

Despite SIDS being one of the leading causes of post-neonatal infant death, it is a relatively rare event and thus the optimal study design is the observational case-control study. With this design, rare events can be captured as they happen (cases) and compared to suitable controls, although it is often difficult to establish whether significant associations are causal or whether the observations collected are subject to bias. With SIDS investigations in particular, the importance of the final sleeping environment and lack of an immediate causal explanation means recall and misclassification bias can be problematic. Both the CESDI and the SWISS studies were therefore designed with certain features in mind to reduce the potential of bias:

- Both studies were conducted in a specified geographical area over a set period of time to monitor whether we could achieve high case ascertainment and how much the findings could be generalized to the wider population.

- A notification network was set up (including general practitioners, midwives, health visitors, pediatricians, neonatal units, emergency departments, ambulance control, pathologists, mortuary attendants, coroners and coroners' officers, and parent support groups), so that most deaths would be reported within 24 hours of the death. This rapid system of notification would both reduce recall bias and help initiate bereavement support for the parents.

- A wide umbrella of sudden unexpected deaths in infancy (SUDI) was included in the study and families interviewed. A multidisciplinary panel was set up to decide whether the cause of each death was eventually explained or remained unexplained (i.e. SIDS). This not only reduced the chances of misclassification, but also provided an important group of explained deaths that we could compare to the unexplained SIDS deaths.

- The bereaved families received two home visits: initially, within days of the death to document a narrative account of events leading up to the infant's death, and a second visit within two weeks of the death to complete the rest of the questionnaire. This allowed families to first explain what happened in their own words before obtaining a detailed standardized response to the rest of our questions.

- Control families received one home visit. A period of sleep, termed the "reference sleep", was identified in the 24 hours before the interview, which corresponded to the time of day in which the index infant had died, with emphasis on the index parents' view of whether it had been a night- or daytime sleep. Thus recall bias was minimized and a direct "event" comparison could be recorded.

- The same standardized questionnaire was used for case and control families and the consistency of approach was maintained by regular training meetings amongst the researchers. The anonymity of the data collected was also emphasized to the families so as to allow collection of sensitive information.

## The CESDI SUDI Study

### Study methodology and ascertainment

The CESDI SUDI case-control study was conducted between February 1993 and March 1996, in five former Health Regions of England (South West, Wessex, Trent, Northern, and Yorkshire Regions; see Figure 15.1). It included a mixture of rural and urban communities populated by 17.7 of the 58 million people living in England at that

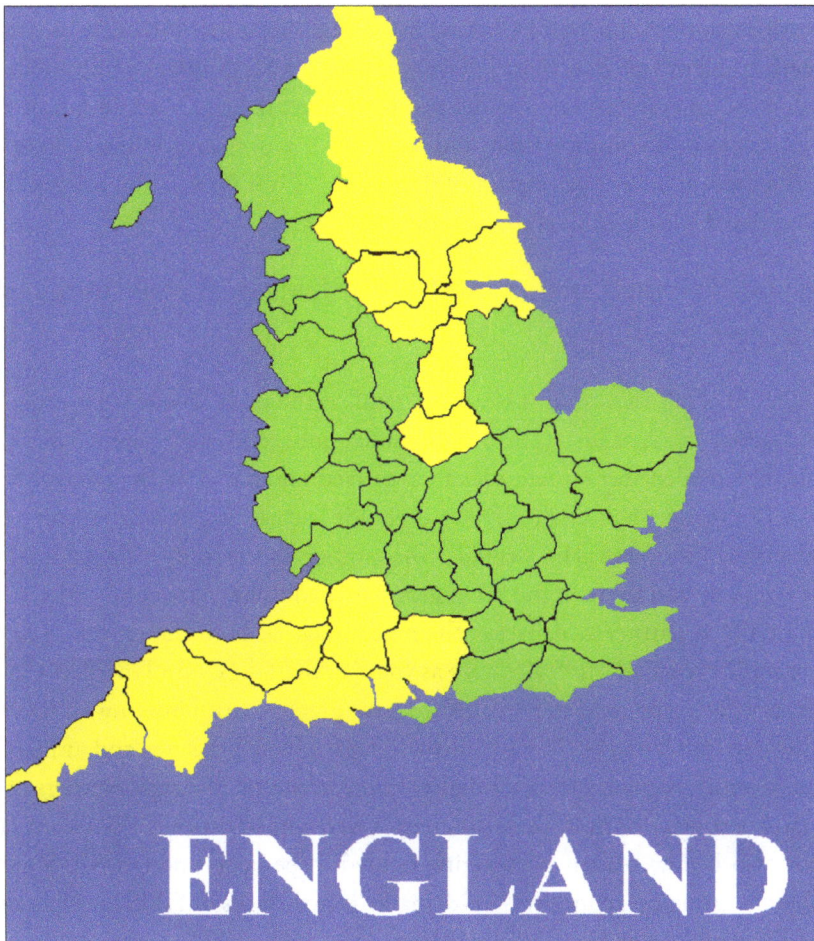

Figure 15.1: CESDI SUDI study map. (Authors' own work.)

time. This was a study of all SUDI deaths from 1 week to 1 year of age, from which the primary analysis focused on the unexplained SIDS deaths. For the controls, the health visitor (a locally based community nurse) for the infant who died was asked to identify four surviving infants in his/her caseload born within two weeks of the index infant, two older and two younger. Home visits to control families soon after the death of the index infant meant that the control infants were matched closely for age and broadly matched for geographical area, time of year, as well as whether the final sleep was a night- or daytime sleep. Information was collected both about the family's usual practices by day and by night and about the period when the infant died.

During the study period, a total of 456 SUDI cases were identified, of which 93 were later fully explained and 363 were classified as SIDS. Cross-checking of death notifications with national records two years after the end of the study period identified just 8 missed deaths, yielding 98.3% ascertainment of eligible cases. The median time from death to notification was 14 hours; from death to initial interview, 4 days; and from death to follow-up interview, 7 days. Of the 363 SIDS infants, 325 (90%) were included in the analysis (24 families did not wish to participate; 7 could not be traced; 4 were subject to police investigation; and 3 did not live in the study area), along with a full set of 4 control infants per case (1,300 controls). Over 90% of the control families were interviewed within 12 days of the index death.

## Background characteristics and identifying high-risk families
### Background characteristics

The families of SIDS victims in this study straddled the social divide from professional and managerial occupations (16%) to manual jobs and never employed (25%), although they tended to be more socially deprived compared to the control families (Table 15.1). Nearly a half of all SIDS households had no waged income compared to less than a fifth of the control households. The mothers in the study were predominantly of white ethnicity and those in the SIDS group tended to be more poorly educated and unsupported by a partner at delivery. The median age of both the mothers (23 years) and partners (27 years) of SIDS victims was younger than the control mothers (26 years) and partners (29 years), and they tended to have greater parity in terms of live births, stillbirths, and miscarriages. Whilst anemia, high blood pressure, and urinary tract infections during pregnancy were all slightly more common amongst mothers of SIDS infants than amongst controls, these differences were not statistically significant (and so are not shown below). Antenatal booking tended to be later amongst SIDS mothers, and smoking during pregnancy was quite marked: two-thirds of SIDS mothers smoked compared to a quarter of the control mothers.

Table 15.1: CESDI SUDI study — Significant family characteristics.

| Characteristic | Category | SIDS | | Controls | | p-value |
|---|---|---|---|---|---|---|
| | | n/N | % | n/N | % | |
| Social class[1] | I, II | 50/322 | 15.5% | 443/1,296 | 34.2% | <0.001 (3df) |
| | IIIN | 80/322 | 24.8% | 402/1,296 | 31.0% | |
| | IIIM, IV | 113/322 | 35.1% | 344/1,296 | 26.5% | |
| | V, Never employed | 79/322 | 24.5% | 107/1,296 | 8.3% | |
| Waged income | None in household | 158/323 | 48.9% | 237/1,298 | 18.3% | <0.001 |
| Maternal ethnicity | White | 299/324 | 92.3% | 1217/1,298 | 93.8% | 0.02 (3 df) |
| | Black | 7/324 | 2.2% | 20/1,298 | 1.5% | |
| | Asian | 11/324 | 3.4% | 55/1,298 | 4.2% | |
| | Other | 7/324 | 2.2% | 6/1,298 | 0.4% | |
| Maternal education | No qualification | 129/316 | 40.8% | 245/1,293 | 18.9% | <0.001 |
| Marital status | Supported[2] | 283/325 | 87.1% | 1237/,1300 | 95.2% | <0.001 |
| Maternal age | <26 years | 197/325 | 60.6% | 484/1,300 | 37.2% | <0.001 |
| Paternal age | <26 years | 103/285 | 36.1% | 283/1,256 | 22.5% | <0.001 |
| Number of children[3] | 1 child | 90/325 | 27.7% | 558/1,300 | 42.9% | <0.001 (3df) |
| | 2 children | 94/325 | 28.9% | 454/1,300 | 34.9% | |
| | 3 children | 85/325 | 26.2% | 188/1,300 | 14.5% | |
| | 4 or more | 56/325 | 17.3% | 100/1,300 | 7.7% | |
| Previous stillbirth | 1 or more | 10/325 | 3.1% | 15/1,300 | 1.2% | 0.01 |
| Previous miscarriage | 1 or more | 90/325 | 27.7% | 261/1,291 | 20.2% | 0.003 |
| Antenatal booking | Late or none[4] | 17/309 | 5.5% | 22/1,268 | 13.1% | <0.001 |
| Maternal smoking | During pregnancy | 212/322 | 65.8% | 348/1,299 | 26.8% | <0.001 |

[1]Based on occupation (I: professional to V: manual) of both parents including previous occupation if currently unemployed.
[2]Mother supported by a partner at delivery (whether or not they were married or living together).
[3]Including the child in the study.
[4]Third trimester or did not book care.

Risk scoring systems to identify families with infants at high risk of SIDS have previously been attempted but with little success (11-13). We modeled the above significant characteristics in Table 15.1 on the first two years of the CESDI data and tested the sensitivity and specificity of the resulting algorithm on the third-year data set. There were four significant predictors: maternal smoking during pregnancy, low maternal age (<26 years), larger families (three or more children), and poor socioeconomic status (social class IV, V, or unemployed). Three or more of these predictors identified 42% of SIDS families from just 8% of the population. This scoring system was subsequently used to identify high-risk control families in the SWISS study (10).

## Matching factors and infant characteristics

### Matching factors

The median age of SIDS infants was 13 weeks (Interquartile range: 8 weeks to 21 weeks). The median age of the control infants was slightly older (11 days), given the unanticipated time lag of arranging a home interview that suited the control families (Figure 15.2).

There was no significant seasonal pattern amongst the SIDS deaths (27.4% occurred in the colder winter months of December, January, and February), and control interviews did not significantly differ by month. Deaths occurred in both urban (83.4%) and rural (17.6%) locations; controls were matched exactly to this broad geographical locality, although, as Table 15.1 shows, this does not mean sociodeprivation markers were matched. The proportion of daytime deaths (16.9%) was similar to the proportion of daytime sleeps from which the control infant woke (15.8%).

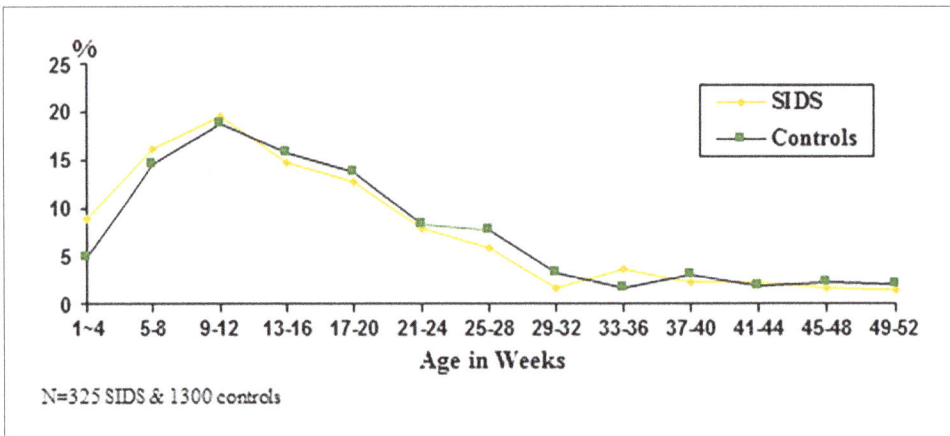

Figure 15.2: CESDI SUDI study — Age distribution of SIDS infants and controls. (Authors' own work.)

There was a male preponderance of SIDS deaths; the median birth weight (3,053 g) was significantly lower compared to the controls (3,399 g); and preterm births were much more common among the SIDS infants (Table 15.2). The median birth percentile (which takes account of weight by gestational age and gender) for SIDS cases was the 38th percentile compared to the 50th percentile for controls. When the birth weight percentile variable and the variables for gestational age and sex were put into a multiple logistical regression model, all three variables remained significant, hence the lower birth weight of the SIDS infants was not due solely to their shorter gestational age. A detailed analysis of subsequent weight measurements showed that poor postnatal weight gain was independently associated with an increased risk of SIDS, although there was no evidence of increased growth retardation before death (14). Almost twice as many SIDS infants were delivered by emergency cesarean section and significantly more of the SIDS infants had an Apgar score of below 8 at one minute and five minutes. Multiple births were far more common amongst SIDS infants than controls and nearly a quarter of the SIDS infants were admitted to a Special Care Baby Unit compared to 7% of the control infants; the main reasons were breathing difficulties, infection, problems with blood sugar levels, poor feeding, hypothermia, and growth retardation.

Table 15.2: CESDI SUDI study — Significant infant characteristics.

| Characteristic | Category | SIDS | | Controls | | p-value |
|---|---|---|---|---|---|---|
| | | n/N | % | n/N | % | |
| Gender | Male | 205/325 | 63.1% | 672/1,300 | 51.7% | <0.001 |
| Birth weight | <2,500 g | 74/325 | 22.8% | 66/1,292 | 5.1% | <0.001 |
| Gestation | <37 weeks | 63/323 | 19.5% | 70/1,288 | 5.4% | <0.001 |
| Birth percentile | <14th percentile[1] | 71/323 | 22.0% | 169/1,286 | 13.1% | <0.001 |
| Delivery by CS[2] | Emergency | 44/321 | 13.7% | 167/1,290 | 8.3% | 0.003 |
| Multiple birth | Twin or triplet | 17/325 | 5.2% | 12/1,300 | 0.9% | <0.001 |
| Apgar score at 1 min | <8 | 79/311 | 25.4% | 250/1,263 | 19.8% | 0.03 |
| Apgar score at 5 min | <8 | 16/311 | 5.1% | 27/1,258 | 2.1% | 0.004 |
| Admission to SCBU[3] | Yes | 80/323 | 24.8% | 92/1,291 | 7.1% | <0.001 |

[1]Standard deviation below the mean.
[2]Cesarian Section.
[3]Special Care Baby Unit.

During their short lives, SIDS infants were significantly more likely to experience an episode of lifelessness (Table 15.3). Of those who had experienced such an episode, a similar proportion were reported to have experienced the cessation of breathing and a change in color, and the parents of a similar proportion had contacted a doctor. However, more SIDS infants (44%) than control infants (28%) were reported to have had more than one episode, to have experienced apparent cessation of breathing for more than 10 seconds (56% vs 22% controls), and to have been taken to hospital (47% vs 33% controls).

Table 15.3: CESDI SUDI study — Significant risk factors during life.

| Factors | Category | SIDS | | Controls | | p-value |
|---|---|---|---|---|---|---|
| | | n/N | % | n/N | % | |
| Episode of lifelessness | At least one | 37/317 | 11.7% | 39/1,299 | 3.0% | <0.001 |
| Postnatal depression | Severe[1] | 7/312 | 2.2% | 10/1,283 | 0.8% | 0.03[2] |
| Moving house in last year | Once | 100/323 | 31% | 219/1,297 | 16.9% | <0.001 |
| | Twice | 29/323 | 9.1% | 34/1,297 | 2.6% | <0.001 |
| | Three or more | 23/323 | 7.1% | 20/1,297 | 1.5% | <0.001 |
| Postnatal exposure to smoke | 1-2 hrs | 43/308 | 14.0% | 137/1,288 | 10.6% | <0.001 |
| | 3-5 hrs | 33/308 | 10.7% | 72/1,288 | 5.6% | <0.001 |
| | 6-8 hrs | 29/308 | 9.4% | 34/1,288 | 2.6% | <0.001 |
| | 9 or more hrs | 60/308 | 19.5% | 55/1,288 | 4.3% | <0.001 |
| Maternal drug consumption[3] | Yes | 27/314 | 8.6% | 34/1,296 | 2.6% | <0.001 |
| Paternal drug consumption[3] | Yes | 42/322 | 13.0% | 52/1,298 | 4.0% | <0.001 |
| Infant breastfed | Ever | 141/323 | 43.7% | 774/1,298 | 59.6% | <0.001 |
| Length of previous infant sleep | >10 hrs | 40/303 | 13.2% | 302/1,297 | 23.3% | 0.007 |
| | <5 hrs | 87/303 | 28.7% | 192/1,297 | 14.8% | <0.001 |

[1]From the Health Visitor Records.
[2]Using Fisher's Exact Test.
[3]After the pregnancy.

A very small, but significant, proportion of SIDS mothers were recorded as having severe postnatal depression by the health visitor. As well as differences in social deprivation, there were differences in social disruption, as families of SIDS infants experienced moving house more often over the previous year with increasing risk associated with greater numbers of changes of accommodation. As Table 15.1 shows, maternal smoking during pregnancy was very common amongst the SIDS mothers; a detailed analysis showed there was a clear dose-response effect of higher risk with more cigarettes smoked, and this difference was apparent whether smoking was measured before, during, or after pregnancy (9). We also found that smoke exposure from partners and other people living in the household was significant in contributing to postnatal daily exposure, with a clear dose response effect: at 1-2 hours the risk was 2.4 [95% CI: 1.5 to 3.9]; at 3-5 hours the risk was 3.8 [95% CI: 2.2 to 6.6]; at 6-8 hours the risk was 5.9 [95% CI: 3.2 to 10.9]; and at 9 or more hours the risk was 8.3 [95% CI: 4.9 to 14.0]. The parents were asked whether they had used illegal substances (glue, amphetamines, barbiturates, cannabis, speed, LSD, cocaine, ecstasy, methadone, heroin, or crack) on more than one occasion. Before, during, and after pregnancy both SIDS parents were more likely to use illegal drugs compared to the controls, the main drug of choice being cannabis. A greater proportion of control infants were breastfed, suggesting the possibility of a protective effect, although this association and any dose-response effect was lost when post-matching the control families to the same socioeconomic status (15). The parents were asked to recall the longest period for which their infant slept in the 24 hours prior to the last sleep; a greater proportion of control infants had slept for longer than 10 hours and a greater proportion of SIDS infants had slept for less than 5 hours.

## Risk factors in the final sleep environment

Infants put down on their side (odds ratio (OR) = 2.2 [95% CI: 1.6-3.0]) or front (OR = 10.2 [95% CI: 5.9-17.7]) for sleep were at risk and the associated risk doubled if they were found in either of these two positions. Infants placed on their side and found on their front tended to be younger, suggesting that the change from the side position may reflect the instability of the younger infants. The presumed stability of infants with their lower arm extended whilst in the side position (recommended in the initial "Back to Sleep" campaign) had little effect. Table 15.4 also shows that more of the SIDS mothers worried that the infant was too cold whilst more of the control mothers were worried the infant was too hot; significantly more of the SIDS infants were wrapped too warmly and used a duvet. Using a pillow in the infant cot was a rare event but more common amongst SIDS infants. A small proportion of SIDS (4.4%) and control infants (2.7%) had, on several occasions, previously been found with bed covers over their heads after a sleep; however, for this last sleep a larger proportion of SIDS (16%) were found with covers over their head or face. Significantly more SIDS infants slept with a parent in the parental bed or on a sofa, and significantly more slept unobserved outside the parental bedroom. Further analysis also showed that lack of parental observation during daytime sleeps was also a risk factor (16). Although the majority of both SIDS and control infants were generally well in the 24 hours prior to the last sleep, a retrospective Baby Check score (17) suggested significantly more SIDS infants (11%) needed a doctor or emergency medical attention compared to the controls (4%). There was no identifiable difference in the frequency of use of a dummy (pacifier) for usual night-time or daytime sleeps between cases and controls, but significantly fewer SIDS infants used a dummy for the last sleep. The parents in the study were asked whether they had any change in routine which would have involved the infant prior to the last sleep. The changes identified were similar in both groups (and included going out for the first time in a while; visiting friends; going on holiday; or going out socializing) but were more common amongst the SIDS parents. Usual weekly alcohol consumption was greater for both SIDS parents and binge drinking (more than four units of alcohol in any on session) was more common. Prior to the last sleep, more of the SIDS mothers consumed three or more units of alcohol compared to the controls. This finding was similar but did not quite reach significance amongst the SIDS partners.

Table 15.4: CESDI SUDI study — Significant risk factors in the final sleep environment.

| Factors | Category | SIDS | | Controls | | p-value |
|---|---|---|---|---|---|---|
| | | n/N | % | n/N | % | |
| Position but down[1] | Side | 129/317 | 40.7% | 361/1,295 | 27.9% | <0.001 |
| | Front | 47/317 | 14.8% | 39/1,295 | 3.0% | <0.001 |
| Position found[1] | Side | 76/306 | 24.8% | 134/1,248 | 10.7% | <0.001 |
| | Front | 114/306 | 37.3% | 77/1,248 | 6.2% | <0.001 |
| Mother worried that infant was | … Too cold | 88/317 | 27.8% | 205/1,298 | 15.8% | 0.007 |
| | … Too hot | 81/317 | 25.6% | 564/1,298 | 43.5% | <0.001 |
| Infant wrapped too warm | >10 togs | 45/320 | 14.1% | 65/1,299 | 5.0% | <0.001 |
| Used a duvet | For last sleep | 128/323 | 39.6% | 265/1,299 | 20.4% | <0.001 |
| Used a pillow in the cot | For last sleep | 26/318 | 8.2% | 29/1,297 | 2.2% | <0.001 |
| Head covered by bedding | Yes | 49/303 | 16.2% | 38/1,289 | 2.9% | <0.001 |
| Where infant slept | Separate room | 114/321 | 35.5% | 420/1,299 | 32.2% | <0.001 |
| | Parent's bed | 82/321 | 25.5% | 189/1,299 | 14.5% | <0.001 |
| | Sofa with parent | 20/321 | 6.2% | 6/1,299 | 0.5% | <0.001 |
| Required doctor last 24 hrs[2] | Yes | 36/318 | 11.3% | 47/1,299 | 3.6% | <0.001 |
| Infant health in last 24 hrs[3] | Only fair | 80/321 | 24.9% | 182/1,299 | 14.0% | <0.001 |
| | Poor | 19/321 | 5.9% | 20/1,299 | 1.5% | <0.001 |

| Infant used a dummy | Yes | 124/313 | 39.6% | 664/1,296 | 51.2% | <0.001 |
|---|---|---|---|---|---|---|
| Change in routine | Time of last sleep | 66/321 | 20.6% | 165/1,299 | 12.7% | <0.001 |
| Maternal alcohol consumption | >2 units | 37/314 | 11.8% | 41/1,297 | 3.2% | <0.001 |

[1]Reference sleep: those infants put down prone or found prone.
[2]Using a Baby Check score of 12 or more.
[3]Reference group: those infants to be considered healthy in the last 24 hours before the last sleep

## The multivariable model

All associations significant in the univariable analysis were modeled to determine which factors generated the greatest risk when adjusted together. Twenty factors remained significant in the final model (Table 15.5). Infants found after the last sleep with bedding over their face or head were relatively rare amongst the control infants (3%) but occurred amongst a sixth of SIDS deaths (16%). Parental narrative accounts of the deaths, and the wider epidemiological evidence, do not lend support to the idea that head covering is simply a consequence of some terminal struggle (18). Advice to place the feet of the infant at the foot of the cot, to tuck in covering, and to use infant sleeping bags is now given to reduce the risk of this particular factor. Infant vulnerability before birth (short gestational age at birth and exposure to tobacco smoke during pregnancy), during life (low birth percentile, episodes of lifelessness, and postnatal tobacco exposure), and prior to the final sleep (poor infant health, shorter previous sleep duration, and feeding less than usual) are all represented in the model, as were both social deprivation (no waged income) and social disruption in terms of moving house and change in routine.

There was a significant risk associated with bed sharing, but a higher risk when the infant slept in a separate room to the parents, and the risk was an order of magnitude higher if the infant co-slept on a sofa. A subsequent in-depth analysis of the sleeping environment showed the risk associated with being found in the parental bed was not significant for older infants or for infants of parents who did not smoke, and became non-significant after adjustment for recent maternal alcohol consumption and use of duvets (both included in this model) as well as parental tiredness and overcrowded housing conditions (19). The initial "Back to Sleep" campaign both in the United Kingdom (UK) and the United States (US) advised that infants could be slept on their side but data from this study suggests that the side position still put infants at risk. Further analysis highlighted that infants of low birth weight, who were placed on their side, were at particularly increased risk (20). The proportion of control infants put down in the prone position was just 3%, suggesting that the "Back to Sleep" campaign was effective; however, the proportions amongst SIDS infants were higher (15%), thus being placed prone was still a risk factor. The campaign prior to the study also identified infants being wrapped too warmly as a risk factor; this was still apparent but now represented by the protective factor of control mothers being worried that the infant was too hot. The apparent protective effect of dummies has been found in previous studies (21), although it is not clear what the physiological mechanism might be or whether the lack of any difference in usual practice suggests that the absence of a dummy for the final sleep is a proxy marker for some change in routine not measured (22).

Table 15.5: CESDI SUDI study — Multivariable model.

| Factors | Non-ref group | OR [95% CI]2 | p-value |
|---|---|---|---|
| Head covered | Yes | 33.22 [9.46, 116.69] | <0.001 |
| Gestational age | 36 weeks or less | 10.91 [3.90, 30.50] | <0.001 |
| Where infant slept[1] | separate room | 12.80 [5.00, 32.76] | <0.001 |
| | parent's bed | 4.09 [1.84, 9.11] | <0.001 |
| | sofa with parent | 53.85 [7.13, 406.94] | <0.001 |
| Postnatal exposure to tobacco smoke | 6 to 8 hours | 7.03 [1.71, 28.98] | 0.007 |
| | 9 or more hours | 12.37 [3.79, 40.38] | <0.001 |
| Length of previous infant sleep | >10 hours | 0.22 [0.09, 0.52] | <0.001 |
| Sleep position for last sleep | put down side | 2.19 [1.23, 3.91] | 0.008 |
| | put down front | 6.78 [2.10, 21.92] | 0.001 |
| Episode of lifelessness | at least one | 7.59 [2.14, 26.93] | 0.002 |
| Waged income | none in household | 2.76 [1.45, 5.25] | 0.002 |
| Maternal alcohol consumption | >2 units last 24hrs | 7.83 [2.13, 28.73] | 0.002 |
| Maternal smoking | during pregnancy | 2.58 [1.38, 4.82] | 0.002 |
| No. of children (including study child) | 2 or 3 | 2.78 [1.45, 5.34] | 0.002 |
| | 4 or more | 3.65 [1.36, 9.82] | 0.01 |
| Moving house | twice in last year | 4.76 [1.30, 17.47] | 0.02 |
| | three times or more | 8.93 [2.08, 38.29] | 0.003 |
| Used dummy (pacifier) | for last sleep | 0.41 [0.22, 0.77] | 0.006 |
| Birth weight percentiles | continuous var. | 1.55 [1.12, 2.14]2 | 0.008 |
| Infant health last 24 hrs | only fair | 2.33 [1.11, 4.90] | 0.03 |
| | poor | 4.71 [1.24, 17.91] | 0.02 |
| Pillow in cot | for the last sleep | 5.72 [1.40, 23.30] | 0.02 |

| Mother worried that infant was[3] | ... too hot | 0.44 [0.23, 0.87] | 0.02 |
|---|---|---|---|
| Feeding last 24 hrs | less than usual | 3.10 [1.09, 8.80] | 0.03 |
| Used a duvet | for last sleep | 2.00 [1.03, 3.85] | 0.04 |
| Change in routine | in last 24 hours | 2.35 [1.03, 5.36] | 0.04 |

The model includes 277 cases and 1,261 controls (95% of the data).

[1] Reference group: those infants who shared a room with the parents but not the parental bed.

[2] OR based on units of one standard deviation.

[3] Reference group: those mothers not anxious about infant's thermal environment or those anxious about infant being too cold.

Risk factors that were significant in the univariate analysis but not significant when added to the above model include gender, young maternal age, paternal smoking and drug abuse, multiple births, stillbirths, admission to SCBU, housing tenure, reduced income support, mode of infant feeding and duration, maternal postnatal depression, other people smoking in the household, usual maternal alcohol consumption, usual and recent alcohol consumption of the partner, maternal use of illegal substances, the number of infant hospital admissions, infant health and medication in the last week; and for the last sleep: non-parental care, tog values of bedding and clothing, whether the heating was on or door was ajar, whether infant wore a hat, use of a cot bumper, whether the infant was sweating, how the bed covers were tucked, softness of the mattress, the number of toys in the cot, use of listening devices.

Of the four predictors selected prior to birth to identify high-risk families, socioeconomic deprivation (in terms of no waged income), maternal smoking during pregnancy, and high parity remained in the model, while low maternal age was borderline (p=0.06).

## Factors not associated with SIDS

The age at which infants receive their primary course of immunization in the UK corresponds to the peak age for the incidence of the SIDS; sporadic reports promoted speculation that these two events might be related (23-25). However, we found that after confounding was controlled for, immunization uptake was lowest among the infants who died, with no temporal relationship or correlation with signs and symptoms of illness (26). A detailed re-analysis of time-dependent variables showed in this, and similar, studies that the risk of SIDS in vaccinated cases and controls neither increased nor reduced during the early post-vaccination period (27).

In the CESDI SUDI study, we tested a theory postulated at the time that toxic gas emanating from the infant mattress may be associated with SIDS; specifically, the production of toxic trihydride gases, arsine, stibine, and phosphene by fungal degradation of flame retardants or plasticizers added to the PVC of mattress covers. There was no evidence that colonization of mattresses by the particular fungus implicated (Scopularis brevicaulis) was common, no association between mattress concentrations of antimony and those in tissue or hair samples (28), and no evidence that the use of mattresses with integral PVC covers was associated with an increased risk of SIDS — in fact, the association of such mattress covers was with a significantly lower risk of SIDS (29).

We asked about apnea monitors only in the third year of the study and found that these were used more for the last sleep by the families of SIDS infants (6/121 or 5%) compared to the controls (11/512 or 2.1%). This finding was not significant (Fisher's Exact test: p=0.11) but neither was it in the direction of a protective effect. This suggests that the infants using such monitors were at higher risk of SIDS, and the use of the monitor had no effect on the outcome.

## Comparison of SIDS and explained SUDI deaths

Of the 93 explained SUDI deaths, we managed to conduct home interviews for 72. The major causes of death among those considered by the multidisciplinary panel to be fully explained were infection (46%), accidental death (15%), congenital anomalies (14%), and non-accidental injury (13%). The remaining deaths included metabolic disorders, bowel obstruction, bronchopulmonary dysplasia, and cardiomyopathy. Many of the background and clinical characteristics associated with fetal and infant vulnerability amongst SIDS infants were similar amongst the explained deaths (30, 31). The explained SUDI infants were older (median age 127 days) but there were more deaths in the first month of life; they had a higher frequency of neonatal problems and congenital malformations; and there were lower rates of maternal smoking during pregnancy (49% compared to 66% amongst the SIDS mothers).

# The SWISS Study

## Study methodology and ascertainment

The SWISS Study was conducted across six counties in the South West region of England (study population 4.9 million; see Figure 15.3) between January 2003 and December 2006. This was a study of all SUDI deaths from birth to 2 years old, although the primary focus was the SIDS cases. Controls were chosen from St Michael's maternity hospital in Bristol during the third trimester of pregnancy. Two control groups were used: a random sample (those who did not give consent were replaced by parents with a similar socioeconomic classification based on occupation) and a high-risk group based on the scoring system described above from the CESDI study. The timing of the home interviews for the control groups was weighted to reflect the age distribution of the SIDS cases.

During the study period, the study identified 157 SUDI cases, of which 90 met the criteria for SIDS (a rate of 0.49 deaths per 1,000 live births, which was similar to the national rate at that time). Of the 90 SIDS cases identified, 80 (89%) were included for analysis — four families did not consent to the study; three deaths occurred before the study had full ethics permission; two families moved out of the study area; and one death was initially suspicious. The study team carried out reference sleep interviews with

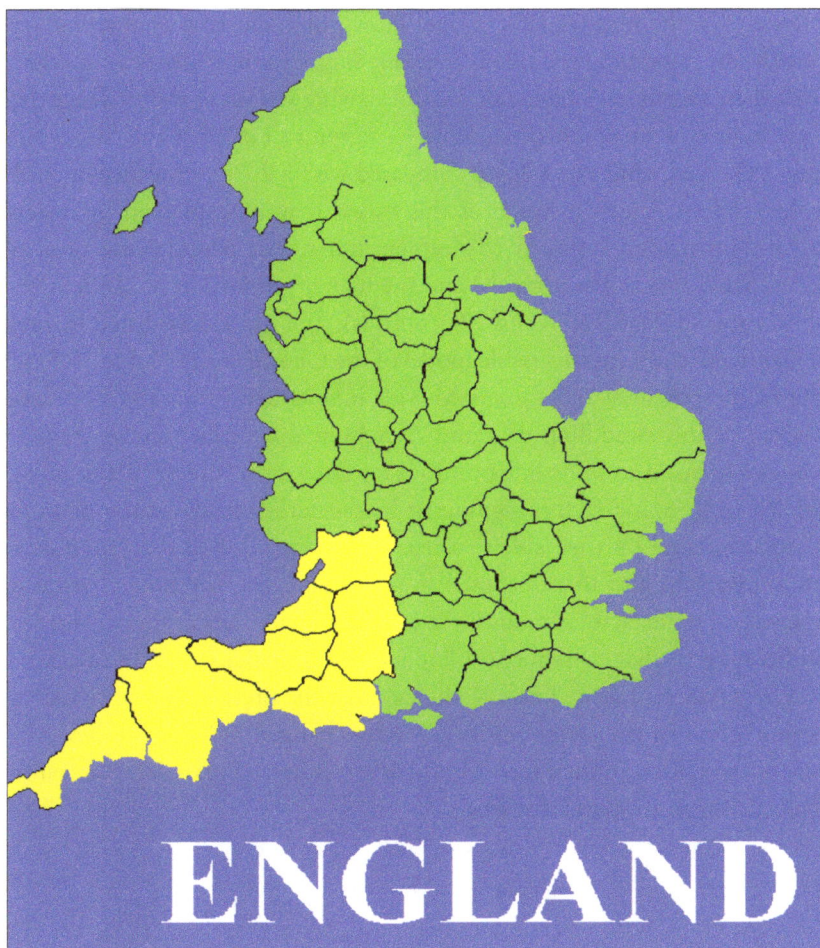

Figure 15.3: SWISS study map. (Authors' own work.)

87 random control families and 82 high-risk families. The median time from death to notification was just two hours, and a joint agency approach was used to interview the majority of parents (75%) within 24 hours of the death (32).

## Main findings

The age distribution of the SIDS infants was significantly different from the CESDI study with a median age of 66 days, almost a month younger than the SIDS infants from 10 years earlier (median 91 days). Given the smaller size of the SWISS study, compared to its predecessor, some of the categorical variables were collapsed (notably, bed sharing and sofa sharing were added together), and the focus on the main findings was directional shifts away from the main findings of the CESDI study rather than the size of point estimates and wide confidence intervals in the SWISS study.

Interestingly, the multivariable model shown in Table 15.6 comparing the SIDS infants with the randomly sampled controls was virtually identical to the model comparing these deaths with high-risk controls, giving weight to the evidence that these factors are independent of socioeconomic background (10). Of the SIDS infants in this study, 54% died while co-sleeping compared with a 20% prevalence of co-sleeping among the random controls. Much of this excess may be explained by a significant multivariable interaction between co-sleeping and recent parental use of alcohol or drugs (31% SIDS versus 3% controls) and the higher proportion of SIDS infants who co-slept on a sofa (17% SIDS versus 1% controls). The risk factors listed in Table 15.6 were all identified in the multivariable model of the CESDI study (Table 15.5) with the exception of the potential risk associated with infants being swaddled. A subsequent meta-analysis of this swaddling data and data from three other studies suggests that current advice to avoid front or side positions for sleep especially applies to infants who are swaddled (33). Some factors significant in the earlier study were not as marked, notably infants placed on their side to sleep, infants found with their head covered or wrapped too warmly, and those exposed to postnatal tobacco smoke. The decrease in the prevalence of these factors amongst the control populations in the 10 years between these studies suggests that subsequent risk reduction campaigns after the "Back to Sleep" campaign may have had some impact. The fact that the prevalence and risk association with infants found in the prone position hardly changed between studies, whilst the SIDS rate in the UK continued to fall in the intervening 10 years (after accounting for any diagnostic shift), supports this idea.

Table 15.6: SWISS study — Multivariable model.

| Factors | Non-Ref Group | SIDS | | Random Controls | | OR [95% CI][1] | p-value |
|---|---|---|---|---|---|---|---|
| | | n/N | % | n/N | % | | |
| Maternal alcohol | >2 units consumed | 19/77 | 24.7% | 2/87 | 2.3% | 41.62 [5.45-318.09] | 0.0003 |
| Where infant slept[2] | parental bed/ sofa | 43/79 | 54.4% | 18/87 | 20.7% | 21.77 [3.79-125.00] | 0.001 |
| | separate room | 21/79 | 26.6% | 21/87 | 24.1% | 21.34 [2.99-152.56] | 0.002 |
| Maternal smoking | during pregnancy | 47/79 | 59.5% | 12/87 | 13.8% | 13.36 [3.07-58.83] | 0.001 |
| Infant swaddled | for the last sleep | 19/78 | 24.4% | 5/87 | 5.7% | 31.06 [4.21-228.94] | 0.001 |

| Maternal education | no qualifications | 28/80 | 35.0% | 12/87 | 13.8% | 15.55 [2.59-93.50] | 0.003 |
|---|---|---|---|---|---|---|---|
| Sleep position for last sleep | found prone | 23/79 | 29.1% | 9/86 | 10.5% | 6.61 [1.57-27.88] | 0.010 |
| Gestational age | 36 weeks or less | 21/80 | 26.3% | 4/87 | 4.6% | 11.52 [1.64-80.82] | 0.014 |
| Number of children[3] | 4 or more children | 18/80 | 22.5% | 5/87 | 5.7% | 11.64 [1.57-86.05] | 0.016 |
| Used a pillow[4] | for the last sleep | 16/78 | 20.5% | 3/87 | 3.4% | 10.59 [1.43-78.39] | 0.021 |
| Infant health last 24 hrs | only fair or poor | 22/79 | 27.8% | 5/87 | 5.7% | 8.06 [1.11-58.42] | 0.039 |

Multivariable logistic regression model includes 74/80 SIDS cases (92.5%) and 86/87 random controls (98.9%).

[1]Adjusted for infant age (p=0.70) and day or night sleep (p=0.74) as well as the significant factors shown in the above multivariable model.

[2]Multi-categorical variable, infants sleeping in a cot next to the parental bed used as the reference group.

[3]Including the study child.

[4]Either the head or whole body of the infant was on the pillow.

## Combining Data from the CESDI and SWISS Studies

The "Back to Sleep" campaign had a dramatic effect on the number of SIDS deaths occurring in a cot but less effect on co-sleeping deaths, which accounted for over 50% of SIDS deaths in the SWISS study (34). Previously, we have demonstrated both that a proportion of these co-sleeping deaths occurred while the parent and infant slept on a sofa or chair, and that there was a significant interaction between co-sleeping and parents recently consuming alcohol or drugs or being smokers. However, the question remains as to whether there is still a residual risk of bed sharing in the absence of these hazardous circumstances. Data from both the CESDI and SWISS studies were combined to answer this question (35).

Of the 405 SIDS infants and 1,387 controls in the two studies, we had data on the sleep environment in which the infant was found for 400 SIDS infants (98.8%) and 1,386 controls (99.9%). Over a third of SIDS infants (36%) were found co-sleeping with an adult at the time of death compared to 15% of the controls after reference sleep. The overall risk of SIDS for infants who co-slept was more than threefold and almost fourfold when adjusted for other factors associated with SIDS (Table 15.7). When categorized by co-sleeping environment, the multivariable risk of co-sleeping with an adult on a sofa or chair, or with an adult who had consumed more than two units of alcohol, was 18 times greater than for those who did not co-sleep; and four times greater for those who slept next to a parent who smoked. There was no significant multivariable risk of bed sharing in the absence of these hazards (OR = 1.1 [95% CI: 0.6-2.0]). Splitting the data into younger and older infants increased the risk in all co-sleeping environments, although it was not quite significant if the infant was bed sharing in the absence of these hazards (OR = 1.6 [95% CI: 0.96-2.7]), and it was in the direction of protection for older bed-sharing infants (OR = 0.1 [95% CI: 0.01-0.5]). These findings support a public health strategy that both acknowledges that bed sharing happens, rather than simply advising against such practice, and emphasizes specific hazardous co-sleeping environments that parents should avoid. Sofa sharing is not a safe alternative to bed sharing, and bed sharing should be avoided if parents consume alcohol, smoke, or take drugs, or if the infant was born preterm.

Table 15.7: CESDI and SWISS data combined — the risk associated with co-sleeping for last sleep.

| Overall | SIDS | | Controls | | Multivariable Risk[1] | |
|---|---|---|---|---|---|---|
| | N | % | N | % | OR [95% CI] | p-value |
| Did not co-sleep | 255 | 63.8% | 1173 | 84.6% | 1.00 [Ref Group] | |
| Co-slept | 145 | 36.3% | 213 | 15.4% | 3.91 [2.72-5.62] | <0.0001 |
| By different co-sleeping environments | | | | | | |
| Did not co-sleep | 255 | 63.8% | 1173 | 84.6% | 1.00 [Ref Group] | |
| Co-slept on a sofa or chair | 33 | 8.3% | 7 | 0.5% | 18.34 [7.10-47.35] | <0.0001 |
| Bed shared next to adult (>2 units of alcohol) | 29 | 7.3% | 12 | 0.9% | 18.29 [7.68-43.54] | <0.0001 |
| Bed shared next to adult who smoked | 59 | 14.8% | 63 | 4.5% | 4.04 [2.41-6.75] | <0.0001 |
| Bed shared in the absence of these hazards | 24 | 6.0% | 131 | 9.5% | 1.08 [0.58-2.01] | 0.82 |

[1]Adjusted for infant age and whether the last sleep was a day or night sleep, as well as for infant characteristics: birth weight <2,500 g, preterm, male gender and currently breastfeeding; maternal characteristics: larger families (≥3 children), younger mothers (≤21 years), and poor maternal education (<GCSE or no qualification); factors at the time of the last sleep: infant unwell (scoring 8 or more on the Baby Check), infant placed prone or side, infant swaddled, use of a duvet, use of a dummy, and infant found with head covered.

The logistic regression model used 1,700/1,786 (95.4%) individuals.

Interestingly, dummy use was only associated with a lower risk of SIDS among co-sleepers rather than among infants sleeping in cots. This lends weight to the idea that the absence of a dummy may be a marker for a change in routine such as parents deciding to bed share rather than in itself conferring any protective effect to the infant. Sleeping prone was largely a risk factor amongst infants sleeping in cots, suggesting that more sensitive pathology investigations are needed to establish the causal mechanisms of death for infants who co-sleep in hazardous circumstances.

## Lessons Learnt for Future Investigations

- Any future investigation needs to include all SUDI deaths. Classification of SIDS is difficult, and recent diagnostic shifts suggest that all unexpected deaths should be captured and classification decided by multidisciplinary panel. Explained SUDI deaths can serve as additional controls for both the epidemiologist and pathologist, especially in terms of whether related factors are unique to SIDS deaths or infant deaths in general.

- A rapid notification network reporting the deaths and joint agency approach can work and gives families the best support at a difficult time as well as reducing recall bias in research studies. The experience from both studies was that bereaved families wanted contact sooner rather than later to help comprehend what had happened.

- Given the welcome reduction in SIDS rates, a conventional case-control study design may be difficult to implement, suggesting that increased efforts should focus on collecting detailed data regionally or nationally when SUDI infants die. Such data can be used both for monitoring purposes and (given the potential wider study population) for periodically conducting observational studies if suitable control infants can be found. International consensus of what data should be collected, and in what format, needs to be agreed so that these data can be both monitored and pooled in future investigations.

- Any such data collection needs to focus on the specific environment in which the infant is found, including details of all those who share that environment. This will both improve classification of SUDI deaths and provide evidence for the future direction of risk reduction campaigns.

- Any significant association found with established infant care practices and SIDS needs careful scrutiny of whether the link is causal or a marker for something else potentially unmeasured. In considering subsequent risk reduction advice, one needs to take account of the wider implications beyond SIDS research in terms of the benefit or harm of an infant care practice and the cultural expectations surrounding it.

- We use several proxy markers to measure social deprivation but find it more difficult to measure social disruption and the potential chaos that can increase vulnerability for young infants. Future investigations need to try and capture changes in routine, especially those that may interfere with usual infant care practices.

- Control families should be randomly chosen and research ethics permission obtained for the research team to approach these families. This approach was used in the CESDI study (recruitment rate over 90%) but not obtained for the SWISS study, where the initial approach was via the mother's usual midwife (recruitment rate 25%).

- The timing of interviewing control families should be chosen such that the reference sleep is comparable to the time the SIDS infant died, in terms of infant age, day of the week, and time of the day (so that infant care practices and associated parental activity can be adjusted for).

- There is a potential for future intervention studies to reduce deaths further, but as any intervention will probably be labor-intensive on a one-to-one basis of hard-to-reach groups, such an endeavor at the population level will need to be targeted. At the moment, more work needs to be done to improve the sensitivity and specificity of the algorithms so far proposed to identify high-risk families.

# References

1. Beal S, Blundell H. Sudden infant death syndrome related to position in the cot. Med J Australia. 1978;2:217-18.

2. Saturnus KS. Plötzicher Kindstod — Eine Folge der Bauchlage? In: Festschrift Professor Leithoff. Kriminalstatistik, Heidelberg. 1985;67-81.

3. Davies DP. Cot death in Hong Kong: A rare problem? Lancet. 1985;ii:1346-25. https://doi.org/10.1016/S0140-6736(85)92637-6.

4. de Jonge GA, Engleberts AC, Koomen-Liefting AJ, Kostense PJ. Cot death and prone sleeping position in the Netherlands. BMJ. 1989;298:722. https://doi.org/10.1136/bmj.298.6675.722.

5. Fleming PJ, Gilbert R, Azaz Y, Berry PJ, Rudd PT, Stewart AW, et al. Interaction between bedding and sleeping position in the sudden infant death syndrome: A population based case-control study. BMJ. 1990;301:85-9. https://doi.org/10.1136/bmj.301.6743.85.

6. Mitchell EA, Scragg R, Stewart AW, Becroft DMO, Taylor BJ, Ford RP, et al. Results from the first year of the New Zealand cot death study. NZ Med J. 1991;104(906)71-6.

7. Dattani N, Cooper N. Trends in cot death. Health Statistics Quarterly. 2000;5:10-16.

8. Fleming PJ, Blair PS, Bacon C, Bensley D, Smith I, Taylor E, et al. Environment of infants during sleep and risk of the sudden infant death syndrome: Results from 1993-5 case-control study for confidential inquiry into stillbirths and deaths in infancy. BMJ. 1996;313:191-5. https://doi.org/10.1136/bmj.313.7051.191.

9. Blair PS, Fleming PJ, Bensley D, Bacon C, Smith I, Taylor E, et al. Smoking and the sudden infant death syndrome: Results from 1993-5 case-control study for confidential inquiry into stillbirths and deaths in infancy. BMJ. 1996;313:195-8. https://doi.org/10.1136/bmj.313.7051.195.

10. Blair PS, Sidebotham P, Evason-Coombe C, Edmonds M, Heckstall-Smith EM, Fleming P. Hazardous cosleeping environments and risk factors amenable to change: Case-control study of SIDS in south west England. BMJ. 2009;339:b3666. https://doi.org/10.1136/bmj.b3666.

11. Carpenter RG, Gardner A, Mcweeny P, Emery JL. Multistage scoring system for identifying infants at risk of unexpected death. Arch Dis Child. 1977;52:606-12. https://doi.org/10.1136/adc.52.8.606.

12. Oakley JR, Tavare CJ, Stanton AN. Evaluation of the Sheffield system for identifying children at risk from unexpected death in infancy. Arch Dis Child. 1978;53:649-52. https://doi.org/10.1136/adc.53.8.649.

13. d'Espaignet ET, Dwyer T, Newman NM, Ponsonby A-L, Candy SG. The development of a model for predicting infants at high risk of sudden infant death syndrome in Tasmania. Paediatr Perinat Epidemiol. 1990;4:422-35. https://doi.org/10.1111/j.1365-3016.1990.tb00670.x.

14. Blair PS, Nadin P, Cole TJ, Fleming PJ, Smith IJ, Ward Platt M, et al. Weight gain and sudden infant death Syndrome: Changes in weight z-scores may identify infants at increased risk. Arch Dis Child. 2000;82:462-9. https://doi.org/10.1136/adc.82.6.462.

15. Fleming PJ, Blair PS, Ward Platt M, Tripp J, Smith IJ, & the CESDI SUDI Research Group. Sudden infant death syndrome and social deprivation: Assessing epidemiological factors after post-matching for deprivation. Paediatr Perinat Epidemiol. 2003;17:272-80. https://doi.org/10.1046/j.1365-3016.2003.00465.x.

16. Blair PS, Platt MW, Smith IJ, Fleming PJ. Sudden infant death syndrome and the time of death: Factors associated with night-time and day-time deaths. Int J Epidemiol. 2006;35(6):1563-9. https://doi.org/10.1093/ije/dyl212.

17. Morley CJ, Thornton AJ, Cole TJ, Hewson PH, Fowler MA. Baby Check: A scoring system to grade the severity of acute illness in babies under 6 months old. Arch Dis Child. 1991;66:100-6. https://doi.org/10.1136/adc.66.1.100.

18. Blair PS, Mitchell EA, Heckstall-Smith EM, Fleming PJ. Head covering — A major modifiable risk factor for sudden infant death syndrome: A systematic review. Arch Dis Child. 2008;93(9):778-83. https://doi.org/10.1136/adc.2007.136366.

19. Blair PS, Fleming PJ, Smith IJ, Ward Platt M, Young J, Nadin P, et al. Babies sleeping with parents: Case-control study of factors influencing the risk of sudden infant death syndrome. BMJ. 1999;319:1457-62. https://doi.org/10.1136/bmj.319.7223.1457.

20. Blair PS, Platt MW, Smith IJ, Fleming PJ. Sudden infant death syndrome and sleeping position in pre-term and low birthweight infants: An opportunity for targeted intervention. Arch Dis Child. 2006;91(2):101-6. https://doi.org/10.1136/adc.2004.070391.

21. Mitchell EA, Blair PS, L'Hoir MP. Should pacifiers be used to prevent SIDS? Pediatrics. 2006 May;117(5):1755-8. https://doi.org/10.1542/peds.2005-1625.

22. Fleming PJ, Blair PS, Pollard K, Ward Platt M, Leach C, Smith I, et al. Pacifier use and sudden infant death syndrome: Results from the CESDI/SUDI case control study. Arch Dis Child. 1999;81:112-16. https://doi.org/10.1136/adc.81.2.112.

23. Solberg LK. DTP vaccination, visit to child care health centre and sudden infant death syndrome (SIDS): Evaluation of DPT vaccination. Oslo Health Council. 1985;1-19.

24. Roberts SC. Vaccination and cot deaths in perspective. Arch Dis Child. 1987;62:7549. https://doi.org/10.1136/adc.62.7.754.

25. Flahault A, Messiah A, Jougla E, Bouvet E, Perin J, Hatton F. Sudden infant death syndrome and diphtheria/tetanus toxoid/pertussis/poliomyelitis immunisation [letter]. Lancet. 1988;1:5823-6. https://doi.org/10.1016/S0140-6736(88)91369-4.

26. Fleming PJ, Blair PS, Platt MW, Tripp J, Smith IJ, Golding J. The UK accelerated immunisation programme and sudden unexpected death in infancy: Case-control study. BMJ. 2001;322(7290):822. https://doi.org/10.1136/bmj.322.7290.822.

27. Kuhnert R, Schlaud M, Poethko-Müller C, Vennemann M, Fleming P, Blair PS, et al. Reanalyses of case-control studies examining the temporal association between

sudden infant death syndrome and vaccination. Vaccine. 2012;30(13):2349-56. https://doi.org/10.1016/j.vaccine.2012.01.043.

28. Lyon TDB, Patriarca M, Howatson AG, Fleming PJ, Blair PS, Fell GS. Age dependence of potentially toxic elements (Sb, Cd, Pb, Ag) in human liver tissue from paediatric subjects. J Environ Monit. 2002;4:1034-1039. https://doi.org/10.1039/b205972j.

29. Expert group to investigate cot death theories: Toxic gas hypothesis. Report. London: Department of Health, 1998.

30. Leach CEA, Blair PS, Fleming PJ, Smith IJ, Ward Platt M, Berry PJ, et al. Epidemiology of SIDS and explained sudden infant deaths: CESDI SUDI research group. Pediatrics. 1999;104(4)e43.

31. Ward Platt M, Blair PS, Fleming PJ, Smith IJ, Cole TJ, Leach CEA, et al. A clinical comparison of SIDS and explained sudden infant deaths. How healthy and how normal? Arch Dis Child. 2000;82(2):98-106. https://doi.org/10.1136/adc.82.2.98.

32. Sidebotham P, Blair PS, Evason Coombe C, Edmond M, Heckstall-Smith E, Fleming P. Responding to unexpected infant deaths: Experience in one English region. Arch Dis Child. 2010;95(4):291-5.

33. Pease AS, Fleming PJ, Hauck FR, Moon RY, Horne RS, L'Hoir MP, et al. Swaddling and the risk of sudden infant death syndrome: A meta-analysis. Pediatrics. 2016;137(6):e20153275. https://doi.org/10.1542/peds.2015-3275.

34. Blair PS, Sidebotham P, Berry PJ, Evans M, Fleming PJ. Major changes in the epidemiology of sudden infant death syndrome: A 20 year population based study of all unexpected deaths in infancy. Lancet. 2006;367(9507):314-19. https://doi.org/10.1016/S0140-6736(06)67968-3.

35. Blair PS, Sidebotham P, Pease A, Fleming PJ. Bed-sharing in the absence of hazardous circumstances: Is there a risk of sudden infant death syndrome? An analysis from two case-control studies conducted in the UK. PLoS One. 2014;9(9):e107799. https://doi.org/10.1371/journal.pone.0107799.

# 16

# An Australian Perspective

Jane Freemantle, PhD[1] and
Louise Ellis, BA, DipEd[2]

[1]*Melbourne School of Population and Global Health,*
*The University of Melbourne, Victoria, Australia*
[2]*Red Nose, Melbourne, Victoria, Australia*

## Introduction

An accurate picture of mortality informs a society as to its social progress within each community, as mortality is a key indicator of effective public health policies and programs. Data on the causes of sudden infant and childhood mortality also reflect a broader set of social, economic, and political issues (1). As an example, sudden infant and child mortality is a key indicator of an important public health issue, given that some of the causes of infant and childhood mortality are potentially preventable. Effective prevention strategies and relevant health policy require a comprehensive and accurate profile of mortality, which, in turn, requires a better understanding of the epidemiology and mechanisms involved. This profile should include not only the patterns and trends of mortality over time, but also measurements of the indicators that have the potential to contribute to premature mortality among infants and children. These factors should include perinatal, maternal, and infant indicators; the specific causes of death; and the role of the geographical location as an indicator of excess sudden infant and child mortality (2).

This chapter will outline the Australian perspective associated with sudden infant death syndrome (SIDS) and sudden infant and early childhood death. It will comment on the patterns and trends of sudden infant and early childhood mortality reported for all Australians and then focus on the First Peoples of Australia, the Aboriginal and Torres Strait Islander population, within the limitations of the availability of an accurate ascertainment of the Indigenous population. With respect to Aboriginal and Torres Strait Islander peoples, in this chapter the authors follow the Australian Institute of Health and Welfare (AIHW) principal that "[t]o acknowledge the separate Indigenous peoples of Australia, the term 'Aboriginal and Torres Strait Islander people' is preferred … [H]owever, the term 'Indigenous' is used interchangeably when referring to Indigenous status or when assists readability" (3).

The chapter will conclude with a case study that describes a health promotion project that was introduced in Western Australia (WA) in 2005: Reducing the Risks of SIDS in Aboriginal Communities (RROSIAC). This project addresses the high rates of sudden unexpected death in infants (SUDI) in WA Aboriginal and Torres Strait Islander people in rural and remote communities, which have continued despite decreasing rates among non-Indigenous communities following the Red Nose SUDI risk reduction campaigns. It also provides an example of the use of linked population data to more accurately ascertain the impact of public health interventions among minority populations.

## SUDI, Including SIDS in Australia

In the 10th (current) edition of the International Classification of Diseases (ICD-10), code R95 refers to SIDS (previous editions of ICD: ICD-8 in 1965: code 795; ICD-9 in 1979: 798.00). The term SUDI has recently become more widely used for deaths that occur suddenly and unexpectedly, usually in otherwise healthy infants (4). These deaths are often listed under the ICD-10 code R99 (other ill-defined and unspecified causes), which refers to sudden deaths that are unexpected and initially unexplained. The Australian official statistics agency, the Australian Bureau of Statistics (ABS), provides annual cause of death data showing deaths under 12 months of age classified as ICD-10 codes R95-R99. This chapter refers to SIDS (R95) or SUDI (R95-99) persons aged under 12 months.

Australia has been at the forefront internationally in the field of knowledge regarding SUDI. Australian researchers were among the first to provide data linking prone (face-down) sleep position to an increased risk of SIDS(5), and Australia's state and national "Reduce the Risks" campaigns were responsible for the dramatic and continued decrease in SUDI(6), from 500 cases in 1989 (1.97 per 1,000 live births) (7) to 113 cases in 2015 (0.4 per 1,000 live births) (8).

### International comparisons

At 0.50 per 1,000 live births, Australia's SUDI rate for the years 2002-10 is considered mid-range (0.4-0.6 per 1,000 live births). This rate is a little higher than England and Wales and Canada, which had a rate of 0.45 per 1,000 live births during the same period, and a little lower than Germany (0.53 per 1,000 live births) and Japan (0.60 per 1,000 live births) (9).

## History in Australia

Apart from some noteworthy exceptions (10), it appears that sudden and unexpected deaths of infants were not at the forefront of medical research in Australia until around the time that Adelaide pediatrician Susan Beal was asked to investigate the incidence of SIDS in South Australia in 1970 (11). Between 1973 and 1990 she visited more than 500 families whose babies had died suddenly and unexpectedly, gathering information from the scene in which the baby died and having discussions with the bereaved families. Beal (12) is quoted as having said a decade later: "All I learned about SIDS I learned from the families" (p. 128). (See Figure 16.9.) In 1986, Beal concluded that "abandoning prone sleeping for infants in Adelaide should reduce the incidence of SIDS" (13) (p. 13). Although an association between prone sleep and SIDS was reported in the medical literature in the 1940s (14), Beal is credited with being the first person anywhere to recommend avoidance of prone sleep (11), and her study is the first one cited on the list compiled by Peter Blair for the International Society for the Study and Prevention of Perinatal and Infant Death (ISPID) of all SIDS case-control studies with parental contact that have collected data on or after 1985 (15).

At around this time, studies of SIDS were underway at the Menzies Centre for Population Health Research in Tasmania, where the annual rate of SIDS was twice the national average (16). Aware that case-control studies from around the world had already shown that prone sleeping position might be a major factor in SIDS, the authors pointed out that the research was retrospective, raising concern that recall bias might explain the findings. The Menzies Centre had unique prospective data that demonstrated that the association between prone sleeping and SIDS was equally strong, ruling out recall bias (16). In 1991, they published their findings (17), prompting a meeting of Australian and overseas experts to discuss the relationship between prone sleeping and SIDS (18). The experts recommended that healthy infants should not be placed in the prone position, should not be exposed to smoking (either in utero or after birth), should be breastfed, and should avoid overheating (19). The community-

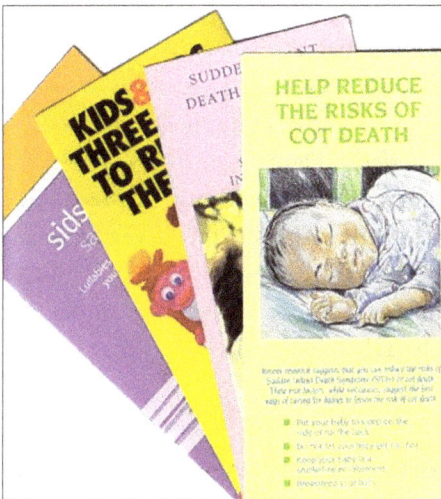

Figure 16.1: SIDS and SUDI Risk reduction literature 1990-2002 (20).

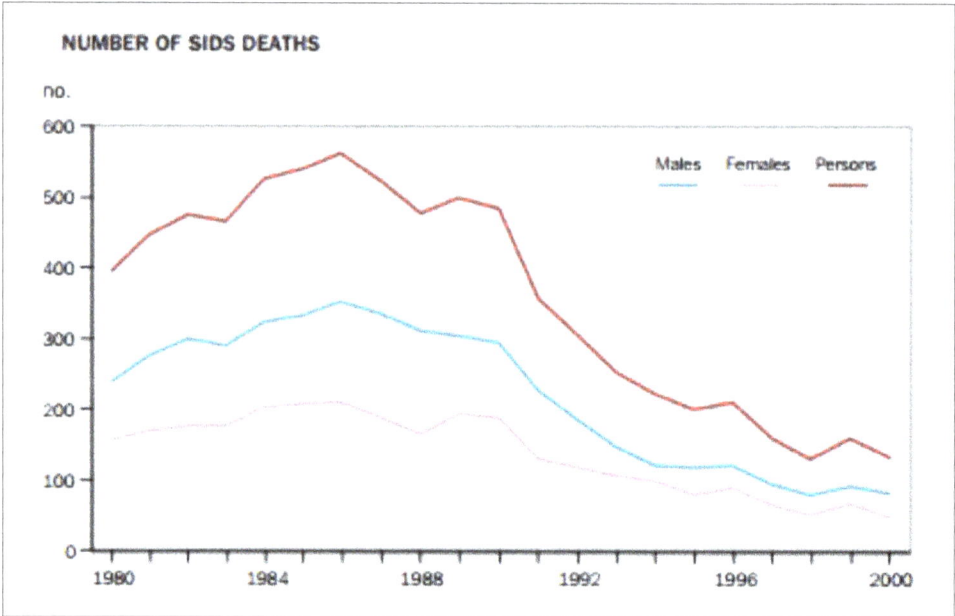

Figure 16.2: Number of SIDS deaths pre- and post the "Reduce the Risk" campaigns in Australia (7). (Reproduced with permission from Louise Ellis and Red Nose (formerly SIDS and Kids).)

funded mass education campaign known as the "Reduce the Risks" (RTR) campaign was launched to inform medical professionals and families of these recommendations (Figure 16.1). The first policy change recorded for health professionals was in July 1990, when Community Services Victoria (Australia) requested all their maternal and child health nurses to advise parents to place their babies on their sides or backs to sleep and to avoid overheating (20). The RTR campaign led to a significant decline of almost 40% when contrasting the pre- and post-campaign periods (Figure 16.2) (19). Australia's first RTR campaign was developed, and subsequent campaigns initiated, by the Sudden Infant Death Research Foundation (SIDRF). The ABS conducted a survey of infant sleeping positions in July 1992 which showed that only a minority of infants (40%) were placed on their back to sleep (21). Much work needed to be done to educate parents and carers on ways to reduce the risk of SUDI.

The history and achievements of the Red Nose organization

The Sudden Infant Death Research Foundation (SIDRF) was founded in 1977 in response to the sudden and unexpected death of 8-month-old Glenn Fitzgerald. Glenn was one of the 18 Victorian babies who died suddenly and unexpectedly in infancy in Victoria that month (22). His devastated parents established the SIDRF in their lounge room the following day (23). The SIDRF subsequently became known as SIDS and Kids and is now known as Red Nose.

Funds for the risk reduction programs were generated by the Red Nose Day campaign, launched in 1988 by SIDRF. Red Nose Day was the first signature day of its kind in Australia (24), characterized by the clown-like red nose shown in Figure 16.9. Other achievements of the organization have included funding research nationally since 1988 and providing professional and peer support of families bereaved by the sudden unexpected death of a child (25). Currently, the three main agendas of Red Nose are bereavement, research, and education.

The founder of SIDRF, Kaarene Fitzgerald, did not restrict her endeavors to reducing SIDS to Australia — in fact, she co-founded SIDS International and chaired the group from 1989 to 1992. Other international collaborative efforts included the Global Strategy Task Force (GSTF) and the European Society for the Study and Prevention of Infant Death (ESPID) (26). This co-ordinated, multinational SUDI reduction effort grew from the home of a bereaved family, the members of whom dedicated the rest of their lives to reducing the impact and incidence of SUDI.

## Sustaining the reductions of infant deaths during the 1990s and over time

SUDI deaths in Australia plummeted at the beginning of the 21st century but increased between 2004-07, and plateaued for the next decade (Figure 16.3).

During this time, SUDI risk reduction efforts continued in earnest. The nine member organizations (MOs) of SIDRF ensured representation in each state or territory of Australia. While there were individual differences, all MOs offered bereavement support and risk reduction education. The organization appointed a librarian to search for, retrieve, and summarize the research from Australia and around the world on sudden unexpected death in infancy and childhood. The collection, known as the Australian SIDS Online Catalogue (ASOC), predated widely accessible alternatives such as the US National Library of Medicine database, PubMed (launched 1996) (27), and Google Scholar (launched 2004) (28). Furthermore, the organization broadened its goal of SIDS reduction to include sudden deaths in early childhood, such as fatal sleep accidents. The recommendations of the Safe Sleeping Program were:

- Put baby on back to sleep, from birth.
- Sleep baby with face uncovered.
- Cigarette smoke is bad for babies.

These recommendations were based on the consensus of a Scientific Forum, convened in 2000 by SIDS and Kids to review the risk factors for SIDS. The forum was attended by Australasian SIDS researchers, pediatricians, pathologists, and child health experts (29).

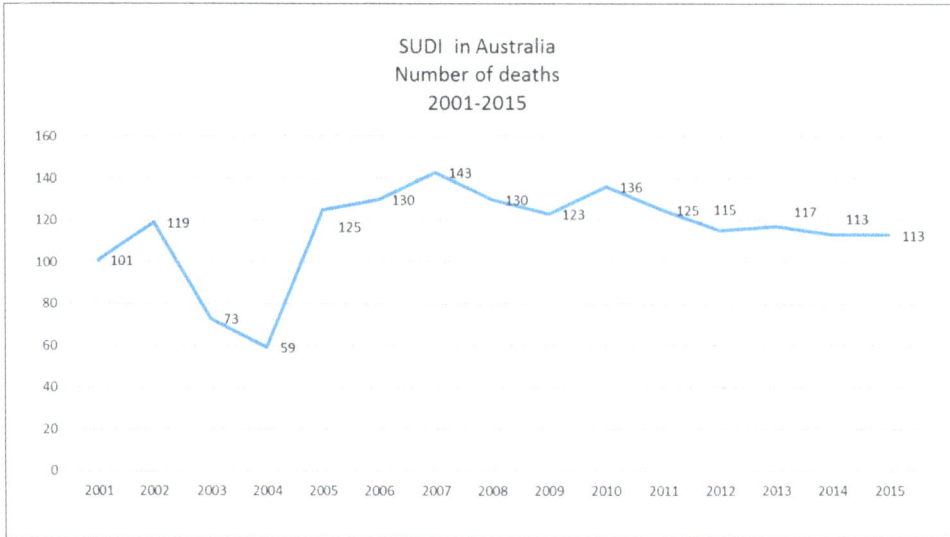

Figure 16.3: SUDI in Australia, 2001-15. (Source: Australian Bureau of Statistics.) X-axis = year; Y-axis = number of cases.

A National Advisory Scientific Group (NSAG) was formed to discuss the research and ensure that the SUDI risk reduction recommendations and safe sleeping advice were all supported by a solid body of evidence (30). The recommendations were made available in posters, brochures, and information statements (31).

In 2002, two further recommendations were added:

- Provide a safe sleeping environment, day and night: safe cot, safe mattress, safe bedding, and safe sleeping place.
- Sleep baby in their own cot in the same room as their parents for the first 6 to 12 months of life.

A one-day scientific consensus forum was held in Sydney in 2010, where Australian and international researchers reviewed the evidence underpinning the Australian Safe Sleeping Health Promotion Programme. The focus was on each of the potentially modifiable risk factors for SUDI. The participants recommended that future "Reducing the Risk" campaign messages should focus on back to sleep, face uncovered, avoidance of cigarette smoke before and after birth, safe sleeping environment, room sharing, and sleeping baby in own cot (Figure 16.4) (29).

Breastfeeding had been included as a "Reducing the Risk" of SIDS message in 1991 but removed for the 1997 campaign due to lack of evidence of its role in RTR. Evidence subsequently accumulated and a sixth recommendation, breastfeed baby, was included in the 2012 Red Nose national public health campaign (32).

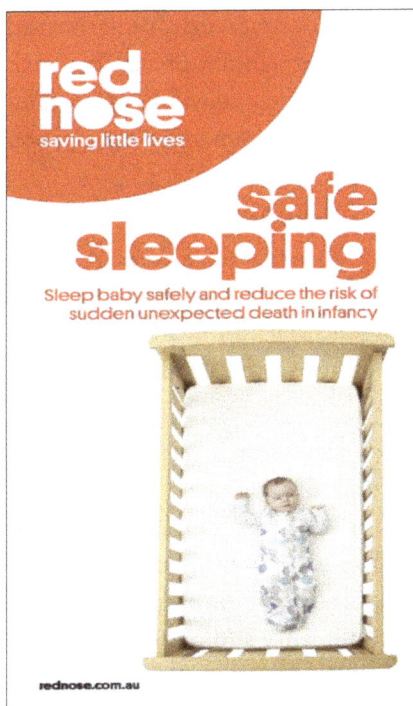

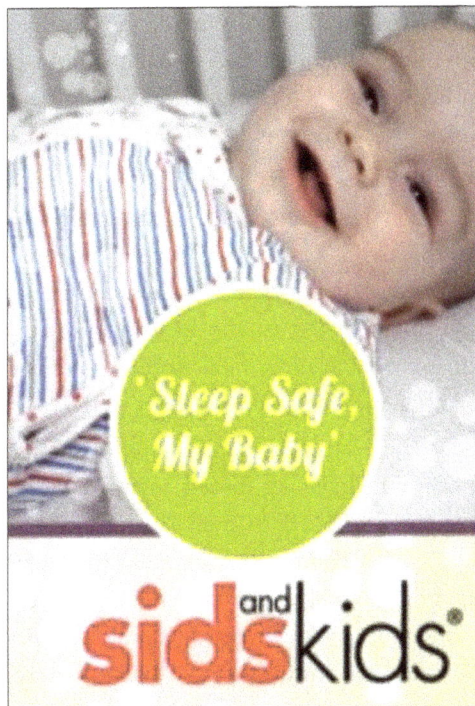

Figure 16.4: Sleep Safe My Baby public health campaign launched 2012. (Reproduced with permission from Louise Ellis and Red Nose (formerly SIDS and Kids).)

## Present day

Australia continues to contribute significantly to world research into sudden unexpected death in infancy and childhood, with significant research being undertaken, at institutions including but not limited to Monash University and the University of Melbourne, the University of Sydney, the University of Tasmania Menzies Institute for Medical Research, the Children's Hospital at Westmead, and the Institute of Forensic Medicine in New South Wales. Researchers from the University of Adelaide, for example, have made significant contributions to the global understanding of SUDI, such as the recent work on the amyloid precursor protein, known as APP, in the brains of infants who died suddenly and unexpectedly, described as "a world breakthrough in the fight against SIDS" (33).

Coronial investigation and recommendations have also made an impact on the rate of SUDI in Australia. The national database of coronial information launched in July 2000, known as the National Coronial Information System (NCIS), placed Australia as the only country in the world at that time to have developed a national collection of coronial information (34). Australian coroners have drawn national attention to SUDI risk factors such as co sleeping with young babies (35).

Recommendations made by pathologists also demonstrate that pediatric and forensic pathologists have a vital role to play in the risk prevention of sudden death in infancy or childhood through forensic examination and their contribution to child death review. Their reports provide forensic evidence that contributes to the formulation of public health strategies (36).

Of significance is the information derived from mandatory reporting under Australian Consumer Law, which mandates suppliers to report any product-related death, serious injury, or serious illness associated with a consumer product (37). This reporting has led to the identification of unsafe products on the market that may, for example, lead to fatal sleep accidents in childhood in Australia (38), which have devastated families for centuries (39).

These successes in policy, child death investigation and research, and public health promotion have combined to make significant impacts on the rate of infant death attributed to SIDS or fatal sleep accidents in Australia: the SUDI rate since 1990 has fallen by 80% and it is estimated that 9,500 infant lives have been saved as a result of the infant safe sleeping campaigns.[1] Tragically, however, the significant progress that has been made in reducing sudden and unexpected death in infancy and early childhood in Australia has not been seen equally in all sectors of the population.

## Sudden Aboriginal and Torres Strait Islander Infant and Early Childhood Death

### Data quality

At the outset it is important to note that accurate information describing Australian Indigenous infant and early childhood mortality has not always been available. In 1984, the Australian Government initiated moves nationally to improve the identification of Indigenous people in births and deaths data collections (2). Prior to 1976, no Australian jurisdiction separately identified Indigenous people in vital statistics or hospital-based collections. By the end of 1999, all major vital statistics and hospital-based collections included the Aboriginal or Torres Strait Islander status of people who were born, died, or admitted to hospital in every Australian state and territory, although the collection of these data was not necessarily mandatory. The AIHW and the ABS continue to strive to collect and present accurate data, as well as to promote the vital importance of collecting accurate Indigenous status information to service providers. Indeed, the Registrars-General have

---

1   Red Nose staff calculations using ABS causes of death data. Calculations confirmed as correct by the ABS.

implemented a number of education programs to encourage Indigenous populations to self-identify in the registration of births and deaths.

However, it is generally acknowledged that, for various reasons, not all Indigenous people are accurately identified in the different data sets. Also, delays in registration of births and deaths are more common for Indigenous people. For example, of all the deaths of Indigenous people which occurred in Australia in 2011, 87% were registered in 2011 compared with 95% of non-Indigenous deaths (40). This results in an under-identification and subsequent under-count of Indigenous people in statutory and administrative data collections, and thus the complete ascertainment of Indigenous infant and early childhood mortality is questionable. The states/territory where ascertainment continues to be of concern are Victoria (Vic), the Australian Capital Territory (ACT), and Tasmania (TAS) (41).

The data described in the following sections will reflect data sourced from reported aggregated data derived from the five jurisdictions (four states and one territory) for which the quality of Indigenous identification in the data was considered to be adequate: New South Wales (NSW), Queensland (Qld), South Australia (SA), Western Australia (WA), and the Northern Territory (NT).

## SIDS rate in Aboriginal and Torres Strait Islander peoples

Data published by the AIHW in 2015 reported that SIDS was the second most prominent cause of death among all Aboriginal and Torres Strait Islander infants and accounted for 6.7% of deaths in the years 2010-12. The AIHW further reported that SIDS deaths in this population had more than halved since 1997-99, from 58 deaths per 100,000 population to 25 per 100,000 in the years 2010-12 (42). More recent data published by AIHW in 2017 reported that SIDS accounted for 5.0% of deaths in the years 2011-15, which was 18.0 per 100,000 population (for the five reported jurisdictions) (43).

SUDI has been reported as a predominant cause of Indigenous infant mortality along with injuries, the rates reported being between three and seven times higher for Indigenous infants compared to the non-Indigenous population (Figure 16.5). For example, the most recent data reported that deaths due to injury accounted for half of the deaths for children aged between 1 and 4 years, the rate of death due to injury being four times higher in the Indigenous compared with the non-Indigenous population in the period 2011-15: 20.1 per 100,000 compared with 5.1 per 100,000 (44). The trend

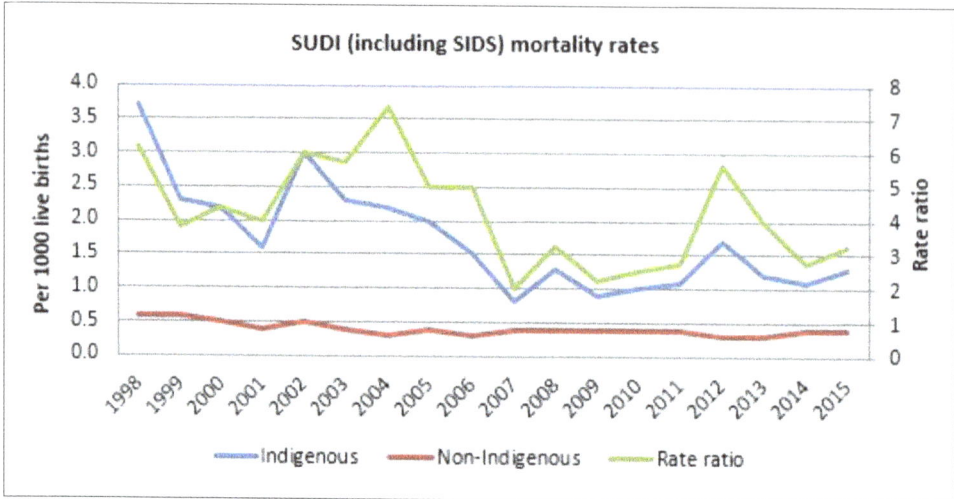

**SUDI (including SIDS) mortality rates**

Figure 16.5: SUDI mortality rates in Indigenous populations 1998-2015. (Source: (44). Licensed from the Commonwealth of Australia under a Creative Commons Attribution 3.0 Australia Licence.)

in SUDI deaths being higher in Indigenous populations continued across the period of 1998 to 2015. In the years 2011-15, the rate of SUDI was 1.3 per 1,000 compared to 0.3 for non-Indigenous infants. The ABS and AIHW reported in 2017 that SUDI comprised 21% of the total deaths of Indigenous infants from the five jurisdictions in years 2011-15 (44). It is worth noting that patterns of causes of death vary significantly between infants and young children. While "external" causes of death (for example, injury and poisoning) make up less than 4% of infant deaths, they account for more than half (53%) of the deaths of Aboriginal and Torres Strait Islander children aged 1 to 4, with these deaths mainly due to transport accidents (18% of deaths), and accidental drowning or accidental threats to breathing (17%). Indeed, the leading cause of death among Aboriginal children aged between 1 to 4 years is injury and poisoning.

Figure 16.6 shows rates of SIDS and SUDI by Indigenous status. When considering the above rates, it is important to note that many of the sudden and unexpected deaths of Indigenous infants in Australia are not classified as SIDS (R-95). Issues such as isolation and rurality may cause difficulty in the performance of adequate examinations (44), and some bereaved families have sought permission for an autopsy not to be performed on cultural or religious grounds (45). These sudden and unexpected infant deaths would therefore be classified R96-R99, or SUDI.

Using linked Victorian statutory administrative birth and death population data, the Victorian Aboriginal Child Mortality Study (VACMS) reported that the cumulative mortality rate (CMR) attributed to SIDS for Victorian-born Indigenous infants was

| Cause of death | Deaths | | Rate per 1,000 live births | | Rate ratio | Rate differe nce |
| --- | --- | --- | --- | --- | --- | --- |
| | Indigenous | Non-Indigenous | Indigenous | Non-Indigenous | | |
| Certain conditions originating in the perinatal period (P00–P96) | 256 | 1,774 | 3.1 | 1.7 | 1.8 | 1.4 |
| Signs, symptoms & ill-defined conditions (R00-R99) | 103 | 357 | 1.3 | 0.3 | 3.6 | 0.9 |
| SIDS (R95) | 39 | 157 | 0.5 | 0.2 | 3.1 | 0.3 |
| SUDI (R99) | 64 | 199 | 0.8 | 0.2 | 4.1 | 0.6 |
| Congenital malformations (Q00–Q99) | 67 | 816 | 0.8 | 0.8 | 1.0 | — |
| Diseases of the respiratory system (J00–J99) | 20 | 48 | 0.2 | — | 5.2 | 0.2 |
| Injury & poisoning (V01–Y98) | 19 | 84 | 0.2 | 0.1 | 2.8 | 0.2 |
| Infectious and parasitic diseases (A00–B99) | 11 | 51 | 0.1 | — | 2.7 | 0.1 |
| Diseases of the circulatory system (I00–I99) | 5 | 51 | 0.1 | — | 1.2 | — |
| Other conditions | 19 | 212 | 0.2 | 0.2 | 1.1 | — |
| All causes | 500 | 3,393 | 6.1 | 3.3 | 1.9 | 2.8 |

Figure 16.6: Causes of infant death, by Indigenous status, NSW, Qld, WA, SA, and NT 2011-15. (Source: Australian Institute of Health and Welfare. See also: https://www.pmc.gov.au/resource-centre/indigenous-affairs/health-performance-framework-2017-report.)

five times greater than for non-Indigenous infants between 1999-2008 (RR [relative risk] = 5.0: CI [confidence interval] 2.9-8.6, p<0.0001). The CMR attributed to SIDS decreased among the non-Indigenous infant population (RR = 0.9, 0.6-1.1), but increased nearly twofold among the Indigenous population (RR = 1.8, 0.6-5.7). The risk of an Indigenous infant dying due to SIDS compared with a non-Indigenous infant was significantly higher and doubled across the birth year groups (1999-2003 RR = 3.2: CI 1.2-8.6; 2004-08 RR = 6.6: 3.5-12.8). Although the difference between the two cohorts did not reach statistical significance, the direction of the estimates, and the magnitude of effect, have significant public health relevance, particularly with regards to the relevance and acceptance of the "Back to Sleep" campaign within the Victorian Indigenous community.

There is no single factor that can predict SUDI. However, there are a number of factors that have been identified as being associated with increased risk of sudden unexplained and unexpected death in infancy. These include (but are not limited to) sharing a sleep surface (29, 46, 47, 48, 49), sleep position (29, 50), tobacco smoking (29, 50, 51, 52, 53), drinking/drug use (29), prematurity (50, 54, 55, 56, 57), low birth weight (59), age (45, 58, 59, 60), gender (61), race (1, 29, 62, 63, 64), and teenage mothers (65, 66). Protective factors include antenatal care (55, 67), breastfeeding (32, 68), and room sharing (69). However, current and comparative data of the status of these risk factors in Indigenous and non-Indigenous Australian populations are not readily available. Table 16.1 includes the available and identified data associated with a number of the risk factors outlined above and the source of these data. For Indigenous infants, the second most common cause of infant mortality was SUDI, accounting for 21% of Indigenous infant deaths.

Table 16.1: Contributing factors associated with deaths attributed to SUDI in Indigenous and non-Indigenous populations, year as identified.

| Contributing factor | Indigenous rate | Non-Indigenous rate | Reference/s | Notes |
|---|---|---|---|---|
| Smoking, drinking, or drug use during pregnancy | Smoking: 45.6%<br><br>Alcohol consumption: 9.8%<br><br>Used drug: 4.9% | Smoking: 12.5%<br><br>Alcohol consumption: none identified<br><br>Used drugs: none identified | AHMAC 2017 (47) | Age-standardized rates for 2014, based on AIHW analysis of the National Perinatal Data Collection |
| Poor antenatal care — proxy, women who attended:<br>• at least one antenatal visit in the first trimester<br>• five or more antenatal visits during pregnancy | One visit in first trimester: 53.2%<br><br>Five or more antenatal visits during pregnancy: 85.5% | One visit in first trimester: 60.2%<br><br>Five or more antenatal visits during pregnancy: 95.3% | SCRGSP (Steering Committee for the Review of Government Service Provision) 2016, *National Agreement Performance Information 2015-16: National Indigenous Reform Agreement*, Productivity Commission, Canberra | Age-standardized rates for 2014, based on analysis by AIHW of National Perinatal Data Collection |
| Prematurity | Babies born preterm: 14% | Babies born preterm: 8% | AIHW 2016 (70) | |
| Low birth weight | Babies with low birth weight: 11.8% | Babies with low birth weight: 6.2% | AHMAC 2017 (47) | Low birth weight live-born babies, by Indigenous status of the mother and state/territory, 2014 |
| Mothers younger than 20 (teenage pregnancy) | Proportion of babies born to teenage mothers: 16.9% | Proportion of babies born to teenage mothers: 2.1% | SCRGSP 2016, *Overcoming Indigenous Disadvantage: Key Indicators 2016*, Productivity Commission, Canberra | Based on data from ABS Births, Australia, 2014 |
| Sex (boys are more likely to die of SIDS) | Proportion of live births that are for male babies: 52.2% | Proportion of live births that are for male babies: 51.5% | AHMAC 2017 (47) | Estimated based on data for 2011-15 on live births by sex |

# Factors contributing to sudden infant and early childhood deaths in Indigenous communities

The key risk factors associated with sudden infant and child mortality for Indigenous Australians include low birth weight preterm births, maternal health and behaviors (smoking, alcohol, nutrition during pregnancy), socioeconomic status, and access to health services. There have been improvements for Indigenous Australians for several of these risk factors in recent years — for example, a 9% decline in low birth weight between 2000 and 2011 (see measure 1.01, Tier 1, in the Australian Institute of Health and Welfare's Aboriginal and Torres Strait Islander health performance framework 2017 report) (71). However, there remains a significant disparity between the Indigenous and non-Indigenous rates of low birth weight (two times higher for Indigenous infants), smoking during pregnancy (four times higher), and antenatal care in the first trimester (15% lower) (72). Data derived from the 2011 census describing socioeconomic status associated with SIDS reported that the proportion of Indigenous deaths in the most disadvantaged quintiles (1 and 2) was 72%, which compared with non-Indigenous deaths at 39% (47). Geographical factors have been reported to be associated with increased prevalence: in 2011, the AIHW reported that the proportion of Indigenous deaths occurring in major cities and inner regional areas was 57% compared with non-Indigenous infant deaths, which was 90% (47).

## Low birth weight

In 2014, the average weight of a live-born baby of an Indigenous mother was 140 g less than a baby of a non-Indigenous mother (3,215 g and 3,355 g respectively); 11% (1,514) of Indigenous live-born were low birth weight, compared with 6.2% (18,276) of babies with non-Indigenous mothers. There was a slight decrease in the proportion of low birth weight babies born to Indigenous mothers between 2004 and 2014, from 13% in 2004 to 12% in 2014; the proportion remained similar for babies born to non-Indigenous mothers — that is, 6% in the same period. Babies of Indigenous mothers were also 1.5 times as likely to be small for gestational age (14.1%) compared with babies of non-Indigenous mothers (9.1%) (72).

## Preterm birth

In 2014, the average gestational age of babies of Indigenous mothers was 38.2 weeks, which was similar to those born to non-Indigenous mothers (38.6 weeks). Around 1 in 7 babies born to Indigenous mothers (14%) were born preterm, compared with 8% of babies born to non-Indigenous mothers. Babies of Indigenous mothers who smoked were 1.3 times as likely to be born preterm compared with babies born to non-Indigenous mothers who smoked (72).

In 2014, Indigenous mothers accounted for 17% of mothers who smoked tobacco at any time during pregnancy, despite accounting for only 4% of births. Almost 1 in 2 Aboriginal and Torres Strait Islander mothers reported smoking during pregnancy (45%, compared with 13% of non-Indigenous mothers) (72).

## Antenatal care

Regular antenatal care has been found to have a positive effect on, and provide the foundation for, good health outcomes for mothers and babies. Earlier and more regular attendance for antenatal care is required in order to improve outcomes for Aboriginal and Torres Strait Islander mothers and their babies, as well as continued improvements in the quality of antenatal care received. Antenatal care occurs later and less frequently for Indigenous women compared with non-Indigenous women. The most recent Health Performance Framework reported that in 2014, only 53.2% of Indigenous mothers attended at least one antenatal session in the first trimester. The age-standardized proportion of Indigenous mothers was 7% lower than for non-Indigenous women (47).

A study in Western Australia in 2006 using population-linked data reported that the CMR for both populations was highest among infants whose mothers resided in remote locations: Indigenous 23.5/1,000 live births; non-Indigenous 6.8 per 1,000 live births. The RR of infant mortality for Aboriginal and Torres Strait Islander infants (compared with non-Indigenous) was also highest in remote locations: RR = 3.5 (95% CI 3.1, 4.0) (1).

## Risk reduction programs for Aboriginal and Torres Strait Islander families

### Background

The report from the Closing the Gap Clearinghouse examined what works and conversely, what does not work, in closing the gap of Indigenous disadvantage in Australia. Among the things that do not work were short-term, one-off programs. The report called for Indigenous community involvement and engagement, adequate resourcing, and planned and comprehensive interventions that included respect for language and culture, and development of initiatives through partnerships, networks, and shared leadership (73).

A report prepared for Red Nose by researchers from Griffith University aimed to evaluate safe sleeping practices and knowledge in three different Indigenous communities in Queensland (74). The researchers noted that established or Western initiatives aimed at minimizing the risk factors of SIDS sometimes conflicted with cultural practices and traditions (e.g. co-sleeping) and/or required costly investments from families (e.g. purchasing certain types of "approved" cots). Culturally sensitive alternatives were promulgated and recommendations suggested that included advocating the findings of the report to the full range of services, organizations, and people concerned with infant and maternal care; considering initiatives that had the potential to impact on socioeconomic factors that act as determinants of health for Indigenous infants and their mothers; recruitment of Indigenous staff within services and organizations dedicated to more inclusive practices; and engaging with Indigenous communities in Queensland.

## Case study: Reducing the Risks of SIDS in Aboriginal Communities (RROSIAC)

This project was initiated in 2005, as a result of a report using data derived from linked population data that identified the continuing high mortality rate attributed to SUDI in WA 1992-2006 (2). The data reported that Indigenous infant deaths were primarily attributed to SUDI (18.6%). While the rate of SUDI had fallen over this period, due to the national risk reduction education campaigns, the difference in the decline was substantially different between the Indigenous and the non-Indigenous population (16% per grouped year period in the former and 29% in the latter population). This roughly equated to a CMR in Indigenous infants of approximately eight times higher than that calculated for non-Indigenous infants.

These unacceptably high rates of SUDI, the relatively slow decline, and the corresponding increasing disparities between the two populations strongly suggested that the available health promotion and education messages identifying SUDI risk factors were not reaching Indigenous communities, and this provided the impetus for the development of the RROSIAC. The RROSIAC developed a culturally appropriate safe sleeping program that included Indigenous-specific resources and training programs for the prevention of SUDI. The resources (Figure 16.7) were developed in consultation with community members and Indigenous and non-Indigenous experts and aimed to

- identify Indigenous knowledge and awareness of SUDI and the associated risk factors
- identify Indigenous-specific education resources, training packages, and programs, and develop community-led strategies to ensure safe sleeping
- disseminate these resources to Indigenous communities and evaluate the effectiveness of the implementation of these resources in conjunction with the Indigenous communities and associated with the review of population-linked data.

The RROSIAC program has continued and has been extended to other rural and remote communities in WA; and a similar project, Safe Sleeping in Victorian Aboriginal Communities (SSIVAC), is currently being developed in Victoria.

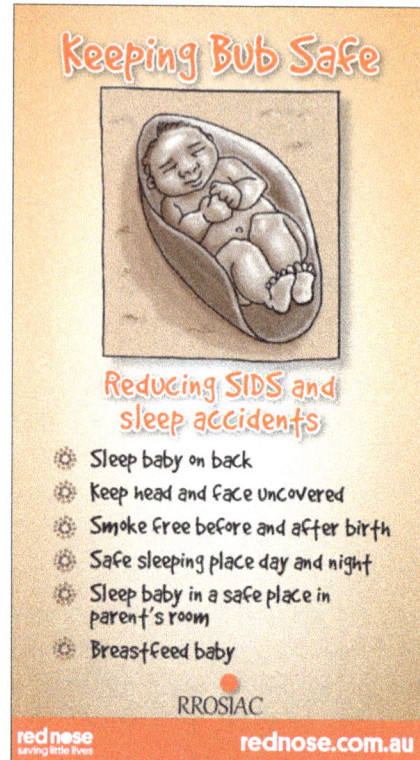

Figure 16.7: RROSIAC brochure. Reducing the risk of SUDI in Aboriginal communities. (Reproduced with permission from Louise Ellis and Red Nose (formerly SIDS and Kids). Available from: https://rednose.com.au/page/reducing-the-risk-of-sudi-in-aboriginal-communities.)

## Future

While currently it is not possible to provide a complete and accurate national profile of Indigenous infant and early childhood mortality, recent advances in the use of population data linkage has improved the ascertainment of Indigenous vital statistics data. One example is the AIHW's "Enhanced Mortality Database" project, which uses data linkage to improve estimates of deaths and life expectancy of Indigenous populations (75). Death and birth registrations are linked with hospital and perinatal data to investigate opportunities to improve the measurement of Indigenous infant and early childhood deaths. Another example of the use of population data linkage to improve the ascertainment of the Indigenous population and therefore more accurate reporting of vital statistics is the VACMS, conducted in Victoria between 2008 and 2012 (76). The linked data resulted in a reclassification of the Indigenous status of births and identified a further 4,333 births to mothers and/or fathers who identified as Aboriginal and/or Torres Strait Islander (representing an 87% increase in Indigenous birth numbers). The VACMS also, for the first time, reported cause-specific infant mortality rates for the Victorian Indigenous population from 1998 to 2009 inclusive: 4.6 per 1,000 live births, with the rate of SIDS increasing over the years studied (77).

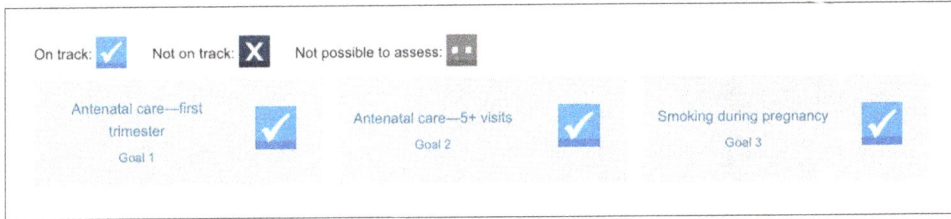

Figure 16.8: AIHW tracking progress. (Source: Australian Institute of Health and Welfare.)

Another measure of the progress in closing the gap is the Australian government's Implementation Plan goals for the Aboriginal and Torres Strait Islander Health Plan 2013-2023 (78). The Implementation Plan has set goals to be achieved by 2023 for 20 indicators, including the maternal health and parenting domain goals, which include:

- Increase the rate of Aboriginal and Torres Strait Islander women attending at least one antenatal visit in the first trimester to 60% by 2023 (age-standardized rates).

- Increase the rate of Aboriginal and Torres Strait Islander women attending at least five antenatal care visits to 90% by 2023 (age-standardized rates).

- Decrease the rate of Aboriginal and Torres Strait Islander women who smoke during pregnancy to 37% by 2023 (age-standardized rates).

The data in the Australian Institute of Health and Welfare's web report tracking the Implementation Plan's progress (79) indicate that several goals are currently on track (Figure 16.8).

## Conclusions

Australia has had a long history of significant contribution to the study and prevention of SUDI worldwide. Bereaved families have provided information that has been meticulously investigated (12). These findings have combined with solid medical/scientific research to inform risk reduction public programs that have had direct impact on the incidence of SUDI in Australia (19).

There is one birth in Australia every 1 minute and 41 seconds (80). Efforts continue to reach these babies' families with information on ways to reduce the risk of SUDI and sleep baby safely. Successful public health campaigns are those designed to reach the various communities that comprise the population, including high-risk groups such as the Indigenous population. Despite the significant progress that has been made in addressing the SUDI incidence in these high-risk populations, gaps persist. Future efforts must address this gap through providing carefully developed and targeted education programs for the parents, carers, and healthcare providers of all babies

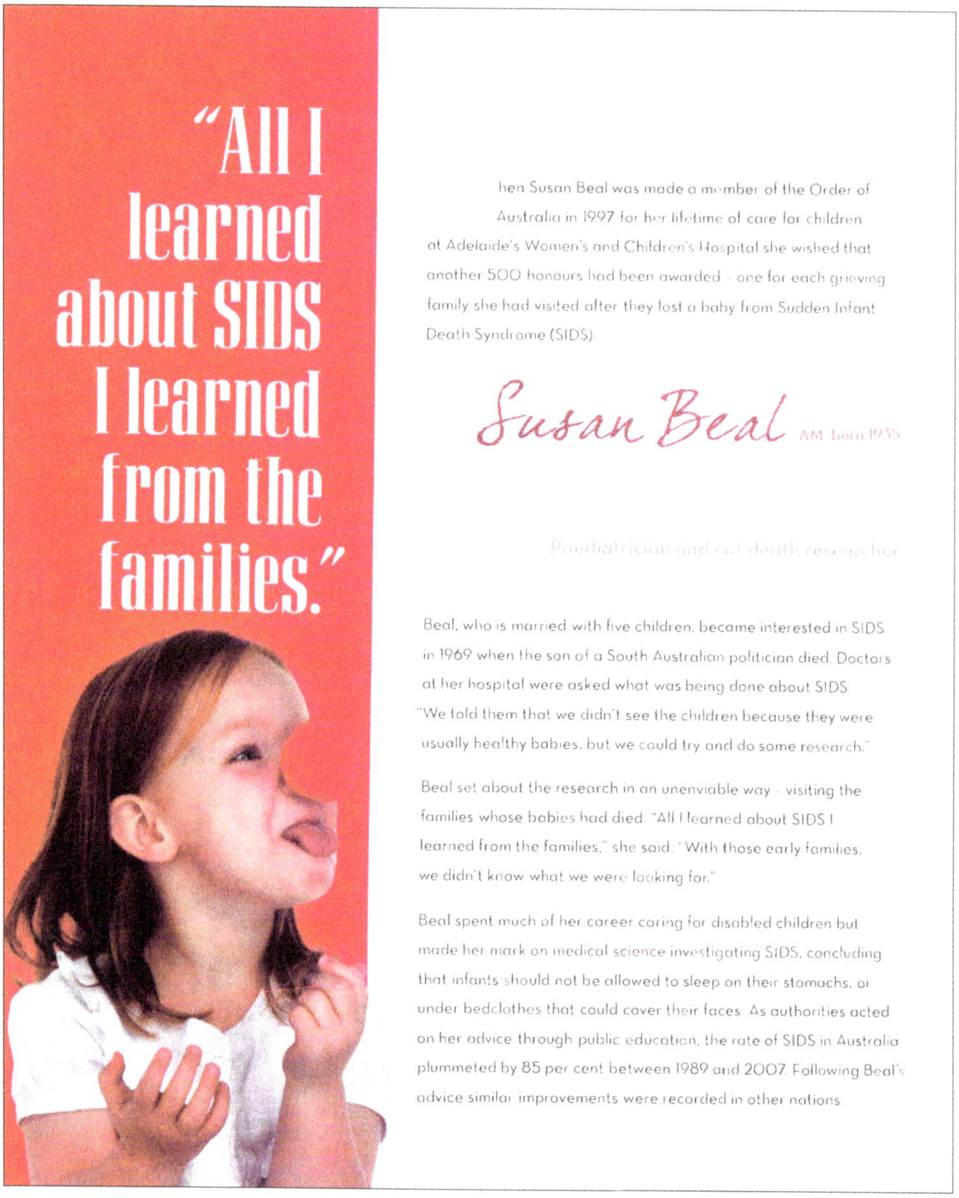

"All I learned about SIDS I learned from the families."

hen Susan Beal was made a member of the Order of Australia in 1997 for her lifetime of care for children at Adelaide's Women's and Children's Hospital she wished that another 500 honours had been awarded — one for each grieving family she had visited after they lost a baby from Sudden Infant Death Syndrome (SIDS).

*Susan Beal* AM, born 1935

Paediatrician and cot death researcher

Beal, who is married with five children, became interested in SIDS in 1969 when the son of a South Australian politician died. Doctors at her hospital were asked what was being done about SIDS. "We told them that we didn't see the children because they were usually healthy babies, but we could try and do some research."

Beal set about the research in an unenviable way — visiting the families whose babies had died. "All I learned about SIDS I learned from the families," she said. "With those early families, we didn't know what we were looking for."

Beal spent much of her career caring for disabled children but made her mark on medical science investigating SIDS, concluding that infants should not be allowed to sleep on their stomachs, or under bedclothes that could cover their faces. As authorities acted on her advice through public education, the rate of SIDS in Australia plummeted by 85 per cent between 1989 and 2007. Following Beal's advice similar improvements were recorded in other nations.

Figure 16.9: The role of bereaved families in the investigation of SIDS in Australia and depiction of a Red Nose. (Reproduced with permission from Louise Ellis and Red Nose (formerly SIDS and Kids).)

and young children in Australia, regardless of cultural/racial background. In order to ensure a sound evidence base, it is imperative that research continue to be funded to produce the evidence to inform public health programs for families of ways to reduce the risk of SUDI and to sleep baby safely. Indeed, it is through families that much of our knowledge about SIDS has been learned and the drive to reduce the number of SIDS deaths achieved (Figure 16.9). Although the incidence of SUDI in Australia has significantly reduced in the non-Indigenous population since the start of risk reduction campaigns in the early 1990s, it remains a tragic and continuing issue, especially among Australia's Indigenous population.

Over its history, Red Nose has been an innovator in bereavement support and community education on both the national and international stage and this will continue into the future.

To quote a long time employee, *All of this is the monumental outcome from the death of one very small, very loved baby* (Judith Rochester) (81).

# References

1. Freemantle CJ, Read AW, de Klerk NH, McAullay D, Anderson IP, Stanley FJ. Patterns, trends, and increasing disparities in mortality for Aboriginal and non-Aboriginal infants born in Western Australia, 1980-2001: Population database study. Lancet. 2006;367(9524):1758-66. https://doi.org/10.1016/S0140-6736(06)68771-0.

2. Freemantle CJ. Indicators of infant and childhood mortality for Indigenous and non-Indigenous infants and children born in Western Australia from 1980 to 1997 inclusive [PhD]. Perth: University of Western Australia (Perth), 2003.

3. Australian Institute of Health and Welfare. Australia's health 2014: Indigenous health. [Available from: http://www.aihw.gov.au/australias-health/2014/indigenous-health/]. Accessed 7 November 2017.

4. Taylor BJ, Garstang J, Engelberts A, Obonai T, Cote A, Freemantle J, et al. International comparison of sudden unexpected death in infancy rates using a newly proposed set of cause-of-death codes. Arch Dis Child. 2015;100:1018-23. https://doi.org/10.1136/archdischild-2015-308239.

5. Byard RW. Inaccurate classification of infant deaths in Australia: A persistent and pervasive problem. Med J Aust. 2001;175(1):5-7.

6. d'Espaignet ET, Bulsara M, Wolfenden L, Byard RW, Stanley FJ. Trends in sudden infant death syndrome in Australia from 1980 to 2002. Forensic Sci Med Pathol. 2008;4(2):83-90. https://doi.org/10.1007/s12024-007-9011-y.

7. Australian Bureau of Statistics. SIDS in Australia 1980-2000: A statistical overview. [Available from: https://web.archive.org/web/20080721212951/http://www.sidsandkids.org/documents/finalsidspaper2003_002.pdf]. Accessed 7 November 2017.

8. Australian Bureau of Statistics (ABS). 3303.0 — Causes of death, Australia, 2015. [Available from: http://www.abs.gov.au/ausstats]. Accessed 7 November 2017.

9. Taylor BJ, Garstang J, Engelberts A, Obonai T, Cote A, Freemantle J, et al. International comparison of sudden unexpected death in infancy rates using a newly proposed set of cause-of-death codes. Arch Dis Child. 2015;100:1018-23. https://doi.org/10.1136/archdischild-2015-308239.

10. Bowden K. Sudden death or alleged accidental suffocation in babies. Med J Aust. 1950;1(3):65.

11. Australian Women's Archives Project. The Australian women's register: Beal, Susan (1935- ). [Available from: http://www.womenaustralia.info/biogs/AWE0951b.htm]. Accessed 7 November 2017.

12. Livingstone T. The power of 100: One hundred women who have shaped Australia. Sydney: Focus, 2010.

13. Beal SM. Sudden infant death syndrome: Epidemiological comparisons between South Australia and communities with a different incidence. Aust Paediatr J. 1986;22:13-16.

14. Abramson H. Accidental mechanical suffocation in infants. J Pediatr. 1944;25(5):404-13. https://doi.org/10.1016/S0022-3476(44)80005-1.

15. Blair P. References to SIDS case-control studies from 1985 to 2012: Epidemiological studies with parental contact. [Available from: https://www.ispid.org/fileadmin/user_upload/textfiles/SIDS_case-control_studies.pdf]. Accessed 7 November 2017.

16. Dwyer T. The Menzies Centre for Population Health Research. Med J Aust. 2001;175(11-12):617-20.

17. Dwyer T, Ponsonby A, Newman N, Gibbons L. Prospective cohort study of prone sleeping position and sudden infant death syndrome. Lancet. 1991;337:1244-7.

18. A scientific review of the association between prone sleeping position and sudden infant death syndrome. J Paediatr Child Health. 1991;27:323-4. https://doi.org/10.1111/j.1440-1754.1991.tb00411.x.

19. Tursan d'Espaignet E, Bulsara M, Wolfenden L, Byard RW, Stanley FJ. Trends in sudden infant death syndrome in Australia from 1980 to 2002. Forensic Sci Med Pathol. 2008;4(2):83-90. https://doi.org/10.1007/s12024-007-9011-y.

20. Fitzgerald K. History: SIDS groups and organisations. Unpublished document: Melbourne, 2001.

21. Australian Bureau of Statistics (ABS). Survey of infant sleeping positions. ABS Cat. No. 4386.0. Canberra: ABS, July 1992.

22. Red Nose. Our history. [Available from: https://rednose.com.au/page/our-history]. Accessed 7 November 2017.

23. Jerums G. The gift of life. Melbourne Weekly Magazine. 2002;June 23-29:16-18.

24. SIDS and Kids. Annual report 2016. [Available from: https://rednose.com.au/downloads/Annual_Report_2016.pdf]. Accessed 7 November 2017.

25. Red Nose. Guiding light. [Available from: https://rednosegriefandloss.com.au/]. Accessed 7 November 2017.

26. Fitzgerald K. The "Reduce the Risks" Campaign, SIDS International, the Global Strategy Task Force and the European Society for the Study and Prevention of Infant Death. In: Sudden infant death syndrome: Problems, progress, and possibilities. Eds Byard RW, Krous HF. New York: Arnold, Co-published by Oxford University Press, London, 2001. p.310-18.

27. Canese K. PubMed celebrates its 10th anniversary! NLM Tech Bull. 2006;352:e5. [Available from: https://www.nlm.nih.gov/pubs/techbull/so06/so06_pm_10.html]. Accessed 7 November 2017.

28. Van Noorden R. Google Scholar pioneer on search engine's future. [Available from: http://www.nature.com/news/google-scholar-pioneer-on-search-engine-s-future-1.16269]. Accessed 7 November 2017.

29. Mitchell EA, Freemantle J, Young J, Byard RW. Scientific consensus forum to review the evidence underpinning the recommendations of the Australian SIDS and Kids Safe Sleeping Health Promotion Programme — October 2010. J Paediatr Child Health. 2012;48(8):626-33. https://doi.org/10.1111/j.1440-1754.2011.02215.x.

30. Red Nose. National Scientific Advisory Group. [Available from: https://rednose.com.au/team/C106]. Accessed 7 November 2017.

31. Red Nose. Education. [Available from: https://rednose.com.au/resources/education]. Accessed 17 January 2018.

32. Young J, Watson K, Ellis L, Raven L. Responding to evidence: Breastfeed baby if you can — The sixth public health recommendation to reduce the risk of sudden and unexpected death in infancy. Breastfeed Rev. 2012;20(1):7-15.

33. Jensen LL, Banner J, Ulhøi BP, Byard RW. The development of a technique for assessing the distribution of APP staining in sudden infant and early childhood

death. Neuropathol Appl Neurobiol. 2014;40:385-97. https://doi.org/10.1111/nan.12109.

34. National Coronial Information System (NCIS). About NCIS: History. [Available from: http://www.ncis.org.au/data-collection/history/]. Accessed 7 November 2017.

35. Bugeja L, Dwyer J, McIntyre S-J. Sleep-related infant deaths and the role of co-sleeping: A case series study in Victoria Australia. Melbourne: Coroners Court of Victoria, c. 2011.

36. Byard R. Accidental childhood death and the role of the pathologist. Pediatr Dev Pathol. 2000;3(5):405-18. https://doi.org/10.1007/s100240010089.

37. Australian Competition and Consumer Commission. A guide to the mandatory reporting law in relation to consumer goods. [Available from: https://www.productsafety.gov.au/publication/a-guide-to-the-mandatory-reporting-law-in-relation-to-consumer-goods]. Accessed 7 November 2017.

38. Australian Competition & Consumer Commission. Regulation impact statement (RIS) for consumer product safety standard — Children's portable folding cots (Consumer protection notice no. 4 of 2008). Available from: [https://www.legislation.gov.au/Details/F2008L00550/Explanatory%20Statement/Text]. Accessed 7 November 2017.

39. Fatalities and casualties: A child's death. Sydney Morning Herald [internet]; 3 January 1902. [Available from: http://nla.gov.au/nla.news-article14446995]. Accessed 7 November 2017.

40. Australian Bureau of Statistics. Life tables for Aboriginal and Torres Strait Islander Australians, 2010-2012: ABS cat. no. 3302.0.55.003. Available from: [http://www.abs.gov.au/ausstats/abs@.nsf/mf/3302.0.55.003]. Accessed 7 November 2017.

41. Australian Institute of Health and Welfare. Mortality and life expectancy of Indigenous Australians 2008 to 2012: AIHW cat. no. IHW 140. [Available from: http://www.aihw.gov.au/publication-detail/?id=60129548470]. Accessed 7 November 2017.

42. Australian Institute of Health and Welfare. Premature mortality in Australia 1997-2012: AIHW web report. [Available from: http://www.aihw.gov.au/deaths/premature-mortality/]. Accessed 7 November 2017.

43. AHMAC (Australian Health Ministers' Advisory Council). Aboriginal and Torres Strait Islander health performance framework 2017: Online data tables: Measure 1.20: Infant and child mortality. [Available from: http://www.aihw.gov.au/indigenous-data/health-performance-framework/data/]. Accessed 7 November 2017.

44. Byard RW, Krous HF. Diagnostic and medicolegal problems with sudden infant death syndrome. In: Forensic pathology reviews. Ed Tsokos M. Totowa, NJ: Humana Press, 2004. pp.189-98. https://doi.org/10.1007/978-1-59259-786-4_7.

45. Arnold BB. A more respectful autopsy? Digital technologies and case law. Aust Health Law Bull. 2016;24(1):6-10.

46. Moon RY, & Task Force on Sudden Infant Death Syndrome. SIDS and other sleep-related infant deaths: Evidence base for 2016 updated recommendations for a safe infant sleeping environment. Pediatrics. 2016;138(5):pii:e20162940.

47. Red Nose. Sharing a sleep surface with a baby. [Available from: https://rednose.com.au/article/sharing-a-sleep-surface-with-a-baby]. Accessed 7 November 2017.

48. Carlin RF, Moon RY. Risk factors, protective factors, and current recommendations to reduce sudden infant death syndrome: A review. JAMA Pediatr. 2017;171(2):175-80. https://doi.org/10.1001/jamapediatrics.2016.3345.

49. Fleming P, Pease A, Blair P. Bed-sharing and unexpected infant deaths: What is the relationship? Paediatr Respir Rev. 2015;16(1):62-7. https://doi.org/10.1016/j.prrv.2014.10.008.

50. Red Nose. Why back to sleep is the safest position for your baby. [Available from: https://rednose.com.au/article/why-back-to-sleep-is-the-safest-position-for-your-baby]. Accessed 7 November 2017.

51. Mitchell EA, Thompson JM, Zuccollo J, MacFarlane M, Taylor B, Elder D, et al. The combination of bed sharing and maternal smoking leads to a greatly increased risk of sudden unexpected death in infancy: The New Zealand SUDI nationwide case control study. NZ Med J. 2017;130(1456):52-64.

52. Red Nose. Smoking. [Available from: https://rednose.com.au/article/smoking]. Accessed 7 November 2017.

53. Getahun D, Amre D, Rhoads GG, Demissie K. Maternal and obstetric risk factors for sudden infant death syndrome in the United States. Obstet Gynecol. 2004;103(4):646-52. https://doi.org/10.1097/01.AOG.0000117081.50852.04.

54. Witcombe NB, Yiallourou SR, Sands SA, Walker AM, Horne RSC. Preterm birth alters the maturation of baroreflex sensitivity in sleeping infants. Pediatrics. 2012;129(1):e89-96. https://doi.org/10.1542/peds.2011-1504.

55. Halloran DR, Alexander GR. Preterm delivery and age of SIDS death. Ann Epidemiol. 2006;16(8):600-6. https://doi.org/10.1016/j.annepidem.2005.11.007.

56. Fyfe KL, Yiallourou SR, Wong FY, Odoi A, Walker AM, Horne RSC. Gestational age at birth affects maturation of baroreflex control. J Pediatr. 2015;166(3):559-65. https://doi.org/10.1016/j.jpeds.2014.11.026.

57. Blair PS, Platt MW, Smith IJ, Fleming PJ. Sudden infant death syndrome and sleeping position in pre-term and low birth weight infants: An opportunity for targeted intervention. Arch Dis Child. 2006;91:101-6. https://doi.org/10.1136/adc.2004.070391.

58. Möllborg P, Alm B. Sudden infant death syndrome during low incidence in Sweden 1997-2005. Acta Paediatr. 2010;99(1):94-8.

59. Chang R-KR, Keens TG, Rodriguez S, Chen AY. Sudden infant death syndrome: Changing epidemiologic patterns in California 1989-2004. J Pediatr. 2008;153(4):498-502. https://doi.org/10.1016/j.jpeds.2008.04.022.

60. Malloy MH, Freeman DH. Age at death, season, and day of death as indicators of the effect of the back to sleep program on sudden infant death syndrome in the United States, 1992-1999. Arch Pediatr Adolesc Med. 2004;158(4):359-65. https://doi.org/10.1001/archpedi.158.4.359.

61. Mage DT, Donner EM. Is excess male infant mortality from sudden infant death syndrome and other respiratory diseases x-linked? Acta Paediatr. 2014;103(2):188-93. https://doi.org/10.1111/apa.12482.

62. Blackwell CC, Moscovis SM, Gordon AE, Al Madani OM, Hall ST, Gleeson M, et al. Ethnicity, infection and sudden infant death syndrome. FEMS Immunol Med Microbiol. 2004;42(1):53-65. https://doi.org/10.1016/j.femsim.2004.06.007.

63. Baddock SA, Tipene-Leach D, Williams SM, Tangiora A, Jones R, Iosua E, et al. Wahakura versus bassinet for safe infant sleep: A randomized trial. Pediatrics. 2017;139(2):e20160162. https://doi.org/10.1542/peds.2016-0162.

64. Knight J, Webster V, Kemp L, Comino E. Sudden infant death syndrome in an urban Aboriginal community. J Paediatr Child Health. 2013;49(12):1025-31. https://doi.org/10.1111/jpc.12306.

65. Caraballo M, Shimasaki S, Johnston K, Tung G, Albright K, Halbower AC. Knowledge, attitudes, and risk for sudden unexpected infant death in children of adolescent mothers: A qualitative study. J Pediatr. 2016;174:78-83.e2. https://doi.org/10.1016/j.jpeds.2016.03.031.

66. Siva N. Risk of cot death in babies of British teen mothers is still high. BMJ. 2010;341:c4673. https://doi.org/10.1136/bmj.c4673.

67. van Nguyen JM, Abenhaim HA. Sudden infant death syndrome: Review for the obstetric care provider. Am J Perinatol. 2013;30(9):703-14. https://doi.org/10.1055/s-0032-1331035.

68. Red Nose. Breastfeeding and the risk of sudden unexpected death in infancy. Available from: https://rednose.com.au/article/

breastfeeding-and-the-risk-of-sudden-unexpected-death-in-infancy]. Accessed 7 November 2017.

69. Red Nose. Room sharing with baby. [Available from: https://rednose.com.au/article/room-sharing-with-baby]. Accessed 7 November 2017.

70. AIHW. Australia's mothers and babies 2014 — In brief. [Available from: http://www.aihw.gov.au/publication-detail/?id=60129557656]. Accessed 7 November 2017.

71. AIHW. Aboriginal and Torres Strait Islander health performance framework 2017 report: Detailed analyses. [Available from: http://www.aihw.gov.au/indigenous-data/health-performance-framework]. Accessed 7 November 2017.

72. Australian Health Ministers' Advisory Council (AHMAC). Aboriginal and Torres Strait Islander health performance framework 2014. Available from: [https://www.pmc.gov.au/sites/default/files/publications/indigenous/Health-Performance-Framework-2014/tier-1-health-status-and-outcomes/120-infant-and-child-mortality.html]. Accessed 11 January 2018.

73. Osborne K, Baum F, Brown L. What works? A review of actions addressing the social and economic determinants of Indigenous health. Issues Paper no. 7. [Available from: https://aifs.gov.au/publications/what-works]. Accessed 7 November 2017.

74. Demosthenous C, Demosthenous H. The Indigenous Safe Sleeping Project: Closing the gap on knowledge, resources and access in Queensland. Brisbane: SIDS & Kids Queensland, 2011.

75. Australian Institute of Health and Welfare. An enhanced mortality database for estimating Indigenous life expectancy: A feasibility study. [Available from: http://www.aihw.gov.au/publication-detail/?id=10737422286]. Accessed 7 November 2017.

76. Freemantle J, Ritte R, Heffernan B, Cutler T, Iskandar D. Victorian Aboriginal Child Mortality Study. Phase 1: The birth report — Patterns and trends in births to Victorian Aboriginal and Torres Strait Islander and Non-Aboriginal and Torres Strait Islander mothers and/or fathers 1988-2008 inclusive. Melbourne: The Lowitja Institute, 2013.

77. Freemantle J, Ritte R, Smith K, Iskandar D, Cutler T, Heffernan B, et al. Victorian Aboriginal child mortality study: Patterns, trends and disparities in mortality between Aboriginal and Non-Aboriginal infants and children, 1999-2008. Melbourne: The Lowitja Institute, 2014.

78. Australian Government: Department of Health. National Aboriginal and Torres Strait Islander health plan 2013-2023. [Available from: http://www.health.gov.au/natsihp]. Accessed 7 November 2017.

79. Australian Institute of Health and Welfare. Tracking progress against the implementation plan goals for the Aboriginal and Torres Strait Islander health plan 2013-2023: First monitoring. [Available from: https://www.aihw.gov.au/reports/indigenous-health-welfare-services/tracking-progress-against-implementation-plan-goal/contents/summary]. Accessed 7 November 2017.

80. Australian Bureau of Statistics. Population clock. [Available from: http://www.abs.gov.au/ausstats/abs%40.nsf/94713ad445ff1425ca25682000192af2/1647509ef7e25faaca2568a900154b63?]. Accessed 7 November 2017.

81. Red Nose: Statement regarding history & future. [Available from: https://rednose.com.au/page/our-history]. Accessed 7 November 2017.

# 17 A South African Perspective

Johan J Dempers, MBChB, Dip For Med Path[1],
Elsie H Burger, MBChB, MMed (Forens Path)[2],
Lorraine Du Toit-Prinsloo, MBChB, Dip For Med
Path, MMed (Forens Path)[3] and
Janette Verster, MBChB, Dip For Med Path,
MMed (Forens Path)[1,4]

[1]*Department of Pathology, Faculty of Health Sciences,
University of Stellenbosch, Tygerberg, South Africa*
[2]*Department of Forensic Medicine, Forensic and Analytical
Science Service, New South Wales Health Pathology, Sydney, Australia*
[3]*Department of Forensic Medicine, University of Pretoria, Pretoria, South Africa*
[4]*NSW Forensic Institute, NSW Government, Sydney, Australia*

## Introduction

South Africa, at the southern tip of the African continent, is often referred to as "a world in one country" — a multicultural, biodiverse country with a vibrant economy. It is home to eight World Heritage Sites and seven different biomes. The country is divided into nine provinces, each with its own legislature, premier, and executive council. Eleven official languages are recognized (1).

The country covers some 1,219,602 km² and is home to around 55.91 million people, of which close to 11% are under 4 years of age. The infant mortality rate is estimated at 33.7 per 1,000 live births (2016), a figure which has seen a steady decline from around 48.2 per 1,000 live births in 2002. Similarly, the under-5 mortality rate declined from 70.8 child deaths per 1,000 live births to 44.4 child deaths per 1,000 live births between 2002 and 2016 (2). Despite the decline in these rates over the years, South Africa is still faced with an immense challenge if it wishes to decrease the high death rate in infants. Investigation into unexpected deaths in children are complicated by multiple factors, however, including a significant variation in population density in different regions of the country, a lack of standardized national death investigation protocols, language and culture barriers, and a paucity of resources and funding for medico-legal death investigation and qualified forensic pathologists, especially in the rural regions of the country.

It is nearly impossible to understand the medico-legal death investigation process in South Africa without being mindful of the political history and development of the country, specifically the most recent 100 years or so. The South African political arena is most significantly marked by the process of segregation and the ideology of apartheid, which was consolidated after the 1948 general election, won by the National Party. Government regulated the job market, often with only the white minority being allowed skilled work opportunities. Legislation culminated in the *Natives (Urban Areas) Act 1923*, entrenching urban segregation. Pass laws controlled African mobility. The introduction of apartheid policies coincided with the adoption by the African National Congress in 1949 of its program of action, expressing the renewed militancy of the 1940s. Mass resistance to white minority and colonial rule in neighboring states led to Portuguese decolonization in the mid-1970s and the abdication to the Zimbabwean regime in 1980. South Africa became increasingly more isolated internationally, with pressure in the form of financial, trade, sport, and cultural sanctions eventually resulting in the announcement of the unbanning of liberation movements and release of political prisoners by FW de Klerk at the opening of Parliament in 1989. This marked the beginning of the end of apartheid and the start of the process of reconciliation and the establishment of a true democracy. This eventually led to South Africa's first democratic election in April 1994. Currently, South Africa has a constitutional multiparty, three-tier (local, provincial, national) democracy. It is inevitable that policies of segregation, restriction of free movement of citizens, discrepant economic isolation, and governmental oppression will have an influence on the profile of death in infancy. However, despite the progress made over the 21 years since the first democratic election in the country, the legacy of apartheid can still be seen in the profile of medico-legal death investigation in the country.

## Medico-legal Death Investigation in South Africa — Overview

The medico-legal death investigation system in South Africa is a hybrid system. This system shares characteristics with the coroner and medical examiner systems in other parts of the world, yet maintains characteristics unique to the South African environment and legal practice. Players in the death investigation process are the South African Police Service (SAPS), Forensic Pathology Service (FPS), and the National Prosecuting Authority (NPA). Unnatural deaths are investigated under the auspices of the *Inquests Act 58 of 1959* ("*Inquests Act*"). Under this act, the responsibility to conduct an investigation into the circumstances and cause of death is that of the SAPS. Under the act, any person who has reason to believe that any other person has died due to other than natural causes is compelled to report this suspicion to a police officer. This police officer is compelled to investigate the circumstances of the death or alleged death, and report the death to the magistrate of the district concerned. The act furthermore stipulates that if the body of a person who has allegedly died from other than natural causes is available, it shall be examined by the district surgeon or any other medical practitioner, who may, if he or she deems it necessary for the purpose of ascertaining with greater certainty the cause of death, examine any internal organ or any part or any of the contents of the body (3). By implication, therefore, consent from the next of kin to perform a medico-legal autopsy, and to retain specimens, is not required, as long as the process serves the purpose of determining the cause of, and circumstances around, the death of the individual.

Consequently, medico-legal autopsies are mandated in all suspected unnatural deaths in an attempt to establish the cause of death with greater certainty. Unnatural deaths are defined by the Regulations Regarding the Rendering of Forensic Pathology Service (reg 636) in terms of the *National Health Act 2003* (4), as well as the *Health Professions Act*[1], as follows:

- any death due to physical or chemical influence, direct or indirect, or related complications
- any death, including those deaths which would normally be considered to be a death due to natural causes, which in the opinion of a medical practitioner, has been the result of an act of commission or omission which may be criminal in nature
- where the death is sudden and unexpected, or unexplained, or where the cause of death is not apparent.

Section 56 of the above act further states that "where the death is of a person undergoing, or is itself a result of, a procedure of a therapeutic, diagnostic, or palliative nature, or of which any aspect of such a procedure has been a contributory cause", such a death will also be determined unnatural.

Sudden unexpected death in infants and children is therefore specifically mandated by law to be investigated in South Africa (3, 4).

All medico-legal post-mortem examinations are performed by a forensic medical practitioner (FMP), who could be a qualified forensic pathologist, registrar (resident,

---

1 More details of the *Health Professions Act 1974* (South Africa) are available at: https://www.acts.co.za/health-professions-act-1974/index.html.

or forensic pathologist-in-training), or a medical officer, to establish the cause of, and circumstances surrounding, death. The determination of the manner of death, however, is not considered to fall within the responsibility of the forensic medical practitioner, but rather with the presiding judicial officer — that is, an inquest magistrate (5, 6).

## The Forensic Pathology Service

Prior to 2006, the SAPS were the legal custodians of the dead, and the responsibility for facilitating the examination of the remains in cases of suspected unnatural death was that of the police service. Even though the medical practitioners conducting medico-legal autopsies (District Surgeons) had always been in the employment of the Department of Health for this service, their assistants had been employed by the SAPS. In 2006, the FPS was established within the Department of Health. Since then, the assistants, or Forensic Pathology Officers (FPO), have been in the employ of the Department of Health, which opened new possibilities with regards to the development of practice standards, and specifically death scene investigation, in forensic pathology. Forensic Pathology Officers who attend the scene have the opportunity to assist the scene police officer, as well as the forensic medical practitioner, with the preliminary death scene investigation and with transport of the remains to the forensic pathology laboratory (7), as well as to assist the forensic medical practitioner with the autopsy.

## Death scene investigation in South Africa

In the case of a sudden and unexpected death, the SAPS will be called to the scene of death and will notify the FPS of the case. The forensic medical practitioner may be requested by the police scene officer or the investigating officer to attend the scene of death as part of a complete medico-legal investigation into the circumstances of death. However, attendance of the scene is generally deemed to be at the discretion of the forensic medical practitioner, as no protocol exists for the attendance and investigation of the scene of death by a forensic medical practitioner. The scene officer may also request specialist investigators employed by the SAPS to attend death scenes, in order to assist with the examination of the scene and collection of specimens at the scene. This includes photographers and forensic scientists, such as experts in dactyloscopy, blood splatter analysis, ballistics, DNA analysis, and so on.

There are, however, only a limited number of forensic scientists in the employment of the SAPS, who are mostly prioritized to assist in the investigation of violent crimes. Due to high case volumes, it is impossible for these scientists to also investigate cases of sudden unexpected death. Thus, specialized death scene investigation in cases of sudden and unexpected death in infancy (SUDI) is not performed as a rule and these scenes are not readily attended by a forensic medical practitioner or forensic science team. This holds potentially dire consequences for the investigation into cases of sudden death, specifically of infants, as important information is often lost if a comprehensive scene investigation does not precede the physical autopsy. In an effort to inform the autopsy process with a scene investigation, the FPS in some provinces have started in-house training programs for FPOs. The fact that there are no formally trained, dedicated death scene examiners within the FPS in South Africa significantly complicates the investigation of cases of sudden death in children, and specifically SUDI cases. Currently, the responsibility of gathering contemporaneous information regarding the deceased infant, the circumstances of death, and the scene of death rests with the non-medically-trained Forensic Pathology and Police Officers.

It has been known for some years that a formal training course for FPOs will imply a significant improvement in the quality of medico-legal death scene investigation, and avenues have been investigated since 2014 to establish a formal training course for FPS personnel. This has culminated in the development of a training course aligned with the South African Qualifications Authority, Health Professions Council of South Africa, and Higher Education Qualifications Sub-Framework, which is currently in the final stages of curriculum development. It is expected that the course will see its first intake of trainees in 2019/2020.

## The Decade of Awakening

Accurate, contemporary statistics pertaining to the incidence of sudden infant death syndrome (SIDS) in South Africa are not available. In 1983, Molteno et al. reported the rate of unexplained infant deaths in Cape Town as 3.05/1,000 live births (8). Following this important report on the wellbeing of infants in the Cape Town rural and urban areas, there followed a relatively uneventful period of approximately 20 years during which there were almost no scientific publications that evaluated specifically the profile of SUDI/SIDS in the country.

Four seminal events were to encourage a renewed vigor in the investigation of sudden infant death in South Africa, thereby introducing a decade from early 2000 during which an increased awareness of the importance of research into sudden death in the young can only be described as an awakening.

In September 1990, the United Nations Millennium Declaration was adopted. The Declaration committed nations to a global partnership to reduce extreme poverty, and set out a series of targets with a deadline of 2015 — the Millennium Development Goals (MDGs) (9). MDGs Four and Five focused attention on the problems of child mortality and maternal health, and in South Africa the goal was to decrease the under-5 mortality rate by two-thirds (10). This set the scene for a blossoming awareness of the role of forensic pathologists, not only in determining the cause of death in infancy, but in making valuable contributions in the arenas of healthcare administration and mortality prevention.

In 2007, the initiation of an international collaborative research investigation of SIDS by the Prenatal Alcohol in SIDS and Stillbirth (PASS) Network in high-risk communities (including the East Metropole of the City of Cape Town), called the Safe Passage Study, marked the second major influence in the development of a research ethos into sudden death in South Africa (11). This prospective study focused on the relationship between prenatal alcohol exposure, SIDS, and stillbirth. The aim of the study was to enroll 12,000 pregnant women, who were at high risk of consuming alcohol during pregnancy, in two areas, namely Cape Town, South Africa (7,000 cases) and the Northern Plains (NP), United States of America (5,000 cases). All live-born infants to study participants were followed up at 1 month and 1 year of age, with a number of clinical investigations carried out during pregnancy and at each postnatal visit (11). All study participants who suffered fetal or infant demises during the first year of life were approached regarding consent for a research autopsy. In addition to the usual histology, microbiology, and virology samples collected during SUDI autopsies at the Tygerberg Forensic Pathology Laboratory, brain samples were also collected for tissue receptor autoradiography and other analyses. The last baby born to this study was born in August 2015, with follow-up continuing for another year.

One of the first publications to emanate from this collaboration suggested a classification schema for SUDI deaths which incorporates possible asphyxia (12). This schema was also used in the adjudication of SUDI deaths that followed in the PASS study. In 2011 two case studies, demonstrating unusual causes of SUDI and the value of full autopsies in SUDI cases, were published (13, 14). The experiences of the PASS network researchers and social workers led to a thoughtful publication on the process of obtaining consent for autopsy research in SUDI and fetal death cases. Recommendations were made regarding the timing, setting, and content of interviews for this purpose (15), especially in socioeconomically disadvantaged populations.

In 2016 a feasibility assessment of serotonin receptor binding in the medulla oblongata, using autoradiography (See Chapter 26), was published, and showed great promise for further use of this analysis in the PASS study (16). Future analyses from this rich database, specifically with regards to the risks for SIDS and pathophysiological understanding of SIDS, are eagerly awaited.

The third event to significantly influence the focus with which infant deaths were to be investigated was the establishment of the National Forensic Pathology Service in 2006. With the responsibility of death investigation now vested in the FPS, in-house training resulted in a greater awareness of the importance of improving the standard of scene investigation and autopsy practice. These factors culminated in the first National SUDI/SIDS mini-symposium, held as part of the 50th annual congress of the Federation of South African Societies of Pathology, in 2010.

As attention was being increasingly focused on the examination and investigation of sudden death in children, a significant shortcoming in the process of research into infant and child mortality proved to be the paucity of current information on mortality in the young. This sparked collaborative investigation into the status quo of death investigation in infants, and culminated in the publication of two important papers; these and other resultant studies and subsequent publications marked the fourth important event that stimulated increased research into death in the young in the country.

The first project was conducted as a collaboration between the Tygerberg and Pretoria Forensic Pathology Laboratories in the Western Cape and Gauteng Provinces respectively. This analysis, investigating deaths from 2000 to 2004, included 512 infants who died suddenly and unexpectedly, of which 171 cases (33.4%) were classified as SIDS (17). The follow-up, or so-called multicenter study, was conducted at five large academic centers and included eight mortuaries. In the 2005 to 2009 period, 2,704 cases of sudden unexpected infant deaths were investigated, with 224 cases (8.3%) classified as SIDS (18). In a further 383 cases (14.2%), the cause of death was unascertained at autopsy (18). Death scene investigations were conducted by the pathologists in only 14 cases — seven of these incorporating doll re-enactments.

In 2015, research into findings from death notification by Statistics South Africa indicated that 0.6% of all deaths in South African children under 1 year (excluding obvious fetal deaths) were reported to be due to SIDS (19). However, a further 10.4% of cases were assigned to "other ill-defined and unspecified causes of mortality" (19) (p. 20). This large percentage of ill-defined causes of death demonstrated not only the problem of poor death certification practice in South Africa, but also the variation in the terminology used to capture causes of SUDI deaths. Terms such as "undetermined" and "unascertained" may be used by some, while other forensic medical practitioners may have diagnosed SIDS in the same cases.

In Cape Town, partly because of the collaboration between the PASS study, the Western Cape FPS, and the University of Stellenbosch, it was apparent that investigation of SIDS/SUDI cases, including the collection of accurate data around the death of the infant, was further complicated by the lack of standardization of infant death investigation and autopsy protocols (8, 20). This may very well also have interfered with potential intervention programs in communities that are already challenged by socioeconomic and infrastructure issues. The implementation of a Death Scene Investigation (DSI) protocol meeting high international standards was deemed of the utmost importance if South Africa was to address the high reported SIDS rate (8). However, it was not clear if the implementation of such a protocol was feasible against the background of a lack of formally trained death scene investigators, personnel and budgetary constraints, and a significant case load.

In order to test the potential for the institution of a standardized investigation protocol in the Eastern Metropole of Cape Town in the Western Cape, a feasibility study was undertaken, whereby a standardized autopsy and infant DSI was instituted through a collaborative effort of local FPOs and clinical providers. The standardized DSI published by the Centers for Disease Control (CDC), Atlanta, United States (US) (21), was selected. Forensic pathologists and clinical investigators from the US conducted training workshops in SUDI protocols for FPOs attached to the Western Cape Forensic Pathology Service, forensic medical practitioners attached to the Faculty of Medicine and Health Science (FMHS) of the University of Stellenbosch, and healthcare practitioners in obstetrics and pediatrics at local clinics. All autopsies included detailed external examination, histology, bacteriologic and viral cultures, HIV testing, and toxicology screening where indicated. The brain was not fixed, but standardized, representative histology was taken at autopsy. Financial constraints hindered routine testing for metabolic and genetic screening, unless specifically indicated.

Virtually all infants were found dead after a sleep period, mainly in the early morning by their mothers, and were co-sleeping on the night of death. This interesting finding further illustrated the tendency for co-sleeping, a tendency which was already evident in a study on sleeping positions of infants in the Cape Peninsula in 1992. In this study, it was reported that 94% of infants from the local population co-slept with their parents (22).

This feasibility study demonstrated that implementation of a SIDS/SUID death investigation, meeting high international standards, can be achieved in the Eastern Metropole of the city of Cape Town, a region with a high SIDS rate and significant infrastructure challenges (20). The study also marked the implementation of a SUDI questionnaire that has been adapted and developed over the years to include more relevant locally important information at the Forensic Pathology Laboratories in the Western Cape. This questionnaire is completed by FPOs, both when attending the death scene, as well as when interviewing the families of deceased infants.

## The medico-legal autopsy in sudden death in infants and children in South Africa

Depending on the circumstances of death, financial and technical constraints in a specific region, and the forensic medical practitioner's experience, the ancillary investigations to a full autopsy performed in SUDI autopsies in South Africa include the following:

### Histological examination of tissue

In cases where the cause of death remains obscure after autopsy, the taking of tissue for histological examination remains the standard. In the multicenter study, it was apparent that histology was only performed in 43.5% of cases; however, inclusion of histological examination varied significantly between the different centers (Pretoria: 71.4% of cases; Cape Town-Tygerberg: 58.7% of cases; Bloemfontein: 44.5% of cases; Johannesburg: 16.6% of cases; and Durban: 15.7% of cases) (18). In academic centers, histology is reviewed by the forensic pathologist who performed the autopsy, and in the case of a junior registrar, the sections are usually reviewed in conjunction with a qualified forensic pathologist. Service delivery constraints do not allow for formal histological review of the slides by an expert panel.

## Microbiology

Microscopy and culture mainly form part of the SUDI death investigation protocol in Cape Town, South Africa. No microbiology studies were reported to have been included in two of the major centers in South Africa, with very limited microbiology screening in two other centers, as part of the findings of the multicenter study (18).

## Virology

Virology screening also mainly forms part of SUDI death investigation in Cape Town. No reports of any virological screening tests were found at three of the major centers in the SUDI study population reviewed during the multicenter study (18).

## Radiology

The multicenter study between 2005-09 showed that radiological screening was only performed in 31 cases (1.2%) in four major centers in South Africa (18). With the international development of forensic radiology and imaging, some of the large medico-legal laboratories in the country have acquired the LODOX® Statscan® full-body digital X-ray machine in recent years. Full-body digital radiography screening prior to the autopsy examination has thus proven much more accessible; however, mainly due to the heavy case load, radiological screening is still not performed in all cases at all medico-legal facilities. Although high-resolution imaging modalities such as Computerized Tomography (CT) and Magnetic Resonance Imaging (MRI) are not yet readily available on the premises of any medico-legal laboratory in South Africa, some academic centers have agreements in place that ensure access to high-resolution imaging modalities at affiliated academic hospitals.

## Toxicology

Due to financial and resource constraints, toxicological screening is not usually performed as part of the SUDI death investigation protocol in most centers in South Africa. Toxicological screening is only requested in cases where a suspicion of poisoning or ingestion of a substance is forthcoming in the case history. Establishment of dedicated toxicological laboratories within FPSs, an incentive with which the Cape Town West Metro FPS is leading the way, will hopefully see an increase in this valuable investigative screening modality in SUDI death investigation.

## Biochemistry

All Forensic Pathology Laboratories have access to the services of the National Health Laboratory Service. Biochemical investigations are requested as indicated by the history and findings in the case; none are performed routinely.

In the multicenter study, metabolic screening was performed in only one autopsy examination at Tygerberg-Cape Town (18). Molecular studies are currently not routine practice in any mortuary in South Africa, mainly as a result of budgetary constraints (23).

# Recent Advances in Investigation into Death in Infancy and Childhood in South Africa

## Child death review

The child death review (CDR) trend internationally started in the late 20th century, and CDRs are being conducted in First World countries like the US, the United Kingdom, New Zealand, Australia, and Canada (24). Besides the diagnostic challenges posed by the multitude of SUDI and other sudden unexpected deaths in children in South Africa, it was realized that caution must be exercised not to miss cases of child neglect, abuse, and homicide. Of cases presenting as SUDI, 10% are found to be infanticide (25). The difficulty in recognizing cases of child abuse and neglect probably results in under-reporting of these cases in high-income communities, and it is feared that the problem may even be of a greater magnitude in a Third World setting. A study conducted in 2009 found that the homicide rate in children younger than 18 years in South Africa was 5.5 per 100,000, compared to 2.4 homicidal deaths per 100,000 reported internationally. The age group most at risk for fatal child abuse in South Africa was found to be the 0-4 age group (24).

For this purpose, CDR meetings have been instituted in two provinces in South Africa. The CDR process is now well underway in two major centers in Cape Town, (Metro East and Metro West), two peripheral centers in the Western Cape Province (namely George and Paarl), a major center in Durban, as well as one peripheral center in Pietermaritzburg in Kwazulu-Natal. The CDR team consists of forensic pathologists, representatives from the Children's Institute, Department of Social Development, National Prosecuting Authority, SAPS, district pediatricians, as well as pediatric epidemiologists, where available.

The current child death review structure comprehensively evaluates the social circumstances of each child who dies under presumed unnatural circumstances, including the ante- and postnatal history, living arrangements and family structure, available records of visits to health facilities, and autopsy findings, by means of completion of a comprehensive questionnaire for each case and multiagency case discussion (26).

## Findings of the child death review pilot study

The CDR pilot reviewed 711 cases at two different facilities in two different provinces from 1 January 2014 to 31 December 2014. Deaths due to natural causes were found in more than half of the total study population (10). Infant deaths constituted 374 of these cases, of which more than 80% were finally diagnosed with a natural cause of death (10). Some of the main findings include that most of these children succumb to lower respiratory tract infections, mainly in the neonatal period, and although some of the affected neonates were delivered prematurely, it would appear as though their caretakers do not seem to recognize signs of distress timeously (10, 26). The accuracy in formulating the cause of death was enhanced through the interdisciplinary CDR discussions, especially in cases of sudden and unexpected death. The CDR also serves as an effective audit tool in forensic medical practice (26). It did come to light that not all health agencies adhere to the regulations stipulating referral of cases of SUDI to the SAPS as potential cases of other-than-natural death, due to a discrepancy in the case referral and admission pattern in the different provinces. Of all cases of neglect or omission of care, the CDR pilot identified 33 which would otherwise probably have been overlooked (10).

## Additional benefits of the child death review process
### Facilitation of judicial process

For the short period during which the CDR has been running, it has already impacted the judicial process significantly. Cases of child homicide and neglect are brought to the attention of the senior state prosecutors in the region within a month after the death of the deceased. The further death investigation, in such cases, can then be guided by the state prosecutor and the legal proceedings expedited. In all cases where a suspicion with regards to the death arises from the CDR discussion, the pathologist is alerted to complete the case as a matter of urgency and the SAPS can be instructed to obtain further information or witness statements, where indicated. Previously, the state prosecutor often only became aware of a criminal case after the case was deemed fully investigated, the autopsy report completed, and the docket presented to the state prosecutor by the investigating officer.

### Identification of cases that require department of social development (DSD) intervention

The inclusion of a social worker in the CDR/SUDI death review team aids in identifying families with poor socioeconomic circumstances in need of intervention, especially where morbidity might be prevented in siblings of deceased infants, who are potentially subjected to the same dire circumstances. The social worker could also play an important role in counseling bereaved family members and possibly could also, in the future, assist in genetic counseling.

### Quality control of medical services

The multidisciplinary case discussions are not only geared at evaluating the social and medical care that the deceased child received, but also the deceased's access to care and possible health systems failures, which could be addressed at a regional level. Health system failures were thought to have played a role in 11.2% of deaths in the CDR pilot case population (10).

*Community feedback and development*

In some areas, community health workers are available, who can greatly assist in health education for high-risk families. This is especially so where lack of insight, a low level of education, or young age of the parents/guardians of the deceased child are deemed to have influenced the case outcome. Factors like regular clinic visits, immunization, and danger signs in acutely ill children are being addressed.

*Multidisciplinary case overview and diagnostic review*

One of the major advantages of the CDR process for the forensic medical practitioner is the fact that specialists in other fields may be consulted in order to formulate a more detailed cause of death cascade, especially in cases where no clear macro- or microscopic diagnosis is forthcoming. Unfortunately, the high case load, which results in having between 30 to 50 cases for discussion at each monthly review meeting at each facility, precludes one from in-depth discussion with regards to the diagnostic process, specifically in SUDI cases. For this reason, formulating a SUDI death investigation review process in South Africa is imperative. A SUDI investigative panel could ensure that the diagnosis in each case is formulated according to a standard format if the panel adheres to structured diagnostic criteria (27, 28). A SUDI death review process would address inconsistencies in SUDI death investigation and region-specific case investigation, and would also provide guidance in formulating consistent diagnoses, thus enabling research into the field specific to the South African population. Once CDR has been established in all provinces in South Africa, the optimal opportunity will arise to correlate investigation protocols and introduce a standardized national SUDI death investigation protocol.

## Establishment of a national forensic pathology training course

The imminent implementation of the long-anticipated Forensic Pathology Officer training course is eagerly awaited. The finalization of the curriculum and registration of the course with South African accreditation mark significant progress towards expert death scene investigation, which ultimately serves the process of cause of death determination.

## Challenges to the Investigation of Sudden Childhood Death in South Africa

### Priority of investigating sudden childhood death

In 2015, 11.5% of all deaths recorded in South Africa were of children under 18 years of age, with children under 1 year representing 70% of these deaths (19). According to this report by Statistics South Africa on mortality and causes of death in South Africa, non-natural causes of death constituted 6.7% of the total number of childhood deaths (2).

In a relatively resource-strapped environment such as Forensic Pathology, competing for funding within the budget of the department of health — in a country where infections such as tuberculosis, HIV, pneumonia, and gastroenteritis, as well as malnutrition, still cause significant child deaths — proves to be challenging.

## Lack of a standardized, national, SUDI death investigation protocol

One of the major problems that has hampered SUDI/SIDS death investigation and research in South Africa is the fact that no national SUDI death investigation protocol currently exists. This has the unfortunate result that there are major differences between centers pertaining to autopsy protocols, as well as ancillary investigations performed during the SUDI autopsy, even at the academic (university-affiliated) centers. Currently, histological tissue processing and microscopy examination are also not readily available in some rural centers, especially in provinces and service areas in the periphery, where no qualified forensic pathologists are employed.

## Molecular autopsy

The association between possible channelopathies and SIDS has been documented since 1976 (35). It has been suggested that channelopathies may be responsible for up to 5% to 10% of deaths in SUDI cases (36, 37). Mutations in genes associated with prolonged QT syndrome in the SIDS population have been studied by a number of authors. Brink et al. reported on prolonged QT syndrome in the South African population and documented a founder effect for the *KCNQ1*-A341V gene (31). In 2017, an international collaboration led by South African researchers identified a novel genetic cause of arrhythmogenic right ventricular cardiomyopathy from a South African family (32).

Mutations in the SCN5A gene (associated with cardiac channelopathies) were retrospectively analyzed in Pretoria in a SUDI population (38). The findings indicated possibly significant positive mutations of varying significance (38). Currently, it is not routine practice to conduct molecular testing on SUDIs in South Africa.

Major challenges in molecular testing include cost implications, deciding which mutations to test for, and ultimately determining whether or not the mutation did indeed cause the death. The interpretation of the genetic results should be done by a multidisciplinary team and must include pediatric geneticists, cardiologists, and the forensic pathologist. Despite the obstacles, driven by research to identify population-specific "hotspot" regions which will drastically reduce the costs, selective and directed implementation of molecular autopsy techniques is looming in the future of infant death investigation.

## Broadening the research footprint in forensic pathology

While the *Inquests Act* affords the forensic medical practitioner significant privilege and freedom to determine the cause and circumstances surrounding the death, this does not come without disadvantages. Distrust in the medico-legal process may very well cause the public and next of kin to be hesitant to consent to research on deceased family members, where the research does not fall within the ambit of diagnosing the cause of death. Revision and updating of the antiquated *Inquests Act* is a priority, and discussion around the issue has been raised at academic meetings and the National Forensic Pathology Service Committee.

## The Road Ahead

### Implementation of a standardized national SUDI death investigation protocol

The importance and value of implementing a standardized SUDI death investigation protocol cannot be overstated. This applies to the complete investigation process, including the scene investigation, history taking and ancillary investigations, and protocols for evidence and sample collection.

### Formal and in-house forensic pathology officer training program

All efforts must be made to establish the planned forensic pathology officer training course. In the interim, in-house training programs will continue, as the materials taught are in essence the contents of the formal course as proposed. A death scene investigation protocol should form part of all SUDI investigations.

### Imaging guidelines for the evaluation of infant deaths

Currently, infant cases are only referred for a "baby gram" when non-accidental injury is suspected from the case history and/or external examination of the body. Dedicated forensic CT scanners are not currently available, even though forensic radiology and imaging is a fast-growing specialty field in forensic pathology. The development of forensic imaging protocols has been earmarked as an important investigation modality and field of research in many of the country's academic forensic pathology divisions (33).

### Finding novel ways of establishing community rapport and interaction

The SIDS rate in the United States decreased from 1.2 per 1,000 live births to 0.53 per 1,000 live births over 8 years due to safe sleep recommendations. Similar success rates have been obtained in Norway and Otago, New Zealand, through supine sleep campaigns (39). It was suggested that, by simply advising parents to place preterm or low birth weight babies in a supine position in a separate sleeping environment in the parents' room, the SIDS rate in England and Wales could possibly be reduced by 20% or up to 100 infant lives per year. This could also greatly reduce the impact of SIDS in South Africa (34). The FPS is ideally placed to communicate issues pertaining to safe sleeping environments and other risk factors to the community. The FPS is represented well in rural, as well as urban, regions, and through contact with clinicians, information can be disseminated to parents about safe sleep practices prior to discharging neonates from the hospital or clinic in the postnatal period as part of a standard care package.

The community should also be actively informed about other potential risk factors through community initiatives, whilst still respecting traditional beliefs, as was seen in the New Zealand Wahakura program, where traditional skills were utilized to create safe sleep baskets for infants of parents who prefer their infants to be placed in the parental bed to sleep (39).

## Multidisciplinary approach to infant and childhood sudden death

Apart from the CDR of pediatric cases in selected centers in South Africa, a multidisciplinary evaluation and audit of cases of SUDI and SIDS is not commonplace in South African Forensic Pathology. The positive outcome of multidisciplinary approach was readily apparent in the PASS collaboration, but again challenges around expertise, staff numbers, service burden, and resources make this a difficult proposition at most facilities. Solutions have to be explored in order for committees to review all records, including the post-mortem report and results of ancillary investigations according to a standard protocol, as well as information from the scene of death, preferably including a doll re-enactment, and any additional clinical history obtained. This will ultimately also result in improved monitoring of the SUDI cases in South Africa. Review committees can also identify shortfalls in the current investigation protocol and, by eliminating the missing elements found during case review, in the forensic investigation, including scene investigation.

## Conclusions

Despite significant political and social challenges, both in the past and more recently, South African is known as the "Rainbow Nation" — not just because of the ethnic diversity of the inhabitants, but also because of the air of positivity and happiness that pervades communities. It is a country with a beautiful, progressive constitution and human rights culture, where the African philosophy of Ubuntu, or "humanity towards others", signifies a belief in a universal bond of sharing which connects all humanity. At Nelson Mandela's memorial, President Barack Obama spoke about Ubuntu, saying: "There is a word in South Africa — Ubuntu — a word that captures Mandela's greatest gift: his recognition that we are all bound together in ways that are invisible to the eye; that there is a oneness to humanity; that we achieve ourselves by sharing ourselves with others, and caring for those around us" (40).

It is because of this attitude of caring, of being bound together, that South Africans are taking note of the high burden of SUDI. It is also why the past two decades have seen a sharp focus on practices and protocols that address the finding of causes of death in our young, so that intervention strategies may be implemented in order to further decrease the mortality rate in this vulnerable portion of the population.

# References

1. South African Government. Geography and Climate. [Available from: http://www.gov.za/about-sa/geography-and-climate]. Accessed 27 October 2017.

2. Statistics South Africa. P0302 — Mid-year population estimates 2016. [Available from: http://www.statssa.gov.za/publications/P0302/P03022016.pdf]. Accessed 27 October 2017.

3. *Inquests Act 58 of 1959* (South Africa). [Available from: http://www.justice.gov.za/legislation/acts/1959-58.pdf]. Accessed 27 October 2017.

4. *National Health Act 2003* (South Africa) reg 636. Regulations Regarding the rendering of Forensic Pathology Service. [Available from: http://www.gov.za/sites/www.gov.za/files/30075n.pdf]. Accessed 27 October 2017.

5. Godwin TA. End of life: Natural or unnatural death investigation and certification. Dis Mon. 2005;51(4):218-77. https://doi.org/10.1016/j.disamonth.2005.06.001.

6. Committee for the Workshop on the Medicolegal Death Investigation System. Medicolegal Death Investigation System: Workshop summary. Washington, DC: The National Academies Press, 2003.

7. Bernitz H, Kenyhercz M, Kloppers B, L'Abbé EN, Labuschagnes GN, Olckers A, et al. The history and current status of forensic science in South Africa. In: The global practice of forensic science. Chichester: John Wiley & Sons, 2015. p. 241-60.

8. Molteno MA. Early childhood mortality in Cape Town. South Afr Med J. 1989;75(12):570-4.

9. United Nations Development Program. Millennium Development Goals. [Available from: http://www.undp.org/content/undp/en/home/sdgoverview/mdg_goals.html]. Accessed 27 October 2017.

10. Mathews S, Martin LJ, Coetzee D, Scott C, Naidoo T, Brijmohun Y, et al. The South African child death review pilot: A multiagency approach to strengthen healthcare and protection for children. South Afr Med J. 2016;106(9):895-9. https://doi.org/10.7196/SAMJ.2016.v106i9.11234.

11. Dukes KA, Burd L, Elliott AJ, Fifer WP, Folkerth RD, Hankins GD, et al. The Safe Passage study: Design, methods, recruitment, and follow-up approach. Paediatr Perinat Epidemiol. 2014;28(5):455-65. https://doi.org/10.1111/ppe.12136.

12. Randall BB, Wadee SA, Sens MA, Kinney HC, Folkerth RD, Odendaal HJ, et al. A practical classification schema incorporating consideration of possible asphyxia in cases of sudden unexpected infant death. Forensic Sci Med Pathol. 2009;5(4):254. https://doi.org/10.1007/s12024-009-9083-y.

13. Dempers J, Wadee SA, Boyd T, Wright C, Odendaal HJ, Sens MA. Hepatic hemangioendothelioma presenting as sudden unexpected death in infancy: A case report. Pediatr Dev Pathol. 2011;14(1):71-4. https://doi.org/10.2350/10-01-0776-CR.1.

14. Dempers J, Sens MA, Wadee SA, Kinney HC, Odendaal HJ, Wright CA. Progressive primary pulmonary tuberculosis presenting as the sudden unexpected death in infancy: A case report. Forensic Sci Int. 2011;206(1):e27-30. https://doi.org/10.1016/j.forsciint.2010.07.018.

15. Odendaal HJ, Elliott A, Kinney HC, Human M, Gaspar D, Petersen D, et al. Consent for autopsy research for unexpected death in early life. Obstet Gynecol. 2011;117(1):167. https://doi.org/10.1097/AOG.0b013e318200cb17.

16. Haynes RL, Folkerth RD, Paterson DS, Broadbelt KG, Dan Zaharie S, Hewlett RH, et al. Serotonin receptors in the medulla oblongata of the human fetus and infant: The analytic approach of the international Safe Passage study. J Neuropathol Exp Neurol. 2016;75(11):1048-57. https://doi.org/10.1093/jnen/nlw080.

17. du Toit-Prinsloo L, Dempers JJ, Wadee SA, Saayman G. The medico-legal investigation of sudden, unexpected and/or unexplained infant deaths in South Africa: Where are we — and where are we going? Forensic Sci Med Pathol. 2011;7(1):14-20. https://doi.org/10.1007/s12024-010-9184-7.

18. du Toit-Prinsloo L, Dempers J, Verster J, Hattingh C, Nel H, Brandt VD, et al. Toward a standardized investigation protocol in sudden unexpected deaths in infancy in South Africa: A multicenter study of medico-legal investigation procedures and outcomes. Forensic Sci Med Pathol. 2013;9(3):344-50. https://doi.org/10.1007/s12024-013-9427-5.

19. Statistics South Africa. Mortality and causes of death in South Africa, 2015: Findings from death notification. Statistical release no. P0309.3. Pretoria, South Africa: Statistics South Africa, 2017.

20. Dempers JJ, Coldrey J, Burger EH, Thompson V, Wadee SA, Odendaal HJ, et al. The institution of a standardized investigation protocol for sudden infant death in the eastern metropole, Cape Town, South Africa. J Forensic Sci. 2016;61(6):1508-14. https://doi.org/10.1111/1556-4029.13204.

21. Hanzlick RL, Jentzen JM, Clark SC. Sudden, unexplained infant death investigation: Guidelines for the scene investigator. Atlanta, GA: Centers for Disease Control and Prevention, 2007.

22. Potgieter ST, Kibel MA. Sleeping positions of infants in the Cape Peninsula. SAMJ. 1992;81(7):355-7.

23. van Deventer BS, Rossouw SH, du Toit-Prinsloo L. Sudden and unexpected childhood deaths investigated at the Pretoria medico-legal laboratory, South Africa, 2007-2011. SAMJ. 2016;106(10):983-5. https://doi.org/10.7196/SAMJ.2016.v106i10.11170.

24. Mathews S, Abrahams N, Martin LJ. Child death reviews in the context of child abuse fatalities — Learning from international practice. [Available from: http://137.158.155.94/bitstream/handle/11427/3969/CI_misc_childdeaths_2013.pdf?sequence=1]. Accessed 31 October 2017.

25. Levene S, Bacon CJ. Sudden unexpected death and covert homicide in infancy. Arch Dis Child. 2004;89(5):443-7. https://doi.org/10.1136/adc.2003.036202.

26. Mathews S, Martin LJ, Coetzee D, Scott C, Brijmohun Y. Child deaths in South Africa: Lessons from the child death review pilot. South Afr Med J. 2016;106(9):851-2. https://doi.org/10.7196/SAMJ.2016.v106i9.11382.

27. Shapiro-Mendoza CK, Camperlengo L, Ludvigsen R, Cottengim C, Anderson RN, Andrew T, et al. Classification system for the sudden unexpected infant death case registry and its application. Pediatrics. 2014;134(1):e210-19. https://doi.org/10.1542/peds.2014-0180.

28. Sauber-Schatz EK, Sappenfield WM, Shapiro-Mendoza CK. Comprehensive review of sleep-related sudden unexpected infant deaths and their investigations: Florida 2008. Matern Child Health J. 2015;19(2):381-90. https://doi.org/10.1007/s10995-014-1520-1.

29. Krous HF, Nadeau JM, Silva PD, Blackbourne BD. A comparison of respiratory symptoms and inflammation in sudden infant death syndrome and in accidental or inflicted infant death. Am J Forensic Med Pathol. 2003;24(1):1-8. https://doi.org/10.1097/01.PAF.0000051520.92087.C3.

30. Mathews S, Abrahams N, Jewkes R, Martin LJ, Lombard C. The epidemiology of child homicides in South Africa. Bull World Health Organ. 2013;91(8):562-8. https://doi.org/10.2471/BLT.12.117036.

31. Brink PA, Corfield VA. The long QT syndrome in South Africa: Long QT syndrome. SA Heart. 2008;5(4):160-3.

32. Mayosi BM, Fish M, Shaboodien G, Mastantuono E, Kraus S, Wieland T, et al. Identification of Cadherin 2 (CDH2) mutations in arrhythmogenic right ventricular cardiomyopathy. Circulation: Cardiovascular Genetics. 2017;10(2):e001605. https://doi.org/10.1161/CIRCGENETICS.116.001605.

33. Aalders MC, Adolphi NL, Daly B, Davis GG, de Boer HH, Decker SJ, et al. Research in forensic radiology and imaging; identifying the most important issues. JOFRI. 2017;8:1-8. https://doi.org/10.1016/j.jofri.2017.01.004.

34. Blair PS, Platt MW, Smith IJ, Fleming PJ. Sudden infant death syndrome and sleeping position in pre-term and low birth weight infants: An opportunity for targeted intervention. Arch Dis Child. 2006;91(2):101-6. https://doi.org/10.1136/adc.2004.070391.

35. Schwartz PJ. Cardiac sympathetic innervation and sudden infant death syndrome. A possible pathogenic link. Am J Med. 1976;60:167-72. https://doi.org/10.1016/0002-9343(76)90425-3.

36. Ackerman MJ, Siu BL, Sturner WQ. Postmortem molecular analysis of SCN5A defects in sudden infant death syndrome. J Am Med Assoc. 2001;286:2264-9. https://doi.org/10.1001/jama.286.18.2264.

37. Ackerman MJ, Tester DJ, Bell CM, Towbin JA, January CT, Makielski JC, et al. Cardiac channel mutations in SIDS: A population-based molecular autopsy study. Circulation. 2002;106(19):167.

38. van Niekerk C, van Deventer BS, du Toit-Prinsloo L. Long QT syndrome and sudden infant death. J Clin Pathol. 2017;70(9):808-13.

39. Ball HL, Volpe LE. Sudden infant death syndrome (SIDS) risk reduction and infant sleep location — Moving the discussion forward. Soc Sci Med. 2013;79:84-91. https://doi.org/10.1016/j.socscimed.2012.03.025.

40. LoGiruato B. Here is Barack Obama's powerful tribute to Nelson Mandela. Business Insider [internet]; 10 December 2013. [Available from: http://www.businessinsider.com/obama-nelson-mandela-memorial-service-speech-full-text-2013-12#ixzz2n55J7Sv8]. Accessed 27 October 2017.

# 18

# A United Kingdom Perspective

Joanna Garstang, MBChB, MSc, PhD[1]
and Anna S Pease, MA, MSc, PhD[2]

[1]*Warwick Medical School, University of Warwick, Coventry, UK*
[2]*The University of Bristol, Bristol, UK*

## Introduction

Sudden infant death syndrome (SIDS) is still a leading cause for infant mortality in the United Kingdom (UK) despite the significant reduction in cases since the 1990s. Currently, there are ongoing public health campaigns aimed at promoting safer sleep, as the majority of SIDS cases in the UK occur in unsafe sleep environments. There is little uniformity of practice nationally about which deaths should be classified as SIDS or "unascertained", with very few deaths recognized as being due to accidental asphyxia. The investigation of sudden and unexpected death in infancy (SUDI) has changed considerably since the early 2000s. Joint agency investigation by police, healthcare, and social care is now standard, with local review of all child deaths mandatory.

## Incidence

### UK rates

SIDS is a prominent cause of death for infants in the UK (1). There were 247 unexplained deaths of children under 2 years of age in 2014; of these, 230 were unexplained infant deaths, giving a rate of 0.30 deaths per 1,000 live births, the lowest on record (2). There were 17 unexplained deaths of children aged between 12 and 24 months, accounting

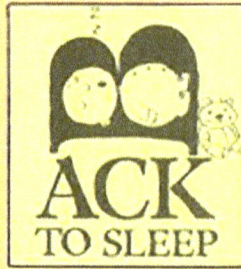

Figure 18.1: Front cover of the first "Back to Sleep" leaflet, Department of Health, 1991.

for 6.9% of all unexplained deaths of children younger than 2 years. Much higher rates of deaths in the 1970s and 1980s (2.30 deaths per 1,000 live births, or 1,593 deaths in 1988) (3) led to a concerted effort to identify modifiable risk factors and translate these into advice for parents. As in other countries, associations between unexplained infant deaths and the prone sleeping position, smoking during pregnancy, and overwrapping led to educational campaigns for parents, the successful implementation of which has led to a rapid decline in these deaths in the last 25 years.

## The UK "Back to Sleep" campaign

The introduction of the "Back to Sleep" campaign in the UK in 1991 (see Figure 18.1) led to a dramatic fall in the number of infants dying (see Figures 18.2 and 18.3). The campaign in the UK was promoted at a national level and included a strong media element, as well as guidance for health professionals, to change their recommendations to parents. Anne Diamond, who was a popular TV presenter at the time, had a son, Sebastian, who died of SIDS in 1991. She campaigned strongly for the changes to advice (4), which eventually included a television advertisement in collaboration with the Department of Health (5). Beginning in October 1991, there were three main components of the original campaign: sleeping position, smoking, and thermal stress.

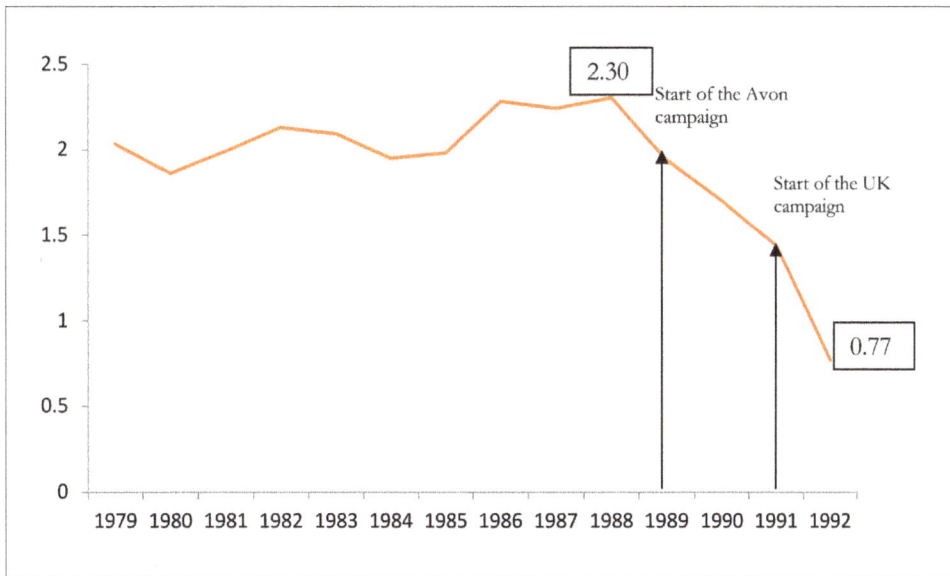

Figure 18.2: SIDS rates (deaths per 1,000 live births) in the UK from 1979-92. Note: y-axis represents number of cases per 1,000 live births; x-axis represents year. (Authors' own work.)

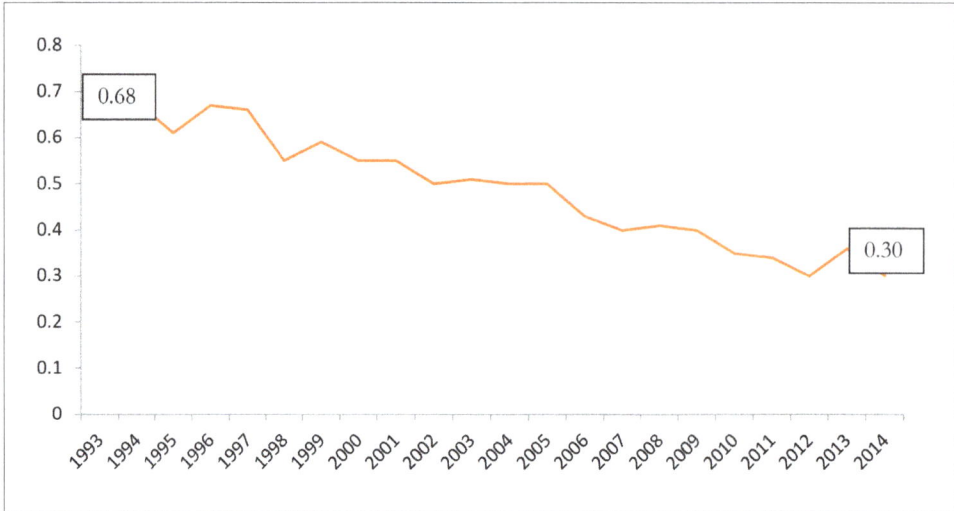

Figure 18.3: SIDS rates in the UK from 1993-2014. Note: y-axis represents number of cases per 1,000 live births; x-axis represents year. (Authors' own work.)

The success of the "Back to Sleep" campaign brought about a staggering decrease in SIDS incidence in the UK, reducing the number of SIDS deaths by up to 40% within the first year of the campaign (6). Figure 18.2 shows the death rates from 1979, well before the start of the campaigns, up to 1992, the year following the national campaign. SIDS rates had already started to decline from 1989 when Fleming led a regional "Back to Sleep" campaign in Avon in the South West region of England, and this advice began to be taken up unofficially in other areas of the UK. The rates shown are adjusted to include all SIDS and unascertained deaths in infants between 28 days and 12 months.

In some countries, such as the US and Australia, after an initial dramatic fall the SIDS rate has plateaued, but this is not the case in the UK. The initial 67% fall from 1988-92 has been followed by a further 56% fall from 1993 to 2014. Figure 18.3 shows the decline in rates in the UK from 1993-2014.

## Changing profile of risk factors

A study looking at the epidemiological changes over the last 20 years (7) charted the prevalence of known risk factors over this time period and found that rates of prone sleeping between 1994 and 2003 had remained relatively stable (23%-24%), following a fall from 89% before the "Back to Sleep" campaign. This suggested that the subsequent fall in SIDS deaths was not due to steadily decreasing rates of prone positioning, but rather was due to the importance of other risk factors. This point was further clarified in a study comparing two major UK SIDS case-control studies 10 years apart (8). This noted the stability of prone sleeping across this time period, as well as steep falls in the use of side position for sleep, postnatal smoke exposure, and head covering, alongside increases in using the feet-to-foot position and attempts to breastfeed. The further halving of the SIDS rate for this time period is attributed more to the increase in the importance of these other risk factors. Table 18.1 below shows the changes in care practices across this time period, as measured by the two studies.

Table 18.1: Impact of risk reduction advice in the 10 years between CESDI and SWISS studies. (Adapted from (8).) CESDI = Confidential Enquiry into Stillbirths and Deaths in Infancy Study. SWISS = South West Infant Sleep Scene Study.

| Risk (R) or Protective (P) Factor | CESDI Study | | | |
|---|---|---|---|---|
| | Fleming & Blair (1993-96) | | SWISS Study Blair & Fleming (2003-06) | |
| | SIDS % | Controls % | SIDS % | Controls % |
| R-Placed prone to sleep | 15% | 3% | 14% | 6% |
| R-Placed on side to sleep | 41% | 28% | 18% | 10% |
| R-Postnatal exposure to smoke | 54% | 23% | 16% | 6% |
| R-Head covered by bedding | 16% | 3% | 5% | 0% |
| P-Feet placed at foot of cot | 3% | 4% | 50% | 60% |
| P-Mother attempted to breastfeed | 44% | 60% | 70% | 79% |

As the incidence of SIDS has declined, the association with social deprivation has become more marked. In the Avon region of South West England, during 1984-88, 23% of SIDS occurred in the 10% most deprived communities, whereas by 1999-2003 this had risen to 48% of SIDS cases (7).

## Diagnostic Difficulties in the UK

In the UK the term SUDI is generally used according to the Confidential Enquiry for Stillbirths and Deaths in Infancy (CESDI) SUDI Study definition: the death of an infant which was not anticipated as a significant possibility 24 hours before the death or where there was a similarly unexpected collapse leading to or precipitating the events which led to the death (9). SUDI may therefore be used to describe the presentation of any unexpected infant death; typically in the UK one-third of SUDI are subsequently found to have a medical cause determined.

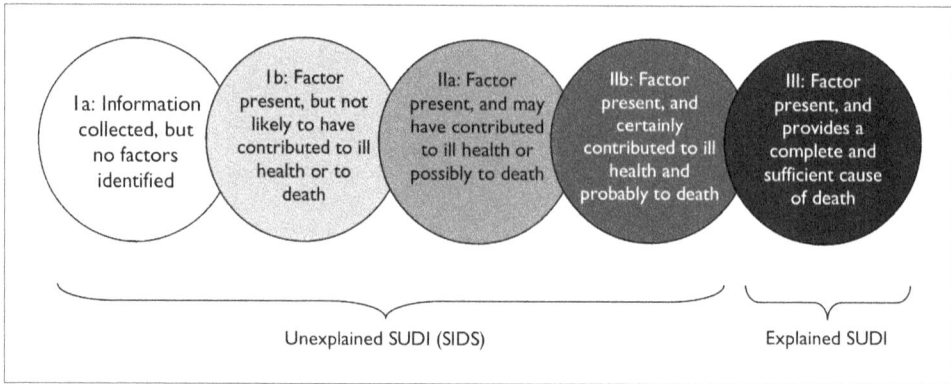

Figure 18.4: Avon classification of SUDI framework. (Adapted from (16).)

Deaths that remain unexplained after complete investigation may be classified as SIDS, as per the San Diego definition (10), although frequently this term is not used and often unexplained deaths are labeled "unascertained" instead. All unexpected deaths in the UK are investigated by coroners, who are responsible for issuing medical certificates of cause for death. Coroners usually rely on pathologists' conclusions from the post-mortem examination to inform death certification; however, many pathologists are reluctant to use the term SIDS if there are risk factors for accidental asphyxia (11, 12). For this reason, official statistics on SIDS have under-reported the death rates. Combining both SIDS and unascertained death classifications provides a more accurate rate of infant deaths with no known cause and this is the approach now taken by the UK Office for National Statistics (13).

The UK also has low rates of accidental asphyxia in SUDI compared to many other countries (14). The reasons for this are unclear but may include professionals investigating SUDI failing to recognize asphyxial deaths or their reluctance to make the diagnosis given that this cannot be diagnosed conclusively at post-mortem examination (15).

Given these diagnostic difficulties, and the need to recognize relevant risk factors in SUDI, the Avon Classification system was proposed following the work of the CESDI Study (9). This is now beginning to be an internationally recognized system for the appropriate classification of unexpected infant deaths, although it is not often used in routine clinical practice. This classification of SUDI deaths provides for both explained and unexplained causes of death. There are five broad subgroups describing the unexplained SUDI deaths, presented in Figure 18.4. This system acknowledges the role of known risk factors without assigning them incorrectly as a cause of death.

## Current UK Advice

The dominant method of communicating SIDS risk reduction advice was previously through national campaigns. Television advertisements and national leaflets were produced and conversations with health professionals supported the effort. In a climate of fear where SIDS was much more common, a simple change such as putting infants to sleep face up was palatable to the general population (especially since prone sleep had only been recently advised without an underlying tradition) and once adopted, SIDS rates plummeted. This type of intervention promotes rapid change but it needs a specific context within which to work. Today, SIDS is a much rarer event, and while most parents are still concerned about it, this same kind of campaign would not be likely to bring the rates down further, especially since most of these deaths now occur in poorer families rather than across the spectrum of social classes. It is also more difficult to advise against practices which have a traditional or cultural basis — for example, bed sharing — and promote those that do not — for example, pacifier use.

The only routine, national SIDS risk reduction intervention in the UK is currently provided by midwives and health visitors. This advice is usually in the form of a brief face-to-face discussion with mothers who have either recently given birth, or who are attending antenatal classes where information on safe sleep is included. However, as local child death review has become established there is more awareness of the number of SUDI cases occurring in the context of unsafe sleep environments. As a result, there are numerous local campaigns led by child death review teams focusing on safe sleeping. Some areas have introduced safe sleep assessments, where health visitors or midwives see where infants sleep, suggest necessary changes, and document an action plan with parents which is recorded within the parent-held child health record. Some areas have also introduced "Baby boxes" similar to those used in Finland; these provide parents with both clothing and other infant items and a safe sleep environment for the infant.

Programs to reduce the risk of SIDS for specific populations also exist embedded within other programs — for example, the Baby Steps (17) program for young parents, aimed at preventing abuse and neglect (run by the NSPCC), or the "Baby Buddy" mobile app (18), aimed at improving knowledge and uptake of health advice (developed by Best Beginnings).[1] Such programs exist in specific locations in the UK and are not currently widespread.

Two main charities in the UK promote SIDS risk reduction messages, as well as supporting bereaved families. These are The Lullaby Trust in England and Wales, and the Scottish Cot Death Trust in Scotland. Advice in Northern Ireland is distributed via the Department of Health, Social Service and Public Safety. The following list details

---

1   The Baby Buddy app can be downloaded from the Best Beginnings website: https://www.bestbeginnings. org.uk/baby-buddy.

the current SIDS risk reduction messages, correct at the time of writing and produced by The Lullaby Trust (19).

- Always place your baby on their back to sleep
- Keep your baby smoke free during pregnancy and after birth
- Breastfeed your baby, if you can
- Place your baby to sleep in a separate cot or Moses basket in the same room as you for the first 6 months
- Use a firm, flat, waterproof mattress in good condition
- Never sleep on a sofa or in an armchair with your baby
- Don't sleep in the same bed as your baby if you smoke, drink, take drugs or are extremely tired, or if your baby was born prematurely or was of low birth weight
- Avoid letting your baby get too hot
- Don't cover your baby's face or head while sleeping or use loose bedding

## Co-sleeping advice

In the UK, current advice is that the safest place for infants to sleep is their own cot, in their parents' room, but this advice does not recommend specifically that parents do not co-sleep. The National Institute for Health and Care Excellence (NICE) Guidelines for postnatal care (20) recommend that parents should be made aware of the associations between co-sleeping and SIDS and be informed that the risks from co-sleeping may be greater when parents smoke or consume alcohol or drugs, or where babies are born with low birth weight or premature. The guidelines, however, do not separate sofa sharing and bed sharing, but use the term "co-sleeping" to include both, despite the increased risk of any co-sleeping on a sofa.

# Investigation of SUDI

## The Kennedy Report

> It is every family's right to have their baby's death investigated thoroughly. (Baroness Helena Kennedy QC (23))

In the early 2000s, two mothers, Sally Clark and Angela Cannings, who had been convicted of murdering their infants, were subsequently released on appeal. Sally Clark's conviction was considered unsafe due to the failure of the pathologist conducting the post-mortem examination to disclose microbiology results; these results may or may not have been relevant to the death (21). Angela Cannings's conviction was unsafe due to a genuine disagreement between expert witnesses, therefore guilt could not be proved beyond all reasonable doubt (22). The incidence of SIDS had fallen dramatically in the 1990s following the recognition of the risks of prone sleeping and the "Reduce the

Risks" public health campaign; as a result, SUDI was much rarer and child protection issues occurred in a greater proportion of cases (7). Pediatricians had begun to feel ill-equipped to manage SUDI cases and there were concerns about the overall low standards of investigation that had led to the acquittals. As a result, a Working Group was established, chaired by Baroness Kennedy, to determine new standards for investigating unexpected infant deaths; this Working Group consisted of pediatricians, pathologists, coroners, police officers, and parent support groups. The Kennedy Report detailed a joint agency protocol for the management of SUDI (23). This protocol was based upon evidence from the CESDI SUDI study (9) and the investigative practices for SUDI that had been used in Avon for many years, led by Fleming.

## The joint agency approach

The joint agency approach (JAA) is based on the guidelines in the Kennedy Report (23) which have recently been revised and updated (24). Since 2008, in England and Wales, national statutory guidance requires that all unexpected child deaths are investigated using the JAA (25) and this process is being developed in Scotland and Northern Ireland. The aims of the JAA are to establish the complete cause of death and address the needs of family; these needs include those of emotional support, as well as potentially the safeguarding of other children. The JAA is described in detail in a previous chapter (Chapter 5) but is summarized here. The investigation is led by experienced pediatricians and the police response is provided by specialist teams with particular expertise in managing child death and child safeguarding enquiries. Key elements include taking the deceased infant to an Emergency Department, a pediatrician (possibly accompanied by the police) taking a detailed medical history from the parents, a joint examination of the scene of death by police and pediatrician, and follow-up for the parents. There is inter-agency communication throughout the JAA with a case conference to discuss the full causes of death. Coroners' investigations run independently of the JAA, although it is expected that both coroners and JAA professionals share information and assist each other's enquiries.

A recent evaluation of the JAA found that parents viewed it positively, particularly valuing the information the process provided them about why their child had died, although many wanted more emotional support to be available for them. Professionals found the joint working practices very helpful, especially the joint home visit and death scene analysis by specialist police and pediatrician (26, 27).

## Child Death Overview Panels

Since 2008, all child deaths in England and Wales are subject to scrutiny by local Child Death Overview Panels (CDOP) with the aim of improving the welfare and safety of all children in the locality (25). When any child dies, from birth to 18 years, all agencies involved with the child or family are required to provide information to the CDOP. This information is then anonymized and reviewed by a local multi-agency CDOP team. Typically, a CDOP consists of representatives from Public Health, pediatrics, maternity services, local government, police, education, and social care. Cases are discussed and a standard outcome template is completed for each child, summarizing the case and detailing cause and risk factors for death. These risk factors include those intrinsic to the child, in the family or environment, parenting capacity, and service provision. Panel members also determine whether the death is considered preventable; this is defined in the CDOP statutory guidance (25) as "those in which modifiable factors may have contributed to the death. These are factors defined as those, where, if actions could be taken through national or local interventions, the risk of future child deaths could be reduced" (p. 85).

As yet there has been no national analysis of CDOP data, although there are plans to establish a national database. An analysis of CDOP outcome data from 10 different CDOPs in the West Midlands region of England highlighted a wide variation in practice between CDOPs (15). However, in many areas, learning from CDOP has led to public health campaigns, particularly concerning safe sleep environments.

In addition to the JAA and CDOP, a Serious Case Review (SCR) is held if a child dies or is seriously harmed and child abuse or neglect may have been a factor in the death. The focus of the SCR, however, is on the involvement of different agencies with the family and on interagency processes rather than on causes or risk factors for death.

## Conclusions

As SIDS has declined dramatically in the UK, it has become more associated with social deprivation. Unsafe sleep environments remain a significant factor in the majority of SIDS cases despite public health campaigns and recommendations for healthcare professionals to promote safe sleeping with parents. Since 2008, all unexpected child deaths are investigated jointly by police, healthcare, and social care, with the aims of establishing complete causes of death as well as supporting the bereaved families. There is also local review of all child deaths in order to learn from these to improve the health and welfare of all children.

## References

1.  Sidebotham P, Fraser J, Fleming P, Ward Platt M, Hain R. Patterns of child death in England and Wales. Lancet. 2014;384(9946):904-14. https://doi.org/10.1016/S0140-6736(13)61090-9.

2.  Office for National Statistics. Unexplained deaths in infancy, England and Wales, 2013. London: Office for National Statistics, 2015.

3.  Mitchell EA. The changing epidemiology of SIDS following the national risk reduction campaigns. Pediatr Pulmonol Suppl. 1997;16:117-19. https://doi.org/10.1002/ppul.1950230865.

4.  Diamond A. "I just couldn't let go": Anne Diamond recalls the awful day she lost her son to cot death. The Daily Mail [internet]; 16 August 2011. [Available from: http://www.dailymail.co.uk/femail/article-2026392/Anne-Diamond-recalls-awful-day-lost-son-cot-death.html]. Accessed 31 October 2017.

5.  Department of Health. Back to Sleep [TV advertisement]. 1991. [Available from: https://www.youtube.com/watch?v=8Bzcsl8qlg0]. Accessed 11th Jan 2018.

6.  Her Majesty's Stationery Office. Report of the chief medical officer's expert group on the sleeping position of infants and cot death. London: Her Majesty's Stationery Office, 1993.

7.  Blair PS, Sidebotham P, Berry PJ, Evans M, Fleming PJ. Major epidemiological changes in sudden infant death syndrome: A 20-year population-based study in the UK. Lancet. 2006;367(9507):314-19. https://doi.org/10.1016/S0140-6736(06)67968-3.

8.  University of Bristol. Bristol research leads to a worldwide fall in the number of cot deaths. [Available from: http://results.ref.ac.uk/DownloadFile/ImpactCaseStudy/pdf?caseStudyId=40166. Accessed 16 September 2015.

9.  Fleming P, Blair P, Bacon C, Berry J, editors. Sudden unexpected deaths in infancy: The CESDI-SUDI Studies, 1993-1996. London: The Stationery Office, 2000.

10. Krous HF, Beckwith JB, Byard RW, Rognum TO, Bajanowski T, Corey T, et al. Sudden infant death syndrome and unclassified sudden infant deaths: A definitional and diagnostic approach. Pediatrics. 2004;114(1):234-8. https://doi.org/10.1542/peds.114.1.234.

11. Gould SJ, Weber MA, Sebire NJ. Variation and uncertainties in the classification of sudden unexpected infant deaths among paediatric pathologists in the UK: Findings of a National Delphi Study. J Clin Pathol. 2010;63(9):796-9. https://doi.org/10.1136/jcp.2010.079715.

12. Limerick SR, Bacon CJ. Terminology used by pathologists in reporting on sudden infant deaths. J Clin Pathol. 2004;57(3):309-11. https://doi.org/10.1136/jcp.2003.013052.

13. Office for National Statistics. Unexplained deaths in infancy, England and Wales, 2012. London: Office for National Statistics, 2014.

14. Taylor BJ, Garstang J, Engelberts A, Obonai T, Cote A, Freemantle J, et al. International comparison of sudden unexpected death in infancy rates using a newly proposed set of cause-of-death codes. Arch Dis Child. 2015;100(11):1018-23. https://doi.org/10.1136/archdischild-2015-308239.

15. Garstang J, Ellis C, Griffiths F, Sidebotham P. Unintentional asphyxia, SIDS, and medically explained deaths: A descriptive study of outcomes of child death review (CDR) investigations following sudden unexpected death in infancy. Forensic Sci Med Pathol. 2016;12(4):407-15. https://doi.org/10.1007/s12024-016-9802-0.

16. Blair PS, Byard RW, Fleming PJ. Sudden unexpected death in infancy (SUDI): Suggested classification and applications to facilitate research activity. Forensic Sci Med Pathol. 2012;8(3):312-15. https://doi.org/10.1007/s12024-011-9294-x.

17. NSPCC. Baby Steps: Helping parents cope with the pressures of a new baby. [Available from: http://www.nspcc.org.uk/services-and-resources/services-for-children-and-families/baby-steps/]. Accessed 31 October 2017.

18. Best Beginnings. Baby Buddy, the multi-award winning free app for parents and parents to be. [Available from: http://www.bestbeginnings.org.uk/babybuddy]. Accessed 31 October 2017.

19. The Lullaby Trust. Safer sleep for babies: A guide for parents. [Available at: https://www.lullabytrust.org.uk/wp-content/uploads/safer-sleep-for-parents.pdf]. Accessed 31 October 2017.

20. National Institute for Health and Care Excellence. Addendum to clinical guideline 37, Postnatal Care: Routine postnatal care of women and their babies. UK: National Institute for Health and Care Excellence, 2014.

21. *R v Clark* [2003] EWCA Crim 1020.

22. *R v Cannings* [2004] EWCA Crim 01.

23. Royal College of Pathologists, Royal College of Paediatrics and Child Health. Sudden unexpected death in infancy: A multi-agency protocol for care and investigation. UK: Royal College of Pathologists, Royal College of Paediatrics and Child Health, 2004.

24. Royal College of Pathologists, Royal College of Paediatrics and Child Health. Sudden unexpected death in infancy and childhood: Multi-agency guidelines for care and investigation. [Available from: https://www.rcpath.org/discover-pathology/news/new-guidelines-for-the-investigation-of-sudden-unexpected-death-in-infancy-launched.html]. Accessed 12 January 2018.

25. HM Government. Working together to safeguard children. London: Department for Education, 2015.

26. Garstang J. Why did my baby die? An evaluation of parental and professional experiences of joint agency investigations following sudden unexpected death in infancy [PhD]. [Available from: http://wrap.warwick.ac.uk/view/author_id/18088.html]. Accessed 12 January 2018.

27. Garstang J, Griffiths F, Sidebotham P. Rigour and rapport: A qualitative study of parents' and professionals' experiences of joint agency infant death investigation. BMC Pediatrics. 2017;17(1):48. https://doi.org/10.1186/s12887-017-0803-2.

# 19 A United States Perspective

Kawai O Tanabe, MPH and
Fern R Hauck, MD, MS

*Department of Family Medicine, University of Virginia
School of Medicine, Charlottesville, Virginia, USA*

## Introduction

Sudden infant death syndrome (SIDS) rates have declined significantly in the United States (US) as a result of the "Back to Sleep" campaign. Despite this and many state and local risk reduction campaigns, rates still remain high in the African American and American Indian/Alaska Native populations. The American Academy of Pediatrics (AAP) recently released (2016) updated guidelines and recommendations for a safe sleep environment (12). However, certain recommendations, especially the advice against infant bed sharing, continue to be controversial and are not followed by some groups. Further research on the reasons for non-adherence and identification of culturally acceptable and safe alternatives that address parental concerns are needed to help in targeting educational interventions in high-risk populations. In this chapter, we will address SIDS from a US perspective, covering rates and trends, interventions to reduce risk, the bed-sharing controversy, and current laws and regulations in the US.

## SIDS Rates in the US

Sudden unexpected infant death (SUID), also known as sudden unexpected death in infancy (SUDI), is defined as the sudden and unexpected death of an infant regardless of cause (1). The largest proportion of SUID deaths among all racial/ethnic groups is attributed to sudden infant death syndrome (SIDS). SIDS, a subset of SUID, is defined as "the sudden and unexpected death of an infant under 12 months of age that remains unexplained after a review of the clinical history, complete autopsy and death scene investigation" (1) (p. 681). In 2014, there were approximately 3,500 SUID deaths in the US, and 44% of them (1,500 deaths) were attributed to SIDS (2). Despite continued efforts to promote safe sleep, the SIDS mortality rates in the US have plateaued.

## Trends

In 1994, in response to studies from Europe and Australia, the *Eunice Kennedy Shriver* National Institute of Child Health and Human Development (NICHD) initiated the "Back to Sleep" campaign to help educate millions of caregivers in the US on ways to reduce the risk of SIDS (3). The campaign promoted placing babies on their back to sleep. In 2012, the NICHD expanded the campaign to emphasize safe sleep environments and back sleeping as ways to reduce SIDS and other sleep-related deaths, renaming it the "Safe to Sleep" campaign. In the years following the initial campaign, SIDS rates decreased by 50% in the US (3). This decline was consistent with the decline in prone sleeping (4). However, despite ongoing efforts to promote safe sleep, recent declines in SIDS mortality rates have been smaller, and, as of 2014, the SIDS mortality rate is 39 deaths per 100,000 live births (5).

## Racial/ethnic disparities

SUID and SIDS mortality rates, like other infant mortality causes, have substantial racial and ethnic disparities (3). For example, the SUID death rates in the US from 2010-13 were 190.5 deaths per 100,000 live births for American Indian/Alaska Natives and 171.8 deaths per 100,000 live births for non-Hispanic black infants, which were more than two times those for non-Hispanic white infants (84.4 deaths per 100,000 live births) (6). The mortality rate due to SIDS was 83% higher (73.3 deaths per 100,000 live births) in non-Hispanic black infants and 95% higher (78.3 deaths per 100,000 live births) in American Indian/Alaskan Native infants compared to non-Hispanic white infants (40.1 deaths per 100,000 live births) (7). This may in part be explained by the difference in prevalence of supine sleep position and other sleep environments among the different racial and ethnic groups (8). The National Infant Sleep Position Study (NISP) found that the prevalence of supine positioning was 53% among black infants, 73% among Hispanic infants, and 75% among white infants (4, 8). Similarly, bed sharing and the use of soft bedding were also more common among black families (3, 9, 10). A recent study showed that there is an overall increasing trend in the number of infants who usually share a bed or other sleep surface (11). The same study found that black infants are 3.5 times more likely to share a bed than white infants (11), and that this trend is increasing for black infants while remaining unchanged among white infants.

# Recommendations for a Safe Infant Sleep Environment, Controversies and Barriers to Adherence

## Recommendations

The AAP Task Force on SIDS recently released its updated 2016 recommendations for a safe sleep environment (Table 19.1) (12). The guidelines include supine sleep for every sleep; using a firm sleep surface; room sharing without bed sharing; and avoiding soft bedding and overheating. Additional recommendations include using a pacifier; avoiding smoke exposure, alcohol and illicit drug use; breastfeeding; obtaining regular prenatal care; and receiving routine immunizations (12).

Table 19.1: Summary of 2016 AAP Safe Sleep Recommendations. (Based on the recommendations of the AAP and adapted from Table 2 in (12).)

| Safe Sleep Recommendations | |
|---|---|
| 1. | Back to sleep for every sleep |
| 2. | Use a firm sleep surface |
| 3. | Breastfeeding is recommended |
| 4. | Room sharing without bed sharing ideally for the first year of life, but at least for the first 6 months |
| 5. | Keep soft objects and loose bedding away from the infant's sleep area |
| 6. | Consider offering a pacifier at naptime and bedtime |
| 7. | Avoid smoke exposure during pregnancy and after birth |
| 8. | Avoid alcohol and illicit drug use during pregnancy and after birth |
| 9. | Avoid overheating and head covering in infants |
| 10. | Pregnant women should obtain regular prenatal care |
| 11. | Infants should be immunized in accordance with AAP and CDC recommendations |
| 12. | Do not use home cardiorespiratory monitors as a strategy to reduce the risk of SIDS |
| 13. | Healthcare providers and childcare providers should endorse and model the SIDS risk reduction recommendations from birth |
| 14. | Media and manufacturers should follow safe sleep guidelines in their messaging and advertising |
| 15. | Continue the "Safe to Sleep" campaign, focusing on ways to reduce the risk of all sleep-related infant deaths |

| 16. | Avoid the use of commercial devices that are inconsistent with safe sleep recommendations |
|-----|---|
| 17. | Supervised, awake tummy time is recommended |
| 18. | Continue research and surveillance on the risk factors, causes, and pathophysiologic mechanisms of SIDS and other sleep-related deaths |
| 19. | No evidence to recommend swaddling as a strategy to reduce the risk of SIDS |

## Common controversies

There has been considerable controversy in the US regarding the AAP recommendations advising against parent-infant bed sharing. The epidemiologic evidence supports this recommendation (13). Adult beds are not designed for infant safety, and often contain other bedding materials, such as pillows and comforters, which may increase the risk of SIDS as well as death due to other causes, including asphyxia and suffocation, and unintentional injuries, such as falls. There is growing concern among public health and SIDS program professionals about bed sharing because of the rising number of deaths attributed to accidental strangulation and suffocation in bed (14). Nonetheless, bed sharing is common; up to 60% of mothers of infants reported bed sharing at least once within the infant's first year of life (15). In a national survey of mothers of infants under 8 months of age, 14% reported routinely bed sharing in the prior two weeks (3).

There are many reasons given by mothers for sleeping with their infants, including facilitating feeding (breastfeeding or formula), comforting a fussy or sick infant, helping with sleep for mother and infant, bonding, cultural tradition, and feeling that babies are safest when close to their mother. Some breastfeeding advocacy groups encourage bed sharing to promote breastfeeding, including longer duration and exclusivity (3). They argue that bed sharing is safe among infants who are breastfed (a protective factor for SIDS) and infants whose mothers do not smoke, drink alcohol, or use illicit substances. However, this issue is still being debated; two recent analyses (from studies outside the US) reached different conclusions and recommendations (see Chapter 10) (3, 16, 17).

The new AAP guidelines recognize that mothers often fall asleep while nursing their infants, and that it is safer to fall asleep while nursing in bed than on a couch, sofa, or armchair (12). It is recommended that mothers return their infants to their own sleep surface once they awaken. It is also recommended that bedding that could cause head covering or airway obstruction should be removed from the adult bed.

## Barriers to adherence

The barriers determining infant sleeping practices are complex and often involve behavioral, environmental, and biological factors. Most parents base their decisions about sleep location on their perception of the infant's comfort and convenience for the parent. However, a large study of African American mothers in Washington, DC found that they had different views about what they considered comfortable (18). Some thought that infants who slept longer were most comfortable while others thought the surface should not be too thin or too hard. Many mothers also had different definitions for what was considered a "firm" sleep surface, with some believing that a taut surface equaled a firm surface, so it would be acceptable to place pillows or blankets on top of a taut sheet (18). Parents may also opt to bed share in order to monitor the infant more closely or breastfeed and bond with the infant (19, 20).

Some of the socioeconomic and environmental factors discussed by these mothers for bed sharing involved not having space to put a crib, not having money to buy a crib, or worrying about dangers from insects, kidnappings, or stray gunfire (20). Other reasons for not adhering to the recommended safe sleep practices included not trusting the guidelines due to the inconsistencies in the recommendations over the years, as well as observing the practices and behaviors of their healthcare providers, who did not endorse or model safe sleep guidelines (19, 21). In another study that included African American and American Indian mothers in Michigan, similar barriers were identified, including concerns for infant safety and the perception that an infant placed in the supine position will choke, despite evidence against this (19, 22).

Further discussion with these two cohorts of mothers examined their beliefs and behaviors related to SIDS and safe sleep (19, 22). The investigators found that regardless of socioeconomic backgrounds, there were three major themes that explained their beliefs regarding SIDS: [1] lack of plausibility (not understanding how recommendations to reduce the risk of SIDS could be defined for an entity that has an "unknown cause"; [2] randomness ("God's will"); and [3] parental vigilance (the belief that as long as the parent was near the infant, SIDS would not happen) (19, 22). Many of the mothers did not see the usefulness of following safe sleep practices unless they could be guaranteed that SIDS would not occur if they followed the guidelines.

Results from these studies suggest that education about safe sleep recommendations needs to go hand in hand with detailed explanations about the reasons behind the recommendations and more definitive descriptions about our understanding of SIDS causation (18-22). In addition, the meaning of terms that are used in the recommendations, such as "firm sleep surface", needs to be better explained, and mothers should be asked by healthcare providers about their understanding of the recommendations, to allow clarification if any misunderstandings exist.

## Interventions to Reduce the Risk of SIDS

Healthcare providers play an important role in modeling AAP recommendations and influencing parents and caregivers on safe sleep behaviors (23). Unfortunately, a recent study showed that more than half of healthcare providers are inconsistent with modeling safe sleep practices in the hospital and teaching safe sleep recommendations to parents (24). There have been multiple interventions implemented to reduce the risk of SIDS by encouraging parents to follow safe sleep guidelines. A recent systematic review of safe sleep interventions internationally from 1990-2015 found 29 studies that met the inclusion criteria, 22 of which were based in the US (25). Of the 29 studies, 19 targeted families and infant caregivers, 8 targeted healthcare professionals, and 2 targeted childcare professionals. Some of the more commonly targeted behaviors for the interventions included SIDS knowledge, sleep location, and infant sleep position. Out of the 8 US studies measuring SIDS knowledge, 7 of them found significant differences in knowledge while 1 found no significant difference after the intervention (25). Of the 10 US studies that measured sleep location (use of crib in the parents' room), only 3 of them reported that their interventions were successful in increasing the rates of using a crib (25). Of the 14 US studies, 7 that measured infant sleep position concluded that their interventions were successful in changing the rates of, or intention to use, supine sleep position (25); 6 found no significant differences, while 1 study reported increased rates of supine sleep position, but did not report statistical significance (25). However, a recent study conducted in Ohio that was not included in the systematic review found that by implementing a statewide quality improvement collaborative and providing Maintenance of Certification (MOC) Part IV participation (part of the process required for US physicians to retain specialty board certification), they were able to show an improvement in infant safe sleep practices across their six children's hospitals (23).

There are many national, statewide and local efforts to educate mothers and nurses on safe sleep. A recent review discussed several safe sleep interventions and examined evidence of their effectiveness (26). Interventions that focused on health messaging include a public health campaign in 2009 on safe sleep in the city of Baltimore, Maryland, called 'B'more for Healthy Babies' (BHB). Up until then, Baltimore had one of the highest infant mortality rates in the US (27). The city created a video, with testimonials from three Baltimore parents who lost their infants while bed sharing, called "SLEEP SAFE: Alone, Back, Crib. No Exceptions". The video is shown to all mothers while they are in the hospital, in addition to other sites including the Special Supplemental Nutrition Program for Women, Infants and Children (WIC) sites, city detention centers, Department of Social Services, and jury duty locations (26). BHB's SLEEP SAFE initiative includes media campaigns, community outreach, and provider education. In addition to declining infant mortality rates, Baltimore has also seen a 40% decrease in the racial disparities between African American and white infants from 2009-12 (27).

One of the more provocative health messaging campaigns regarding safe sleep came from the Milwaukee, Wisconsin's Department of Health. The city had 89 infant deaths related to SIDS or SUID, and, of those, 52% were bed sharing at the time of their death (28). In response to these statistics, Milwaukee public health officials developed a campaign that used extreme fear-invoking messages to generate attention. Much like the anti-smoking campaigns that show images of diseased lungs, the city in 2010 showed a photograph of a tombstone instead of a headboard at the top of an adult bed, with the phrase "For too many babies last year, this was their final resting place". In 2011, another ad of an infant sleeping in an adult bed next to a butcher's knife with the slogan "Your baby sleeping with you can be just as dangerous" was posted. No formal evaluation of this campaign was conducted; however, the Department of Health reported that the requests for free cribs increased in the years following the campaign (26, 28).

Other interventions focus on breaking down barriers and increasing accessibility. The Cribs for Kids National Infant Safe Sleep Initiative is a national coalition of non-profit organizations that provide free cribs to low-income families that may not be able to afford one. The program also provides education on safe sleep to parents and caregivers. The Women, Infants and Children (WIC) programs in several states also provide books, brochures, and vouchers with safe sleep messages (29). One study surveyed a sample of crib recipients in Pennsylvania and found that 38% of infants would have slept in the same bed as an adult had they not received a crib (30). Bedtime Basics for Babies was another program that provided free cribs and safe sleep education to high-risk families in Washington, DC, Indiana, and Washington state (31). Eligible families received a portable crib, a crib sheet, a wearable blanket, a pacifier, and safe sleep education. Families also watched an informational video on safe sleep and were asked to participate in a survey before and after crib receipt. Knowledge of recommended infant sleep position improved from 76% to 94% (p<0.001), and intended use of supine position also increased from 80% to 87% (p<0.001) after receipt of the intervention (31). The study found that crib distribution and safe sleep education together successfully changed the participants' knowledge about safe sleep and the placement of infants on their backs in their own crib for sleep (31).

There continues to be resistance to safe sleep guidelines among professionals; therefore, interventions have been developed that focus on the education of healthcare professionals (26). Cribs for Kids supports a Safe Sleep Hospital Initiative, which is a "hospital certification program awarding recognition to hospitals that demonstrate a commitment to community leadership for best practices and education on infant sleep safety" (32). The program was developed in 2008 and aims to reduce the risk of injury and death to infants while sleeping. The program's goal is to provide accurate and consistent safe sleep information to all hospital personnel, enable hospitals to model safe sleep practices, and provide consistent and repeated safe sleep information to parents and caregivers (33).

Breastfeeding is recommended to reduce the risk of SIDS. The Baby Friendly Hospital Initiative is an international program that was launched by the World Health Organization (WHO) and the United Nations Children's Fund (UNICEF). The initiative recognizes hospitals that offer the best possible care for infant feeding and mother-infant bonding. The program is a comprehensive model including education, policy change, and training of all hospital personnel using tools such as the Ten Steps to Successful Breastfeeding (34). Currently, there are more than 450 US hospitals and birthing centers in all 50 states, the District of Columbia and the Commonwealth of Puerto Rico that are designated as Baby-Friendly facilities (34).

## Laws and Regulations

Many states have laws related to SIDS and protocols for autopsies of SIDS cases. At least 12 states have laws requiring firefighters, emergency medical technicians, law enforcement officials, or childcare workers to take special training on SIDS (35). Studies have estimated that 20% of SIDS deaths in the US occur in childcare settings where they have been placed prone to sleep (36, 37). Approximately 17 states have required SIDS risk reduction education for all childcare providers; however, these regulations are only applicable to licensed childcare centers and not to family childcare homes, which are difficult to identify (26).

In addition to legislation and regulations around childcare professionals, a recent area of focus has been around the use of crib bumpers. Maryland's Department of Health and Mental Hygiene (DHMH) and the city of Chicago, Illinois have laws that ban the sale of crib bumpers. Crib bumpers, which are designed to wrap around the crib slats, were initially developed to prevent entrapment of an infant's head between the slats of the crib. However, crib standards now require the width between the slats to be less than 2 3/8" (approximately 6 cm), which removed the need for crib bumpers (3). Crib bumpers have been implicated in deaths attributed to suffocation, strangulation, and entrapment (38). The Maryland DHMH and the city of Chicago concluded that the crib bumpers offer no benefit and pose a risk of suffocation and death. The recent AAP guidelines also state that they do not recommend the use of crib bumpers because of the potential for suffocation, entrapment, and strangulation (3).

There are other commercially available products on the market today, such as special mattresses, sleep devices, sleep surfaces, wedges, and positioners, which are labeled as protective against the risk of SIDS. However, they are often made of soft, compressible material which may increase the risk of suffocation (3). Furthermore, there is no scientific evidence to back up these claims. Due to the lack of scientific evidence and the potential risk of suffocation, entrapment, and strangulation with these products, the AAP, along with the Consumer Product Safety Commission (CPSC) and the Food and Drug Administration (FDA), warns against their use, unless they meet CPSC safety standards — for example, in the case of special crib mattresses or sleep surfaces (3).

## Conclusions

Deaths from SIDS in the US have declined by over 50% as a result of national guidelines and campaigns, as well as many other interventions at the state and local levels. However, certain recommendations, especially the advice against infant bed sharing, continue to be controversial and are not followed by certain groups within the population. Research is needed to further understand the reasons for non-adherence to recommendations and to identify, where possible, culturally acceptable, safe alternatives and prudent policies.

## Acknowledgements

Ms Tanabe and Dr Hauck are grateful to their families for their support and encouragement, and to the SIDS community for their tireless work on behalf of infants and families.

## References

1.  Willinger M, James LS, Catz C. Defining the sudden infant death syndrome (SIDS): Deliberations of an expert panel convened by the National Institute of Child Health and Human Development. Pediatr Pathol. 1991;11:677-84. https://doi.org/10.3109/15513819109065465.

2.  Centers for Disease Control and Prevention. Sudden unexpected infant death and sudden infant death syndrome: About SUID and SIDS. [Available at: http://www.cdc.gov/sids/aboutsuidandsids.htm]. Accessed 17 November 2016.

3.  Moon RY. SIDS and other sleep-related infant deaths: Evidence base for 2016 updated recommendations for a safe infant sleeping environment. Pediatrics. 2016;138(5):e20162940. https://doi.org/10.1542/peds.2016-2940.

4.  Colson ER, Rybin D, Smith LA, Colton T, Lister G, Corwin MJ. Trends and factors associated with infant sleeping position: The National Infant Sleep Position study, 1993-2007. Arch Pediatr Adolesc Med. 2009;163(12):1122-8. https://doi.org/10.1001/archpediatrics.2009.234.

5.  Centers for Disease Control and Prevention. CDC wonder. [Available at: https://wonder.cdc.gov/]. Accessed 9 January 2017.

6.  Centers for Disease Control and Prevention. Sudden unexpected infant death and sudden infant death syndrome: Data and statistics. [Available at: https://www.cdc.gov/sids/data.htm]. Accessed 17 November 2016.

7.  Mathews TJ, MacDorman MF, Thoma ME. Infant mortality statistics from the 2013 period linked birth/infant death data set. Natl Vital Stat Rep. 2015;64(9):1-30.

8.  Hauck FR, Moore CM, Herman SM, Donovan M, Kalelkar M, Christoffel KK, et al. The contribution of prone sleeping position to the racial disparity in sudden infant death syndrome: The Chicago infant mortality study. Pediatrics. 2002;110(4):772-80. https://doi.org/10.1542/peds.110.4.772.

9.  Shapiro-Mendoza CK, Colson ER, Willinger M, Rybin DV, Camperlengo L, Corwin MJ. Trends in infant bedding use: The National Infant Sleep Position Study, 1993-2010. Pediatrics. 2015;135(1):10-17. https://doi.org/10.1542/peds.2014-1793.

10. Flick L, White DK, Vemulapalli C, Stulac BB, Kemp JS. Sleep position and the use of soft bedding during bed sharing among African American infants at increased risk for sudden infant death syndrome. J Pediatr. 2001;138(3):338-43. https://doi.org/10.1067/mpd.2001.111428.

11. Colson ER, Willinger M, Rybin D, Heeren T, Smith LA, Lister G, et al. Trends and factors associated with infant bed sharing, 1993-2010: The National Infant Sleep Position Study. JAMA Pediatr. 2013;167(11):1032-7. https://doi.org/10.1001/jamapediatrics.2013.2560.

12. Moon RY, & Task Force on Sudden Infant Death Syndrome. SIDS and other sleep-related infant deaths: Updated 2016 recommendations for a safe infant sleeping environment. Pediatrics. 2016;138(5):e20162940. https://doi.org/10.1542/peds.2016-2940.

13. Vennemann MM, Hense HW, Bajanowski T, Blair PS, Complojer C, Moon RY, et al. Bed sharing and the risk of sudden infant death syndrome: Can we resolve the debate? J Pediatr. 2012;160(1):44-8.e2. https://doi.org/10.1016/j.jpeds.2011.06.052.

14. Shapiro-Mendoza CK, Kimball M, Tomashek KM, Anderson RN, Blanding S. US infant mortality trends attributable to accidental suffocation and strangulation in bed from 1984 through 2004: Are rates increasing? Pediatrics. 2009;123(2):533-9. https://doi.org/10.1542/peds.2007-3746.

15. Kendall-Tackett K, Cong Z, Hale TW. Mother-infant sleep locations and nighttime feeding behavior: US data from the survey of mothers' sleep and fatigue. Clinical Lactation. 2010;1(1):27-31. https://doi.org/10.1891/215805310807011837.

16. Blair PS, Sidebotham P, Pease A, Fleming PJ. Bed-sharing in the absence of hazardous circumstances: Is there a risk of sudden infant death syndrome? An analysis from two case-control studies conducted in the UK. PLoS One. 2014;9(9):e107799. https://doi.org/10.1371/journal.pone.0107799.

17. Carpenter R, McGarvey C, Mitchell EA, Tappin DM, Vennemann MM, Smuk M, et al. Bed sharing when parents do not smoke: Is there a risk of SIDS? An individual level analysis of five major case-control studies. BMJ Open. 2013;3(5):e002299. https://doi.org/10.1136/bmjopen-2012-002299.

18. Ajao TI, Oden RP, Joyner BL, Moon RY. Decisions of black parents about infant bedding and sleep surfaces: A qualitative study. Pediatrics. 2011;128:494-502. https://doi.org/10.1542/peds.2011-0072.

19. Moon RY, Oden RP, Joyner BL, Ajao TI. Qualitative analysis of beliefs and perceptions about sudden infant death syndrome in African-American mothers: Implications for safe sleep recommendations. J Pediatr. 2010;157(1):92-7.e2. https://doi.org/10.1016/j.jpeds.2010.01.027.

20. Joyner BL, Oden R, Ajao TI, Moon R. Where should my baby sleep? A qualitative study of African-American infant sleep location decisions. J Natl Med Assoc. 2010;102:881-9. https://doi.org/10.1016/S0027-9684(15)30706-9.

21. Oden R, Joyner BL, Ajao TI, Moon R. Factors influencing African-American mothers' decisions about sleep position: A qualitative study. J Natl Med Assoc. 2010;102:870-80. https://doi.org/10.1016/S0027-9684(15)30705-7.

22. Herman S, Adkins M, Moon RY. Knowledge and beliefs of African-American and American Indian parents and supporters about infant safe sleep. J Community Health. 2015;40(1):12-19. https://doi.org/10.1007/s10900-014-9886-y.

23. Macklin JR, Gittelman MA, Denny SA, Southworth H, Arnold MW. The EASE quality improvement project: Improving safe sleep practices in Ohio children's hospitals. Pediatrics. 2016;138(4):e20154267. https://doi.org/10.1542/peds.2015-4267.

24. Bullock LF, Mickey K, Green J, Heine A. Are nurses acting as role models for the prevention of SIDS? Am J Matern Child Nurs. 2004;29(3):172-7. https://doi.org/10.1097/00005721-200405000-00008.

25. Salm Ward TC, Balfour GM. Infant safe sleep interventions, 1990-2015: A review. J Community Health. 2016;41(1):180-96. https://doi.org/10.1007/s10900-015-0060-y.

26. Moon RY, Hauck FR, Colson ER. Safe infant sleep interventions: What is the evidence for successful behavior change? Curr Pediatr Rev. 2016;12(1):67-75. https://doi.org/10.2174/1573396311666151026110148.

27. Baltimore City Health Department. B'more for healthy babies: Infant mortality statistics and research. [Available at: http://www.healthybabiesbaltimore.com/about-bhb/infant-mortality-statistics-and-research]. Accessed 17 November 2016.

28. Milwaukee Health Department. Safe sleep campaign. [Available at: http://city.milwaukee.gov/health/Safe-Sleep-Campaign#.WHOmj7mTUg4]. Accessed 17 November 2016.

29. Association of State and Territorial Health Officials. Safe sleep factsheet. [Available at: http://www.astho.org/Maternal-and-Child-Health/Safe-Sleep/]. Accessed 17 November 2016.

30. Carlins EM, Collins KS. Cribs for kids: Risk and reduction of sudden infant death syndrome and accidental suffocation. Health Soc Work. 2007;32(3):225-9. https://doi.org/10.1093/hsw/32.3.225.

31. Hauck FR, Tanabe KO, McMurry T, Moon RY. Evaluation of bedtime basics for babies: A national crib distribution program to reduce the risk of sleep-related sudden infant deaths. J Community Health. 2015;40(3):457-63. https://doi.org/10.1007/s10900-014-9957-0.

32. Bannon JA. The National Safe Sleep Hospital certification program. [Available at: http://www.cribsforkids.org/hospitalinitiative/registration/]. Accessed 18 November 2016.

33. Bannon JA, Goodstein MH. Safe sleep hospital certification. [Available at: http://www.cribsforkids.org/instructions-starting-a-hospital-based-safe-sleep-program/]. Accessed 18 November 2016.

34. Baby-Friendly USA. Baby-friendly hospital initiative. [Available at: https://www.babyfriendlyusa.org/]. Accessed 5 March 2018.

35. National Conference of State Legislatures. Sudden unexpected infant death legislation. [Available at: http://www.ncsl.org/research/health/sudden-infant-death-syndrome-laws.aspx]. Accessed 18 November 2016.

36. Moon RY, Sprague BM, Patel KM. Stable prevalence but changing risk factors for sudden infant death syndrome in child care settings in 2001. Pediatrics. 2005;116(4):972-7. https://doi.org/10.1542/peds.2005-0924.

37. Moon RY, Patel KM, Shaefer JM. Sudden infant death syndrome in child care settings. Pediatrics. 2000;106(2):295-300. https://doi.org/10.1542/peds.106.2.295.

38. Thach BT, Rutherford GW Jr, Harris K. Deaths and injuries attributed to infant crib bumper pads. J Pediatr. 2007;151(3):271-4. https://doi.org/10.1016/j.jpeds.2007.04.028.

# 20 A Scandinavian Perspective

Torleiv Ole Rognum, MD, MHA, PhD[1,2],
Åshild Vege, MD, PhD[1,2],
Arne Stray-Pedersen, MD, PhD[1,2] and
Lillian Bøylestad[1]

[1]Section of Pediatric Forensic Medicine, Department of Forensic Sciences,
Oslo University Hospital, Norway
[2]Department of Forensic Medicine, Division of Laboratory Medicine,
University of Oslo, Norway

## Introduction

In the 1980s, sudden infant death syndrome (SIDS) in Norway made up half of all post-neonatal deaths, and more than 80% of all sudden unexpected deaths during the first year after birth. As in most Western countries, the rate of SIDS in Scandinavian countries dropped dramatically after 1990 (the era of safe sleep campaigns). Before 1990 the police attended the death scene following a sudden death in an infant, as in all other cases of sudden unexpected deaths, regardless of age. Due to massive criticisms from parents who felt incriminated, the Prosecutor General in 1991 withdrew the police from the scene of death in infants. Since the diagnosis of SIDS requires performance of a death scene investigation, an initiative was necessary. This chapter discusses SIDS in Scandinavia and the issues faced regarding death scene investigations.

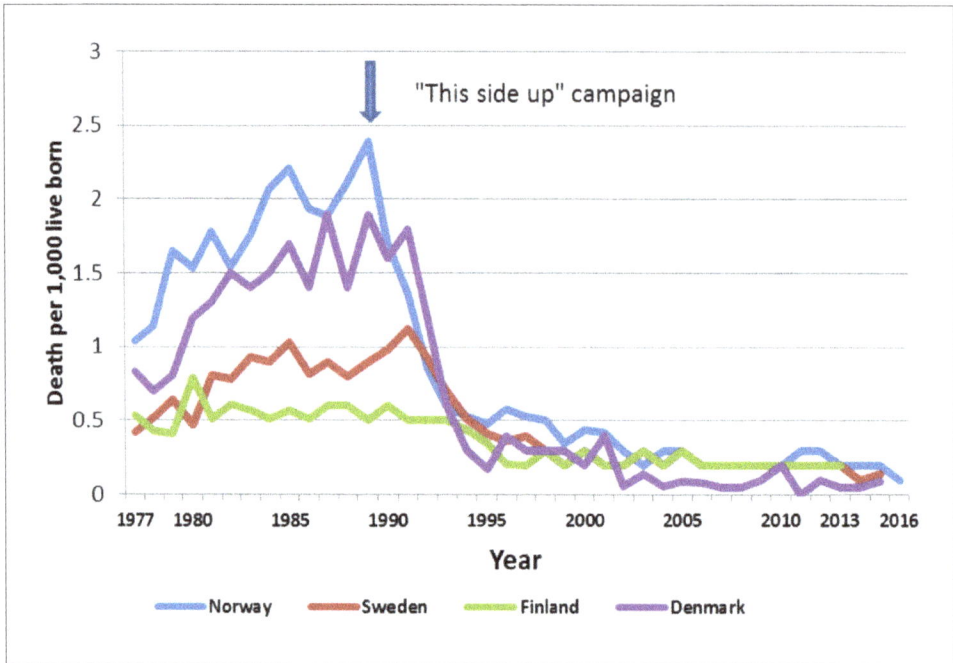

Figure 20.1: SIDS rates in the Nordic countries 1977-2013. (Reproduced with permission from Statistics Norway and the National Boards of Health in Sweden, Denmark and Finland.)

## SIDS Epidemic

Of the Scandinavian countries, Norway and Denmark were most severely hit by the SIDS epidemic in the 1980s (1). In Sweden and Finland the epidemic was less dramatic (1). As in all Western countries, the "this side up" campaign led to a dramatic drop in the SIDS rate. In Norway the SIDS rate has dropped from 2.4 per 1,000 live-born to 0.15 per 1,000 live-born in 2016 (Figure 20.1).

### The SIDS epidemic: Real or due to a diagnostic shift?

The question as to whether the dramatic reduction in SIDS rate might partly be due to a change in diagnostic practice has been ruled out in Norway. Looking at the total post-neonatal mortality, there was an increase during the 1980s and a decline during the 1990s, in parallel with the drop in SIDS rates (Figure 20.2).

## The SIDS Diagnosis

Since SIDS is a diagnosis of exclusion (2), it is necessary to perform an extensive autopsy, including comprehensive histology, microbiology, X-ray examination, toxicology, genetic

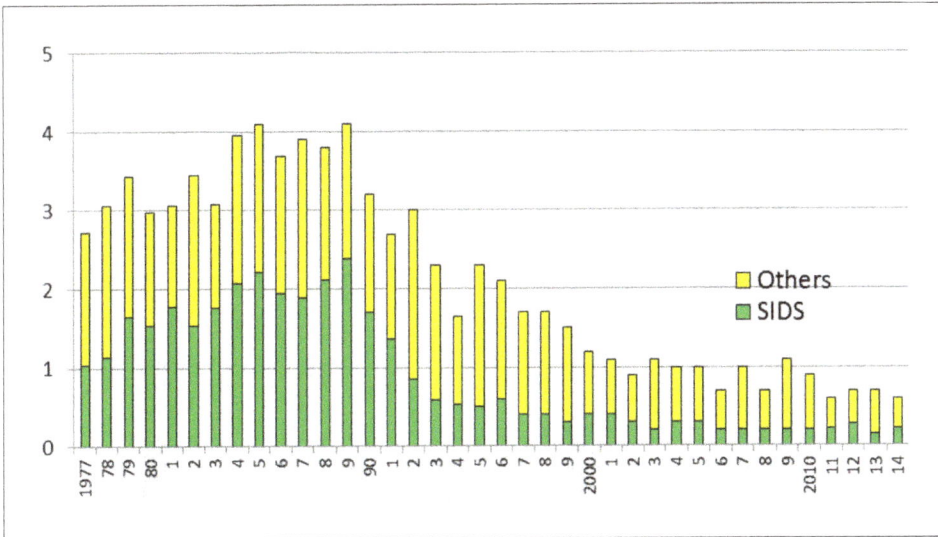

Figure 20.2: Post-neonatal death rate in Norway 1977-2015. (Reproduced with permission from Statistics Norway.) Green column = SIDS. Yellow column = other causes of death. Post-neonatal death rates increase and decline in parallel with the increase and decline in SIDS rate. Thus the SIDS epidemic was not due to shift in diagnostic practice.

testing, and metabolic screening before concluding that SIDS is the cause of death. It is also mandatory to perform a death scene investigation. In Norway all of these diagnostic tools, in addition to a CT scan, are included. Full metabolic screening is not yet operative. We do, however, perform testing for medium-chain acyl-CoA dehydrogenase deficiency (MCAD) mutation, and plan to add full metabolic screening in the future. The result of the autopsy is discussed in an interdisciplinary case conference and the final diagnosis given. The case conference also discusses whether the death could have been prevented.

## Controversy about death scene investigations

Death scene investigation has been a matter of controversy in Norway. Before 1990 the police would go to the death scene in all cases of sudden death in infants. Due to some unfortunate episodes in which uniformed police had been interrogating the parents in their homes immediately after the infant had been found dead, there were protests in the media. The grief process was further disturbed when the family would receive a letter from the police three months after the loss of their child informing them that the criminal case was dismissed (3).

The public protest regarding this situation resulted in the withdrawal of the police from the scene of sudden death in infants in 1991. The police were instructed to order a

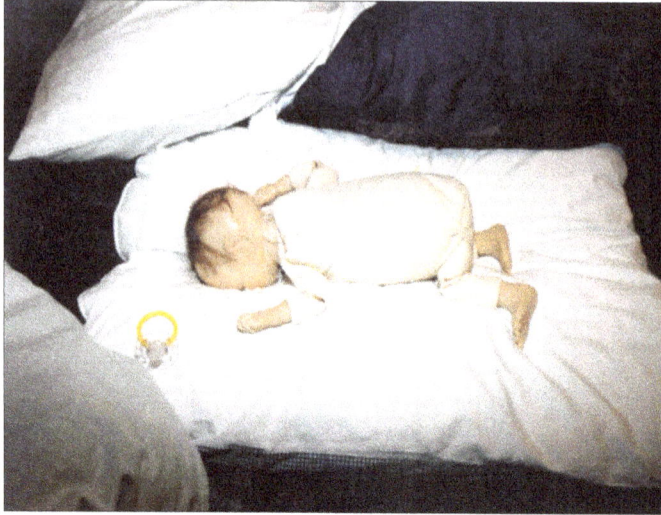

Figure 20.3: Doll reconstruction during death scene investigation: the position in which an infant was found dead, placed between the parents in a double bed with an adult duvet on the top. The infant's own duvet had served as a mattress. (Authors' photograph.)

forensic autopsy in all cases, and the nearest department of pediatrics together with the primary healthcare became responsible for the follow-up of the family.

Pilot study of the effectiveness of death scene investigations

It turned out that the withdrawal of the police from the death scene, not replacing them with other personnel, was a mistake. Thus in the period 2001-04 a research project with voluntary death scene visits was launched. The visit was performed by the forensic pathologist who had performed the autopsy, together with an expert with a police background. This visit was to take place within 48 hours after the infant was found dead. There were 69 deaths in the test period and 46 death scene investigations were performed (4).

During the death scene visit, a thorough history was obtained, including information about the pregnancy, birth, and newborn period, as well as what happened during the last week before death. The position in which the infant was put to sleep and how he or she was found dead were reconstructed by means of a doll (Figure 20.3). After the autopsy was finished and all laboratory findings were available, there was a multidisciplinary case conference in which a conclusion was made as to the cause of death.

Death scene investigation was of significance for the diagnosis in 32% of the cases (4). The most important finding of the pilot project was disclosure of seven cases of neglect. In the four years prior to the pilot project, we only discovered two cases of neglect. Conversely, in 14 cases with initial suspicion of a criminal act, the case could be immediately dismissed as non-criminal after the death scene visit (4). Evaluation by a crisis psychologist, who performed a qualitative interview study of the families five weeks after the death scene visit, was very favorable for the project (5).

## Assessing associated risk factors

Risk factors, such as prone sleeping, parental smoking, and overheating were registered, scored, and compared to scores based on information from age- and sex-matched controls from the same area. The control study was performed by means of a questionnaire asking families about housing, smoking habits, and sleeping position of their infants during the day of the SIDS death. The risk factor scores were significantly higher in the SIDS cases than in the controls (4).

## Lessons learned regarding death scene investigations from the pilot study

The pilot study concluded that death scene investigations should be mandatory (4). This recommendation induced an intense debate in Norway. In the end, Parliament decided that the death scene investigation of sudden deaths in infants and small children (0 to 4 years) should be voluntary and should be organized as a health service. The voluntary death scene investigation in infants and small children should be offered after the police had finished their initial investigation. Moreover, the police were instructed to investigate all cases of sudden unexpected deaths in children from birth to 18 years of age.

The handling of these deaths is complicated by a paragraph in the Norwegian constitution saying that house examination may only be performed in criminal cases. This means that the police are not allowed to enter a family's home without consent from the parents, after the dead child has been moved from the scene — that is, brought to the nearest hospital. Otherwise, police need a reason for suspicion of a criminal nature and a decision by the court. The result is that in a proportion of cases there will be no death scene investigation, either by the police or by health services (represented by the forensic pathologist and the expert with police background).[1] This is a challenge that has yet to be solved.

## New legislation and regulations of the investigation in sudden unexpected deaths in children in Norway

After several years of debate, the Norwegian Parliament decided that voluntary death scene visits should be offered to all families who have lost an infant or small child suddenly and unexpectedly. The service was operative by 1 November 2010. The

---

1   This result comes from unpublished observation.

Institute of Forensic Medicine in Oslo became responsible for the death scene visits. Three people with police education serve the whole country. They perform the visits in co-operation with the forensic pathologist who performed the autopsy.

After a revision of the *Criminal Procedure Act 2011* (*"Criminal Procedure Act"*), it has become police duty to investigate all sudden unexpected deaths in children up to 18 years of age. If the police do not find anything of a criminal nature, the family of children aged from birth to 4 years are offered a voluntary death scene visit. If the forensic pathologist and the death scene examiner discover suspicious findings, they have to report to the police without regard to professional secrecy. To many medical doctors and jurists, this method seems odd. A mandatory death scene investigation performed by police and medical experts in all cases of sudden unexpected deaths in children would have been preferable.

## Experience with the new legislation

By December 2015 there had been 173 sudden unexpected deaths in the age group from birth to 4 years in Norway. A voluntary death scene visit was offered to 86 families and

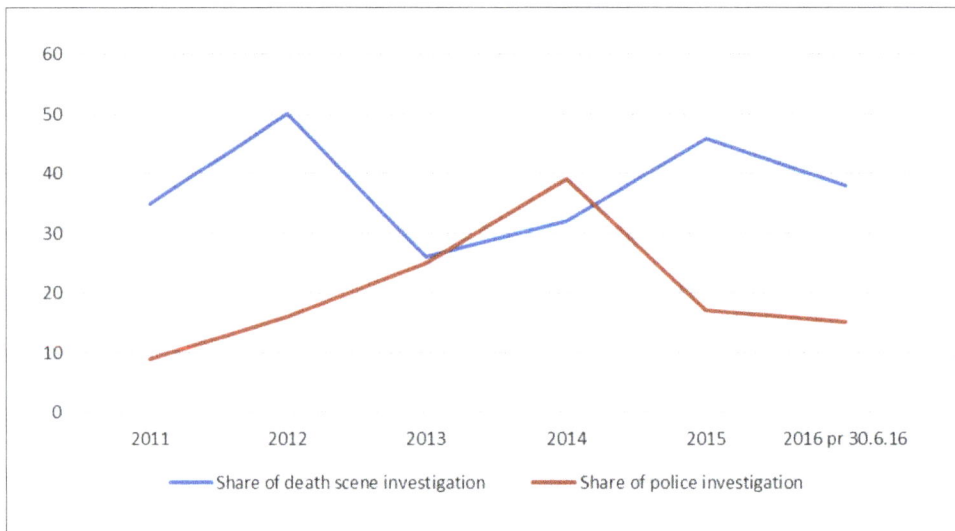

Figure 20.4: Development in the proportion of cases of police investigation and voluntary death scene investigation as a percentage of all cases in the period 2011 to 30 June 2016. X-axis represents year; Y-axis represents percentage of all cases. In sudden unexplained deaths or suspected maltreatment occurring in hospitals, death scene investigations are usually not performed. This figure shows the distribution of sudden unexpected deaths in infants and small children (0-4 years) and the proportion of voluntary death scene visits in the different parts of Norway. The Oslo region has 55% of the total population of 5.2 million. (Authors' own work.)

67 gave informed consent. The proportion of cases with a voluntary death scene visit has varied between 30% and 50% (Figure 20.4). The highest proportion of voluntary death scene visits was seen in the north of Norway, whereas Oslo had the highest number of visits (Figure 20.5). No visits were performed in Trondheim, probably due to a lack of dedicated forensic pathologists in this region.

The distribution of police investigation and voluntary death scene visits has varied throughout the period since 2010 (Figure 20.4). After a revision of the *Criminal Procedure Act* in 2011, death scene investigations by the police increased from 10% to 40% in 2014 (Figure 20.4). Since 2014 there has been a decline in death scene investigations by the police (Figure 20.4). Approximately 10% of the families do not have a death scene investigation by the police nor by health services. In sudden unexplained deaths in newborns occurring in hospital, there is most often no scene examination.

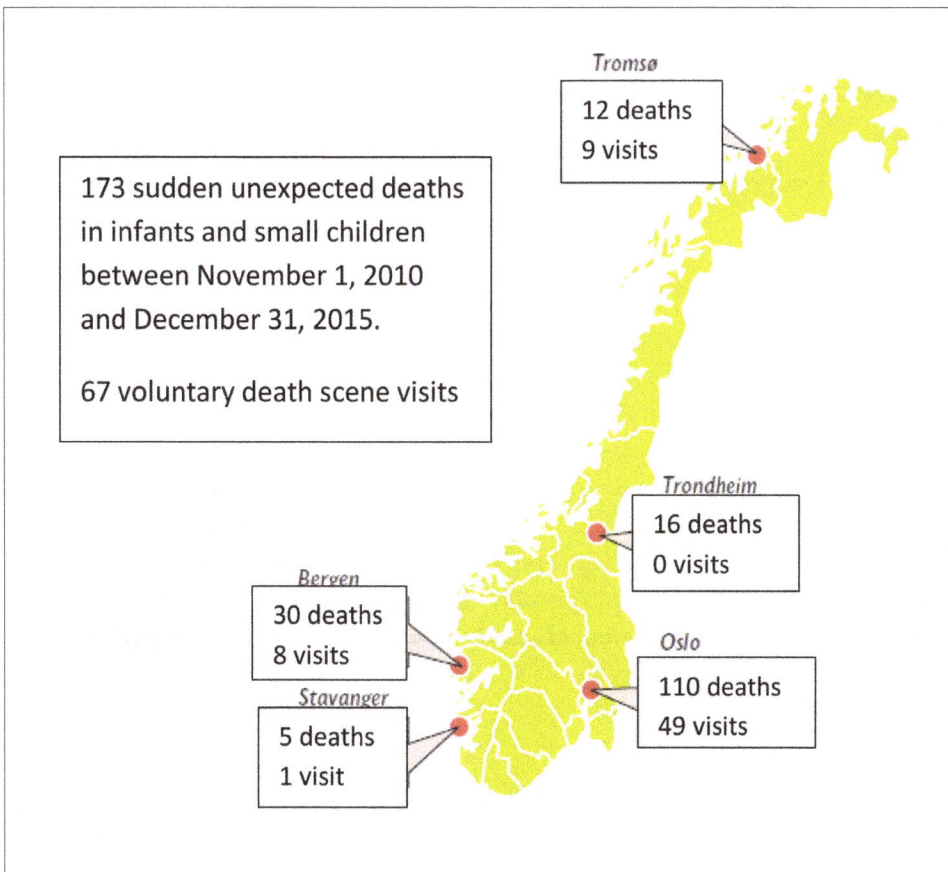

Figure 20.5: Distribution of sudden unexpected deaths in youngsters and the proportion of voluntary death scene visits. (Authors' own work.)

In 166 cases, both cause and classification of death could be established. Seven cases had to be excluded due to lack of sufficient information. Of the 166 with established diagnosis, 36% were classified as SIDS or SUDC, whereas 38% were due to disease, 8% to accidents, and 5% due to neglect, maltreatment/abuse, or homicide. Finally, 9% were deemed "undetermined" (Table 20.1).

Table 20.1: Classifications in 166 cases of sudden unexpected deaths in children under 4 years of age in Norway from 1 November 2010 to 31 December 2015. (Authors' own work.) Note that 7 cases have been excluded due to lack of sufficient information.

| Modes of death | SIDS/ SUDC | Disease | Neglect | Abuse | Homicide | Medical mal-treatment | Undeter-mined | Accident |
|---|---|---|---|---|---|---|---|---|
| Total group | 59 (36%) | 63 (38%) | 4 (2%) | 2 (1%) | 3 (2%) | 7 (4%) | 15 (9%) | 13 (8%) |

## Sudden Unexpected Death in Infants in Demark and Sweden

### Denmark

Denmark has a low SIDS rate (0.09 per 1,000 live births in 2015) (Figure 20.1). In cases of sudden unexpected infant death, a thorough autopsy is performed, including comprehensive tissue sampling for histology and usually (but not always) a neuropathologic examination. CT scanning of the whole body is always included, and in cases where there are suspicions of child abuse, a full-body X-ray is performed as well. Toxicological analyses are not always performed, but adequate material for such examination, as well as for genetic analyses, is sampled and stored for at least one year. The death scene is always examined by the police, but the forensic pathologist may request to participate in the examination and possibly also to take part in a reconstruction. In cases where there is suspicion of a criminal act, the police will ask the forensic pathologist to take part in the examination.

### Sweden

Sweden has a very low SIDS rate (0.14 per 1,000 live births in 2015) (Figure 20.1). In cases of sudden unexpected infant death, a thorough autopsy including both a comprehensive histological examination of all organs and a neuropathological examination is performed. A full-body X-ray and a CT scan is included in the protocol, as well as microbiological examination of body fluids and lung tissue and toxicological analysis. The death scene is examined by the police in cases of possible criminal activity.

## Conclusions

The Scandinavian countries experienced a SIDS epidemic in the 1980s. Norway and Denmark had the highest rates (Norway 2.4 per 1,000 live births in 1989). Risk factor campaigns launched in 1990 have been very effective. In 2015, all Scandinavian countries have rates below 0.2. SIDS is a diagnosis per exclusion and requires death scene investigation and autopsy with a large number of additional tests. In Finland, Sweden, and Denmark death scene investigations are performed by the police. In Norway, new legislation requires police investigation in all cases of sudden unexpected deaths in children under 18 years of age. If nothing of a criminal nature is disclosed in cases of death in infants and toddlers, the families are offered a voluntary death scene visit by the forensic pathologist and an expert with police education. This health service has been evaluated by crisis psychologists and found to be helpful for the families. Whereas SIDS constituted approximately 80% of all sudden unexpected deaths in infants in the 1980s, they now only constitute 33%. The diagnostic work is demanding. Therefore, all cases are discussed in an interdisciplinary case conference, where the final diagnosis is decided and where there is discussion about whether the death could have been prevented and what can be learned for future prevention.

## References

1. Byard RW, Rognum TO. Autopsy findings: Sudden infant death syndrome — Epidemiology and etiology. In: Encyclopedia of forensic and legal medicine. Eds Payne James J, Byard RW. London: Elsevier, 2016. https://doi.org/10.1016/B978-0-12-800034-2.00049-5.

2. Krous HF, Beckwith JB, Byard RW, Rognum TO, Bajanowski T, Corey T, et al. Sudden infant death syndrome and unclassified sudden infant deaths: A definitional and diagnostic approach. Pediatrics. 2004;114(1):234-8. https://doi.org/10.1542/peds.114.1.234.

3. Rognum TO, Lier LA. Police investigation and SIDS: An improved system of cooperation between health personnel, forensic pathologists, and the police? In: Sudden infant death syndrome — New trends in the nineties. Ed Rognum TO. Oslo: Scandinavian University Press, 1995.

4. Rognum TO, Wille-Sveum L, Arnestad M, Stray-Pedersen A, Vege Å. Death scene investigation in infants and small children. The Norwegian experiment. Scand J Forens Sci. 2010;16:20-3.

5. Heltne U, Dyregrov A, Dyregrov K. Death scene investigation: Parents' experiences. Scand J Forens Sci. 2017;23 [Epub ahead of print]. https://doi.org/10.1515/sjfs-2016-0009.

# 21

# Neonatal Monitoring: Prediction of Autonomic Regulation at 1 Month from Newborn Assessments

Michael M Myers, PhD[1,2,3],
Nina Burtchen, MD, PhD[5],
Maria Ordonez Retamar, BS[1],
Maristella Lucchini, MS[4] and
William P Fifer, PhD[1,2,3]

[1]Division of Developmental Neuroscience, New York State
Psychiatric Institute, New York, USA
[2]Department of Pediatrics, Columbia University, New York, USA
[3]Department of Psychiatry, Columbia University, New York, USA
[4]DEIB, Politecnico di Milano, Milano, Italy
[5]Department of Psychosomatic Medicine and Psychotherapy,
University of Freiburg, Freiburg, Germany

## Introduction

It has been nearly 30 years since the publication of a seminal book that defined the state of knowledge related to the epidemiology of, and mechanisms underlying, sudden infant death syndrome (SIDS) (1). Despite decades of subsequent research, much of which is summarized in other chapters in this book, we must acknowledge that SIDS remains an enigma. Indeed, two longstanding definitions of SIDS (2, 3) are testament to our lack of understanding of why infants die of SIDS — that is, these deaths remain unexplained after thorough investigation. Although infrequent, SIDS remains the most common cause of infant death between 1 month and 1 year of age, and the deaths of 2,000 infants annually in the United States (US) alone are unimaginable tragedies for these 2,000 families. At the heart of the reason why we have such an incomplete understanding of SIDS is, fortunately, its rarity. In the US, the 2014 estimates suggest that SIDS is the cause of death for about 3.9 of every 10,000 infants born each year (4). Over the past few decades, our understanding of the external factors that contribute to why infants die of SIDS has come from numerous, worldwide, epidemiological studies. Associations gleaned from these studies have led to recommendations including strong discouragement for mothers not to smoke during pregnancy paired with specific guidance for safe sleeping practices. Subsequent to these recommendations, the rate of SIDS was reduced in many countries (5). However, the physiological mechanisms that underlie SIDS remain unknown.

By definition, SIDS deaths are unexpected. While there may be evidence of low-grade infection prior to the time of death (6) in general, there are no overt, chronic signs of the impending demise. These deaths do not seem to be "programmed", in the sense that they are inevitable; rather, they appear to be due to suboptimal physiological regulatory responses to what may be rather common challenges faced by infants during the first year of life. Nonetheless, these deaths are not random. Some infants are more likely to experience the failure of adequate physiological responses to environmental challenges than others, hence the concept of the vulnerable infant. Infants born prematurely are at greater risk for SIDS (7), as are infants of mothers who smoked or drank during pregnancy (8, 9). Yet we still do not understand how such factors create physiological vulnerability, and investigations of risk factor mechanisms remain a mainstay of SIDS research.

An extremely important area of SIDS research that reinforces the non-random nature of SIDS deaths is based on anatomical and biochemical differences between SIDS infants and infants dying of known causes (10). Results from post-mortem studies, reviewed in other chapters of this book, provide compelling evidence for differences in brain structure and function that are linked to vulnerability for SIDS. These studies have largely focused on brainstem anomalies, with many revealing differences in serotonergic systems within brainstem areas associated with the regulation of breathing, the cardiovascular system, temperature regulation, and sleep-wake cycles (11). These findings strongly support the hypothesis that SIDS is the result of dysregulation of the autonomic nervous system (ANS). However, it is important to note that anomalies also are found in other regions of the brain, including the forebrain, suggesting deficits in brain development of SIDS infants that may be quite widespread (12).

The major function of the ANS is to provide organisms with integrated physiological responses to a wide variety of environmental challenges, requiring adjustments to body temperature, blood pressure, and respiratory activity. These challenges frequently occur during sleep and the transitions between sleep states. While population-based research strategies have sought to identify specific environmental factors that place infants at greater risk, other researchers have worked to identify physiological markers linked to the vulnerability to SIDS. In general, it is believed that SIDS infants appear to have increased vulnerability to triggering events which ordinarily should not be life-threatening (13). During specific critical periods of development, characterized by major changes in sleep organization and autonomic balance, all infants, particularly those with adverse prenatal histories, may have a diminished capacity to adequately respond to autonomic challenges (14). As examples, physiologic deficits associated with this risk status may be the inability to mount adequate cardiovascular responses to hypotensive and thermal challenges during the vulnerable period for SIDS (15-17), adequate respiratory activation in response to hypoxic and/or hypercarbic challenges (18, 19), and appropriate cortical arousals from sleep to a variety of physiologic challenges (20, 21). Thus, many SIDS researchers have proposed that the maturation of brainstem regions involved in the integration of cardiac and respiratory functions underlies these vulnerabilities.

The overall premise of our own research is that at least some SIDS victims are unable to mount rescue responses to homeostatic challenges in the extrauterine environment, and that assessments of ANS activity will reveal vulnerabilities in this system prior to death. Our working model is that many SIDS cases, and infants at the greatest risk, will exhibit altered baseline autonomic activity and atypical responses to cardiorespiratory challenges. Several years ago we published the case of a SIDS infant with abnormalities in the brainstem serotonergic system who also exhibited extreme values for cardiorespiratory variables measured on the second day of life (22). This was the first reported case of a SIDS infant with a documented brainstem abnormality and clear evidence of neonatal dysfunction in cardiorespiratory respiratory control. Consistent with this finding, infants who subsequently die of SIDS have been shown to have higher heart rates, reduced heart rate variability, disturbed co-ordination between cardiac and respiratory measures, increased variability and rate of breathing during quiet sleep, fewer short respiratory pauses, and abnormalities in the beat-to-beat dynamics of cardiac control (23-29). Several studies have assessed the ability of infants to respond to respiratory, thermal, and autonomic challenges (30-32). Based on studies demonstrating the presence of functioning baroreceptor reflexes during the neonatal period in many species (33), we and others have studied heart rate and electrocortical responses associated with blood pressure changes following postural adjustment and have shown that these baroreceptor-mediated reflexes are present in newborn infants within the first few days after birth (32, 34-40). These homeostatic responses, which can be assessed in the neonate, provide measures of the competence of neural mechanisms to process, and respond to, a frequently encountered stimulus.

Unfortunately, there are still no widely accepted animal models with the determining characteristics of SIDS. Nonetheless, as reviewed in other chapters of this volume, animal model studies can provide important information about mechanisms and risk factors that influence cardiorespiratory control during early development. As examples, much has been learned from animal models about how cardiorespiratory control mechanisms are affected by nicotine exposure (41, 42), various neurotransmitter systems (including serotonin and gamma-aminobutyric acid [GABA]) (43-49), repeated hypoxic experiences (50), chemo- and baroreceptor feedback (51, 52), and interactions with endotoxins (53, 54). Despite the impressive advances in understanding that animal models have provided about cardiorespiratory control during early development, we still do not know exactly how these mechanisms are related to SIDS. However, as noted previously, there is wide agreement that deficits in regulation of these systems underlie the vulnerability to SIDS.

Dysfunction in autonomic control may underlie SIDS, with a window of increased risk starting as early as 1 month of age (1). A central question is, however, whether measurements of autonomic function, including heart rate and heart rate variability at an age prior to the age of increased risk for SIDS, can be used to predict possible deficits in autonomic function and response to environmental challenge during the high-risk period. As mentioned above, in a report of a single case of SIDS, we found evidence of parasympathetic/sympathetic imbalance during sleep, as well as several cardiorespiratory variables with extreme values (22). The remainder of this chapter focuses on results of a study where we explored data from a set of infants collected over the past few years in which such measurements were made in newborns and again at 1-month postnatal age. These new longitudinal analyses suggest that extremes in certain measures of ANS function at the beginning of the high-risk window for SIDS (1 month) may be predicted by the same measurements in the neonatal period, prior to the time of increased risk for SIDS.

## Study Design and Findings

This study focused on a cohort of infants born between 35 and 41 weeks of gestation (n=55) (Table 21.1). The Institutional Review Boards of the New York State Psychiatric Institute and of the Columbia University Medical Center (CUMC) approved all procedures used in this study. Newborns were assessed 12-84 hours after birth and, when possible, again at 1 month (±1 week) postnatal age. None of the infants were admitted to the NICU or had any major illness or known genetic disorder. All infants had a minimum Apgar score of 8 after 5 minutes of life and weighed between 2,010 and 4,525 g. Mothers were at least 18 years of age (average of 31±7 years) and were fluent in English and/or Spanish. Review of the maternal medical chart revealed no evidence of major illness, genetic disorders, or past/present medicated/non-medicated psychiatric complaints.

Physiological assessments of these infants were conducted between 8 am and 4 pm in a quiet room near to the newborn nursery. Infants were gently swaddled and transferred to a bassinet with a soft memory-foam pillow in the supine position. The time since the last feeding of infants ranged from 15 to 30 minutes. Three electrocardiography (ECG) leads were placed on the infant's chest (left abdominal, and left and right scapula) and a respiratory inductance belt was placed around the infant's abdomen. ECG and respiration signals were acquired at 500 and 200 samples per second, respectively. The physiological signals were filtered to eliminate 60Hz noise, and R-wave and respiratory peaks were marked with automated marking software. Since cardiorespiratory variables differ as a function of sleep state (55, 56), prior to analyses, an algorithm based on respiratory rate variability was used to code for one of four sleep states (active sleep (AS), quiet sleep (QS), indeterminate, and awake). Details of the validation of this method have been recently published (57). Only data from AS and QS were used for the current analyses. Sleep state coding was supplemented by behavioral codes entered throughout the study and review of study videos to determine when infants were awake, crying, or fussy.

Table 21.1: Summary of the characteristics of the study cohort of infants.

| Gestational Age, weeks, mean ± SD | 38 ± 2 |
|---|---|
| Birth Weight, g, mean ± SD | 2,620 ± 364 |
| Sex, % female | 54.5 |
| 5 minute Apgar, range | 8-9 |
| Newborn test age (hours), mean ± SD | 42 ± 19 |
| one month test age (days), mean ± SD | 33 ± 4 |

The following parameters were computed in 30-second epochs during a 10-minute undisturbed period of sleep: mean heart rate (HR, bpm), standard deviation of R-wave to R-wave intervals (SD-RRI, sec), the interquartile range of R-wave to R-wave intervals (IQR-RRi, sec), sustained beat-to-beat changes in RRi (% of all consecutive changes in RRi that were either two consecutive increases or two consecutive decreases, SUS, %), the square root of the mean squared successive differences in R-wave intervals (rMSSD-RRi, sec), high frequency RRi (integrated spectral power of RRi over the frequency range of normal infant breathing rates, 0.5-1.5Hz, loge, sec2) and breathing rate (f, breaths/minute). The median values for all 30-second epochs in each sleep state for each of these measures were then computed. A minimum of four epochs in each sleep state was required for the analyses.

Table 21.2 summarizes the mean values for cardiorespiratory parameters by sleep state, i.e. AS and QS, at the two ages of assessment (newborn, NB, and 1 month, 1M). These analyses showed that significant effects of state during the newborn period were found only for breathing rate, whereas at 1 month all parameters, except HR and SUS, were higher in AS than in QS. Effects of age were found in QS measures except for SUS and breathing rate and, in AS, all parameters except breathing rate were different in 1-month-old infants compared to newborns. At 1 month, HR is higher and HRV measures are lower than in newborns.

Table 21.2: Physiological measures by age and sleep state: Heart rate, 5 measures of heart rate (RRi) variability, and respiratory frequency in Quiet Sleep (QS) and Active Sleep (AS) during the newborn (NB) period and at approximately 1 month (1M) postnatal age (means ± SE). ns = not significant. For effects of state (repeated measures comparing AS vs QS) there were 10 newborn subjects and 17 subjects at 1M with data in both states. The number of subjects for comparisons between ages (repeated measures comparing NB vs 1M) was 21 for QS and 28 for AS.

| Variable | NB | | 1M | | Effects of Age | |
|---|---|---|---|---|---|---|
| | QS (n=22) | AS (n=44) | QS (n=41) | AS (n=32) | QS | AS |
| HR | 120.8 | $126.6^{(state,ns)}$ | 143.4 | $148.3^{ns}$ | <0.001 | <0.001 |
| (bpm) | ± 2.5 | ± 1.7 | ± 1.5 | ± 2.1 | | |
| SD-RRi | 0.018 | $0.023^{ns}$ | 0.012 | $0.019^{<0.001}$ | <0.001 | <0.001 |
| (sec) | ± 0.002 | ± 0.002 | ± 0.001 | ±0.001 | | |
| IQR-RRi | 0.026 | $0.033^{ns}$ | 0.015 | $0.027^{<0.001}$ | <0.02 | <0.02 |
| (sec) | ± 0.003 | ± 0.003 | ± 0.001 | ± 0.002 | | |
| SUS changes | 20.0 | $18.6^{ns}$ | 14.6 | $14.6^{ns}$ | ns | <0.007 |
| in-RRi (%) | ± 2.1 | ± 1.2 | ± 1.7 | ± 1.1 | | |
| rMSSD-RRi | 0.015 | $0.012^{ns}$ | 0.008 | $0.009^{<0.001}$ | <0.005 | <0.005 |
| (sec) | ± 0.002 | ± 0.001 | ± 0.001 | ± 0.001 | | |
| loge HF-RRi | -15.6 | $-15.7^{ns}$ | -16.4 | $-16.1^{<0.01}$ | <0.01 | <0.05 |
| $(sec^2)$ | ± 0.2 | ± 0.1 | ± 0.2 | ± 0.1 | | |
| f | 41.6 | $51.0^{<0.02}$ | 42.7 | $53.4^{<0.001}$ | ns | ns |
| (breaths/min) | ± 2.0 | ± 1.7 | ± 1.2 | ±1.5 | | |

Despite the fact that measures of autonomic function change substantially with age, it is nonetheless possible that values obtained during the newborn period are correlated with, and are predictive of, values at an older age. Thus, we next asked if there were significant correlations between measures of cardiorespiratory function taken during the newborn period versus those at 1 month. Table 21.3 shows the results of these analyses. Two variables showed significant across-age correlations, both reflecting variation in heart rate at high frequencies, rMSSD and HF-RRi.

Although there are significant correlations between newborn and 1-month data, especially for measures of beat-to-beat variability (rMSSD and HF-RRi), the significant effects of sleep state (shown in Table 21.2) present an early risk assessment problem — particularly when recording lengths are short and thereby often preclude obtaining data in both active and quiet sleep states. Specifically, this presents an issue when trying to estimate values at 1 month or older from those obtained shortly after birth.

Table 21.3: Correlations between ages by sleep state. Shown are partial correlations, controlling for differences in gestational age at birth, between physiological measures obtained during the newborn period and those obtained at 1 month of age for active sleep and quiet sleep. ns = not significant, * $p < 0.05$, **$p < 0.01$, ***$p < 0.001$.

| | Active Sleep (n=27) | Quiet Sleep (n=21) |
|---|---|---|
| Variable | r | r |
| HR | $0.27^{ns}$ | $0.25^{ns}$ |
| SD-RRi | $0.35^{ns}$ | $0.05^{ns}$ |
| IQR-RRi | $0.33^{ns}$ | $-0.02^{ns}$ |
| SUS-RRi | $0.40^{*}$ | $0.19^{ns}$ |
| rMSSD | $0.51^{**}$ | $0.49^{*}$ |
| $\log_e$ HF-RRi | $0.49^{**}$ | $0.55^{**}$ |
| f | $0.44^{*}$ | $0.30^{ns}$ |

However, if data from both sleeps could be combined, this would improve the chances of obtaining early values with predictive validity. To determine the feasibility of this approach we computed the correlations between values obtained during AS versus those obtained during QS at each age. Table 21.4 contains the results of these computations. Consistent with prior studies by Harper and colleagues (56), our analyses show a very high degree of stability in individual differences in autonomic measures across sleep states for most variables. The lowest correlation between AS and QS values during the newborn period was for IQR-RRi (0.65), which was also the variable with the lowest correlation at 1 month (0.39). However, rMSSD, a time domain measure of beat-to-beat, i.e. high frequency heart rate variability, was very highly correlated between sleep states at both ages (newborn r = 0.95, 1 month r = 0.86).

Based on these high correlations between sleep states it was appropriate to devise a strategy for combining data across sleep states. To do this, we first transformed values within each sleep state to z-scores and then averaged z-scores across sleep states. Then, controlling for age at birth, correlations between values obtained at the two ages were computed. For each of these regression analyses a small number of outliers (Studentized residuals >2 or <-2) were removed, resulting in the between-age correlations shown in Table 21.5.

Table 21.4: Correlations between sleep states by age. Partial correlations between physiological measures obtained during quiet sleep versus those obtained during active sleep, controlling for gestational age at birth, at the newborn and 1 month (1M) ages. ns = not significant, * p<0.05, **p<0.01, ***p<0.001.

| | Newborn (n=10) | 1 month (n=17) |
|---|---|---|
| Variable | r | r |
| HR | 0.92*** | 0.85*** |
| SD-RRi | 0.89*** | 0.55* |
| IQR-RRi | 0.65* | 0.39$^{ns}$ |
| SUS-RRi | 0.80** | 0.80*** |
| rMSSD-RRi | 0.95*** | 0.86*** |
| log$_e$ HF-RRi | 0.83** | 0.72** |
| f | 0.84** | 0.86*** |

Table 21.5: Correlations between ages combining data across sleep states. Correlations between the average of active and quiet sleep z-scores for physiological measures obtained during the newborn period versus those obtained at 1 month of age after removing outliers (see text).

| Variable | n | r | p |
|---|---|---|---|
| HR | 52 | 0.27 | 0.06 |
| SD-RRi | 52 | 0.24 | 0.09 |
| IQR-RRi | 52 | 0.27 | 0.06 |
| SUS-RRi | 51 | 0.27 | 0.07 |
| rMSSD-RRi | 50 | 0.62 | <0.001 |
| log$_e$ HF-RRi | 52 | 0.56 | <0.001 |
| f | 51 | 0.27 | 0.06 |

Together, these procedures produced a data set with significantly increased numbers of subjects (50-52 vs 27 in AS alone or 21 in QS alone). These results support the conclusion that the variables with the most robust stability from the newborn to the 1-month period are those which quantify beat-to-beat or high-frequency variation in heart rate. To show

how individual subjects contribute to these correlations, Figure 21.1 presents a scatter plot of the standardized values, averaged over sleep states, for the newborn and 1 month data.

The data set used in these analyses contained infants with a wide range of gestational age at birth, ranging from what is considered to be late preterm (gestational age (GAs) 35-36 weeks), to term age (GAs 39-41 weeks). As further tests of our approach, we divided the infants into these two groups and repeated the statistical procedures described above. The results shown in Figure 21.2 show that the significant stability in rMSSD across ages is clearly evident regardless of gestational age at birth (late preterm correlation = 0.67, p<0.003; term correlation = 0.56, p<0.004).

As one final test of our approach, we divided the infants according to sex and repeated the standardization procedure and averaging across sleep states. Figure 21.3 presents these results. For both males and females, the age-to-age correlations of the time domain measure of beat-to-beat heart rate variability were significant. Together, these results show that a subset of measures of autonomic function taken near the time of birth can be used to predict individual values weeks later, as the infants near the time of increased vulnerability for SIDS.

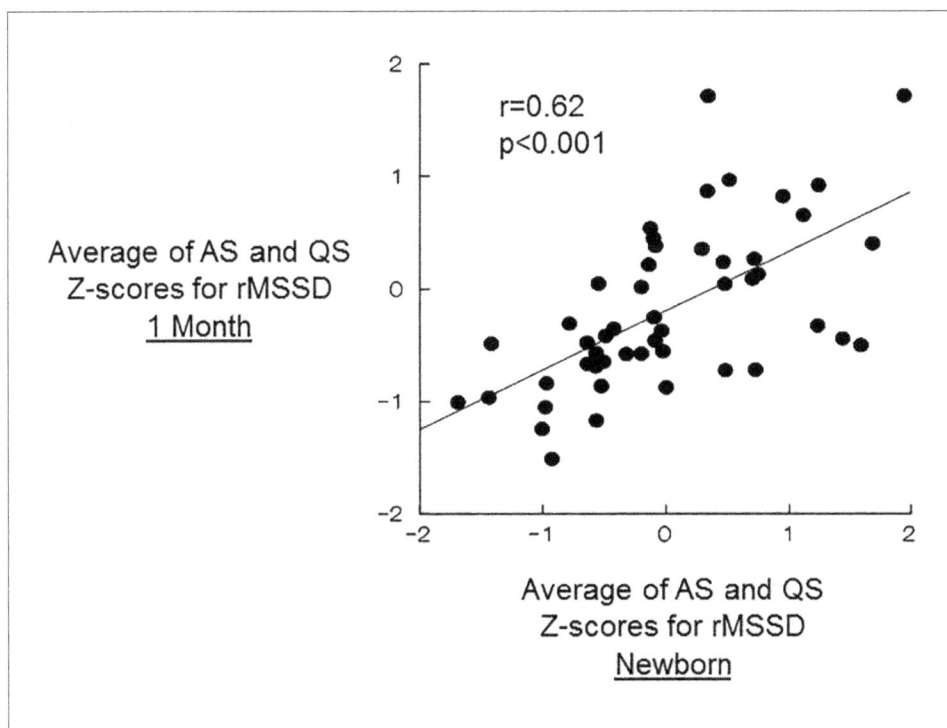

Figure 21.1: Newborn rMSSD versus rMSSD at 1 month of age. Values within each age are the averages of within state (active sleep, quiet sleep) z-scores.

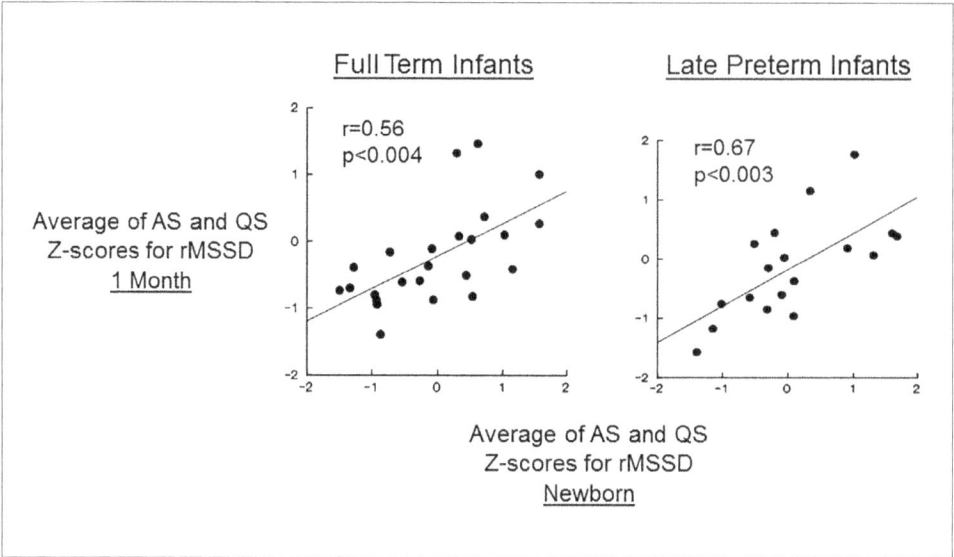

Figure 21.2: Newborn rMSSD versus rMSSD at 1 month of age: Full term and late preterm. Values within each age are the averages of within state (active sleep, quiet sleep) z-scores. The left panel shows the plot for full term infants (GAs 39-41), the right panel for late preterm infants (GAs 35-36).

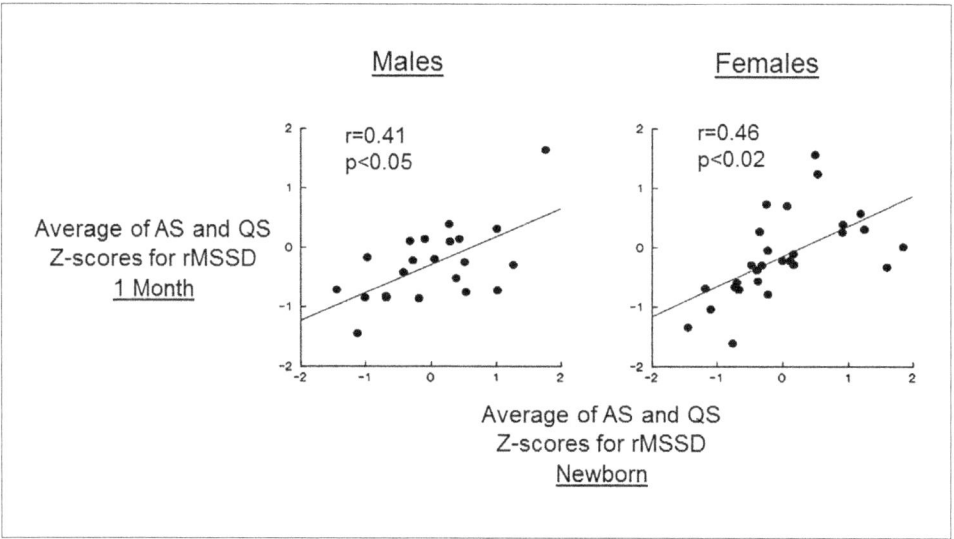

Figure 21.3: Newborn rMSSD versus rMSSD at 1 month of age: Males and females. Values within each age are the averages of within state (active sleep, quiet sleep) z-scores. The left panel shows the plot for male infants, the right panel for females.

# Discussion

Finding measures of physiological function that reflect vulnerability to SIDS, and that provide markers of subsequent risk, remains a major focus of SIDS research. In this chapter we present new evidence showing that certain measures of autonomic function, particularly those reflecting high-frequency, beat-to-beat variability, are highly correlated across sleep states. This allowed us to combine, using standardized scores within an age, values for AS and QS. Thus, if a newborn infant only had data from one sleep state, that data point could be used to predict 1-month values. This approach should facilitate physiological risk assessment as early as the first few days of life.

The finding that high-frequency variability in heart rate provides the most consistent prediction of subsequent values from the newborn to 1 month of age is important for two reasons. First, from decades of both animal and human studies we know that much of the beat-to-beat variability in heart rate is created by changes in heart rate linked to the respiratory cycle (58, 59). With inspiration, heart rate increases, whereas with exhalation, heart rate slows down. This variation in heart rate, known as respiratory sinus arrhythmia, is mediated by variation in parasympathetic (vagal) nerve activity impinging on the sinus node (60-62). Measures of this so-called high-frequency heart rate (or heart period) variability, including spectral power integrated over the normal range of breathing rates or the time domain measure rMSSD, provide indirect indices of parasympathetic control of heart rate (63, 64). Accordingly, our analyses suggest that it is possible to predict, from as little as 10 minutes of data during the newborn period, which infants are most likely to have atypical (low or high) levels of parasympathetic control weeks later, when infants enter a period of increased risk for SIDS.

The second reason why finding age stability of high-frequency heart rate variability is particularly important is that from reports based on two prior prospective studies of SIDS, measures of heart rate variability, including those of high-frequency heart rate variability, were found to be lower in infants who subsequently die of SIDS (23, 24, 26, 65, 66). It remains unknown whether alterations in parasympathetic control of heart rate are actually contributors to SIDS deaths, or whether they are markers linked to other physiological processes that are the proximal mechanisms for SIDS. However, the ability to identify, even in the newborn period, infants on the extremes of this key regulatory function provides new hope for early identification of increased risk.

SIDS researchers all share three goals: to understand the mechanisms underlying SIDS; to be better able to identify, prospectively, which infants are at greatest risk; and, based on this knowledge, to design strategies to reduce SIDS. Although early prediction of which infants will exhibit extreme values in cardiorespiratory values during the window of vulnerability for SIDS affords an important research strategy, this approach is constrained by our knowledge of which parameters are most closely linked to SIDS. This is a limitation due to the paucity of prospectively obtained physiological data on infants who subsequently die of SIDS. Remarkably, this number has remained at 46 cases for over 25 years, with 16 such cases being obtained prospectively in the groundbreaking studies of Southhall and colleagues (67) and 30 cases in the illuminating studies conducted by Kahn and colleagues (27).

By the end of 2017 it is expected that a new cohort of SIDS infants, with prospectively obtained data during both gestation and early infancy, will become available for analysis. The Prenatal Alcohol in SIDS and Stillbirth (PASS) Network was formed to investigate prenatal alcohol exposure and risk for SIDS, stillbirth, and fetal alcohol spectrum disorders (FASD) (68). The PASS network's Safe Passage Study recruited nearly 12,000 subjects from sites in North and South Dakota and in Cape Town, South Africa. The Safe Passage Study assessed participants from pregnancy through 1 year of age to test the primary hypothesis that prenatal alcohol exposure increases risk for SIDS, stillbirth, and fetal alcohol spectrum disorders. A major goal of the Safe Passage Study was to obtain physiological data on as many of the ~12,000 enrolled subjects as possible during gestation and early infant time periods. Normative cardiorespiratory data from the newborn and 1-month periods have been published (69). In the Safe Passage Study, which took over 10 years to complete, heart rates, breathing rates, and blood pressures were obtained on most infants near the time of birth and/or at 1 month of age. These measurements were made using a standardized protocol in which, while the infants were sleeping, data were collected during a baseline period and following three 45o head-up tilts. For many of these infants, measurements of electroencephalogram and hearing were also conducted. The physiological goals embedded in the Safe Passage Study were to characterize autonomic control during the first month of life in the hope that new information would lead to early identification of risk for later ANS dysfunction and SIDS, thus enabling timely interventions and more effective prevention strategies. While results from this new prospective study were not available in time for the publication of this chapter, the reader should be encouraged that the search for answers as to why SIDS occurs continues.

# References

1. Schwartz PJ, Southall DP, Valdes-Dapena M. The sudden infant death syndrome. In: Cardiac and respiratory mechanisms and interventions. Vol. 533. New York: New York Academy of Sciences, 1988.

2. Willinger M, James LS, Catz C. Defining the sudden infant death syndrome (SIDS): Deliberations of an expert panel convened by the National Institute of Child Health and Human Development. Pediatr Pathol. 1991;11(5):677-84. https://doi.org/10.3109/15513819109065465.

3.  Krous HF, Beckwith JB, Byard RW, Rognum TO, Bajanowski T, Corey T, et al. Sudden infant death syndrome and unclassified sudden infant deaths: A definitional and diagnostic approach. Pediatrics. 2004;114(1):234-8. https://doi.org/10.1542/peds.114.1.234.

4.  Mathews TJ, Driscoll AK. Trends in infant mortality in the United States, 2005-2014. NCHS Data Brief, no. 279. Hyattsville, MD: National Center for Health Statistics, 2017.

5.  Moon RY, Hauck FR, Colson ER. Safe infant sleep interventions: What is the evidence for successful behavior change? Curr Pediatr Rev. 2016;12(1):67-75. https://doi.org/10.2174/1573396311666151026110148.

6.  Goldwater PN. Infection: The neglected paradigm in SIDS research. Arch Dis Child. 2017;102:767-72. https://doi.org/10.1136/archdischild-2016-312327.

7.  Malloy MH, Hoffman HJ. Prematurity, sudden infant death syndrome, and age of death. Pediatrics. 1995;96(3 Pt 1):464-71.

8.  Moon RY, Horne RS, Hauck FR. Sudden infant death syndrome. Lancet. 2007;370(9598):1578-87. https://doi.org/10.1016/S0140-6736(07)61662-6.

9.  Odendaal HJ, Steyn DW, Elliott A, Burd L. Combined effects of cigarette smoking and alcohol consumption on perinatal outcome. Gynecol Obstet Invest. 2009;67(1):1-8. https://doi.org/10.1159/000150597.

10.  Kinney HC, Rognum TO, Nattie EE, Haddad GG, Hyma B, McEntire B, et al. Sudden and unexpected death in early life: Proceedings of a symposium in honor of Dr Henry F Krous. Forensic Sci Med Pathol. 2012;8(4):414-25. https://doi.org/10.1007/s12024-012-9376-4.

11.  Kinney HC, Richerson GB, Dymecki SM, Darnall RA, Nattie EE. The brainstem and serotonin in the sudden infant death syndrome. Annu Rev Pathol. 2009;4:517-50. https://doi.org/10.1146/annurev.pathol.4.110807.092322.

12.  Kinney HC, Poduri AH, Cryan JB, Haynes RL, Teot L, Sleeper LA, et al. Hippocampal formation maldevelopment and sudden unexpected death across the pediatric age spectrum. J Neuropathol Exp Neurol. 2016;75(10):981-97. https://doi.org/10.1093/jnen/nlw075.

13.  Filiano JJ, Kinney HC. A perspective on neuropathologic findings in victims of the sudden infant death syndrome: The triple-risk model. Biol Neonate. 1994;65(3-4):194-7. https://doi.org/10.1159/000244052.

14.  Fifer WP, Myers MM. Sudden fetal and infant deaths: Shared characteristics and distinctive features. Semin Perinatol. 2002;26(1):89-96. https://doi.org/10.1053/sper.2002.29854.

15. Harper RM, Bandler R. Finding the failure mechanism in sudden infant death syndrome. Nat Med. 1998;4(2):157-8. https://doi.org/10.1038/nm0298-157.

16. Harper RM. Sudden infant death syndrome: A failure of compensatory cerebellar mechanisms? Pediatr Res. 2000;48(2):140-2. https://doi.org/10.1203/00006450-200008000-00004.

17. Matthews T. SIDS — A defect in circulatory control. Ir Med J. 2000;93(6):164-5.

18. Neary MT, Breckenridge RA. Hypoxia at the heart of sudden infant death syndrome? Pediatr Res. 2013;74(4):375-9. https://doi.org/10.1038/pr.2013.122.

19. Darnall RA. The carotid body and arousal in the fetus and neonate. Respir Physiol Neurobiol. 2013;185(1):132-43. https://doi.org/10.1016/j.resp.2012.06.005.

20. Kahn A, Groswasser J, Franco P, Scaillet S, Sawaguchi T, Kelmanson I, et al. Sudden infant deaths: Arousal as a survival mechanism. Sleep Med. 2002;3 Suppl 2:S11-14. https://doi.org/10.1016/S1389-9457(02)00157-0.

21. Kahn A, Groswasser J, Franco P, Scaillet S, Sawaguchi T, Kelmanson I, et al. Sudden infant deaths: Stress, arousal and SIDS. Early Hum Dev. 2003;75 Suppl:S147-66. https://doi.org/10.1016/j.earlhumdev.2003.08.018.

22. Kinney HC, Myers MM, Belliveau RA, Randall LL, Trachtenberg FL, Fingers ST, et al. Subtle autonomic and respiratory dysfunction in sudden infant death syndrome associated with serotonergic brainstem abnormalities: A case report. J Neuropathol Exp Neurol. 2005;64(8):689-94. https://doi.org/10.1097/01.jnen.0000174334.27708.43.

23. Schechtman VL, Raetz SL, Harper RK, Garfinkel A, Wilson AJ, Southall DP, et al. Dynamic analysis of cardiac R-R intervals in normal infants and in infants who subsequently succumbed to the sudden infant death syndrome. Pediatr Res. 1992;31(6):606-12. https://doi.org/10.1203/00006450-199206000-00014.

24. Schechtman VL, Harper RM, Kluge KA, Wilson AJ, Hoffman HJ, Southall DP. Heart rate variation in normal infants and victims of the sudden infant death syndrome. Early Hum Dev. 1989;19(3):167-81. https://doi.org/10.1016/0378-3782(89)90077-7.

25. Schechtman VL, Harper RM, Wilson AJ, Southall DP. Sleep apnea in infants who succumb to the sudden infant death syndrome. Pediatrics. 1991;87(6):841-6.

26. Kluge KA, Harper RM, Schechtman VL, Wilson AJ, Hoffman HJ, Southall DP. Spectral analysis assessment of respiratory sinus arrhythmia in normal infants and infants who subsequently died of sudden infant death syndrome. Pediatr Res. 1988;24(6):677-82. https://doi.org/10.1203/00006450-198812000-00005.

27. Kahn A, Groswasser J, Rebuffat E, Sottiaux M, Blum D, Foerster M, et al. Sleep and cardiorespiratory characteristics of infant victims of sudden death: A prospective case-control study. Sleep. 1992;15(4):287-92. https://doi.org/10.1093/sleep/15.4.287.

28. Kahn A, Sawaguchi T, Sawaguchi A, Groswasser J, Franco P, Scaillet S, et al. Sudden infant deaths: From epidemiology to physiology. Forensic Sci Int. 2002;130 Suppl:S8-20. https://doi.org/10.1016/S0379-0738(02)00134-2.

29. Kato I, Franco P, Groswasser J, Scaillet S, Kelmanson I, Togari H, et al. Incomplete arousal processes in infants who were victims of sudden death. Am J Respir Crit Care Med. 2003;168(11):1298-303. https://doi.org/10.1164/rccm.200301-134OC.

30. Thach BT. The role of respiratory control disorders in SIDS. Respir Physiol Neurobiol. 2005;149(1-3):343-53. https://doi.org/10.1016/j.resp.2005.06.011.

31. Fox GP, Matthews TG. Autonomic dysfunction at different ambient temperatures in infants at risk of sudden infant death syndrome. Lancet. 1989;2(8671):1065-7. https://doi.org/10.1016/S0140-6736(89)91080-5.

32. Myers MM, Gomez-Gribben E, Smith KS, Tseng A, Fifer WP. Developmental changes in infant heart rate responses to head-up tilting. Acta Paediatr. 2006;95(1):77-81. https://doi.org/10.1080/08035250500325074.

33. Gootman PM. Developmental aspects of reflex control of the circulation. In: Reflex control of the circulation. Eds Zucker IH, Gilmore JP. Boca Raton, FL: CRC Press, 1991.

34. Fifer WP, Greene M, Hurtado A, Myers MM. Cardiorespiratory responses to bidirectional tilts in infants. Early Hum Dev. 1999;55(3):265-79. https://doi.org/10.1016/S0378-3782(99)00026-2.

35. Grieve PG, Myers MM, Stark RI, Housman S, Fifer WP. Topographic localization of electrocortical activation in newborn and two- to four-month-old infants in response to head-up tilting. Acta Paediatr. 2005;94(12):1756-63. https://doi.org/10.1080/08035250510042933.

36. Grieve PG, Stark RI, Isler JR, Housman SL, Fifer WP, Myers MM. Electrocortical functional connectivity in infancy: Response to body tilt. Pediatr Neurol. 2007;37(2):91-8. https://doi.org/10.1016/j.pediatrneurol.2007.04.004.

37. Thoresen M, Cowan F, Walloe L. Cardiovascular responses to tilting in healthy newborn babies. Early Hum Dev. 1991;26(3):213-22. https://doi.org/10.1016/0378-3782(91)90161-U.

38. Finley JP, Hamilton R, MacKenzie MG. Heart rate response to tilting in newborns in quiet and active sleep. Biol Neonate. 1984;45(1):1-10. https://doi.org/10.1159/000241756.

39. Chen CM, Tsai TC, Lan MC. Effect of body tilting on physiological functions in healthy term neonates. Acta Paediatr. 1995;84(5):474-7. https://doi.org/10.1111/j.1651-2227.1995.tb13677.x.

40. Andrasyova D, Kellerova E. Blood pressure and heart rate response to head-up position in full-term newborns. Early Hum Dev. 1996;44(3):169-78. https://doi.org/10.1016/0378-3782(95)01706-2.

41. Slotkin TA, Saleh JL, McCook EC, Seidler FJ. Impaired cardiac function during postnatal hypoxia in rats exposed to nicotine prenatally: Implications for perinatal morbidity and mortality, and for sudden infant death syndrome. Teratology. 1997;55(3):177-84. https://doi.org/10.1002/(SICI)1096-9926(199703)55:3<177::AID-TERA2>3.0.CO;2-#.

42. Hafstrom O, Milerad J, Sandberg KL, Sundell HW. Cardiorespiratory effects of nicotine exposure during development. Respir Physiol Neurobiol. 2005;149(1-3):325-41. https://doi.org/10.1016/j.resp.2005.05.004.

43. Nattie E. Sudden infant death syndrome and serotonIn: Animal models. Bioessays. 2009;31(2):130-3. https://doi.org/10.1002/bies.200800200.

44. Duncan JR, Garland M, Myers MM, Fifer WP, Yang M, Kinney HC, et al. Prenatal nicotine-exposure alters fetal autonomic activity and medullary neurotransmitter receptors: Implications for sudden infant death syndrome. J Appl Physiol. 2009;107(5):1579-90. https://doi.org/10.1152/japplphysiol.91629.2008.

45. Duncan JR, Garland M, Stark RI, Myers MM, Fifer WP, Mokler DJ, et al. Prenatal nicotine exposure selectively affects nicotinic receptor expression in primary and associative visual cortices of the fetal baboon. Brain Pathol. 2015;25(2):171-81. https://doi.org/10.1111/bpa.12165.

46. Cummings KJ, Commons KG, Hewitt JC, Daubenspeck JA, Li A, Kinney HC, et al. Failed heart rate recovery at a critical age in 5-HT-deficient mice exposed to episodic anoxia: Implications for SIDS. J Appl Physiol. 2011;111(3):825-33. https://doi.org/10.1152/japplphysiol.00336.2011.

47. Cummings KJ, Hewitt JC, Li A, Daubenspeck JA, Nattie EE. Postnatal loss of brainstem serotonin neurones compromises the ability of neonatal rats to survive episodic severe hypoxia. J Physiol. 2011;589(Pt 21):5247-56. https://doi.org/10.1113/jphysiol.2011.214445.

48. Darnall RA, Schneider RW, Tobia CM, Zemel BM. Arousal from sleep in response to intermittent hypoxia in rat pups is modulated by medullary raphe GABAergic mechanisms. Am J Physiol Regul Integr Comp Physiol. 2012;302(5):R551-60. https://doi.org/10.1152/ajpregu.00506.2011.

49. Cerpa VJ, Aylwin Mde L, Beltran-Castillo S, Bravo EU, Llona IR, Richerson GB, et al. The alteration of neonatal raphe neurons by prenatal-perinatal cicotine. Meaning for sudden infant death syndrome. Am J Respir Cell Mol Biol. 2015;53(4):489-99. https://doi.org/10.1165/rcmb.2014-0329OC.

50. Darnall RA, Chen X, Nemani KV, Sirieix CM, Gimi B, Knoblach S, et al. Early postnatal exposure to intermittent hypoxia in rodents is proinflammatory, impairs white matter integrity, and alters brain metabolism. Pediatr Res. 2017;82:164-72. https://doi.org/10.1038/pr.2017.102.

51. Hofer MA. Lethal respiratory disturbance in neonatal rats after arterial chemoreceptor denervation. Life Sci. 1984;34(5):489-96. https://doi.org/10.101 6/0024-3205(84)90505-8.

52. Curran AK, Leiter JC. Baroreceptor-mediated inhibition of respiration after peripheral and central administration of a 5-HT1A receptor agonist in neonatal piglets. Exp Physiol. 2007;92(4):757-67. https://doi.org/10.1113/expphysiol.2007.037481.

53. Blood-Siegfried J, Nyska A, Geisenhoffer K, Lieder H, Moomaw C, Cobb K, et al. Alteration in regulation of inflammatory response to influenza a virus and endotoxin in suckling rat pups: A potential relationship to sudden infant death syndrome. FEMS Immunol Med Microbiol. 2004;42(1):85-93. https://doi.org/10.1016/j.femsim.2004.06.004.

54. Voss LJ, Bolton DP, Galland BC, Taylor BJ. Endotoxin effects on markers of autonomic nervous system function in the piglet: Implications for SIDS. Biol Neonate. 2004;86(1):39-47. https://doi.org/10.1159/000077452.

55. Horne RS, Witcombe NB, Yiallourou SR, Scaillet S, Thiriez G, Franco P. Cardiovascular control during sleep in infants: Implications for sudden infant death syndrome. Sleep Med. 2010;11(7):615-21. https://doi.org/10.1016/j.sleep.2009.10.008.

56. Harper RM, Hoppenbrouwers T, Sterman MB, McGinty DJ, Hodgman J. Polygraphic studies of normal infants during the first six months of life. I. Heart rate and variability as a function of state. Pediatr Res. 1976;10(11):945-8. https://doi.org/10.1203/00006450-197611000-00008.

57. Isler JR, Thai T, Myers MM, Fifer WP. An automated method for coding sleep states in human infants based on respiratory rate variability. Dev Psychobiol. 2016;58(8):1108-15. https://doi.org/10.1002/dev.21482.

58. Spyer KM. Central nervous mechanisms responsible for cardio-respiratory homeostasis. Adv Exp Med Biol. 1995;381:73-9. https://doi.org/10.1007/978-1-4615-1895-2_8.

59. Grossman P, Taylor EW. Toward understanding respiratory sinus arrhythmia: Relations to cardiac vagal tone, evolution and biobehavioral functions. Biol Psychol. 2007;74(2):263-85. https://doi.org/10.1016/j.biopsycho.2005.11.014.

60. McCabe PM, Yongue BG, Ackles PK, Porges SW. Changes in heart period, heart-period variability, and a spectral analysis estimate of respiratory sinus arrhythmia in response to pharmacological manipulations of the baroreceptor reflex in cats. Psychophysiology. 1985;22(2):195-203. https://doi.org/10.1111/j.1469-8986.1985.tb01585.x.

61. Berntson GG, Bigger JT Jr., Eckberg DL, Grossman P, Kaufmann PG, Malik M, et al. Heart rate variability: Origins, methods, and interpretive caveats. Psychophysiology. 1997;34(6):623-48. https://doi.org/10.1111/j.1469-8986.1997.tb02140.x.

62. Eckberg DL. Human sinus arrhythmia as an index of vagal cardiac outflow. J Appl Physiol Respir Environ Exerc Physiol. 1983;54(4):961-6.

63. Hedman AE, Hartikainen JE, Tahvanainen KU, Hakumaki MO. The high frequency component of heart rate variability reflects cardiac parasympathetic modulation rather than parasympathetic "tone". Acta physiologica Scandinavica. 1995;155(3):267-73. https://doi.org/10.1111/j.1748-1716.1995.tb09973.x.

64. Spiers JP, Silke B, McDermott U, Shanks RG, Harron DW. Time and frequency domain assessment of heart rate variability: A theoretical and clinical appreciation. Clin Auton Res. 1993;3(2):145-58. https://doi.org/10.1007/BF01819000.

65. Schechtman VL, Harper RM, Kluge KA, Wilson AJ, Hoffman HJ, Southall DP. Cardiac and respiratory patterns in normal infants and victims of the sudden infant death syndrome. Sleep. 1988;11(5):413-24. https://doi.org/10.1093/sleep/11.5.413.

66. Franco P, Szliwowski H, Dramaix M, Kahn A. Polysomnographic study of the autonomic nervous system in potential victims of sudden infant death syndrome. Clin Auton Res. 1998;8(5):243-9. https://doi.org/10.1007/BF02277969.

67. Southall DP, Richards JM, Stebbens V, Wilson AJ, Taylor V, Alexander JR. Cardiorespiratory function in 16 full-term infants with sudden infant death syndrome. Pediatrics. 1986;78(5):787-96.

68. Dukes KA, Burd L, Elliott AJ, Fifer WP, Folkerth RD, Hankins GD, et al. The safe passage study: Design, methods, recruitment, and follow-up approach. Paediatr Perinat Epidemiol. 2014;28(5):455-65. https://doi.org/10.1111/ppe.12136.

69. Myers MM, Elliott AJ, Odendaal HJ, Burd L, Angal J, Groenewald C, et al. Cardiorespiratory physiology in the Safe Passage Study: Protocol, methods and normative values in unexposed infants. Acta Paediatr. 2017;106: 1260-72. https://doi.org/10.1111/apa.13873.

# 22

# Autonomic Cardiorespiratory Physiology and Arousal of the Fetus and Infant

Rosemary SC Horne, PhD, DSc

*The Ritchie Centre, Monash University and Hudson Institute of Medical Research, Melbourne, Australia*

## Introduction

Despite intensive research over the past decades, the mechanisms which lead to sudden infant death syndrome (SIDS) still remain elusive. SIDS is presumed to occur in an apparently healthy infant during a period of sleep (1). A failure of cardiorespiratory control mechanisms, together with an impaired arousal from sleep response, are believed to play an important role in the final event of SIDS. Sleep has a marked influence on respiratory and cardiovascular control in both adults and infants, although sleep states, sleep architecture, and arousal from sleep processes in infants are very different from those of adults and undergo significant maturation during the first year of life, particularly in the first six months when SIDS risk is greatest (2).

Arousal from sleep involves both physiological and behavioral responses and has long been considered a vital survival response for restoring homeostasis in reaction to various life-threatening situations, such as prolonged hypoxia or hypotension (3). There are two distinct arousal types defined in infants, subcortical activation and full cortical arousal, which reflect the hierarchical activation from the brainstem (including heart rate, blood pressure, and ventilation changes) to the cortex (4). Any impairment of these protective responses may render an infant vulnerable to the respiratory and cardiovascular instabilities that are common during infancy and that have been postulated to occur in SIDS. In support of this possibility, extensive physiological and neuropathological studies have provided compelling evidence that impaired cardiovascular control, with a concomitant failure to arouse from sleep, are involved in the final events leading to SIDS. The first six months of life are a critical period of development when rapid maturation of the brain, cardiorespiratory system, and sleep state organization are all taking place (2, 5). Thus, the investigation of sleep physiology in healthy infants during this high-risk period provides important insights into the likely mechanisms involved in the pathogenesis of SIDS.

## Development of Sleep

The maturation of sleep is one of the most important physiological processes occurring during the first year of life and is particularly rapid during the first six months after birth (5). Behavioral states in infants are defined by physiological and behavioral variables that are stable over time and occur repeatedly in an individual infant and also across infants (6). The emergence of sleep states is dependent on the central nervous system and is a good and reliable indicator of normal and abnormal development (7).

Sleep states and sleep architecture in infants are quite different from those in adults. In adults, the definition of the two sleep states, rapid eye movement (REM) sleep and non-rapid eye movement (NREM) sleep, requires the recording of brain activity (electroencephalogram or EEG), muscle tone (submental electromyogram or EMG), and eye movements (electro-occulogram or EOG). In infants, sleep states are defined using both electrophysiological and behavioral criteria as active sleep (AS) and quiet sleep (QS), which are the precursors of adult REM sleep and NREM sleep, respectively. QS is characterized by high-voltage, low-amplitude EEG activity, the absence of eye movements, and regular heart rate and respiration. In contrast, AS is characterized by low-amplitude, high-frequency EEG activity, eye movements, reduced EMG, and irregular heart rate and respiration (Figure 22.1). In addition, a third state, that of indeterminate sleep (IS), is defined when criteria for AS and QS are not met. IS is usually considered a sign of immaturity and the incidence decreases with increasing postnatal age.

Rhythmic cyclical rest activity patterns can be observed in the human fetus from 28 weeks of gestation (8). In infants born preterm the infant sleep states cannot be distinguished in infants younger than 26 weeks of gestation (9). By 28-30 weeks of gestation AS can be recognized by the presence of eye movements, body movements, and irregular breathing and heart rate. At this gestational age QS is difficult to identify, as submental hypotonia is difficult to evaluate, and the majority of the sleep period is spent in AS. QS does not become clearly identifiable until about 36 weeks of gestational age (8). The percentage of time spent in QS increases with gestational age and by term equal amounts of time are spent in both AS and QS, with the two states alternating throughout each sleep period. The proportion of AS decreases across the first six months

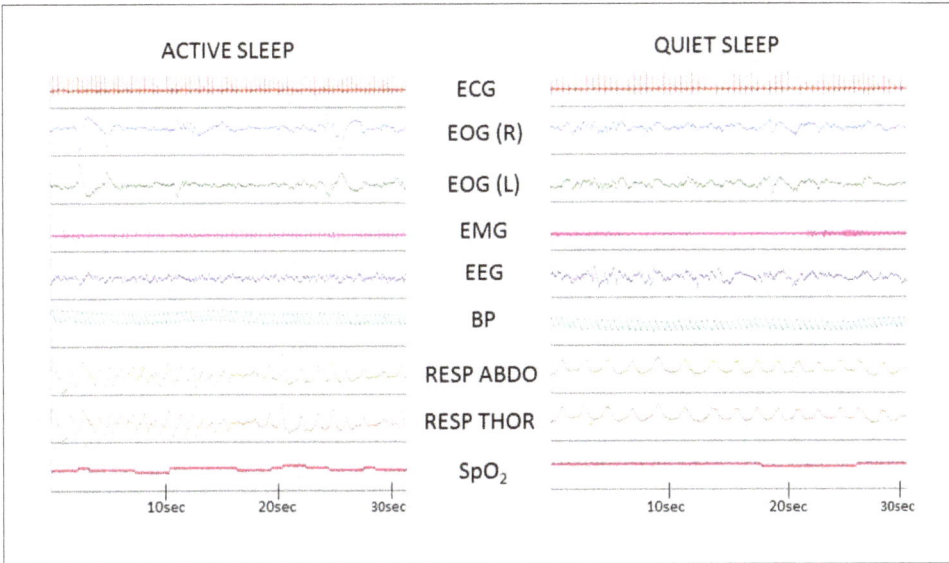

Figure 22.1: Cardiorespiratory parameters in active and quiet sleep in an infant. ECG: electrocardiograph. EOG: electrooculogram. EMG: electromyogram. EEG: electroencephalogram. BP: blood pressure. RESP ABDO: abdominal respiratory effort. RESP THOR: thoracic respiratory effort. SpO$_2$: oxygen saturation. HR: heart rate. Note regular breathing and heart rate in quiet sleep compared to active sleep. (Author's own work.)

of life to make up approximately 25% of total sleep time, similar to that in adults (10). In contrast, the proportion of QS increases with age to make up about 75% of total sleep time by 6 months of age (10).

At term, infants sleep for about 16-17 hours out of every 24 (8). There is a gradual decrease in total sleep time, with infants sleeping 14-15 hours at 16 months of age and 13 to 14 hours by 6 to 8 months of age. In the neonatal period, infants awaken every two to six hours for feeding, regardless of the time of day and stay awake for one to two hours (11). The major change in sleep-wake pattern occurs between six weeks and three months post-term age (11). During the first six months after term, consolidation and entrainment of sleep at night develops and sleep periods lengthen. At 3 weeks of age the mean length of the longest sleep period has been reported to be 211.7 minutes, increasing to 358.0 minutes by 6 months of age (12). The longest sleep period was randomly distributed between daytime and night time at 3 months but had moved to night time by 6 months (12).

Dramatic changes in the sleep EEG patterns of infants occur during early infancy as the brain matures. The EEG patterns of QS and AS differ with a relatively continuous pattern in AS and a relatively discontinuous pattern in QS. A continuous pattern is defined by the presence of background activity throughout each 30-second epoch scored, while a discontinuous pattern is defined by the presence of higher-amplitude EEG waves during <50% of each epoch (13). A semi-discontinuous EEG pattern of depressions and continuous delta activity during ≤70% of each epoch is called a tracé alternant pattern and can be identified at 32-34 weeks of gestational age (13). This pattern is prominent in preterm infants, but it also occurs in infants born at term and disappears one month after term-equivalent age. Sleep spindles appear coincidentally with the disappearance of tracé alternant (14). True continuous delta frequency does not appear until 8-12 weeks of age, and it is not until this age that adult criteria for determining the stages of NREM sleep can be used (15).

In summary, during infancy sleep is at a lifetime maximum and significant changes, which reflect maturation of the central nervous system, occur in the maturation of sleep. Sleep has a marked effect on cardiorespiratory control. Cardiorespiratory disturbances occur predominantly in AS, so the predominance of AS in early infancy may increase the risk of cardiorespiratory disturbances during this period of development.

## Effects of sleep state on cardiorespiratory control

There are marked differences in cardiorespiratory control between the two sleep states (AS and QS) (Table 22.1). Assessment of cardiovascular control is commonly made by studies of heart rate and heart rate patterning or variability (HRV) and blood pressure and its variability (16). The short-term, or high-frequency (HF), variability in heart rate is related to parasympathetic vagal activity, while long-term or low-frequency (LF) variability depends on both sympathetic and parasympathetic branches of the autonomic nervous system. The parasympathetic, or vagal, and sympathetic activities constantly interact; however, under resting conditions vagal tone dominates. Vagal afferent stimulation leads to reflex excitation of vagal efferent activity and inhibition of sympathetic efferent activity, resulting in a decrease in heart rate and blood pressure. The opposite reflex effects are mediated by the stimulation of sympathetic afferent activity. Analysis of the changes in heart rate pattern has been used to assess the state and function of the central oscillators, sympathetic and parasympathetic vagal activity, humoral factors, and the sinus node (16).

In infants, heart rate is higher in AS compared to QS, and this sleep state difference is evident as early as two to three weeks after birth in term infants (17). HRV is also higher in AS compared to QS, as a result of the predominance of sympathetic activity in AS (17). Sleep state also affects blood pressure, with higher values in AS and increased variability (18). Respiratory control is also affected by sleep state. In infants, respiratory rate decreases from wake to sleep, and breathing is more variable in AS, with short apneas occurring more frequently in this state than in QS (5). In infants the majority of apneas are central, and obstructive events are uncommon.

Table 22.1: The effects of sleep state on cardiorespiratory variables in infants.

| Cardiorespiratory Variable | Active Sleep | Quiet Sleep |
|---|---|---|
| Heart rate | increased | decreased |
| Blood pressure | increased | decreased |
| Heart rate variability | elevated | decreased |
| Blood pressure variability | elevated | decreased |
| Baroreflex sensitivity | similar | similar |
| Respiratory rate | increased | decreased |
| Respiratory variability | increased | decreased |
| Hypoxic ventilatory response | immature | immature |

Periodic breathing is common in newborn infants and decreases with increasing postnatal age. Respiratory instability is more common in preterm infants, and the vast majority of these infants will suffer from recurrent prolonged pauses in breathing associated with arterial desaturation and bradycardia, termed apnea of prematurity. Preterm infants also have significantly more episodes of periodic breathing (defined as three or more sequential apneas lasting more than 3 seconds) than those born at term. This immature pattern of breathing is associated with less severe desaturation than apnea of prematurity, but may be very frequent during sleep. Recent studies have shown that periodic breathing is associated with clinically significant falls in cerebral oxygenation which can persist up to six months post-term corrected age (19). Respiratory rate and variability decrease during the first six months of postnatal life (5). An increased respiratory rate in younger infants may be necessary due to the increased demand for carbon dioxide clearance (due to increased metabolic rate), while permitting the infant to maintain ventilation with minimal effort (20). Attempting to modulate ventilation by changing tidal volume would require increased effort due to the highly pliable ribcage and decreased diaphragmatic efficacy (20).

## SIDS Risk Factors and Autonomic Control and Arousal

It is currently believed that SIDS is not due to a single factor but is multifactorial in origin. Over the past four decades several models have been proposed to explain the multifactorial nature of SIDS, including the three interrelated causal spheres of influence model (21), the Quadruple Risk Model (22) and the Triple Risk Model (23). The most widely accepted model is the Triple Risk Model for SIDS, which provides useful means for organizing SIDS knowledge. This model proposes that SIDS occurs when three

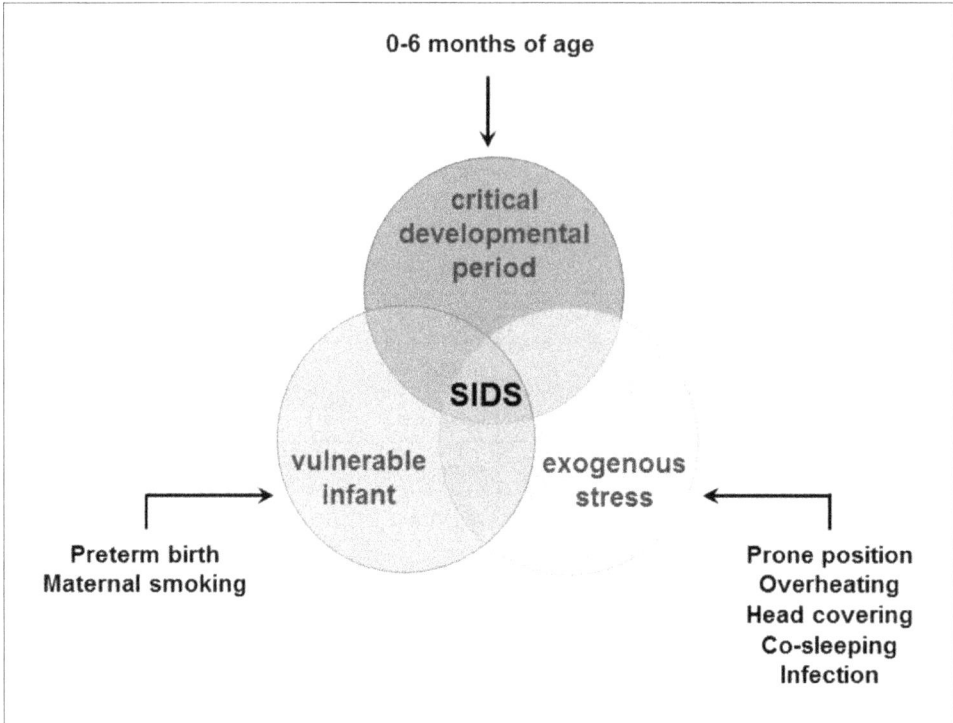

Figure 22.2: Triple Risk Model for SIDS, illustrating the three overlapping factors: [1] a vulnerable infant; [2] a critical developmental period; and [3] an exogenous stress. (Adapted from (23).)

This model proposes that when a vulnerable infant, such as one born preterm or exposed to maternal smoking, is at a critical but unstable developmental period in homeostatic control and is exposed to an exogenous stressor — such as being placed prone to sleep, being overheated, having their head covered, being in a co-sleeping situation, or having recently had an infection — then SIDS may occur. The model proposes that infants will die of SIDS only if all three factors are present, and that the vulnerability lies dormant until they enter the critical developmental period and are exposed to an exogenous stressor. SIDS usually occurs during sleep, and the peak incidence is between 2 to 4 months of age, when sleep patterns are rapidly maturing. The final pathway to SIDS is widely believed to involve immature cardiorespiratory control, in conjunction with a failure of arousal from sleep (24).

factors occur simultaneously: [1] a vulnerable infant; [2] a critical developmental period for homeostatic control; and [3] an exogenous stressor (23) (Figure 22.2).

In an attempt to understand how the Triple Risk Hypothesis is related to infant cardiorespiratory physiology, many researchers have examined how the known risk and protective factors for SIDS alter infant physiology and arousal, particularly during sleep.

The remainder of this chapter discusses the association between the three components of the Triple Risk Hypothesis and major risk factors for SIDS, such as prone sleeping and maternal smoking, together with three "protective" factors and cardiovascular control and arousability from sleep in infants, along with their potential involvement in SIDS.

## Vulnerable infant

Neuropathologic findings from SIDS victims show significant deficits in brainstem and cerebellar structures involved in the regulation of both respiratory drive, cardiovascular control, sleep/wake transition, and arousal from sleep (25-32). Furthermore, genetic polymorphisms have been identified in SIDS victims which affect genes involved in autonomic function, neurotransmission, energy metabolism, and the response to infection (33-37). Infants with certain genetic polymorphisms are believed to be more vulnerable to SIDS, particularly when these are associated with challenges caused by suspected suboptimal intrauterine and postnatal environments (24).

### Exposure to cigarette smoke, alcohol, and illicit drugs

Prenatal and/or postnatal exposure to cigarette smoke is one factor which increases infant vulnerability to SIDS (38, 39), with over 40 studies showing a positive association with risk ratios of between 0.7 and 4.85 (40-43). This increased SIDS risk is likely to be due to the effects of nicotine exposure on autonomic control and arousal (32, 44-48). In support of this idea, Duncan and colleagues (49) found that chronic exposure to nicotine in the prenatal baboon fetus altered serotonergic and nicotinic acetylcholine receptor binding in regions of the medulla, critical to cardiorespiratory control. Furthermore, they identified that these alterations were associated with abnormalities in fetal heart rate variability, indicating altered cardiovascular control (49). Studies in infants exposed to maternal smoking have demonstrated altered heart rate and blood pressure control compared with control infants (50-56). Maternal tobacco smoking also decreases both total arousability and the proportion of cortical arousals. Arousal impairment was observed for both spontaneous arousals from sleep and responses induced by various stimuli (57-63). Few mothers change their smoking behavior postpartum (64); it is therefore difficult to ascertain whether these physiological effects are caused by prenatal or postnatal smoke exposure. Environmental smoke (in the same room) independently increases the risk of SIDS (65, 66). Importantly, it has been shown that before discharge from hospital, preterm infants of smoking mothers already exhibited disruptions in sleep patterns prior to any postnatal smoke exposure (67).

Exposure to alcohol is also a risk for SIDS (68, 69). Animal studies have shown that arousal latency to hypoxia is increased when rat pups were exposed to prenatal alcohol (70). Furthermore, a number of studies have identified that prenatal exposure to illicit drugs also increases the risk for SIDS (71-73). Studies have shown that infants exposed to illicit drugs had an impaired response to a hypoxic challenge at the peak age for SIDS (74). However, another study found no differences in arousal responses to auditory stimuli in methamphetamine-exposed infants; however, infants in both groups were also exposed to maternal smoking (75).

In summary, there is considerable evidence from both animal and human studies suggesting that prenatal exposure to cigarette smoke, alcohol, and illicit drugs has deleterious effects on the developing brain and cardiorespiratory system. It is suggested that these effects increase infant vulnerability to SIDS.

## Preterm birth

Maternal smoking may also be a confounding risk factor for SIDS due to its association with other risk factors, such as preterm birth and intrauterine growth restriction (IUGR) (76-79), which likely result from suboptimal intrauterine environments. Regardless of prenatal exposure to maternal smoking, infants born both preterm and IUGR are at increased risk for SIDS (80-87). The proportion of infants who die suddenly and unexpectedly and who are preterm is approximately four times as great as those born at term (20% compared to 5%). These proportional differences have remained unchanged since the introduction of public campaigns for reducing the risks, and the risk factors for preterm infants are similar to those born at term (84, 85). Despite more than halving the rate for preterm infant deaths attributed to SIDS over the last 20 years, the risk for SIDS deaths among preterm infants compared with infants born at term remains elevated (87).

The risk for SIDS in preterm infants has also been shown to be inversely related to gestational age (88-95), with one study demonstrating that the incidence of SIDS in infants born at 24-28 weeks, 29-32 weeks, 33-36 weeks, and more than 37 weeks was 3.52, 3.01, 2.27, and 1.06 deaths per 1,000 live births respectively (83).

Impaired heart rate control, manifesting as shorter cardiac R-R intervals and higher resting sympathetic tone, has been reported in term-born IUGR infants when compared with infants of appropriate size for gestational age (96, 97). Similarly, preterm infants demonstrated impaired autonomic control compared with term infants studied at, or before, term-equivalent age, and this pattern was inversely related to gestational age at birth (98-103). Longitudinal studies after term-equivalent age have identified that preterm infants exhibited lower blood pressure, delayed blood pressure recovery following head-up tilting, and impaired baroreflex control of blood pressure and heart rate across the first six months corrected age, when compared with age-matched term infants (104-108). Furthermore, maturation of baroreflex control of blood pressure is affected by gestational age at birth, with infants born very preterm (<32 weeks of gestation) having reduced increases in baroreflex sensitivity compared to both preterm and term infants (109). Recently, studies have also identified that cerebral oxygenation is also lower in preterm, compared to term, infants across the first six months corrected age (110) and that cerebrovascular control after a head-up tilt is more variable (111), indicating immature or impaired control.

When compared with term infants at matched conceptional ages, preterm infants also exhibit decreased frequencies and durations of spontaneous arousals from sleep (112-114), together with decreased heart rate responses following arousal (115). Furthermore, preterm infants exhibited longer arousal latencies after exposure to mild hypoxia (15% inspired $O_2$), reaching significantly lower oxygen saturations than term infants (116). Cardiorespiratory complications commonly associated with prematurity, apnea and bradycardia, have also been shown to suppress total arousability when these infants were compared to preterm infants with no history of apnea (117).

In summary, infants born preterm and growth-restricted are at increased risk for SIDS, and alterations in cardiorespiratory control and arousability during sleep likely underpin this vulnerability. Such physiological disturbances may be further exacerbated during a critical developmental period within infancy and by exposure to exogenous stressors.

## Critical developmental period

Approximately 90% of SIDS deaths occur in infants aged less than 6 months (24, 118). During this period, the central nervous system undergoes dramatic maturational changes which are reflected in extensive alterations to sleep architecture, EEG characteristics, and autonomic cardiorespiratory control. The 2- to 4-month period, in particular, has been described as a "developmental window of vulnerability" (119, 120), and coincides with the age where a distinct peak in SIDS incidence occurs (24, 118). The age of peak SIDS incidence has been reported to have remained constant at 2 to 4 months of age following the introduction of safe sleeping campaigns in some studies (118, 121). However, other studies have reported that the peak SIDS incidence may now occur at an earlier age (122), with a decrease in the median peak age from 80 to 64 days in Sweden (123) and 91 to 66 days in South West England (124) since the initiation of "Back to Sleep" campaigns.

### Autonomic control

Autonomic function increases with gestational age in the fetus during pregnancy (125, 126). Both parasympathetic and sympathetic activities increase during gestation, but not in the same manner. The largest increase in parasympathetic activity occurs during the last trimester, while the largest increase in sympathetic activity occurs early on, with smaller changes occurring during the last trimester (127). After birth at term, heart rate increases initially over the first month of life before declining gradually, as a result of an increase in parasympathetic dominance of autonomic control of heart rate (18, 128). Studies of the maturation of heart rate control using HRV have shown an increasing dominance of parasympathetic control across the first six months of life (17). Preterm birth has been associated with immaturity of autonomic nervous system control of the cardiovascular system. This manifests as higher heart rates (98, 99), reduced heart rate variability (99, 129, 130), and decreased baroreflex sensitivity compared to infants born at term (131, 132). Longitudinal studies examining the maturation of blood pressure and its control during sleep in healthy term infants are limited, primarily because of the difficulty of measuring blood pressure continuously and non-invasively. From large studies using intermittent blood pressure measurements, it has been identified that during the first six weeks after birth, systolic blood pressure rises rapidly to reach a steady level which is maintained during infancy (133). Diastolic blood pressure has been shown to fall after birth, reaching a nadir at approximately 2 months of age, followed by a gradual increase until 1 year of life (133).

A number of significant developmental factors may make an infant more vulnerable to a cardiorespiratory challenge during this critical developmental period from birth to 6 months of age, and particularly between 2 to 4 months when the risk of SIDS peaks. Studies in both preterm (105, 110) and term (18) infants have identified a nadir in basal blood pressure during sleep at 2 to 4 months of age, when compared to both earlier (2 to 4 weeks) and later (5 to 6 months) ages studied; a nadir in physiological anemia also occurs at this age. Blood pressure responses to a cardiovascular challenge (head-up tilting) are also impaired at 2 to 4 months compared to younger (2 to 4 weeks) and older (5 to 6 months) ages (134). Studies have also shown that there is a maturational reduction in cerebral oxygenation, which is most marked between 2 to 4 weeks and 2 to 4 months of age, which may be due to limited or inadequate flow-metabolism coupling at this age (135). Thus, the 2- to 4-month age could represent a critical time period when effects of low blood pressure could accentuate decrements in oxygen-carrying capacity and delivery to critical organs (18).

There are even fewer studies of maturation of blood pressure variability (BPV) in infants. BPV decreases with increasing gestational age until term, suggesting a reduction in sympathetic modulation to term-equivalent age (136). BPV continues to decrease with postnatal age after term (137). Taken together these findings suggest that, while sympathetic vascular control is predominant in the newborn period, there is a shift to that of predominantly parasympathetic control with increasing postnatal age, with critical maturational changes occurring when the risk of SIDS is greatest.

The arterial baroreflex is the most important autonomic regulatory mechanism for the short-term control of blood pressure, heart rate, and cardiac contractility. This reflex minimizes changes in blood pressure primarily by altering heart rate and arterial vascular tone. Thus, when there is an increase in blood pressure, it is countered by a decrease in both heart rate and arterial vascular tone. The responses of heart rate and vascular tone are mediated by the efferent parasympathetic and sympathetic limb of the baroreflex respectively. As both systems are involved, studies of the baroreflex provide information on the sympathovagal balance of control of the autonomic nervous system.

The baroreflex is present and functional from early fetal life and undergoes significant maturation in utero. The effectiveness of the baroreflex, termed baroreflex sensitivity, increases significantly with postnatal age from 5 to 6 ms/mmHg at 2 to 4 weeks of age to 11-16 ms/mmHg at 5 to 6 months of age, a value similar to that reported in adults (138). Whilst immature, infants may be at increased vulnerability to hypotensive or hypertensive events.

## Effects of postnatal age on respiratory control

In order to maintain blood oxygen levels, adult humans exposed to lowered oxygen levels experience a prompt increase in ventilation that peaks within 3 to 5 minutes. This period of hyperventilation is sustained for approximately 15 to 30 minutes before a subsequent decline to pre-hypoxic baseline values. This response is referred to as the hypoxic ventilatory response (HVR). The HVR in infants is quite different to that of adults. Following exposure to low oxygen levels, infants exhibit a "biphasic" HVR response which typically consists of a transient hyperventilation (within the first 2 minutes) termed the augmented phase, followed by a sustained reduction in ventilation towards or below normoxic levels, termed the depressive phase. This biphasic HVR has been demonstrated in term and preterm infants during both wakefulness and sleep and some studies have observed the immature HVR in human infants up to two months after birth (139, 140), while others have shown that it remains immature up to 6 months of age (141).

## Arousal responses

Infant arousal responses are also affected by postnatal age, although these maturational effects are sleep-state-dependent. Previous studies have demonstrated that in response to respiratory (mild hypoxia), tactile (nasal air-jet) and auditory stimulation, total arousability is reduced with increasing age during quiet sleep, whilst remaining unchanged in active sleep (142-144). Following the introduction of standard scoring criteria for sub-cortical activation and cortical arousal as separate entities, a recent study noted that spontaneous sub-cortical activations decreased with increasing postnatal age, whilst cortical arousals increased (145). Conversely, another study analyzed both spontaneous and nasal air-jet induced arousability during supine sleep, and found no change in the percentage of cortical arousals (from total responses) throughout the first six months of life (146). Interestingly, when the same infants slept in the prone position, an increased propensity of cortical arousal was identified at 2 to 3 months, the age when SIDS is most common (63, 146). This increase in cortical arousals may reflect an innate protective response to ensure an appropriate level of arousal for restoring homeostasis, not only during a vulnerable period of development, but also in the presence of an exogenous stressor (e.g. the prone sleeping position).

In summary, a large body of work has demonstrated that both autonomic control of the cardiovascular system and arousal responses from sleep are maximally affected by the major risk factors for SIDS, at 2 to 4 months of age when SIDS risk is greatest.

## Exogenous stressor(s)

An exogenous stressor constitutes the third aspect of the Triple Risk Model for SIDS. Epidemiological studies have identified numerous factors common to SIDS victims, such as the prone sleeping position, overheating, and recent infection, which may disrupt homeostasis (24, 33, 147, 148).

### Prone sleeping

The prone sleeping position has long been considered the major risk factor for SIDS (78, 149-152), with some studies suggesting a causal relation between prone sleep and SIDS (153, 154). Several physiological changes ensue when infants sleep prone, including increased peripheral skin temperature and baseline heart rate, together with decreased heart rate variability (18, 155-163). In an effort to identify changes in autonomic cardiovascular control with sleeping position, studies examining heart rate responses to auditory and nasal air-jet stimuli have suggested an increase in sympathetic, and a decrease in parasympathetic, tone in the prone sleeping position (164, 165). Furthermore, sympathetic effects on blood pressure and vasomotor tone are decreased in the prone sleeping position. Lower resting blood pressure and altered cardiovascular responses to head-up tilting have also been identified in term infants when sleeping in the prone position, compared with the supine position (18, 134). Cerebral oxygenation is reduced and cerebrovascular control impaired in the prone position in both term (135, 166) and preterm infants (110, 167). In addition, prone sleeping infants exhibit reduced cardiac and respiratory responses when arousing from sleep, when compared to sleeping in the supine position (164, 165).

Previous studies of both term and preterm infants have consistently identified increases in sleep time, with significant reductions in spontaneous arousability associated with prone sleeping when compared with the supine position (168-171). Furthermore, in other studies the prone sleeping position depressed arousal responses provoked by postural change (155), auditory (172), and somatosensory challenges (62, 156, 173). It has been demonstrated that both spontaneous and induced arousal responses are similarly affected by sleep state and SIDS risk factors, suggesting that they are mediated through the same pathways (174). Despite this well-documented decrease in total arousability, examining subcortical and cortical responses separately has produced conflicting results. Although one study reported a decreased frequency of spontaneous cortical arousals in the prone position (171), more recent studies have found an increased proportion of cortical arousals (of total responses) in both infants not exposed to cigarette smoke and those exposed to cigarette smoke when sleeping prone (63, 146). This apparent promotion of full cortical arousal, demonstrated for both spontaneous and stimulus-induced responses, may protectively compensate against the threat of altered autonomic control and the already blunted total arousability imposed by the prone position.

The prone sleeping position also potentiates the risk of overheating, by reducing the exposed surface area available for radiant heat loss and reducing respiratory heat loss when the infants face is covered (175). Both physiological studies in healthy infants and theoretical model studies of heat balance have observed a decreased ability to lose heat when in the prone position (176-178). Early studies observed decreased variation in behavior and respiratory pattern, increased heart rate, and increased peripheral skin temperature during prone, compared with supine, sleep (177). These studies suggest that infants are less able to maintain adequate respiratory and metabolic homeostasis when sleeping prone.

Increased sweating occurs in SIDS victims, regardless of whether infants slept prone or supine; these cases were predominantly associated with a covered face (118, 179). A history of profuse sweating in SIDS victims has been postulated to be a phenomenon representing an abnormality of function of the autonomic nervous system (180). The involvement of thermal stress with SIDS is further supported by the finding of similar odds ratios for both too much and too little bedding (181), and the suggestion that future SIDS victims may have had atypical temperature regulation (182). Infant arousability is also affected by body and room temperature: decreased sleep continuity and increased body movements have been associated with exposure to cooler temperatures (183), whilst infants sleeping in warmer environments (28 °C vs 24 °C) exhibited increased arousal thresholds to auditory stimuli (184). Furthermore, based on studies assessing blood pressure control in infants (157, 162), it has been suggested that in response to the increased peripheral skin temperature when infants sleep prone, thermoregulatory vasodilatation of the peripheral microvasculature occurs, resulting in a decrease in blood pressure and a reduction in vasomotor tone. Recent studies in preterm infants have shown that increased ambient temperature led to significant changes in autonomic control with elevated heart rate and lower heart rate variability compared to thermoneutral or cooler temperature (185).

## Head covering

Head covering has been identified as a major risk for SIDS, with between 16-28% of SIDS infants found with their heads covered. Although a causal relationship with SIDS has not been established (186, 187), it appears likely that rebreathing and impaired arousal are involved. It has been suggested that the increased SIDS risk associated with head covering may result from hypoxia and hypercapnia via rebreathing of expired air (186, 188). Head covering in healthy infants has profound effects on autonomic control during sleep (189). Franco and colleagues (189) found that infants sleeping supine with their head covered by a bedsheet exhibited decreased parasympathetic activity, increased sympathetic activity, and increased body temperature when compared with head-uncovered periods. In addition, arousal responses in active sleep were also depressed when the head was covered (190).

## Bed sharing

Bed sharing or co-sleeping has also been reported to significantly increase the risk of SIDS, particularly when the mother smokes (118, 124, 191, 192), with more than 50% of SIDS deaths occurring in this situation between 1997 and 2006 (193, 194). There have been few studies investigating the physiology behind this risk factor. In infants from non-smoking families who were studied on successive bed-sharing and solitary-sleeping nights, bed sharing was associated with increased awakenings and transient arousals during slow-wave sleep compared to solitary nights (195). In contrast, another study found that bed-sharing infants spent less time moving and were more likely to have their heads partially or fully covered by bedding than cot-sleeping infants (196). Thus more studies are required to identify the exact physiological changes which occur during bed sharing.

## Swaddling

Swaddling, or firm wrapping, is a traditional infant care practice which, according to an extensive historical review, has been used in some form or another by various cultures since medieval times (197). Low incidences of SIDS in populations where swaddling is common has led to the proposal that swaddling may be protective (198, 199) and on this basis a number of SIDS prevention organizations recommend it. Several studies have documented a "tranquil" behavioral state with longer sleep periods in swaddled infants. Therefore, despite a disparity between studies on the risk for SIDS (124, 200, 201), swaddling has become increasingly popular as a soothing technique throughout the world (202, 203).

Swaddling is a common practice in infants throughout the first six months of life, during the period of increased SIDS risk. The duration of swaddling and the age of initiation of the practice vary widely. The average duration of swaddling has been reported to be 35 days in infants in Yunnan Province in China (204) and to be for the entire first year of life in rural Turkish children (205). The age of initiation of swaddling also varies, with reports of commencing swaddling in the first month of life in Mongolia (206) and immediately after birth in Russia (207). Currently it is unclear if swaddling is protective against SIDS or if it is indeed a risk. In the United Kingdom during the mid-1990s, swaddling during the last sleep was more common amongst SIDS infants than age-matched controls (14% vs. 9%); furthermore, a more recent study showed that this difference has since become more marked (19% vs. 6%) (124). However, a recent meta-analysis has concluded that swaddling was not protective and that placing an infant prone when swaddled significantly increased the risk of death (208). That there is no evidence to recommend swaddling as a strategy to reduce the risk of SIDS has now been endorsed by the American Academy of Pediatrics (209).

Studies investigating the effect of swaddling on cardiovascular control are limited. Swaddling elicits a mild increase in respiratory frequency, most likely due to restricted tidal volumes imposed by the firm wrapping (210-212). No significant effects have been documented on baseline heart rate, skin temperature, or oxygen saturation in term infants when swaddled during sleep (211, 213). Studies which compared infants who were routinely swaddled to those who were unused to this practice found that sleep time and heart rate variability were only altered in those infants naïve to swaddling (214). Several studies investigated the effects of swaddling in relation to infant arousability; however, divergent results have been published. The commonly observed decreases in spontaneous movements and startle responses with swaddling are in contrast to effects of other protective factors for SIDS (197, 215). One study reported that when infants were swaddled, fewer startle responses progressed to a full awakening, indicating an inhibition of the cortical arousal process (216). More recent studies reported that swaddled infants exhibited increased arousal thresholds in response to nasal air-jet stimulation. Furthermore, a decreased frequency of full cortical arousals was observed primarily in infants who were unaccustomed to being swaddled, at 3 months of age (211). Spontaneous cortical arousals were also decreased in those infants unaccustomed to being swaddled, at 3 months of age (214).

These arousal differences between routinely swaddled and naïve-to-swaddling infants, only at this age of peak SIDS risk, may explain the contradictory findings of another group which found decreased auditory arousal thresholds in swaddled infants when compared to infants who were free to move (213). The authors attributed these effects of swaddling on arousal to the greater autonomic changes found after auditory stimulation in swaddled conditions (217). As with the other risk factors discussed above, the mechanisms whereby swaddling may increase the risk for SIDS remain unclear, and further research is required.

### Other external stressors

Other external stressors, such as infection, fever, and minor respiratory and gastrointestinal illnesses, commonly occur in the days to weeks preceding death of SIDS victims (218-220). Although not identified as an independent risk factor for SIDS, minor infections have been associated with an increased likelihood of SIDS when combined with head covering or prone sleeping (122, 200). In the prone sleeping position, minor infection, in combination with fever, could further exacerbate thermoregulatory effects on peripheral vasculature, which could increase the susceptibility of a hypotensive episode. Thus, hypotension, in combination with a decreased ability to arouse from sleep, which has been documented in term infants immediately following an infection

(221), could potentially further impair an infant's ability to appropriately respond to a life-threatening challenge such as circulatory failure or an asphyxial insult.

In summary, numerous studies have shown that exposure to exogenous stressors which have been associated with increased SIDS risk, such as prone sleeping and head covering, impair autonomic cardiorespiratory control and infant arousal responses from sleep. The mechanism of increased risk for other factors, such as bed sharing and swaddling, is less clear and further research is required.

## SIDS-"Protective" Factors and Autonomic Control and Arousal

Some studies have suggested that infant care practices such as breastfeeding, dummy/pacifier use, and immunization decrease the risk of SIDS. These potentially protective factors for SIDS have all been associated with alterations to both cardiovascular autonomic control and arousal responses during sleep. However, results are often inconsistent, and supporting evidence is less extensive than for the risk factors discussed above; thus, these potentially preventative factors remain controversial amongst researchers.

### Breastfeeding

Breastfeeding reduces the incidence of SIDS by approximately half (odds ratio (OR) 0.52, 95% CI: 0.46-0.60), even after multivariate analyses accounted for potentially confounding socioeconomic factors (218, 222, 223). This apparent protection may be a biological effect, given that breastfeeding has been associated with a decreased incidence of diarrhea, vomiting, colds, and other infections; in addition, breast milk is rich in antibodies and many micronutrients (218, 224, 225). Only one study has assessed the effects of breastfeeding on the cardiovascular system during sleep in term infants, and this study found that heart rate was significantly lower in breastfed infants when compared with formula-fed infants (226). Although little is known about the effects of breastfeeding compared to formula feeding on cardiovascular control in infants, physiological studies have demonstrated an apparent promotion of arousal from sleep associated with breastfeeding. One study found that breastfed infants spent more time awake during the night, thus requiring more frequent parental visits (227). Another study showed that healthy breastfed infants aroused more readily from active sleep than formula-fed infants in response to nasal air-jet stimulation at 2 to 3 months postnatal age (228). Although there is a general consensus that breastfeeding should be encouraged, the relationship between breastfeeding for SIDS prevention remains unclear.

### Dummy/Pacifier use

The finding that use of a dummy/pacifier has a protective effect for SIDS has consistently emerged from epidemiological studies, with significant associations being described for both usage during the final sleep and "dummy ever used" (OR: 0.46. CI 0.36-0.59) (118, 229-234). Studies have suggested that a likely mechanism for this protection against SIDS is increased heart rate variability, which has been demonstrated during sucking periods in term (235, 236) and preterm infants (237). Conversely, dummy sucking has also been shown to have no effect on heart rate, heart rate variability, respiratory frequency, or oxygen saturation in term infants (238, 239). In addition, pacifier sucking has been shown to elicit increases in blood pressure in quietly awake or sleeping term infants (236, 240) and in preterm infants (237). Another potential mechanism for the protective nature of dummy use against SIDS is an enhanced arousability from sleep. However, results of the few studies which have been conducted are conflicting, with one study reporting decreased arousal thresholds to auditory stimulation observed in infants who regularly used a dummy, when compared with those who did not use a dummy (241). In contrast, other studies have reported no effect of dummy use on either the frequency or duration of spontaneous arousals in sleeping infants, when studied both with and without a dummy in the mouth (242, 243). It has also been hypothesized that sucking on a dummy during sleep may assist in maintaining airway patency, thus preventing a pharyngeal vacuum and the consequent sealing of the airway (244, 245). Thus the risk of oropharyngeal obstruction may be reduced due to the forward positioning of the tongue when sucking on a dummy (245). Although epidemiological studies have provided strong support for dummy/pacifier use to be protective for SIDS, the physiological mechanisms responsible for this protection remain uncertain.

## Immunization

The peak incidence of SIDS coincides at the time when infants are receiving their first triple antigen vaccinations. In the 1970s there were case reports of infant deaths shortly after the diphtheria-tetanus-pertussis immunization and there were concerns that there was a causal relationship. In 2003 the National Academy of Sciences in the USA reviewed the available data and rejected the idea that there was a causal relationship (246). Additionally, large population case-control studies have found that fewer immunized infants die from sudden and unexpected death in infancy (SUDI), and thus immunization is protective (247-249). A more recent meta-analysis found a multivariate OR for immunization and SUDI to be 0.54 (95% CI: 0.31-0.76); in other words the risk of SUDI is halved in immunized infants (250, 251). There have been limited studies on the physiological benefits of vaccination; however, one study showed that arousal responses and sleep patterns were not affected in the immediate post-vaccination period, despite elevated temperature and heart rate (252).

In summary, factors which have been shown to be protective against SIDS show increases in autonomic control and arousability, as in the case of dummy/pacifier use and breastfeeding, or no change, as in the case of immunization.

## Conclusions

Assessment of cardiovascular control and arousal processes during sleep is important in understanding sleep-related pathologies such as SIDS. In otherwise healthy infants, studies have demonstrated impairment of these physiological mechanisms in association with all three aspects of the Triple Risk Model, thus demonstrating the heterogeneous nature of SIDS. Altered cardiovascular and cerebrovascular control, in conjunction with a failure to arouse from sleep, could potentially impair an infant's ability to appropriately compensate for life-threatening challenges, such as prolonged hypotension or asphyxia during sleep. The concept of a close relationship between SIDS and autonomic dysfunction becomes more compelling with the demonstration of an apparent promotion of arousal from sleep by protective factors for SIDS. Despite successful public awareness campaigns dramatically reducing SIDS rates, this decline in SIDS incidence may have stabilized (253-256). Thus, further research is imperative to elucidate the exact mechanisms involved in the final events of SIDS, allowing identification of "at-risk" infants in the future. The ability to identify these infants would have the potential to increase awareness in both parents and clinicians, whilst minimizing the incidence of SIDS with close monitoring and early intervention.

## References

1.  Krous HF, Beckwith JB, Byard RW, Rognum TO, Bajanowski T, Corey T, et al. Sudden infant death syndrome and unclassified sudden infant deaths: A definitional and diagnostic approach. Pediatrics. 2004;114:234-8. https://doi.org/10.1542/peds.114.1.234.

2.  Curzi-Dascalova L, Peirano P, Morel-Kahn F. Development of sleep states in normal premature and full-term newborns. Dev Psychobiol. 1988;21(5):431-44. https://doi.org/10.1002/dev.420210503.

3.  Phillipson EA, Sullivan CE. Arousal: The forgotten response to respiratory stimuli. Am Rev Respir Dis. 1978;118:807-9.

4.  International Paediatric Work Group on Arousals. The scoring of arousals in healthy term infants (between the ages of 1 and 6 months). J Sleep Res. 2005;14:37-41. https://doi.org/10.1111/j.1365-2869.2004.00426.x.

5.  Gaultier C. Cardiorespiratory adaptation during sleep in infants and children. Pediatr Pulmonol. 1995;19(2):105-17. https://doi.org/10.1002/ppul.1950190206.

6.  Prechtl HF. The behavioral states of the newborn infant (a review). Brain Res. 1974;76(2):185-212. https://doi.org/10.1016/0006-8993(74)90454-5.

7. Curzi-Dascalova L, Challamel MJ. Neurophysiological basis of sleep development. In: Sleep and breathing in children: A developmental approach. Eds Loughlin GM, Carroll JL, Marcus CL. New York: Marcel Dekker, 2000.

8. Parmelee AH, Stern E. Development of states in infants. In: Sleep and the maturing nervous system. Eds Clemente CD, Purpura DP, Mayer FE. New York: Academic, 1972. p. 199-228.

9. Dreyfus-Brisac C. Sleep ontogenesis in early human prematurity from 24 to 27 weeks conceptual age. Dev Psychobiol. 1968;1:162-9. https://doi.org/10.1002/dev.420010303.

10. de Weerd AW, van den Bossche RA. The development of sleep during the first months of life. Sleep Med Rev. 2003;7(2):179-91. https://doi.org/10.1053/smrv.2002.0198.

11. Coons SC, Guilleminault C. Development of sleep-wake patterns and non-rapid eye movement sleep stages during the first six months of life in normal infants. Pediatrics. 1982;69(6):793-8. https://doi.org/10.1097/00004583-198211000-00028.

12. Coons S. Development of sleep and wakefulness during the first 6 months of life. Ed Guilleminault C. New York: Raven Press, 1987. p. 17-27.

13. Curzi-Dascalova L, Mirmiran M. Manual of methods for recording and analysing sleep-wakefulness states in preterm and full term infants. Paris: Les Editions INSERM, 1996.

14. Metcalf D. The ontogenesis of sleep-awake states from birth to 3 months. Electroencephalogr Clin Neurophysiol. 1970;28(4):421.

15. Grigg-Damberger M, Gozal D, Marcus CL, Quan SF, Rosen CL, Chervin RD, et al. The visual scoring of sleep and arousal in infants and children. J Clin Sleep Med. 2007;3(2):201-40.

16. Task Force of the European Society of Cardiology and the North American Society of Pacing and Electrophysiology. Heart rate variability: Standards of measurement, physiological interpretation, and clinical use. Circulation. 1996;93(5):1043-65. https://doi.org/10.1161/01.CIR.93.5.1043.

17. Horne RS. Cardio-respiratory control during sleep in infancy. Paediatr Respir Rev. 2014;15(2):163-9. https://doi.org/10.1016/j.prrv.2013.02.012.

18. Yiallourou SR, Walker AM, Horne RSC. Effects of sleeping position on development of infant cardiovascular control. Arch Dis Child. 2008;93(10):868-72. https://doi.org/10.1136/adc.2007.132860.

19. Decima PF, Fyfe KL, Odoi A, Wong FY, Horne RS. The longitudinal effects of persistent periodic breathing on cerebral oxygenation in preterm infants. Sleep Med. 2015;16(6):729-35. https://doi.org/10.1016/j.sleep.2015.02.537.

20. Kerem E. Why do infants and small children breathe faster? Pediatr Pulmonol. 1996;21(1):65-8. https://doi.org/10.1002/1099-0496(199601)21:1<65::AID-PPUL1950210104>3.0.CO;2-R.

21. Emery JL. A way of looking at the causes of crib death. In: Proceedings of the International Research Conference on the Sudden Infant Death Syndrome. Eds Tildon JT, Roeder LM, Steinschneider A. New York, USA: Academic Press, 1983.

22. Mage DT, Donner M. A unifying theory for SIDS. Int J Pediatr. 2009:1-10. https://doi.org/10.1155/2009/368270.

23. Filiano J, Kinney HC. A perspective on neuropathologic findings in victims of the sudden infant death syndrome: The Triple-Risk Model. Biol Neonate. 1994;65:194-7. https://doi.org/10.1159/000244052.

24. Moon RY, Horne RSC, Hauck FR. Sudden infant death syndrome. Lancet. 2007;370:1578-87. https://doi.org/10.1016/S0140-6736(07)61662-6.

25. Paterson DS, Trachtenberg FL, Thompson EG, Belliveau RA, Beggs AH, Darnall BA, et al. Multiple serotonergic brainstem abnormalities in sudden infant death syndrome. JAMA. 2006;286(17):2124-32. https://doi.org/10.1001/jama.296.17.2124.

26. Kinney HC, Cryan JB, Haynes RL, Paterson DS, Haas EA, Mena OJ, et al. Dentate gyrus abnormalities in sudden unexplained death in infants: Morphological marker of underlying brain vulnerability. Acta Neuropathol. 2015;129(1):65-80. https://doi.org/10.1007/s00401-014-1357-0.

27. Kinney HC, Filiano JJ, Sleeper LA, Mandell F, Valdes-Dapena M, White WF. Decreased muscarinic receptor binding in the arcuate nucleus in sudden infant death syndrome. Science. 1995;269(5229):1446-50. https://doi.org/10.1126/science.7660131.

28. Panigrahy A, Filiano J, Sleeper LA, Mandell F, Valdes-Dapena M, Krous HF, et al. Decreased serotonergic receptor binding in rhombic lip-derived regions of the medulla oblongata in the sudden infant death syndrome. J Neuropathol Exp Neurol. 2000;59(5):377-84. https://doi.org/10.1093/jnen/59.5.377.

29. Panigrahy A, Filiano JJ, Sleeper LA, Mandell F, Valdes-Dapena M, Krous HF, et al. Decreased kainate receptor binding in the arcuate nucleus of the sudden infant death syndrome. J Neuropathol Exp Neurol. 1997;56(11):1253-61. https://doi.org/10.1097/00005072-199711000-00010.

30. Machaalani R, Say M, Waters KA. Serotinergic receptor 1A in the sudden infant death syndrome brainstem medulla and associations with clinical risk factors. Acta Neuropathologica. 2009;117(3):257-65. https://doi.org/10.1007/s00401-008-0468-x.

31. Machaalani R, Waters KA. Neuronal cell death in the sudden infant death syndrome brainstem and associations with risk factors. Brain. 2008;131:218-28. https://doi.org/10.1093/brain/awm290.

32. Machaalani R, Waters KA. Neurochemical abnormalities in the brainstem of the sudden infant death syndrome (SIDS). Paediatr Respir Rev. 2014;15(4):293-300. https://doi.org/10.1016/j.prrv.2014.09.008.

33. Kinney HC, Thach BT. The sudden infant death syndrome. N Engl J Med. 2009;361(8):795-805. https://doi.org/10.1056/NEJMra0803836.

34. Lavezzi AM, Casale V, Oneda R, Weese-Mayer DE, Matturri L. Sudden infant death syndrome and sudden intrauterine unexplained death: Correlation between hypoplasia of raphe nuclei and serotonin transporter gene promoter polymorphism. Pediatr Res. 2009;66(1):22-7. https://doi.org/10.1203/PDR.0b013e3181a7bb73.

35. Weese-Mayer DE, Ackerman MJ, Marazita ML, Berry-Kravis EM. Sudden infant death syndrome: Review of implicated genetic factors. Am J Med Genet A. 2007;143A:771-88. https://doi.org/10.1002/ajmg.a.31722.

36. Filonzi L, Magnani C, Lavezzi AM, Rindi G, Parmigiani S, Bevilacqua G, et al. Association of dopamine transporter and monoamine oxidase molecular polymorphisms with sudden infant death syndrome and stillbirth: New insights into the serotonin hypothesis. Neurogenetics. 2009;10:65-72. https://doi.org/10.1007/s10048-008-0149-x.

37. Courts C, Madea B. Genetics of the sudden infant death syndrome. Forensic Sci Int. 2010;203(1-3):25-33. https://doi.org/10.1016/j.forsciint.2010.07.008.

38. Mitchell E, Scragg R, Stewart AW, Becroft DMO, Taylor B, Ford RPK, et al. Results from the first year of the New Zealand cot death study. NZ Med J. 1991;104:71-6.

39. Matturri L, Ottaviani G, Lavezzi AM. Maternal smoking and sudden infant death syndrome: Epidemiological study related to pathology. Virchows Arch. 2006;449:697-706. https://doi.org/10.1007/s00428-006-0308-0.

40. Anderson HR, Cook DG. Passive smoking and sudden infant death syndrome: Review of the epidemilogical evidence. Thorax. 1997;52:1003-9. https://doi.org/10.1136/thx.52.11.1003.

41. Blair PS, Bensley D, Smith I, Bacon C, Taylor B, Berry J. Smoking and the sudden infant death syndrome: Results from 1993-5 case-control study for confidential

inquiry into stillbirths and deaths in infancy. BMJ. 1996;313:195-8. https://doi.org/10.1136/bmj.313.7051.195.

42. Dwyer T, Ponsonby A, Couper D. Tobacco smoke exposure at one month of age and subsequent risk of SIDS — A prospective study. Am J Epidemiol. 1999;149:593-602. https://doi.org/10.1093/oxfordjournals.aje.a009857.

43. Haglund B. Cigarette smoking and sudden infant death syndrome: Some salient points in the debate. Acta Paediatrica Supplement. 1993;389:37-9. https://doi.org/10.1111/j.1651-2227.1993.tb12872.x.

44. Machaalani R, Say M, Waters KA. Effects of cigarette smoke exposure on nicotinic acetylcholine receptor subunits alpha7 and beta2 in the sudden infant death syndrome (SIDS) brainstem. Toxicol Appl Pharmacol. 2011;257(3):396-404. https://doi.org/10.1016/j.taap.2011.09.023.

45. Machaalani R, Ghazavi E, Hinton T, Waters KA, Hennessy A. Cigarette smoking during pregnancy regulates the expression of specific nicotinic acetylcholine receptor (nAChR) subunits in the human placenta. Toxicol Appl Pharmacol. 2014;276(3):204-12. https://doi.org/10.1016/j.taap.2014.02.015.

46. Lavezzi AM, Mecchia D, Matturri L. Neuropathology of the area postrema in sudden intrauterine and infant death syndromes related to tobacco smoke exposure. Auton Neurosci. 2012;166(1-2):29-34. https://doi.org/10.1016/j.autneu.2011.09.001.

47. Hunt NJ, Russell B, Du MK, Waters KA, Machaalani R. Changes in orexinergic immunoreactivity of the piglet hypothalamus and pons after exposure to chronic postnatal nicotine and intermittent hypercapnic hypoxia. Eur J Neurosci. 2016;43(12):1612-22. https://doi.org/10.1111/ejn.13246.

48. Vivekanandarajah A, Chan YL, Chen H, Machaalani R. Prenatal cigarette smoke exposure effects on apoptotic and nicotinic acetylcholine receptor expression in the infant mouse brainstem. Neurotoxicology. 2016;53:53-63. https://doi.org/10.1016/j.neuro.2015.12.017.

49. Duncan JR, Garland M, Myers MM, Fifer WP, Yang M, Kinney HC, et al. Prenatal nicotine-exposure alters fetal autonomic activity and medullary neurotransmitter receptors: Implications for sudden infant death syndrome. J Appl Physiol. 2009;107(5):1579-90. https://doi.org/10.1152/japplphysiol.91629.2008.

50. Browne CA, Colditz PB, Dunster KR. Infant autonomic function is altered by maternal smoking during pregnancy. Early Hum Develop. 2000;59:209-18. https://doi.org/10.1016/S0378-3782(00)00098-0.

51. Dahlstrom A, Ebersjo C, Lundell B. Nicotine in breast milk influences heart rate variability in the infant. Acta Paediatrica. 2008;97(8):1075-9. https://doi.org/10.1111/j.1651-2227.2008.00785.x.

52. Fifer WP, Fingers ST, Youngman M, Gomez-Gribben E, Myers MM. Effects of alcohol and smoking during pregnancy on infant autonomic control. Dev Psychobiol. 2009;51:234-42. https://doi.org/10.1002/dev.20366.

53. Cohen G, Vella S, Jeffery H, Lagercrantz H, Katz-Salamon M. Cardiovascular stress hyperreactivity in babies of smokers and in babies born preterm. Circulation. 2008;118(18):1848-53. https://doi.org/10.1161/CIRCULATIONAHA.108.783902.

54. Thiriez G, Bouhaddi M, Mourot L, Nobili F, Fortrat JO, Menget A, et al. Heart rate variability in preterm infants and maternal smoking during pregnancy. Clin Auton Res. 2009;19(3):149-56. https://doi.org/10.1007/s10286-009-0003-8.

55. Viskari-Lahdeoja S, Hytinantti T, Andersson S, Kirjavainen T. Heart rate and blood pressure control in infants exposed to maternal cigarette smoking. Acta Paediatrica. 2008;97(11):1535-41. https://doi.org/10.1111/j.1651-2227.2008.00966.x.

56. Franco P, Chabanski S, Szliwowski H, Dramaix M, Kahn A. Influence of maternal smoking on autonomic nervous system in healthy infants. Pediatr Res. 2000;47(2):215-20. https://doi.org/10.1203/00006450-200002000-00011.

57. Sawnani H, Jackson T, Murphy T, Beckerman R, Simakajornboon N. The effect of maternal smoking on respiratory and arousal patterns in preterm infants during sleep. Am J Respir Crit Care Med. 2004;169:733-8. https://doi.org/10.1164/rccm.200305-692OC.

58. Tirosh E, Libon D, Bader D. The effect of maternal smoking during pregnancy on sleep respiratory and arousal patterns in neonates. J Perinatol. 1996;16(6):435-8.

59. Franco P, Groswasser J, Hassid S, Lanquart J, Scaillet S, Kahn A. Prenatal exposure to cigarette smoking is associated with a decrease in arousal in infants. J Pediatr. 1999;135(1):34-8. https://doi.org/10.1016/S0022-3476(99)70324-0.

60. Chang AB, Wilson SJ, Masters IB, Yuill M, Williams G, Hubbard M. Altered arousal response in infants exposed to cigarette smoke. Arch Dis Child. 2003;88:30-3. https://doi.org/10.1136/adc.88.1.30.

61. Lewis KW, Bosque EM. Deficient hypoxia awakening response in infants of smoking mothers: Possible relationship to sudden infant death syndrome. J Pediatr. 1995;127(5):691-9. https://doi.org/10.1016/S0022-3476(95)70155-9.

62. Horne RSC, Ferens D, Watts A-M, Vitkovic J, Andrew S, Cranage SM, et al. Effects of maternal tobacco smoking, sleeping position and sleep state on arousal

in healthy term infants. Arch Dis Child Fetal Neonatal Ed. 2002;87:F100-F5. https://doi.org/10.1136/fn.87.2.F100.

63. Richardson HL, Walker AM, Horne RSC. Maternal smoking impairs arousal patterns in sleeping infants. Sleep. 2009;32(4):515-21. https://doi.org/10.1093/sleep/32.4.515.

64. Johansson A, Halling A, Hermansson G. Indoor and outdoor smoking. Impact on children's health. Eur J Public Health. 2003;13(1):61-6. https://doi.org/10.1093/eurpub/13.1.61.

65. Schoendorf KC, Kiely JL. Relationship of sudden infant death syndrome to maternal smoking during and after pregnancy. Pediatrics. 1992;90(6):905-8.

66. Klonoff-Cohen HS, Edelstein SL, Lefkowitz ES, Srinivasan IP, Kaegi D, Chang JC, et al. The effect of passive smoking and tobacco exposure through breast milk on sudden infant death syndrome. JAMA. 1995;273(10):795-8. https://doi.org/10.1001/jama.1995.03520340051035.

67. Stephan-Blanchard E, Telliez F, Leke A, Djeddi D, Bach V, Libert J, et al. The influence of in utero exposure to smoking on sleep patterns in preterm neonates. Sleep. 2008;31(12):1683-9. https://doi.org/10.1093/sleep/31.12.1683.

68. Strandberg-Larsen K, Gronboek M, Andersen AM, Andersen PK, Olsen J. Alcohol drinking pattern during pregnancy and risk of infant mortality. Epidemiology. 2009;20(6):884-91. https://doi.org/10.1097/EDE.0b013e3181bbd46c.

69. O'Leary CM, Jacoby PJ, Bartu A, D'Antoine H, Bower C. Maternal alcohol use and sudden infant death syndrome and infant mortality excluding SIDS. Pediatrics. 2013;131(3):e770-8. https://doi.org/10.1542/peds.2012-1907.

70. Sirieix CM, Tobia CM, Schneider RW, Darnall RA. Impaired arousal in rat pups with prenatal alcohol exposure is modulated by GABAergic mechanisms. Physiol Rep. 2015;3(6):e12424. https://doi.org/10.14814/phy2.12424.

71. Rajegowda BK, Kandall SR, Falciglia H. Sudden unexpected death in infants of narcotic-dependent mothers. Early Hum Dev. 1978;2(3):219-25. https://doi.org/10.1016/0378-3782(78)90026-9.

72. Chavez CJ, Ostrea EM Jr., Stryker JC, Smialek Z. Sudden infant death syndrome among infants of drug-dependent mothers. J Pediatr. 1979;95(3):407-9. https://doi.org/10.1016/S0022-3476(79)80517-X.

73. Williams SM, Mitchell EA, Taylor BJ. Are risk factors for sudden infant death syndrome different at night? Arch Dis Child. 2002;87(4):274-8. https://doi.org/10.1136/adc.87.4.274.

74. Ali K, Rossor T, Bhat R, Wolff K, Hannam S, Rafferty GF, et al. Antenatal substance misuse and smoking and newborn hypoxic challenge response. Arch Dis Child Fetal Neonatal Ed. 2016;101(2):F143-8. https://doi.org/10.1136/archdischild-2015-308491.

75. Galland BC, Mitchell EA, Thompson JM, Wouldes T, Group NIS. Auditory evoked arousal responses of 3-month-old infants exposed to methamphetamine in utero: A nap study. Acta Paediatrica. 2013;102(4):424-30. https://doi.org/10.1111/apa.12136.

76. Andriessen P, Koolen AMP, Berendsen RCM, Wijn PFF, ten Broeke EDM, Oei SG, et al. Cardiovascular fluctuations and transfer function analysis in stable preterm infants. Pediatr Res. 2003;53(1):89-97. https://doi.org/10.1203/00006450-200301000-00016.

77. Mitchell EA, Ford RPK, Stewart AW, Taylor BJ, Becroft DMO, Thompson JMD, et al. Smoking and the sudden infant death syndrome. Pediatrics. 1993;91:893-6.

78. Brooke H, Gibson A, Tappin D, Brown H. Case control study of sudden infant death syndrome in Scotland, 1992-5. BMJ. 1997;314:1516-20. https://doi.org/10.1136/bmj.314.7093.1516.

79. Schellscheidt J, Oyen N, Jorch G. Interactions between maternal smoking and other perinatal risk factors for SIDS. Acta Paediatrica. 1997;86:857-63. https://doi.org/10.1111/j.1651-2227.1997.tb08612.x.

80. Bergman AB, Ray CG, Pomeroy MA, Wahl PW, Beckwith JB. Studies of the sudden infant death syndrome in King County, Washington. 3. Epidemiology. Pediatrics. 1972;49(6):860-70.

81. Grether JK, Schulman J. Sudden infant death syndrome and birth weight. J Pediatr. 1989;114:561-7. https://doi.org/10.1016/S0022-3476(89)80694-8.

82. Adams MM, Rhodes PH, McCarthy BJ. Are race and length of gestation related to age at death in the sudden infant death syndrome? Paediatr Perinat Epidemiol. 1990;4(3):325-39. https://doi.org/10.1111/j.1365-3016.1990.tb00655.x.

83. Malloy MH, Hoffman HJ. Prematurity, sudden infant death syndrome, and age of death. Pediatrics. 1995;96(3):464-71.

84. Blair PS, Platt MW, Smith IJ, Fleming PJ, & CESDI SUDI Research Group. Sudden infant death syndrome and sleeping position in pre-term and low birth weight infants: An opportunity for targeted intervention. Arch Dis Child. 2006;91:101-6. https://doi.org/10.1136/adc.2004.070391.

85. Thompson JM, Mitchell EA, & New Zealand Cot Death Study Group. Are the risk factors for SIDS different for preterm and term infants? Arch Dis Child. 2006;91(2):107-11. https://doi.org/10.1136/adc.2004.071167.

86. Gilbert NL, Fell DB, Joseph KS, Liu S, Leon JA, Sauve R, et al. Temporal trends in sudden infant death syndrome in Canada from 1991 to 2005: Contribution of changes in cause of death assignment practices and in maternal and infant characteristics. Paediatr Perinat Epidemiol. 2012;26(2):124-30. https://doi.org/10.1111/j.1365-3016.2011.01248.x.

87. Malloy MH. Prematurity and sudden infant death syndrome: United States 2005-2007. J Perinatol. 2013;33(6):470-5. https://doi.org/10.1038/jp.2012.158.

88. Peterson DR. Sudden, unexpected death in infants. An epidemiologic study. Am J Epidemiol. 1966;84(3):478-82. https://doi.org/10.1093/oxfordjournals.aje.a120660.

89. Standfast SJ, Jereb S, Janerich DT. The epidemiology of sudden infant death in upstate New York. JAMA. 1979;241(11):1121-4. https://doi.org/10.1001/jama.1979.03290370025021.

90. Hoffman HJ, Damus K, Hillman L, Krongrad E. Risk factors for SIDS: Results of the National Institute of Child Health and Human Development SIDS cooperative epidemiology study. Ann N Y Acad Sci. 1988;533:13-30. https://doi.org/10.1111/j.1749-6632.1988.tb37230.x.

91. Hoffman HJ, Hillman LS. Epidemiology of the sudden infant death syndrome: Maternal, neonatal, and postneonatal risk factors. Clin Perinatol. 1992;19(4):717-37.

92. Grether JK, Schulman J. Sudden infant death syndrome and birth weight. J Pediatrics. 1989;114:561-7. https://doi.org/10.1016/S0022-3476(89)80694-8.

93. Malloy MH, Hoffman MA. Prematurity, sudden infant death syndrome and age of death. Pediatrics. 1995;96(3):464-71.

94. Malloy MH, Freeman DH Jr. Birth weight- and gestational age-specific sudden infant death syndrome mortality: United States, 1991 versus 1995. Pediatrics. 2000;105(6):1227-31. https://doi.org/10.1542/peds.105.6.1227.

95. Halloran DR, Alexander GR. Preterm delivery and age of SIDS death. Ann Epidemiol. 2006;16(8):600-6. https://doi.org/10.1016/j.annepidem.2005.11.007.

96. Galland BC, Taylor B, Bolton DPG, Sayers RM. Heart rate variability and cardiac reflexes in small for gestational age infants. J Appl Physiol. 2006;100(3):933-9. https://doi.org/10.1152/japplphysiol.01275.2005.

97. Spassov L, Curzi-Dascalova L, Clairambault J, Kauffmann F, Eiselt M, Medigue C, et al. Heart rate and heart rate variability during sleep in small-for-gestational age newborns. Pediatr Res. 1994;35(4 Pt 1):500-5. https://doi.org/10.1203/0000 6450-199404000-00022.

98. Katona PG, Frasz A, Egbert J. Maturation of cardiac control in full-term and preterm infants during sleep. Early Hum Dev. 1980;4(2):145-59. https://doi.org/ 10.1016/0378-3782(80)90018-3.

99. Eiselt M, Curzi-Dascalova L, Clairambault J, Kauffmann F, Medigue C, Peirano P. Heart rate variability in low-risk prematurely born infants reaching normal term: A comparison with full-term newborns. Early Hum Dev. 1993;32:183-95. https:// doi.org/10.1016/0378-3782(93)90011-I.

100. Eiselt M, Zwiener U, Witte H, Curzi-Dascalova L. Influence of prematurity and extrauterine development on the sleep state dependant heart rate patterns. Somnologie. 2002;6(3):116-23. https://doi.org/10.1046/j.1439-054X.2002.02189.x.

101. Patural H, Barthelemy JC, Pichot V, Mazzocchi C, Teyssier G, Damon G, et al. Birth prematurity determines prolonged autonomic nervous system immaturity. Clin Auton Res. 2004;14:391-5. https://doi.org/10.1007/s10286-004-0216-9.

102. Patural H, Pichot V, Jaziri F, Teyssier G, Gaspoz JM, Roche F, et al. Autonomic cardiac control of very preterm newborns: A prolonged dysfunction. Early Hum Dev. 2008;84(10):681-7. https://doi.org/10.1016/j.earlhumdev.2008.04.010.

103. Longin E, Gerstner T, Schaible T, Lanz T, Konig S. Maturation of the autonomic nervous system: Differences in heart rate variability in premature vs term infants. J Perinat Med. 2006;34:303-8. https://doi.org/10.1515/JPM.2006.058.

104. Witcombe NB, Yiallourou SR, Walker AM, Horne RSC. Delayed blood pressure recovery after head-up tilting during sleep in preterm infants. J Sleep Res. 2010(19):93-102. https://doi.org/10.1111/j.1365-2869.2009.00793.x.

105. Witcombe NB, Yiallourou SR, Walker AM, Horne RSC. Blood pressure and heart rate patterns during sleep are altered in preterm-born infants: Implications for sudden infant death syndrome. Pediatrics. 2008;122(6):1242-8. https://doi. org/10.1542/peds.2008-1400.

106. Witcombe NB, Yiallourou SR, Sands SA, Walker AM, Horne RS. Preterm birth alters the maturation of baroreflex sensitivity in sleeping infants. Pediatrics. 2012;129(1):e89-96. https://doi.org/10.1542/peds.2011-1504.

107. Fyfe KL, Yiallourou SR, Wong FY, Odoi A, Walker AM, Horne RS. The effect of gestational age at birth on post-term maturation of heart rate variability. Sleep. 2015;38(10):1635-44. https://doi.org/10.5665/sleep.5064.

108. Yiallourou SR, Witcombe NB, Sands SA, Walker AM, Horne RS. The development of autonomic cardiovascular control is altered by preterm birth. Early Hum Dev. 2013;89(3):145-52. https://doi.org/10.1016/j.earlhumdev.2012.09.009.

109. Fyfe KL, Yiallourou SR, Wong FY, Odoi A, Walker AM, Horne RS. Gestational age at birth affects maturation of baroreflex control. J Pediatr. 2015;166(3):559-65. https://doi.org/10.1016/j.jpeds.2014.11.026.

110. Fyfe KL, Yiallourou SR, Wong FY, Odoi A, Walker AM, Horne RS. Cerebral oxygenation in preterm infants. Pediatrics. 2014;134(3):435-45. https://doi.org/10.1542/peds.2014-0773.

111. Fyfe K, Odoi A, Yiallourou SR, Wong F, Walker AM, Horne RS. Preterm infants exhibit greater variability in cerebrovascular control than term infants. Sleep. 2015;38(9):1411-21. https://doi.org/10.5665/sleep.4980.

112. Horne RSC, Cranage SM, Chau B, Adamson TM. Effects of prematurity on arousal from sleep in the newborn infant. Pediatr Res. 2000;47:468-74. https://doi.org/10.1203/00006450-200004000-00010.

113. Scher MS, Steppe DA, Dahl RE, Asthana S, Guthrie RD. Comparison of EEG sleep measures in healthy full-term and preterm infants at matched conceptional ages. Sleep. 1992;15(5):442-8. https://doi.org/10.1093/sleep/15.5.442.

114. Richardson HL, Horne RS. Arousal from sleep pathways are affected by the prone sleeping position and preterm birth: Preterm birth, prone sleeping and arousal from sleep. Early Hum Dev. 2013;89(9):705-11. https://doi.org/10.1016/j.earlhumdev.2013.05.001.

115. Tuladhar R, Harding R, Adamson TM, Horne RSC. Comparison of postnatal development of heart rate responses to trigeminal stimulation in sleeping preterm and term infants. J Sleep Res. 2005;14:29-36. https://doi.org/10.1111/j.1365-2869.2004.00434.x.

116. Verbeek MMA, Richardson HL, Parslow PM, Walker AM, Harding R, Horne RSC. Arousal and ventilatory responses to mild hypoxia in sleeping preterm infants. J Sleep Res. 2008;17:344-53. https://doi.org/10.1111/j.1365-2869.2008.00653.x.

117. Horne RSC, Andrew S, Mitchell K, Sly DJ, Cranage SM, Chau B, et al. Apnoea of prematurity and arousal from sleep. Early Hum Dev. 2001;61:119-33. https://doi.org/10.1016/S0378-3782(00)00129-8.

118. Carpenter RG, Irgens LM, Blair PS, Fleming PJ, Huber J, Jorch G, et al. Sudden unexplained infant death in 20 regions in Europe: Case control study. Lancet. 2004;363:185-91. https://doi.org/10.1016/S0140-6736(03)15323-8.

119. Kohyama J. Sleep as a window on the developing brain. Curr Probl Pediatr. 1998;28(3):69-92. https://doi.org/10.1016/S0045-9380(98)80054-6.

120. Carroll JL. Developmental plasticity in respiratory control. J App Physiol. 2003;94:375-89. https://doi.org/10.1152/japplphysiol.00809.2002.

121. Blair PS, Sidebotham P, Berry PJ, Evans M, Fleming PJ. Major epidemiological changes in sudden infant death syndrome: A 20-year population-based study in the UK. Lancet. 2006;367:314-19. https://doi.org/10.1016/S0140-6736(06)67968-3.

122. Hunt CE, Hauck FR. Sudden infant death syndrome. CMAJ. 2006;174(13):1861-9. https://doi.org/10.1503/cmaj.051671.

123. Mollborg P, Alm B. Sudden infant death syndrome during low incidence in Sweden 1997-2005. Acta Paediatrica. 2010;99(1):94-8.

124. Blair PS, Sidebotham P, Evason-Coombe C, Edmonds M, Heckstall-Smith EMA, Fleming P. Hazardous co-sleeping environments and risk factors amenable to change: Case-control study of SIDS in south west England. BMJ. 2009;339:b3666. https://doi.org/10.1136/bmj.b3666.

125. Gagnon R, Campbell K, Hunse C, Patrick J. Patterns of human fetal heart rate accelerations from 26 weeks to term. Am J Obstet Gynecol. 1987;157:743-8. https://doi.org/10.1016/S0002-9378(87)80042-X.

126. Karin J, Hirsch M, Akselrod S. An estimate of fetal autonomic state by spectral analysis of fetal heart rate fluctuations. Pediatr Res. 1993;34:134-8. https://doi.org/10.1203/00006450-199308000-00005.

127. Wakai RT. Assessment of fetal neurodevelopment via fetal magnetocardiography. Exp Neurol. 2004;190:S65-S71. https://doi.org/10.1016/j.expneurol.2004.04.019.

128. Harper R, Hoppenbrouwers T, Sterman M, McGinty D, Hodgman J. Polygraphic studies of normal infants during the first six months of life. I. Heart rate and variability as a function of state. Pediatr Res. 1976;10:945-51. https://doi.org/10.1203/00006450-197611000-00008.

129. de Beer NA, Andriessen P, Berendsen RC, Oei SG, Wijn PF, Oetomo SB. Customized spectral band analysis compared with conventional Fourier analysis of heart rate variability in neonates. Physiol Meas. 2004;25(6):1385-95. https://doi.org/10.1088/0967-3334/25/6/004.

130. Andriessen P, Janssen B, Berendsen RC, Oetomo SB, Wijn PF, Blanco CE. Cardiovascular autonomic regulation in preterm infants: The effect of atropine. Pediatr Res. 2004;56(6):939-46. https://doi.org/10.1203/01.PDR.0000145257.75072.BB.

131. Waldman S, Krauss AN, Auld PA. Baroreceptors in preterm infants: Their relationship to maturity and disease. Dev Med Child Neurol. 1979;21(6):714-22. https://doi.org/10.1111/j.1469-8749.1979.tb01692.x.

132. Gournay V, Drouin E, Roze JC. Development of baroreflex control of heart rate in preterm and full term Infants. Arch Dis Childhood Fetal Neonatal Ed. 2002;86(3):151-4. https://doi.org/10.1136/fn.86.3.F151.

133. Task Force on Blood Pressure Control in Children. Report of the second task force on blood pressure control in children — 1987. Pediatrics. 1987;19(1):1-25.

134. Yiallourou SR, Walker AM, Horne RSC. Prone sleeping impairs circulatory control during sleep in healthy term infants; implications for sudden infant death syndrome. Sleep. 2008;31(8):1139-46.

135. Wong FY, Witcombe NB, Yiallourou SR, Yorkston S, Dymowski AR, Krishnan L, et al. Cerebral oxygenation is depressed during sleep in healthy term infants when they sleep prone. Pediatrics. 2011;127(3):e558-65. https://doi.org/10.1542/peds.2010-2724.

136. Andriessen P, Oetomo SB, Peters C, Vermeulen B, Wijn PFF, Blanco CE. Baroreceptor reflex sensitivity in human neonates: The effect of postmenstrual age. J Physiol. 2005;568:333-41. https://doi.org/10.1113/jphysiol.2005.093641.

137. Yiallourou SR, Sands SA, Walker AM, Horne RS. Maturation of heart rate and blood pressure variability during sleep in term-born infants. Sleep. 2012;35(2):177-86. https://doi.org/10.5665/sleep.1616.

138. Yiallourou SR, Sands SA, Walker AM, Horne RS. Postnatal development of baroreflex sensitivity in infancy. J Physiol. 2010;588(Pt 12):2193-203. https://doi.org/10.1113/jphysiol.2010.187070.

139. Cohen G, Malcolm G, Henderson-Smart D. Ventilatory response of the newborn infant to mild hypoxia. Pediatr Pulmonol. 1997;24:163-72. https://doi.org/10.1002/(SICI)1099-0496(199709)24:3<163::AID-PPUL1>3.0.CO;2-O.

140. Martin RJ, DiFiore JM, Jana L, Davis RL, Miller MJ, Coles SK, et al. Persistence of the biphasic ventilatory response hypoxia in preterm infants. J Pediatr. 1998;132(6):960-4. https://doi.org/10.1016/S0022-3476(98)70391-9.

141. Parslow PM, Cranage SM, Adamson TM, Harding R, Horne RSC. Arousal and ventilatory responses to hypoxia in sleeping infants: Effects of maternal smoking. Respir Physiol Neurobiol. 2004;140:77-87. https://doi.org/10.1016/j.resp.2004.01.004.

142. Parslow PM, Harding R, Cranage SM, Adamson TM, Horne RSC. Ventilatory responses preceding hypoxia-induced arousal in infants: Effects of sleep-state.

Respir Physiol Neurobiol. 2003;136:235-47. https://doi.org/10.1016/S1569-9048(03)00085-5.

143. Trinder J, Newman NM, Le Grande M, Whitworth F, Kay A, Pirkis J, et al. Behavioral and EEG responses to auditory stimuli during sleep in newborn infants and in infants aged 3 months. Biological Psychology. 1990;90:213-27. https://doi.org/10.1016/0301-0511(90)90035-U.

144. Parslow PM, Harding R, Cranage SM, Adamson TM, Horne RSC. Arousal responses to somatosensory and mild hypoxic stimuli are depressed during quiet sleep in healthy term infants. Sleep. 2003;26(6):739-44.

145. Montemitro E, Franco P, Scaillet S, Kato I, Groswasser J, Villa MP, et al. Maturation of spontaneous arousals in healthy infants. Sleep. 2008;31(1):47-54. https://doi.org/10.1093/sleep/31.1.47.

146. Richardson HL, Walker AM, Horne RSC. Sleep position alters arousal processes maximally at the high-risk age for sudden infant death syndrome. J Sleep Res. 2008;17:450-7. https://doi.org/10.1111/j.1365-2869.2008.00683.x.

147. Blackwell C, Moscovis S, Hall S, Burns C, Scott RJ. Exploring the risk factors for sudden infant deaths and their role in inflammatory responses to infection. Front Immunol. 2015;6:44. https://doi.org/10.3389/fimmu.2015.00044.

148. Galland BC, Elder DE. Sudden unexpected death in infancy: Biological mechanisms. Paediatr Respir Rev. 2014;15(4):287-92. https://doi.org/10.1016/j.prrv.2014.09.003.

149. Oyen H, Markstead T, Skjaerven R, Irgens LM, Helweg-Larsen K, Alm B, et al. Combined effects of sleeping position and the perinatal risk factors in sudden infant death syndrome: The Nordic epidemiological study. Pediatrics. 1997;100(4):613-21. https://doi.org/10.1542/peds.100.4.613.

150. Mitchell EA. Sleeping position of infants and the sudden infant death syndrome. Acta Paediatrica. 1993;389:26-30. https://doi.org/10.1111/j.1651-2227.1993.tb12870.x.

151. Ponsonby AL, Dwyer T. The Tasmanian SIDS case-control study: Univariate and multivariate risk factor analysis. Paediatr Perinat Epidemiol. 1995;9:256-72. https://doi.org/10.1111/j.1365-3016.1995.tb00141.x.

152. Taylor JA, Krieger JW, Reay DT, David RL, Harruff R, Cheney LK. Prone sleeping position and sudden infant death syndrome in King County, Washington: A case control study. Pediatrics. 1996;128:626-30. https://doi.org/10.1016/S0022-3476(96)80126-0.

153. Beal SM, Finch CF. An overview of retrospective case-control studies investigating the relationship between prone sleeping position and SIDS. J Paediatr Child Health. 1991;27:334-9. https://doi.org/10.1111/j.1440-1754.1991.tb00414.x.

154. Fleming PJ, Gilbert R, Azaz Y, Berry PJ, Rudd PT, Stewart A, et al. Interaction between bedding and sleeping position in the sudden infant death syndrome: A population based case-control study. BMJ. 1990;301(6743):85-9. https://doi.org/10.1136/bmj.301.6743.85.

155. Galland BC, Reeves H, Taylor B, Bolton DPG. Sleep position, autonomic function, and arousal. Arch Dis Child Fetal Neonatal Ed. 1998;78:189-94. https://doi.org/10.1136/fn.78.3.F189.

156. Horne R, Ferens D, Watts A, Vitkovic J, Lacey B, Andrew S, et al. The prone sleeping position impairs arousability in term infants. J Pediatr. 2001;138:811-16. https://doi.org/10.1067/mpd.2001.114475.

157. Galland B, Taylor B, Bolton D, Sayers R. Vasoconstriction following spontaneous sighs and head-up tilts in infants sleeping prone and supine. Early Hum Dev. 2000;58:119-32. https://doi.org/10.1016/S0378-3782(00)00070-0.

158. Ariagno RL, Mirmiran M, Adams MM, Saporito AG, Dubin AM, Baldwin RB. Effect of position on sleep, heart rate variability, and QT interval in preterm infants at 1 and 3 months' corrected age. Pediatrics. 2003;111:622-5. https://doi.org/10.1542/peds.111.3.622.

159. Sahni R, Schulz H, Kashyap S, Ohira-Kist K, Fifer WP, Myers MM. Postural differences in cardiac dynamics during quiet and active sleep in low birthweight infants. Acta Paediatrica. 1999;88:1396-401. https://doi.org/10.1111/j.1651-2227.1999.tb01058.x.

160. Gabai N, Cohen A, Mahagney A, Bader D, Tirosh E. Arterial blood flow and autonomic function in full-term infants. Clin Physiol Funct Imaging. 2006;26:127-31. https://doi.org/10.1111/j.1475-097X.2006.00661.x.

161. Kahn A, Grosswasser J, Sottiaux M, Rebuffat E, Franco P, Dramaix M. Prone or supine body position and sleep characteristics in infants. Pediatrics. 1993;91:1112-15.

162. Chong A, Murphy N, Matthews T. Effect of prone sleeping on circulatory control in infants. Arch Dis Child. 2000;82:253-6. https://doi.org/10.1136/adc.82.3.253.

163. Ammari A, Schulze KF, Ohira-Kist K, Kashyap S, Fifer WP, Myers MM, et al. Effects of body position on thermal, cardiorespiratory and metabolic activity in low birth weight infants. Early Hum Dev. 2009;85:497-501. https://doi.org/10.1016/j.earlhumdev.2009.04.005.

164. Franco P, Grosswasser J, Sottiaux M, Broadfield E, Kahn A. Decreased cardiac responses to auditory stimulation during prone sleep. Pediatrics. 1996;97:174-8.

165. Tuladhar R, Harding R, Cranage SM, Adamson TM, Horne RSC. Effects of sleep position, sleep state and age on heart rate responses following provoked arousal in term infants. Early Hum Dev. 2003;71:157-69. https://doi.org/10.1016/S0378-3782(03)00005-7.

166. Wong F, Yiallourou SR, Odoi A, Browne P, Walker AM, Horne RS. Cerebrovascular control is altered in healthy term infants when they sleep prone. Sleep. 2013;36(12):1911-18. https://doi.org/10.5665/sleep.3228.

167. Fyfe KL, Yiallourou SR, Wong FY, Horne RS. The development of cardiovascular and cerebral vascular control in preterm infants. Sleep Med Rev. 2014;18(4):299-310. https://doi.org/10.1016/j.smrv.2013.06.002.

168. Ariagno R, van Liempt S, Mirmiran M. Fewer spontaneous arousals during prone sleep in preterm infants at 1 and 3 months corrected age. J Perinatol. 2006;26:306-12. https://doi.org/10.1038/sj.jp.7211490.

169. Goto K, Maeda T, Mirmiran M, Ariagno R. Effects of prone and supine position on sleep characteristics in preterm infants. Psychiatry Clin Neurosci. 1999;53:315-17. https://doi.org/10.1046/j.1440-1819.1999.00549.x.

170. Bhat RY, Hannam S, Pressler R, Rafferty GF, Peacock JL, Greenough A. Effect of prone and supine position on sleep, apneas, and arousal in preterm infants. Pediatrics. 2006;118:101-7. https://doi.org/10.1542/peds.2005-1873.

171. Kato I, Scaillet S, Groswasser J, Montemitro E, Togari H, Lin J, et al. Spontaneous arousability in prone and supine position in healthy infants. Sleep. 2006;29(6):785-90. https://doi.org/10.1093/sleep/29.6.785.

172. Franco P, Pardou A, Hassid S, Lurquin P, Groswasser J, Kahn A. Auditory arousal thresholds are higher when infants sleep in the prone position. J Pediatr. 1998;132:240-3. https://doi.org/10.1016/S0022-3476(98)70438-X.

173. Horne RSC, Bandopadhayay P, Vitkovic J, Cranage SM, Adamson TM. Effects of age and sleeping position on arousal from sleep in preterm infants. Sleep. 2002;25:746-50. https://doi.org/10.1093/sleep/25.7.746.

174. Richardson HL, Walker AM, Horne R. Stimulus type does not affect infant arousal response patterns. J Sleep Res. 2010;19:111-15. https://doi.org/10.1111/j.1365-2869.2009.00764.x.

175. Ponsonby A, Dwyer T, Gibbons LE, Cochrane JA, Jones ME, McCall MJ. Thermal environment and sudden infant death syndrome: Case-control study. BMJ. 1992;304:279-91. https://doi.org/10.1136/bmj.304.6822.277.

176. Tuffnell CS, Peterson SA, Wailoo MP. Prone sleeping infants have a reduced ability to lose heat. Early Human Dev. 1995;43:109-16. https://doi.org/10.1016/0378-3782(95)01659-7.

177. Skadberg BT, Markstead T. Behavior and physiological responses during prone and supine sleep in early infancy. Arch Dis Child. 1997;76:320-4. https://doi.org/10.1136/adc.76.4.320.

178. Bolton DPG, Nelson EAS, Taylor BJ, Weatherall IL. Thermal balance in infants. J Appl Physiol. 1996;80(6):2234-42.

179. L'Hoir MP, Engelberts AC, van Well GTJ, McClelland S, Westers P, Dandachli T, et al. Risk and preventive factors for cot death in The Netherlands, a low-incidence country. Eur J Pediatr. 1998;157:681-8. https://doi.org/10.1007/s004310050911.

180. Kahn A, Wachholder A, Winkler M, Rebuffat E. Prospective study on the prevalence of sudden infant death and possible risk factors in Brussels: Preliminary results (1987-1988). Eur J Pediatr. 1990;149:284-6. https://doi.org/10.1007/BF02106296.

181. Williams SM, Taylor BJ, Mitchell EA, & Other members of the National Cot Death Study Group. Sudden infant death syndrome: Insulation from bedding and clothing and its effect modifiers. Int J Epidemiology. 1996;25(2):366-75. https://doi.org/10.1093/ije/25.2.366.

182. Naeye RL, Ladis B, Drage JS. Sudden infant death syndrome: A prospective study. Am J Dis Child. 1976;130:1207-10. https://doi.org/10.1001/archpedi.1976.02120120041005.

183. Bach V, Bouferrache B, Kremp O, Maingourd Y, Libert JP. Regulation of sleep and body temperature in response to exposure to cool and warm environments in neonates. Pediatrics. 1994;93(5):789-96.

184. Franco P, Scaillet S, Valente F, Chabanski S, Groswasser J, Kahn A. Ambient temperature is associated with changes in infants' arousability from sleep. Sleep. 2001;24:325-9. https://doi.org/10.1093/sleep/24.3.325.

185. Stephan-Blanchard E, Chardon K, Leke A, Delanaud S, Bach V, Telliez F. Heart rate variability in sleeping preterm neonates exposed to cool and warm thermal conditions. PloS One. 2013;8(7):e68211. https://doi.org/10.1371/journal.pone.0068211.

186. Blair PS, Mitchell EA, Heckstall-Smith EMA, Fleming PJ. Head covering a major modifiable risk factor for sudden infant death syndrome: A systematic review. Arch Dis Child. 2008;93:778-83. https://doi.org/10.1136/adc.2007.136366.

187. Mitchell EA, Thompson JM, Becroft DM, Bajanowski T, Brinkmann B, Happe A, et al. Head covering and the risk for SIDS: Findings from the New Zealand and German SIDS case-control studies. Pediatrics. 2008;121(6):e1478-e83. https://doi.org/10.1542/peds.2007-2749.

188. Paluszynska DA, Harris KA, Thach BT. Influence of sleep position experience on ability of prone-sleeping infants to escape from asphyxiating microenvironments by changing head position. Pediatrics. 2004;114(6):1634-9. https://doi.org/10.1542/peds.2004-0754.

189. Franco P, Lipshut W, Valente F, Adams M, Grosswasser J, Kahn A. Cardiac autonomic characteristics in infants sleeping with their head covered by bedclothes. J Sleep Res. 2003;12(2):125-32. https://doi.org/10.1046/j.1365-2869.2003.00340.x.

190. Franco P, Lipshutz W, Valente F, Adams S, Scaillet S, Kahn A. Decreased arousals in infants who sleep with the face covered by bedclothes. Pediatrics. 2002;109(6):1112-17. https://doi.org/10.1542/peds.109.6.1112.

191. Carpenter R, McGarvey C, Mitchell EA, Tappin DM, Vennemann MM, Smuk M, et al. Bed sharing when parents do not smoke: Is there a risk of SIDS? An individual level analysis of five major case-control studies. BMJ Open. 2013;3(5):e002299. https://doi.org/10.1136/bmjopen-2012-002299.

192. Blair PS, Sidebotham P, Pease A, Fleming PJ. Bed-sharing in the absence of hazardous circumstances: Is there a risk of sudden infant death syndrome? An analysis from two case-control studies conducted in the UK. PloS One. 2014;9(9):e107799. https://doi.org/10.1371/journal.pone.0107799.

193. Escott AS, Elder DE, Zuccollo JM. Sudden unexpected infant death and bedsharing: Referrals to the Wellington Coroner 1997-2006. N Z Med J. 2009;122(1298):59-68.

194. Hauck FR, Signore C, Fein SB, Raju TNK. Infant sleeping arrangements and practices during the first year of life. Pediatrics. 2008;122:S113-20. https://doi.org/10.1542/peds.2008-1315o.

195. McKenna JJ, Mosko SS. Sleep and arousal synchrony and independence among mothers and infants sleeping apart and together (same bed): An experiment in evolutionary medicine. Acta Paediatr Suppl. 1994;397:94-102. https://doi.org/10.1111/j.1651-2227.1994.tb13271.x.

196. Baddock SA, Galland BC, Bolton DP, Williams SM, Taylor BJ. Differences in infant and parent behaviors during routine bed sharing compared with cot sleeping in the home setting. Pediatrics. 2006;117(5):1599-607. https://doi.org/10.1542/peds.2005-1636.

197. Lipton EL, Steinschneider A, Richmond JB. Swaddling, a child care practice: Historical, cultural, and experimental observations. Pediatrics. 1965;35:521-67.

198. van Sleuwen BE, L'Hoir MP, Engleberts AC, Westers P, Schulpen TWJ. Infant care practices related to cot death in Turkish and Moroccan families in the Netherlands. Arch Dis Child. 2003;88:784-8. https://doi.org/10.1136/adc.88.9.784.

199. Beal SM, Porter C. Sudden infant death syndrome related to climate. Acta Paediatrica Scand. 1991;80:278-87. https://doi.org/10.1111/j.1651-2227.1991.tb11850.x.

200. Ponsonby A-L, Dwyer T, Gibbons LE, Cochrane JA, Wang Y-G. Factors potentiating the risk of sudden infant death syndrome associated with the prone position. New Eng J Med. 1993;329(6):377-82. https://doi.org/10.1056/NEJM199308053290601.

201. Wilson CA, Taylor BJ, Laing RM, Williams SM, Mitchell EA. Clothing and bedding and its relevance to sudden infant death syndrome: Further results from the New Zealand Cot Death Study. Journal of Paediatrics and Child Health. 1994;30:506-12. https://doi.org/10.1111/j.1440-1754.1994.tb00722.x.

202. Karp H. The happiest baby on the block. New York: Bantam, 2002.

203. van Sleuwen BE, Engelberts AC, Boere-Boonekamp MM, Kuis W, Schulpen TWJ, L'Hoir MP. Swaddling: A systematic review. Pediatrics. 2007;120:e1097-106. https://doi.org/10.1542/peds.2006-2083.

204. Li Y, Liu J, Liu F, Guo G, Anme T, Ushijima H. Maternal child-rearing behaviors and correlates in rural minority areas of Yunnan, China. J Dev Behav Pediatr. 2000;21:114-22. https://doi.org/10.1097/00004703-200004000-00005.

205. Caglayan S, Yaprak I, Seckin E, Kansoy S, Aydinlioglu H. A different approach to sleep problems of infancy: Swaddling above the waist. Turk J Pediatr. 1991;33(2):117-20.

206. Urnaa V, Kizuki M, Nakamura K, Kaneko A, Inose T, Seino K, et al. Association of swaddling, rickets onset and bone properties in children in Ulaanbaatar, Mongolia. Public Health. 2006;120:834-40. https://doi.org/10.1016/j.puhe.2006.05.009.

207. Bystrova K, Matthiesen AS, Widstrom AM, Ransjo-Arvidson AB, Welles-Nystrom B, Vorontsov I, et al. The effect of Russian Maternity Home routines on breastfeeding and neonatal weight loss with special reference to swaddling. Early Hum Dev. 2007;83:29-39. https://doi.org/10.1016/j.earlhumdev.2006.03.016.

208. Pease AS, Fleming PJ, Hauck FR, Moon RY, Horne RS, L'Hoir MP, et al. Swaddling and the risk of sudden infant death syndrome: A meta-analysis. Pediatrics. 2016;137(6):e20153275. https://doi.org/10.1542/peds.2015-3275.

209. Moon RY, & Task Force On Sudden Infant Death Syndrome. SIDS and other sleep-related infant deaths: Evidence base for 2016 updated recommendations for a safe infant sleeping environment. Pediatrics. 2016;138(5):e20162940. https://doi.org/10.1542/peds.2016-2940.

210. Gerard CM, Harris KA, Thach BT. Physiologic studies on swaddling: An ancient child care practice, which may promote the supine position for infant sleep. J Pediatr. 2002;141(3):398-403. https://doi.org/10.1067/mpd.2002.127508.

211. Richardson HL, Walker AM, Horne RSC. Minimizing the risk of sudden infant death syndrome: To swaddle or not to swaddle? J Pediatr. 2009;155:475-81.

212. Narangerel G, Pollock J, Manaseki-Holland S, Henderson J. The effects of swaddling on oxygen saturation and respiratory rate of healthy infants in Mongolia. Acta Paediatrica. 2007;96:261-5. https://doi.org/10.1111/j.1651-2227.2007.00123.x.

213. Franco P, Seret N, van Hees J, Scaillet S, Grosswasser J, Kahn A. Influence of swaddling on sleep and arousal characteristics of healthy infants. Pediatrics. 2005;115:1307-11. https://doi.org/10.1542/peds.2004-1460.

214. Richardson HL, Walker AM, Horne RS. Influence of swaddling experience on spontaneous arousal patterns and autonomic control in sleeping infants. J Pediatr. 2010;157(1):85-91. https://doi.org/10.1016/j.jpeds.2010.01.005.

215. Chisholm JS. Swaddling, cradleboards and the development of children. Early Hum Dev. 1978;2(3):255-75. https://doi.org/10.1016/0378-3782(78)90029-4.

216. Gerard CM, Harris KA, Thach BT. Spontaneous arousals in supine infants while swaddled and unswaddled during rapid eye movement and quiet sleep. Pediatrics. 2002;110(6):70-6. https://doi.org/10.1542/peds.110.6.e70.

217. Franco P, Scaillet S, Grosswasser J, Kahn A. Increased cardiac autonomic responses to auditory challenges in swaddled infants. Sleep. 2004;27(8):1527-32. https://doi.org/10.1093/sleep/27.8.1527.

218. Hoffman HJ, Damus K, Hillman L, Krongrad E. Risk factors for SIDS. Results of the National Institute of Child Health and Human Development SIDS cooperative epidemiological study. Ann N Y Acad Sci. 1988;533:13-30. https://doi.org/10.1111/j.1749-6632.1988.tb37230.x.

219. Leach CE, Blair PS, Fleming PJ, Smith IJ, Platt MW, Berry PJ, et al. Epidemiology of SIDS and explained sudden infant deaths. Pediatrics. 1999;104:43-53. https://doi.org/10.1542/peds.104.4.e43.

220. Heininger U, Kleemann WJ, Cherry JD, & Sudden Infant Death Syndrome Study Group. A controlled study of the relationship between bordetella pertussis

infections and sudden unexplained deaths among German infants. Pediatrics. 2004;114(1):9-15. https://doi.org/10.1542/peds.114.1.e9.

221. Horne RS, Osborne A, Vitkovic J, Lacey B, Andrew S, Chau B, et al. Arousal from sleep in infants is impaired following an infection. Early Hum Dev. 2002;66(2):89-100. https://doi.org/10.1016/S0378-3782(01)00237-7.

222. Vennemann MM, Bajanowski T, Brinkmann B, Jorch G, Yucsesan K, Sauerland C, et al. Does breastfeeding reduce the risk of sudden infant death syndrome? Pediatrics. 2009;123(3):e406-10. https://doi.org/10.1542/peds.2008-2145.

223. Hauck FR, Thompson JM, Tanabe KO, Moon RY, Vennemann MM. Breastfeeding and reduced risk of sudden infant death syndrome: A meta-analysis. Pediatrics. 2011;128(1):103-10. https://doi.org/10.1542/peds.2010-3000.

224. Gordon AE, Saadi AT, MacKenzie DAC, Molony N, James VS, Weir DM, et al. The protective effect of breast feeding in relation to sudden infant death syndrome (SIDS): III. Detection of IgA antibodies in human milk that bind to bacterial toxins implicated in SIDS. FEMS Immunol Med Microbiol. 1999;25(1-2):175-82. https://doi.org/10.1111/j.1574-695X.1999.tb01341.x.

225. McVea KLSP, Turner PD, Peppler DK. The role of breastfeeding in sudden infant death syndrome. J Human Lactation. 2000;16(1):13-20. https://doi.org/10.1177/089033440001600104.

226. Butte NF, Smith EO, Garza C. Heart rate of breast-fed and formula-fed infants. J Pediatr Gastroenterol Nutr. 1991;13(4):391-6. https://doi.org/10.1097/00005176-199111000-00009.

227. Elias MF, Nicolson NA, Bora C, Johnston J. Sleep/wake patterns of breast-fed infants in the first 2 years of life. Pediatrics. 1986;77(3):322-9.

228. Horne R, Franco P, Adamson T, Grosswasser J, Kahn A. Influences of maternal cigarette smoking on infant arousability. Early Hum Dev. 2004;79(1):49-58. https://doi.org/10.1016/j.earlhumdev.2004.04.005.

229. Fleming PJ, Blair PS, Pollard K, Platt MW, Leach C, Smith I, et al. Pacifier use and sudden infant death syndrome: Results from the CESDI/SUDI case control study. Arch Dis Child. 1999;81:112-16. https://doi.org/10.1136/adc.81.2.112.

230. Hauck FR, Omojokun OO, Siadaty MS. Do pacifiers reduce the risk of sudden infant death syndrome? A meta-analysis. Pediatrics. 2005;116:e716-23. https://doi.org/10.1542/peds.2004-2631.

231. Li D, Willinger M, Petiti DB, Odouli R, Liu L, Hoffman HJ. Use of a dummy (pacifier) during sleep and risk of sudden infant death syndrome (SIDS): Population

based case-control study. BMJ. 2006;332:18-22. https://doi.org/10.1136/bmj.38671.640475.55.

232. Mitchell EA, Blair PS, L'Hoir MP. Should pacifiers be recommended to prevent sudden infant death syndrome? Pediatrics. 2006;117(5):1755-8. https://doi.org/10.1542/peds.2005-1625.

233. Vennemann MM, Bajanowski T, Brinkmann B, Jorch G, Sauerland C, Mitchell EA, et al. Sleep environment risk factors for sudden infant death syndrome: The German Sudden Infant Death Syndrome Study. Pediatrics. 2009;123(4):1162-70. https://doi.org/10.1542/peds.2008-0505.

234. Horne RS, Hauck FR, Moon RY, L'Hoir MP, Blair PS, Physiology and Epidemiology Working Groups of the International Society for the Study and Prevention of Perinatal and Infant Death. Dummy (pacifier) use and sudden infant death syndrome: Potential advantages and disadvantages. J Paediatr Child Health. 2014;50(3):170-4. https://doi.org/10.1111/jpc.12402.

235. Franco P, Chabanski S, Scaillet S, Grosswasser J, Kahn A. Pacifier use modifies infant's cardiac autonomic controls during sleep. Early Hum Dev. 2004;77:99-108. https://doi.org/10.1016/j.earlhumdev.2004.02.002.

236. Yiallourou SR, Poole H, Prathivadi P, Odoi A, Wong FY, Horne RS. The effects of dummy/pacifier use on infant blood pressure and autonomic activity during sleep. Sleep Med. 2014;15(12):1508-16. https://doi.org/10.1016/j.sleep.2014.07.011.

237. Horne RS, Fyfe KL, Odoi A, Athukoralage A, Yiallourou SR, Wong FY. Dummy/pacifier use in preterm infants increases blood pressure and improves heart rate control. Pediatr Res. 2016;79(2):325-32. https://doi.org/10.1038/pr.2015.212.

238. Lappi H, Valkonen-Korhonen M, Georgiadis S, Tarvainen MP, Tarkka IM, Karjalainen PA, et al. Effects of nutritive and non-nutritive sucking on infant heart rate variability during the first 6 months of life. Infant Behav Dev. 2007;30:546-56. https://doi.org/10.1016/j.infbeh.2007.04.005.

239. Hanzer M, Zotter H, Sauseng W, Pichler G, Mueller W, Kerbl R. Non-nutritive sucking habits in sleeping infants. Neonatol. 2010;97:61-6. https://doi.org/10.1159/000231518.

240. Cohen M, Brown DR, Myers MM. Cardiovascular responses to pacifier experience and feeding in newborn infants. Dev Psychobiol. 2001;39:34-9. https://doi.org/10.1002/dev.1025.

241. Franco P, Scaillet S, Wermenbol V, Valente F, Groswasser J, Kahn A. The influence of a pacifier on infants' arousals from sleep. J Pediatr. 2000;136:775-9.

242. Hanzer M, Zotter H, Sauseng W, Pichler G, Pfurtscheller K, Mueller W, et al. Pacifier use does not alter the frequency or duration of spontaneous arousals in sleeping infants. Sleep Med. 2009;10:464-70. https://doi.org/10.1016/j.sleep.2008.03.014.

243. Odoi A, Andrew S, Wong FY, Yiallourou SR, Horne RS. Pacifier use does not alter sleep and spontaneous arousal patterns in healthy term-born infants. Acta Paediatrica. 2014;103(12):1244-50. https://doi.org/10.1111/apa.12790.

244. Tonkin SL, Lui D, McIntosh CG, Rowley S, Knight DB, Gunn AJ. Effect of pacifier use on mandibular position in preterm infants. Acta Paediatrica. 2007;96(10):1433-6. https://doi.org/10.1111/j.1651-2227.2007.00444.x.

245. Cozzi F, Albani R, Cardi E. A common pathophysiology for sudden cot death and sleep apnoea. "The vacuum-glossoptosis syndrome". Med Hypoth. 1979;5(3):329-38. https://doi.org/10.1016/0306-9877(79)90013-6.

246. Stratton K, Almario DA, Wizemann TM, McCormick MC. Immunization safety review: Vaccinations and sudden unexpected death in infancy. Washington DC: National Academies Press, 2003.

247. Mitchell EA, Stewart AW, Clements M. Immunisation and the sudden infant death syndrome. New Zealand Cot Death Study Group. Arch Dis Child. 1995;73(6):498-501. https://doi.org/10.1136/adc.73.6.498.

248. Jonville-Bera AP, Autret-Leca E, Barbeillon F, Paris-Llado J. Sudden unexpected death in infants under 3 months of age and vaccination status — A case-control study. Br J Clin Pharmacol. 2001;51(3):271-6. https://doi.org/10.1046/j.1365-2125.2001.00341.x.

249. Fleming PJ, Blair PS, Platt MW, Tripp J, Smith IJ, Golding J. The UK accelerated immunisation programme and sudden unexpected death in infancy: Case-control study. BMJ. 2001;322(7290):822. https://doi.org/10.1136/bmj.322.7290.822.

250. Vennemann MM, Butterfass-Bahloul T, Jorch G, Brinkmann B, Findeisen M, Sauerland C, et al. Sudden infant death syndrome: No increased risk after immunisation. Vaccine. 2007;25(2):336-40. https://doi.org/10.1016/j.vaccine.2006.07.027.

251. Vennemann MM, Hoffgen M, Bajanowski T, Hense HW, Mitchell EA. Do immunisations reduce the risk for SIDS? A meta-analysis. Vaccine. 2007;25(26):4875-9. https://doi.org/10.1016/j.vaccine.2007.02.077.

252. Loy CS, Horne RS, Read PA, Cranage SM, Chau B, Adamson TM. Immunization has no effect on arousal from sleep in the newborn infant. J Paediatr Child Health. 1998;34(4):349-54. https://doi.org/10.1046/j.1440-1754.1998.00244.x.

253. Leiter JC, Bohm I. Mechanisms of pathogenesis in the sudden infant death syndrome. Respir Physiol Neurobiol. 2007;159:127-38. https://doi.org/10.1016/j.resp.2007.05.014.

254. Chang RR, Keens TG, Rodriguez S, Chen AY. Sudden infant death syndrome: Changing epidemiologic patterns in California 1989-2004. J Pediatr. 2008;153(4):498-502. https://doi.org/10.1016/j.jpeds.2008.04.022.

255. Hauck FR, Tanabe KO. International trends in sudden infant death syndrome: Stabilization of rates requires further action. Pediatrics. 2008;122(3):660-6. https://doi.org/10.1542/peds.2007-0135.

256. Fleming PJ, Blair PS, Pease A. Sudden unexpected death in infancy: Aetiology, pathophysiology, epidemiology and prevention in 2015. Arch Dis Child. 2015;100:984-8. https://doi.org/10.1136/archdischild-2014-306424.

# 23

# The Role of the Upper Airway in SIDS and Sudden Unexpected Infant Deaths and the Importance of External Airway-Protective Behaviors

Bradley T Thach, MD

*Washington University, School of Medicine, St Louis, USA*

## Introduction

Upper airway obstruction causing sudden death is well recognized. Examples include food aspiration, infectious disease such as diphtheria, and intentional or accidental suffocation.

Obstructive sleep apnea (OSA) has often been suggested as a cause of sudden and unexpected infant death (SUID). The fact that sudden infant death syndrome (SIDS)/SUID is believed to occur during sleep lends support for this theory. The cause of death in such a case would not be evident at post-mortem examination and so would be consistent with a SUID death. The severity of OSA increases with viral infections of the upper airway which increase nasal resistance. Additionally, epidemiological studies have found that a family history of OSA is a risk factor for SUID (1). However, were OSA to be a major cause of infant deaths, it would not explain the beneficial effect of back sleeping in reducing SUID/SIDS deaths. Significantly, brief episodes of upper airway obstruction during sleep are more common in infants who ultimately died of SIDS/SUID than in infants who survived (2).

## The Role of Upper Airway Infection, Laryngeal Chemoreflex, Apnea, and Brain Cytokines in SUID/SIDS

It has been suggested that prolonged apnea, associated with the normally airway-protective laryngeal chemoreflex (LCR) reflexes, might be causal in SIDS/SUID (3-6). The LCR combined responses are initiated when low chloride or acidic liquids stimulate intra-epithelial receptors in the inter-arytenoid space of the larynx (5, 7, 8). Such stimulation results in swallowing, apnea, vocal cord constriction, cough, and arousal from sleep (4, 8, 10). The apnea component of the LCR is particularly prominent in preterm infants, and later diminishes with maturation (8, 11). Stimulation of the LCR by introducing a drop of water onto the larynx can cause prolonged apnea, especially in preterm infants (12, 13).

The interaction between the LCR, infection, and circulating cytokines is particularly relevant to SIDS causal theories. Hypothetically, upper airway infection, particularly with respiratory syncytial virus (RSV), can result in a fatal course of events that leads to SIDS/SUID. Like the apnea caused by introducing water into an infant's larynx, RSV-related prolonged apnea is characterized by central apnea associated with obstructed inspiratory efforts, as with LCR apnea or prolonged central apnea during periodic breathing (14). Infants between 2 and 4 months of age are at highest risk for SIDS and normally have transient "physiologic" anemia. This is usually more prominent in preterm than in term infants.

These findings are particularly relevant to the pathogenesis of SIDS/SUID in this regard. First, anemia increases activity of LCR-associated prolonged apnea (15). Second, it has been shown that neonatal exposure to cigarette smoke, a risk factor for SIDS, prolongs LCR apnea in lambs during winter months (16). Third, the age for first acquiring an RSV infection coincides with the peak in SIDS incidence. Thus, several risk factors for SIDS, including prematurity, are associated with enhancement of LCR apnea. Together, these findings suggest that viral infection with RSV, or other viruses, could be a cause of SIDS by virtue of the effects of infection in potentiating LCR apnea (17). Several studies in infants and animal models indicate links between upper respiratory viral infection, LCR reflexes, brainstem or cerebrospinal fluid (CSF) cytokines, and SIDS. A recent study found that cytokines including interlukin-1beta (IL-1B) are increased in the brainstems of SIDS compared with control (accidental death) infants (18). Yet another study showed that interleukin cytokines associated with laryngeal inflammation are on average elevated in the CSF of SIDS infants compared to control infants (19). The mechanisms underlying increased interleukin cytokines are unclear. Cytokines can be transported to the brain from peripheral tissues by a hematogenous route (20, 21). Studies in animals have found that intravenous or intrathecal injection of IL-1B augments LCR reflexes and the associated prolonged apnea. All in all, these studies reinforce the theory that upper airway viral infection could possibly potentiate LCR prolonged apnea and this could be involved in the sequence of events leading to SIDS/SUID.

## Airway-Protective Behaviors

Since many deaths formerly diagnosed as SIDS are now attributed to accidental suffocation, it is relevant to consider inadequate external airway protection behaviors in suffocation deaths. Studies in primates have shown that animals can learn and perfect reflex-like subconscious beneficial motor behaviors. Such "motor learning" is thought to involve cerebellar and midbrain sites (22, 23). Many activities, such as crawling and walking, are finally learned as a result of trial and error, at which time those activities become subconscious reflexive behaviors. It has been suggested that a defect in the acquisition of learned head turning and other avoidance behaviors may underlie the increased risk for SIDS when the face is occluded by soft bedding in prone sleeping infants (24, 25).

In fact, failure to acquire protective escape behaviors, such as head turning, has been documented in infants who are inexperienced in prone sleeping (26). These infants, who are accustomed to back sleeping, have a great deal of difficulty in gaining access to fresh air when sleeping face down on soft bedding (26). Studies have also shown that such inexperienced infants are very much at increased risk for accidental suffocation if they are placed prone by a caretaker (27). An infant's ability to lift and turn his/her head to the side is dependent on prior experience (26). Infants who have experience in prone sleeping frequently have brief episodes of asphyxia due to rebreathing of expired air when they turn to a face-down position during sleep (28). Therefore, it is likely that the majority of prone sleeping infants "learn" how to avoid asphyxiation. However, some infants who are experienced in prone sleeping have not acquired adequate escape maneuvers when exposed to hypoxic situations (25). Therefore, inadequate "motor learning" may underlie the well-documented increased risk for sudden death in prone sleeping infants. Studies have shown that learned escape behaviors are independent of postnatal age, which confirms the importance of learning through prior experience, rather than acquisition of the escape ability simply as a result of normal maturation (26). We conclude that developmental deficits in central neural pathways that contribute to motor learning might increase the risk of accidental suffocation in infants.

## Conclusions

In summary, we have considered several factors relating to upper airway pathology and its role in SIDS/SUID infant deaths. This includes obstructive sleep apnea, and aberrant airway reflexes potentiated by viral infection. The success of back sleeping in SIDS/SUID rate reduction suggests that obstructive sleep apnea is not a common cause of SIDS/SUID. In addition, since many infant deaths formerly attributed to SIDS are now being diagnosed as accidental suffocation, we have addressed the issue of failure of external airway-protective responses contributing to suffocation, especially when in the prone sleep position.

# References

1. Tishler P, Redline S, Ferrette V, Hans MG, Altose MD. The association of sudden unexpected infant death with obstructive sleep apnea. Am J Respir Crit Care Med. 1996;153:1857-63. https://doi.org/10.1164/ajrccm.153.6.8665046.

2. Kahn A, Groswasser J, Rebuffat E, Sottiaux M, Blum D, Foerster M, et al. Sleep and cardiorespiratory characteristics of infant victims of sudden death: A prospective case-control study. Sleep. 1992;15:287-92. https://doi.org/10.1093/sleep/15.4.287.

3. Downing SE, Lee JC. Laryngeal chemo sensitivity: A possible mechanism for sudden infant death. Pediatrics. 1975;55:640-9.

4. Harding R, Johnson P, Johnson BE, McClelland ME, Wilkerson AR. Proceedings: Cardiovascular changes in newborn lambs induced by stimulation of laryngeal receptors with water. J Physiol. 1976;256:35-6.

5. Harding, R, Johnson P, McClelland ME. Liquid-sensitive laryngeal receptors in the developing sheep, cat and monkey. J Physiol. 1978;279:409-22. https://doi.org/10.1113/jphysiol.1978.sp012281.

6. Stoltenberg L, Sundar T, Almaas R, Storm H, Rognum TO, Saugstad OD. Changes in apnea and autoresuscitation in piglets after intravenous and intrathecal interleukin-1 beta injection. J Perinat Med. 1994;22(5):421-32. https://doi.org/10.1515/jpme.1994.22.5.421.

7. Boggs DF, Bartlett D Jr. Chemical specificity of a laryngeal apneic reflex in puppies. J Appl Physiol Respir Environ Exerc Physiol. 1982 Aug;53(2):455-62.

8. Pickens DL, Schefft GL, Thach BT. Pharyngeal fluid clearance and aspiration: Preventive mechanisms in sleeping infants. J Appl Physiol. 1989;66(3):1164-71.

9. Davies AM, Koenig JS, Thach BT. Upper airway chemoreflex responses to saline and water in preterm infants. J Appl Physiol. 1988;64(4):1412-20.

10. St Hilaire M, Samson N, Nsegbe E, Duvareille C, Moreau-Bussiere F, Micheau P, et al. Postnatal maturation of laryngeal chemoreflexes in the preterm lamb. J Appl Physiol. 2007;102:1492-38.

11. Davies AM, Koenig JS, Thach BT. Characteristics of upper airway chemoreflex prolonged apnea in human infants. Am Rev Respir Dis. 1989;139(3):668-73. https://doi.org/10.1164/ajrccm/139.3.668.

12. Pickens DL, Schefft G, Thach BT. Prolonged apnea associated with upper airway protective reflexes in apnea of prematurity. Am Rev Respir Dis. 1988;137(1):113-18. https://doi.org/10.1164/ajrccm/137.1.113.

13. Pickens Dl, Shefft GL, Thach BT. Characterization of prolonged apneic episodes associated with respiratory syncytial virus infection. Pediatr Pulmonol. 1989;6(3):195-201. https://doi.org/10.1002/ppul.1950060314.

14. Fagenholz SA, Lee AJC, Downing SE. Association of anemia with reduced central respiratory drive in the piglet. Yale J Biol Med. 1979;52(3):263-70.

15. St-Hillaire M, Duvareille C, Avoine O, Samson N, Micheau P, Douek A, et al. Effects of postnatal smoke exposure on laryngeal chemoreflexes in newborn lambs. J Appl Physiol. 2010;109(6):1820-6. https://doi.org/10.1152/japplphysiol.01378.2009.

16. Lindgren C, Jing L, Graham B, Grøgaard J, Sundell H. Respiratory syncytial virus infection reinforces reflex apnea in young lambs. Pediatr Res. 1992;31(4 Pt 1):381-5. https://doi.org/10.1203/00006450-199204000-00015.

17. Kadhim H, Kahn A, Sebire G. Distinct cytokine profile in SIDS braIn: A common denominator in a multifactorial syndrome? Neurology. 2003;61(9):1256-9. https://doi.org/10.1212/01.WNL.0000092014.14997.47.

18. Vege A, Rognum TO, Scott H, Aasen AO, Saugstad OD. SIDS cases have increased levels of interleukin-6 in cerebrospinal fluid. Acta Paediatr. 1995;84(2):193-6. https://doi.org/10.1111/j.1651-2227.1995.tb13608.x.

19. Banks WA, Ortiz L, Plotkin SR, Kastin AJ. Human interleukin (IL) 1 alpha and murine IL-beta are transported from blood to brain in the mouse by a shared saturable mechanism. J Pharmacol Exp Ther. 1991;259(3):988-96.

20. Maehken J, Olsson T, Zachau A, Klareskog L. Local enhancement of major histocompatibility complex (MHC) class I and II expression and cell infiltration in experimental allergic encephalomyelitis around axotomized motor neurons. J Neuroimmunol. 1989;23(2):125-32. https://doi.org/10.1016/0165-5728(89)90031-3.

21. Gilbert PF, Thach WT. Purkinje cell activity during motor learning. Brain Res. 1977;128(2):309-28. https://doi.org/10.1016/0006-8993(77)90997-0.

22. Thach WT, Goodkin HP, Keating JG. The cerebellum and the adaptive coordination of movement. Annu Rev Neurosci. 1992;15:403-42. https://doi.org/10.1146/annurev.ne.15.030192.002155.

23. Burns B, Lipsett LP. Behavioral factors in crib death: Toward an understanding of the sudden infant death syndrome. J Appl Deve Psych. 1991;12(2): 150-84. https://doi.org/10.1016/0193-3973(91)90009-S.

24. Lipsett LP. Crib death: A behavioural phenomenon? Curr Dir Psychol Sci. 2003;12(5):164-70. https://doi.org/10.1111/1467-8721.01253.

25. Paluszynska DA, Harris KA, Thach BT. Influence of sleep position experience on ability of prone-sleeping infants to escape from asphyxiating microenvironments by changing head position. Pediatrics. 2004;114(6):1634-9. https://doi.org/10.1542/peds.2004-0754.

26. Mitchell EA, Thach BT, Thompson JM, Williams S. Changing infants' sleep position increases risk of sudden infant death syndrome. New Zealand Cot Death Study. Arch Pediatr Adolesc Med. 1999;153(11):1136-41. https://doi.org/10.1001/archpedi.153.11.1136.

27. Waters KA., Gonzalez A, Jean C, Mortielli A, Brouillette RT. Face-straight-down and face-near-straight-down position, prone-sleeping infants. J Pediatr. 1996;128:616-25. https://doi.org/10.1016/S0022-3476(96)80125-9.

# 24 The Autopsy and Pathology of Sudden Infant Death Syndrome

Roger W Byard, MBBS, MD

*School of Medicine, The University of Adelaide, Adelaide, Australia and Florey Institute of Neuroscience and Mental Health, Victoria, Australia*

*There are no facts, only interpretations.*
Friedrich Nietzsche (1844-1900)

## Introduction

In Chapter 1 the various definitions of sudden infant death syndrome (SIDS) were discussed, with the one common theme being the lack of diagnostic features. In a way, pathology represents the weak link in the SIDS chain, as there have never been consistent and reproducible diagnostic tissue markers (1, 2). Thus, current definitions of SIDS are generally of exclusion, which means that the term "SIDS" can only be used for an infant death once other causes of sudden death have been excluded. This requires very careful interpretation of the autopsy findings to determine whether tissue changes are causative or coincidental, or whether they are merely epiphenomena. Other problems also involve the history and circumstances, which may be typical but are also not diagnostic (3, 4).

As there are no pathognomonic markers at autopsy in SIDS deaths, there is a danger that the "diagnosis" will be used inappropriately for natural deaths, accidents, and homicides — John Emery's "diagnostic dustbin" (5, 6). The degree of certainly with which alternative diagnoses can be made varies and the Avon system grades this from Ia for completely unexplained deaths, to grade III when a definite cause can be established (7).

Another issue which has arisen many times is the lack of a control population with which to compare the findings in SIDS autopsies. Examples of this include the reported changes in the heart in SIDS infants which were subsequently considered to be part of normal growth and development of an immature organ, and the ubiquitous finding of minor inflammatory infiltrates in various organs that are often more common in controls and do not, therefore, indicate significant lethal occult infection (8, 9).

Despite recommendations for decades that autopsies are a mandatory part of the work-up of SIDS cases, they have not always been performed in cases that have still been classified as "SIDS". For example, in publications from the 1990s the autopsy rate was less than 25% in Belgium (10) and autopsies occurred in only 50 to 60% of infants in the Netherlands (11). In Australia, in the not-too-distant past, infant and toddler autopsies were either not being done, or were being undertaken by physicians without pathology training. On occasion, cranial cavities were not opened or neuropathology was not undertaken (12, 13). Autopsy rates in infants have ranged from 0 to 100% globally (14). Clearly, without autopsies the causes of death in these cases must be considered undetermined. The quality of autopsy investigations should also be considered, as autopsies may be quite limited in their scope due to differences in local practices. This may not always be obvious when accrued data are being analyzed.

A question that is frequently asked is: how often could a definitive alternative diagnosis be made following a properly performed autopsy? This has varied over the years, with reduced numbers of sudden deaths in infancy from organic diseases now, most likely due to better antenatal screening, postnatal testing, and therapeutic interventions. Alternative diagnoses to SIDS were made in approximately 8 to 18% of cases of sudden infant death as the "Reduce the Risks" campaigns were launched (15-17). This percentage rose to more than 25% subsequently (18), in part due to improved death scene examinations as part of standard autopsy evaluations (19, 20).

If autopsies are not part of the standard work-up for SIDS deaths, then epidemiological and other research data derived from such populations must be treated very circumspectly. Given that the macro- and microscopic features of SIDS have been well illustrated in standard texts (1, 2, 8), and given the sensitivity of such images, this chapter will instead focus on protocols and controversies in the interpretation of autopsy findings rather than on morphology.

## Death Scene Investigation

Although death scene examinations are a requirement of all of the major current definitions of SIDS (21, 22), this has not been met with universal acceptance (23), as was noted in Chapter 1. However, it is now generally accepted that the term SIDS cannot be used unless there has been an examination of the circumstances of death, including the death scene by trained personnel (24, 25). The reality is that it is vital to obtain as much information as soon after death as possible, as it may not be possible to retrieve accurate information at a later date. While more information may make evaluations more complex, it does help in delineating particular subsets of infant deaths and it also enables subsequent meaningful peer review.

A good example of mistakes that may be made if there is not a proper death scene examination involves cases of accidental asphyxia. As both asphyxia and SIDS may have identical autopsy findings (26), cases of wedging or overlaying may only be identified after the death scene has been examined and a doll has been used to reconstruct the infant's position (8, 27, 28). Scene examination may be crucial in identifying broken or poorly constructed cribs. In addition, other information that can be acquired at the time of scene examination includes the time the infant was put to bed and last seen alive, the time when found, the sleeping position, numbers of sleeping partners, softness/firmness of the sleeping surface, and the quantity and quality of bedding and/or clothing.

The Centers for Disease Control have published a comprehensive death scene checklist known as the Sudden Unexplained Infant Death Investigation (SUIDI) reporting forms (www.cdc.gov/SIDS) (see Table 24.1).

Before an autopsy is undertaken, the examining pathologist should have full information from the death scene, which has been compiled by trained police officers and medical personnel (29). All features at the scene should be recorded photographically and on video. It is often extremely useful to take parents/carers through the scene using a doll substitute to demonstrate how and where the infant was put to sleep and found. On occasion, it may be necessary to bring the infant's bedding and sleeping surface (e.g. crib, pram, or stroller) to the morgue for scene reconstruction and evaluation.

## Issues with Shared Sleeping

One area that death scene examination has shed some light on is shared or co-sleeping. The significance of sharing a sleeping surface with an infant has been the subject of protracted debate now for decades (30-36). There is certainly evidence that sleeping near parents/carers will reduce the risk of SIDS, most likely due to increased arousals (37-41). However, there is also compelling evidence that certain infants will not survive the night if they are placed to sleep within the parental bed (42) and that this is particularly so with sofa sleeping and breastfeeding (43-46).

Examination of the literature shows that an adult sharing a bed with an infant increases the risk of SIDS/infant death with an odds ratio of 1.7. This is particularly so where infants are aged between 1 and 12 weeks and where mothers have smoked (8). However, it is clear that there are many societies around the world where shared sleeping with infants is the usual practice. This may mean that Western cultures make shared sleeping dangerous by using soft mattresses and placing infants between obese, sedated, or intoxicated parents (28, 33).

An Irish study showed that the risk of death with shared sleeping was increased with low birth weight, more bedding, and more than one adult in the bed (47), all factors that increase risks of suffocation. Co-sleeping "SIDS" deaths increased in the United Kingdom from 12% to 50% over a 20-year period (1984-2003) (48). A similar finding was made in South Australia in the early 1990s, with co-sleeping deaths increasing from 7.5% (1983-90) to 32.3% (1991-93) (49). The Triple Risk Model for shared sleeping summarizes the factors that may contribute to these trends and their potential interactions (50).

Another component to this equation is infant vulnerability. It has been clearly demonstrated that some infants are very susceptible to the effects of upper airway occlusion (51, 52). This may explain why certain infants have suffocated under a maternal breast while breastfeeding (28, 44, 53).

It is difficult to determine the exact mechanisms of death in infants who are dying in parental beds, as the pathological findings at autopsy are entirely nonspecific. However, despite all of these deaths (whether co-sleeping or not) being labeled "SIDS" (30-32), differences in the sex ratios between infants who die while co-sleeping compared to infants who die alone would suggest that there are differences between these two groups that should be explored further (54). Neuropathological findings are also different, with increased levels of β-amyloid precursor proteins being found in the brains of alone, compared to shared, sleepers (55).

## Medical History Review

As specified in current definitions (20, 22), a thorough review of the medical history of the deceased infant is required before the autopsy is commenced, checking for any evidence of potentially lethal medical conditions such as congenital heart disease. It is important to review the immediate ante-mortem history for evidence of potentially significant disease such as a fever indicating possible fatal infection.

Information should be obtained regarding the pregnancy, delivery, type of feeding, and immunization status. Family histories should include information on parental illnesses and addictions, including smoking habits. Details of illnesses, injuries, and deaths of siblings may be an indication of inherited disease such as a channelopathy, one of the many inborn errors of metabolism, or of inflicted injury. However, minimal differences in the history have been noted between SIDS infants and infants who have died unexpectedly from an established diagnosis (56).

# Autopsy Findings

One of the most useful developments in recent years in the pathological evaluation of unexpected infant and early childhood deaths has been the development and adoption of autopsy protocols (18, 57) — in particular, the International Standardized Autopsy Protocol (ISAP) (see Table 24.2), which was developed by SIDS International and the NICHD (58). The aim of the protocol was to standardize autopsy practices and improve diagnostic accuracy, provide additional information to supplement information obtained from the clinical history review and death scene examination, enhance opportunities to further reduce infant death rates, enable more meaningful comparisons of infant death rates between populations, and improve the quality of research into unexpected infant death. The protocol has been endorsed by the National Association of Medical Examiners (NAME) and the Society for Pediatric Pathology (SPP) in the USA and has been implemented in a number of countries (8).

Thus protocols provide recommendations and details on the conduct of infant autopsies covering radiological, external, and internal examinations, with specifications for histologic, toxicologic, electrolyte/metabolic, microbiologic, and molecular/genetic testing. Increased numbers of deaths due to dangerous sleeping environments and drug effects have provided endorsement for the effectiveness of these protocols (18, 59-63). Another effect of providing recommendations for standardized approaches to cases is to reduce differences among pathologists within the same institution (64). However, merely providing protocols is not enough, as they must be adhered to. This unfortunately does not always occur, with, for example, almost 10% of US pathologists still not ordering formal skeletal surveys, and 30% favoring "babygrams" over formal skeletal surveys (65). The role of post-mortem computed tomography (CT) and magnetic resonance imaging (MRI) "virtopsy" in sudden infant and early childhood deaths is yet to be established. An example of an autopsy checklist is provided in Table 24.3 (8).

Table 24.3: An example of a checklist for cases of unexplained infant death. (Adapted from (8).)

| CASE NUMBER | Date |
|---|---|
| **Attending personnel** | |
| Police | ( ) |
| Physical evidence officers | ( ) |
| Child protection physician | ( ) |
| Pediatric pathologist | ( ) |
| Others (specify) | ( ) |

**Photographs**

| | |
|---|---|
| Front, back, face | ( ) |
| Eyes, mouth | ( ) |
| Soft tissue dissections | ( ) |
| Body cavities | ( ) |
| Other | ( ) |

**Specimens**

| | |
|---|---|
| Brain for neuropathology | ( ) |
| Spinal cord for neuropathology | ( ) |
| Eyeballs | ( ) |

Samples

| | |
|---|---|
| Blood/urine/liver for toxicology | ( ) |
| Blood/CSF for microbiological culture | ( ) |
| Lung/spleen swabs for microbiological culture | ( ) |
| Blood/vitreous/liver/skin for metabolic study | ( ) |
| Blood for DNA | ( ) |
| Heart tissue for virology | ( ) |
| Vitreous humor for electrolytes | ( ) |
| ±Liver/blood/gastric contents for storage (-20°C) | ( ) |

Filter paper storage:

| | |
|---|---|
| blood spot | ( ) |
| urine spot (optional) | ( ) |
| hair (optional) | ( ) |

## CONTACT DETAILS/PHONE NUMBERS

| | |
|---|---|
| Forensic technician | _____ |
| Police communications | _____ |
| Child protection physician | _____ |
| Child abuse report line/crisis care | _____ |
| Pediatric pathologist | _____ |
| Local SIDS Association | _____ |
| Ambulance officers | _____ |

## External findings

A full external examination of all body surfaces including the anogenital region, nose, and ears should be undertaken as soon as possible after death. The major reasons for this are to check for any unexplained injuries or lesions that may raise suspicions of accidental or inflicted injury, such as bruises (66), and also to compare patterns of lividity with the reported position of the body. Lividity results from pooling of blood in the dependent parts of the body after death. This examination should be done as quickly as possible, with photographs, as lividity will shift for a number of hours after death, resulting in most cases having supine-dependent lividity with buttock and mid-back blanching at the time of autopsy due to positioning on their backs after death (67). Mismatch in lividity patterns may indicate that parents have incorrectly reported the position of their infant when found (68).

Facial, cervical, and conjunctival petechial hemorrhages are not found in SIDS cases and may suggest underlying sepsis from meningococcal disease, recent forceful vomiting or coughing from pertussis, hematological disease, or chest/neck compression (69-72). Dysmorphic features may indicate an underlying congenital condition that may have adversely effected survival (73). While dysmorphic lesions, such as talipes, polydactyly and pectus excavatum, and hemangiomas and nevi were once reported in SIDS infants (8, 74), these are usually absent. Once the initial external examination has been completed, the body should be transferred for a full skeletal survey by trained pediatric radiographers in order to exclude recent and remote occult bony injury.

Infants who die of SIDS generally do not have external abnormalities; that is, they appear normally formed and well nourished. The only markings or signs of injury are those associated with attempted resuscitation such as impressions on the chest from electrocardiography (ECG) stickers, minor abrasions around the mouth and nose from endotracheal tubes, oozing venipuncture wounds around the wrists, elbows, and feet, and intraosseous puncture wounds over the tibia (75-78). The fingers may be flexed holding fibers from bedding, and blanching and folding of the skin of the neck should not be mistaken for a ligature mark (2).

Occasionally, there may be frothy white pulmonary edema fluid in the mouth and nares from agonal left ventricular failure, but this is uncommon (79). It may be blood-tinged due to rupturing of small vessels in the distal airspaces, but should not be frankly bloody unless there has been attempted resuscitation. Blood around the mouth and nares in the absence of medical intervention raises the possibility of suffocation and so may necessitate examination of bedding more closely (80, 81). Purulent mucus in the upper airway indicates ante-mortem upper respiratory tract infection.

## Internal findings

The abdominal cavity is normal in appearance with glistening, non-dehydrated organs located in their usual positions. There is no evidence of injury or hemorrhage and the scant amount of intraperitoneal fluid that is present is clear and non-purulent. Within the chest cavity the most striking finding is of numerous petechiae within the thymus gland and sometimes over the epicardium and plural visceral surfaces. Their etiology remains unclear and, although they are not specific to SIDS, they tend to be found in greater numbers than in infants dying from other entities (82). The distribution of petechiae is not affected by sleeping position (67), although reduced numbers are found in the dorsal portions of the cervical lobes of the thymus — so-called Beckwith's sign (8, 83). They occur in 68% to 95% of cases (84). The lungs tend to be edematous, and congested, and as with other findings of no urine within the bladder and liquid blood within the heart, this is not diagnostic (85).

## Microscopic findings

By definition, the histologic findings in SIDS infants are unremarkable, as significant disease would warrant an alternative diagnosis (86). Sections from the thymus and lungs show areas of interstitial hemorrhage corresponding to the macroscopically noted petechiae. The lungs are congested and edematous, sometimes with foci of incidental submucosal chronic inflammatory cells (87, 88). Although it has been suggested that these small minor inflammatory aggregates are markers of significant lethal infections (89, 90), there is no evidence for this (91). The possibility that cytokines associated with these foci of inflammation are involved in the fatal episode is purely hypothetical (92-96). It should also be noted that such areas of minor chronic inflammation are commonly found in lung sections from a wide range of non-infectious cases, accidents, or homicides (97).

Over the years there have been several contentious markers that have been put forward to differentiate SIDS cases from accidental or homicidal suffocation. It is worthwhile exploring two of these in detail to show that they are no longer considered reliable.

First, it was suggested that intra-alveolar hemorrhage indicated airway obstruction from overlaying or smothering (98). However, it was subsequently noted that intra-alveolar hemorrhage is a very common finding in the very young that may be influenced by attempts at resuscitation, the position of the infant's body after death, and the post-mortem interval (99). If sections have been taken from dependent areas of the lungs there may also be marked congestion with intra-alveolar hemorrhage. Asphyxial episodes from smothering may show marked congestion with areas of hemorrhage (98), but these changes are very variable and subject to the influence of a number of other factors (99). It has been very pithily put that "pulmonary haemorrhage … is neither a necessary nor a specific marker of deliberate or accidental suffocation" (100).

Second, the other finding that was used to suggest previous trauma or suffocation was that of hemosiderin within intra-alveolar macrophages (101-104). However, intra-alveolar hemosiderin may be found in otherwise unremarkable SIDS cases that have typical clinical, historical, and autopsy features (105). Hemosiderin may also be deposited in the lungs following episodes of aspiration of blood, or as a result of medical conditions with chronic pulmonary congestion such as congestive cardiac failure or mitral valve stenosis. It has been stated that "the available literature has very little supporting evidence for using pulmonary haemosiderin as grounds for suspicion of previous asphyxic abuse" (106), and so it will not usually be possible for the etiology of the previous hemorrhage to be determined simply from this histologic finding (107). Various criteria have been proposed to assist in the histologic evaluation of these cases (108, 109).

## Conclusions

The autopsy investigation of cases of sudden and unexpected infant deaths should be undertaken in an organized and comprehensive manner according to established protocols. The investigation of these deaths cannot rely purely on the pathological findings, but must integrate clinical and family histories with death scene findings. The crucial role of infant mortality committees in monitoring these deaths cannot be underestimated. Finally, it must be recognized that the pathological findings in SIDS infants are by its very nature nonspecific and it is vital that not too much emphasis is placed on incidental findings such as low-grade chronic inflammation, intra-alveolar hemorrhage, and hemosiderin deposition.

Table 24.1: The Sudden Unexplained Infant Death Investigation Report form (SUIDIRF). (From http://www.cdc.gov/SIDS.)

**Reporting Form**

**SUIDI**
Sudden Unexp ained nfant Death nvestigation

**INVESTIGATION DATA**

**Infant's Information:** Last: _____ First: _____ M. _____ Case# _____

Sex: ☐ Male ☐ Female Date of Birth ___/___/___ Age _____ SS# _____
Month Day Year

Race: ☐ White ☐ Black/African Am. ☐ Asian/Pacific Islander ☐ Am. Indian/Alaskan Native ☐ Hispanic/Latino ☐ Other

**Infant's Primary Residence Address:**

Address _____ City _____ Zip _____

**Incident Address:**

Address _____ City _____ Zip _____

**Contact Information for Witness:**

**Relationship to the deceased:** ☐ Birth Mother ☐ Birth Father ☐ Grandmother ☐ Grandfather

☐ Adoptive or Foster Parent ☐ Physician ☐ Health Records ☐ Other:

Last _____ First _____ M. _____ SS# _____

Home Address _____ City _____ State _____ Zip _____

Place of Work _____ City _____ State _____ Zip _____

Phone (H) _____ Phone (W) _____ Date of Birth _____

**WITNESS INTERVIEW**

**1** Are you the usual caregiver? ☐ Yes ☐ No _____

**2** Tell me what happened:
_____
_____
_____

**3** Did you notice anything unusual or different about the infant in the last 24 hrs? ☐ No ☐ Yes ⇨ Describe: _____

**4** Did the infant experience any falls or injury within the last 72 hrs? ☐ No ☐ Yes ⇨ Describe: _____

When was the infant LAST PLACED? ................. ___/___/___ : _____
Month Day Year Military Time Location (room)

**6** When was the infant *LAST KNOWN ALIVE (LKA)*? ___/___/___ : _____
Month Day Year Military Time Location (room)

**7** When was the infant *FOUND*? ........... ............. ___/___/___ : _____
Month Day Year Military Time Location (room)

**8** Explain how you knew the infant was still alive. _____

**9** Where was the infant - (P)laced, (L)ast known alive, (F)ound (circle P, L, or F in front of appropriate response)?

| P L F Bassinet | P L F Bedside co-sleeper | P L F Car seat | P L F Chair |
| P L F Cradle | P L F Crib | P L F Floor | P L F In a person's arms |
| P L F Mattress/box spring | P L F Mattress on floor | P L F Playpen | P L F Portable crib |
| P L F Sofa/couch | P L F Stroller/carriage | P L F Swing | P L F Waterbed |

P L F Other _____

**10** In what position was the infant LAST PLACED? ☐ Sitting ☐ On back ☐ On side ☐ On stomach ☐ Unknown
Was this the infant's usual position? ☐ Yes ☐ No ⇨ What was the infant's usual position? _____

**11** In what position was the infant *LKA*? ☐ Sitting ☐ On back ☐ On side ☐ On stomach ☐ Unknown
Was this the infant's usual position? ☐ Yes ☐ No ⇨ What was the infant's usual position? _____

**12** In what position was the infant *Found*? ☐ Sitting ☐ On back ☐ On side ☐ On stomach ☐ Unknown
Was this the infant's usual position? ☐ Yes ☐ No ⇨ What was the infant's usual position? _____

**13** FACE position when *LAST PLACED*? ☐ Face down on surface ☐ Face up ☐ Face right ☐ Face left

**14** NECK position when *LAST PLACED*? ☐ Hyperextended (head back) ☐ Flexed (chin to chest) ☐ Neutral ☐ Turned

**15** FACE position when *LKA*? ☐ Face down on surface ☐ Face up ☐ Face right ☐ Face left

**16** NECK position when *LKA*? ☐ Hyperextended (head back) ☐ Flexed (chin to chest) ☐ Neutral ☐ Turned

**17** FACE position when *FOUND*? ☐ Face down on surface ☐ Face up ☐ Face right ☐ Face left

**18** NECK position when *FOUND*? ☐ Hyperextended (head back) ☐ Flexed (chin to chest) ☐ Neutral ☐ Turned

**19** What was the infant wearing? *(ex. t-shirt, disposable diaper)* _____

**20** Was the infant tightly wrapped or swaddled? ☐ No ☐ Yes ⇨ Describe: _____

**21** Please indicate the types and numbers of layers of bedding both over and under infant (not including wrapping blanket):

| Bedding UNDER Infant | None | Number | Bedding OVER Infant | None | Number |
|---|---|---|---|---|---|
| Receiving blankets | ☐ | _____ | Receiving blankets | ☐ | _____ |
| Infant/child blankets | ☐ | _____ | Infant/child blankets | ☐ | _____ |
| Infant/child comforters (thick) | ☐ | _____ | Infant/child comforters *(thick)* | ☐ | _____ |
| Adult comforters/duvets | ☐ | _____ | Adult comforters/duvets | ☐ | _____ |
| Adult blankets | ☐ | _____ | Adult blankets | ☐ | _____ |
| Sheets | ☐ | _____ | Sheets | ☐ | _____ |
| Sheepskin | ☐ | _____ | Pillows | ☐ | _____ |
| Pillows | ☐ | _____ | Rubber or plastic sheet | ☐ | _____ |
| Rubber or plastic sheet | ☐ | _____ | Other, specify: | | _____ |
| Other, specify: | | _____ | | | |

Which of the following devices were operating in the infant's room?
☐ None ☐ Apnea monitor ☐ Humidifier ☐ Vaporizer ☐ Air Purifier ☐ Other _____

**24** What was the temperature of the infant's room? ☐ Hot ☐ Cold ☐ Normal ☐ Other _____

**25** Which of the following items were near the infant's face, nose, or mouth?
☐ Bumper pads ☐ Infant pillows ☐ Positional supports ☐ Stuffed animals ☐ Toys ☐ Other

**26** Which of the following items were within the infant's reach? ☐ Blankets ☐ Toys ☐ Pillows
☐ Pacifier ☐ Nothing ☐ Other

**27** Was anyone sleeping with the infant? ☐ No ☐ Yes ⇨ Name these people.

| Name | Age | Height | Weight | Location in Relation to Infant | Impaired (intoxicated, tired) |
|---|---|---|---|---|---|
| | | | | | |
| | | | | | |

**28** Was there evidence of wedging? ☐ No ☐ Yes ⇨ Describe: _____

**29** When the infant was found, was s/he: ☐ Breathing ☐ Not breathing
If not breathing, did you witness the infant stop breathing? ☐ No ☐ Yes

**30** What had led you to check on the infant? _____

**31** Describe infant's appearance when found.

| | Unknown | No | Yes | Describe and specify location: |
|---|---|---|---|---|
| a) Discoloration around face/nose/mouth | ☐ | ☐ | ☐ ⇨ | _____ |
| b) Secretions (foam, froth) | ☐ | ☐ | ☐ ⇨ | _____ |
| c) Skin discoloration (livor mortis) | ☐ | ☐ | ☐ ⇨ | _____ |
| d) Pressure marks (pale areas, blanching) | ☐ | ☐ | ☐ ⇨ | _____ |
| e) Rash or petechiae (small, red blood spots on skin, membranes, or eyes) | ☐ | ☐ | ☐ ⇨ | _____ |
| f) Marks on body (scratches or bruises) | ☐ | ☐ | ☐ ⇨ | _____ |
| g) Other | | | ⇨ | _____ |

**32** What did the infant feel like when found? *(Check all that apply.)*
☐ Sweaty ☐ Warm to touch ☐ Cool to touch
☐ Limp, flexible ☐ Rigid, stiff ☐ Unknown
☐ Other ⇨ Specify: ....................

**33** Did anyone else other than EMS try to resuscitate the infant? ☐ No ☐ Yes ⇨ Who and when?

Who _____     ___/___/___   ___:___
                                  Month  Day  Year   Military Time

**34** Please describe what was done as part of resuscitation:
_____
_____
_____

**35** Has the parent/caregiver ever had a child die suddenly and unexpectedly? ☐ No ☐ Yes ⇨ Explain
_____

**1** Source of medical information: ☐ Doctor ☐ Other healthcare provider ☐ Medical record
☐ Mother/primary caregiver ☐ Family ☐ Other:

**2** In the 72 hours prior to death, did the infant have:

| | Unknown | No | Yes | | Unknown | No | Yes |
|---|---|---|---|---|---|---|---|
| a) Fever | ☐ | ☐ | ☐ | h) Diarrhea | ☐ | ☐ | ☐ |
| b) Excessive sweating | ☐ | ☐ | ☐ | i) Stool changes | ☐ | ☐ | ☐ |
| c) Lethargy or sleeping more than usual | ☐ | ☐ | ☐ | j) Difficulty breathing | ☐ | ☐ | ☐ |
| d) Fussiness or excessive crying | ☐ | ☐ | ☐ | k) Apnea (stopped breathing) | ☐ | ☐ | ☐ |
| e) Decrease in appetite | ☐ | ☐ | ☐ | l) Cyanosis (turned blue/gray) | ☐ | ☐ | ☐ |
| f) Vomiting | ☐ | ☐ | ☐ | m) Seizures or convulsions | ☐ | ☐ | ☐ |
| g) Choking | ☐ | ☐ | ☐ | n) Other, specify: _____ | | | |

**3** In the 72 hours prior to death, was the infant injured or did s/he have any other condition(s) not mentioned?
☐ No ☐ Yes ⇨ Describe:

**4** In the 72 hours prior to the infants death, was the infant given any vaccinations or medications?
*(Please include any home remedies, herbal medications, prescription medicines, over-the-counter medications.)*
☐ No ☐ Yes ⇨ List below

| Name of vaccination or medication | Dose last given | Date given | | | Approx. time | | Reasons given/ |
|---|---|---|---|---|---|---|---|
| | | Month | Day | Year | Military | Time | comments: |
| 1 _____ | _____ | __/__/__ | | | ___:___ | | _____ |
| 2 _____ | _____ | __/__/__ | | | ___:___ | | _____ |
| 3 _____ | _____ | __/__/__ | | | ___:___ | | _____ |
| 4 _____ | _____ | __/__/__ | | | ___:___ | | _____ |

**5** At any time in the infant's life, did s/he have a history of?

|  | Unknown | No | Yes | Describe: |
|---|---|---|---|---|
| a) Allergies (food, medication, or other) | ☐ | ☐ | ☐ ⇨ | _____ |
| b) Abnormal growth or weight gain/loss | ☐ | ☐ | ☐ ⇨ | _____ |
| c) Apnea (stopped breathing) | ☐ | ☐ | ☐ ⇨ | _____ |
| d) Cyanosis (turned blue/gray) | ☐ | ☐ | ☐ ⇨ | _____ |
| e) Seizures or convulsions | ☐ | ☐ | ☐ ⇨ | _____ |
| f) Cardiac (heart) abnormalities | ☐ | ☐ | ☐ ⇨ | _____ |
| g) Metabolic disorders | ☐ | ☐ | ☐ ⇨ | _____ |
| h) Other | ☐ | ☐ | ☐ ⇨ | _____ |

**6** Did the infant have any birth defects(s)?      ☐ No      ☐ Yes

Describe: _____

**7** Describe the two most recent times that the infant was seen by a physician or health care provider:
(Include emergency department visits, clinic visits, hospital admissions, observational stays, and telephone calls)

|  | First most recent visit | Second most recent visit |
|---|---|---|
| a) Date | ___/___/___ <br> Month  Day  Year | ___/___/___ <br> Month  Day  Year |
| b) Reason for visit | _____ | _____ |
| c) Action taken | _____ | _____ |
| d) Physician's name | _____ | _____ |
| e) Hospital/clinic | _____ | _____ |
| f) Address | _____ | _____ |
| g) City, ZIP | _____ | _____ |
| h) Phone number | (____)____-____ | (____)____-____ |

**8** Birth hospital name:

Street

City _____ State _____ ZIP _____

Date of discharge ___/___/___
Month  Day  Year

**9** What was the infant's length at birth?      _____ inches _____ or _____ centimeters

**10** What was the infant's weight at birth?      _____ pounds _____ ounces _____ or _____ grams

**11** Compared to the delivery date, was the infant born on time, early, or late?

☐ On time      ☐ Early - How many weeks early?      ☐ Late - How many weeks late? _____

**12** Was the infant a singleton, twin, triplet, or higher gestation?

☐ Singleton      ☐ Twins      ☐ Triplet      ☐ Quadruplet or higher gestation

**13** Were there any complications during delivery or at birth? *(emergency c-section, child needed oxygen)*

☐ No      ☐ Yes ⇨ Describe the complications: _____

_____

_____

**14** Are there any alerts to pathologist? *(previous infant deaths in family, newborn screen results)*

☐ No      ☐ Yes ⇨ Specify: _____

_____

_____

## INFANT DIETARY HISTORY

**1** On what day and at what approximate time was the infant last fed?

_____ / _____ / _____
Month   Day   Year

_____ : _____
Military   Time

**2** What is the name of the person who last fed the infant? _____

**3** What is his/her relationship to the infant? _____

**4** What foods and liquids was the infant fed in the last 24 hours *(include last fed)*?

| | Unknown | No | Yes | | Quantity | Specify: *(type and brand if applicable)* |
|---|---|---|---|---|---|---|
| a) Breast milk (one/both sides, length of time) | ☐ | ☐ | ☐ | ⇨ | _____ ounces | _____ |
| b) Formula (brand, water source - ex. Similac, tap water) | ☐ | ☐ | ☐ | ⇨ | _____ ounces | _____ |
| c) Cow's milk | ☐ | ☐ | ☐ | ⇨ | _____ ounces | _____ |
| d) Water (brand, bottled, tap, well) | ☐ | ☐ | ☐ | ⇨ | _____ ounces | _____ |
| e) Other liquids (teas, juices) | ☐ | ☐ | ☐ | ⇨ | _____ ounces | _____ |
| f) Solids | ☐ | ☐ | ☐ | ⇨ | | _____ |
| g) Other | ☐ | ☐ | ☐ | ⇨ | | _____ |

**5** Was a new food introduced in the 24 hours prior to his/her death?

☐ No   ☐ Yes ⇨ Describe *(ex. content, amount, change in formula, introduction of solids)*

_____
_____
_____

**6** Was the infant last placed to sleep with a bottle?

☐ Yes   ☐ No ⇨ Skip to question **9** below

**7** Was the bottle propped? *(i.e., object used to hold bottle while infant feeds)*

☐ No   ☐ Yes ⇨ What object was used to prop the bottle? _____

**8** What was the quantity of liquid (in ounces) in the bottle? _____

**9** Did death occur during?   ☐ Breast-feeding   ☐ Bottle-feeding   ☐ Eating solid foods   ☐ Not during feeding

**10** Are there any factors, circumstances, or environmental concerns that may have impacted the infant that have not yet been identified? *(ex. exposed to cigarette smoke or fumes at someone else's home, infant unusually heavy, placed with positional supports or wedges)*

☐ No   ☐ Yes ⇨ Describe concerns: _____

_____
_____

## PREGNANCY HISTORY

**1** Information about the infant's birth mother:

First name _____   Middle name _____

Last name _____   Maiden name _____

Date of birth: _____ / _____ / _____
Month   Day   Year

SS # _____ - _____ - _____

Current Address _____   City _____

Previous Address   State   ZIP

How long has the birth mother been a resident at this address?   _____ and _____
Years   Months   City   State

**2** At how many weeks or months did the birth mother begin prenatal care?

_____ Weeks   _____ Months   ☐ No prenatal care   ☐ Unknown

**3** Where did the birth mother receive prenatal care? *(Please specify physician or other health care provider name and address.)*

Physician/provider _____ Hospital/clinic _____ Phone ( ___ ) _____ - _____

Street _____ City _____ State _____ ZIP _____

**4** During her pregnancy with the infant, did the biological mother have any complications?
*(ex. high blood pressure, bleeding, gestational diabetes)*

☐ No  ☐ Yes ⇨ Specify  _____

**5** Was the biological mother injured during her pregnancy with the infant? *(ex. auto accident, falls)*

☐ No  ☐ Yes ⇨ Specify  _____

**6** During her pregnancy, did she use any of the following?

|  | Unknown | No | Yes | Daily consumption |  | Unknown | No | Yes | Daily consumption |
|---|---|---|---|---|---|---|---|---|---|
| a) Over the counter medications | ☐ | ☐ | ☐ | _____ | d) Cigarettes | ☐ | ☐ | ☐ | _____ |
| b) Prescription medications | ☐ | ☐ | ☐ | _____ | e) Alcohol | ☐ | ☐ | ☐ | _____ |
| c) Herbal remedies | ☐ | ☐ | ☐ | _____ | f) Other | ☐ | ☐ | ☐ | |

**7** Currently, does any caregiver use any of the following?

|  | Unknown | No | Yes | Daily consumption |  | Unknown | No | Yes | Daily consumption |
|---|---|---|---|---|---|---|---|---|---|
| a) Over the counter medications | ☐ | ☐ | ☐ | _____ | d) Cigarettes | ☐ | ☐ | ☐ | _____ |
| b) Prescription medications | ☐ | ☐ | ☐ | _____ | e) Alcohol | ☐ | ☐ | ☐ | _____ |
| c) Herbal remedies | ☐ | ☐ | ☐ | | f) Other | ☐ | ☐ | ☐ | |

**INCIDENT SCENE INVESTIGATION**

**1** Where did the incident or death occur?  _____

**2** Was this the primary residence?  ☐ Yes  ☐ No

**3** Is the site of the incident or death scene a daycare or other childcare setting?

☐ Yes  ☐ No ⇨ Skip to question **8** below

**4** How many children were under the care of the provider at the time of the incident or death? _____ *(under 18 years or older)*

**5** How many adults were supervising the child(ren)?  _____ *(18 years or older)*

**6** What is the license number and licensing agency for the daycare?

License number: _____  Agency: _____

**7** How long has the daycare been open for business? _____

**8** How many people live at the site of the incident or death scene?

_____ Number of adults (18 years or older)  _____ Number of children (under 18 years old)

**9** Which of the following heating or cooling sources were being used? (Check all that apply.)

| | | | |
|---|---|---|---|
| ☐ Central air | ☐ Gas furnace or boiler | ☐ Wood burning fireplace | ☐ Open window(s) |
| ☐ A/C window unit | ☐ Electric furnace or boiler | ☐ Coal burning furnace | ☐ Wood burning stove |
| ☐ Ceiling fan | ☐ Electric space heater | ☐ Kerosene space heater | |
| ☐ Floor/table fan | ☐ Electric baseboard heat | ☐ Other ⇨ Specify | _____ |
| ☐ Window fan | ☐ Electric *(radiant)* ceiling heat | ☐ Unknown | |

**10** Indicate the temperature of the room where the infant was found unresponsive:

_____ Thermostat setting  _____ Thermostat reading  _____ Actual room temp.  _____ Outside temp.

**11** What was the source of drinking water at the site of the incident or death scene? *(Check all that apply.)*

| | | |
|---|---|---|
| ☐ Public/municipal water source | ☐ Bottled water | ☐ Other ⇨ Specify _____ |
| ☐ Well | ☐ Unknown | |

**12** The site of the incident or death scene has: (check all that apply)

| | | |
|---|---|---|
| ☐ Insects | ☐ Mold growth | ☐ Odors or fumes ⇨ Describe: |
| ☐ Smoky smell (like cigarettes) | ☐ Pets | ☐ Presence of alcohol containers |
| ☐ Dampness | ☐ Peeling paint | ☐ Presence of drug paraphenalia |
| ☐ Visible standing water | ☐ Rodents or vermin | ☐ Other ⇨ Specify _____ |

**13** Describe the general appearance of incident scene: *(ex. cleanliness, hazards, overcrowding, etc.)*

_____
_____

THE PAST, THE PRESENT AND THE FUTURE

**1** Are there any factors, circumstances, or environmental concerns about the incident scene investigation that may have impacted the infant that have not yet been identified?

_____

_____

**2** Arrival times:   Law enforcement at scene: _____ : _____   DSI at scene: _____ : _____   Infant at hospital: _____ : _____

        Military   Time                        Military   Time                      Military   Time

**Investigator's Notes**

Indicate the task(s) performed.

☐ Additional scene(s)? (forms attached)      ☐ Doll reenactment/scene re-creation      ☐ Photos or video taken and noted

☐ Materials collected/evidence logged        ☐ Referral for counseling                ☐ EMS run sheet/report

☐ Notify next of kin or verify notification  ☐ 911 tape

If more than one person was interviewed, does the information differ?

☐ No      ☐ Yes ⇨ Detail any differences, inconsistencies of relevant information: (ex. placed on sofa, last known alive on chair.)

_____

_____

_____

_____

**INVESTIGATION DIAGRAMS**

**1** Scene Diagram:          **2** Body Diagram:

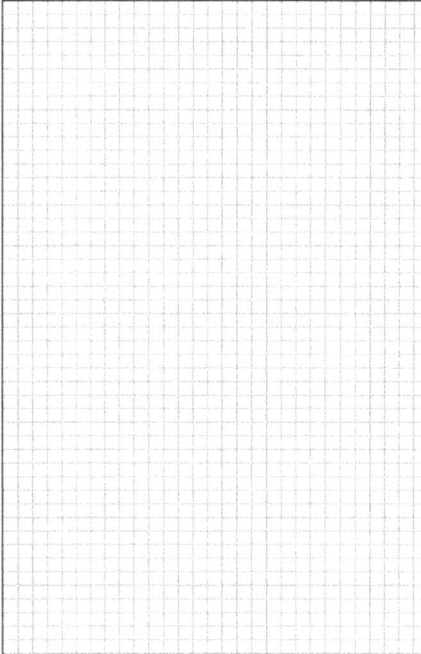

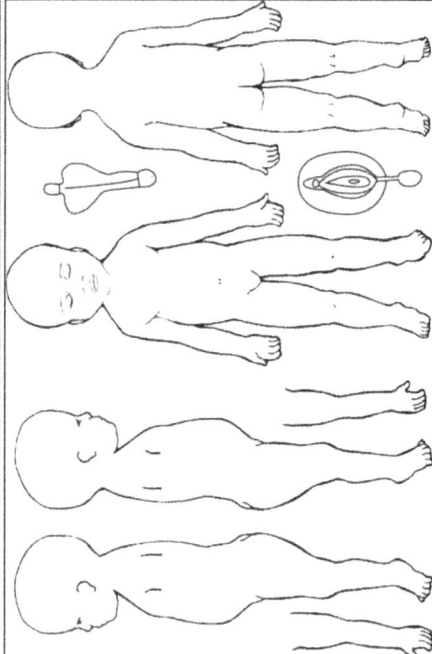

## SUMMARY FOR PATHOLOGIST

**Case Information**

Investigator Information: Name _____ Agency _____ Phone _____

Investigated: ____/____/_____    _____:_____    Pronounced Dead: _____/____/_____    _____:_____
           Month  Day  Year   Military Time                Month  Day  Year   Military Time

Infant's Information:   Last _____   First _____   M. _____   Case # _____

Sex:  ☐ Male   ☐ Female        Date of Birth    ____/____/_____        Age _____
                                        Month  Day  Year               Months

Race:  ☐ White   ☐ Black/African Am.   ☐ Asian/Pacific Islander   ☐ Am. Indian/Alaskan Native   ☐ Hispanic/Latino   ☐ Other

**1** | Indicate whether preliminary investigation suggests any of the following:

**Sleeping Environment**

| Yes | No | |
|-----|----|---|
| ☐ | ☐ | Asphyxia *(ex. overlying, wedging, choking. nose/mouth obstruction, re-breathing. neck compression, immersion in water)* |
| ☐ | ☐ | Sharing of sleeping surface with adults, children, or pets |
| ☐ | ☐ | Change in sleeping condition *(ex. unaccustomed stomach sleep position, location, or sleep surface)* |
| ☐ | ☐ | Hyperthermia/Hypothermia *(ex. excessive wrapping, blankets, clothing, or hot or cold environments)* |
| ☐ | ☐ | Environmental hazards *(ex. carbon monoxide, noxious gases, chemicals, drugs, devices)* |
| ☐ | ☐ | Unsafe sleeping conditions *(ex. couch/sofa, waterbed, stuffed toys, pillows, soft bedding)* |

**Infant History**

| Yes | No | |
|-----|----|---|
| ☐ | ☐ | Diet *(ex. solids introduction etc.)* |
| ☐ | ☐ | Recent hospitalization |
| ☐ | ☐ | Previous medical diagnosis |
| ☐ | ☐ | History of acute life-threatening events *(ex. apnea, seizures, diffi culty breathing)* |
| ☐ | ☐ | History of medical care without diagnosis |
| ☐ | ☐ | Recent fall or other injury |
| ☐ | ☐ | History of religious, cultural, or ethnic remedies |
| ☐ | ☐ | Cause of death due to natural causes other than SIDS *(ex. birth defects, complications of preterm birth)* |

**Family Info**

| Yes | No | |
|-----|----|---|
| ☐ | ☐ | Prior sibling deaths |
| ☐ | ☐ | Previous encounters with police or social service agencies |
| ☐ | ☐ | Request for tissue or organ donation |
| ☐ | ☐ | Objection to autopsy |

**Exam**

| Yes | No | |
|-----|----|---|
| ☐ | ☐ | Pre-terminal resuscitative treatment |
| ☐ | ☐ | Death due to trauma (injury), poisoning, or intoxication |

**Investigator Insight**

| Yes | No | |
|-----|----|---|
| ☐ | ☐ | Suspicious circumstances |
| ☐ | ☐ | Other alerts for pathologist's attention |

Any "Yes" answers should be explained and detailed.

Brief description of circumstances: _____

_____

_____

_____

_____

_____

_____

_____

**Pathologist**

**2** | Pathologist Information:

Name _____   Agency _____

Phone ( _____ ) _____-_____   Fax ( _____ ) _____-_____

Table 24.2: International Standardized Autopsy Protocol. The International Standardized Autopsy Protocol for cases of unexpected infant death represents the first attempt to provide an international protocol aimed at standardizing autopsy practices and diagnoses. The protocol was developed by a working group set up by SIDS International and the NICHD in the 1990s (58, 19).

**INTERNATIONAL STANDARDIZED AUTOPSY PROTOCOL**

**FOR SUDDEN UNEXPECTED INFANT DEATH**

| Decedent's Name | | Local Accession Number |
|---|---|---|
| Age/Sex | Ethnicity | |
| Date Of Birth | Date/Time of Death | |
| Date/Time of Autopsy | Pathologist | |
| County/District | Country | |

**FINAL ANATOMIC DIAGNOSES**

MICROBIOLOGY RESULTS:

TOXICOLOGY RESULTS:

CHEMISTRY RESULTS:

PATHOLOGIST----------------------------------------------------------------

DECEDENT'S NAME----------------------------------------------

ACCESSION NUMBER-----------------------------------------

1

**COUNTY & COUNTRY**----------------------------------------------

**PATHOLOGIST**------------------------------------------------------

|  | YES | NO | |
|---|---|---|---|
| **MICROBIOLOGY** Date/Time |  |  | |
| **Done before autopsy,** |  |  | |
| VIRUSES trachea stool, |  |  | |
| BACTERIA blood CSF fluids, |  |  | |
| FUNGI discretionary, |  |  | |
| MYCOBACTERIA discretionary, |  |  | |
| Done during autopsy, |  |  | |
| BACTERIA liver lung and myocardium, |  |  | |
| VIRUSES liver lung and myocardium, |  |  | |
| **PHOTOGRAPHS** include, |  |  | |
| Name Case number County Country Date, |  |  | |
| Measuring device Color reference, |  |  | |
| Consider front & back, |  |  | |
| Gross abnormalities, |  |  | |
| **RADIOGRAPHIC STUDIES** consider, |  |  | |
| Whole body, |  |  | |
| Thorax and specific lesions, |  |  | |
| **EXTERNAL EXAMINATION,** |  |  | |
| Date & Time of autopsy |  |  | |
| Date & Time of Autopsy, |  |  | |
| Sex (circle) Male Female, |  |  | |

2

| | | | |
|---|---|---|---|
| Observed race (circle), | | | |
| White | Black | | |
| Asian | Arab | | |
| Pacific Islander | Gypsy, | | |
| Hispanic, Other (specify), | | | |
| Rigor mortis: describe distribution, | | | |
| Livor mortis: describe distribution and if fixed, | | | |
| **WEIGHTS AND MEASURES,** | | | |
| Body Weight, | | | gm |
| Crown-Heel Length, | | | cm |
| Crown-Rump Length | | | cm |
| Occipitofrontal Circumference, | | | cm |
| Chest Circumference at Nipples, | | | cm |
| Abdominal Circumference at Umbilicus, | | | cm |

3

**DECEDENT'S NAME**-----------------------------------------------------

**ACCESSION NUMBER**-------------------------------------------------

**COUNTY & COUNTRY**-------------------------------------------------

**PATHOLOGIST**---------------------------------------------------------

| GENERAL APPEARANCE/DEVELOPMENT | YES | NO | NO EXAM |
|---|---|---|---|
| Development normal | | | |
| Nutritional status | | | |
| Normal | | | |
| Poor | | | |
| Obese | | | |
| Hydration | | | |
| Normal | | | |
| Dehydrated | | | |
| Edematous | | | |
| Pallor | | | |
| **HEAD** | | | |
| Configuration normal | | | |
| Scalp and hair normal | | | |
| Bone consistency normal | | | |
| Other | | | |
| **TRAUMA EVIDENCE** | | | |
| Bruises | | | |
| Lacerations | | | |
| Abrasions | | | |
| Burns | | | |
| Other | | | |
| **PAST SURGICAL INTERVENTION** | | | |
| Scars | | | |

4

| | | | |
|---|---|---|---|
| Other | | | |
| **RESUSCITATION EVIDENCE** | | | |
| Facial mask marks | | | |
| Lip abrasions | | | |
| Chest ecchymoses | | | |
| EKG monitor pads | | | |
| Defibrillator marks | | | |
| Venipunctures | | | |
| Other | | | |
| **CONGENITAL ANOMALIES** | | | |
| **EXTERNAL** | | | |
| **INTEGUMENT** | | | |
| Jaundice | | | |
| Petechiae | | | |
| Rashes | | | |
| Birthmarks | | | |
| Other abnormalities | | | |
| **EYES** (remove when indicated and legal) | | | |
| Color circle Brown Blue Green Hazel | | | |
| Cataracts | | | |
| Position abnormal | | | |
| Jaundice | | | |
| Conjunctiva abnormal | | | |
| Petechiae | | | |
| Other abnormalities | | | |
| **EARS** | | | |
| Low set | | | |
| Rotation abnormal | | | |
| Other abnormalities | | | |

5

| NOSE | | | |
|---|---|---|---|
| Discharge (describe if present) | | | |
| Configuration abnormal | | | |
| Septal deviation | | | |
| Right choanal atresia | | | |
| Left choanal atresia | | | |
| Other abnormalities | | | |
| **MOUTH** | | | |
| Discharge (describe if present) | | | |
| Labial ffenulum abnormal | | | |
| Teeth present | | | |
| Number of upper | | | |
| Number of lower | | | |
| **TONGUE** | | | |
| Abnormally large | | | |
| Frenulum abnormaL | | | |
| Other abnormalities | | | |
| **PALATE** | | | |
| Cleft | | | |
| High arched | | | |
| Other abnormalities | | | |
| **MANDIBLE** | | | |
| Micrognathia | | | |
| Other abnormalities | | | |
| **NECK** | | | |
| abnormal | | | |
| **CHEST** | | | |
| abnormal | | | |
| **ABDOMEN** | | | |

6

| | | | |
|---|---|---|---|
| Distended | | | |
| Umbilicus abnormal | | | |
| Hernias | | | |
| Other abnormal | | | |
| **EXTERNAL GENITALIA** Abnormal | | | |
| **ANUS abnormal** | | | |
| **EXTREMITIES abnormal** | | | |
| **INTERNAL EXAMINATION** | | | |
| Subcutis Thickness 1cm below umbilicus: | | | |
| Subcutaneous emphysema | | | |
| Situs inversus | | | |
| **PLEURAL CAVITIES** abnormal | | | |
| Fluid describe if present | | | |
| Right, ml | | | |
| Left, ml | | | |
| **PERICARDIAL CAVITY** abnormal | | | |
| Fluid, describe if present, ml | | | |
| Other abnormalities | | | |
| **PERITONEAL CAVITY** abnormal | | | |
| Fluid, describe if present, ml | | | |
| **RETROPERITONEUM** abnormal | | | |
| **PETECHIAE** (indicate if dorsal and/or ventral) | | | |
| Parietal pleura | | | |
| Right | | | |
| Left | | | |
| Visceral pleura | | | |
| Right | | | |
| Left | | | |
| Pericardium | | | |

7

| | | | |
|---|---|---|---|
| Epicardium | | | |
| Thymus | | | |
| Parietal peritoneum | | | |
| Visceral peritoneum | | | |
| **UPPER AIRWAY OBSTRUCTION** | | | |
| Foreign body | | | |
| Mucus plug | | | |
| Other | | | |
| **NECK SOFT TISSUE HEMORRHAGE** | | | |
| **HYOID BONE** abnormal | | | |
| **THYMUS** | | | |
| Weight, gms | | | |
| Atrophy | | | |
| Other abnormalities | | | |
| **EPIGLOTTIS** abnormal | | | |
| **LARYNX** abnormal | | | |
| Narrowed lumen | | | |
| **TRACHEA** abnormal | | | |
| Stenosis | | | |
| Obstructive exudates | | | |
| Aspirated gastric contents | | | |
| ET tube tip location | | | |
| **MAINSTEM BRONCHI** abnormal | | | |
| Edema fluid | | | |
| Mucus plugs | | | |
| Gastric contents | | | |
| Inflammation | | | |
| **LUNGS** | | | |
| Weight | | | |

8

| | | | |
|---|---|---|---|
| Right | | | gm |
| Left | | | gm |
| Abnormal | | | |
| Congestion, describe location, severity | | | |
| Hemorrhage, describe location, severity | | | |
| Edema, describe location | | | |
| Severity (circle) | | | |
| Consolidation, describe location, severity | | | |
| Anomalies | | | |
| Pulmonary artery | | | |
| Thromboembolization | | | |
| **PLEURA** abnormal | | | |
| **RIBS** abnormal | | | |
| Fractures | | | |
| with hemorrhages | | | |
| Callus formation | | | |
| Configuration abnormal | | | |
| **DIAPHRAGM** abnormal | | | |
| **CARDIOVASCULAR SYSTEM** | | | |
| Heart weightgm | | | gm |
| Left ventricular thickness | | | cm |
| Right ventricular thickness | | | cm |
| Septal thickness maximum | | | cm |
| Mitral valve circumference | | | cm |
| Aortic valve circumference | | | cm |
| Tricuspid valve circumference | | | cm |
| Pulmonary valve circumference | | | cm |
| Myocardium abnormal | | | |
| Ventricular inflow/outflow tracts narrow | | | |

9

| | | | |
|---|---|---|---|
| Valvular vegetations/thromboses | | | |
| Aortic coarctation | | | |
| Patent ductus arteriosus | | | |
| Chamber blood (circle) fluid clotted | | | |
| Congenital heart disease | | | |
| Atrial septal defect | | | |
| Ventricular septal defect | | | |
| Abnormal pulmonary venous connection | | | |
| Other | | | |
| Location of vascular cathether tips | | | |
| Occlusive vascular thrombosis locations | | | |
| Other abnormalities | | | |
| **ESOPHAGUS** abnormal | | | |
| **STOMACH** abnormal | | | |
| Describe contents and volume | | | |
| **SMALL INTESTINE** abnormal | | | |
| Hemorrhage | | | |
| Volvulus | | | |
| Describe contents | | | |
| **COLON** abnormal | | | |
| Congestion | | | |
| Hemorrhage | | | |
| Describe contents | | | |
| **APPENDIX** abnormal | | | |
| **MESENTERY** abnormal | | | |
| **LIVER** abnormal | | | |
| Weight | | gm | |
| **GALLBLADDER** abnormal | | | |
| **PANCREAS** abnormal | | | |

10

| | | | |
|---|---|---|---|
| **SPLEEN** abnormal | | | |
| Weight | | | |
| **KIDNEYS** abnormal | | | |
| Weight | | | |
| Right | | | gm |
| Left gm | | | gm |
| **URETERS** abnormal | | | |
| **BLADDER** abnormal | | | |
| Contents, volume | | | |
| **PROSTATE** abnormal | | | |
| **UTERUS, F. TUBES, and OVARIES** abnormal | | | |
| **THYROID** abnormal | | | |
| **ADRENALS** abnormal | | | |
| Right | | | gm |
| Left | | | gm |
| Combined | | | gm |
| **PITUITARY** abnormal | | | |
| **CONGENITAL ANOMALIES, INTERNAL** | | | |
| **CENTRAL NERVOUS SYSTEM** | | | |
| Whole brain weight | | | |
| Fresh | | | gm |
| Fixed | | | gm |
| Combined cerebellum/brainstem weight | | | |
| Fresh | | | gm |
| Fixed | | | gm |
| Evidence of trauma | | | |
| Scalp abnormal | | | |
| Galea abnormal | | | |
| Fractures | | | |

11

| | | | |
|---|---|---|---|
| Anterior fontanelle abnormal | | | |
| Dimensions | | | |
| Calvarium abnormal | | | |
| Cranial sutures abnormal | | | |
| Closed (fused) | | | |
| Overriding | | | |
| Widened | | | |
| Base of skull abnormal | | | |
| Configuration abnormal | | | |
| Middle ears abnormal | | | |
| Foramen magnum abnormal | | | |
| Hemorrhage, estimate volumes (ml) | | | |
| Epidural | | | |
| Dural | | | |
| Subdural | | | |
| Subarachnoid | | | |
| Intracerebral | | | |
| Cerebellum | | | |
| Brainstem | | | |
| Spinal cord | | | |
| Intraventricular | | | |
| Other | | | |
| Dural lacerations | | | |
| Dural sinus thrombosis | | | |
| **BRAIN: IF EXTERNALLY ABNORMAL** | | | |
| **FIX BEFORE CUTTING** | | | |
| Configuration abnormal | | | |
| Hydrocephalus | | | |
| Gyral pattern abnormal | | | |

12

| | | | |
|---|---|---|---|
| Cerebral edema | | | |
| Herniation | | | |
| Uncal | | | |
| Tonsillar | | | |
| Tonsillar necrosis | | | |
| Leptomeningeal exudates (culture) | | | |
| Cerebral contusions | | | |
| Malformations | | | |
| Cranial nerves abnormal | | | |
| Circle of Willis/basilar arteries abnormal | | | |
| Ventricular contours abnormal | | | |
| Cerebral infarction | | | |
| Contusional tears | | | |
| Other abnormalities | | | |
| **SPINAL CORD** | | | |
| Inflammation | | | |
| Contusion(s) | | | |
| Anomalies Other abnormalities | | | |

13

DECEDENT'S NAME------------------------------------------------

ACCESSION NUMBER---------------------------------------------

COUNTY & COUNTRY---------------------------------------------

PATHOLOGIST-----------------------------------------------------

|  | YES | NO |
|---|---|---|
| **MANDATORY SECTIONS TAKEN** | | |
| Skin, if lesions | | |
| Thymus | | |
| Lymph node | | |
| Epiglottis, vertical | | |
| Larynx, supraglottlc, transverse | | |
| Larynx, true cords, transverse | | |
| Trachea and thyroid, transverse | | |
| Trachea at carina, transverse | | |
| Lungs, all lobes | | |
| Diaphragm | | |
| Heart, septum and ventricles | | |
| Esophagus, distal 3 cm | | |
| Terminal ileum | | |
| Rectum | | |
| Liver | | |
| Pancreas with duodenum | | |
| Spleen | | |
| Kidney with capsule | | |
| Adrenal | | |
| Rib with costochondral junction | | |
| Submandibular gland | | |
| Cervical spinal cord | | |

14

| | | |
|---|---|---|
| Rostral medulla junction | | |
| Pons | | |
| Midbrain | | |
| Hippocampus | | |
| Frontal lobe Cerebellum Choroid Plexus | | |
| **OIL RED O STAINED SECTIONS, IF INDICATED** | | |
| Heart | | |
| Liver | | |
| Muscle | | |
| **DISCRETIONARY MICROSCOPIC SECTIONS** | | |
| Supraglottic soft tissue | | |
| Lung hilum | | |
| Pancreatic tail | | |
| Mesentery | | |
| Stomach | | |
| Colon | | |
| Appendix | | |
| Testes or ovaries | | |
| Urinary bladder | | |
| Psoas muscle | | |
| Palatine tonsils | | |
| Basal ganglia | | |
| **METABOLIC DISORDERS** | | |
| **RETAIN ON FILTER PAPER IN ALL CASES** | | |
| Whole blood (I drop) Urine (I drop) | | |
| Hair (taped down) | | |
| **TOXICOLOGY AND ELECTROLYTES** | | |
| **FLUID AND TISSUES SAVED FOR 1 YEAR** | | |
| Whole blood and serum, save at −70°C and + 4°C | | |

15

| | | |
|---|---|---|
| Liver, save 100 gms at −700°C | | |
| Frontal lobe, save at−70°C | | |
| Urine, save at −700°C Bile | | |
| Vitreous humor | | |
| Serum | | |
| Gastric contents | | |
| **Analyses performed, but not limited to:** | | |
| Cocaine and metabolites | | |
| Morphine and metabolites | | |
| Amphetamine and metabolites | | |
| Volatiles (ethanol, acetone, etc.) | | |
| Other indicated by history and exam | | |
| **FROZEN TISSUES, SAVE AT−70°C** | | |
| Lung | | |
| Heart | | |
| Liver | | |
| Lymph node | | |

## REFERENCES

Krous, H. An international standardised autopsy protocol for sudden unexpected infant death. In: Sudden infant death syndrome. New trends in the nineties. Ed Rognum TO. Oslo: Scandinavian University Press, 1995. p. 81-95.

Krous, HF, Byard RW. International standardized autopsy protocol for sudden unexpected infant death. In: *Sudden infant death syndrome. Problems, progress and possibilities.* Ed Byard RW, Krous HF. London: Arnold, 2001. p. 319-33.

16

# References

1. Byard RW, Rognum TO. Autopsy findings — Sudden infant death syndrome — Epidemiology and etiology. In: Encyclopedia of forensic and legal medicine. 2nd ed. Vol. 1. Eds Payne-James J, Byard RW. Oxford: Academic Press, 2016. p. 354-67. https://doi.org/10.1016/B978-0-12-800034-2.00049-5.

2. Byard RW, Rognum TO. Autopsy findings — Sudden infant death syndrome — Pathological findings and autopsy approach. In: Encyclopedia of forensic and legal medicine. 2nd ed. Vol. 1. Eds Payne-James J, Byard RW. Oxford: Academic Press, 2016. p. 368-82. https://doi.org/10.1016/B978-0-12-800034-2.00401-8.

3. Sturner WQ. Sudden infant death syndrome — The medical examiner's viewpoint. Perspect Pediatric Pathol. 1995;19:76-86.

4. Byard RW. Possible mechanisms responsible for the sudden infant death syndrome. J Paediatr Child Health. 1991;27:147-57. https://doi.org/10.1111/j.1440-1754.1991.tb00376.x.

5. Emery JL. A way of looking at the causes of crib death. In: Sudden infant death syndrome. Eds Tildon JT, Roeder LM, Steinschneider A. Academic Press: New York, 1983. p. 123-32.

6. Emery JL. Is sudden infant death syndrome a diagnosis? Or is it just a diagnostic dustbin? Brit Med J. 1989;299:1240. https://doi.org/10.1136/bmj.299.6710.1240.

7. Blair PS, Byard RW, Fleming PJ. Sudden unexpected death in infancy (SUDI): Suggested classification and applications to facilitate research activity. Forensic Sci Med Pathol. 2012;8:312-15. https://doi.org/10.1007/s12024-011-9294-x.

8. Byard RW. Sudden death in the young. 3rd ed. Cambridge, UK: Cambridge University Press, 2010. https://doi.org/10.1017/CBO9780511777783.

9. Collins KA, Byard RW. Forensic pathology of infancy and childhood. New York: Springer Publishers, 2014. https://doi.org/10.1007/978-1-61779-403-2.

10. Kahn A, Wachholder A, Winkler M, Rebuffat E. Prospective study on the prevalence of sudden infant death and possible risk factors in Brussels: Preliminary results (1987-1988). Eur J Pediatrics. 1990;149:284-6. https://doi.org/10.1007/BF02106296.

11. Engelberts AC, de Jonge GA, Kostense PJ. An analysis of trends in the incidence of sudden infant death in The Netherlands 1969-89. J Paediatr Child Health. 1991;27:329-33. https://doi.org/10.1111/j.1440-1754.1991.tb00413.x.

12. Byard RW. Inaccurate classification of infant deaths in Australia: A persistent and pervasive problem. Med J Aust. 2001;175:5-7.

13. Armstrong KL, Wood D. Can infant death from child abuse be prevented? Med J Aust. 1991;155:593-6.

14. Fitzgerald K. The "Reduce the Risks" campaign, SIDS International, the Global Strategy Task Force and the European Society for the Study and Prevention of Infant Death. In: Sudden infant death syndrome. Problems, progress and possibilities. Eds Byard RW, Krous HF. London: Arnold, 2001. p. 310-18.

15. Byard RW, Carmichael E, Beal S. How useful is post-mortem examination in sudden infant death syndrome? Pediatr Pathol. 1994;14:817-22. https://doi.org/10.3109/15513819409037679.

16. Emery JL, Chandra S, Gilbert-Barness EF. Findings in child deaths registered as sudden infant death syndrome (SIDS) in Madison, Wisconsin. Pediatr Pathol. 1988;8:171-8. https://doi.org/10.3109/15513818809022294.

17. Fleming PJ, Berry PJ, Gilbert R, Golding J, Rudd PT, Hall E, et al. Categories of preventable unexpected infant deaths. Arch Dis Child. 1991;66:171-2. https://doi.org/10.1136/adc.66.1.170-b.

18. Mitchell E, Krous HF, Donald T, Byard RW. An analysis of the usefulness of specific stages in the pathological investigation of sudden infant death. Am J Forensic Med Pathol. 2000;21:395-400. https://doi.org/10.1097/00000433-200012000-0002.

19. Byard RW, Krous HF. Sudden infant death syndrome. Problems, progress and possibilities. London: Arnold, 2001.

20. Krous HF, Beckwith JB, Byard RW, Rognum TO, Bajanowski T, Corey T, et al. Sudden infant death syndrome and unclassified sudden infant deaths: A definitional and diagnostic approach. Pediatrics. 2004;114:234-8. https://doi.org/10.1542/peds.114.1.234.

21. Byard RW. Changing infant death rates: Diagnostic shift, success story, or both? Forensic Sci Med Pathol. 2013;9:1-2. https://doi.org/10.1007/s12024-012-9350-1.

22. Willinger M, James LS, Catz C. Defining the sudden infant death syndrome (SIDS): Deliberations of an expert panel convened by the National Institute of Child Health and Human Development. Pediatr Pathol. 1991;11:677-84. https://doi.org/10.3109/15513819109065465.

23. Becroft DMO. An international perspective [letter]. Arch Pediatr Adol Med. 2003;157:292.

24. Byard RW, Becker LE, Berry PJ, Campbell P, Fitzgerald K, Hanzlick R. Death scene investigation. In: Sudden infant death syndrome. Problems, progress and possibilities. Eds Byard RW, Krous HF. London: Arnold, 2001. p. 58-65.

25. Byard RW, Becker LE, Berry, PJ, Campbell PE, Fitzgerald K, Hilton JMN, et al. The pathological approach to sudden infant death — Consensus or confusion? Recommendations from the 2nd SIDS Global Strategy Meeting, Stavangar, Norway, August 1994, and the 3rd Australasian SIDS Global Strategy Meeting, Gold Coast, Australia, May 1995. Am J Forensic Med Pathol. 1996;17:103-5. https://doi.org/10.1097/00000433-199606000-00003.

26. Byard RW, Jensen L. Fatal asphyxial episodes in the very young — Classification and diagnostic issues. Forensic Sci Med Pathol. 2007;3:177-81. https://doi.org/10.1007/s12024-007-0020-7.

27. Bass M, Kravath RE, Glass L. Death-scene investigation in sudden infant death. N Engl J Med. 1986;315:100-5. https://doi.org/10.1056/NEJM198607103150206.

28. Byard RW, Hilton J. Overlaying, accidental suffocation, and sudden infant death. J Sud Infant Death Synd Infant Mort. 1997;2:161-5.

29. Byard RW. Hazardous infant and early childhood sleeping environments and death scene examination. J Clin Forensic Med. 1996;3:115-22. https://doi.org/10.1016/S1353-1131(96)90000-0.

30. Vennemann MM, Hense H-W, Bajanowski T, Blair PS, Complojer C, Moon RY, et al. Bed sharing and the risk of sudden infant death syndrome: Can we resolve the debate? J Pediatr. 2012;160:44-8. https://doi.org/10.1016/j.jpeds.2011.06.052.

31. Carpenter R, McGarvey C, Mitchell EA, Tappin DM, Vennemann MM, Smuk M, et al. Bed sharing when parents do not smoke: Is there a risk of SIDS? An individual level analysis of five major case-control studies. BMJ Open. 2013;3:e002299. https://doi.org/10.1136/bmjopen-2012-002299.

32. Horne RSC, Hauck FR, Moon RY. Sudden infant death syndrome and advice for safe sleeping. Brit Med J. 2015;350:h1989. https://doi.org/10.1136/bmj.h1989.

33. Byard RW. Is co-sleeping in infancy a desirable or dangerous practice? J Paediatr Child Health. 1994;80:198-9. https://doi.org/10.1111/j.1440-1754.1994.tb00618.x.

34. Byard RW. Should infants and adults sleep in the same bed together? Med J Aust. 2012;196:10-11. https://doi.org/10.5694/mja11.11358.

35. Byard RW. Bed sharing and sudden infant death syndrome [letter]. J Pediatr. 2012;160:1063. https://doi.org/10.1016/j.jpeds.2012.03.006.

36. Byard RW. Sofa sleeping and infant death. Brit Med J. 2015;350:h1989. https://doi.org/10.1136/bmj.h1989.

37. McKenna JJ, Mosko S. Evolution and infant sleep: An experimental study of infant-parent co-sleeping and its implications for SIDS. Acta Paediatrica. 1993;389 (Suppl):31-6. https://doi.org/10.1111/j.1651-2227.1993.tb12871.x.

38. McKenna JJ, Mosko S. Mother-infant cosleeping: Toward a new scientific beginning. In: Sudden infant death syndrome. Problems, progress and possibilities. Eds Byard RW, Krous HF. London: Arnold, 2001. p. 258-74.

39. McKenna JJ, McDade T. Why babies should never sleep alone: A review of the co-sleeping controversy in relation to SIDS, bedsharing and breast feeding. Paediatr Resp Rev. 2005;6:134-52. https://doi.org/10.1016/j.prrv.2005.03.006.

40. Mitchell EA, Thompson JMD. Co-sleeping increases the risk of SIDS, but sleeping in the parents' bedroom lowers it. In: Sudden infant death syndrome. New trends in the nineties. Ed Rognum TO. Oslo: Scandinavian University Press, 1995. p. 266-9.

41. Scragg RKR, Mitchell EA, Stewart AW, Ford RP, Taylor BJ, Hassall IB, et al. Infant room-sharing and prone sleep position in sudden infant death syndrome. Lancet. 1996;347:7-12. https://doi.org/10.1016/S0140-6736(96)91554-8.

42. Byard RW. Overlaying, co-sleeping, suffocation, and sudden infant death syndrome: The elephant in the room. Forensic Sci Med Pathol. 2015;11:273-4. https://doi.org/10.1007/s12024-014-9600-5.

43. Byard RW, Beal S, Blackbourne B, Nadeau JM, Krous HF. Specific dangers associated with infants sleeping on sofas. J Paediatrics Child Health. 2001;37:476-8. https://doi.org/10.1046/j.1440-1754.2001.00747.x.

44. Byard RW. Is breast feeding in bed always a safe practice? J Paediatrics Child Health. 1998;234:418-19. https://doi.org/10.1046/j.1440-1754.1998.00264.x.

45. Byard RW. Breast feeding and unexpected neonatal and infant death [letter]. Arch Dis Child. Fetal Neonat Ed. 2012;97:F75.

46. Byard RW. Breastfeeding and sudden infant death syndrome [letter]. J Paediatrics Child Health. 2013;49:E353. https://doi.org/10.1111/jpc.12139.

47. McGarvey C, McDonnell M, Hamilton K, O'Regan M, Matthews T. An eight-year study of risk factors for SIDS: Bed-sharing vs non bed-sharing. Arch Dis Child. 2005;91:318-23. https://doi.org/10.1136/adc.2005.074674.

48. Blair PS, Sidebotham P, Berry PJ, Evans M, Fleming PJ. Major epidemiological changes in sudden infant death syndrome: A 20-year population-based study in the UK. Lancet. 2006;367:314-19. https://doi.org/10.1016/S0140-6736(06)67968-3.

49. Bourne AJ, Beal SM, Byard RW. Bed sharing and sudden infant death syndrome. Brit Med J. 1994;308:537-8. https://doi.org/10.1136/bmj.308.6927.537c.

50. Byard RW. The triple risk model for shared sleeping [letter]. J Paediatr Child Health. 2012;48:947-8. https://doi.org/10.1111/j.1440-1754.2012.02565.x.

51. Byard RW, Burnell RH. Apparent life threatening events and infant holding practices. Arch Dis Child. 1995;73:502-4. https://doi.org/10.1136/adc.73.6.502.

52. Parkins KJ, Poets CF, O'Brien LM, Stebbens VA, Southall DP. Effect of exposure to 15% oxygen on breathing patterns and oxygen saturation in infants: Interventional study. Brit Med J. 1998;316:887-91. https://doi.org/10.1136/bmj.316.7135.887.

53. Anonymous. The prevention of overlaying. Lancet. 1892;i:45.

54. Byard RW, Elliott J, Vink R. Infant gender, cosleeping and sudden death. J Paediatr Child Health. 2012;48:517-19. https://doi.org/10.1111/j.1440-1754.2011.02226.x.

55. Jensen LL, Banner J, Byard RW. Does β-APP staining of the brain in infant bed sharing deaths differentiate these cases from sudden infant death syndrome? J Forensic Leg Med. 2014;27:46-9. https://doi.org/10.1016/j.jflm.2014.07.006.

56. Bartholomew SEM, MacArthur BA, Bain AD. Sudden infant death syndrome in south east Scotland. Arch Dis Child. 1987;62:951-6. https://doi.org/10.1136/adc.62.9.951.

57. Byard RW, Mackenzie J, Beal SM. Formal retrospective case review and sudden infant death. Acta Paediatrica. 1997;86:1011-12. https://doi.org/10.1111/j.1651-2227.1997.tb15191.x.

58. Krous HF. The International Standardised Autopsy Protocol for sudden unexpected infant death. In: Sudden infant death syndrome. New trends in the nineties. Ed Rognum TO. Oslo: Scandinavian University Press, 1995. p. 81-95.

59. McGraw EP, Pless JE, Pennington DJ, White SJ. Postmortem radiography after unexpected death in neonates, infants, and children: Should imaging be routine? Am J Roentgen. 2002;178:1517-21. https://doi.org/10.2214/ajr.178.6.1781517.

60. Arnestad M. Sudden unexpected death in intrauterine life, infancy and early childhood in southeast Norway 1984-1999. Oslo: University of Oslo Press, 2002.

61. Arnestad M, Vege Å, Rognum TO. Evaluation of diagnostic tools applied in the examination of sudden unexpected deaths in infancy and early childhood. Forensic Sci Int. 2002;125:262-8. https://doi.org/10.1016/S0379-0738(02)00009-9.

62. Berry J, Allibone E, McKeever P, Moore I, Wright C, Fleming P. The pathology study: The contribution of ancillary pathology tests to the investigation of unexpected infant death. In: Sudden unexpected deaths in infancy. The CESDI SUDI studies 1993-1996. Eds Fleming P, Blair P, Bacon C, Berry J. London: The Stationary Office, 2000. p. 97-112.

63. Langlois NEI, Ellis PS, Little DL, Hulewicz B. Toxicologic analysis in cases of possible sudden infant death syndrome. A worthwhile exercise? Am J Forensic Med Pathol. 2002;23:162-6. https://doi.org/10.1097/00000433-200206000-00010.

64. Ballenden NR, Laster K, Lawrence JA. Pathologist as gatekeeper: Discretionary decision-making in cases of sudden infant death. Aust J Soc Issues. 1993;28:124-39. https://doi.org/10.1002/j.1839-4655.1993.tb00921.x.

65. Laskey AL, Haberkorn KL, Applegate KE, Catellier MJ. Postmortem skeletal survey practice in pediatric forensic autopsies: A national survey. J Forensic Sci. 2009;54:189-91. https://doi.org/10.1111/j.1556-4029.2008.00922.x.

66. Ingham AI, Langlois NEI, Byard RW. The significance of bruising in infants — A forensic postmortem study. Arch Dis Child. 2011;96:218-20. https://doi.org/10.1136/adc.2009.177469.

67. Byard RW, Stewart WA, Beal SM. Pathological findings in SIDS infants found in the supine position compared to the prone. J Sud Infant Death Synd Infant Mort. 1996;1:45-50.

68. Byard RW, Jensen LL. How reliable is reported sleeping position in cases of unexpected infant death? J Forensic Sci. 2008;53:1169-71. https://doi.org/10.1111/j.1556-4029.2008.00813.x.

69. Byard RW, Krous HF. Petechial hemorrhages and unexpected infant death. Leg Med. 1999;1:193-7. https://doi.org/10.1016/S1344-6223(99)80037-6.

70. Hilton JMN. The pathology of the sudden infant death syndrome. In: Paediatric forensic medicine and pathology. Ed Mason JK. London: Chapman & Hall, 1989. p. 156-64. https://doi.org/10.1007/978-1-4899-7160-9_10.

71. Knight B. The coroner's autopsy. A guide to non-criminal autopsies for the general pathologist. Edinburgh: Churchill Livingstone, 1983.

72. Oehmichen M, Gerling I, Meissner C. Petechiae of the baby's skin as differentiation symptom of infanticide versus SIDS. J Forensic Sci. 2000;45:602-7. https://doi.org/10.1520/JFS14735J.

73. Byard RW. Forensic issues in Down syndrome fatalities. J Forensic Legal Med. 2007;14:475-81. https://doi.org/10.1016/j.jflm.2007.01.001.

74. Biering-Sørensen F, Jorgensen T, Hilden J. Sudden infant death in Copenhagen 1956-71. I. Infant feeding. Acta Paediatrica. 1978;67:129-37. https://doi.org/10.1111/j.1651-2227.1978.tb16292.x.

75. Berry PJ. Pathological findings in SIDS. J Clin Pathol. 1992;46(Suppl):11-16.

76. Rognum TO. Definition and pathologic features. In: Sudden infant death syndrome. Problems, progress and possibilities. Eds Byard RW, Krous HF. London: Arnold, 2001. p. 4-30.

77. Valdes-Dapena M. A pathologist's perspective on the sudden infant death syndrome — 1991. Path Ann. 1992;27(Pt 1):133-64.

78. Valdes-Dapena M. The sudden infant death syndrome: Pathologic findings. Clin Perinatol. 1992;19:701-16.

79. Byard RW, Krous HF. Sudden infant death syndrome: Overview and update. Pediatr Dev Pathol. 2003;6:112-27. https://doi.org/10.1007/s10024-002-0205-8.

80. Becroft DMO, Thompson JMD, Mitchell EA. Epidemiology of intrathoracic petechial hemorrhages in sudden infant death syndrome. Pediatr Dev Pathol. 1998;1:200-9. https://doi.org/10.1007/s100249900027.

81. Krous HF, Nadeau JM, Byard RW, Blackbourne BD. Oronasal blood in sudden infant death. Am J Forensic Med Pathol. 2001;22:346-51. https://doi.org/10.1097/00000433-200112000-00003.

82. Byard RW, Moore L. Can thymic petechiae be used to separate SIDS infants from controls? Pathology. 1993;25(Suppl):7.

83. Beckwith JB. Intrathoracic petechial hemorrhages: A clue to the mechanism of death in sudden infant death syndrome? Ann NY Acad Sci. 1988;533:37-47. https://doi.org/10.1111/j.1749-6632.1988.tb37232.x.

84. Beckwith JB. The mechanism of death in sudden infant death syndrome. In: Sudden infant death syndrome. Medical aspects and psychological management. Eds Culbertson JL, Krous HF, Bendell RD. London: Edward Arnold, 1989. p. 48-61.

85. Valdes-Dapena M. The morphology of the sudden infant death syndrome: An overview. In: Sudden infant death syndrome. Eds Tildon JA, Roeder LM, Steinschneider A. New York: Academic Press, 1983. p. 169-82.

86. Byard RW. Sudden infant death syndrome — A "diagnosis" in search of a disease. J Clin Forensic Med. 1995;2:121-8. https://doi.org/10.1016/1353-1131(95)90079-9.

87. Emery JL, Dinsdale F. Increased incidence of lymphoreticular aggregates in lungs of children found unexpectedly dead. Arch Dis Child. 1974;49:107-11. https://doi.org/10.1136/adc.49.2.107.

88. Williams AL. Tracheobronchitis and sudden infant death syndrome. Pathology. 1980;12:73-8. https://doi.org/10.3109/00313028009060055.

89. Rambaud C, Cieuta C, Canioni D, Rouzioux C. Cot death and myocarditis. Cardiol Young. 1992;2:266-71. https://doi.org/10.1017/S1047951100001025.

90. Shatz A, Hiss J, Arensburg B. Myocarditis misdiagnosed as sudden infant death syndrome (SIDS). Med Sci Law. 1997;37:16-18. https://doi.org/10.1177/002580249703700104.

91. Byard RW, Krous HF. Minor inflammatory lesions and sudden infant death: Cause, coincidence or epiphenomena? Pediatr Pathol. 1995;15:649-54. https://doi.org/10.3109/15513819509027003.

92. Blackwell CC, Weir DM, Busuttil A, Saadi AT, Raza MW, Zorgani AA, et al. Infection, inflammation, and the developmental stage of infants: A new hypothesis for the aetiology of SIDS. In: Sudden infant death syndrome. New trends in the nineties. Ed Rognum TO. Oslo: Scandinavian University Press, 1995. p. 189-96.

93. Blackwell CC, Moscovis SM, Gordon AE, Al Madani OM, Hall ST, Gleeson M, et al. Cytokine responses and sudden infant death syndrome: Genetic, developmental and environmental risk factors. J Leuko Biol. 2005;78:1242-54. https://doi.org/10.1189/jlb.0505253.

94. Blackwell CC, Weir DM, Busuttil A. A microbiological perspective. In: Sudden infant death syndrome. Problems, progress and possibilities. Eds Byard RW, Krous HF. London: Arnold, 2001. p. 182-208.

95. Guntheroth WG. Interleukin-1 as intermediary causing prolonged sleep apnea and SIDS during respiratory infections. Med Hypoth. 1989;28:121-3. https://doi.org/10.1016/0306-9877(89)90025-X.

96. Summers AM, Summers CW, Drucker DB, Hajeer AH, Barson A, Hutchinson IV. Association of IL-10 genotype with sudden infant death syndrome. Hum Immunol. 2000;61:1270-3. https://doi.org/10.1016/S0198-8859(00)00183-X.

97. Krous HF, Nadeau JM, Silva PD, Blackbourne BD. A comparison of respiratory symptoms and inflammation in sudden infant death syndrome and in accidental or inflicted infant death. Am J Forensic Med Pathol. 2003;24:1-8. https://doi.org/10.1097/01.PAF.0000051520.92087.C3.

98. Yukawa N, Carter N, Rutty G, Green MA. Intra-alveolar haemorrhage in sudden infant death syndrome: A cause for concern? J Clin Pathol. 1999;52:581-7. https://doi.org/10.1136/jcp.52.8.581.

99. Hanzlick R. Pulmonary hemorrhage in deceased infants. Baseline data for further study of infant mortality. Am J Forensic Med Pathol. 2001;22:188-92. https://doi.org/10.1097/00000433-200106000-00016.

100. Berry PJ. Intra-alveolar haemorrhage in sudden infant death syndrome: A cause for concern? J Clin Pathol. 1999;52:553-4. https://doi.org/10.1136/jcp.52.8.553.

101. Becroft DM, Lockett BK. Intra-alveolar pulmonary siderophages in sudden infant death: A marker for previous imposed suffocation. Pathology. 1997;29:60-3. https://doi.org/10.1080/00313029700169554.

102. Hanzlick R, Delaney K. Pulmonary hemosiderin in deceased infants: Baseline data for further study of infant mortality. Am J Forensic Med Pathol. 2000;21:319-22. https://doi.org/10.1097/00000433-200012000-00004.

103. Milroy CM. Munchausen syndrome by proxy and intra-alveolar haemosiderin. Int J Leg Med. 1999;112:309-12. https://doi.org/10.1007/s004140050255.

104. Schluckebier DA, Cool CD, Henry TE, Martin A, Wahe JW. Pulmonary siderophages and unexpected infant death. Am J Forensic Med Pathol. 2002;23:360-3. https://doi.org/10.1097/00000433-200212000-00012.

105. Byard RW, Stewart WA, Telfer S, Beal SM. Assessment of pulmonary and intrathymic hemosiderin deposition in sudden infant death syndrome. Pediatr Pathol Lab Med. 1997;17:275-82. https://doi.org/10.1080/15513819709168572.

106. Forbes A, Acland P. What is the significance of haemosiderin in the lungs of deceased infants? Med Sci Law. 2004;44:348-52. https://doi.org/10.1258/rsmmsl.44.4.348.

107. Weber MA, Ashworth MT, Risdon RA, Malone M, Sebire NJ. The frequency and significance of alveolar haemosiderin-laden macrophages in sudden infant death. Forensic Sci Int. 2009;187:51-7. https://doi.org/10.1016/j.forsciint.2009.02.0.

108. Bajanowski T, Vege Å, Byard RW, Krous HF, Arnestad M, Bachs L, et al. Sudden infant death syndrome (SIDS) — Standardised investigations and classification: Recommendations. Forensic Sci Int. 2007;165:129-43. https://doi.org/10.1016/j.forsciint.2006.05.028.

109. Rognum TO, Arnestad M, Bajanowski T, Banner J, Blair P, Borthne A, et al. Consensus on diagnostic criteria for the exclusion of SIDS. Scand J Forensic Sci. 2003;9:62-73.

# 25

# Natural Diseases Causing Sudden Death in Infancy and Early Childhood

Victoria A Bryant, BPharm(Hons), MBBS[1] and
Neil J Sebire, BClinSci, MBBS, MD[1,2]

*[1]UCL Great Ormond Street Institute of Child Health
London, London, UK
[2]Camelia Botnar Laboratories, Great Ormond Street
Hospital for Children, London, UK*

## Introduction

Global childhood mortality rates in the under-5s were 44 per 1,000 live births in 2013, ranging from 2.3 in Singapore to 152.5 in Guinea-Bissau (Western sub-Saharan Africa), with rates of 4.9 per 1,000 live births in the United Kingdom (UK) (1). In England and Wales there are >5,000 deaths annually in children aged 0-19 years (2) from an estimated population of 12.9 million in this age group (3). Around 3,000 of these deaths are in infants (less than 1 year) with the majority having known serious medical conditions; such deaths are hence "expected". Most are due to perinatal and immaturity-related conditions, which account for around 40% of cases, followed by congenital anomalies. Many of these deaths occur in the early (less than 7 days) or late neonatal (7 to 27 days) period (2). The next most commonly affected age group is adolescents, who account for around 1,000 deaths annually, with more than half being due to external, non-natural causes (2).

Unexpected death occurring in an apparently healthy infant is termed "sudden unexpected death in infancy (SUDI)" and refers to such a presentation in an infant 7-365 days of age. According to most definitions, unexpected deaths in infants under 7 days of age are excluded from the SUDI category, and instead have been termed "sudden unexpected early neonatal death (SUEND)". All cases of SUDI and SUEND require investigation to determine the cause of death. In England and Wales such cases are referred to Her Majesty's Coroner (HMC), who will direct a post-mortem examination by a specialist pediatric pathologist. The primary rationale of the post-mortem examination, including its components and ancillary investigations, is to diagnose or exclude those natural (and non-natural) causes of death which are identifiable and to allow a specific cause of death to be provided (the specific details of the autopsy procedure are detailed in Chapter 24). Whilst many cases will subsequently be found to have died from previously unrecognized medical conditions, such as congenital anomalies or acquired natural diseases, a significant number will remain unexplained despite a complete autopsy including ancillary investigations (microbiology, virology, radiology, and metabolic studies). These cases are referred to as "unexplained SUDI", "unascertained", or "sudden infant death syndrome (SIDS)" according to the precise circumstances of the case and local practice, these terms by definition being diagnoses of exclusion.

Excluding SIDS cases and neonatal deaths (0-27 days), for infants and children in England and Wales the most common acquired causes of natural deaths are neoplasms, diseases affecting the neurological, cardiovascular or respiratory systems, and infections (2) (Figure 25.1). It is likely that >50% of these cases may occur in infants and children with known life-limiting conditions. However, similar to in infancy, sudden unexpected death in childhood (SUDC; >1 year) also occurs, albeit less frequently than SUDI, with cases referred to the Coroner in the same manner. Following investigation, unexplained SUDC is less common than SIDS but remains a significant proportion of all childhood deaths; in England and Wales, for example, there were 212 registered SIDS cases compared to 27 unexplained SUDC cases in 2014 (4). However, globally, accurate figures regarding the proportions of explained and unexplained deaths following autopsy are difficult to establish. This is, in part, due to wide variability in the death certification process, making epidemiological evaluation unreliable (5), and a lack of large population-based studies, in particular those investigating SUDC. A recent review identified 24 published studies investigating 25 cohorts (17 in infants, 4 including both infants and children, and 4 children only) from 11 different countries; following full investigation the cause of death was found in 9-67% of SUDI and 22-86% of SUDC cases (6). In the same study, infection was reported as the commonest explanation for death overall in SUDI (52% of all the cases reported across studies) and variably reported in individual studies to account for between 15-86% of the explained cases. Of the studies in children >1 year, 36-68% of explained deaths were due to infectious causes (6).

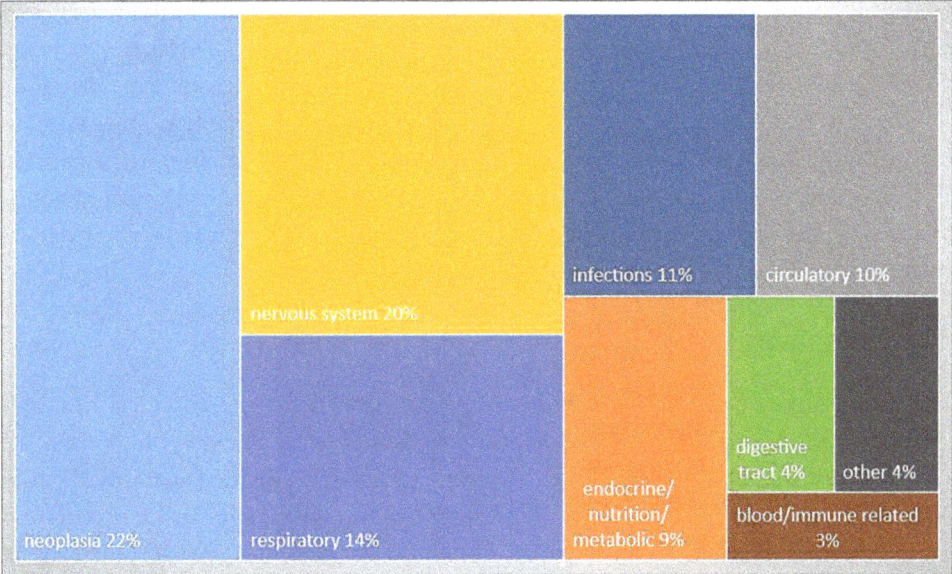

Figure 25.1: Treemap demonstrating the major causes of natural death in children (aged 28 days to 19 years) by disease/organ system in England and Wales (based on yearly average from 2009-11) (2).)

## Natural Disease and Unexplained Deaths

Much research over the last 40 years into SIDS has identified various environmental risk factors (7) and has led to changes in sleeping practices, with dramatic reductions in the reported incidence (8). Despite this, a significant number of deaths remain unexplained in both infants and children, and various hypotheses have been suggested to explain such cases. Developmental anomalies of the hippocampus, specifically the dentate gyrus, sometimes associated with a personal or family history of febrile seizures, are thought to represent a developmental vulnerability in infants and young children who die during sleep (9). Sudden arrhythmic deaths are considered in cases where the autopsy reveals no pathology to account for the death (10). In such cases genetic testing to identify possible channelopathies is undertaken in both the index case and close relatives, but often the yield is poor (11). It has also been suggested that clinically undiagnosed infections may be associated with apparently unexplained deaths since parents/carers often report a history of mild illness leading up to the sudden death (12); and it has been suggested that an atypical systemic inflammatory response may trigger a final common pathway in the absence of a traditional established and recognizable host-response.

This chapter will focus on the autopsy features of the spectrum of natural diseases which can cause sudden death in infancy and childhood. Since a myriad of diseases could theoretically lead to death, it is not possible to describe all such entities. Therefore, we describe the more frequently encountered diseases identified at post-mortem examination, in addition to some less common but diagnostically important entities. For convenience, the chapter is divided into subsections by major organ systems/ anatomical location, with the final section discussing a number of specific bacterial infections implicated in sudden death.

## The Respiratory System

The complexity of the respiratory tract is such that there are many anatomical areas that may be affected by abnormal developmental or pathological changes which have the potential to cause death in childhood. The respiratory tract is divided anatomically into the upper and lower respiratory tract (URT, LRT). The URT starts at the nostrils and mouth through the nasal passages, paranasal sinuses, pharynx, and the part of the larynx superior to the vocal cords; the LRT is defined as the portion of the larynx inferior to the vocal cords, trachea, bronchi, and acini (comprising the bronchiole, alveolar ducts, and alveoli as the functional unit of lungs). The lungs are limited by the thoracic cage and diaphragm from which they are normally separated by the pleural space. A wide range of disorders may affect any of these sites and respiratory pathology represents one of the most common organ systems responsible for natural deaths in infancy and childhood (13).

### Congenital and developmental anomalies

Congenital and developmental anomalies may affect any part of the respiratory tract. Some are identifiable macroscopically at autopsy whilst others require microscopic tissue examination. Gross anomalies are most likely to cause death by airway compromise (14) (Table 25.1). Histological anomalies predominantly represent abnormal development of lung parenchyma leading to death secondary to impairment of gaseous exchange (discussed in more detail later). Many gross anomalies are likely to be detected or suspected at antenatal screening and so can be managed at birth. However, some are not apparent and may present as sudden death in the early neonatal period, during infancy, or in later childhood. Congenital anomalies may be associated with malformation syndromes or may be isolated findings.

Table 25.1: Examples of congenital anomalies associated with airway obstruction. (Adapted from (14).)

| Anomaly | Age and presentation |
|---|---|
| Choanal atresia | Birth — if complete, airway obstruction |
| Laryngeal atresia | Birth, immediate treatment required for survival, often syndromic |
| Laryngomalacia | Infancy — airway collapse/obstruction |
| Laryngeal clefts | Infancy with stridor, respiratory distress, often syndromic |
| Laryngeal stenosis | Early infancy with airway obstruction |
| Tracheal agenesis | Birth with no cry and failure of intubation |
| Tracheal stenosis | Commonly acquired following endotracheal intubation |
| Tracheomalacia | Any age with airway collapse and obstruction |
| Tracheal stenosis | Sudden airway occlusion (inflamed, mucus plug) |
| Bronchomalacia | Airway collapse/obstruction |
| Other | |
| Lingual thyroglossal duct cyst | Any age with upper airway obstruction |
| Macroglossia | Any age with upper airway obstruction |
| Micrognathia | Any age with acute airway obstruction |
| Lingual lymphangioma | Airway obstruction if involves base of the tongue |
| Vascular ring | Early infancy with airway obstruction due to tracheal compression |

***Primary diffuse developmental pulmonary disorders (Congenital lung dysplasia).*** These represent a group of lethal, developmental lung diseases of uncertain etiology which usually present in the neonatal period.

*Acinar Dysplasia* (AD) appears to represent major arrest of lung development, the lungs being abnormally small with apparent maturation arrest at the pseudoglandular or early canalicular stage (15). Lack of normal acini renders adequate gas exchange impossible, and affected infants are refractory to ventilation and die shortly after birth. The underlying cause remains unclear, but case reports revealing positive family history suggest a genetic basis in at least some cases (16).

*Congenital Alveolar Dysplasia* (CAD) is a primary malformation of alveoli due to retardation and disturbance of normal lung growth. The lungs may be of normal size, but histological examination reveals arrest of development at the late canalicular or early saccular stage (Figure 25.2). Neonates show signs of respiratory failure and pulmonary hypertension shortly after birth. Although resuscitation is possible, they remain ventilator-dependent and die due to respiratory failure (15).

*Alveolar Capillary Dysplasia with misalignment of pulmonary veins* (ACD/MPV) is characterized by abnormal development of the pulmonary vasculature (17), with pulmonary veins, which normally sit in the interlobular septa, displaced alongside arteries and bronchioles in the bronchovascular bundles. There is an associated striking reduction in the normal subepithelial capillary bed, with capillaries being centrally positioned within widened alveolar septa, resulting in increased diffusion distance for gaseous exchange. Most infants develop progressive respiratory failure, cyanosis, and early signs of persistent pulmonary hypertension of the newborn (PPHN, see below) within 48 hours of birth; however, delayed presentation may be weeks or months later. Regardless of the age at presentation, mortality approaches 100%, with most reported cases diagnosed at autopsy (17). Most cases appear to be due to de novo heterozygous point mutations or deletions in the FOXF1 transcription factor gene or its distant enhancer region on chromosome 16q24.1 (18). Around 10% of cases also involve siblings, suggesting an inherited form of the disease (17).

*Congenital pulmonary lymphangectasia* is a rare anomaly of the lymphatic system of the lungs which may be associated with a more generalized lymphatic maldevelopment. It is characterized by dilated lymphatic channels in the bronchovascular bundles, interlobular septa, and pleura. It can be complicated by development of chylothorax, with subsequent lung hypoplasia if occurring in utero but typically presents with

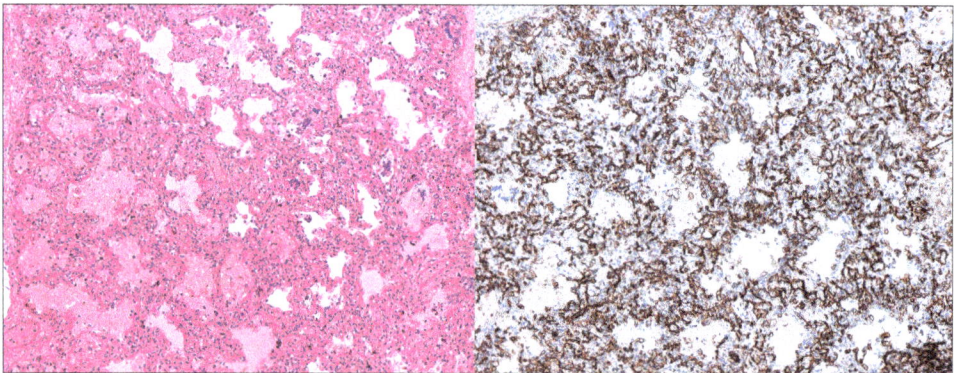

Figure 25.2: Congenital alveolar dysplasia in a 21-day-old term male. Noted to be wheezy for two weeks with some feeding difficulties and found dead in his crib. Left panel: Hematoxylin- and eosin- (H&E-) stained lung showing alveolar immaturity and alveolar damage (x 10). Right panel: Staining with CD31 highlights double capillary loops. (From the autopsy archives at Great Ormond Street Hospital.)

respiratory distress in newborns due to recurrent chylous effusions and is uniformly fatal (15). On gross examination the lungs have a subtle cobblestone appearance with prominent interlobular septa.

*Inborn errors of surfactant metabolism* are rare and present predominantly in infancy. More than 30 inherited autosomal recessive mutations of genes affecting surfactant production and processing have been identified, and clinical presentation and histological manifestations very much depend on the causative gene (19). The three major causative genes are those encoding for *surfactant protein B* (SFTPB), *ATP-binding cassette transporter A3* (ABCA3), and *surfactant protein C* (SFTPC). *SFTPB deficiency* is a lethal disease of neonates resulting in a histological pattern of variant pulmonary alveolar proteinosis (PAP) with Periodic acid-Schiff (PAS)-positive granular alveolar material. Autosomal dominant *ABCA3 mutations* have been found to cause fatal surfactant deficiency in newborns and infants <3 months of age. Histology may show a PAP or desquamative interstitial pneumonia (DIP) pattern characterized by numerous macrophages in the alveolar spaces. The PAS-positive PAP deposits are described as being more granular in *SFTPB deficiency* compared to the "glassy" deposits in *ABCA3 mutations* (15). *SFTPC deficiency* typically affects older infants and shows a pattern of chronic pneumonitis of infancy (CPI) with interstitial thickening, mild inflammatory infiltrate, edema, and diffuse type II pneumocyte hyperplasia (15).

## Other respiratory causes of sudden neonatal death

*Persistent pulmonary hypertension of the newborn (PPHN)* occurs following the failure of normal pulmonary vascular relaxation during the cardiopulmonary transition from fetal to independent circulation. PPHN is associated with perinatal asphyxia, meconium aspiration syndrome, pneumonia, and pulmonary hypoplasia, with mortality rates reaching near 50%, even when treated (20). Presentation as sudden death is unusual but well described; it has been reported to account for 10% of sudden deaths in the first week of life (21). Idiopathic PPHN has normal lung parenchyma with remodeled pulmonary vasculature, and it accounts for 10-20% of all cases of PPHN (20).

*Massive pulmonary hemorrhage (MPH)* causes death within the first few days after birth. It is more frequent in babies of low birth weight (<2,500 g) who develop severe respiratory distress, often with blood-stained secretions, immediately after birth or within the first 48 hours of life. Many associations have been described including sepsis, hyaline membrane disease, perinatal asphyxia, and cardiac defects (22). The pathogenesis of MPH remains unknown, but it is suggested to reflect a non-specific reaction to acute lung injury or reperfusion injury. Other theories include a terminal event precipitated by acute left ventricular failure (23). At autopsy the lungs are heavy and hemorrhagic (Figure 25.3) and microscopic examination reveals blood-filled alveoli with confluent hemorrhage.

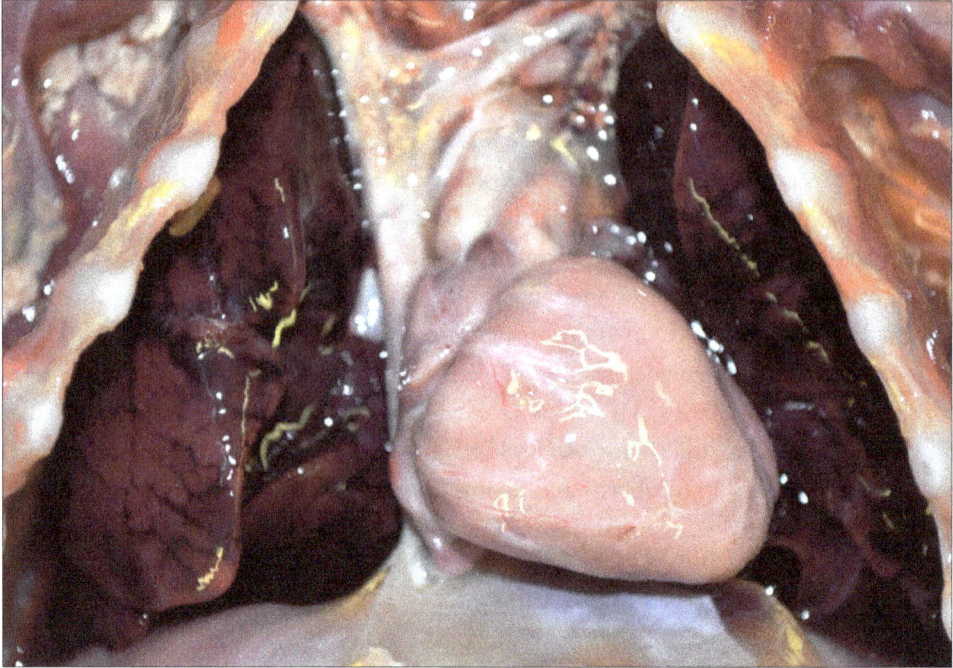

Figure 25.3: Massive pulmonary hemorrhage in a live-born term male who rapidly developed respiratory distress and died shortly after birth. Note the relative pallor of the heart. (From the autopsy archives at Great Ormond Street Hospital.)

*Meconium aspiration syndrome (MAS)* is rare, occurring in around 10% of neonates born through meconium-stained amniotic fluid (MSAF). MSAF is unusual before 38 weeks' gestation, but the incidence increases with longer gestations (24). MAS is defined clinically as respiratory distress in a neonate born through MSAF, requiring supplemental oxygen during the first two hours of life and lasting for at least 12 hours in the absence of congenital malformations of airways, lungs, or heart (25). The pathophysiology is not completely clarified but is thought to be associated with fetal distress, hence meconium passage in utero. Fetal distress induces gasping, leading to aspiration of large volumes of MSAF with rapid developmental of severe respiratory distress at birth. Aspiration of MSAF may lead to plugging of airways and surfactant dysfunction, with resultant pulmonary arterial hypertension and inflammation, all of which have a role in development of MAS (26). Histological examination of the lungs reveals meconium, vernix, abundant squames, and cellular debris in both distal and proximal airspaces. There may also be hyaline membranes, pulmonary hemorrhage, and necrosis (24). In some cases of apparently unexpected early infant deaths, histological features suggestive of MAS may be present in the absence of a definite history of MSAF and the diagnosis may not have been made prior to death.

## Respiratory tract infections

*Upper respiratory tract infections (URTI)* are commonly caused by viruses, and although they are generally mild, severe cases and complications can occur in children and rapidly lead to death. *Epiglottitis* and *bacterial tracheitis* are commonly caused by *Hemophilus influenza type b* (in non-vaccinated individuals), *Streptococcus*, and *Staphylococcus* infection. *Bacterial tracheitis* causes exudative pseudomembrane formation; and in *epiglottitis*, there is diffuse edema of the epiglottis, which develops a cherry-red discoloration. Both may cause acute obstruction of the upper airways and rapid death without prompt medical attention (27). Diagnosis at autopsy is usually straightforward with macroscopic and histological abnormalities.

*Acute laryngotracheobronchitis (Croup)* is the commonest cause of infectious upper airway obstruction in children up to 6 years old, but most cases are in those aged 1 to 2 years (27). Croup is a viral illness characterized by stridor due to subglottic edema and exudative inflammation. *Parainfluenza virus (types 1, 2, 3)* and *Rhinovirus* are the commonest etiologies followed by *Enterovirus, Respiratory Syncytial virus* (RSV), *Influenza virus*, and *Human bocavirus*. *Measles* is a rare but important cause in unvaccinated individuals (28). Aside from airway obstruction, other major risks to children are fatigue from increased work of breathing, secondary bacterial infection, and plugging of smaller airways by the inflammatory exudate, which can lead to obliterative bronchiolitis.

*Lower respiratory tract infections (LRTI)* may be caused by bacteria, viruses, or fungal infections. *Acute bronchiolitis* is a major concern in infants, especially those <6 months of age. Winter epidemics occur due to RSV but other etiologies include *Mycoplasma, Human Metapneumovirus, Parainfluenza virus*, and *Adenoviruses*.

*Pneumonia* can cause acute respiratory failure and is a relatively frequent cause of death in infants and pre-school age children, many of which are apparently "unexpected", in that the child may not have seemed severely unwell prior to the collapse/death. Infection may be viral, bacterial, or fungal in origin. *Streptococcus pneumoniae, Hemophilus influenzae*, and *RSV* are the major life-threatening causes of pneumonia in young children worldwide. Other viral causes include *Human Metapneumovirus, Parainfluenza, Measles*, and *Adenovirus*, with death often due to secondary bacterial infection, for example with *Staphylococcus aureus*. This is an important cause of secondary pneumonia following viral respiratory illness and is associated with a high incidence of complications such as lung abscess and empyema.

*Whooping cough* is caused by *Bordetella pertussis*, a gram-negative coccobacillus only found in humans. Globally it is ranked amongst the 10 leading causes of childhood mortality (29). It is most severe during the first six months of life, particularly in premature, non- or incompletely immunized infants, with >60% of all deaths from pertussis in infants less than 1 year. The bacterium causes direct damage to the respiratory epithelium, causing it to shed and obstruct the airways, whilst the toxin can suppress the immune response in the lung, delaying recruitment of neutrophils (29). Infection can take a fulminant course with rapid onset of respiratory distress, pulmonary hypertension, and refractory hypoxemia. Histological examination reveals a necrotizing bronchiolitis, hemorrhage, and fibrinous edema.

*Congenital pneumonia* is caused by aspiration of infected amniotic fluid in utero from ascending genital tract infection and is commonly associated with premature rupture of membranes, chorioamnionitis, and prolonged labor. In live births it is reported in up to 20% of neonates dying within the first 48 hours of life, with premature infants being most susceptible. *Escherichia coli* and *Group B streptococcus* (GBS) are amongst the most frequently responsible organisms. Histological diagnosis requires a mononuclear cell infiltrate within the interstitium, in addition to the presence of squames and maternal neutrophils in alveolar spaces (from infected amniotic fluid).

*Aspiration pneumonia* may cause destruction of the upper respiratory mucosa and necrotizing inflammation of the lung parenchyma due to the acidity of gastric contents. In infants it has been associated with diaphragmatic hernia, pyloric stenosis, and gastroesophageal reflux disease. In older children it is commonly associated with neurological conditions such as cerebral palsy.

Diagnosis of LRTI at autopsy is based primarily on identification of significant airway or airspace inflammatory cell infiltration, with or without positive microbiological findings. It should be noted that there is some controversy regarding assessment of "severity" of such changes and their relationship to cause of death, with some providing LRTI as the likely cause in all cases in which any definite evidence is present, whereas others may interpret the findings as present but insufficient to explain the death. At present, until further "gold standard" tests are available for evaluating mechanisms of death, definitive determination of clinical significance remains impossible.

*Respiratory papillomatosis* is associated with maternal condylomata (HPV 6 and 11 have been implicated) with vertical transmission during vaginal delivery (30). Multiple squamous papillomas usually become apparent in childhood, although they may begin in infancy. Extension into the tracheobronchial tree may lead to airway obstruction and sudden death. Histological examination reveals epithelial hyperplasia and koilocytosis. A complication of surgical management of aggressive disease is airway stenosis (31).

## Acquired respiratory conditions

Bronchial asthma is the commonest chronic lung disease of childhood and is characterized by hypersensitivity of the airways to allergens, irritants, or viral infections, as well as cold air, exercise, and emotional upset. Exacerbations result in bronchospasm and hypersecretion of mucus, with "plugging" of airways leading to reduced gaseous exchange and ventilation-perfusion mismatch with subsequent hypoxemia. Acute exacerbations may lead to status asthmaticus, defined as asthma refractory to treatment, which is a well-recognized cause

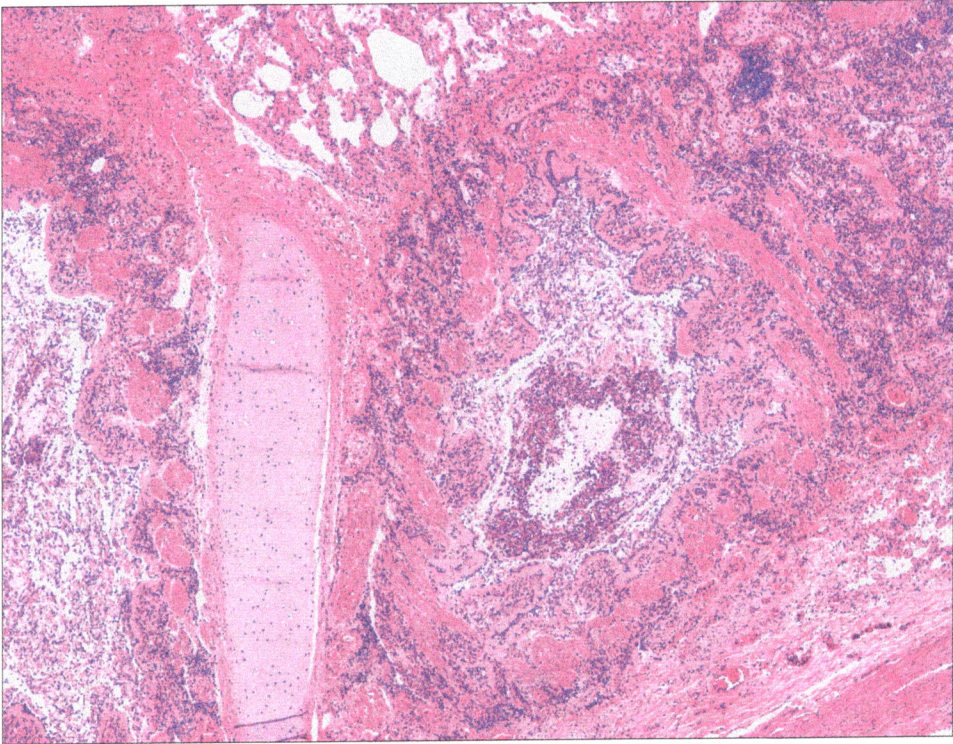

Figure 25.4: Acute asthma in a 9-year-old female. H&E-stained lung (x 4) showing mucus plugging of a bronchiole and chronic changes of thickened basement membrane and smooth muscle hypertrophy. (From the autopsy archives at Great Ormond Street Hospital.)

of death. However, sudden death may also occur in children previously thought to have mild disease or with minimal symptoms prior to death (32). Rarely, the first diagnosis of asthma may be made at autopsy. On macroscopic examination, typically the lungs appear hyperinflated and will often obscure the heart when viewed anteriorly. Thick mucus plugs may be seen on the cut surface with emphysematous changes due to distal air-trapping. On histological examination (Figure 25.4), mucosal edema, bronchospasm, and thick mucus plugging with eosinophils in the airways may all be seen to varying extents, all contributors to worsening hypoxia. Remodeling changes commensurate to the chronicity of the disease may be present, including smooth muscle hypertrophy, basement membrane thickening, goblet cell hyperplasia, and hypertrophy of submucosal mucus glands. There are no pathognomonic changes unique to fatal cases.

*Follicular bronchitis* is characterized by lymphoid hyperplasia of bronchus-associated lymphoid tissue (BALT), causing narrowing of bronchioles by external compression (Figure 25.5). It is rare in childhood and the etiology is unknown (33). Onset of symptoms may be in early infancy through to adolescence, and individuals may present

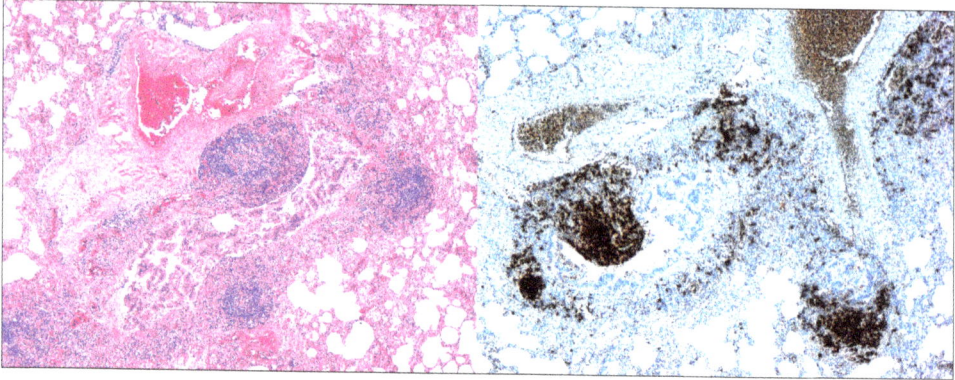

Figure 25.5: Follicular bronchitis in a 17-month-old male with symptoms of URTI, being treated with antibiotics, found dead in his cot. Left panel: H&E-stained lung (x 4). Right panel: Staining with CD20 highlights reactive lymphoid follicles encroaching into a bronchiole (x 4). (From the autopsy archives at Great Ormond Street Hospital.)

with cough, dyspnea, recurrent or massive hemoptysis, failure to thrive (34), or sudden death. In adults follicular bronchitis has been associated with collagen vascular disorders, immunodeficiency, and hypersensitivity reactions.

*Plastic bronchitis (cast bronchitis)* is characterized by the formation of gelatinous cohesive branching airway casts (35). In children it may occur in association with asthma, cystic fibrosis, or respiratory tract infections. Usually expectorated, casts may rarely lead to death from airway obstruction. Plastic bronchitis is a recognized, albeit rare, complication in children with congenital heart disease after single-ventricle palliation. In this scenario it is believed to be associated with increased pulmonary lymphatic flow, although the pathogenesis is unclear (36).

## Anaphylaxis

Anaphylaxis is an acute life-threatening reaction to an allergen in a susceptible individual. In children it is most commonly triggered by foods, followed by insect venom (37). In those under 2 years, allergies to cows' milk and eggs are the most frequent causes. Older children are more affected by reaction to nuts, including hazelnuts and cashews, in the pre-school years. Peanut allergy can occur at any age. Clinical signs of mucosal edema affecting the lips and tongue and bronchospasm can rapidly lead to death without prompt medical treatment. Diagnosis of anaphylaxis is, however, difficult at autopsy since there may be no specific gross or histological features, so details of the circumstances of death and medical history are essential. The most useful confirmatory test is blood showing increased levels of mast cell tryptase (samples remain useful for up to three days following death) and increased levels of total IgE or specific IgE to known or suspected allergens (38).

# The Cardiovascular System

## Congenital heart disease

Congenital heart disease (CHD) is the most common birth defect, affecting around 1% of live births (39): it has an estimated prevalence of 6-8 per 1,000 live births (40). With advances in antenatal diagnosis over the last 30 years, many congenital heart defects are identified prior to birth allowing time for preparation and early management of the neonate. Despite this, undiagnosed congenital heart disease still remains an important cause of sudden unexpected death, particularly during early infancy, with reports indicating that as many as 25% of babies with severe congenital heart disease may be discharged from hospital undiagnosed, and in some of these the diagnosis will first be made at autopsy (41). Most defects that are life-threatening in the neonatal period (0-27 days) have a duct-dependent systemic or pulmonary circulation issue, with signs becoming apparent on closure of the ductus arteriosus. Detailed discussion of CHD is beyond the scope of this chapter, but we present selected examples based on the types of cases more frequently encountered as sudden unexpected deaths in infancy and childhood. In general, it is recommended that the heart is examined in a systematic manner based on sequential segmental analysis, in which all connections, chambers, and relationships are evaluated and described. It should also be noted that anomalous pulmonary venous drainage may demonstrate unusual anatomical features and hence the heart, or at least its connections, should be examined in situ prior to removal.

*Coarctation of the Aorta* (CoA) describes a narrowed segment of the aortic arch which can be of any length. The narrowing may be pre-ductal, juxta-ductal or post-ductal in location and may be part of a more complex heart defect or may occur in isolation (42). Newborn infants with CoA may be stable initially, but rapid deterioration ensues with closure of the ductus arteriosus. CoA is a particularly challenging prenatal diagnosis, even in experienced centers (41).

*Aortic stenosis* accounts for approximately 5% of CHD (24) and may be above, below, or at the aortic valve when it may be secondary to abnormalities of the cusps. *Critical aortic stenosis* is life-threatening, causing obstruction to the left ventricular outflow tract and rendering the systemic circulation duct-dependent (42). At the severe end of the spectrum, aortic stenosis merges with *Hypoplastic left heart syndrome* (HLHS) with underdevelopment of the left side of the heart, with or without, mitral stenosis or atresia. HLHS accounts for up to 25% of all neonatal deaths from CHD (43). The etiology of HLHS is unknown and, whilst severe cases may be diagnosed during mid-trimester ultrasound scan, HLHS can evolve later in pregnancy and remain undetected until presentation shortly after birth. In these cases it has been hypothesized that an intrauterine insult in a genetically susceptible fetus occurs after embryogenesis; it may be immunological, infectious, or autoimmune in nature (43).

*Transposition of the great arteries* (TGA) is one of the most common cyanotic congenital heart diseases in newborns and is associated with early death if untreated. If there is a co-existing large ventricular septal defect (VSD), infants may be stable initially, developing heart failure after a few weeks of life (42). TGA is a difficult antenatal diagnosis as it is usually associated with a normal four-chamber view on ultrasound and, as such, low detection rates have been reported in routine antenatal anomaly scans (41).

*Total anomalous pulmonary venous connection* occurs when there is no connection between the pulmonary veins and the left atrium; instead the pulmonary veins drain to a common anomalous vein which joins directly to the superior or inferior vena cava or the portal vein. A patent foramen ovale or atrial septal defect is essential to provide a right-to-left shunt, allowing admixed oxygenated and deoxygenated blood to reach the left side of the heart (44). The condition is unlikely to be detected on routine prenatal anomaly scan (45) and may only become apparent in infancy. Surgical reconnection is essential in all cases (44). Sudden death may occur before diagnosis is made, where there is obstruction to pulmonary venous return as with infradiaphragmatic connection.

## Cardiomyopathies

Cardiomyopathy is defined as "a myocardial disorder in which the heart muscle is structurally and functionally abnormal in the absence of CAD, hypertension, valvular or congenital heart disease sufficient to cause the abnormality" (46). Pediatric cardiomyopathies are a heterogenous group of disorders with an annual incidence of approximately 1.13/100,000 (47). There is a bimodal incidence, with the highest peak in the first year of life and a smaller peak in adolescence (48). They are a rare but well-recognized cause of sudden unexpected death and are reported to account for around 1% of pediatric autopsies (49). Most have a genetic basis and 10-20% of pediatric cardiomyopathies are familial, necessitating referral of close relatives of the deceased for formal cardiology assessment and genetic counseling. *Dilated cardiomyopathy* is the commonest phenotype in childhood and is most frequently secondary to acute myocarditis or neuromuscular disease (50). However, hypocalcemia is a recognized and potentially reversible cause of dilated cardiomyopathy, especially in infants, and it has been seen as a complication of rickets (51, 52) (Figure 25.6).

*Mitochondrial cardiomyopathies* are estimated to occur in 20-40% of children with mitochondrial disease (53). Although cardiac screening is part of the management of individuals known to have mitochondrial disease, the first manifestation may be as sudden death. Mitochondrial cardiomyopathy commonly manifests as hypertrophic cardiomyopathy. Post-mortem diagnosis is made by identification of abnormal mitochondria within cardiac myocytes; this may be suspected on H&E and/or trichrome staining but confirmatory ultrastructure examination of cardiac myocytes is required for diagnosis. Death is most likely due to fatal arrhythmias.

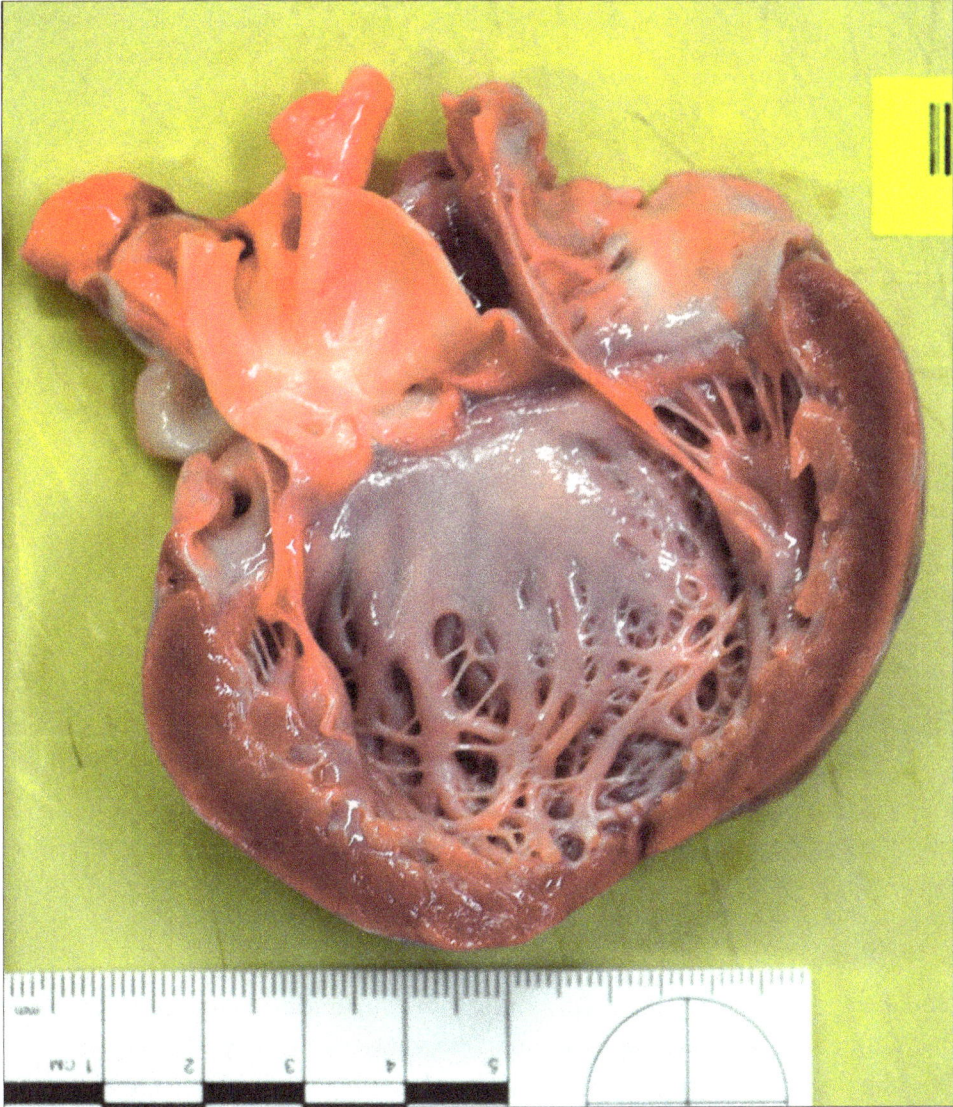

Figure 25.6: Dilated cardiomyopathy with endocardial fibroelastosis caused by rickets in a 9-month-old black female. (From the autopsy archives at Great Ormond Street Hospital.)

*Histiocytoid cardiomyopathy* is a rare arrhythmogenic disorder which occurs in the first two years of life and has a strong female predominance (female-to-male ratio 3:1) (54). Previously regarded as a developmental anomaly or neoplastic process, it has had many synonyms including "Purkinje cell tumor" and "oncocytic cardiomyopathy". It has since been reclassified by the American Heart Association as a primary genetic cardiomyopathy with mitochondrial, X-linked, and autosomal recessive inheritance

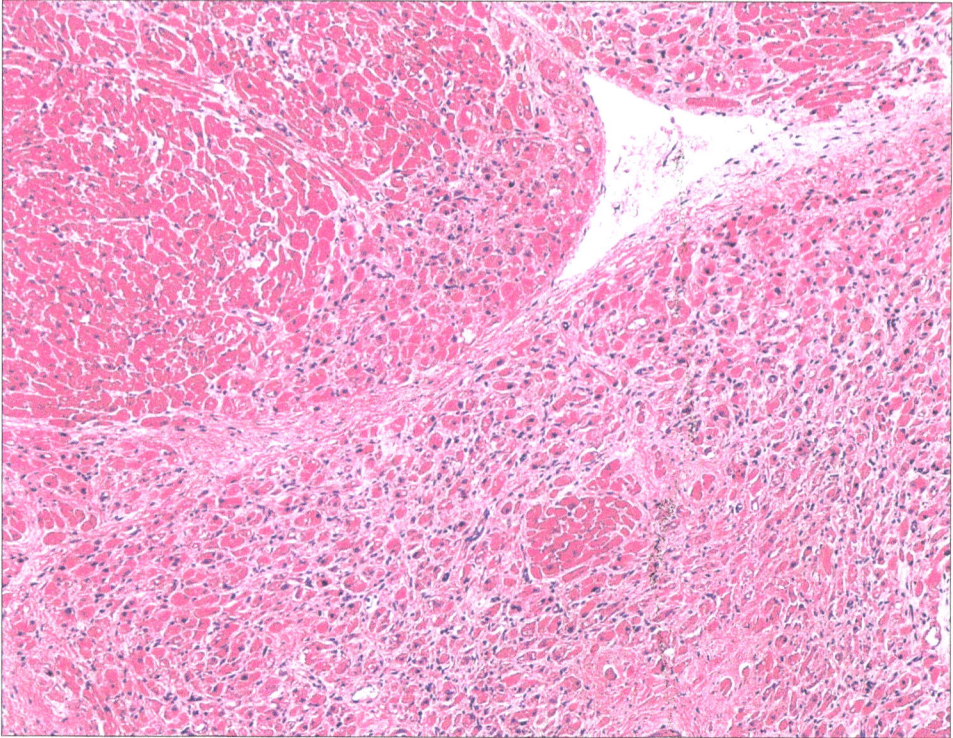

Figure 25.7: Histiocytoid cardiomyopathy in a 14-month-old female with symptoms of mild URTI for two to three weeks. H&E-stained myocardium showing histiocytoid cells in the lower right aspect compared to normal-appearing myocytes in the upper left corner (x 10). (From the autopsy archives at Great Ormond Street Hospital.)

described (55). Clinical presentation may be with arrhythmias, dilated cardiomyopathy, and heart failure, or as sudden death. At autopsy the heart may appear grossly normal but histological examination reveals nodules of variably sized eosinophilic cells with granular cytoplasm that resemble histiocytes (Figure 25.7).

*Mitogenic cardiomyopathy* is a recently described, distinctive form of dilated cardiomyopathy which manifests in early infancy and is invariably fatal (48). Presentation is commonly between 1 and 3 months of age with general lethargy, poor feeding, and respiratory distress, or sudden death. Histological examination reveals myocyte hypertrophy with hyperchromatic nuclei and occasional "caterpillar" nuclei. Mitotic activity is markedly increased, with a reported proliferation index of 10-20% with Ki67 immunohistochemistry compared to <1% in age-matched controls (48).

*Arrythmogenic right ventricular cardiomyopathy* (ARVC) is a disease of the desmosomal complex which results in fibro-fatty myocardial infiltration of either ventricle leading to

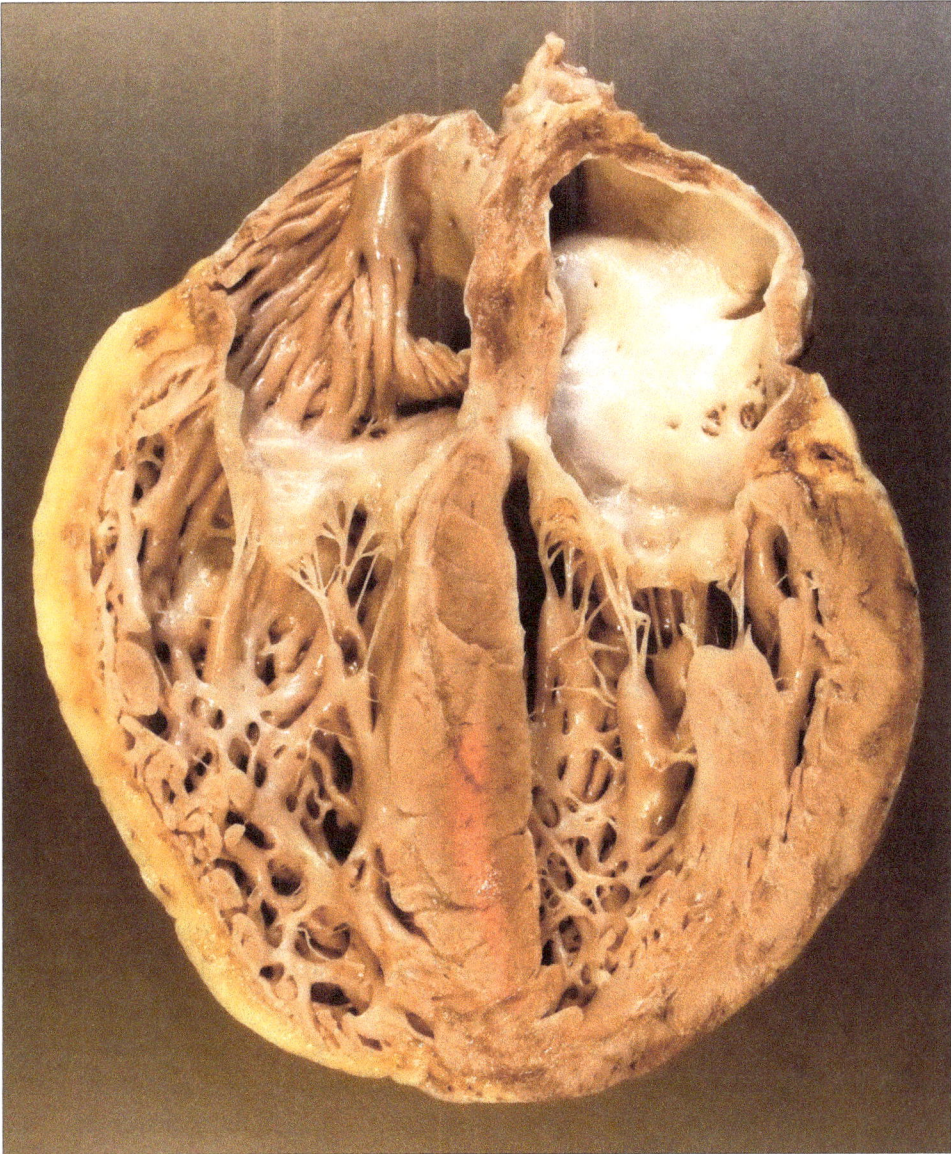

Figure 25.8: Fatty replacement of the right ventricular wall of the heart (left side of the photograph) in a 14-year-old male who collapsed whilst playing football. (From the autopsy archives at Great Ormond Street Hospital.)

ventricular arrhythmias, usually manifesting in adolescence and young adulthood (56). Frequency in the general population is estimated to be 1 in 5,000, with many cases remaining asymptomatic (57). Examination of the heart reveals extensive replacement of the cardiac myocytes by adipose tissue and fibrosis (Figure 25.8).

## Cardiac channelopathies

Abnormalities in the ion channels in myocardial cell membranes can give rise to cardiac arrhythmias and can increase the risk of sudden death. Major channelopathies include long QT syndrome (LQTS), short QT syndrome (SQTS), Brugada syndrome (BS), and catecholamingeric polymorphic ventricular tachycardia (CPVT) (58). In such cases the heart appears structurally and histologically normal at autopsy and no other cause of death is identified. Suggestive factors in the medical history or circumstances of death which raise the suspicion of a channelopathy-related death include a history of syncopal episodes or palpitations, or a witnessed collapse during normal daily activities. Gene sequencing is required for diagnosis, as the channelopathies are caused by mutations in genes associated with ion channels (in the case of LQTS, SQTS, and BS) or those involved with cellular metabolism of calcium ions (in the case of CPVT) (58). More than 100 mutations have been detected and most have an autosomal-dominant inheritance pattern which has implications for other family members. Genetic testing in unselected cases remains problematic, however, since the mere finding of a "variant" or "mutation" in one of the many channelopathy genes does not necessarily indicate that this was associated with functional effects or death, and in such cases evaluation of family members is also required.

## Acute myocarditis

Acute myocarditis is inflammation of the cardiac myocytes which can result in heart failure, dilated cardiomyopathy, and sudden death, representing approximately 2% of all unexpected pediatrics deaths referred for autopsy (59). Most commonly of viral etiology, the majority were thought to be due to *Enteroviruses (Coxsackie B)* and *Adenovirus*. However, *Parvovirus B19* is increasingly recognized as a cause of fatal acute myocarditis in childhood (60) and other viruses such as *Influenza viruses*, *Cytomegalovirus* (CMV), and *Varicella zoster* have also been implicated. Autopsy diagnosis is based on histological features, with the Dallas criteria generally accepted as the gold standard, requiring cardiac myocyte necrosis and/or degeneration with an associated inflammatory infiltrate (50) (Figure 25.9). Virology studies may be negative, particularly where the clinical course was protracted.

## Primary cardiac tumors

Primary cardiac tumors are rare, having an overall incidence of 0.02-0.04% in the pediatric population, with 50% diagnosed in the first year of life (61). Most cases are asymptomatic and the majority of tumors will spontaneously regress. However, if the tumors are positioned in critical areas, such as the conducting system, or if they are obstructing inflow or outflow tracts, there is a high risk of sudden death. The commonest

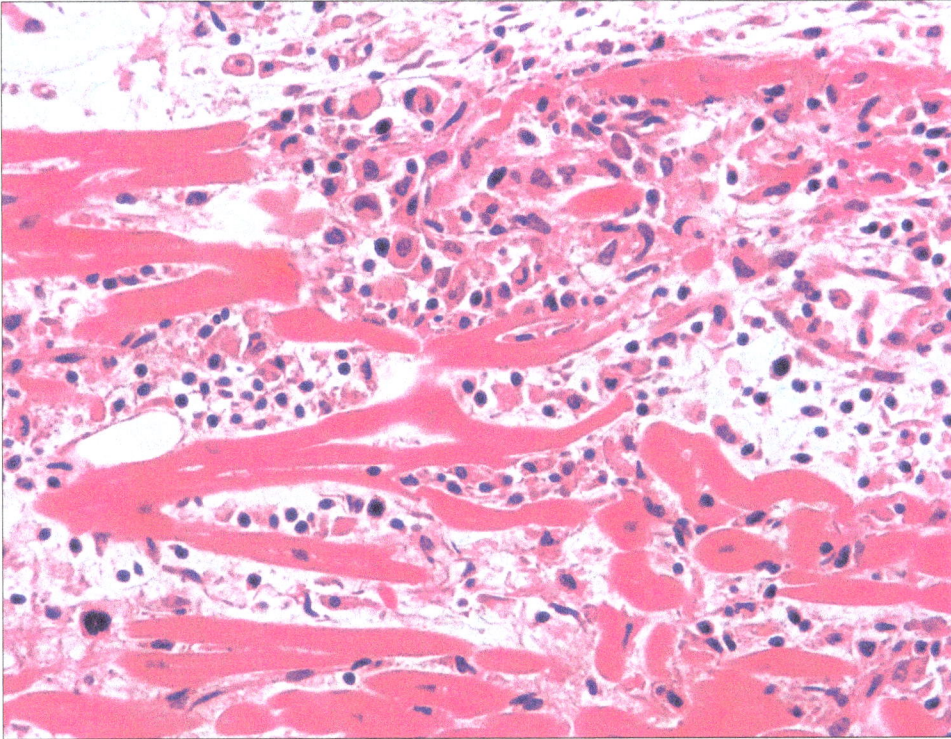

Figure 25.9: Acute myocarditis showing edema and extensive infiltration by chronic inflammatory cells and myocyte destruction, from a 14-year-old female with a one-week history of chest pain, fever, and dyspnea (H&E x 40). (From the autopsy archives at Great Ormond Street Hospital.)

are *rhabdomyomas*, which account for 45% of primary cardiac tumors in children; they are often associated with tuberous sclerosis but may occur in isolation. *Cardiac fibromas* (Figure 25.10) account for 25-30%; these rarely regress and their infiltrative nature makes complete resection difficult, if not impossible. More than one-third of cardiac fibromas are diagnosed in infancy, presenting with congestive heart failure or cyanosis. Conduction anomalies occur in 13% of cases and sudden cardiac death is reported in 10-30% (61). *Cardiac myxomas* are exceedingly rare in childhood (although they represent the commonest primary cardiac tumor in adults) and diagnosis raises the possibility of Carney complex, an autosomal-dominant multiple neoplasia syndrome characterized by multiple skin lentigines, neuronal, endocrine, and multiple cardiac myxomas. Other less common tumors include cardiac *lipomas* and *teratomas* (61).

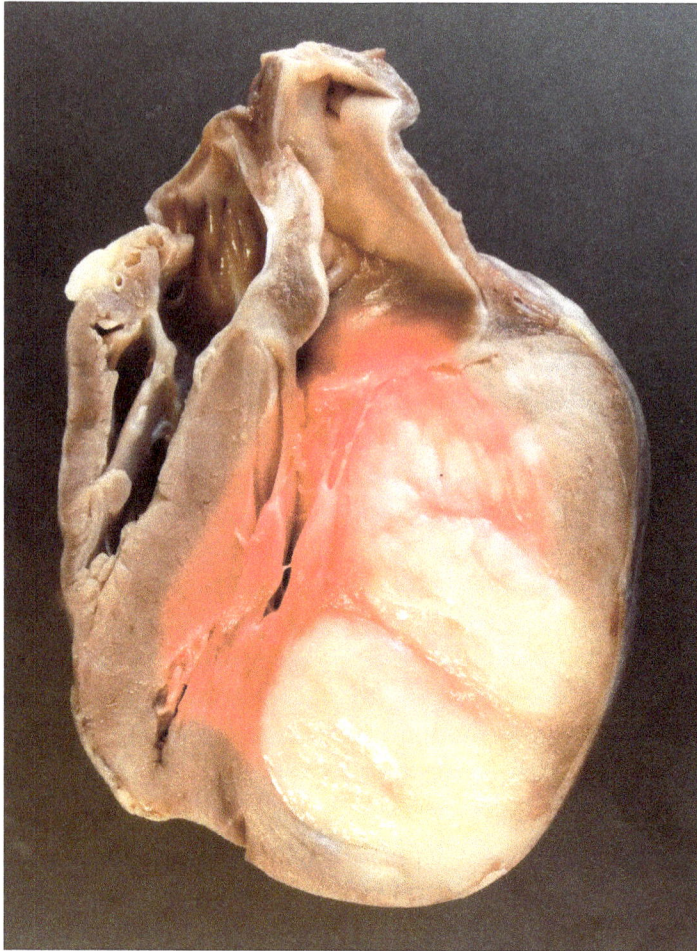

Figure 25.10: Cardiac fibroma effacing the left ventricle in a 4-month-old male. (From the autopsy archives at Great Ormond Street Hospital.)

## Vascular causes of sudden death

*Coronary artery disease (CAD)* is an uncommon cause of death in childhood and may be congenital or acquired. In contrast to adult practice, most cases are due to congenital anomalies often involving the origin of the left coronary artery (LCA) (62). *Coronary artery anomalies* are relatively common, occurring in up to 1.2% of population, but most are of no clinical significance. They may be part of complex structural congenital heart disease or they may occur in isolation. Sudden death may transpire at any age and is thought to be due to compression of the aberrant artery at some point along its course, with restriction of coronary blood flow resulting in infarction and cardiac arrest. Post-mortem examination may reveal areas of infarcts of varying age in the distribution of the affected artery due to previous, non-lethal restriction to myocardial perfusion.

*Atherosclerotic CAD* in childhood is only seen in homozygotes for familial hypercholesterolemia, leading to death from myocardial infarction. Individuals commonly present in infancy and childhood, with typical skin manifestations such as xanthelasma (yellowish plaques of cholesterol around the inner canthus of the eyelid), and lipid-lowering treatment can be instigated. If untreated, CAD manifests by the age of 10 years and sudden unexpected death from myocardial infarction has been reported in children as young as 3 years old (63).

*Kawasaki disease* is a vasculitis of unknown etiology which affects small- and medium-sized muscular vessels with a predilection for coronary arteries. It is a disease of childhood, with the highest incidence in children of Asian origin and most cases occurring in those under 5 years old (64). Coronary complications may be acute, such as myocardial infarction, or chronic, such as stenosis, dilatation, and aneurysm formation; giant aneurysms (>6mm diameter) are a high risk for stenosis. Chronic complications occur in 15-25% of untreated patients compared to <10% of treated individuals (65). Sudden unexpected death can occur due to thrombotic occlusion of a giant aneurysm, and diagnosis of Kawasaki disease has been made at autopsy (66) (Figure 25.11).

*Aortic dissection* is generally regarded as a disease of adulthood, but rare cases occur in children, most often associated with congenital heart disease, chronic hypertension, or connective tissue disorders (Marfan, Ehlers-Danlos, and Loeys-Dietz syndromes, for example) (67). Inherent or acquired weakness in the medial layer of the aorta predisposes the tissue to dissection; the aorta may rupture and, depending on the site, result in cardiac tamponade, hemothorax, or hemoperitoneum. Cases have been reported in patients with no known risk factors (68).

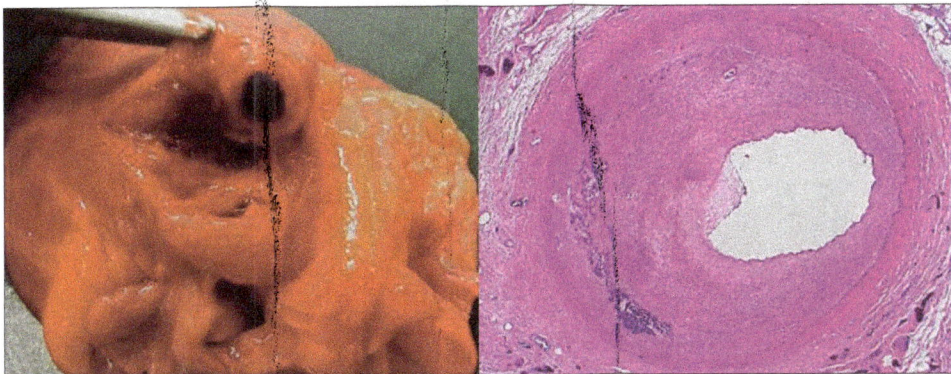

Figure 25.11: Kawasaki disease with thrombotic occlusion of a giant aneurysm. Left panel: Kawasaki disease with thrombotic occlusion of a giant aneurysm in the left coronary artery. Right panel: Intimal thickening and calcification seen on histology. From a previously undiagnosed case in a 3-year-old boy who died suddenly and unexpectedly at home. (Reproduced with permission from Dr Simi George, St Thomas' Hospital, London, UK.)

# Natural Intracranial Causes of Sudden Death

## Central nervous system (CNS) infections

*Meningitis* is inflammation of the leptomeninges surrounding the brain and spinal cord; it can be due to bacterial, viral, fungal, or parasitic infections. Bacterial causes are very much dependent on the age of the child; for example, neonatal meningitis is most commonly caused by GBS (Figure 25.12), *Escherichia coli*, and other gram-negative organisms (69). In contrast, *Neisseria meningitidis* is a greater risk for children >1 year old and adolescents (70) (various organisms are discussed in more detail in the infectious diseases section). Fungal meningitis is usually due to yeast-producing fungi such as *Cryptococcus* or *Coccidiodomycosis*, although it may occur with *Candida sp.* (71).

*Primary amebic meningoencephalitis (PAM)* is a rare and invariably fatal disease caused by *Naegleria fowleri*, which is a free-living ameba found in freshwater habitats

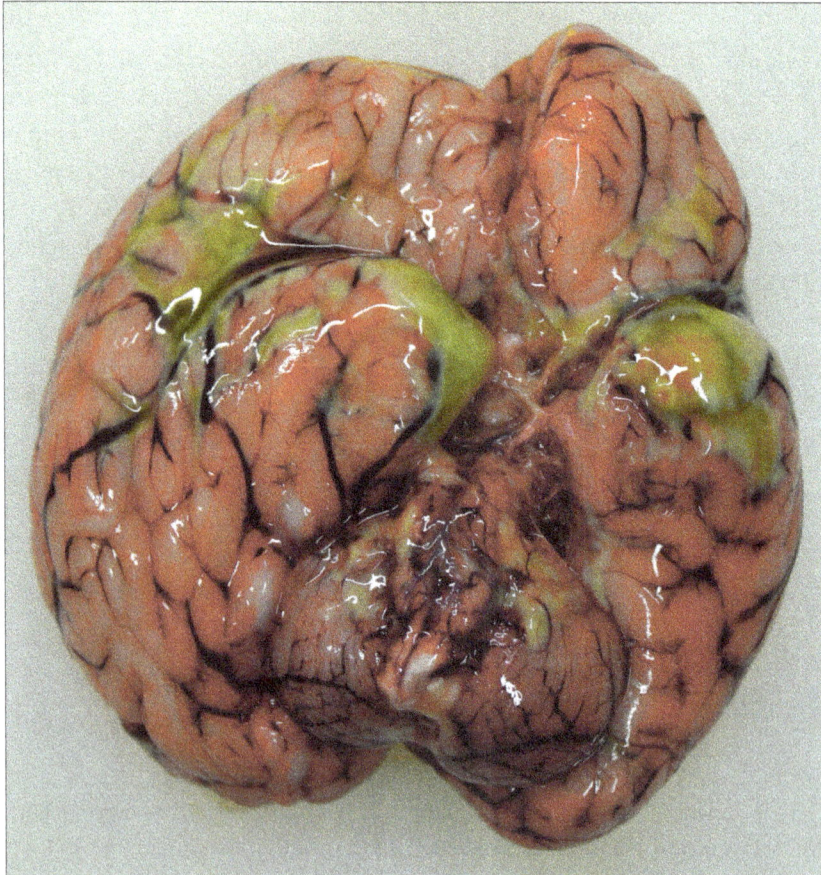

Figure 25.12: Purulent meningitis caused by Group B streptococcal infection in a 3-day old neonate. (From the autopsy archives at Great Ormond Street Hospital.)

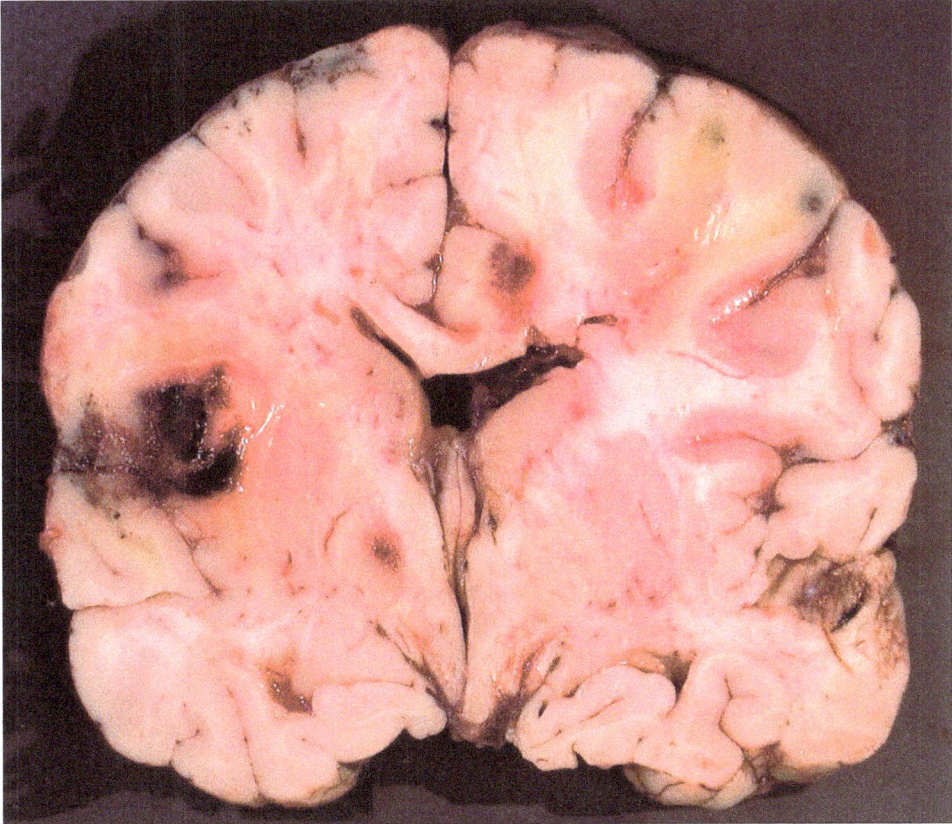

Figure 25.13: Aspergillus infection. Coronal section of brain showing hemorrhagic foci secondary to disseminated aspergillus infection in an 11-year-old female, following chemotherapy for non-hodgkin lymphoma. (From the autopsy archives at Great Ormond Street Hospital.)

worldwide (72). Infection is via the nasal route, with ameba migration along the olfactory nerve and into the brain, with rapid development of cerebral edema leading to cerebellar herniation and death (73). PAM is rapidly fatal and diagnosis is usually made after death (72).

*Cerebritis* describes a poorly defined area of acute inflammation within the brain, usually caused by pyogenic (pus-producing) bacteria such as staphylococci, streptococci, and mycobacteria, or by hyphae-producing fungi such as *Aspergillus sp.* and *Mucormycosis*. Cerebritis may progress to *cerebral abscess* if left untreated, and it may cause death by mass effect, with cerebral edema and herniation with compression of vital brainstem structures. Sometimes, depending on the site of the abscess, there may be rupture into the ventricles, rapidly leading to death (71). Fungal brain infections are more commonly associated with immunocompromised individuals, such as those receiving chemotherapy (Figure 25.13).

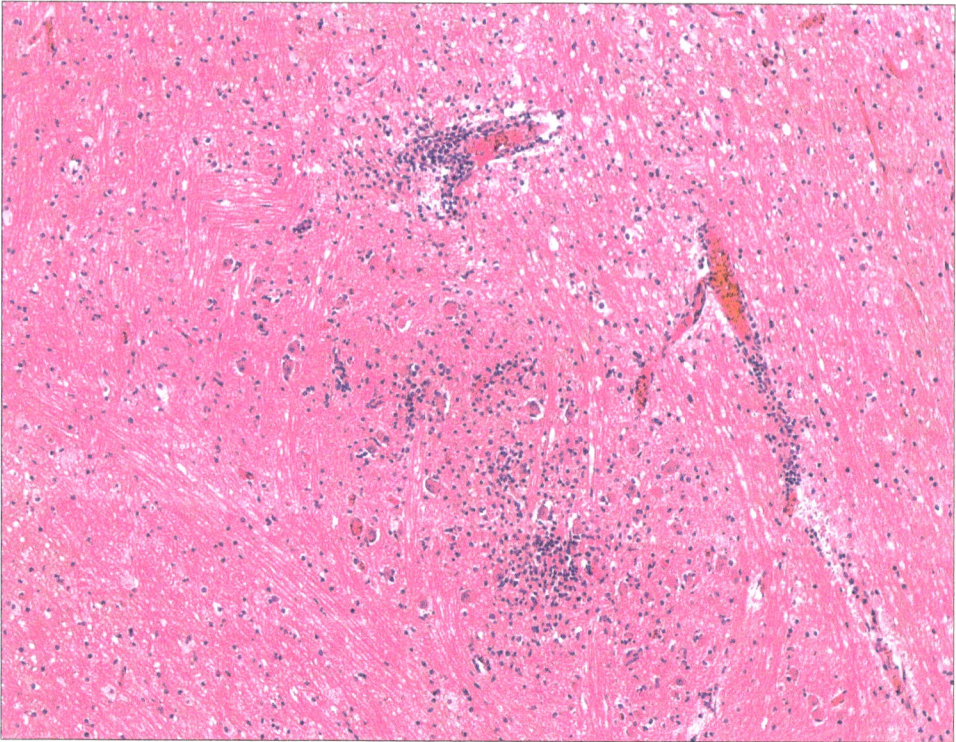

Figure 25.14: Brainstem encephalitis in an 18-month-old boy with history of mild URTI symptoms, found dead in his cot. H&E-stained medulla showing microglial nodules and cuffing of blood vessels by lymphocytes (x 10). (From the autopsy archives at Great Ormond Street Hospital.)

*Encephalitis* refers to inflammation of the substance of the brain. It is further classified as "leukoencephalitis" when only the white matter is involved, "polio encephalitis" when only the grey matter is affected, and "panencephalitis" where there is both white and grey matter involvement. There are multiple etiologies, with infection being the commonest, but also autoimmune disease and paraneoplastic syndromes. *Brainstem encephalitis* (Figure 25.14) specifically refers to inflammation of the hindbrain and is used interchangeably with the term *rhomboencephalitis* (which strictly speaking pertains to the pons, cerebellum, and medulla) (74).

Of infectious causes, *Listeria* is the commonest, primarily affecting healthy young adults. However, certain enteroviral causes are becoming increasingly recognized worldwide, such as *Enterovirus 71* (EV71) (74). EV71 causes outbreaks of hand, foot and mouth disease in children as well as upper respiratory tract infections and gastroenteritis. Neurological complications are reported in up to 25% of cases and occur around one to three weeks following the initial illness. Presentation can be precipitous, with collapse and rapid deterioration to death. Survivors may suffer long-term functional morbidity due to focal paresis, causing it to be dubbed as the "new polio" (75). *Herpes simplex virus* (HSV), *Epstein-Barr virus* (EBV), and *Human herpesvirus 6* (HHV-6) are also known etiologies.

## Spontaneous intracranial hemorrhages

Non-traumatic intracranial hemorrhage is an uncommon cause of sudden unexpected death in infancy and childhood. Vascular anomalies, brain tumors, and congenital heart disease are the more frequently identified causes (76), but underlying hematological and connective tissue disorders may also be implicated, and in some cases no cause is identified (77) (Figure 25.15). Important vascular anomalies include *arteriovenous malformations* (AVM) which are defined as abnormal connections between arteries

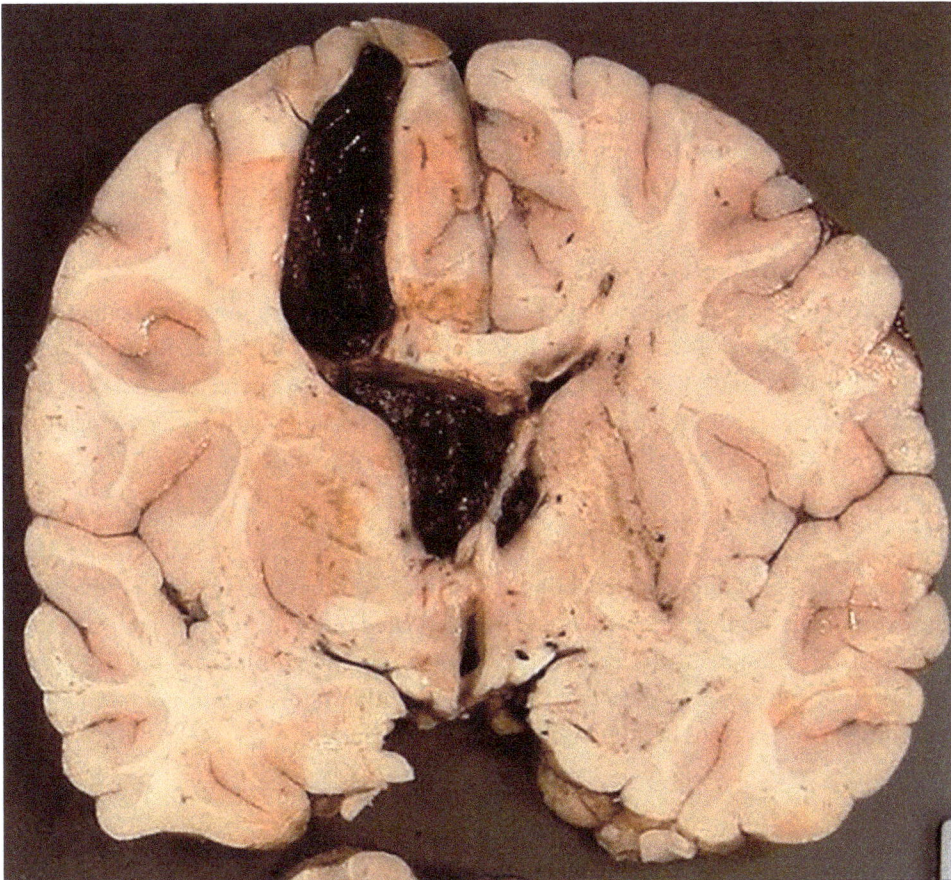

Figure 25.15: Intraventricular hemorrhage. Coronal section of the brain showing extensive spontaneous intraventricular hemorrhage in a 6-year-old female, previously fit and well, who presented with sudden collapse. No structural cause for the hemorrhage was identified. (From the autopsy archives at Great Ormond Street Hospital.)

and veins. They present with hemorrhage in up to 80% of affected children (78), of whom 25% die from the initial rupture (79). AVMs are presumed to be congenital malformations, with only a small number found in association with genetic mutations such as hereditary hemorrhagic telangiectasia, which accounts for around 3% of all cases (79).

*Cavernous malformations* (*cavernoma*) are formed from a compact mass of contiguous vessels with no intervening normal parenchyma, and may occur in the brain or spinal cord. They are rare, with an estimated prevalence of 0.4-0.5% in autopsy and MRI studies, and 50-80% are sporadic (80). Most cavernomas present in young adulthood, but some cases affect children. In childhood there is a bimodal age presentation, infancy through to 3 years and early puberty, 12-16 years (80).

*Aneurysm of the vein of Galen* is very rare and often detected antenatally or in the early neonatal period, typically presenting with high-output cardiac failure, pulmonary hypertension or, in more severe cases, multi-organ failure. Management is with endovascular intervention which is timed according to physiological variables; however, sudden death may occur prior to diagnosis/ treatment and is usually associated with cardiac decompensation during an infective episode. Infants may develop hydrocephalus and seizures, whereas older children and adults may present with intracranial hemorrhage (81).

*Subarachnoid hemorrhage* (SAH) is caused by ruptured intracranial (berry) aneurysms in 85% of cases across all ages, with the most common location being within the circle of Willis. Most aneurysmal SAHs are sporadic, but their discovery raises the possibility of underlying connective tissue disorders and polycystic renal disease. The 15% of cases that are non-aneurysmal may be associated with AVMs, Moyamoya syndrome (discussed below), arterial dissection, and coagulopathies (82).

## Arterial ischemic stroke

Although rare in childhood, arterial ischemic stroke (AIS) has the same pathophysiology and evolution in children as in adults and the associated mortality is 7-28% (83). Around half of all affected individuals have predisposing conditions and some of the risk factors are shown in Table 25.2 (84). In contrast to adults, atherosclerosis is a very rare cause of childhood AIS. At least 10% of childhood cases remain idiopathic (83).

Table 25.2: Risk factors for AIS in children.

| Arteriopathies | Vasculitis, infectious, post-infectious, Moyamoya disease/syndrome |
|---|---|
| Cardiac | Congenital heart disease, acquired heart disease |
| Prothrombotic states | Thrombophilias, combined oral contraceptive pill |
| Hematological disease | Sickle cell disease, thrombotic thrombocytopenic purpura |
| Acute systemic conditions | Sepsis, hypovolemic shock, dehydration |
| Chronic head and neck disorders | Migraine, brain tumor, ventriculo-peritoneal (VP) shunt |

*Moyamoya disease* is caused by progressive bilateral stenosis of the internal carotid arteries causing multiple AIS of variable ages, mostly affecting the anterior circulation. Collaterals develop from enlarged perforating vessels in the base of the brain which give a "puff of smoke" appearance on angiography, hence the Japanese term "moyamoya" (85). The etiology is unknown but it predominantly affects people of Asian origin. *Moyamoya syndrome* has the same pathological features but is associated with predisposing conditions such as neurofibromatosis type 1, Trisomy 21, sickle cell disease, and cranial irradiation, to name but a few (85).

## Sudden unexpected death in epilepsy

Sudden unexpected death in epilepsy (SUDEP) is a well-known complication of any seizure disorder, with rates in childhood reported as 1.1-4.3/10,000 patient years (86). It is a diagnosis of exclusion after detailed post-mortem examination reveals no anatomical or toxicological cause of death in an individual with a known history of epilepsy. Structural brain lesions may be identified as the underlying cause of epilepsy, such as cortical malformations, hippocampal sclerosis, cerebral atrophy, and hydrocephalus, but often there is no obvious pathology identified. A number of mechanisms have been proposed, including cardiac arrhythmias and central apnea (86).

## Neurometabolic disorders

Neurometabolic diseases are rare, but they account for a significant number of diseases that affect the pediatric brain and probably a significant proportion of neurodegenerative diseases in childhood (87). Approximately 25% of cases present during the neonatal period, often with acute encephalopathies which can be rapidly fatal. Older infants and children can present with slowly progressive symptoms, allowing time for investigation and diagnosis, and they are less likely to be encountered in the context of sudden unexpected death.

*Aminoacidopathies* and *organic acidemias* can present within days of birth, due to postnatal accumulation of toxic metabolites which in utero would have crossed the placenta to be metabolized by the mother.

*Lysosomal* and *Peroxisomal storage disorders* result in intracellular accumulation of macromolecules, often causing slowly progressive symptoms; the exception is *Zellweger syndrome*, which typically presents in the neonatal period with failure to thrive and neurological signs leading to early death.

*Neurotransmitter diseases* present early with severe encephalopathy and drug-resistant seizures; these often involve monoamine synthesis and gamma-Aminobutyric acid (GABA) metabolism pathways (88).

## Occult CNS tumors

These are extremely rare causes of sudden death in childhood. Various neoplasms have been described including aggressive tumors such as *medulloblastoma* (89-91) and *glioblastoma* (92), as well as tumors regarded as indolent such as *pilocytic astrocytoma* (90, 91). In such cases there may be vague preceding symptoms or the child may present acutely with sudden onset of severe headache or collapse just prior to death. Death may be due to mass effect or intra-tumoral hemorrhage leading to cerebral edema and raised intracranial pressure with herniation, leading to compression of vital cardiorespiratory centers.

# Intra-abdominal Causes of Sudden Death

## Gastroenteritis

Usually there is a preceding history of diarrheal/vomiting illness, but sudden death may occur, presumably due to severe dehydration and serum electrolyte disturbance, with younger children and infants particularly at risk. Autopsy examination may reveal non-specific signs of dehydration, including sunken eyes and sunken fontanelles in infants, although these can be difficult to assess post-mortem. Stool cultures and virology may reveal the causative etiology.

## Gastrointestinal bleeding

**Upper gastrointestinal (GI) bleeds** cause hematemesis with subsequent melena, and any delay in treatment may rapidly lead to hypovolemic shock and death. Depending on the cause, the bleeding point may be found in the esophagus, stomach, or duodenum. *Gastro-esophageal varices* develop secondary to portal hypertension from any cause (e.g. portal vein thrombosis or cirrhosis with bleeding being the most serious complication (93)).

*Spontaneous rupture of the esophagus (Boerhaave syndrome)* is very rare in children, with few cases reported in the literature (94). It is associated with intractable vomiting and may occur on the background of gastroesophageal reflux disease, as in Figure 25.16.

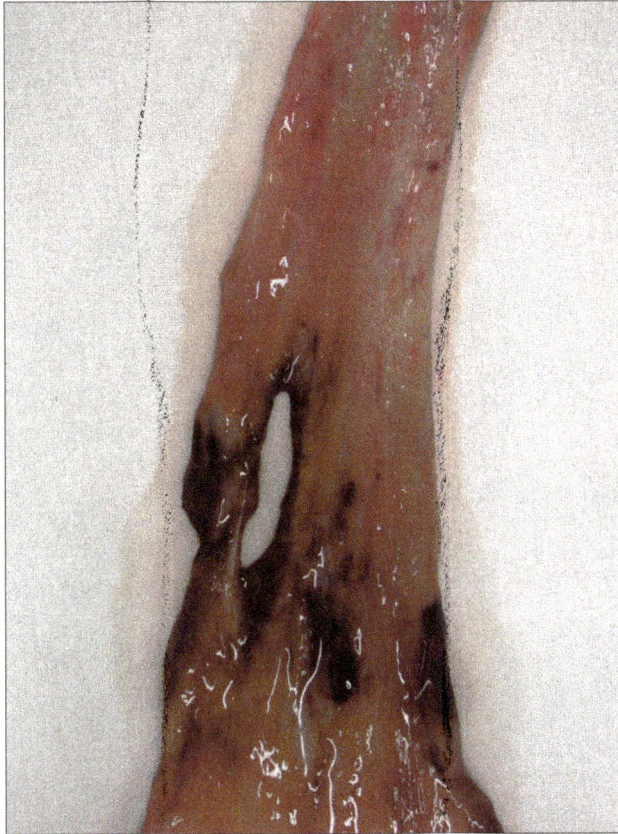

Figure 25.16: Ruptured esophagus in a 13-year-old female with cerebral palsy and gastroesophageal reflux disease, found unresponsive after a three-day history of cough and fever. (From the autopsy archives at Great Ormond Street Hospital.)

*Gastric and duodenal ulcers*, although uncommon in children, are most frequently caused by *Helicobacter pylori* infection but are also associated with chronic use of non-steroidal anti-inflammatory drugs (NSAIDs). Deep ulcers may erode through the stomach or duodenal wall causing death due to peritonitis, or through local arteries resulting in massive hemorrhage.

*Lower GI bleeds* may cause hematochezia (fresh blood in the stool) or melena. Massive bleeds may rapidly lead to death if untreated.

*Intussusception* is probably the commonest cause of GI bleeding in infants. It occurs when the proximal intestine telescopes into the more distal part, most frequently involving the terminal ileum. The lead point may be due to lymphoid hyperplasia in response to viral infection, such as *Adenovirus* or *Rotavirus*, or may occur as a complication of a *Meckel's diverticulum*, intestinal duplication cyst, or, rarely, a

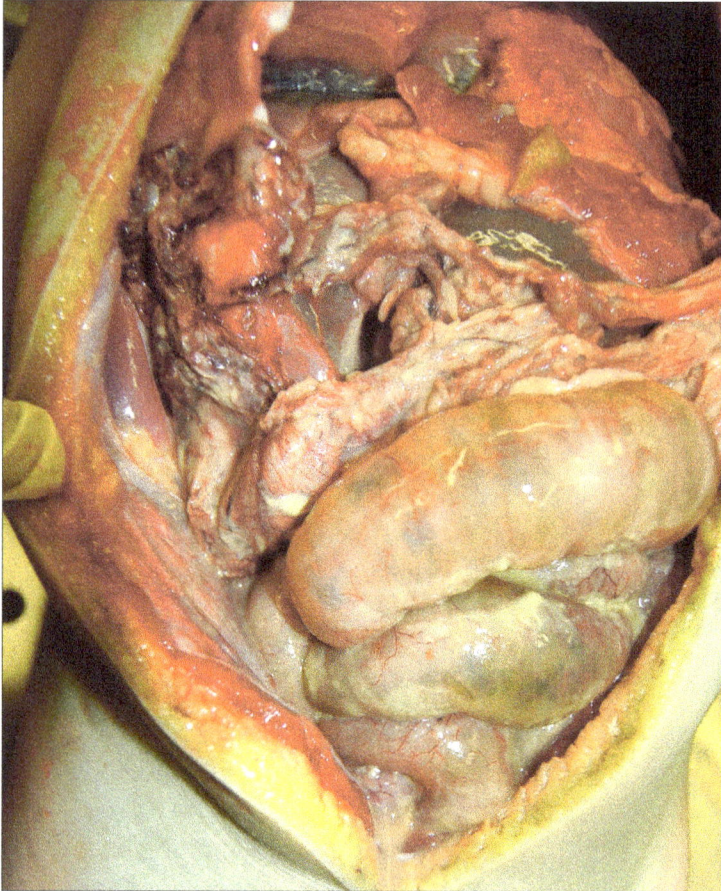

Figure 25.17: Ruptured appendix. Peritonitis secondary to a ruptured appendix abscess in a 4-year-old female with attention deficit disorder. (From the autopsy archives at Great Ormond Street Hospital.)

neoplasm. *Meckel's diverticulum* is the commonest congenital anomaly of the intestine and is due to incomplete obliteration of the vitelline (omphalomesenteric) duct during fetal life. Located in the distal small intestine, proximal to the ileocecal valve, it can cause life-threatening hemorrhage when ectopic gastric mucosa is present. Although a common cause of lower GI bleeding in the <2-year-olds, symptoms may present at any age.

## Peritonitis

*Acute appendicitis* may occur at any age. Although uncommon in infancy it may be difficult to diagnose in life; the same is also true for older children with communication difficulties such as those with cerebral palsy or severe autism. Late presentation and or diagnosis may result in perforation, acute peritonitis, and death (Figure 25.17).

## Intestinal obstruction

*Volvulus* is the twisting of the gut around its mesentery, causing infarction and rapidly leading to death if untreated. It may occur at any age but classically presents in infancy. It usually occurs in the context of malrotation of the intestines during fetal life. This results in abnormal positioning and fixation of the intestines and principally involves the midgut.

*Mesenteric defects* are a rare cause of intestinal obstruction from internal herniation of the ileum, and may be acquired or congenital. Acquired defects are due to traumatic injury or previous intra-abdominal surgery in which the mesentery has been incised and incompletely closed. Congenital defects are rare and their cause is unknown (95); typically, they occur near the terminal ileum and are round to oval with a diameter of 2-10 cm. They remain asymptomatic until herniation occurs; this may be intermittent, making ante-mortem diagnosis difficult.

*Hirschsprung's disease* is commonly diagnosed in the neonatal period with bowel obstruction and failure to pass meconium, or it can present later in childhood with chronic constipation. It is caused by failure of migration of neural crest cells within the colon leading to aganglionosis, and may involve the rectum and distal colon or may affect the entire colon. Life-threatening complications associated with bowel obstruction include perforation and enterocolitis. Another rare association is *Ondine's curse*, which is a central hypoventilation syndrome which has been implicated in sudden death (96). Such disorders rarely present with sudden death in contemporary practice.

# Disorders of Metabolism

Metabolic disorders may be congenital (inborn errors of metabolism/inherited metabolic diseases) or acquired, such as diabetes mellitus or vitamin D deficiency (due to poor diet and lack of sunlight). Metabolic defects all have the potential to cause sudden unexpected death. Often it is the age at presentation, together with the medical history and events leading up to death, that raise the suspicion for metabolic disease.

At present, in the UK, six inherited metabolic diseases are screened for after birth as part of the neonatal Blood Spot (Guthrie) test, which involves taking a small blood sample via a heel prick within the first few days of life (97). These include *phenylketonuria* (PKU), *medium chain acyl CoA dehydrogenase deficiency* (MCADD), *maple syrup urine disease* (MSUD), *isovaleric acidemia* (IVA), *glutaric aciduria type 1* (GA1), and *homocystinuria, pyridoxine unresponsive* (HCU). All are rare, with PKU and MCADD affecting around 1 in 10,000 babies born in UK and the others occurring in 1 in 100,000-150,000 live births; but all are amenable to treatment by dietary modification or supplementation and/or drug treatment (97). However, the list of other known metabolic diseases is legion and new diagnoses are constantly being added.

Metabolic disorders were first identified as a possible cause of sudden unexpected death in the pediatric population in the mid-1980s. Subsequently, a range of suitable specimens to be taken prospectively as part of the autopsy were recommended which could be stored frozen for further investigation if required (98). For suspected inherited metabolic disorders, bodily fluid samples include urine, blood, bile, vitreous fluid, and CSF. (It should be noted that for metabolic investigation it is advisable to obtain samples as soon as possible after death to avoid interpretive difficulties as a consequence of post-mortem change.) Blood and bile spots can be stored on a Guthrie card but urine, vitreous, and CSF require freezing at -80 °C. A sample of skin, taken under sterile conditions, for fibroblast culture also requires freezing; fibroblasts will often grow from skin taken after a child has been dead for several days and are used for many enzyme assays. Macroscopic autopsy findings that raise the possibility of a metabolic disorder include dysmorphic features, a pale and enlarged liver, hypertrophic or dilated cardiomyopathy, and cerebral edema. Histological findings include severe fatty change in the liver, heart, skeletal muscle, or kidney, with identification aided by staining frozen tissue samples with oil red-O or osmium. Electron microscopy is a very useful adjunct to identify certain pathologies, such as multicore myopathy in skeletal muscle.

Mitochondrial fatty acid oxidation (FAO) disorders are amongst the most common inborn errors of metabolism affecting infants and children (99) and may mimic SIDS. Fatty acid oxidation is essential for energy production and homeostasis, especially during periods of fasting. Fatty acids are metabolized in the liver, cardiac, and skeletal muscles by mitochondria, and the process involves numerous enzymes, co-enzymes, and transporters. Normally, partial oxidation of fatty acids in the liver produces ketones which are used as an alternative energy substrate to glucose, and metabolic intermediates of FAO are used for gluconeogenesis to maintain homeostasis during periods of fasting (100). Defects in any of the involved enzymes, co-enzymes, or transporters are responsible for the development of FAO disorders which ultimately prevent the effective use of fat during times of stress: when fasting or exercising, during cold temperatures, or when there is increased metabolic demand due to illness. Metabolic decompensation results in acidosis, hypoglycemia, coma, and rapid deterioration to death. Inheritance of FAO disorders is in an autosomal recessive manner, with the age at presentation dependent on the particular enzyme/transporter involved (6). Detailed description of individual FAO disorders is beyond the scope of this chapter; however, some of the defects associated with sudden death in infancy and childhood are listed in Table 25.3.

Table 25.3: Fatty acid oxidation disorders. (Adapted from (100-102).

| Deficiency states | Usual age at presentation and signs/symptoms | Autopsy tissue and biochemical findings | Confirmatory tests/ genetics |
|---|---|---|---|
| **Medium chain acyl CoA dehydrogenase deficiency (MCADD)** | • Infancy to 2 years (can be in first days of life or up to 6 years) — often viral illness, fasting triggers, hypoglycemia, vomiting, lethargy, apnea, encephalopathy. 20-25% may die during first episode. | • Myoglobinuria<br>• Blood spot — decreased/normal free carnitine, increased medium chain acylcarnitines | • Fibroblast confirmatory<br>• ACADM mutation in 85% |
| **Carnitine transporter deficiency (OCTN2 transporter)** | • Infancy with poor feeding, irritability, and lethargy<br>• Childhood with progressive cardiomyopathy and limb girdle myopathy | • Cardiomyopathy with endocardial fibroelastosis, muscle, hepatomegaly<br>• Blood spot — low plasma carnitine and acylcarnitine | • Fibroblast culture — decreased carnitine transport<br>• SLC22A5 — heterogenous mutations |
| **Carnitine palmitoyl transferase (CPT) 1A deficiency** | • Newborn and early infancy after illness/prolonged fasting, seizures, recurrent hypoketotic-hypoglycemia | • Lipid deposition in kidney<br>• Blood spot — increased free carnitine, decreased long-chain acyl carnitine | • Fibroblast culture — decreased enzyme activity<br>• CPT1A-heterogenous mutations |
| **CPT II deficiency** | • Perinatal (rapidly fatal) — hypoketotic-hypoglycemia, hepatomegaly, seizures<br>• Infants and young children 6-24 months — hypoglycemia, encephalopathy, respiratory distress, cardiomyopathy<br>• (Classic adult CPT II deficiency — adolescent onset: recurrent myoglobinuria following exercise/fasting but normal inbetween) | • Dysmorphism, hepatomegaly, cardiomyopathy; lipid storage in heart, liver, skeletal muscle and kidney; neuronal migration defects in perinatal deaths<br>• Blood spot — elevated long chain acyl carnitine | • Fibroblast confirmation required<br>• CPT2 — heterogenous mutations |
| **Carnitine acyl-transferase (CACT)** | • Neonates — episodic hypoketotic-hypoglycemia, hyperammonemia, seizures, cardiomyopathy, arrhythmias, apnea, progressive neurological, cardiac and hepatic damage | • Blood spot — low levels of free carnitine, elevated long-chain acyl carnitines | • Gene sequence analysis<br>• SLC25A20 — heterogenous mutations |
| **Very long chain acyl CoA dehydrogenase (VLCAD)** | • Neonates — most severe, fasting hypoglycemia, cardiomyopathy<br>• Infants — less severe, hypoglycemia without cardiomyopathy | • Cardiomyopathy, hepatomegaly<br>• Blood spot — low serum carnitine, raised acylcarnitines | • Fibroblast culture confirms enzyme deficiency<br>• ACADVL heterogenous mutations |
| **Short chain acyl CoA dehydrogenase (SCAD)** | • 2-24 months — hypoglycemia during illness, developmental delay, hypotonia, seizures, failure to thrive, vomiting | • Dysmorphism, hepatomegaly; lipid storage in liver, muscle, heart<br>• Blood spot — elevated C4 carnitine | • Fibroblasts confirmatory<br>• ACADS mutations |

*Persistent hyperinsulinemic hypoglycemia of infancy (PHHI, "nesidioblastosis")* is a rare genetic disorder thought to affect 1 in 50,000 births but with increased incidence in communities where there is a high level of consanguineous marriage (103). Neonates may present with seizures, somnolence, and motor abnormalities and there may be macrosomia or hypertrophic cardiomyopathy (104). There is a high risk of brain damage and death. First-line treatment is with diazoxide, but this is ineffective in some forms, in which octreotide may be used. Many mutations have been identified, but the commonest and most severe monogenic form is caused by mutations of the subunits of the beta-cell plasma membrane K+ ATP channels, leading to focal islet cell adenomatosis (104). Diagnosis in life depends on a high index of suspicion, and pre-operative [18]Fluoro-DOPA-PET scans are used to localize lesions prior to surgery. In some cases of diffuse disease, total pancreatectomy may be required. Diagnosis at autopsy can be difficult and depends on adequate examination and sampling of the pancreas. Different morphological types are identified at microscopy including focal adenomatosis/adenomatous hyperplasia and diffuse PHHI in which careful analysis of morphology of islet of Langerhans reveals large B cells with abnormally large, hyperchromatic nuclei (103). Immunohistochemistry with a cocktail of pancreatic enzymes is helpful to highlight overactive cells. Genetic testing of suspected cases and family counseling is essential.

*Type 1 diabetes mellitus (T1DM)* is caused by failure of the endocrine pancreas to produce insulin. If poorly controlled, and especially during inter-current illness (usually infection), diabetic ketoacidosis may ensue. Ketoacidosis results from high concentrations of ketone bodies formed by the breakdown of fatty acids and amino acids which are used as an alternative energy source in the absence of utilizable glucose (insulin is essential for the cellular uptake of glucose from the blood). Without prompt treatment, ketoacidosis rapidly leads to coma and death, but even with treatment there remains a significant risk of cerebral edema, usually between 4 to 12 hours of initiation (105). "Dead in bed syndrome" is a poorly understood cause of sudden unexpected death in T1DM, the cause of which is unknown but has been postulated to be associated with cardiac arrhythmia (106).

## Bacterial Infections

### Sepsis and septic shock

Sepsis is defined as a systemic inflammatory response (SIRS) in the presence of invasive infection. Severe sepsis requires cardiovascular dysfunction or acute respiratory distress syndrome or dysfunction in two or more other organs (107). Septic shock is a subset of sepsis with cardiovascular dysfunction and is associated with a greater risk of mortality than sepsis alone. In pediatric sepsis a wide variety of organisms have been implicated including *Staphylococcus aureus*, *Streptococcus pneumoniae*, *Neisseria meninigitis*, *Hemophilus influenza*, *Pseudomonas aeruginosa*, *Escherichia coli*, and *Klebsiella sp.*, some of which will be described in more detail below. Viral pathogens may also manifest as severe sepsis or septic shock including *RSV*, *Influenza*, *Parainfluenza*, and *Adenovirus*, although the mortality is usually less than with bacterial infection.

Diagnosis of sepsis as the cause of death can be difficult at autopsy, especially when a clear macroscopic or histological focus of infection cannot be identified. The clinical history may, or may not, be helpful, as often children are reported to be "snuffly" or as having signs or symptoms which suggest mild infection. In all cases of sudden unexpected death, microbiology samples from "sterile sites" are taken routinely as part of the autopsy protocol. This is regardless of any history of clinical signs or symptoms leading up to the death, as children, especially infants, may exhibit no or very non-specific signs of infection prior to death. Before opening the cadaver, and with particular care to optimize sterility, cerebrospinal fluid (CSF) and other samples such as nasopharyngeal or rectal swabs may be obtained for virology and bacteriology. On opening the thorax, blood cultures can be obtained from the internal jugular vein or right ventricle and tissue samples/swabs from the lung and spleen for bacteriology, again using a sterile technique. Tissue samples/swabs for virology include heart, lung, spleen, bowel, and, in some cases, brain. Additional fluids which may also be collected for microbiology studies include urine, pleural, pericardial, and peritoneal fluid if applicable.

There are various signs which may be identified at autopsy which raise the possibility, but are not pathognomic, of sepsis. A generalized hemorrhagic/purpuric rash may be present as a consequence of disseminated intravascular coagulation. Bilateral adrenal hemorrhages are often striking in appearance, with both adrenal glands appearing enlarged and almost black in color; this finding is classically associated with the Waterhouse-Friderichsen syndrome secondary to fulminant meningococcal disease but may be present in sepsis from any cause. However, non-sepsis-related causes are also described, including coagulopathies, hypotension, and any cause of physiological stress (108). It is quite obvious that if a clear focus of infection is identified on macroscopic examination — for example, empyema or purulent meningitis (Figure 25.12) — this helps in establishing an accurate cause of death. If no focus of infection is identified macroscopically or on histological examination of tissue, but microbiology cultures from three separate sites grow a recognized pathogen in pure culture, this is generally accepted to be causative of death. However, it should be emphasized that difficulties in the interpretation of the significance of post-mortem microbiological results persist, especially when multiple organisms are present which may be due to "post-mortem translocation" often of "gut-type flora". Post-mortem translocation or overgrowth is a difficult concept, however, because it is not universal and does not appear to be clearly dependent on post-mortem interval.

*Toxic shock syndrome* (TSS) is a severe and potentially fatal condition, typically caused by toxin-producing strains of *Staphylococcus aureus* and *Streptococcus pyogenes*. The toxins act as super-antigens by bypassing the usual antigen presentation pathway; they cause massive T-cell activation with an uncontrolled release of inflammatory mediators (109) and resultant massive vasodilation, capillary leak, and hypotension (toxic shock). It has been associated with tampon use (110), burns, and secondary bacterial infection in chicken pox. In the UK the incidence in children is reported to be 0.38 per 100,000 and mortality estimated at 28% (109). Clinical manifestations may include pharyngitis or skin infections with progression to fever, generalized maculopapular rash with desquamation, profound hypotension, and multi-organ failure (111), but onset may be abrupt, making diagnosis challenging early on. Many streptococci and staphylococci contain the genes for toxin production, and molecular subtyping allows for identification of the presence of these genes. However, despite having the gene, toxins will only be expressed under certain conditions, and most people develop immunity to these "super-antigens early in life" (110). Streptococcal TSS has been shown to affect younger children more commonly than staphylococcal TSS (109).

*Neisseria meningitidis (meningococcus)* is the leading cause of infection-related death in early childhood (112), with a mortality rate of >20% in children with meningococcal sepsis (70). *Meningococcus* is a gram-negative diplococcus of which there are 12 serogroups, with most invasive diseases caused by groups A, B, C, W, X, and Y, of which groups B and C are the major disease-causing strains in the UK (112). There is a bimodal age distribution, with most cases occurring during the first year of life and in adolescence. Rare cases occur in the neonatal period (<28 days old) (113). Meningococci are normally carried in the nasopharynx of healthy individuals, with disease occurring when bacteria are transmitted to susceptible individuals and outbreaks ensuing when large groups of young people come together, such as at the start of university semester.

Clinical presentation of meningococcal disease is with septicemia or meningitis or as a combination of the two (114); however, rapid onset means that sudden death may occur before any clinical diagnosis is established. In such cases there may only be subtle findings at autopsy rather than the classic signs of meningococcal septicemia described above. Tissue and fluid samples may be sterile if the individual has received antibiotics ante-mortem, and PCR analysis may be required to confirm the diagnosis; results from ante-mortem blood and CSF cultures should be actively sought. Atypical presentations such as septic arthritis, pneumonia, epiglottitis, and endocarditis are well described for the less common meningococcal capsular groups, W and Y, and mainly occur in adults. However, rare cases of adolescents presenting with primarily gastrointestinal symptoms leading rapidly to death have been recently reported in the UK associated with a hypervirulent group W strain; all had multi-organ failure, with one case noted at autopsy to have necrosis of the intestines (115).

*Hemophilus influenzae* is a gram-negative anaerobic coccobacillus that can cause severe infection in infants and children <5 years. Some strains have a polysaccharide capsule and are identified on the basis of antigenic properties (serotypes a-f), of which type b (Hib) is the most pathogenic (116). Unencapsulated or non-type-able (NTHi) strains also exist which are more susceptible to complement mediated bacteriolysis and phagocytosis, rendering them less common causes of invasive infection (116). *H influenza* causes diseases ranging from non-invasive otitis media to severe infections such as pneumonia, meningitis, epiglottitis, septic arthritis, and septicemia (117). Since the introduction of routine vaccination of infants against type b (Hib), there has been a decline in the incidence of Hib-related disease. However, emerging reports indicate an increase in invasive non-Hib infections worldwide, including Hia, Hif, and NTHi (117). Non-Hib infections are reported to be similar, although less severe than those reported with Hib. As always the most vulnerable individuals at the extremes of the age spectrum are likely to be more severely affected. Neonatal NTHi disease is more commonly associated with prematurity and early onset infection (<48 hours) (118).

*Streptococcus infections* cause a wide variety of disease in childhood. *Streptococcus pneumoniae* (*pneumococcus*) is the leading cause of bacterial pneumonia, meningitis, and sepsis in children worldwide (114). *Group A streptococcus* (*GAS/Streptococcus pyogenes*) may cause mild focal infections to severe life-threatening disease or invasive GAS, which has a fatality rate of 7-25% (119). Invasive GAS commonly occurs via an initial skin infection and is well known as a cause of bacterial superinfection during concurrent chicken pox and is also associated with burns. It causes one of three clinical manifestations: septicemia, necrotizing fasciitis, or TSS. Virulent strains of GAS, including M1, 3, 12 and 28, are associated with TSS. *Group B streptococcus (GBS)* is part of normal gut and genital tract flora in 20-40% of women. Maternal colonization may lead to severe neonatal infection and early neonatal death. GBS was previously thought to be the most common cause of bacteremia in febrile infants <90 days of age, but recent data have suggested that it may be superseded by *Escherichia coli* (114). Although rare in infants more than 3 months old, so-called late, late-onset GBS infection (defined as GBS infection in infants >90 days old) is well recognized and is associated with a mortality rate of 20%; at autopsy there may be bacteremia without histological evidence of infection (120). The most virulent serotypes are capsular types Ia, Ib, II, III, and V (121).

*Staphylococcus species* cause a range of disease in children from mild skin infections to severe sepsis. The most important is *Staphylococcus aureus* which, if causing a bacteremia, has a mortality rate of 15-25% (122). Complications include infective endocarditis, CNS embolism, septic arthritis, and empyema. *Staphylococcal scalded skin syndrome* (SSSS) is a potentially life-threatening disease caused by a phage group II *Staphylococcus aureus* infection. More common in children <5 years, it appears abruptly with diffuse erythema and fever; there follows widespread epidermal damage with vesiculobullae and desquamation. Exfoliation of the superficial epidermis occurs at the stratum granulosum due to the effects of circulating bacterial exotoxin acting on desmoglein 1 (123). Potentially fatal complications include secondary infection, pneumonia, and sepsis, but despite this, mortality is less than 10% compared to 40-63%

in adults (123). *Panton-Valentine leucocidin* (PVL) is an important toxin expressed by <2% of clinical isolates of *Staphylococcus aureus*, both methicillin-resistant (MRSA) and methicillin-susceptible strains (124). PVL-expressing strains have been associated with fatal necrotizing pneumonia in young children (125), as well as necrotizing fasciitis, purpura fulminans, and Waterhouse-Friderichsen syndrome (126). PVL proteins have two major actions which cause severe disease in humans: direct effects on white blood cells cause pore formation in the cell membrane, resulting in leakage of intracellular contents with subsequent apoptosis and local tissue necrosis facilitating multiplication of bacteria (127). PVL proteins can also act as super-antigens eliciting a massive immune response, leading to a toxic-shock type picture. *Staphylococcus aureus* is responsible for 70-90% of pediatric osteomyelitis, which is a relatively common condition. PVL-associated cases are much more severe — often involving multiple bones, and sometimes complicated by infective endocarditis, necrotizing pneumonia, cerebral infarcts, rhabdomyolysis, and septic shock and death (127).

*Citrobacter koseri* (formerly *Citrobacter diversus*) is a facultative anaerobic, gram-negative bacillus found in the intestinal tract of humans and animals and also present in soil and water (128). It is recognized as a potential but rare pathogen in infancy and childhood, causing meningitis with concurrent cerebral abscess in 75% of cases (128). The mortality rate is greater than 30% and those who survive are at high risk of severe neurological sequelae (129). The risk of disease is highest in the immunosuppressed and in children with cyanotic congenital heart disease. Other predisposing factors include neurosurgery, middle ear and sinus infections, poor dental hygiene, and congenital lesions of the head and neck. In neonates, early onset infection suggests vertical transmission during delivery; late onset infections also occur and nosocomial outbreak due to umbilical colonization has been reported.

*Salmonella sp.* are the cause of commonly encountered infections manifesting as gastroenteritis and septicemia. Children may develop multisystem infection such as osteomyelitis, liver and splenic abscesses, and overwhelming sepsis, which may be fatal. Children with sickle cell disease are more susceptible to infection.

## Conclusions

Natural causes of sudden unexpected death in infants and children are myriad, and this chapter provides an overview of the most common and/or important entities. The requirement for thorough autopsy by a specialist pediatric pathologist is highlighted by the vast range of conditions that may be encountered, many of which are either unique to this demographic or present with unusual features. In some circumstances, particularly unusual CNS or cardiovascular-related deaths, further super-specialist input may be required and there should be a low threshold for discussion and/or referral to a pediatric neuropathologist or cardiac pathologist. Furthermore, the importance of ancillary investigations is highlighted, including full histological evaluation and the obtaining of appropriate tissue samples for further investigations, such as in cases of suspected metabolic disorders. Given that unexplained deaths represent a significant proportion of sudden unexpected deaths in infancy and childhood (albeit to a lesser extent in childhood), these have important public health and research implications, since these categories are essentially diagnoses of exclusion. This further emphasizes the importance of appropriate specialist pediatric autopsy examination.

# References

1. Wang H, Liddell CA, Coates MM, Mooney MD, Levitz CE, Schumacher AE, et al. Global, regional, and national levels of neonatal, infant, and under-5 mortality during 1990-2013: A systematic analysis for the Global Burden of Disease Study 2013. Lancet. 2014;384(9947):957-79. https://doi.org/10.1016/S0140-6736(14)60497-9.

2. Sidebotham P, Fraser J, Fleming P, Ward-Platt M, Hain R. Patterns of child death in England and Wales. Lancet. 2014;384(9946):904-14. https://doi.org/10.1016/S0140-6736(13)61090-9.

3. Office for National Statistics. Freedom of information: Number of children. [Available from: http://www.ons.gov.uk/aboutus/transparencyandgovernance/freedomofinformationfoi/numberofchildren]. Accessed 12 January 2018.

4. Office for National Statistics. Childhood mortality in England and Wales: 2014. [Available from: http://www.ons.gov.uk/peoplepopulationandcommunity/birthsdeathsandmarriages/deaths]. Accessed 12 January 2018.

5. Taylor BJ, Garstang J, Engelberts A, Obonai T, Cote A, Freemantle J, et al. International comparison of sudden unexpected death in infancy rates using a newly proposed set of cause-of-death codes. Arch Dis Child. 2015;100(11):1018-23. https://doi.org/10.1136/archdischild-2015-308239.

6. Coté A. Investigating sudden unexpected death in infancy and early childhood. Paediatr Respir Rev. 2010;11(4):219-25. https://doi.org/10.1016/j.prrv.2009.12.002.

7. Salm Ward TC, Balfour GM. Infant safe sleep interventions, 1990-2015: A review. J Community Health. 2016;41(1):180-96. https://doi.org/10.1007/s10900-015-0060-y.

8. Adams SM, Ward CE, Garcia KL. Sudden infant death syndrome. Am Fam Physician. 2015;91(11):778-83.

9.    Hefti MM, Cryan JB, Haas EA, Chadwick AE, Crandall LA, Trachtenberg FL, et al. Hippocampal malformation associated with sudden death in early childhood: A neuropathologic study: Part 2 of the investigations of The San Diego SUDC Research Project. Forensic Sci Med Pathol. 2016;12(1):14-25. https://doi.org/10.1007/s12024-015-9731-3.

10.   Santori M, Blanco-Verea A, Gil R, Cortis J, Becker K, Schneider PM, et al. Broad-based molecular autopsy: A potential tool to investigate the involvement of subtle cardiac conditions in sudden unexpected death in infancy and early childhood. Arch Dis Child. 2015;100(10):952-6. https://doi.org/10.1136/archdischild-2015-308200.

11.   Wijeyeratne YD, Behr ER. Sudden death and cardiac arrest without phenotype: The utility of genetic testing. Trends Cardiovasc Med. 2017;27(3):207-213. https://doi.org/10.1016/j.tcm.2016.08.010.

12.   Pryce JW, Bamber AR, Ashworth MT, Klein NJ, Sebire NJ. Immunohistochemical expression of inflammatory markers in sudden infant death; ancillary tests for identification of infection. J Clin Pathol. 2014;67(12):1044-51. https://doi.org/10.1136/jclinpath-2014-202489.

13.   GBD 2015 Child Mortality Collaborators. Global, regional, national, and selected subnational levels of stillbirths, neonatal, infant, and under-5 mortality, 1980-2015: A systematic analysis for the Global Burden of Disease Study 2015. Lancet. 2016;388(10053):1725-74. https://doi.org/10.1016/S0140-6736(16)31575-6.

14.   Gilbert-Barness EF, Spicer DE, Steffensen TS. Handbook of pediatric autopsy pathology. Springer: New York, 2014. https://doi.org/10.1007/978-1-4614-6711-3.

15.   Armes JE, Mifsud W, Ashworth M. Diffuse lung disease of infancy: A pattern-based, algorithmic approach to histological diagnosis. J Clin Pathol. 2015;68(2):100-10. https://doi.org/10.1136/jclinpath-2014-202685.

16.   Chow CW, Massie J, Ng J, Mills J, Baker M. Acinar dysplasia of the lungs: Variation in the extent of involvement and clinical features. Pathology. 2013;45(1):38-43. https://doi.org/10.1097/PAT.0b013e32835b3a9d.

17.   Bishop NB, Stankiewicz P, Steinhorn RH. Alveolar capillary dysplasia. Am J Respir Crit Care Med. 2011;184(2):172-9. https://doi.org/10.1164/rccm.201010-1697CI.

18.   Szafranski P, Herrera C, Proe LA, Coffman B, Kearney DL, Popek E, et al. Narrowing the FOXF1 distant enhancer region on 16q24.1 critical for ACDMPV. Clin Epigenetics. 2016;8:112. https://doi.org/10.1186/s13148-016-0278-2.

19. Dishop MK. Paediatric interstitial lung disease: Classification and definitions. Paediatr Respir Rev. 2011;12(4):230-7. https://doi.org/10.1016/j.prrv.2011.01.002.

20. Steinhorn RH. Neonatal pulmonary hypertension. Pediatric Crit Care Med. 2010;11(Suppl):S79-84. https://doi.org/10.1097/PCC.0b013e3181c76cdc.

21. Weber MA, Ashworth MT, Risdon RA, Brooke I, Malone M, Sebire NJ. Sudden unexpected neonatal death in the first week of life: Autopsy findings from a specialist centre. J Matern Fetal Neonatal Med. 2009;22(5):398-404. https://doi.org/10.1080/14767050802406677.

22. Fedrick J, Butler NR. Certain causes of neonatal death. IV. Massive pulmonary haemorrhage. Biol Neonate. 1971;18(3):243-62. https://doi.org/10.1159/000240366.

23. Chen YY, Wang HP, Lin SM, Chang JT, Hsieh KS, Huang FK, et al. Pulmonary hemorrhage in very low-birthweight infants: Risk factors and management. Pediatr Int. 2012;54(6):743-7. https://doi.org/10.1111/j.1442-200X.2012.03670.x.

24. Pinar H. Postmortem findings in term neonates. Semin Neonatol. 2004;9(4):289-302. https://doi.org/10.1016/j.siny.2003.11.003.

25. Lindenskov PH, Castellheim A, Saugstad OD, Mollnes TE. Meconium aspiration syndrome: Possible pathophysiological mechanisms and future potential therapies. Neonatology. 2015;107(3):225-30. https://doi.org/10.1159/000369373.

26. Mokra D, Calkovska A. How to overcome surfactant dysfunction in meconium aspiration syndrome? Respir Physiol Neurobiol. 2013;187(1):58-63. https://doi.org/10.1016/j.resp.2013.02.030.

27. Mandal A, Kabra SK, Lodha R. Upper airway obstruction in children. Indian J Pediatr. 2015;82(8):737-44. https://doi.org/10.1007/s12098-015-1811-6.

28. Petrocheilou A, Tanou K, Kalampouka E, Malakasioti G, Giannios C, Kaditis AG. Viral croup: Diagnosis and a treatment algorithm. Pediatr Pulmonol. 2014;49(5):421-9. https://doi.org/10.1002/ppul.22993.

29. Rocha G, Soares P, Soares H, Pissarra S, Guimaraes H. Pertussis in the newborn: Certainties and uncertainties in 2014. Paediatri Respir Rev. 2015;16(2):112-18. https://doi.org/10.1016/j.prrv.2014.01.004.

30. Schaab K, Verdile VP. Solitary papilloma of the larynx as the precipitant of sudden death. Am J Emerg Med. 1994;12(5):605-7. https://doi.org/10.1016/0735-6757(94)90282-8.

31. Siegel B, Smith LP. Management of complex glottic stenosis in children with recurrent respiratory papillomatosis. Int J Pediatr Otorhinolaryngol. 2013;77(10):1729-33. https://doi.org/10.1016/j.ijporl.2013.08.003.

32. Champ CS, Byard RW. Sudden death in asthma in childhood. Forensic Sci Int. 1994;66(2):117-27. https://doi.org/10.1016/0379-0738(94)90336-0.

33. Popler J, Wagner BD, Tarro HL, Accurso FJ, Deterding RR. Bronchoalveolar lavage fluid cytokine profiles in neuroendocrine cell hyperplasia of infancy and follicular bronchiolitis. Orphanet J Rare Dis. 2013;8:175. https://doi.org/10.1186/1750-1172-8-175.

34. Uzuner N, Babayigit A, Olmez D, Karaman O, Ozer E, Can D, et al. Follicular bronchiolitis associated with lung abscess in an eight-year-old girl. Turk J Pediatr. 2007;49(2):203-5.

35. Bongaerts D, Wojciechowski M, Suys B, Luijks M, Van Marck E, Jorens PG. Plastic bronchitis in a 5-year-old boy causing asystoly and fatal outcome. J Asthma. 2009;46(6):586-90. https://doi.org/10.1080/02770900902915854.

36. Dori Y, Keller MS, Rome JJ, Gillespie MJ, Glatz AC, Dodds K, et al. Percutaneous lymphatic embolization of abnormal pulmonary lymphatic flow as treatment of plastic bronchitis in patients with congenital heart disease. Circulation. 2016;133(12):1160-70. https://doi.org/10.1161/CIRCULATIONAHA.115.019710.

37. Grabenhenrich LB, Dolle S, Moneret-Vautrin A, Kohli A, Lange L, Spindler T, et al. Anaphylaxis in children and adolescents: The European Anaphylaxis Registry. J Allergy Clin Immunol. 2016;137(4):1128-37.e1. https://doi.org/10.1016/j.jaci.2015.11.015.

38. The 2005 RCPath Working Party on the Autopsy. Guidelines on autopsy practice: Scenario 4: Autopsy for suspected acute anaphylaxis. 2nd ed. London: The Royal College of Pathologists, 2012.

39. Jortveit J, Eskedal L, Hirth A, Fomina T, Dohlen G, Hagemo P, et al. Sudden unexpected death in children with congenital heart defects. Eur Heart J. 2016;37(7):621-6. https://doi.org/10.1093/eurheartj/ehv478.

40. Komisar J, Srivastava S, Geiger M, Doucette J, Ko H, Shenoy J, et al. Impact of changing indications and increased utilization of fetal echocardiography on prenatal detection of congenital heart disease. Congenit Heart Dis. 2017;12(1):67-73. https://doi.org/10.1111/chd.12405.

41. Sharland G. Fetal cardiac screening and variation in prenatal detection rates of congenital heart disease: Why bother with screening at all? Future Cardiol. 2012;8(2):189-202. https://doi.org/10.2217/fca.12.15.

42. Mellander M. Diagnosis and management of life-threatening cardiac malformations in the newborn. Semin Fetal Neonatal Med. 2013;18(5):302-10. https://doi.org/10.1016/j.siny.2013.04.007.

43. Cole CR, Eghtesady P. The myocardial and coronary histopathology and pathogenesis of hypoplastic left heart syndrome. Cardiol Young. 2016;26(1):19-29. https://doi.org/10.1017/S1047951115001171.

44. Stein P. Total anomalous pulmonary venous connection. AORN J. 2007;85(3):509-20; quiz 21-4. https://doi.org/10.1016/S0001-2092(07)60123-9.

45. Olney RS, Ailes EC, Sontag MK. Detection of critical congenital heart defects: Review of contributions from prenatal and newborn screening. Semin Perinatol. 2015;39(3):230-7. https://doi.org/10.1053/j.semperi.2015.03.007.

46. Elliott P, Andersson B, Arbustini E, Bilinska Z, Cecchi F, Charron P, et al. Classification of the cardiomyopathies: A position statement from the European Society of Cardiology Working Group on myocardial and pericardial diseases. Eur Heart J. 2008;29(2):270-6. https://doi.org/10.1093/eurheartj/ehm342.

47. Wilkinson JD, Westphal JA, Bansal N, Czachor JD, Razoky H, Lipshultz SE. Lessons learned from the Pediatric Cardiomyopathy Registry (PCMR) Study Group. Cardiol Young. 2015;25 Suppl 2:140-53. https://doi.org/10.1017/S1047951115000943.

48. Chang KT, Taylor GP, Meschino WS, Kantor PF, Cutz E. Mitogenic cardiomyopathy: A lethal neonatal familial dilated cardiomyopathy characterized by myocyte hyperplasia and proliferation. Hum Pathol. 2010;41(7):1002-8. https://doi.org/10.1016/j.humpath.2009.12.008.

49. Roberts SE, Pryce JW, Weber MA, Malone M, Ashworth MT, Sebire NJ. Clinicopathological features of fatal cardiomyopathy in childhood: An autopsy series. J Paediatr Child health. 2012;48(8):675-80. https://doi.org/10.1111/j.1440-1754.2012.02450.x.

50. Aretz HT. Myocarditis: The Dallas criteria. Hum Pathol. 1987;18(6):619-24. https://doi.org/10.1016/S0046-8177(87)80363-5.

51. Yilmaz O, Olgun H, Ciftel M, Kilic O, Kartal I, Iskenderoglu NY, et al. Dilated cardiomyopathy secondary to rickets-related hypocalcaemia: Eight case reports and a review of the literature. Cardiol Young. 2015;25(2):261-6. https://doi.org/10.1017/S1047951113002023.

52. Fabi M, Gesuete V, Petrucci R, Ragni L. Dilated cardiomyopathy due to hypocalcaemic rickets: Is it always a reversible condition? Cardiol Young. 2013;23(5):769-72. https://doi.org/10.1017/S1047951112001850.

53. El-Hattab AW, Scaglia F. Mitochondrial cardiomyopathies. Front Cardiovasc Med. 2016;3:25. https://doi.org/10.3389/fcvm.2016.00025.

54. Shehata BM, Bouzyk M, Shulman SC, Tang W, Steelman CK, Davis GK, et al. Identification of candidate genes for histiocytoid cardiomyopathy (HC) using whole genome expression analysis: Analyzing material from the HC registry. Pediatr Dev Pathol. 2011;14(5):370-7. https://doi.org/10.2350/10-05-0826-OA.1.

55. Finsterer J. Histiocytoid cardiomyopathy: A mitochondrial disorder. Clin Cardiol. 2008;31(5):225-7. https://doi.org/10.1002/clc.20224.

56. Mazzanti A, Ng K, Faragli A, Maragna R, Chiodaroli E, Orphanou N, et al. Arrhythmogenic right ventricular cardiomyopathy: Clinical course and predictors of arrhythmic risk. J Am Coll Cardiol. 2016;68(23):2540-50. https://doi.org/10.1016/j.jacc.2016.09.951.

57. Castanos Gutierrez SL, Kamel IR, Zimmerman SL. Current concepts on diagnosis and prognosis of arrhythmogenic right ventricular cardiomyopathy/dysplasia. J Thorac Imaging. 2016;31(6):324-35. https://doi.org/10.1097/RTI.0000000000000171.

58. Behere SP, Weindling SN. Inherited arrhythmias: The cardiac channelopathies. Ann Pediatr Cardiol. 2015;8(3):210-20. https://doi.org/10.4103/0974-2069.164695.

59. Weber MA, Ashworth MT, Risdon RA, Malone M, Burch M, Sebire NJ. Clinicopathological features of paediatric deaths due to myocarditis: An autopsy series. Arch Dis Child. 2008;93(7):594-8. https://doi.org/10.1136/adc.2007.128686.

60. Vigneswaran TV, Brown JR, Breuer J, Burch M. Parvovirus B19 myocarditis in children: An observational study. Arch Dis Child. 2016;101(2):177-80. https://doi.org/10.1136/archdischild-2014-308080.

61. Myers KA, Wong KK, Tipple M, Sanatani S. Benign cardiac tumours, malignant arrhythmias. Can J Cardiol. 2010;26(2):e58-61. https://doi.org/10.1016/S0828-282X(10)70009-X.

62. Tavora F, Li L, Burke A. Sudden coronary death in children. Cardiovasc Pathol. 2010;19(6):336-9. https://doi.org/10.1016/j.carpath.2010.06.001.

63. Al-Shaikh AM, Abdullah MH, Barclay A, Cullen-Dean G, McCrindle BW. Impact of the characteristics of patients and their clinical management on outcomes in children with homozygous familial hypercholesterolemia. Cardiol Young. 2002;12(2):105-12. https://doi.org/10.1017/S1047951102000240.

64. Burns JC, Kushner HI, Bastian JF, Shike H, Shimizu C, Matsubara T, et al. Kawasaki disease: A brief history. Pediatrics. 2000;106(2):E27. https://doi.org/10.1542/peds.106.2.e27.

65. McNeal-Davidson A, Fournier A, Scuccimarri R, Dancea A, Houde C, Bellavance M, et al. The fate and observed management of giant coronary artery aneurysms secondary to Kawasaki disease in the Province of Quebec: The complete series since 1976. Pediatr Cardiol. 2013;34(1):170-8. https://doi.org/10.1007/s00246-012-0409-2.

66. Bryant V, George S. Sudden cardiac death in a normally developed male infant: An atypical presentation of Kawasaki Disease. 26th European Congress of Pathology (ECP 2014); 30 August-3 September; London, UK, 2014. Abstract: Virchows Arch. 2014;465(Suppl 1):S196.

67. Fikar CR, Fikar R. Aortic dissection in childhood and adolescence: An analysis of occurrences over a 10-year interval in New York State. Clin Cardiol. 2009;32(6):E23-6. https://doi.org/10.1002/clc.20383.

68. Ngan KW, Hsueh C, Hsieh HC, Ueng SH. Aortic dissection in a young patient without any predisposing factors. Chang Gung Med J. 2006;29(4):419-23.

69. Shah S, Gross JR, Stewart CT. A case report of meningococcal disease in a neonate. WMJ. 2013;112(1):28-30; quiz 1.

70. Esposito S, Tagliabue C, Bosis S. Meningococcal B vaccination (4CMenB) in infants and toddlers. J Immunol Res. 2015;2015:402381. https://doi.org/10.1155/2015/402381.

71. Leestma JE. Intracranial causes of death and their mechanisms. Diagn Histopathol (Oxf). 2016;22(9):327-32. https://doi.org/10.1016/j.mpdhp.2016.08.003.

72. Capewell LG, Harris AM, Yoder JS, Cope JR, Eddy BA, Roy SL, et al. Diagnosis, clinical course, and treatment of primary amoebic meningoencephalitis in the United States, 1937-2013. J Pediatric Infect Dis Soc. 2015;4(4):e68-75. https://doi.org/10.1093/jpids/piu103.

73. Siddiqui R, Ali IK, Cope JR, Khan NA. Biology and pathogenesis of Naegleria fowleri. Acta Trop. 2016;164:375-94. https://doi.org/10.1016/j.actatropica.2016.09.009.

74. Jubelt B, Mihai C, Li TM, Veerapaneni P. Rhombencephalitis/brainstem encephalitis. Curr Neurol Neurosci Rep. 2011;11(6):543-52. https://doi.org/10.1007/s11910-011-0228-5.

75. Teoh HL, Mohammad SS, Britton PN, Kandula T, Lorentzos MS, Booy R, et al. Clinical characteristics and functional motor outcomes of enterovirus 71 neurological disease in children. JAMA Neurol. 2016;73(3):300-7. https://doi.org/10.1001/jamaneurol.2015.4388.

76. Lo WD, Lee J, Rusin J, Perkins E, Roach ES. Intracranial hemorrhage in children: An evolving spectrum. Arch Neurol. 2008;65(12):1629-33. https://doi.org/10.1001/archneurol.2008.502.

77. Meyer-Heim AD, Boltshauser E. Spontaneous intracranial haemorrhage in children: Aetiology, presentation and outcome. Brain Dev. 2003;25(6):416-21. https://doi.org/10.1016/S0387-7604(03)00029-9.

78. Burch EA, Orbach DB. Pediatric central nervous system vascular malformations. Pediatr Radiol. 2015;45 Suppl 3:S463-72. https://doi.org/10.1007/s00247-015-3356-2.

79. Smith ER. Structural causes of ischemic and hemorrhagic stroke in children: Moyamoya and arteriovenous malformations. Curr Opin Pediatr. 2015;27(6):706-11. https://doi.org/10.1097/MOP.0000000000000280.

80. Smith ER, Scott RM. Cavernous malformations. Neurosurg Clin N Am. 2010;21(3):483-90. https://doi.org/10.1016/j.nec.2010.03.003.

81. Recinos PF, Rahmathulla G, Pearl M, Recinos VR, Jallo GI, Gailloud P, et al. Vein of Galen malformations: Epidemiology, clinical presentations, management. Neurosurg Clin N Am. 2012;23(1):165-77. https://doi.org/10.1016/j.nec.2011.09.006.

82. Tilney P. Subarachnoid hemorrhage in a 13-year-old girl. Air Med J. 2010;29(5):198-201. https://doi.org/10.1016/j.amj.2010.06.008.

83. Greenham M, Gordon A, Anderson V, Mackay MT. Outcome in childhood stroke. Stroke. 2016;47(4):1159-64. https://doi.org/10.1161/STROKEAHA.115.011622.

84. Mackay MT, Wiznitzer M, Benedict SL, Lee KJ, Deveber GA, Ganesan V. Arterial ischemic stroke risk factors: The International Pediatric Stroke Study. Ann Neurol. 2011;69(1):130-40. https://doi.org/10.1002/ana.22224.

85. Amlie-Lefond C, Ellenbogen RG. Factors associated with the presentation of moyamoya in childhood. J Stroke Cerebrovasc Dis. 2015;24(6):1204-10. https://doi.org/10.1016/j.jstrokecerebrovasdis.2015.01.018.

86. Milroy CM. Sudden unexpected death in epilepsy in childhood. Forensic Sci Med Pathol. 2011;7(4):336-40. https://doi.org/10.1007/s12024-011-9245-6.

87. Pierre G. Neurodegenerative disorders and metabolic disease. Arch Dis Child. 2013;98(8):618-24. https://doi.org/10.1136/archdischild-2012-302840.

88. Patay Z, Blaser SI, Poretti A, Huisman TA. Neurometabolic diseases of childhood. Pediatr Radiol 2015;45 Suppl 3:S473-84. https://doi.org/10.1007/s00247-015-3279-y.

89. Somers GR, Smith CR, Perrin DG, Wilson GJ, Taylor GP. Sudden unexpected death in infancy and childhood due to undiagnosed neoplasia: An autopsy study. Am J Forensic Med Pathol. 2006;27(1):64-9. https://doi.org/10.1097/01.paf.0000203267.91806.ed.

90. Byard RW, Bourne AJ, Hanieh A. Sudden and unexpected death due to hemorrhage from occult central nervous system lesions. A pediatric autopsy study. Pediatr Neurosurg. 1991;17(2):88-94. https://doi.org/10.1159/000120573.

91. DiMaio SM, DiMaio VJ, Kirkpatrick JB. Sudden, unexpected deaths due to primary intracranial neoplasms. Am J Forensic Med Pathol. 1980;1(1):29-45. https://doi.org/10.1097/00000433-198003000-00007.

92. Sutton JT, Cummings PM, Ross GW, Lopes MB. Sudden death of a 7-year-old boy due to undiagnosed glioblastoma. Am J Forensic Med Pathol. 2010;31(3):278-80. https://doi.org/10.1097/PAF.0b013e3181e8d0ef.

93. McKiernan P, Abdel-Hady M. Advances in the management of childhood portal hypertension. Expert Rev Gastroenterol Hepatol. 2015;9(5):575-83. https://doi.org/10.1586/17474124.2015.993610.

94. Antonis JH, Poeze M, van Heurn LW. Boerhaave's syndrome in children: A case report and review of the literature. J Pediatr Surg. 2006;41(9):1620-3. https://doi.org/10.1016/j.jpedsurg.2006.05.003.

95. Batsis ID, Okito O, Meltzer JA, Cunningham SJ. Internal hernia as a cause for intestinal obstruction in a newborn. J Emerg Med. 2015;49(3):277-80. https://doi.org/10.1016/j.jemermed.2015.04.030.

96. Poceta JS, Strandjord TP, Badura RJ Jr, Milstein JM. Ondine curse and neurocristopathy. Pediatr Neurol. 1987;3(6):370-2. https://doi.org/10.1016/0887-8994(87)90011-7.

97. NHS. Newborn blood spot test: NHS Choices. [Available from: http://www.nhs.uk/conditions/pregnancy-and-baby/pages/newborn-blood-spot-test.aspx]. Accessed 27 November 2017.

98. Emery JL, Howat AJ, Variend S, Vawter GF. Investigation of inborn errors of metabolism in unexpected infant deaths. Lancet. 1988;2(8601):29-31. https://doi.org/10.1016/S0140-6736(88)92955-8.

99. Treem WR. New developments in the pathophysiology, clinical spectrum, and diagnosis of disorders of fatty acid oxidation. Curr Opin Pediatr. 2000;12(5):463-8. https://doi.org/10.1097/00008480-200010000-00008.

100. Tein I. Disorders of fatty acid oxidation. Handb Clin Neurol. 2013;113:1675-88. https://doi.org/10.1016/B978-0-444-59565-2.00035-6.

101. Kompare M, Rizzo WB. Mitochondrial fatty-acid oxidation disorders. Semin Pediatr Neurol. 2008;15(3):140-9. https://doi.org/10.1016/j.spen.2008.05.008.

102. Wang GL, Wang J, Douglas G, Browning M, Hahn S, Ganesh J, et al. Expanded molecular features of carnitine acyl-carnitine translocase (CACT) deficiency by comprehensive molecular analysis. Mol Genet Metab. 2011;103(4):349-57. https://doi.org/10.1016/j.ymgme.2011.05.001.

103. Rahier J, Guiot Y, Sempoux C. Morphologic analysis of focal and diffuse forms of congenital hyperinsulinism. Semin Pediatr Surg. 2011;20(1):3-12. https://doi.org/10.1053/j.sempedsurg.2010.10.010.

104. Stanley CA. Perspective on the genetics and diagnosis of congenital hyperinsulinism disorders. J Clin Endocrinol Metab. 2016;101(3):815-26. https://doi.org/10.1210/jc.2015-3651.

105. Ali Z, Levine B, Ripple M, Fowler DR. Diabetic ketoacidosis: A silent death. Am J Forensic Med Pathol. 2012;33(3):189-93. https://doi.org/10.1097/PAF.0b013e31825192e7.

106. Tu E, Bagnall RD, Duflou J, Lynch M, Twigg SM, Semsarian C. Post-mortem pathologic and genetic studies in "dead in bed syndrome" cases in type 1 diabetes mellitus. Hum Pathol. 2010;41(3):392-400. https://doi.org/10.1016/j.humpath.2009.08.020.

107. Martin K, Weiss SL. Initial resuscitation and management of pediatric septic shock. Minerva Pediatr. 2015;67(2):141-58.

108. Tormos LM, Schandl CA. The significance of adrenal hemorrhage: Undiagnosed Waterhouse-Friderichsen syndrome, a case series. J Forensic Sci. 2013;58(4):1071-4. https://doi.org/10.1111/1556-4029.12099.

109. Adalat S, Dawson T, Hackett SJ, Clark JE. Toxic shock syndrome surveillance in UK children. Arch Dis Child. 2014;99(12):1078-82. https://doi.org/10.1136/archdischild-2013-304741.

110. LeRiche T, Black AY, Fleming NA. Toxic shock syndrome of a probable gynecologic source in an adolescent: A case report and review of the literature. J Pediatr Adolesc Gynecol. 2012;25(6):e133-7. https://doi.org/10.1016/j.jpag.2012.08.011.

111. Nields H, Kessler SC, Boisot S, Evans R. Streptococcal toxic shock syndrome presenting as suspected child abuse. Am J Forensic Med Pathol. 1998;19(1):93-7. https://doi.org/10.1097/00000433-199803000-00018.

112. Ladhani SN, Ramsay M, Borrow R, Riordan A, Watson JM, Pollard AJ. Enter B and W: Two new meningococcal vaccine programmes launched. Arch Dis Child. 2016;101(1):91-5. https://doi.org/10.1136/archdischild-2015-308928.

113. Kiray Bas E, Bulbul A, Comert S, Uslu S, Arslan S, Nuhoglu A. Neonatal infection with Neisseria meningitidis: Analysis of a 97-year period plus case study. J Clin Microbiol. 2014;52(9):3478-82. https://doi.org/10.1128/JCM.01000-14.

114. Pai S, Enoch DA, Aliyu SH. Bacteremia in children: Epidemiology, clinical diagnosis and antibiotic treatment. Expert Rev Anti Infect Ther. 2015;13(9):1073-88. https://doi.org/10.1586/14787210.2015.1063418.

115. Campbell H, Parikh SR, Borrow R, Kaczmarski E, Ramsay ME, Ladhani SN. Presentation with gastrointestinal symptoms and high case fatality associated with group W meningococcal disease (MenW) in teenagers, England, July 2015 to January 2016. Euro Surveill. 2016;21(12). https://doi.org/10.2807/1560-7917. ES.2016.21.12.30175.

116. Gilsdorf JR. What the pediatrician should know about non-typeable Haemophilus influenzae. J Infect. 2015;71 Suppl 1:S10-4. https://doi.org/10.1016/j. jinf.2015.04.014.

117. Desai S, Jamieson FB, Patel SN, Seo CY, Dang V, Fediurek J, et al. The epidemiology of invasive Haemophilus influenzae non-serotype B disease in Ontario, Canada from 2004 to 2013. PloS One. 2015;10(11):e0142179. https://doi.org/10.1371/journal.pone.0142179.

118. Collins S, Litt DJ, Flynn S, Ramsay ME, Slack MP, Ladhani SN. Neonatal invasive Haemophilus influenzae disease in England and Wales: Epidemiology, clinical characteristics, and outcome. Clin Infect Dis. 2015;60(12):1786-92. https://doi. org/10.1093/cid/civ194.

119. Boyd R, Patel M, Currie BJ, Holt DC, Harris T, Krause V. High burden of invasive group A streptococcal disease in the Northern Territory of Australia. Epidemiol Infect. 2016;144(5):1018-27. https://doi.org/10.1017/S0950268815002010.

120. Phares CR, Lynfield R, Farley MM, Mohle-Boetani J, Harrison LH, Petit S, et al. Epidemiology of invasive group B streptococcal disease in the United States, 1999-2005. JAMA. 2008;299(17):2056-65. https://doi.org/10.1001/jama.299.17.2056.

121. Blumberg HM, Stephens DS, Modansky M, Erwin M, Elliot J, Facklam RR, et al. Invasive group B streptococcal disease: The emergence of serotype V. J Infect Dis. 1996;173(2):365-73. https://doi.org/10.1093/infdis/173.2.365.

122. Vogel M, Schmitz RP, Hagel S, Pletz MW, Gagelmann N, Scherag A, et al. Infectious disease consultation for Staphylococcus aureus bacteremia — A systematic review and meta-analysis. J Infect. 2016;72(1):19-28. https://doi. org/10.1016/j.jinf.2015.09.037.

123. Handler MZ, Schwartz RA. Staphylococcal scalded skin syndrome: Diagnosis and management in children and adults. J Eur Acad Dermatol Venereol. 2014;28(11):1418-23. https://doi.org/10.1111/jdv.12541.

124. Spencer DA, Thomas MF. Necrotising pneumonia in children. Paediatr Respir Rev. 2014;15(3):240-5; quiz 5. https://doi.org/10.1016/j.prrv.2013.10.001.

125. Schwartz KL, Nourse C. Panton-Valentine leukocidin-associated Staphylococcus aureus necrotizing pneumonia in infants: A report of four cases and review of the literature. Eur J Pediatr. 2012;171(4):711-17. https://doi.org/10.1007/s00431-011-1651-y.

126. Rougemont AL, Buteau C, Ovetchkine P, Bergeron C, Fournet JC, Bouron-Dal Soglio D. Fatal cases of Staphylococcus aureus pleural empyema in infants. Pediatr Dev Pathol. 2009;12(5):390-3. https://doi.org/10.2350/08-09-0531.1.

127. Sheikh HQ, Aqil A, Kirby A, Hossain FS. Panton-Valentine leukocidin osteomyelitis in children: A growing threat. Br J Hosp Med (Lond). 2015;76(1):18-24. https://doi.org/10.12968/hmed.2015.76.1.18.

128. Vaz Marecos C, Ferreira M, Ferreira MM, Barroso MR. Sepsis, meningitis and cerebral abscesses caused by Citrobacter koseri. BMJ Case Rep. 2012. https://doi.org/10.1136/bcr.10.2011.4941.

129. Chowdhry SA, Cohen AR. Citrobacter brain abscesses in neonates: Early surgical intervention and review of the literature. Childs Nerv Syst. 2012;28(10):1715-22. https://doi.org/10.1007/s00381-012-1746-4.

# 26 Brainstem Neuropathology in Sudden Infant Death Syndrome

Fiona M Bright, PhD[1],
Robert Vink, PhD[2] and
Roger W Byard, MBBS, MD[1,3]

[1]School of Medicine, The University of Adelaide, Adelaide, Australia
[2]Sansom Institute for Health Research, University of South Australia,
Adelaide, Australia
[3]Florey Institute of Neuroscience and Mental Health, Victoria, Australia

## Introduction

Sudden infant death syndrome (SIDS) has a complex and heterogeneous pathogenesis, with multiple abnormalities in a number of physiological functions and systems including neurological, cardiovascular, respiratory, gastrointestinal, nutritional, endocrine, metabolic, infectious, immunological, environmental, and genetic (1-7). Typically, without warning, an apparently healthy infant is found deceased sometime after being placed to sleep (8). There are many theories involving animal and human studies that have attempted to understand the pathophysiology of SIDS. Unfortunately, to date, there are no biomarkers available to aid in the prevention or definitive diagnosis of SIDS. The aim of much scientific research has been to determine the mechanisms of failure in SIDS infants that are undetectable prior to death and that remain just as unclear following death. While the precise cause of death in infants dying of SIDS has not been identified, there is considerable evidence that the syndrome results from a combination of circumstances involving [1] a cardiorespiratory challenge that occurs in [2] a neurologically compromised infant at [3] a specific period of postnatal development (3, 9, 10). The following chapter will focus on the failure of cardiorespiratory and autonomic control associated with neuropathology of the brainstem in SIDS.

An important step in understanding the complex pathophysiology of SIDS was the establishment of the Triple Risk Model, which successfully conceptualized the epidemiological, physiological, and neuropathological data associated with SIDS. The Triple Risk Model proposes three coinciding factors: [1] an underlying vulnerability of the infant; [2] a critical developmental period in homeostatic control that the infant is transitioning through; and [3] the application of an exogenous stressor/s such as an asphyxiating environment (11). The model implies that an infant may be most at risk of SIDS when all three factors are simultaneously present (8, 11). All three factors contribute to the risk of an adverse event that occurs suddenly in an otherwise "healthy" infant. Therefore, consideration of the Triple Risk Model is of key importance to SIDS research, with the model providing a foundation upon which researchers can build in the generation of research hypotheses.

## Underlying Vulnerability and the Brainstem Hypothesis

Multiple neuropathologic studies in SIDS victims have supported the concept that SIDS infants are not entirely "normal" prior to death; instead these infants possess some form of underlying vulnerability exposing them to an increased risk for sudden death (3, 8). Interest in investigation of the brainstem in SIDS began with the findings of Naeye (12), who reported astrogliosis in this region in 50% of SIDS cases, with hypoxia thought to be the underlying cause. Further, research by Kinney et al. (13) showed reactive gliosis in one-fifth of cases. Building upon these observations, research was then directed towards investigation of neurotransmitters in brainstem respiratory related pathways, particularly those located in the medulla oblongata, which controls respiration, chemosensitivity, autonomic function, and arousal (9, 10, 14). As such, there is now sufficient evidence that SIDS, or a certain subset of SIDS, is associated with some form of underlying neural or systematic dysfunction in medullary homeostatic control. This dysfunction is thought to impair critical responses to life-threatening challenges such as hypoxia, hypercarbia, and asphyxia during a sleep period (3, 8, 14), hence the term "brainstem hypothesis". This concept is based on evidence that the brainstem has a crucial role in respiratory, cardiac, and blood pressure control, as well as in central chemosensitivity, thermoregulation, and modulation of upper airway reflexes, particularly during sleep. Additionally, investigations of possible defects in medullary control, consistent with brainstem dysfunction in infants who subsequently died of SIDS, have implicated impaired autoresuscitation (gasping), abnormal respiratory patterning, and episodic obstructive apnea during sleep, autonomic dysfunction (episodic tachycardia/bradycardia, abnormal heart rate variability), and arousal deficits (3, 15-21).

# Brainstem Respiratory Network

Respiration is both a spontaneous and an autonomic physiological function crucial for survival. Respiratory drive plays a critical role in homeostatic control by regulating blood oxygen, carbon dioxide ($CO_2$), and pH levels (22), and it is controlled by rhythmic respiratory signals generated by extensive neural networks located in the medulla oblongata (23, 24). Excitatory amino acids are considered the primary source of neurochemical signals in the generation of respiratory rhythm and inspiratory drive to spinal and cranial motoneurons (25), with basic respiratory rhythm pattern modulated by multiple amine and peptide neurotransmitter and neuromodulator systems (22). Breathing must be constantly adapted to suit metabolic demand and is therefore a highly integrative process. Breathing behaviors are exerted via the integration of multiple respiratory neurons concentrated in the ventral respiratory column, including the prebotzinger (PBC) and botzinger complexes, retrotrapezoid nucleus, parafacial respiratory group, kolliker fuse, and some cortical and cerebellar networks (26, 27). Respiratory rhythm and inspiratory and expiratory motor patterns emerge from the dynamic interactions between these structural and functional components (26).

The core of breathing rhythm generation is the PBC (see Chapter 27). Identified physiologically as an essential part of the medullary respiratory and rhythm-generating network in mammals by Smith et al. in 1991[1], the PBC is well established as a critical region for the generation and co-ordination of respiratory rhythm and breathing cessation (28-30). Three types of respiratory rhythmic control are identified as originating in the PBC — eupnea, sighs, and gasping (10, 31) — and the region is particularly sensitive to hypoxia (31, 32). Lesioning of the PBC results in cessation of breathing in experimental animals (33, 34), and pacemaker neurons within the PBC are postulated to have a role in the control of breathing as a contingency system that may be activated when normal respiratory rhythmogenesis fails (35, 36). Therefore, the structure and function of the PBC is of considerable importance with regards to brainstem respiratory control and failure of such a system in SIDS.

Although well described anatomically in experimental animals, the precise location of the PBC in the human brainstem has remained unclear. However, distinct cytoarchitectural characteristics of neighboring nuclei and fiber tracts, in addition to markers for interneurons of the PBC, may be utilized to help localize the region. Interneurons of the PBC have been shown to express high levels of the tachykinin NK1 receptor (NK1R) (24) and somatostatin (37). Stornetta et al. (37) and Schwarzacher et al. (38) utilized these characteristics to identify a circumscribed region of the ventrolateral medulla containing a high number of NK1R and somatostatin-immunoreactive neurons indicative of the PBC region in experimental animals, and deduced that this region could be the presumptive human homologue (38).

---

1   Smith JC, Ellenberger HH, Ballanyi K, Richter DW, Feldman JL. Pre-Botzinger complex: A brainstem region that may generate respiratory rhythm in mammals. Science. 1991;254(5032):726-9. https://doi. org/10.1126/science.1683005.

# Respiratory Defense Mechanisms and Arousal Failure

Exposure to respiratory challenges occurs frequently during infancy; however, these can usually be overcome because of highly evolved protective respiratory defense mechanisms (36). These mechanisms involve complex feedback pathways at several neuroanatomic levels and are controlled by different underlying neural pathways and neurochemical actions to produce an integrated response (9).

Under normal conditions, increased blood $CO_2$ levels (hypercapnia) or decreased oxygen levels (hypoxia) stimulate an infant to produce respiratory and motor defense mechanisms, including sighs, thrashing, eye opening, head lifting or tilting, and cries, to trigger arousal (39, 40). Arousal from sleep then successfully overcomes the respiratory challenge and restores the network to the normal "eupneic" breathing state (10, 40). This arousal response to harmful stimuli is a key feature of breathing control development in newborns (41), protecting the infant from prolonged respiratory distress (36); thus any interruption or depression of arousal will have significant implications on the normal response to respiratory challenges (40). In the event of arousal failure, the normal breathing state shifts to gasping, which is a strong indicator of exposure to hypoxia. If oxygen becomes available during gasping, recovery from the respiratory challenge is still possible by "autoresuscitation", where complete and rapid return of function of all organs is achieved (36). Gasping and autoresuscitation are, however, the final defenses in overcoming respiratory challenges, and failure of both results in an inability to restore blood oxygen levels with the loss of drive of heart rate (9, 36, 39, 40, 42). A "challenged" infant will therefore experience further respiratory distress, failing to overcome respiratory challenge, and will rapidly succumb to death (10).

SIDS infants also have a markedly reduced ability to turn their faces or to lift their heads away from a dangerous micro-environment, in addition to their inability to produce adequate respiratory musculature activity (43, 44). This suggests that there is an underlying flaw in the control of such mechanisms at the neural and subcellular levels. Studies of infants on monitors who eventually succumbed to SIDS have provided indirect evidence for a sleep-related impairment or a delayed maturation of these defense mechanisms (17, 18). Future SIDS victims from these studies exhibited decreased spontaneous and induced arousals during sleep (18, 45), had altered sleep patterns (20), and had significantly more obstructive and mixed apneas that were associated with altered autonomic responses (18, 21, 45-47). Gasping has also been identified as a common feature of recordings in future SIDS infants, with reports of unusual repeated double and triple gasps that were either completely ineffective or had minimal effects on increasing heart rate (15, 19). Other studies have indicated that SIDS may not always be sudden, but rather that death may be preceded by episodic cycles of tachycardia, bradycardia, or apnea in the hours, to days, before the lethal event (8). This is further supported by markers of chronic tissue hypoxia (48-50), including brainstem gliosis, β-amyloid precursor protein deposition, and apoptosis (12, 13, 51-53).

# Possible Multi-Neurotransmitter Homeostatic Network Dysfunction

Neurochemicals are the mediators of sensory, motor, integrative, and modulatory processing in the respiratory network, including multiple inhibitory and excitatory neurotransmitters and neuromodulators (32, 54). Specifically, in regions of the brainstem involved in the control of respiration, notably the PBC, raphe magnus, and raphe obscurus of the medulla, neurotransmitter amino acids including glutamate, gamma-Aminobutyric acid (GABA), taurine, and glycine, as well as the neurotransmitters serotonin, dopamine, and substance P (SP), and the neuromodulator adenosine are found (55). The respiratory system is controlled by the balance and specific actions of these neurotransmitter and neuromodulator systems, which have diverse roles in regulating the amplitude and frequency of central rhythm generation and respiratory output (32, 56, 57). This is achieved through interaction with motoneurons, sensory neurons, and neurons of the central nervous system (CNS).

Neurotransmitters are expressed in a state-dependent manner and are centrally involved in reconfiguring the respiratory network under normal conditions; they are also involved with the homeostatic response to changes in oxygen and $CO_2$ levels during various states of breathing (55, 57). This occurs through modifying the membrane and synaptic properties of rhythm-generating neurons (58), and by altering their activity during different states, particularly hypoxia (55). Actions of neurochemicals are determined by the concurrent modulation and interaction with one another (29), and any deficiencies in one will be immediately compensated for by the action of others (29, 57). Following the deprivation of a specific modulatory input over a prolonged period, rhythmic activity is restored by the respiratory network functioning in an independent neuromodulator manner (31, 59). Therefore varying networks likely adapt to changes in neurotransmitter and neuromodulator expression by altering the concentration of other endogenously released neurochemicals (58).

As noted, the underlying vulnerability in SIDS infants is thought to be characterized by abnormalities in multiple neurotransmitter networks in the medulla oblongata which control critical homeostatic mechanisms. Indeed, abnormalities in various brainstem neurochemicals, including catecholamines, neuropeptides, indole amines (predominantly serotonin and its receptors), amino acids (predominantly glutamate), growth factors including brain-derived neurotropic growth factor (BDNF), and some cytokine systems, have been reported in infants who died of SIDS (Table 26.1) (60-79).

Observations of abnormal neurochemicals across the medullary network may be the primary defect in SIDS responsible for failure of protective mechanisms to counteract homeostatic imbalances that impinge upon a sleeping infant. While the "multi-transmitter" hypothesis for SIDS acknowledges that neurochemical abnormalities are not limited to one system, it has yet to be established how abnormalities in individual

Table 26.1: Previously published research investigating multiple neurotransmitter and receptor network abnormalities within the brainstem in post-mortem human infant brain tissues in SIDS.

| Neurotransmitter & receptor network studies in SIDS | Brainstem region/nuclei | Method | Key findings & implications for SIDS |
|---|---|---|---|
| **Glutamate/GABA-ergic** | | | |
| Broadbelt et al. 2011 (70) — GABA_A receptor | Medulla | RLB | 25-52% ↓ GABA_A receptor binding |
| Panigrahy et al. 1997 (69) — GABA_Aα3 receptor | GC | WB | 46% ↓ GABA_Aα3 subunit GABA_A receptors abnormality in some SIDS infants in conjunction with 5-HT system deficits |
| Machalaani & Waters 2003 (61) — Glutamate: kainate | Medulla, pons | RLB | ↓ 3H-kainate ARCn. Implications for regulation of CO_2 & blood pressure |
| Machalaani & Waters 2003 (61) — NMDA receptor 1 | Medulla, pons | IHC, non-RISH | ↑ mRNA XII, ION, Cun, vest, DMNV, NSTT, ↑ protein DMNV, ↓ NSTT in SIDS. Implications for cardiorespiratory control |
| **Norepinephrine** | | | |
| Ozawa et al. 2003 (71) — Norepinephrine & epinephrine adrenergic receptor α2A | Midbrain, pons, medulla | IHC | ↓ α2A medullary NTS & VLM nuclei. SIDS may be vulnerable to asphyxia, hypoxia & fail to exhibit brainstem responses |
| Duncan et al. 2010 (72) — Norepinephrine: adrenergic | RO, PGCL | HPLC | ↑ PGCL nuclei. Abnormal NE in conjunction with 5-HT system in SIDS |
| **Neurotensin/Somatostatin** | | | |
| Chigr et al. 1992 (73) — Neurotensin | Medulla | RLB | ↑ NTS. Potentially immature binding sites & abnormal central cardiorespiratory & arousal control |
| Carpentier et al. 1998 (74) — Somatostatin | Medulla, pons | RLB | ↑ medial & lateral parabrachial nuclei. Normal ↓ in receptor binding sites not seen in SIDS, indicates delayed maturation & potential deficit of hyperventilatory response to hypoxia |
| **Acetylcholine: muscarinic & nicotinic receptors** | | | |
| Kinney et al. 1995 (66) — Muscarinic receptors | Medulla, pons | RLB | ↑ ARCn in SIDS may contribute to failure of responses to cardiopulmonary challenges during sleep |
| Kubo et al. 1998 (79) — mAChR muscarinic | Medulla | IHC | ↑ +ve neurons in ARCn. Neuronal changes in ARCn can provide information for PM diagnosis in SIDS |
| Mallard et al. 1999 (62) — mAChR2 muscarinic receptors | Medulla | IHC | ↑ +ve neurons in XII & DMNV, ↓ optical density in XII. Suggest specific defect in cholinergic motor neurons in medulla in SIDS with potentially abnormal cardiorespiratory control |
| Duncan et al. 2008 (60) — nicotinic receptors | Medulla, pons, midbrain | RLB | ↓LC, PAG, RD (controls). ↑ nicotinic receptor binding in (normal) controls not seen in SIDS, suggests SIDS infants are unable to respond to maternal smoking |
| Machalaani et al. 2011 (75) — nicotinic α7 & β2 receptor subunits | Medulla | IHC | ↑ α7 in NTS, gracile & Cun nuclei, ↓ β2 in NTS, ↓ β2 facial nucleus. Suggest SIDS have genetic/environmental defect in molecular regulation of α7 & β2 in response to smoke exposure |
| **Growth factors & cytokines** | | | |
| Kadhim et al. 2003 (78) — IL-1B pro-inflammatory cytokine | Medulla | IHC | ↑ IL-1B in DMNV & ARCn. IL-1 overexpression may contribute to disturbed homeostatic control |
| Rognum et al. 2009 (77) — IL-6R cytokine receptor | Medulla | IHC | ↑ IL-6R in ARCn. Abnormal interactions between IL-6 & ARCn may contribute to impaired responses to hypecapnia |
| Tang et al. 2012 (76) — BDNF & TrkB receptor | Medulla | IHC | ↓ BDNF in DMNV & NTS, ↑ TrkB in DMNV & ARCn. Neuroprotective function of BDNF/TrkB system may be reduced in respiratory nuclei in SIDS |

Abbreviations: 5-HT, serotonin; ARCn, arcuate nucleus; BDNF, brain derived neurotrophic factor; CO_2, carbon dioxide; Cun, cuneate nucleus; DMNV, dorsal motor nucleus of vagus nerve; GC, gigantocellularis lateralis nuclei; HPLC, high performance liquid chromatography; IHC, immunohistochemistry; IL-1B, interleukin 1 beta; IL-6R, interleukin 6 receptor; ION, inferior olivary nucleus; LC, locus coeruleus nuclei; NE, norepinephrine; NMDA, N-methyl D aspartate receptor; NSTT, nucleus of spinal trigeminal nucleus; NTS, nucleus tractus solitarius; PAG, periaqueductal gray; PGCL, paragigantocellularis lateralis nuclei; PM, post-mortem; RISH, non-radioactive in situ hybridization; RD, raphe dorsalis; RLB, radioactive ligand binding; RO, raphe obscurus; TrkB, tropomyosin receptor kinase B; Vest, vestibular nucleus; VLM, ventral lateral medulla; WB, western blotting; XII, hypoglossal nucleus.

systems may influence one another, or what the impact of dysfunction in a particular neurotransmitter might be on other systems within the same, or closely associated, medullary nuclei. This chapter will focus on abnormalities in the monoamine serotonin 5-hydroxytryptamine (5-HT) and neuropeptide substance P (SP) networks within the medulla in SIDS, due to their relationship with cardiorespiratory centers, given that both systems are at the forefront of current investigations into brainstem dysfunction in SIDS.

## Medullary Serotonergic System

There is substantial evidence for multiple neural mechanisms contributing to the fatal event in SIDS. However, the most compelling and reproducible research to date is focused on the hypothesis that SIDS is due to a developmental disorder of medullary serotonergic and related neurotransmitter systems that occurs prenatally but exerts its effects in the postnatal period (9, 72, 80, 81).

Monoaminergic pathways represent a key component of the reticular activating system within the mammalian brain and are involved in multiple physiological functions (82). Serotonin (5-HT) is one of several biologic monoamines located in specific axon terminals that are widely distributed throughout the CNS (83). The 5-HT system is spread throughout the brainstem; however, it is primarily situated in the medulla oblongata where it is referred to as the "medullary 5-HT system" (84-86). The system comprises two core domains, caudal and rostral, which are distinct in their anatomic location, development, functions, and connectivity. The caudal domain projects to the cerebellum and spinal cord and is critical for respiratory and autonomic output. The rostral domain projects to the cerebral cortex, thalamus, hypothalamus, basal ganglia, hippocampus, and amygdala and mediates arousal, cognition, mood, motor activity, and cerebral blood flow (85, 87). The 5-HT system is recognized as a key regulator of the brain's homeostatic control systems, including upper airway control, ventilation and gasping, autonomic control, thermoregulation, chemosensitivity, arousal, and hypoxia-induced plasticity (8, 84, 85).

Serotonin plays a fundamental role in the control and modulation of breathing (23, 56), exhibiting both inhibitory and excitatory effects (57) and acting via a large array of receptors that function to facilitate diverse respiratory effects (88, 89). The synaptic projections of 5-HT neurons are present across all major respiratory nuclei including the PBC, and arise from the midline raphe pallidus and raphe obscurus (90). Several neurotransmitters and neuropeptides are released by 5-HT neurons and directly enhance the excitability of multiple neuron subsets within the respiratory network (85). Serotonergic terminals also contain SP and thyrotropin-releasing hormone (TRH), and receptors for 5-HT, SP, and TRH are localized on neurons across the major respiratory nuclei (91). Activation of these receptors in vitro provokes modulatory effects on respiratory neurons to enhance their excitability and activity of the respiratory network.

There is also considerable evidence recognizing 5-HT neurons as putative central respiratory chemoreceptors that assist in the detection of $CO_2$ and the implementation of ventilatory responses in order to maintain circulatory homeostasis (92).

It is well established that the exogenous release of 5-HT exerts complex modulatory effects on respiratory drive, as observed in in vivo preparations (23, 93). Peña and Ramirez (2002)[2] demonstrated that bursting respiratory neurons rely on endogenously released 5-HT acting on 5-HT$_{2A}$ receptors, and that blockage of these receptors abolishes the critical bursting property of neurons in order to generate normal breathing. Doi and Ramirez (57) found that 5-HT increased and subsequently decreased bursting frequency in pre-inspiratory and inspiratory neurons, highlighting its important modulatory effects. Furthermore, inhibition of 5-HT medullary raphe and extra raphe neurons has been reported to decrease ventilatory sensitivity to C02 and also results in alterations to cardiovascular variables and sleep cycling (94). These observations reinforce the importance of neuromodulators such as 5-HT in adjusting ionic conductance crucial for regulating pacemaker and network properties of the rhythm-generating network.

Serotonergic abnormalities have been reported across multiple SIDS data-sets from varying ethnic, social, and cultural backgrounds (65, 72, 95, 96). These abnormalities involve raphe, extra raphe, and ventral (arcuate) populations of the brainstem containing 5-HT neurons and their projection sites, such as the dorsal motor nucleus of the vagus and the nucleus of the solitary tract (86). Abnormalities identified include alterations in 5-HT receptor binding patterns (5-HT$_{1A}$ and 5-HT$_{2A}$ receptors) (65, 95, 97-99), reduced brainstem levels of 5-HT and tryptophan hydroxylase (TPH2, the rate limiting enzyme-regulating 5-HT synthesis) (72), decreased binding to the 5-HT transporter relative to 5-HT cell density (14, 65), increased 5-HT cell number and density of 5-HT neurons, morphological immaturity of 5-HT neurons (3, 65), and reductions in the level of the 14-3-3 signal transduction family of proteins in regions of the medulla oblongata critically involved in the regulation of homeostatic function (Table 26.2) (100). Given the complex role of 5-HT within the medulla, associated abnormalities are likely responsible for impaired reflexes and responses of critical autonomic respiratory defense mechanisms to exogenous stressors such as hypoxia (9, 14, 101).

While medullary 5-HT abnormalities are the most prominent findings in SIDS research to date, the precise pathogenesis remains unknown, with uncertainty as to whether these abnormalities are associated with the primary event in SIDS or are instead an epiphenomenon. However, it is most likely that the evolution of 5-HT abnormalities is multifactorial, involving a combination of environmental and genetic risk factors (80).

---

2  Peña F, Ramirez JM. Endogenous activation of serotonin-2A receptors is required for respiratory rhythm generation in vitro. J Neurosci. 2002;22(24):11055-64.

| Author/Year | Indole amine target | Brain region/nuclei analyzed | Method | Key findings in SIDS victims |
|---|---|---|---|---|
| Duncan et al. 2010 (72) | 5-HT, 5H1AA | RO, PGCL | HPCL | ↓ 5-HT |
| Paterson et al. 2006 (65) | TPH, converts 5-HT to serotonin, 5-HTT, 5HT1A receptor, 5-HT neurons | Medulla | IHC, RLB | ↑ 5-HT neuron count, density & morphological immaturity, ↓ 5-HT1A in Raphe, ARCn, NTS, MAO & XII, ↓ 5-HTT binding to 5-HT neurons |
| Duncan et al. 2010 (72) | TPH, converts 5-HT to serotonin | RO, PGCL | HPCL | ↓ TPH2 in RO |
| | | RO | WB | |
| Panigrahy et al. 2000 (95) | 5HT1A-D & 5HT2 receptors | Medulla, pons | RLB | ↓ ARCn, ION, GC, RO & IRZ |
| Kinney et al. 2003 (96) | 5HT1A-D & 5HT2 receptors | Medulla, pons | RLB | ↓ ARCn |
| Ozawa & Okado 2002 (97) | 5HT1A receptor | Midbrain, medulla, pons | IHC | ↓ DMNV, NTS, VLM & ↑ PAG |
| Machalaani et al. 2009 (98) | 5HT1A receptor | Medulla | IHC | ↓ DMNV, NTS, Vest, Cun, ION |
| Duncan et al. 2010 (72) | 5HT1A receptor | Medulla | RLB | ↓ DMNV, XII & NTS |
| Ozawa & Okado 2002 (97) | 5HT2A receptor | Midbrain, medulla, pons | IHC | ↓ DMNV, NTS & VLM, ↑ PAG |
| Broadbelt et al. 2012 (100) | 14-3-3 signal transductor, regulator of 5-HT synthesis | Medulla | WB, Mass Spectrometry | ↓ 14-3-3 signal transductor |

Abbreviations: 5-HT, serotonin; 5-HT1A, serotonin receptor 1A; 5H1AA, serotonin metabolite; 5-HT2A, serotonin receptor 2A; 5-HTT, serotonin transporter; ARCn, arcuate nucleus; Cun, cuneate nucleus; DMNV, dorsal motor nucleus of vagus nerve; GC, gigantocellularis lateralis nuclei; HPCL, high performance liquid chromatography; IHC, immunohistochemistry; ION, inferior olivary nucleus; IRZ, intermediate reticular zone; MAO, medial accessory olivary nuclei; NTS, nucleus tractus solitarius; PAG, periaqueductal gray; PGCL, paragigantocellularis lateralis nuclei; RO, raphe obscurus; TPH, tryptophan hydroxylase; TPH2, tryptophan hydroxylase 2; Vest, vestibular nucleus; VLM, ventrolateral medulla; XII, hypoglossal nucleus.

Table 26.2: Previously published research investigating serotonin in post-mortem human infant brain tissue in SIDS.

## Substance P

The neuropeptide SP has also been shown to play an integral role in the modulation of homeostatic function in the medulla, including regulation of respiratory rhythm generation (24, 28, 32), integration of cardiovascular control (102), modulation of the baroreceptor reflex (103), and mediation of the chemoreceptor reflex in response to hypoxia (104, 105). Given the extensive role of SP across multiple homeostatic systems, a number of human conditions have been associated with an altered SP/NK1R system within the CNS (106); therefore it is not unreasonable to hypothesize that abnormalities in SP neurotransmission might also result in autonomic dysfunction during sleep and contribute to SIDS deaths. The role of SP in the pathogenesis of SIDS has been previously explored in a number of studies; however, SP expression in SIDS has been variable, even with respect to the normative distributions of SP and its receptor in the human infant brainstem. Among these studies are reports of increased SP immunoreactivity (64, 107-110), lowered expression of SP in fibers and tracts (111), and reports of no change in SP receptor binding density (112, 113) within various brainstem nuclei in SIDS cases compared to controls (Table 26.3).

The definition of SIDS that has been used in these studies has, however, been a significant confounding factor, as many studies either do not cite a definition or provide explanations as to how cases were classified (114-116). SIDS cases that had extended post-mortem intervals have also been included in analyses in some studies. These factors may explain the differences observed among study results and may unfortunately preclude meaningful comparisons. However, recent work by Bright has identified a significant developmental abnormality of SP and NK1R binding in multiple medullary nuclei related to cardiorespiratory function and autonomic control in SIDS cases compared to controls (117). This research provides support for the hypothesis that abnormalities in a multi-neurotransmitter network, and not simply abnormalities in one neurotransmitter system i.e. 5-HT, underlie the pathogenesis of SIDS deaths. Abnormalities were detected not only in brainstem nuclei that were involved in responses to hypoxia, but also in areas that controlled head and neck movement. The latter findings may explain why SIDS infants are unable to lift their heads out of challenging environments.

Experimental animal studies have contributed to the understanding of a potential functional relationship between 5-HT and SP neurotransmission across brainstem-mediated homeostatic control. As noted, the actions of neurotransmitters are determined by the concurrent modulation and interaction with one another, and so deficiencies in one will likely be immediately compensated for by the actions of others (29). Thus, with respect to the pathogenesis of SIDS, the presence of medullary 5-HT dysfunction within critical brainstem regions such as the raphe nuclei may stimulate a compensatory response by SP or may have adverse affects on SP neurotransmission within the same medullary nuclei. Withdrawal or alteration of the combination of 5-HT and SP-mediated homeostatic control within the developing infant brainstem

Table 26.3: Previously published research investigating substance P in post-mortem human infant brain tissue in SIDS.

| Author/Year | Brain region/nuclei analyzed | Objective & method used | Key findings | Definition of SIDS cited |
|---|---|---|---|---|
| *Bergstrom et al. 1984 (108)* | Cortex, medulla oblongata, pons, hypothalamus | Investigate expression of Met-enkephalin and SP. Radioimmunolabeled assay | Significantly increased SP in medulla oblongata of SIDS cases | 12 SIDS, no definition cited |
| *Takashima et al. 1994 (110)* | Brainstem, ventrolateral medulla | Developmental brainstem pathology in SIDS. Golgi and IHC | Increased SP nerve fibres in pons of SIDS cases | 20 SIDS, No definition cited |
| *Yamanouchi et al. 1993 (64)* | Reticular formation, pontine nuclei | IHC | Increased SP in trigeminal fibres in SIDS cases | 20 SIDS, no definition cited |
| *Obonai et al. 1996 (68)* | Medulla oblongata, dorsal vagal, reticular formation, NTS | IHC, cell count analysis | Increased SP in trigeminal nucleus and NTS in SIDS cases | 15 SIDS, no definition cited |
| *Jordan et al. 1997 (112)* | Raphe magnus obscurus, hypoglossal, locus coeruleus, nucleus cuneiformis, NTS, inferior olive, nucleus parabrachialis | Distribution of SP binding density in medulla oblongata. Autoradiography | No significant change in SP binding site density in SIDS cases | 9 SIDS, classified according to criteria from Taylor et al. 1990: *Minor diseases not normally fatal or essentially unexplained* |
| *Sawaguchi et al. 2003 (113)* | Nuclei spinal, mesencephalic and principal sensory nervi trigemini, nucleus parabrachialis | Correlation of sleep apnoea data and SP expression. Polysomnography sleep data, IHC, cell density | No significant correlation between sleep apnoea and density of SP in SIDS cases | 26 SIDS, no definition cited |
| *Biondo et al. 2004 (107)* | NTS | Investigation of functional and morphological alterations in neurons and glia with SP expression | Significant increase in expression of SP in medulla in SIDS cases | 23 SIDS, no definition cited |
| *Lavezzi et al. 2011 (111)* | Medulla oblongata, spinal trigeminal nucleus | SP expression in medulla oblongata | Negative/low SP expression in fibres and tracts of SIDS in sp. trigeminal | 32 SIDS cases, not defined |

Abbreviations: IHC, Immunohistochemistry; NTS, nucleus tractus solitaries; SP, substance P.

could therefore contribute additively to network dysfunction in a subset of SIDS cases. This may explain the inability of a SIDS infant to execute appropriate responses to life-threatening challenges during sleep.

## Neurotransmitters and the Critical Development Period

Development of respiratory control is complex and begins early in gestation, with the respiratory network continually undergoing extensive refinement and adjustment after birth to reach adult levels of maturity. Humans experience a long gestation and prolonged period of postnatal maturation, and therefore infants are vulnerable to the interaction of a number of environmental factors, both prenatally and postnatally, that may expose them to harmful stimuli, including hypoxia, hyperoxia, and/or potential toxins (118, 119). In addition, during development there is an enhanced sensitivity to $CO_2$ which is thought to be, in part, mediated by the transition from fetal to neonatal patterns of breathing (120). Postnatal developmental changes in networks generating respiratory rhythm are likely to occur concurrently across several brainstem nuclei and, therefore, must be well synchronized to prevent any interruption of breathing (22, 121). Adverse events during this "critical period of development" may result in long-term alterations to the structure and function of the respiratory network, including dysfunction of the ventilatory response to a hypoxic challenge (122-124). Alterations during this period are likely to have a greater effect on respiratory control and maturity than insults later in life (122, 124, 125).

At birth a cascade of neurotransmitters and transcriptional factors are activated and there is increasing evidence that these neurotransmitters, neuromodulators, and their receptors function as developmental signals. These signals are important for the maturation of synapses and formation of neuronal networks, by modulating plasticity of brain circuits (121, 126). Shortly after birth, the respiratory system operates under "alert" conditions, defined by increased excitability in central respiratory networks (127), with a switch in dominance from inhibitory to excitatory neurotransmission (54, 128, 129). The various neurochemicals expressed within the respiratory network have been identified to either increase their expression with age (e.g. glutamate, serotonin, norepinephrine, thyrotropin-releasing hormone) or decrease in expression (e.g. GABA, 5-HT1A receptor, SP, NK1R, somatostatin) with age (54).

Animal studies have provided some insight into what may constitute a critical period in the development of the respiratory network. Wong-Riley and Liu (54) reported that the end of the second postnatal week was the most dynamic in the development of brainstem respiratory control in rat pups. However, at postnatal day 12, a dramatic shift occurred, where a transient dominance of inhibitory over excitatory neurotransmission was observed, in addition to multiple neurochemical and physiological adjustments and switches being simultaneously orchestrated. During this period rat pups had a reduced ability to respond to hypoxia and experienced multifaceted development and adjustment of the respiratory system in order for them to successfully transition from neonatal to adult forms of ventilatory control (125).

Extrapolating from animal studies to that of the developing human infant respiratory network has its challenges; however, these studies assist in potentially explaining why 90% of SIDS deaths occur in the first six months of life (3). The peak incidence in SIDS at 2 to 4 months of age (8, 14) may constitute a period of major brainstem respiratory network development in which an infant's abilities to respond and overcome respiratory insults are diminished. Although abnormalities in neurochemicals and their systems, such as that of the medullary 5-HT network in SIDS, are thought to originate during prenatal development (9), the effects of these abnormalities may only present after birth during the early postnatal period (14). However, exactly when changes in the expression and activity of neurotransmitters and neuromodulators occur in the developing human brain is not known at present, nor the extent to which these changes may impact on normal respiration and contribute to increased vulnerability of a SIDS infant. It is unlikely that a critical developmental period ends abruptly; rather, it is likely to taper off gradually. Therefore, identifying when neurochemical switches occur in the human infant brainstem in particular is necessary to fully understand the critical developmental period and potential abnormalities during this time frame.

## Conclusions

Neuropathological investigations have identified significant abnormalities in the development and function of homeostatic networks in the brainstems of SIDS infants. However, there is a need to broaden the scope of SIDS neuropathology research in order to investigate the interaction of multiple neurotransmitters in the brainstems of infants, in addition to further developing animal models. This will be the challenge of the future in order to prevent SIDS deaths from occurring.

## References

1.  Thach B. Tragic and sudden death. Potential and proven mechanisms causing sudden infant death syndrome. EMBO Rep. 2008;9(2):114-8. https://doi.org/10.1038/sj.embor.7401163.

2.  Weese-Mayer DE, Ackerman MJ, Marazita ML, Berry-Kravis EM. Sudden infant death syndrome: Review of implicated genetic factors. Am J Med Genet. 2007;143A(8):771-88. https://doi.org/10.1002/ajmg.a.31722.

3.  Kinney HC. Neuropathology provides new insight in the pathogenesis of the sudden infant death syndrome. Acta Neuropathol. 2009;117(3):247-55. https://doi.org/10.1007/s00401-009-0490-7.

4. Thach BT. The role of respiratory control disorders in SIDS. Resp Physiol Neurobiol. 2005;149(1-3):343-53. https://doi.org/10.1016/j.resp.2005.06.011.

5. Veereman-Wauters G, Bochner A, van Caillie-Bertrand M. Gastroesophageal reflux in infants with a history of near-miss sudden infant death. J Pediatr Gastroenterol Nutr. 1991;12(3):319-23. https://doi.org/10.1097/00005176-199104000-0000.

6. Byard RW, Krous HF. Sudden infant death syndrome: Overview and update. Pediatr Dev Pathol. 2003;6(2):112-27. https://doi.org/10.1007/s10024-002-0205-8.

7. Byard RW. Sudden death in the young. Cambridge, UK: Cambridge University Press, 2010. https://doi.org/10.1017/CBO9780511777783.

8. Kinney HC, Thach BT. The sudden infant death syndrome. New Engl J Med. 2009;361(8):795-805. https://doi.org/10.1056/NEJMra0803836.

9. Harper RM, Kinney HC. Potential mechanisms of failure in the sudden infant death syndrome. Curr Pediatr Rev. 2010;6(1):39-47. https://doi.org/10.2174/157339610791317214.

10. Garcia AJ, Koschnitzky JE, Ramirez J-MM. The physiological determinants of sudden infant death syndrome. Resp Physiol Neurobiol. 2013;189(2):288-300. https://doi.org/10.1016/j.resp.2013.05.032.

11. Filiano JJ, Kinney HC. A perspective on neuropathologic findings in victims of the sudden infant death syndrome: The triple-risk model. Biol Neonate. 1994;65(3-4):194-7. https://doi.org/10.1159/000244052.

12. Naeye RL. Brain-stem and adrenal abnormalities in the sudden-infant-death syndrome. Am J Clin Pathol. 1976;66(3):526-30. https://doi.org/10.1093/ajcp/66.3.526.

13. Kinney HC, Burger PC, Harrell FE, Hudson RP. "Reactive gliosis" in the medulla oblongata of victims of the sudden infant death syndrome. Pediatrics. 1983;72(2):181-7.

14. Kinney HC. Brainstem mechanisms underlying the sudden infant death syndrome: Evidence from human pathologic studies. Dev Psychobiol. 2009;51(3):223-33. https://doi.org/10.1002/dev.20367.

15. Sridhar R, Thach BT, Kelly DH, Henslee JA. Characterization of successful and failed autoresuscitation in human infants, including those dying of SIDS. Pediatr Pulmonol. 2003;36(2):113-22. https://doi.org/10.1002/ppul.10287.

16. Sawaguchi T, Patricia F, Kadhim H, Groswasser J, Sottiaux M, Nishida H, et al. The correlation between serotonergic neurons in the brainstem and sleep apnea in SIDS victims. Early Hum Dev. 2003;75 Suppl:S31-S40. https://doi.org/10.1016/j.earlhumdev.2003.08.006.

17. Poets CF. Apparent life-threatening events and sudden infant death on a monitor. Paediatr Resp Rev. 2004;5 Suppl A:6.

18. Kato I, Franco P, Groswasser J, Scaillet S, Kelmanson I, Togari H, et al. Incomplete arousal processes in infants who were victims of sudden death. Am J Resp Crit Care Med. 2003;168(11):1298-303. https://doi.org/10.1164/rccm.200301-134OC.

19. Poets CF, Meny RG, Chobanian MR, Bonofiglo RE. Gasping and other cardiorespiratory patterns during sudden infant deaths. Pediatr Res. 1999;45(3):350-4. https://doi.org/10.1203/00006450-199903000-00010.

20. Schechtman VL, Lee MY, Wilson AJ, Harper RM. Dynamics of respiratory patterning in normal infants and infants who subsequently died of the sudden infant death syndrome. Pediatr Res. 1996;40(4):571-7. https://doi.org/10.1203/0 0006450-199610000-00010.

21. Franco P, Pardou A, Hassid S, Lurquin P, Groswasser J, Kahn A. Auditory arousal thresholds are higher when infants sleep in the prone position. J Pediatr. 1998;132(2):240-3. https://doi.org/10.1016/S0022-3476(98)70438-X.

22. Feldman JL, Mitchell GS, Nattie EE. Breathing: Rhythmicity, plasticity, chemosensitivity. Ann Rev Neurosci. 2003;26:239-66. https://doi.org/10.1146/annurev.neuro.26.041002.131103.

23. Bianchi AL, Denavit-Saubié M, Champagnat J. Central control of breathing in mammals: Neuronal circuitry, membrane properties, and neurotransmitters. Physiol Rev. 1995;75(1):1-45.

24. Gray PA, Rekling JC, Bocchiaro CM, Feldman JL. Modulation of respiratory frequency by peptidergic input to rhythmogenic neurons in the preBötzinger complex. Science. 1999;286(5444):1566-8. https://doi.org/10.1126/science.286.5444.1566.

25. Greer JJ, Funk GD, Ballanyi K. Preparing for the first breath: Prenatal maturation of respiratory neural control. J Physiol. 2006;570(Pt 3):437-44. https://doi.org/10.1113/jphysiol.2005.097238.

26. Smith JC, Abdala AP, Rybak IA, Paton JF. Structural and functional architecture of respiratory networks in the mammalian brainstem. Philosophical transactions of the Royal Society of London Series B, Biol Sci. 2009;364(1529):2577-87. https://doi.org/10.1098/rstb.2009.0081.

27. Smith JC, Abdala AP, Borgmann A, Rybak IA, Paton JF. Brainstem respiratory networks: Building blocks and microcircuits. Trends Neurosci. 2013;36(3):152-62. https://doi.org/10.1016/j.tins.2012.11.004.

28. Gray PA, Janczewski WA, Mellen N, McCrimmon DR, Feldman JL. Normal breathing requires preBötzinger complex neurokinin-1 receptor-expressing neurons. Nat Neurosci. 2001;4(9):927-30. https://doi.org/10.1038/nn0901-927.

29. Doi A, Ramirez J-MM. State-dependent interactions between excitatory neuromodulators in the neuronal control of breathing. J Neurosci. 2010;30(24):8251-62. https://doi.org/10.1523/JNEUROSCI.5361-09.2010.

30. Ramirez J-MM. The human pre-Bötzinger complex identified. Brain. 2011;134(Pt 1):8-10. https://doi.org/10.1093/brain/awq357.

31. Lieske SP, Thoby-Brisson M, Telgkamp P, Ramirez JM. Reconfiguration of the neural network controlling multiple breathing patterns: Eupnea, sighs and gasps. Nat Neurosci. 2000;3(6):600-7. https://doi.org/10.1038/75776.

32. Telgkamp P, Cao YQ, Basbaum AI, Ramirez J-MM. Long-term deprivation of substance P in PPT-A mutant mice alters the anoxic response of the isolated respiratory network. J Neurophysiol. 2002;88(1):206-13.

33. Wenninger JM, Pan LG, Klum L, Leekley T, Bastastic J, Hodges MR, et al. Large lesions in the pre-Bötzinger complex area eliminate eupneic respiratory rhythm in awake goats. J Appl Physiol. 2004;97(5):1629-36. https://doi.org/10.1152/japplphysiol.00953.2003.

34. McKay LC, Janczewski WA, Feldman JL. Sleep-disordered breathing after targeted ablation of preBötzinger complex neurons. Nat Neurosci. 2005;8(9):1142-4. https://doi.org/10.1038/nn1517.

35. Nattie E. $CO_2$, brainstem chemoreceptors and breathing. Prog Neurobiol. 1999;59(4):299-331. https://doi.org/10.1016/S0301-0082(99)00008-8.

36. Fewell JE. Protective responses of the newborn to hypoxia. Resp Physiol Neurobiol. 2005;149(1-3):243-55. https://doi.org/10.1016/j.resp.2005.05.006.

37. Stornetta RL, Rosin DL, Wang H, Sevigny CP, Weston MC, Guyenet PG. A group of glutamatergic interneurons expressing high levels of both neurokinin-1 receptors and somatostatin identifies the region of the pre-Bötzinger complex. J Comp Neurol. 2003;455(4):499-512. https://doi.org/10.1002/cne.10504.

38. Schwarzacher SW, Rüb U, Deller T. Neuroanatomical characteristics of the human pre-Bötzinger complex and its involvement in neurodegenerative brainstem diseases. Brain. 2011;134(Pt 1):24-35. https://doi.org/10.1093/brain/awq327.

39. Lijowska AS, Reed NW, Chiodini BA, Thach BT. Sequential arousal and airway-defensive behavior of infants in asphyxial sleep environments. J Appl Physiol. 1997;83(1):219-28.

40. McNamara F, Wulbrand H, Thach BT. Characteristics of the infant arousal response. J Appl Physiol. 1998;85(6):2314-21.

41. Gallego J, Matrot B. Arousal response to hypoxia in newborns: Insights from animal models. Biol Psychol. 2010;84(1):39-45. https://doi.org/10.1016/j.biopsycho.2009.12.001.

42. Garcia AJ 3rd, Rotem-Kohavi N, Doi A, Ramirez JM. Post-hypoxic recovery of respiratory rhythm generation is gender dependent. PLoS One. 2013;8(4):e60695. https://doi.org/10.1371/journal.pone.0060695.

43. Harper RM, Kinney HC, Fleming PJ, Thach BT. Sleep influences on homeostatic functions: Implications for sudden infant death syndrome. Resp Physiol. 2000;119(2-3):123-32. https://doi.org/10.1016/S0034-5687(99)00107-3.

44. Paluszynska DA, Harris KA, Thach BT. Influence of sleep position experience on ability of prone-sleeping infants to escape from asphyxiating microenvironments by changing head position. Pediatrics. 2004;114(6):1634-9. https://doi.org/10.1542/peds.2004-0754.

45. Sawaguchi T, Kato I, Franco P, Sottiaux M, Kadhim H, Shimizu S, et al. Apnea, glial apoptosis and neuronal plasticity in the arousal pathway of victims of SIDS. Forensic Sci Int. 2005;149(2-3):205-17. https://doi.org/10.1016/j.forsciint.2004.10.015.

46. Kahn A, Groswasser J, Sottiaux M, Rebuffat E, Franco P, Dramaix M. Prone or supine body position and sleep characteristics in infants. Pediatrics. 1993;91(6):1112-15.

47. Kato I, Groswasser J, Franco P, Scaillet S, Kelmanson I, Togari H, et al. Developmental characteristics of apnea in infants who succumb to sudden infant death syndrome. Am J Respir Crit Care Med. 2001;164(8 Pt 1):1464-9. https://doi.org/10.1164/ajrccm.164.8.2009001.

48. Vege A, Chen Y, Opdal SH, Saugstad OD, Rognum TO. Vitreous humor hypoxanthine levels in SIDS and infectious death. Acta Paediatr. 1994;83(6):634-9. https://doi.org/10.1111/j.1651-2227.1994.tb13096.x.

49. Cutz E, Perrin DG, Pan J, Haas EA, Krous HF. Pulmonary neuroendocrine cells and neuroepithelial bodies in sudden infant death syndrome: Potential markers of airway chemoreceptor dysfunction. Pediatr Dev Pathol. 2007;10(2):106-16. https://doi.org/10.2350/06-06-0113.1.

50. Jones KL, Krous HF, Nadeau J, Blackbourne B, Zielke HR, Gozal D. Vascular endothelial growth factor in the cerebrospinal fluid of infants who died of sudden infant death syndrome: Evidence for antecedent hypoxia. Pediatrics. 2003;111(2):358-63. https://doi.org/10.1542/peds.111.2.358.

51. Machaalani R, Waters KA. Neuronal cell death in the sudden infant death syndrome brainstem and associations with risk factors. Brain. 2008;131(Pt 1):218-28.

52. Jensen LL, Banner J, Ulhøi BP, Byard RW. β-Amyloid precursor protein staining of the brain in sudden infant and early childhood death. Neuropathol Appl Neurobiol. 2014;40(4):385-97. https://doi.org/10.1111/nan.12109.

53. Jensen LL, Banner J, Byard RW. Does β-APP staining of the brain in infant bed-sharing deaths differentiate these cases from sudden infant death syndrome? J Forensic Leg Med. 2014;27:46-9. https://doi.org/10.1016/j.jflm.2014.07.006.

54. Wong-Riley MTT, Liu Q. Neurochemical development of brain stem nuclei involved in the control of respiration. Resp Physiol Neurobiol. 2005;149(1-3):83-98. https://doi.org/10.1016/j.resp.2005.01.011.

55. Burton MD, Kazemi H. Neurotransmitters in central respiratory control. Resp Physiol. 2000;122(2-3):111-21. https://doi.org/10.1016/S0034-5687(00)00153-5.

56. Bonham AC. Neurotransmitters in the CNS control of breathing. Resp Physiol. 1995;101(3):219-30. https://doi.org/10.1016/0034-5687(95)00045-F.

57. Doi A, Ramirez J-MM. Neuromodulation and the orchestration of the respiratory rhythm. Resp Physiol Neurobiol. 2008;164(1-2):96-104. https://doi.org/10.1016/j.resp.2008.06.007.

58. Telgkamp P, Raman IM. Depression of inhibitory synaptic transmission between Purkinje cells and neurons of the cerebellar nuclei. J Neurosci. 2002;22(19):8447-57.

59. Haji A, Takeda R, Okazaki M. Neuropharmacology of control of respiratory rhythm and pattern in mature mammals. Pharmacol Therap. 2000;86(3):277-304. https://doi.org/10.1016/S0163-7258(00)00059-0.

60. Duncan JR, Paterson DS, Kinney HC. The development of nicotinic receptors in the human medulla oblongata: Inter-relationship with the serotonergic system. Autonom Neurosci. 2008;144(1-2):61-75. https://doi.org/10.1016/j.autneu.2008.09.006.

61. Machaalani R, Waters KA. NMDA receptor 1 expression in the brainstem of human infants and its relevance to the sudden infant death syndrome (SIDS). J Neuropathol Exp Neurol. 2003;62(10):1076-85. https://doi.org/10.1093/jnen/62.10.1076.

62. Mallard C, Tolcos M, Leditschke J, Campbell P, Rees S. Reduction in choline acetyltransferase immunoreactivity but not muscarinic-m2 receptor immunoreactivity in the brainstem of SIDS infants. J Neuropathol Exp Neurol. 1999;58(3):255-64. https://doi.org/10.1097/00005072-199903000-00005.

63. Nachmanoff DB, Panigrahy A, Filiano JJ, Mandell F, Sleeper LA, Valdes-Dapena M, et al. Brainstem 3H-nicotine receptor binding in the sudden infant death syndrome. J Neuropathol Exp Neurol. 1998;57(11):1018-25. https://doi.org/10.1097/00005072-199811000-00004.

64. Yamanouchi H, Takashima S, Becker LE. Correlation of astrogliosis and substance P immunoreactivity in the brainstem of victims of sudden infant death syndrome. Neuropediatr. 1993;24(4):200-3. https://doi.org/10.1055/s-2008-1071539.

65. Paterson DS, Trachtenberg FL, Thompson EG, Belliveau RA, Beggs AH, Darnall R, et al. Multiple serotonergic brainstem abnormalities in sudden infant death syndrome. JAMA. 2006;296(17):2124-32. https://doi.org/10.1001/jama.296.17.2124.

66. Kinney HC, Filiano JJ, Sleeper LA, Mandell F, Valdes-Dapena M, White WF. Decreased muscarinic receptor binding in the arcuate nucleus in sudden infant death syndrome. Science. 1995;269(5229):1446-50. https://doi.org/10.1126/science.7660131.

67. Kopp N, Chigr F, Denoroy L, Gilly R, Jordan D. Absence of adrenergic neurons in nucleus tractus solitarius in sudden infant death syndrome. Neuropediatr. 1993;24(1):25-9. https://doi.org/10.1055/s-2008-1071508.

68. Obonai T, Yasuhara M, Nakamura T, Takashima S. Catecholamine neurons alteration in the brainstem of sudden infant death syndrome victims. Pediatrics. 1998;101(2):285-8. https://doi.org/10.1542/peds.101.2.285.

69. Panigrahy A, Filiano JJ, Sleeper LA, Mandell F, Valdes-Dapena M, Krous HF, et al. Decreased kainate receptor binding in the arcuate nucleus of the sudden infant death syndrome. J Neuropathol Exp Neurol. 1997;56(11):1253-61. https://doi.org/10.1097/00005072-199711000-00010.

70. Broadbelt KG, Paterson DS, Belliveau RA, Trachtenberg FL, Haas EA, Stanley C, et al. Decreased GABAA receptor binding in the medullary serotonergic system in the sudden infant death syndrome. J Neuropathol Exp Neurol. 2011;70(9):799-810. https://doi.org/10.1097/NEN.0b013e31822c09bc.

71. Ozawa Y, Takashima S, Tada H. Alpha2-adrenergic receptor subtype alterations in the brainstem in the sudden infant death syndrome. Early Human Dev. 2003;75 Suppl:129-38. https://doi.org/10.1016/j.earlhumdev.2003.08.016.

72. Duncan JR, Paterson DS, Hoffman JM, Mokler DJ, Borenstein NS, Belliveau RA, et al. Brainstem serotonergic deficiency in sudden infant death syndrome. JAMA. 2010;303(5):430-7. https://doi.org/10.1001/jama.2010.45.

73. Chigr F, Jordan D, Najimi M, Denoroy L, Sarrieau A, de Broca A, et al. Quantitative autoradiographic study of somatostatin and neurotensin binding sites in medulla

oblongata of SIDS. Neurochem Int. 1992;20(1):113-18. https://doi.org/10.1016/0197-0186(92)90134-D.

74. Carpentier V, Vaudry H, Mallet E, Laquerriére A, Leroux P. Increased density of somatostatin binding sites in respiratory nuclei of the brainstem in sudden infant death syndrome. Neurosci. 1998;86(1):159-66. https://doi.org/10.1016/S0306-4522(98)00002-5.

75. Machaalani R, Say M, Waters KA. Effects of cigarette smoke exposure on nicotinic acetylcholine receptor subunits α7 and β2 in the sudden infant death syndrome (SIDS) brainstem. Toxicol Appl Pharmacol. 2011;257(3):396-404. https://doi.org/10.1016/j.taap.2011.09.023.

76. Tang S, Machaalani R, Waters KA. Expression of brain-derived neurotrophic factor and TrkB receptor in the sudden infant death syndrome brainstem. Resp Physiol Neurobiol. 2012;180(1):25-33. https://doi.org/10.1016/j.resp.2011.10.004.

77. Rognum IJ, Haynes RL, Vege A, Yang M, Rognum TO, Kinney HC. Interleukin-6 and the serotonergic system of the medulla oblongata in the sudden infant death syndrome. Acta Neuropathol. 2009;118(4):519-30. https://doi.org/10.1007/s00401-009-0535-y.

78. Kadhim H, Kahn A, Sébire G. Distinct cytokine profile in SIDS braIn: A common denominator in a multifactorial syndrome? Neurology. 2003;61(9):1256-9. https://doi.org/10.1212/01.WNL.0000092014.14997.47.

79. Kubo S, Orihara Y, Gotohda T, Tokunaga I, Tsuda R, Ikematsu K, et al. [Immunohistochemical studies on neuronal changes in brain stem nucleus of forensic autopsied cases. II. Sudden infant death syndrome]. Jap J Leg Med. 1998;52(6):350-4.

80. Kinney HC, Rognum TO, Nattie EE, Haddad GG, Hyma B, McEntire B, et al. Sudden and unexpected death in early life: Proceedings of a symposium in honor of Dr Henry F Krous. Forensic science, medicine, and pathology. 2012;8(4):414-25. https://doi.org/10.1007/s12024-012-9376-4.

81. Paterson DS, Hilaire G, Weese-Mayer DE. Medullary serotonin defects and respiratory dysfunction in sudden infant death syndrome. Resp Physiol Neurobiol. 2009;168(1-2):133-43. https://doi.org/10.1016/j.resp.2009.05.010.

82. Haxhiu MA, Tolentino-Silva F, Pete G, Kc P, Mack SO. Monoaminergic neurons, chemosensation and arousal. Resp Physiol. 2001;129(1-2):191-209. https://doi.org/10.1016/S0034-5687(01)00290-0.

83. Molliver ME. Serotonergic neuronal systems: What their anatomic organization tells us about function. J Clin Psychopharm. 1987;7(6 Suppl):3S-23S. https://doi.org/10.1097/00004714-198712001-00002.

84. Azmitia EC. Serotonin neurons, neuroplasticity, and homeostasis of neural tissue. Neuropsychopharm. 1999;21(2 Suppl):33S-45S. https://doi.org/10.1016/S0893-133X(99)00022-6.

85. Kinney HC, Richerson GB, Dymecki SM, Darnall RA, Nattie EE. The brainstem and serotonin in the sudden infant death syndrome. Ann Rev Pathol. 2009;4:517-50. https://doi.org/10.1146/annurev.pathol.4.110807.092322.

86. Kinney HC, Broadbelt KG, Haynes RL, Rognum IJ, Paterson DS. The serotonergic anatomy of the developing human medulla oblongata: Implications for pediatric disorders of homeostasis. J Chem Neuroanat. 2011;41(4):182-99. https://doi.org/10.1016/j.jchemneu.2011.05.004.

87. Tork IH, Hornung J-P. Raphe nuclei and the serotonergic system. In: The human nervous system. Ed Paxinos G. San Diego: Academic Press, Inc, 1990. p. 1001-22. https://doi.org/10.1016/B978-0-12-547625-6.50035-0.

88. Richter DW, Manzke T, Wilken B, Ponimaskin E. Serotonin receptors: Guardians of stable breathing. Trends Mol Med. 2003;9(12):542-8. https://doi.org/10.1016/j.molmed.2003.10.010.

89. Barnes NM, Sharp T. A review of central 5-HT receptors and their function. Neuropharm. 1999;38(8):1083-152. https://doi.org/10.1016/S0028-3908(99)00010-6.

90. Manaker S, Tischler LJ. Origin of serotoninergic afferents to the hypoglossal nucleus in the rat. J Comp Neurol. 1993;334(3):466-76. https://doi.org/10.1002/cne.903340310.

91. Richerson GB. Serotonergic neurons as carbon dioxide sensors that maintain pH homeostasis. Nat Rev Neurosci. 2004;5(6):449-61. https://doi.org/10.1038/nrn1409.

92. Corcoran AE, Hodges MR, Wu Y, Wang W, Wylie CJ, Deneris ES, et al. Medullary serotonin neurons and central $CO_2$ chemoreception. Resp Physiol Neurobiol. 2009;168(1-2):49-58. https://doi.org/10.1016/j.resp.2009.04.014.

93. Morin D, Hennequin S, Monteau R, Hilaire G. Serotonergic influences on central respiratory activity: An in vitro study in the newborn rat. Brain Res. 1990;535(2):281-7. https://doi.org/10.1016/0006-8993(90)91611-J.

94. Messier ML, Li A, Nattie EE. Inhibition of medullary raphe serotonergic neurons has age-dependent effects on the $CO_2$ response in newborn piglets. J Appl Physiol. 2004;96(5):1909-19. https://doi.org/10.1152/japplphysiol.00805.2003.

95. Panigrahy A, Filiano J, Sleeper LA, Mandell F, Valdes-Dapena M, Krous HF, et al. Decreased serotonergic receptor binding in rhombic lip-derived regions of

the medulla oblongata in the sudden infant death syndrome. J Neuropathol Exp Neurol. 2000;59(5):377-84. https://doi.org/10.1093/jnen/59.5.377.

96. Kinney HC, Randall LL, Sleeper LA, Willinger M, Belliveau RA, Zec N, et al. Serotonergic brainstem abnormalities in Northern Plains Indians with the sudden infant death syndrome. J Neuropathol Exp Neurol. 2003;62(11):1178-91. https://doi.org/10.1093/jnen/62.11.1178.

97. Ozawa Y, Okado N. Alteration of serotonergic receptors in the brain stems of human patients with respiratory disorders. Neuropediatr. 2002;33(3):142-9. https://doi.org/10.1055/s-2002-33678.

98. Machaalani R, Say M, Waters KA. Serotoninergic receptor 1A in the sudden infant death syndrome brainstem medulla and associations with clinical risk factors. Acta Neuropathol. 2009;117(3):257-65. https://doi.org/10.1007/s00401-008-0468-x.

99. Kinney HC. Abnormalities of the brainstem serotonergic system in the sudden infant death syndrome: A review. Pediatr Dev Pathol. 2005;8(5):507-24. https://doi.org/10.1007/s10024-005-0067-y.

100. Broadbelt KG, Rivera KD, Paterson DS, Duncan JR, Trachtenberg FL, Paulo JA, et al. Brainstem deficiency of the 14-3-3 regulator of serotonin synthesis: A proteomics analysis in the sudden infant death syndrome. Mol Cell Proteomics. 2012;11(1). https://doi.org/10.1074/mcp.M111.009530.

101. Panigrahy A, Filiano J, Sleeper LA, Mandell F, Valdes-Dapena M, Krous HF, et al. Decreased serotonergic receptor binding in rhombic lip-derived regions of the medulla oblongata in the sudden infant death syndrome. J Neuropathol Exp Neurol. 2000;59(5):377-84. https://doi.org/10.1093/jnen/59.5.377.

102. Morilak DA, Morris M, Chalmers J. Release of substance P in the nucleus tractus solitarius measured by in vivo microdialysis: Response to stimulation of the aortic depressor nerves in rabbit. Neurosci Lett. 1988;94(1-2):131-7. https://doi.org/10.1016/0304-3940(88)90283-2.

103. Seagard JL, Dean C, Hopp FA. Modulation of the carotid baroreceptor reflex by substance P in the nucleus tractus solitarius. J Auton Nerv Syst. 2000;78(2-3):77-85. https://doi.org/10.1016/S0165-1838(99)00060-0.

104. Lessard A, Coleman CG, Pickel VM. Chronic intermittent hypoxia reduces neurokinin-1 (NK(1)) receptor density in small dendrites of non-catecholaminergic neurons in mouse nucleus tractus solitarius. Exp Neurol. 2010;223(2):634-44. https://doi.org/10.1016/j.expneurol.2010.02.013.

105. Nichols NL, Powell FL, Dean JB, Putnam RW. Substance P differentially modulates firing rate of solitary complex (SC) neurons from control and chronic

hypoxia-adapted adult rats. PloS One. 2014;9(2). https://doi.org/10.1371/journal.pone.0088161.

106. Muñoz M, Coveñas R. Involvement of substance P and the NK-1 receptor in human pathology. Amino Acids. 2014;46(7):1727-50. https://doi.org/10.1007/s00726-014-1736-9.

107. Biondo B, Magagnin S, Bruni B, Cazzullo A, Tosi D, Matturri L. Glial and neuronal alterations in the nucleus tractus solitarii of sudden infant death syndrome victims. Acta Neuropathol. 2004;108(4):309-18. https://doi.org/10.1007/s00401-004-0895-2.

108. Bergström L, Lagercrantz H, Terenius L. Post-mortem analyses of neuropeptides in brains from sudden infant death victims. Brain Res. 1984;323(2):279-85. https://doi.org/10.1016/0006-8993(84)90298-1.

109. Obonai T, Takashima S, Becker LE, Asanuma M, Mizuta R, Horie H, et al. Relationship of substance P and gliosis in medulla oblongata in neonatal sudden infant death syndrome. Pediatr Neurol. 1996;15(3):189-92. https://doi.org/10.1016/S0887-8994(96)00217-2.

110. Takashima S, Mito T, Yamanouchi H. Developmental brain-stem pathology in sudden infant death syndrome. Acta Paediatr Jap. 1994;36(3):317-20. https://doi.org/10.1111/j.1442-200X.1994.tb03191.x.

111. Lavezzi AM, Mehboob R, Matturri L. Developmental alterations of the spinal trigeminal nucleus disclosed by substance P immunohistochemistry in fetal and infant sudden unexplained deaths. Neuropathol. 2011;31(4):405-13. https://doi.org/10.1111/j.1440-1789.2010.01190.x.

112. Jordan D, Kermadi I, Rambaud C, Bouvier R, Dijoud F, Martin D, et al. Autoradiographic distribution of brainstem substance P binding sites in humans: Ontogenic study and relation to sudden infant death syndrome (SIDS). J Neural Trans. 1997;104(10):1101-5. https://doi.org/10.1007/BF01273322.

113. Sawaguchi T, Ozawa Y, Patricia F, Kadhim H, Groswasser J, Sottiaux M, et al. Substance P in the midbrains of SIDS victims and its correlation with sleep apnea. Early Hum Dev. 2003;75(Suppl 9):S51-9. https://doi.org/10.1016/j.earlhumdev.2003.08.008.

114. Krous HF, Beckwith JB, Byard RW, Rognum TO, Bajanowski T, Corey T, et al. Sudden infant death syndrome and unclassified sudden infant deaths: A definitional and diagnostic approach. Pediatrics. 2004;114(1):234-8. https://doi.org/10.1542/peds.114.1.234.

115. Byard RW, Marshall D. An audit of the use of definitions of sudden infant death syndrome (SIDS). J Forensic Leg Med. 2007;14(8):453-5. https://doi.org/10.1016/j.jflm.2006.11.003.

116. Byard RW, Lee V. A re-audit of the use of definitions of sudden infant death syndrome (SIDS) in peer-reviewed literature. J Forensic Leg Med. 2012;19(8):455-6. https://doi.org/10.1016/j.jflm.2012.04.004.

117. Bright F. Expression of substance P and the tachykinin NK1 receptor in the medullary serotonergic network of the human infant during development; implications for sudden infant death syndrome (SIDS) [PhD]. Adelaide: University of Adelaide (Australia), 2017.

118. Carroll JL. Developmental plasticity in respiratory control. J Appl Physiol. 2003;94(1):375-89. https://doi.org/10.1152/japplphysiol.00809.2002.

119. Bavis RW, Olson EB Jr, Mitchell GS. Critical developmental period for hyperoxia-induced blunting of hypoxic phrenic responses in rats. J Appl Physiol. 2002;92(3):1013-18. https://doi.org/10.1152/japplphysiol.00859.2001.

120. Wickström HR, Holgert H, Hökfelt T, Lagercrantz H. Birth-related expression of c-fos, c-jun and substance P mRNAs in the rat brainstem and pia mater: Possible relationship to changes in central chemosensitivity. Brain Res Dev Brain Res. 1999;112(2):255-66. https://doi.org/10.1016/S0165-3806(98)00174-6.

121. Herlenius E, Lagercrantz H. Development of neurotransmitter systems during critical periods. Exp Neurol. 2004;190(Suppl 1):21. https://doi.org/10.1016/j.expneurol.2004.03.027.

122. Carroll JL. Developmental plasticity in respiratory control. J Appl Physiol. 2003;94(1):375-89. https://doi.org/10.1152/japplphysiol.00809.2002.

123. Liu Q, Wong-Riley MTT. Postnatal developmental expressions of neurotransmitters and receptors in various brain stem nuclei of rats. J Appl Physiol. 2005;98(4):1442-57. https://doi.org/10.1152/japplphysiol.01301.2004.

124. Liu Q, Wong-Riley MTT. Postnatal expression of neurotransmitters, receptors, and cytochrome oxidase in the rat pre-Bötzinger complex. J Appl Physiol. 2002;92(3):923-34. https://doi.org/10.1152/japplphysiol.00977.2001.

125. Wong-Riley MTT, Liu Q. Neurochemical and physiological correlates of a critical period of respiratory development in the rat. Resp Physiol Neurobiol. 2008;164(1-2):28-37. https://doi.org/10.1016/j.resp.2008.04.014.

126. Gaspar P, Cases O, Maroteaux L. The developmental role of serotonIn: News from mouse molecular genetics. Nat Rev Neurosci. 2003;4(12):1002-12. https://doi.org/10.1038/nrn1256.

127. Shvarev YN, Lagercrantz H. Early postnatal changes in respiratory activity in rat in vitro and modulatory effects of substance P. Euro J Neurosci. 2006;24(8):2253-63. https://doi.org/10.1111/j.1460-9568.2006.05087.x.

128. Moss IR, Inman JG. Neurochemicals and respiratory control during development. J Appl Physiol. 1989;67(1):1-13.

129. Lagercrantz H. Neuromodulators and respiratory control in the infant. Clin Perinatol. 1987;14(3):683-95.

# 27

# Sudden Infant Death Syndrome, Sleep, and the Physiology and Pathophysiology of the Respiratory Network

Jan-Marino Ramirez, PhD[1,2],
Sanja C Ramirez[1] and
Tatiana M Anderson, PhD[1]

[1]Center for Integrative Brain Research, Seattle Children's
Research Institute, Seattle, USA
[2]Departments of Neurological Surgery, Pediatrics,
University of Washington, Seattle, USA

## Introduction

The identification of risk factors associated with sudden infant death syndrome (SIDS) has led to significant advances in the prevention of this tragic outcome. The discovery of the prone sleeping position and smoking as two of the major risk factors (1-5) led to worldwide awareness campaigns, such as, for example, the "Back to Sleep" campaign launched in the United States in 1996, and various smoking cessation campaigns (6, 7). These initiatives resulted in a dramatic reduction in the number of children succumbing to SIDS (5, 8). Unfortunately, SIDS still remains the number-one cause of death in infants under 1 year of age in many countries, despite epidemiological and pathological studies that continue to identify additional risk factors, such as hearing deficiencies, or various genetic alterations associated with SIDS (9-11, 12, 13). To parents and families, as well as some health professionals and researchers, the sheer number of suggested risk factors and gene mutations can also be bewildering.

The Triple Risk hypothesis by Dr Hannah Kinney and collaborators (14) can partly resolve this confusion. This hypothesis states that SIDS is caused by an incident in which not just one but three risk factors come together to bring an infant into a situation that leads to the sudden death. Specifically, it was proposed that those factors include [1] a vulnerable infant; [2] a critical period of development in homeostatic control; and [3] an exogenous stressor (14, 15). In other words, in the presence of two risk factors, namely being a vulnerable infant in a critical period of development, a third risk factor (e.g. an exogenous stressor) can become the ultimate cause that triggers an irreversible cascade of events leading to the sudden death.

The Triple Risk hypothesis also has important practical implications. The awareness campaigns have shown that it is possible to significantly reduce the risk of an infant being exposed to exogenous stressors. A potentially more challenging task is to identify the infant who is particularly vulnerable, which is clearly one of the major tasks for research. A better understanding of the characteristics of a vulnerable infant would facilitate the development of strategies that target a specific vulnerability. Similarly, it will be important for research to identify and recognize the specific developmental conditions that characterize the critical period for SIDS, especially if they are dysregulated, or to target the important developmental and homeostatic mechanisms to prevent the death. This chapter will describe how different risk factors can contribute to the sudden death, the failure to arouse, the specific conditions associated with sleep, and the neuronal networks controlling cardiorespiratory functions and how they contribute to the events leading to sudden death. In this context we will review the physiology and pathophysiology of important brainstem mechanisms that are critical for survival, but that can sometimes fail. Understanding how these brainstem mechanisms interact with endogenous and exogenous mechanisms can also facilitate understanding of the significance of a variety of risk factors known to contribute to SIDS.

## Sleep and its Implications for SIDS

One of the developmental risk factors for SIDS is sleep, and indeed many SIDS victims die during the morning hours of sleep (16, 17). Infants at the age when SIDS occurs quite frequently spend most of their sleep in a stage known as rapid eye movement or REM sleep. This sleep stage is characterized by the dysregulation of various mechanosensory airway and chemosensory autonomous reflexes that are critical for survival (18, 19). A dysregulation of mechanosensory pathways could be detrimental, since these afferent inputs contribute to a phasic activation of the genioglossus (an extrinsic muscle in the tongue) during inspiration. The phasic activation is critical for keeping the upper airways open during the inspiratory phase and for preventing the pharynx from collapsing during REM sleep (20-24). A role of airway dysfunction and collapse during sleep has been implicated as one of the mechanisms contributing to SIDS (25, 26).

Aside from the effect of sleep on sensory pathways, we know that the release of neurotransmitters and neuromodulators also contributes to the potential complications associated with sleep. The activation of glutamatergic, glycinergic, and gamma-aminobutyric acid (GABA) ergic mechanisms, for example, inhibits premotor neurons projecting to the hypoglossus nucleus in the brainstem, which innervates the genioglossus (27-31). REM sleep is also characterized by decreased activity of neurons that release serotonin (5-HT) or norepinephrine (32). A decrease in activity of noradrenergic and serotonergic neurons (33-35) during REM sleep is particularly significant for understanding SIDS, since disturbances in serotonergic and noradrenergic mechanisms have been implicated as important factors that make a child vulnerable to SIDS (9, 36-39). The REM-specific alterations in reflexes and neuromodulatory control contribute to the vulnerability of an infant to stressors that would not be dangerous in wakefulness or for an older child that developed well-co-ordinated motor behaviors, which allow a child to better cope with dangerous situations occurring during sleep.

Yet not only REM, but also the other sleep stage, namely deep sleep or "slow wave sleep" (SWS), can be challenging to an infant. Specifically, the neuromodulatory milieu during SWS can facilitate the generation of central apneas — that is, periods of breathing cessation that are caused by the central nervous system (40). Indeed, apneas are common in infants, in particular those born prematurely.

Perhaps not surprisingly, healthy children have evolved protective mechanisms that help to overcome dangerous situations which frequently occur during sleep. For example, a child sleeping in a prone position can face a situation in which it breathes into a pillow. This situation, referred to as "rebreathing", will quickly lead to decreased levels of oxygen (hypoxia) and increased levels of carbon dioxide ($CO_2$, hypercapnia) (3, 4, 41, 42) (Figure 27.1).

In response to these conditions, a healthy infant will arouse, and as long as the infant can avoid rebreathing by moving its head into a safe position, it will survive. However, two principle scenarios could lead to an infant's death. First, if the healthy infant cannot escape this situation (e.g. if the infant is covered by heavy blankets), this natural arousal response will not be effective and the infant will suffocate. It should be expected that a suffocation event should not have a gender bias, and could affect male and female infants with a similar likelihood. Alternatively, if the infant is not healthy and/or vulnerable due to various potential risk factors including a genetic brainstem abnormality and/or living in a smoking environment, this vulnerable infant may not arouse and may die in situations that would arouse a healthy infant. It is, for example, conceivable that an infant with a serotonin-abnormality might have a blunted arousal response, which becomes significant if challenged during REM sleep when serotonergic neurons are less active. However, this vulnerable infant would survive if it was never

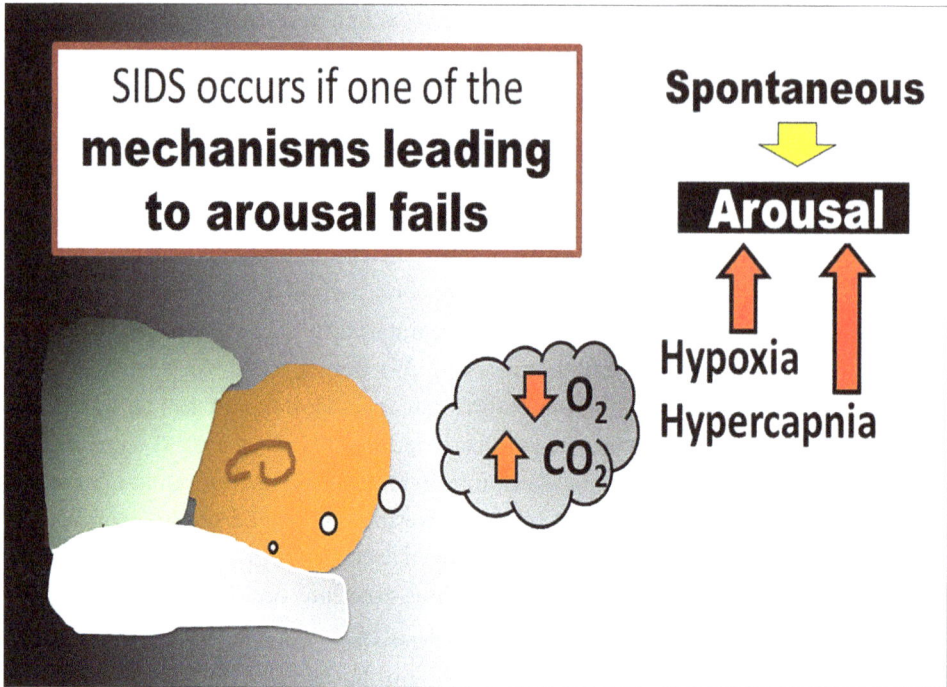

Figure 27.1: The failure to arouse in the presence of a hypoxic challenge can lead to SIDS. Placing an infant in the prone position to sleep increases the risk of the child rebreathing into a pillow or other bedding. Healthy infants employ protective mechanisms to spontaneously arouse and move their head in response to a decrease in oxygen (hypoxia), and the subsequent build-up in carbon dioxide (hypercapnia). However, a vulnerable infant, perhaps one with abnormal serotonin expression in the brainstem or one who is regularly exposed to cigarette smoke, may have a blunted arousal response and fail to autoresuscitate during a hypoxic challenge. A vulnerable child will likely survive if they are never placed in a position in which these protective responses are required. This underscores the importance of placing a child prone on a firm mattress without excessive bedding. (Authors' own work.)

put into a challenging condition that requires those protective arousal responses. These considerations could explain, for example, why a "Back to Sleep" campaign could result in such a dramatic reduction in SIDS deaths, because it reduced the number of vulnerable infants being challenged by the prone sleeping position.

## The Arousal Response

The protective responses leading to arousal have been well studied and they point toward mechanisms that are deeply rooted within the brainstem. These responses are very stereotypic and begin with the generation of a sigh, sometimes also called an "augmented breath". The generation of sighs is followed by increased somatic activity, heart rate change, and often also a sleep state transition (43-45). Thach and colleagues performed a series of experiments on healthy, sleeping infants to demonstrate that arousal from a variety of stimuli begins with a sigh, followed by trashing movements, eye opening, and the repositioning of the head (46-48). Interestingly, these investigators also observed that spontaneous arousals begin with the generation of a sigh (48, 49).

Additionally, studies suggest that infants that succumb to SIDS exhibit a lower frequency of sighs during sleep in contrast to age-matched controls (50). For our understanding of the events leading to SIDS, it is important to emphasize that sighs are very sensitive to changes in blood gases, in particular hypoxia (51-56). As will be described below, this chemical sensitivity seems to be mediated centrally within the lower brainstem in the ventrolateral medulla (56). More recently it has been demonstrated that the mechanisms linking the sigh with arousal involve a close association between the neurons controlling the sigh and the so-called C1-neurons, noradrenergic neurons that mediate arousal, and changes in cortical states (57). These are important considerations for understanding the events leading to SIDS, since we know from prospective studies that spontaneous and induced arousals from sleep are reduced in infants who died of SIDS (16, 58-62).

An important aspect of this behavioral sequence is the coupling between the respiratory behavior and heart rate control. During the inspiratory phase of the sigh, heart rate increases, which is followed by a heart rate decrease during the expiratory phase of the sigh (47, 63-66). Thach and colleagues observed that the larger the heart rate change during the sigh, the more likely it was that an infant would arouse (48, 67). Again, this is a critical finding for understanding the events leading to SIDS, since decreased heart rate variability during the sigh was characteristic for infants that later died of SIDS (50, 68, 69).

Although the link between sigh and arousal is the first line of defense against a hypoxic situation, it is not the last chance to arouse. While sighs are evoked by even slight changes in hypoxia, severe hypoxic conditions will lead to the activation of gasps, which are also associated with heart rate changes and arousal in healthy infants (70). Like the generation of the sigh as the first line of defense, the generation of gasping also follows a very stereotypic transition from normal breathing, also referred to as "eupnea" (71-73). Gasping consists of isolated, rapid inspiratory efforts that are not followed by expirations (71, 72, 74, 75), but like sighs are associated with rapid heart rate changes (73). In some children who died of SIDS, gasping was apparently not associated with heart rate changes, or the number of gasps was very low and ineffective at triggering autoresuscitation (72). Exogenous stressors can further aggravate the situation, such as increased ambient temperature, one of the risk factors for SIDS, which decreases oxygen saturation, increases arousal threshold, and decreases gasping (76-78). Failure to arouse from gasping will result in irreversible events, leading to severe hypoxic damage in the brain, heart failure, and ultimately death.

In conclusion, the defense against a hypoxic exposure follows a two-stage stereotypic sequence of events. At the first sign of hypoxia, sighs are initiated that are followed by movements and arousal. If the arousal is unsuccessful and the hypoxic conditions become more severe, gasps are initiated that are the second and last step to autoresuscitate. However, once gasping occurs any abnormality in the autoresuscitation response will quickly be fatal, as the infant's breathing will cease, followed shortly by cessation of their heartbeat.

## The Control of Breathing and Heart Rate, and the Concept of Brainstem Microcircuits

Ultimately any death is caused by a *loss of cardiorespiratory control* that results in the cessation of breathing and heartbeat. The cardiorespiratory system is controlled by the central nervous system in specific brainstem regions located within the ventrolateral medulla. An emerging concept is that each of these brainstem regions has specialized roles in controlling breathing and heartbeat. Indeed, we refer to each of these regions as a "microcircuit" that is imbued with cellular properties, synaptic and intrinsic membrane properties that generate a specific aspect of cardiorespiratory control (79). Among the microcircuits that have been identified are three networks that each control one particular phase of breathing: the preBötzinger complex (preBötC) which controls inspiration (80), the postinspiratory complex (PiCo) which controls postinspiratory activity (81), and a subset of the parafacial respiratory group (lateral parafacial, $pF_L$) controlling active expiration (82, 83) (Figure 27.2).

Other brainstem areas are specialized to control heartbeat; they include the nucleus ambiguus (NA), a nucleus that contains cardiac vagal neurons and exerts parasympathetic control of the heart, and the retrotrapezoidal nucleus (RTN), containing Phox-2B neurons, which have a strong influence on sympathetic control of the heart. The RTN neurons are also critical for sensing $CO_2$ (84-88). A second area that has also been implicated in the control of $CO_2$ sensing is the raphe nucleus, which contains GABAergic and serotonergic neurons (89, 90). The nucleus tractus solitarius (NTS), in the dorsal medulla, receives important peripheral sensory information (e.g. from the carotid body), which is very sensitive to changes in blood oxygen levels (91-94). Recent findings suggest that the neurons of the NTS are essential for the processing and co-ordination of respiratory and sympathetic responses to hypoxia (95). Furthermore, various noradrenergic nuclei, such as the C1 region, are critical for the control of arousal and the sleep-wake cycle, as mentioned above. Functional cardiorespiratory control requires the tight and operative co-ordination between these important lower brainstem microcircuits.

There are many additional important microcircuits that also play critical roles in the homeostatic regulation of breathing and the heart. These can be found not only in the medulla and the pons, but also in the cerebellum, neocortex, hippocampus, amygdala,

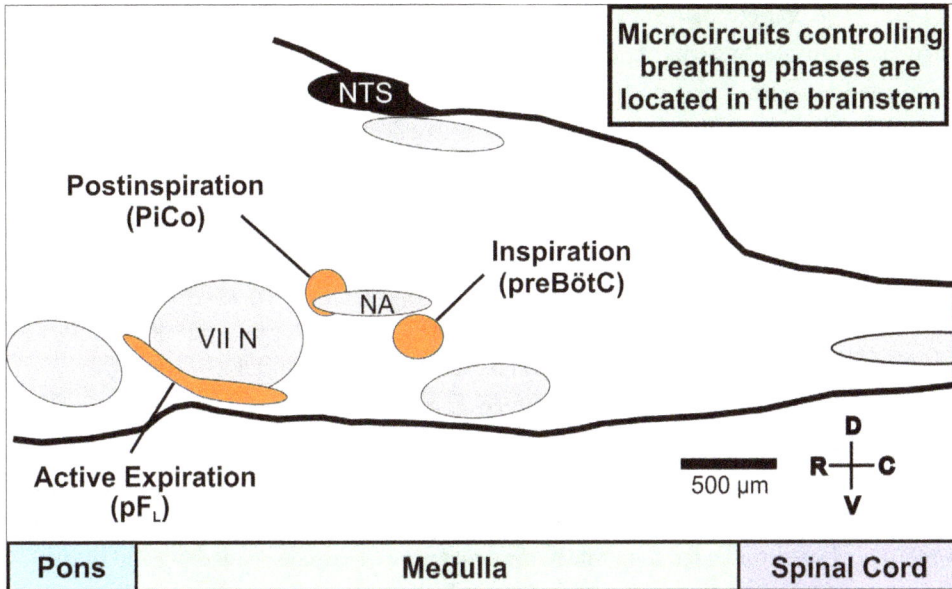

Figure 27.2: Breathing control networks are located in the ventral brainstem. Distinct microcircuits in the ventral lateral medulla of the brainstem are thought to individually control the three phases of breathing. This figure illustrates a schematic from sagittal view of a mouse brainstem. Specifically, the preBötzinger Complex (preBötC) is responsible for controlling inspiration, the postinspiratory complex (PiCo) controls postinspiratory activity, and lateral parafacial neurons ($pF_L$) control active expiration. The breathing networks functionally integrate with cardiac vagal neurons in the nucleus ambiguus (NA), referred to as cardiorespiratory coupling. Additionally, the nucleus tractus solitarius (NTS), located in the dorsal medulla, helps to co-ordinate respiratory and sympathetic responses to hypoxia. Grey shapes represent various motornuclei; VII N = facial motor nucleus. (Authors' own work.)

the hypothalamus, and the periaqueductal gray (PAG) (96-103). Each of these areas has specific roles in the control of breathing and heart rate, but it would exceed the scope of this chapter to discuss all possible interactions of the respiratory network. Suffice to say, respiration is probably one of the most integrated behaviors of all. Indeed, the cerebellum and hippocampus in particular have been implicated in SIDS as well as in sudden unexplained death in childhood (104-109).

## The preBötzinger complex and the control of inspiration

Perhaps the best-understood microcircuit controlling breathing is the so-called preBötC, a well-defined brainstem region known to be critical for the generation of inspiration (80, 110, 111). Lesioning of this microcircuit leads to the cessation of breathing

(112-115). A variety of disorders associated with breathing abnormalities and death, such as Multiple Systems Atrophy (MSA), have been associated with pathological abnormalities within the preBötC (110). Indeed, as early as 1976 Naeye described pathological abnormalities in the form of astrogliosis in SIDS victims in areas that overlap with those now known to co-localize with the preBötC (116).

The preBötC was first anatomically defined by its rich staining for the neurokinin receptor NK1, a receptor that is targeted by endogenously released substance P (117). Another marker was somatostatin, as described by Stornetta et al. (118). With the advance of molecular and genetic techniques, it became possible to identify the neurons critical for the generation of inspiration based on a transcription factor, Dbx1 (119, 120). These Dbx1 neurons seem to be critical for the generation of inspiration (119, 121). A subset of Dbx1 neurons located more dorsal to, and partially overlapping with, the preBötC form the premotor neurons that innervate the hypoglossal nucleus (121, 122). The identification of these neurons allowed the optogenetic manipulation of these neurons, which clearly demonstrated their role in the generation of inspiratory activity and breathing in general (123, 124). However, the preBötC also contains inhibitory neurons, which are important not only for the generation of inspiration, but also for the afferent control of the preBötC (125, 126).

Important for the role of the preBötC in the events leading to SIDS is its ability to reconfigure into different states. Under normal baseline conditions, the preBötC contributes to the generation of normal breathing (also referred to as eupnea). However, the preBötC also spontaneously generates sighs. It is interesting to note that babies sigh every few minutes, and even more frequently right after birth (127, 128). Adult humans continue to sigh in a regular manner, but not as frequently as infants (129, 130, 131). An interesting mechanistic question is how the same neuronal circuitry in the preBötC can generate at the same time both the fast eupneic breathing rhythm and the slow, yet very regular sigh rhythm. Lieske et al. 2000 demonstrated that the majority of neurons in this microcircuit are activated during both eupneic and sigh activity. What seems to drive these differences are cellular mechanisms that differentially control sighs versus eupneic activity (132, 133). It has, for example, been demonstrated that sighs are exquisitely sensitive to a specific calcium channel subtype (P/Q-type channel) that is critical for glutamatergic, i.e. excitatory, synaptic transmission (132). It is noteworthy that mutating this particular channel subtype in an animal model does not affect normal breathing, but abolishes the ability to sigh. These animals ultimately die, which is interesting in the context of SIDS (134). Another aspect worth considering is that eupneic and sigh activity are differentially modulated by neuromodulators that are differentially expressed in sleep. Acetylcholine acting on muscarinic receptors activates sighs but inhibits eupneic activity (135). Serotonin and substance P, which have both been implicated in SIDS, activate sighs (136, 137). However, to what extent a disturbance in serotonin and substance P, as demonstrated for SIDS, also affects the ability to sigh, remains unknown.

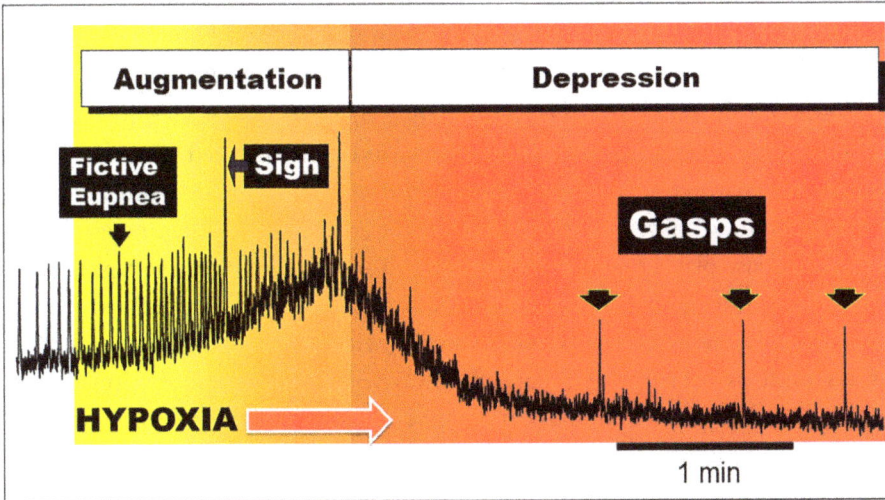

**The hypoxic response of the isolated preBötzinger complex**

Augmentation

Depression

Fictive Eupnea

Sigh

Gasps

HYPOXIA

1 min

Figure 27.3: The isolated preBötzinger complex network reconfigures in response to hypoxia. During normal oxygenation, the preBötzinger complex autonomously generates a rhythmic, fictive eupneic pattern of activity. When exposed to hypoxia, the network responds by initiating an augmentation period typified by an increase in eupneic burst frequency and the generation of sighs. This period is followed by a secondary depressive phase in which gasps are generated. This response pattern of the preBötzinger complex is thought to be the neuronal correlate to the stereotypical hypoxic response observed in humans. (Authors' own work.)

The preBötC also reconfigures in response to hypoxia. Even following isolation, this microcircuit responds to reduced oxygen levels with an initial augmentation and the generation of sighs, followed by a secondary depression and the generation of gasps (Figure 27.3). Thus, the stereotypic response to hypoxia as described above has, to a certain extent, a neuronal correlate within this small neuronal network. Much has been learned about the neurons involved in the generation of the gasps in the preBötC and its underlying cellular mechanisms (70, 138).

## The preBötzinger complex and the raphe nucleus

The preBötC receives important inputs from other microcircuits in other brainstem regions, such as the raphe nucleus, which provides critical neuromodulatory drive to the preBötC. Among the neuromodulators released by the raphe is serotonin, which plays a critical role in stimulating respiratory activity via the 5-HT$_{2A}$ and NK1 receptors, respectively (139). Disturbances in both of these neuromodulators have been implicated in SIDS. It has been specifically hypothesized that a loss of serotonergic drive could lead to the loss of activity in neurons that are required for the generation of gasping or sighing (138, 70). This is a significant observation because sighing and gasping are important behaviors that contribute to the arousal response, as previously mentioned.

However, it is important to emphasize that the raphe nucleus is a microcircuit in itself. This means that the disturbances that have been associated with SIDS cannot be simply summarized as a lack of serotonergic drive. Indeed, too much serotonin, or a dysregulation of different serotonin receptor subtypes or the aminergic transport systems, could also play a role in compromising an arousal response. The raphe contains, for example, autoreceptors for serotonin (the 5-HT$_{1A}$ receptor subtype), which would respond to an increased serotonin concentration with a decreased serotonergic release. Thus, it is perhaps not surprising that different types of serotonergic abnormalities have been implicated in SIDS. Similarly, the raphe contains not only serotonin, but also substance P, a peptidergic neuromodulator which is also critical for respiratory and cardiorespiratory control.

Aside from the raphe, other modulatory nuclei are known to control the preBötC, which includes a variety of noradrenergic nuclei (140, 141), as well as areas releasing orexin or bombesin, which have been implicated in the generation of sighs (142, 143). Sighs are also controlled by cholinergic modulators, which have also been implicated in the control of sleep and wakefulness (135).

## The preBötzinger complex and cardiorespiratory coupling

There is close co-ordination between neuronal circuits controlling the heart and breathing, which is evident in the "biphasic response" to hypoxia. During hypoxia, there is an initial increase in both the heart rate and respiratory rate (144-148). During this initial "augmentation phase" there is also the generation of sighs, which cause further transient increases in heart rate. The augmentation phase is followed by a depression phase during which respiration and heart rate decrease. The general heart rate decrease (bradycardia) is interrupted by transient periods of tachycardia that co-incide with the generation of gasps (71-73). Mechanistically, it is hypothesized that this cardiorespiratory coupling is mediated through an interaction between the preBötzC, the microcircuit controlling inspiration, and the anatomically proximate nucleus ambiguus, a nucleus that contains the cardiac vagal neurons that generate the parasympathetic control of the heart rate. Indeed, these cardiovagal neurons are located at the same level of the nucleus ambiguus as the preBötC (149, 150). It is hypothesized that during each inspiration, inhibitory inspiratory neurons within the preBötC inhibit cardiac vagal neurons in the nucleus ambiguus, which results in the disinhibition at the level of the heart, thus leading to an inspiratory-related heart rate increase. Any disturbance in this core interaction between the respiratory and the cardiac system will result in dysautonomia. Given that arousal is directly linked to the change in heart rate occurring during a sigh and gasp, we expect that a vulnerable infant is likely characterized by a disturbance of this core circuitry. One possible scenario is that in these infants cardiovagal neurons are not as excitable, which would lead to an increased heart rate and decreased cardiorespiratory coupling, all typical signs of dysautonomia (151, 152).

## The postinspiratory complex — A "new kid on the block"

Postinspiration is a distinct phase of breathing that occurs just after an inspiration. It serves as a brake on the passive release of expiratory airflow and protects the larynx and upper airways from aspirating particulate matter and fluid (153). During the postinspiratory phase, laryngeal adductor muscles in the neck are activated and are involved in multiple non-ventilatory behaviors including swallowing, vocalization, and coughing. These behaviors must be tightly co-ordinated with breathing to prevent aspiration. Stimulating sensory laryngeal receptors activates a laryngeal adductor reflex comprising of a prolonged postinspiratory apnea and a dramatic decrease in heart rate (149). While this is normally cardioprotective, in vulnerable individuals exaggeration of the laryngeal adductor reflex can induce a fatal apnea due to prolonged glottal closure (154). This has been proposed as a possible cause of death for SIDS victims (155, 156).

A medullary population rostral to the preBötC was recently identified as an autonomous oscillator thought to control postinspiration (81) (Figure 27.2). This region, termed the PiCo, is also in close proximity to the nucleus ambiguus and has similar rhythm-generating characteristics to the preBötC. Postinspiratory vagal motor output, which innervates the larynx, can be recorded when PiCo neurons are optogenetically excited. Future studies will be necessary to elucidate the PiCo's role in cardiorespiratory coupling, the co-ordination of postinspiratory behaviors, and the laryngeal adductor reflex.

# Conclusions

In conclusion, we have come a long way from identifying the critical risk factors contributing to SIDS to now understanding how these risk factors contribute to pathological changes in the cardiorespiratory response to exogenous stressors such as hypoxia or hypercapnia. Associated with these pathophysiological changes are changes in brainstem anatomy and pathology, as highlighted in Chapter 26. We have also learned how developmental changes in the control of the respiratory system and sleep structure may contribute to the developmental window that characterizes SIDS. These insights suggest that there will not be a unifying explanation for SIDS. Although it is likely that final common pathways involving brainstem dysfunction will lead to the cessation of breathing and heart rate, in the end a multitude of genetic, environmental, behavioral, and metabolic factors will ultimately contribute to SIDS. Thus, every individual will likely have a unique personal history that comes with a unique personal combination of risk factors. New technological advances in genetic screening, management of big data, and the increased ability to measure and monitor physiological states offer unique opportunities that will hopefully help to better identify the individual at risk to succumb to SIDS. These approaches combined will ultimately help to prevent SIDS and thus lower the SIDS risk world-wide.

## Acknowledgement

This publication was supported by grants from the National Institute of Health (PO1HL090554; R01 HL 126523-01), and by the SIDS Fellowship Funds (John Kahan).

## References

1. de Jonge GA, Engelberts AC, Koomen-Liefting AJ, Kostense PJ. Cot death and prone sleeping position in The Netherlands. Brit Med J. 1989;298(6675):722. https://doi.org/10.1136/bmj.298.6675.722.

2. McGlashan ND. Sudden infant deaths in Tasmania, 1980-1986: A seven year prospective study. Soc Sci Med. 1989;29(8):1015-26. https://doi.org/10.1016/0 277-9536(89)90059-2.

3. Chiodini BA, Thach BT. Impaired ventilation in infants sleeping facedown: Potential significance for sudden infant death syndrome. J Pediatr. 1993;123(5):686-92. https://doi.org/10.1016/S0022-3476(05)80841-8.

4. Kemp JS, Kowalski RM, Burch PM, Graham MA, Thach BT. Unintentional suffocation by rebreathing: A death scene and physiologic investigation of a possible cause of sudden infant death. J Pediatr. 1993;122(6):874-80. https://doi. org/10.1016/S0022-3476(09)90010-5.

5. Trachtenberg FL, Haas EA, Kinney HC, Stanley C, Krous HF. Risk factor changes for sudden infant death syndrome after initiation of Back-to-Sleep campaign. Pediatrics. 2012;129(4):630-8. https://doi.org/10.1542/peds.2011-1419.

6. Berard A, Zhao JP, Sheehy O. Success of smoking cessation interventions during pregnancy. Am J Obstet Gynecol. 2016;215(5):611e1-e8.

7. Leung LW, Davies GA. Smoking cessation strategies in pregnancy. J Obstet Gynaecol Can. 2015;37(9):791-7. https://doi.org/10.1016/S1701-2163(15)30149-3.

8. Mage DT, Donner M. A unifying theory for SIDS. Int J Pediatr. 2009;2009:368270.

9.  Paterson DS, Trachtenberg FL, Thompson EG, Belliveau RA, Beggs AH, Darnall R, et al. Multiple serotonergic brainstem abnormalities in sudden infant death syndrome. JAMA. 2006;296(17):2124-32. https://doi.org/10.1001/jama.296.17.2124.

10. Paterson DS, Thompson EG, Kinney HC. Serotonergic and glutamatergic neurons at the ventral medullary surface of the human infant: Observations relevant to central chemosensitivity in early human life. Auton Neurosci. 2006;124(1-2):112-24. https://doi.org/10.1016/j.autneu.2005.12.009.

11. Rubens DD, Vohr BR, Tucker R, O'Neil CA, Chung W. Newborn oto-acoustic emission hearing screening tests: Preliminary evidence for a marker of susceptibility to SIDS. Early Hum Dev. 2008;84(4):225-9. https://doi.org/10.1016/j.earlhumdev.2007.06.001.

12. Carlin RF, Moon RY. Risk factors, protective factors, and current recommendations to reduce sudden infant death syndrome: A review. JAMA Pediatr. 2017;171(2):175-80. https://doi.org/10.1001/jamapediatrics.2016.3345.

13. van Norstrand DW, Ackerman MJ. Genomic risk factors in sudden infant death syndrome. Genome Med. 2010;2(11):86. https://doi.org/10.1186/gm207.

14. Filiano JJ, Kinney HC. A perspective on neuropathologic findings in victims of the sudden infant death syndrome: The triple-risk model. Biol Neonate. 1994;65(3-4):194-7. https://doi.org/10.1159/000244052.

15. Kinney HC, Thach BT. The sudden infant death syndrome. N Engl J Med. 2009;361(8):795-805. https://doi.org/10.1056/NEJMra0803836.

16. Schechtman VL, Harper RM, Wilson AJ, Southall DP. Sleep state organization in normal infants and victims of the sudden infant death syndrome. Pediatrics. 1992;89(5 Pt 1):865-70.

17. Blair PS, Platt MW, Smith IJ, Fleming PJ, Group SSR. Sudden infant death syndrome and the time of death: Factors associated with night-time and day-time deaths. Int J Epidemiol. 2006;35(6):1563-9. https://doi.org/10.1093/ije/dyl212.

18. Douglas NJ, White DP, Weil JV, Pickett CK, Zwillich CW. Hypercapnic ventilatory response in sleeping adults. Am Rev Respir Dis. 1982;126(5):758-62.

19. White DP. Pathogenesis of obstructive and central sleep apnea. Am J Respir Crit Care Med. 2005;172(11):1363-70. https://doi.org/10.1164/rccm.200412-1631SO.

20. Chamberlin NL, Eikermann M, Fassbender P, White DP, Malhotra A. Genioglossus premotoneurons and the negative pressure reflex in rats. J Physiol. 2007;579(Pt 2):515-26. https://doi.org/10.1113/jphysiol.2006.121889.

21. Fogel RB, Malhotra A, Pillar G, Edwards JK, Beauregard J, Shea SA, et al. Genioglossal activation in patients with obstructive sleep apnea versus control subjects. Mechanisms of muscle control. Am J Respir Crit Care Med. 2001;164(11):2025-30. https://doi.org/10.1164/ajrccm.164.11.2102048.

22. Horner RL. Impact of brainstem sleep mechanisms on pharyngeal motor control. Respir Physiol. 2000;119(2-3):113-21. https://doi.org/10.1016/S0034-5687(99)00106-1.

23. Susarla SM, Thomas RJ, Abramson ZR, Kaban LB. Biomechanics of the upper airway: Changing concepts in the pathogenesis of obstructive sleep apnea. Int J Oral Maxillofac Surg. 2010;39(12):1149-59. https://doi.org/10.1016/j.ijom.2010.09.007.

24. Wheatley JR, Mezzanotte WS, Tangel DJ, White DP. Influence of sleep on genioglossus muscle activation by negative pressure in normal men. Am Rev Respir Dis. 1993;148(3):597-605. https://doi.org/10.1164/ajrccm/148.3.597.

25. Krous HF, Haas EA, Chadwick AE, Masoumi H, Stanley C. Intrathoracic petechiae in SIDS: A retrospective population-based 15-year study. Forensic Sci Med Pathol. 2008;4(4):234-9. https://doi.org/10.1007/s12024-008-9054-8.

26. Becher JC, Bhushan SS, Lyon AJ. Unexpected collapse in apparently healthy newborns — A prospective national study of a missing cohort of neonatal deaths and near-death events. Arch Dis Child Fetal Neonatal Ed. 2012;97(1):F30-4. https://doi.org/10.1136/adc.2010.208736.

27. Chase MH, Soja PJ, Morales FR. Evidence that glycine mediates the postsynaptic potentials that inhibit lumbar motoneurons during the atonia of active sleep. J Neurosci. 1989;9(3):743-51.

28. Funk GD, Parkis MA, Selvaratnam SR, Walsh C. Developmental modulation of glutamatergic inspiratory drive to hypoglossal motoneurons. Respir Physiol. 1997;110(2-3):125-37. https://doi.org/10.1016/S0034-5687(97)00078-9.

29. Soja PJ, Morales FR, Baranyi A, Chase MH. Effect of inhibitory amino acid antagonists on IPSPs induced in lumbar motoneurons upon stimulation of the nucleus reticularis gigantocellularis during active sleep. Brain Res. 1987;423(1-2):353-8. https://doi.org/10.1016/0006-8993(87)90862-6.

30. Soja PJ, Lopez-Rodriguez F, Morales FR, Chase MH. The postsynaptic inhibitory control of lumbar motoneurons during the atonia of active sleep: Effect of strychnine on motoneuron properties. J Neurosci. 1991;11(9):2804-11.

31. Yamuy J, Fung SJ, Xi M, Morales FR, Chase MH. Hypoglossal motoneurons are postsynaptically inhibited during carbachol-induced rapid eye

movement sleep. Neuroscience. 1999;94(1):11-15. https://doi.org/10.1016/S0306-4522(99)00355-3.

32. Funk GD, Zwicker JD, Selvaratnam R, Robinson DM. Noradrenergic modulation of hypoglossal motoneuron excitability: Developmental and putative state-dependent mechanisms. Arch Ital Biol. 2011;149(4):426-53.

33. Aston-Jones G, Bloom FE. Activity of norepinephrine-containing locus coeruleus neurons in behaving rats anticipates fluctuations in the sleep-waking cycle. J Neurosci. 1981;1(8):876-86.

34. Jacobs BL, Fornal CA. Activity of brain serotonergic neurons in the behaving animal. Pharmacol Rev. 1991;43(4):563-78.

35. Leung CG, Mason P. Physiological properties of raphe magnus neurons during sleep and waking. J Neurophysiol. 1999;81(2):584-95.

36. Kinney HC. Abnormalities of the brainstem serotonergic system in the sudden infant death syndrome: A review. Pediatr Dev Pathol. 2005;8(5):507-24. https://doi.org/10.1007/s10024-005-0067-y.

37. Duncan JR, Paterson DS, Hoffman JM, Mokler DJ, Borenstein NS, Belliveau RA, et al. Brainstem serotonergic deficiency in sudden infant death syndrome. JAMA. 2010;303(5):430-7. https://doi.org/10.1001/jama.2010.45.

38. Ozawa Y, Obonai T, Itoh M, Aoki Y, Funayama M, Takashima S. Catecholaminergic neurons in the diencephalon and basal ganglia of SIDS. Pediatr Neurol. 1999;21(1):471-5. https://doi.org/10.1016/S0887-8994(99)00033-8.

39. Hilaire G. Endogenous noradrenaline affects the maturation and function of the respiratory network: Possible implication for SIDS. Auton Neurosci. 2006;126-7:320-31. https://doi.org/10.1016/j.autneu.2006.01.021.

40. Ramirez JM, Garcia AJ 3rd, Anderson TM, Koschnitzky JE, Peng YJ, Kumar GK, et al. Central and peripheral factors contributing to obstructive sleep apneas. Respir Physiol Neurobiol. 2013;189(2):344-53. https://doi.org/10.1016/j.resp.2013.06.004.

41. Bolton DP, Taylor BJ, Campbell AJ, Galland BC, Cresswell C. Rebreathing expired gases from bedding: A cause of cot death? Arch Dis Child. 1993;69(2):187-90. https://doi.org/10.1136/adc.69.2.187.

42. Kemp JS, Thach BT. Sudden death in infants sleeping on polystyrene-filled cushions. N Engl J Med. 1991;324(26):1858-64. https://doi.org/10.1056/NEJM199106273242605.

43. Glogowska M, Richardson PS, Widdicombe JG, Winning AJ. The role of the vagus nerves, peripheral chemoreceptors and other afferent pathways in the genesis

of augmented breaths in cats and rabbits. Respir Physiol. 1972;16(2):179-96. https://doi.org/10.1016/0034-5687(72)90050-3.

44. McGinty DJ, London MS, Baker TL, Stevenson M, Hoppenbrouwers T, Harper RM, et al. Sleep apnea in normal kittens. Sleep. 1979;1(4):393-412.

45. Orem J, Trotter RH. Medullary respiratory neuronal activity during augmented breaths in intact unanesthetized cats. J Appl Physiol (1985). 1993;74(2):761-9.

46. Lijowska AS, Reed NW, Chiodini BA, Thach BT. Sequential arousal and airway-defensive behavior of infants in asphyxial sleep environments. J Appl Physiol (1985). 1997;83(1):219-28.

47. McNamara F, Wulbrand H, Thach BT. Characteristics of the infant arousal response. J Appl Physiol (1985). 1998;85(6):2314-21.

48. Thach BT, Lijowska A. Arousals in infants. Sleep. 1996;19(10 Suppl):S271-3. https://doi.org/10.1093/sleep/19.suppl_10.S271.

49. Anderson CA, Dick TE, Orem J. Respiratory responses to tracheobronchial stimulation during sleep and wakefulness in the adult cat. Sleep. 1996;19(6):472-8. https://doi.org/10.1093/sleep/19.6.472.

50. Kahn A, Blum D, Rebuffat E, Sottiaux M, Levitt J, Bochner A, et al. Polysomnographic studies of infants who subsequently died of sudden infant death syndrome. Pediatrics. 1988;82(5):721-7.

51. Bartlett D Jr. Origin and regulation of spontaneous deep breaths. Respir Physiol. 1971;12(2):230-8. https://doi.org/10.1016/0034-5687(71)90055-7.

52. Bell HJ, Haouzi P. The hypoxia-induced facilitation of augmented breaths is suppressed by the common effect of carbonic anhydrase inhibition. Respir Physiol Neurobiol. 2010;171(3):201-11. https://doi.org/10.1016/j.resp.2010.04.002.

53. Bell HJ, Haouzi P. Acetazolamide suppresses the prevalence of augmented breaths during exposure to hypoxia. Am J Physiol Regul Integr Comp Physiol. 2009;297(2):R370-81. https://doi.org/10.1152/ajpregu.00126.2009.

54. Cherniack NS, von Euler C, Glogowska M, Homma I. Characteristics and rate of occurrence of spontaneous and provoked augmented breaths. Acta Physiol Scand. 1981;111(3):349-60. https://doi.org/10.1111/j.1748-1716.1981.tb06747.x.

55. Hill AA, Garcia AJ 3rd, Zanella S, Upadhyaya R, Ramirez JM. Graded reductions in oxygenation evoke graded reconfiguration of the isolated respiratory network. J Neurophysiol. 2011;105(2):625-39. https://doi.org/10.1152/jn.00237.2010.

56. Lieske SP, Thoby-Brisson M, Telgkamp P, Ramirez JM. Reconfiguration of the neural network controlling multiple breathing patterns: Eupnea, sighs and gasps. Nat Neurosci. 2000;3(6):600-7. https://doi.org/10.1038/75776.

57. Burke PG, Abbott SB, Coates MB, Viar KE, Stornetta RL, Guyenet PG. Optogenetic stimulation of adrenergic C1 neurons causes sleep state-dependent cardiorespiratory stimulation and arousal with sighs in rats. Am J Respir Crit Care Med. 2014;190(11):1301-10. https://doi.org/10.1164/rccm.201407-1262OC.

58. Dunne KP, Fox GP, O'Regan M, Matthews TG. Arousal responses in babies at risk of sudden infant death syndrome at different postnatal ages. Ir Med J. 1992;85(1):19-22.

59. Kahn A, Groswasser J, Rebuffat E, Sottiaux M, Blum D, Foerster M, et al. Sleep and cardiorespiratory characteristics of infant victims of sudden death: A prospective case-control study. Sleep. 1992;15(4):287-92. https://doi.org/10.1093/sleep/15.4.287.

60. Kato I, Scaillet S, Groswasser J, Montemitro E, Togari H, Lin JS, et al. Spontaneous arousability in prone and supine position in healthy infants. Sleep. 2006;29(6):785-90. https://doi.org/10.1093/sleep/29.6.785.

61. McCulloch K, Brouillette RT, Guzzetta AJ, Hunt CE. Arousal responses in near-miss sudden infant death syndrome and in normal infants. J Pediatr. 1982;101(6):911-17. https://doi.org/10.1016/S0022-3476(82)80009-7.

62. Sawaguchi T, Kato I, Franco P, Sottiaux M, Kadhim H, Shimizu S, et al. Apnea, glial apoptosis and neuronal plasticity in the arousal pathway of victims of SIDS. Forensic Sci Int. 2005;149(2-3):205-17. https://doi.org/10.1016/j.forsciint.2004.10.015.

63. Haupt ME, Goodman DM, Sheldon SH. Sleep related expiratory obstructive apnea in children. J Clin Sleep Med. 2012;8(6):673-9. https://doi.org/10.1164/ajrccm-conference.2012.185.1_MeetingAbstracts.A6664.

64. Porges WL, Hennessy EJ, Quail AW, Cottee DB, Moore PG, McIlveen SA, et al. Heart-lung interactions: The sigh and autonomic control in the bronchial and coronary circulations. Clin Exp Pharmacol Physiol. 2000;27(12):1022-7. https://doi.org/10.1046/j.1440-1681.2000.03370.x.

65. Weese-Mayer DE, Kenny AS, Bennett HL, Ramirez JM, Leurgans SE. Familial dysautonomia: Frequent, prolonged and severe hypoxemia during wakefulness and sleep. Pediatr Pulmonol. 2008;43(3):251-60. https://doi.org/10.1002/ppul.20764.

66. Wulbrand H, McNamara F, Thach BT. The role of arousal related brainstem reflexes in causing recovery from upper airway occlusion in infants. Sleep. 2008;31(6):833-40. https://doi.org/10.1093/sleep/31.6.833.

67. Thach BT. Graded arousal responses in infants: Advantages and disadvantages of a low threshold for arousal. Sleep Med. 2002;3 Suppl 2:S37-40. https://doi.org/10.1016/S1389-9457(02)00162-4.

68. Franco P, Szliwowski H, Dramaix M, Kahn A. Polysomnographic study of the autonomic nervous system in potential victims of sudden infant death syndrome. Clin Auton Res. 1998;8(5):243-9. https://doi.org/10.1007/BF02277969.

69. Franco P, Verheulpen D, Valente F, Kelmanson I, de Broca A, Scaillet S, et al. Autonomic responses to sighs in healthy infants and in victims of sudden infant death. Sleep Med. 2003;4(6):569-77. https://doi.org/10.1016/S1389-9457(03)00107-2.

70. Pena F, Parkis MA, Tryba AK, Ramirez JM. Differential contribution of pacemaker properties to the generation of respiratory rhythms during normoxia and hypoxia. Neuron. 2004;43(1):105-17. https://doi.org/10.1016/j.neuron.2004.06.023.

71. Hunt CE. The cardiorespiratory control hypothesis for sudden infant death syndrome. Clin Perinatol. 1992;19(4):757-71.

72. Poets CF, Meny RG, Chobanian MR, Bonofiglo RE. Gasping and other cardiorespiratory patterns during sudden infant deaths. Pediatr Res. 1999;45(3):350-4. https://doi.org/10.1203/00006450-199903000-00010.

73. Harper RM, Kinney HC, Fleming PJ, Thach BT. Sleep influences on homeostatic functions: Implications for sudden infant death syndrome. Respir Physiol. 2000;119(2-3):123-32. https://doi.org/10.1016/S0034-5687(99)00107-3.

74. Cherniack NS, Edelman NH, Lahiri S. The effect of hypoxia and hypercapnia on respiratory neuron activity and cerebral aerobic metabolism. Chest. 1971;59:Suppl:29S. https://doi.org/10.1016/S0012-3692(15)31576-2.

75. Pena F, Aguileta MA. Effects of riluzole and flufenamic acid on eupnea and gasping of neonatal mice in vivo. Neurosci Lett. 2007;415(3):288-93. https://doi.org/10.1016/j.neulet.2007.01.032.

76. Serdarevich C, Fewell JE. Influence of core temperature on autoresuscitation during repeated exposure to hypoxia in normal rat pups. J Appl Physiol (1985) . 1999;87(4):1346-53.

77. Franco P, Szliwowski H, Dramaix M, Kahn A. Influence of ambient temperature on sleep characteristics and autonomic nervous control in healthy infants. Sleep. 2000;23(3):401-7.

78. Franco P, Scaillet S, Valente F, Chabanski S, Groswasser J, Kahn A. Ambient temperature is associated with changes in infants' arousability from sleep. Sleep. 2001;24(3):325-9. https://doi.org/10.1093/sleep/24.3.325.

79. Ramirez JM, Dashevskiy T, Marlin IA, Baertsch N. Microcircuits in respiratory rhythm generation: Commonalities with other rhythm generating networks and evolutionary perspectives. Curr Opin Neurobiol. 2016;41:53-61. https://doi.org/10.1016/j.conb.2016.08.003.

80. Smith JC, Ellenberger HH, Ballanyi K, Richter DW, Feldman JL. Pre-Botzinger complex: a brainstem region that may generate respiratory rhythm in mammals. Science. 1991;254(5032):726-9. https://doi.org/10.1126/science.1683005.

81. Anderson TM, Garcia AJ 3rd, Baertsch NA, Pollak J, Bloom JC, Wei AD, et al. A novel excitatory network for the control of breathing. Nature. 2016;536(7614):76-80. https://doi.org/10.1038/nature18944.

82. Janczewski WA, Feldman JL. Distinct rhythm generators for inspiration and expiration in the juvenile rat. J Physiol. 2006;570(Pt 2):407-20. https://doi.org/10.1113/jphysiol.2005.098848.

83. Pagliardini S, Janczewski WA, Tan W, Dickson CT, Deisseroth K, Feldman JL. Active expiration induced by excitation of ventral medulla in adult anesthetized rats. J Neurosci. 2011;31(8):2895-905. https://doi.org/10.1523/JNEUROSCI.5338-10.2011.

84. Ramanantsoa N, Hirsch MR, Thoby-Brisson M, Dubreuil V, Bouvier J, Ruffault PL, et al. Breathing without CO(2) chemosensitivity in conditional Phox2b mutants. J Neurosci. 2011;31(36):12880-8. https://doi.org/10.1523/JNEUROSCI.1721-11.2011.

85. Guyenet PG. Regulation of breathing and autonomic outflows by chemoreceptors. Compr Physiol. 2014;4(4):1511-62. https://doi.org/10.1002/cphy.c140004.

86. Kumar NN, Velic A, Soliz J, Shi Y, Li K, Wang S, et al. Regulation of breathing by CO(2) requires the proton-activated receptor GPR4 in retrotrapezoid nucleus neurons. Science. 2015;348(6240):1255-60. https://doi.org/10.1126/science.aaa0922.

87. Ruffault PL, D'Autreaux F, Hayes JA, Nomaksteinsky M, Autran S, Fujiyama T, et al. The retrotrapezoid nucleus neurons expressing Atoh1 and Phox2b are essential for the respiratory response to CO(2). Elife. 2015;4:e07051. https://doi.org/10.7554/eLife.07051.

88. Guyenet PG, Bayliss DA. Neural control of breathing and $CO_2$ homeostasis. Neuron. 2015;87(5):946-61. https://doi.org/10.1016/j.neuron.2015.08.001.

89. Stornetta RL, Rosin DL, Simmons JR, McQuiston TJ, Vujovic N, Weston MC, et al. Coexpression of vesicular glutamate transporter-3 and gamma-aminobutyric acidergic markers in rat rostral medullary raphe and intermediolateral cell column. J Comp Neurol. 2005;492(4):477-94. https://doi.org/10.1002/cne.20742.

90. Fu W, Le Maitre E, Fabre V, Bernard JF, David Xu ZQ, Hokfelt T. Chemical neuroanatomy of the dorsal raphe nucleus and adjacent structures of the mouse brain. J Comp Neurol. 2010;518(17):3464-94. https://doi.org/10.1002/cne.22407.

91. Mifflin SW. Arterial chemoreceptor input to nucleus tractus solitarius. Am J Physiol. 1992;263(2 Pt 2):R368-75.

92. Chitravanshi VC, Sapru HN. Chemoreceptor-sensitive neurons in commissural subnucleus of nucleus tractus solitarius of the rat. Am J Physiol. 1995;268(4 Pt 2):R851-8.

93. Machado BH. Neurotransmission of the cardiovascular reflexes in the nucleus tractus solitarii of awake rats. Ann N Y Acad Sci. 2001;940:179-96. https://doi.org/10.1111/j.1749-6632.2001.tb03676.x.

94. Accorsi-Mendonca D, Castania JA, Bonagamba LG, Machado BH, Leao RM. Synaptic profile of nucleus tractus solitarius neurons involved with the peripheral chemoreflex pathways. Neuroscience. 2011;197:107-20. https://doi.org/10.1016/j.neuroscience.2011.08.054.

95. Zoccal DB, Furuya WI, Bassi M, Colombari DS, Colombari E. The nucleus of the solitary tract and the coordination of respiratory and sympathetic activities. Front Physiol. 2014;5:238. https://doi.org/10.3389/fphys.2014.00238.

96. Brannan S, Liotti M, Egan G, Shade R, Madden L, Robillard R, et al. Neuroimaging of cerebral activations and deactivations associated with hypercapnia and hunger for air. Proc Natl Acad Sci USA. 2001;98(4):2029-34. https://doi.org/10.1073/pnas.98.4.2029.

97. Burdakov D, Karnani MM, Gonzalez A. Lateral hypothalamus as a sensor-regulator in respiratory and metabolic control. Physiol Behav. 2013;121:117-24. https://doi.org/10.1016/j.physbeh.2013.03.023.

98. Chamberlin NL, Saper CB. Topographic organization of respiratory responses to glutamate microstimulation of the parabrachial nucleus in the rat. J Neurosci. 1994;14(11 Pt 1):6500-10.

99. Liotti M, Brannan S, Egan G, Shade R, Madden L, Abplanalp B, et al. Brain responses associated with consciousness of breathlessness (air hunger). Proc Natl Acad Sci USA. 2001;98(4):2035-40. https://doi.org/10.1073/pnas.98.4.2035.

100. Masaoka Y, Sugiyama H, Katayama A, Kashiwagi M, Homma I. Slow breathing and emotions associated with odor-induced autobiographical memories. Chem Senses. 2012;37(4):379-88. https://doi.org/10.1093/chemse/bjr120.

101. Nattie E, Li A. Respiration and autonomic regulation and orexin. Prog Brain Res. 2012;198:25-46. https://doi.org/10.1016/B978-0-444-59489-1.00004-5.

102. Ramirez JM, Doi A, Garcia AJ 3rd, Elsen FP, Koch H, Wei AD. The cellular building blocks of breathing. Compr Physiol. 2012;2(4):2683-731. https://doi.org/10.1002/cphy.c110033.

103. Subramanian HH, Holstege G. Stimulation of the midbrain periaqueductal gray modulates preinspiratory neurons in the ventrolateral medulla in the rat in vivo. J Comp Neurol. 2013;521(13):3083-98. https://doi.org/10.1002/cne.23334.

104. Cruz-Sanchez FF, Lucena J, Ascaso C, Tolosa E, Quinto L, Rossi ML. Cerebellar cortex delayed maturation in sudden infant death syndrome. J Neuropathol Exp Neurol. 1997;56(4):340-6. https://doi.org/10.1097/00005072-199704000-00002.

105. Lavezzi AM, Ottaviani G, Mauri M, Matturri L. Alterations of biological features of the cerebellum in sudden perinatal and infant death. Curr Mol Med. 2006;6(4):429-35. https://doi.org/10.2174/156652406777435381.

106. Calton MA, Howard JR, Harper RM, Goldowitz D, Mittleman G. The cerebellum and SIDS: Disordered breathing in a mouse model of developmental cerebellar purkinje cell loss during recovery from hypercarbia. Front Neurol. 2016;7:78. https://doi.org/10.3389/fneur.2016.00078.

107. Kinney HC, Cryan JB, Haynes RL, Paterson DS, Haas EA, Mena OJ, et al. Dentate gyrus abnormalities in sudden unexplained death in infants: Morphological marker of underlying brain vulnerability. Acta Neuropathol. 2015;129(1):65-80. https://doi.org/10.1007/s00401-014-1357-0.

108. Kinney HC, Chadwick AE, Crandall LA, Grafe M, Armstrong DL, Kupsky WJ, et al. Sudden death, febrile seizures, and hippocampal and temporal lobe maldevelopment in toddlers: A new entity. Pediatr Dev Pathol. 2009;12(6):455-63. https://doi.org/10.2350/08-09-0542.1.

109. Hefti MM, Kinney HC, Cryan JB, Haas EA, Chadwick AE, Crandall LA, et al. Sudden unexpected death in early childhood: General observations in a series of 151 cases: Part 1 of the investigations of the San Diego SUDC Research Project. Forensic Sci Med Pathol. 2016;12(1):4-13. https://doi.org/10.1007/s12024-015-9724-2.

110. Schwarzacher SW, Rub U, Deller T. Neuroanatomical characteristics of the human pre-Botzinger complex and its involvement in neurodegenerative brainstem diseases. Brain. 2011;134(Pt 1):24-35. https://doi.org/10.1093/brain/awq327.

111. Ramirez JM. The human pre-Botzinger complex identified. Brain. 2011;134(Pt 1):8-10. https://doi.org/10.1093/brain/awq357.

112. Tan W, Janczewski WA, Yang P, Shao XM, Callaway EM, Feldman JL. Silencing preBotzinger complex somatostatin-expressing neurons induces persistent apnea in awake rat. Nat Neurosci. 2008;11(5):538-40. https://doi.org/10.1038/nn.2104.

113. Ramirez JM, Schwarzacher SW, Pierrefiche O, Olivera BM, Richter DW. Selective lesioning of the cat pre-Botzinger complex in vivo eliminates breathing but not gasping. J Physiol. 1998;507(Pt 3):895-907. https://doi.org/10.1111/j.1469-7793.1998.895bs.x.

114. Wenninger JM, Pan LG, Klum L, Leekley T, Bastastic J, Hodges MR, et al. Large lesions in the pre-Botzinger complex area eliminate eupneic respiratory rhythm in awake goats. J Appl Physiol (1985). 2004;97(5):1629-36. https://doi.org/10.1152/japplphysiol.00953.2003.

115. McKay LC, Janczewski WA, Feldman JL. Sleep-disordered breathing after targeted ablation of preBotzinger complex neurons. Nat Neurosci. 2005;8(9):1142-4. https://doi.org/10.1038/nn1517.

116. Naeye RL, Ladis B, Drage JS. Sudden infant death syndrome. A prospective study. Am J Dis Child. 1976;130(11):1207-10. https://doi.org/10.1001/archpedi.1976.02120120041005.

117. Gray PA, Rekling JC, Bocchiaro CM, Feldman JL. Modulation of respiratory frequency by peptidergic input to rhythmogenic neurons in the preBotzinger complex. Science. 1999;286(5444):1566-8. https://doi.org/10.1126/science.286.5444.1566.

118. Stornetta RL, Rosin DL, Wang H, Sevigny CP, Weston MC, Guyenet PG. A group of glutamatergic interneurons expressing high levels of both neurokinin-1 receptors and somatostatin identifies the region of the pre-Botzinger complex. J Comp Neurol. 2003;455(4):499-512. https://doi.org/10.1002/cne.10504.

119. Gray PA, Hayes JA, Ling GY, Llona I, Tupal S, Picardo MC, et al. Developmental origin of preBotzinger complex respiratory neurons. J Neurosci. 2010;30(44):14883-95. https://doi.org/10.1523/JNEUROSCI.4031-10.2010.

120. Bouvier J, Thoby-Brisson M, Renier N, Dubreuil V, Ericson J, Champagnat J, et al. Hindbrain interneurons and axon guidance signaling critical for breathing. Nat Neurosci. 2010;13(9):1066-74. https://doi.org/10.1038/nn.2622.

121. Wang X, Hayes JA, Revill AL, Song H, Kottick A, Vann NC, et al. Laser ablation of Dbx1 neurons in the pre-Botzinger complex stops inspiratory rhythm and impairs output in neonatal mice. Elife. 2014;3:e03427. https://doi.org/10.7554/eLife.03427.

122. Revill AL, Vann NC, Akins VT, Kottick A, Gray PA, Del Negro CA, et al. Dbx1 precursor cells are a source of inspiratory XII premotoneurons. Elife. 2015;4:e12301. https://doi.org/10.7554/eLife.12301.

123. Vann NC, Pham FD, Hayes JA, Kottick A, Del Negro CA. Transient suppression of Dbx1 preBotzinger interneurons disrupts breathing in adult mice. PLoS One. 2016;11(9):e0162418. https://doi.org/10.1371/journal.pone.0162418.

124. Koizumi H, Mosher B, Tariq MF, Zhang R, Koshiya N, Smith JC. Voltage-dependent rhythmogenic property of respiratory pre-Botzinger complex glutamatergic, Dbx1-derived, and somatostatin-expressing neuron populations revealed by graded optogenetic inhibition. eNeuro. 2016;3(3).

125. Winter SM, Fresemann J, Schnell C, Oku Y, Hirrlinger J, Hulsmann S. Glycinergic interneurons are functionally integrated into the inspiratory network of mouse medullary slices. Pflugers Arch. 2009;458(3):459-69. https://doi.org/10.1007/s00424-009-0647-1.

126. Sherman D, Worrell JW, Cui Y, Feldman JL. Optogenetic perturbation of preBotzinger complex inhibitory neurons modulates respiratory pattern. Nat Neurosci. 2015;18(3):408-14. https://doi.org/10.1038/nn.3938.

127. Fleming PJ, Goncalves AL, Levine MR, Woollard S. The development of stability of respiration in human infants: Changes in ventilatory responses to spontaneous sighs. J Physiol. 1984;347:1-16. https://doi.org/10.1113/jphysiol.1984.sp015049.

128. Hoch B, Bernhard M, Hinsch A. Different patterns of sighs in neonates and young infants. Biol Neonate. 1998;74(1):16-21. https://doi.org/10.1159/000014006.

129. Vlemincx E, van Diest I, De Peuter S, Bresseleers J, Bogaerts K, Fannes S, et al. Why do you sigh? Sigh rate during induced stress and relief. Psychophysiology. 2009;46(5):1005-13. https://doi.org/10.1111/j.1469-8986.2009.00842.x.

130. Vlemincx E, Taelman J, De Peuter S, van Diest I, van den Bergh O. Sigh rate and respiratory variability during mental load and sustained attention. Psychophysiology. 2011;48(1):117-20. https://doi.org/10.1111/j.1469-8986.2010.01043.x.

131. Vlemincx E, Abelson JL, Lehrer PM, Davenport PW, van Diest I, van den Bergh O. Respiratory variability and sighing: A psychophysiological reset model. Biol Psychol. 2013;93(1):24-32. https://doi.org/10.1016/j.biopsycho.2012.12.001.

132. Lieske SP, Ramirez JM. Pattern-specific synaptic mechanisms in a multifunctional network. I. Effects of alterations in synapse strength. J Neurophysiol. 2006;95(3):1323-33. https://doi.org/10.1152/jn.00505.2004.

133. Lieske SP, Ramirez JM. Pattern-specific synaptic mechanisms in a multifunctional network. II. Intrinsic modulation by metabotropic glutamate receptors. J Neurophysiol. 2006;95(3):1334-44. https://doi.org/10.1152/jn.00506.2004.

134. Koch H, Caughie C, Elsen FP, Doi A, Garcia AJ 3rd, Zanella S, et al. Prostaglandin E2 differentially modulates the central control of eupnoea, sighs and gasping in mice. J Physiol. 2015;593(1):305-19. https://doi.org/10.1113/jphysiol.2014.279794.

135. Tryba AK, Pena F, Lieske SP, Viemari JC, Thoby-Brisson M, Ramirez JM. Differential modulation of neural network and pacemaker activity underlying eupnea and sigh-breathing activities. J Neurophysiol. 2008;99(5):2114-25. https://doi.org/10.1152/jn.01192.2007.

136. Doi A, Ramirez JM. State-dependent interactions between excitatory neuromodulators in the neuronal control of breathing. J Neurosci. 2010;30(24):8251-62. https://doi.org/10.1523/JNEUROSCI.5361-09.2010.

137. Pena F, Ramirez JM. Substance P-mediated modulation of pacemaker properties in the mammalian respiratory network. J Neurosci. 2004;24(34):7549-56. https://doi.org/10.1523/JNEUROSCI.1871-04.2004.

138. Tryba AK, Pena F, Ramirez JM. Gasping activity in vitro: A rhythm dependent on 5-HT2A receptors. J Neurosci. 2006;26(10):2623-34. https://doi.org/10.1523/JNEUROSCI.4186-05.2006.

139. Pena F, Ramirez JM. Endogenous activation of serotonin-2A receptors is required for respiratory rhythm generation in vitro. J Neurosci. 2002;22(24):11055-64.

140. Viemari JC, Garcia AJ 3rd, Doi A, Ramirez JM. Activation of alpha-2 noradrenergic receptors is critical for the generation of fictive eupnea and fictive gasping inspiratory activities in mammals in vitro. Eur J Neurosci. 2011;33(12):2228-37. https://doi.org/10.1111/j.1460-9568.2011.07706.x.

141. Viemari JC, Garcia AJ 3rd, Doi A, Elsen G, Ramirez JM. Beta-Noradrenergic receptor activation specifically modulates the generation of sighs in vivo and in vitro. Front Neural Circuits. 2013;7:179. https://doi.org/10.3389/fncir.2013.00179.

142. Li A, Nattie E. Antagonism of rat orexin receptors by almorexant attenuates central chemoreception in wakefulness in the active period of the diurnal cycle. J Physiol. 2010;588(Pt 15):2935-44. https://doi.org/10.1113/jphysiol.2010.191288.

143. Li P, Janczewski WA, Yackle K, Kam K, Pagliardini S, Krasnow MA, et al. The peptidergic control circuit for sighing. Nature. 2016;530(7590):293-7. https://doi.org/10.1038/nature16964.

144. Bamford OS, Schuen JN, Carroll JL. Effect of nicotine exposure on postnatal ventilatory responses to hypoxia and hypercapnia. Respir Physiol. 1996;106(1):1-11. https://doi.org/10.1016/0034-5687(96)00051-5.

145. Horne RS, Sly DJ, Cranage SM, Chau B, Adamson TM. Effects of prematurity on arousal from sleep in the newborn infant. Pediatr Res. 2000;47(4 Pt 1):468-74. https://doi.org/10.1203/00006450-200004000-00010.

146. Nock ML, Difiore JM, Arko MK, Martin RJ. Relationship of the ventilatory response to hypoxia with neonatal apnea in preterm infants. J Pediatr. 2004;144(3):291-5. https://doi.org/10.1016/j.jpeds.2003.11.035.

147. Horne RS, Parslow PM, Harding R. Postnatal development of ventilatory and arousal responses to hypoxia in human infants. Respir Physiol Neurobiol. 2005;149(1-3):257-71. https://doi.org/10.1016/j.resp.2005.03.006.

148. Hehre DA, Devia CJ, Bancalari E, Suguihara C. Brainstem amino acid neurotransmitters and ventilatory response to hypoxia in piglets. Pediatr Res. 2008;63(1):46-50. https://doi.org/10.1203/PDR.0b013e31815b4421.

149. Mendelowitz D. Advances in parasympathetic control of heart rate and cardiac function. News Physiol Sci. 1999;14:155-61.

150. Neff RA, Simmens SJ, Evans C, Mendelowitz D. Prenatal nicotine exposure alters central cardiorespiratory responses to hypoxia in rats: Implications for sudden infant death syndrome. J Neurosci. 2004;24(42):9261-8. https://doi.org/10.1523/JNEUROSCI.1918-04.2004.

151. Carroll MS, Kenny AS, Patwari PP, Ramirez JM, Weese-Mayer DE. Respiratory and cardiovascular indicators of autonomic nervous system dysregulation in familial dysautonomia. Pediatr Pulmonol. 2012;47(7):682-91. https://doi.org/10.1002/ppul.21600.

152. Garcia AJ 3rd, Koschnitzky JE, Dashevskiy T, Ramirez JM. Cardiorespiratory coupling in health and disease. Auton Neurosci. 2013;175(1-2):26-37. https://doi.org/10.1016/j.autneu.2013.02.006.

153. Dutschmann M, Jones SE, Subramanian HH, Stanic D, Bautista TG. The physiological significance of postinspiration in respiratory control. Prog Brain Res. 2014;212:113-30. https://doi.org/10.1016/B978-0-444-63488-7.00007-0.

154. Wang X, Guo R, Zhao W, Pilowsky PM. Medullary mediation of the laryngeal adductor reflex: A possible role in sudden infant death syndrome. Respir Physiol Neurobiol. 2016;226:121-7. https://doi.org/10.1016/j.resp.2016.01.002.

155. Leiter JC, Bohm I. Mechanisms of pathogenesis in the sudden infant death syndrome. Respir Physiol Neurobiol. 2007;159(2):127-38. https://doi.org/10.1016/j.resp.2007.05.014.

156. Thach BT. Some aspects of clinical relevance in the maturation of respiratory control in infants. J Appl Physiol (1985). 2008;104(6):1828-34. https://doi.org/10.1152/japplphysiol.01288.2007.

# 28 Neuropathology of Sudden Infant Death Syndrome: Hypothalamus

Karen A Waters, MBBS, PhD[1],
Nicholas J Hunt, BSc(Hons), PhD[2] and
Rita Machaalani, BMedSci(Hons), PhD[2]

[1] *The Children's Hospital at Westmead and The University of Sydney, Camperdown, NSW, Australia*
[2] *The University of Sydney, Camperdown, NSW, Australia*

## Introduction

Since deaths attributed to sudden infant death syndrome (SIDS) occur during sleep, failure to arouse in a stressful situation comprises one component in the proposed mechanism of death. While the infant was previously apparently healthy, the hypothesis underpinning neuropathological studies is that an underlying defect in the infant's brain has contributed to death. The defect in infants who do not arouse may be developmental, inherited, or secondary to previous non-fatal insults. The brainstem and hypothalamus are two regions housing nuclei with important roles in stress responses and arousal mechanisms. This chapter focuses on studies of the hypothalamus and how deficits in this region may contribute to SIDS.

The hypothalamus is a small but complex part of the brain with important roles in the homeostasis of energy balance, circadian rhythms, and stress responses, as well as growth and reproductive behaviors (1). As a regulatory center for so many functions, it receives input from, and transmits output to, a large number of other brain regions. Thus, as the hypothalamus controls many physiological functions, and is highly interconnected with other brain regions, it is an excellent candidate for abnormalities contributing to the pathogenesis of SIDS.

The hypothalamus was evaluated early in the 1990s in SIDS infants (2, 3). At that time, fewer neurotransmitters had been identified compared to today. But even without our current understanding (e.g. of the orexins which were discovered in 1998), the hypothalamus was of interest in SIDS because of its known role in the regulation of sleep. Findings at that time included increased tryptophan content and decreased serotonin, increased serotonin receptor binding, and increased monoamine oxidase-A (MOA) activity, with decreased choline acetyltransferase (ChAT) activity (2) (see Table 28.1).

Updating our knowledge of the hypothalamus and its potential role in SIDS is important, because our understanding of the hypothalamus is now more sophisticated with regards to its structure, functions, and development (1). In addition, a series of recent studies have made important advances in our understanding of abnormalities in the hypothalamus of SIDS infants.

## Structure and Function of the Hypothalamus

The hypothalamus is an integrative center for vital functions that lies above the superior, anterior aspect of the third ventricle, and below the thalamus. It sits in close apposition to central vasculature, with the mammillary bodies and infundibulum "descending through" the center of the circle of Willis (4). The location is vital for some hypothalamic functions, such as the organum vasculosum of the lamina terminalis (OVLT), which detects hypertonicity of the blood to regulate thirst (5).

Descriptive anatomy of the internal structures of the hypothalamus varies, depending on which characteristics are being used to define groups of neurones or regions. These "anatomical" descriptors then tend to cluster in different internal nuclei (Figure 28.1). Studies, particularly in infants, have tended to focus on regions such as those described below, rather than on specific hypothalamic nuclei.

Using anatomical landmarks, the three major regions of nuclear groups and fiber tracts include the lateral, medial, and periventricular hypothalamus, with distinct morphological and functional features. The anatomical landmarks are the anterior column of the *fornix* crossing behind the hypothalamic wall, ending in the lateral part of the homolateral mammillary body, and the mammillo-thalamic tract, which projects from the medial portion of the mammillary body upward to the thalamus (4). Some zones may be more easily defined in non-human species (such as the rat), including pre-optic, tuberal, and posterior regions. The tuberal hypothalamus includes the dorsomedial, ventromedial, paraventricular, supraoptic, and arcuate nuclei (6).

Functional distinctions can also be made, such as the "endocrine hypothalamus", which includes both medial and periventricular anatomical regions and which secretes to the pituitary gland, thus integrating and controlling endocrine functions (7). The medial hypothalamus has more direct control over homeostatic functions such as thirst,

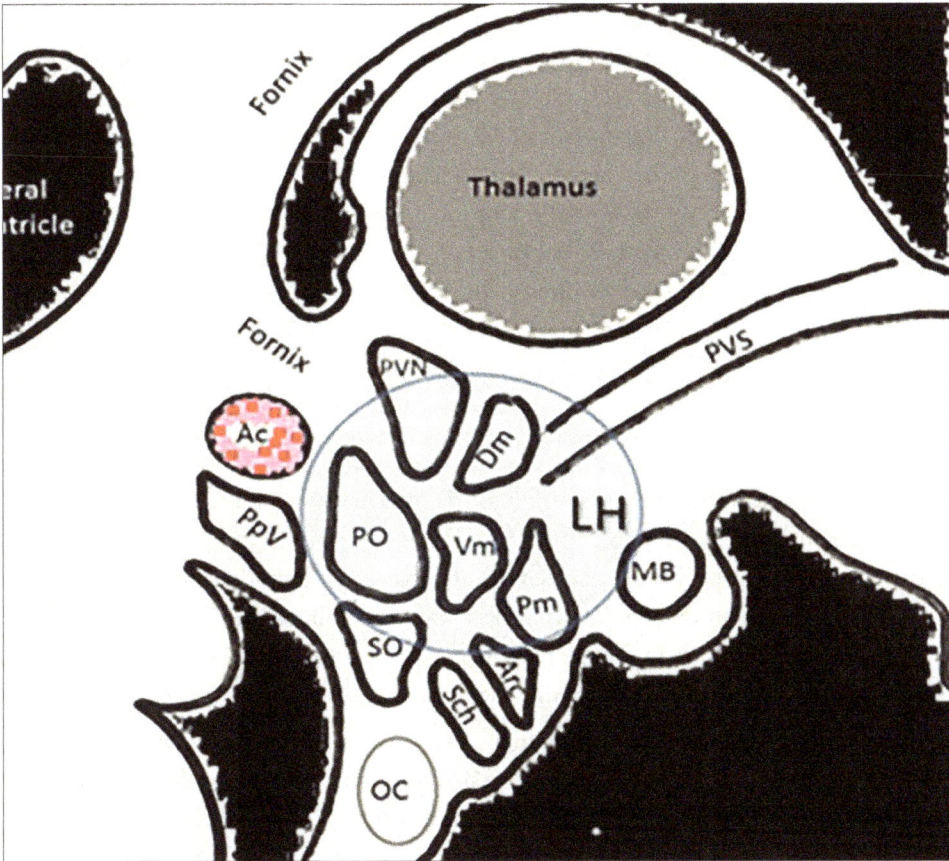

Figure 28.1: Schematic drawing of the anatomy of the human hypothalamus with the majority of the nuclei visible close to the midline section. Fiber tracts: Periventricular system of fiber tracts (PVS). Anatomical structures: Optic chiasm (OC). Anterior carotid artery (Ac) Nuclei: Periventricular nucleus (PVN), Dorsomedial nucleus (Dm), Pre-optic periventricular nucleus (PpV), Pre-optic nucleus (PO), Ventromedical nucleus (Vm), Mammillary body (MB) and Posterior mammillary nucleus (Pm), Suproptic nucleus (SO), Arcuate nucleus (Arc) and Suprachiastmatic nucleus (Sch). The positioning of the lateral hypothalamic (LH) area is indicated by the shadowed region. (Authors' own work.)

hunger, thermoregulation, the sleep-wake cycle, and reproductive behavior, while the lateral hypothalamus has a modulatory role over medial hypothalamic functions.

The hypothalamus can also be divided into four anatomical sections that include the pre-optic area, anterior, tuberal, and posterior areas. Again, functional divisions tend to cross anatomical boundaries, with the anterior segments integrating and controlling energy balance, stress, and reproductive behaviors, as well as mediating autonomic and neuroendocrine responses. The corresponding posterior hypothalamus has important roles in arousal and stress. Using this mode of subdivision, the anterior segments include the anterior pre-optic area with anteroventral components, with nuclei controlling the circadian and sleep-wake systems, including the suprachiasmatic nucleus, anterodorsal with neuroendosecretory functions, and the tuberal hypothalamus (1). The posterior hypothalamus includes the lateral hypothalamus; stimulation of the posterior hypothalamus elicits multiple arousal responses, including cortical activation and motor activity, together with sympathetic responses (8). Neurons in the region have maximum firing during wakefulness and minimum during slow wave sleep. The term "arousal" can be used to indicate an increase in activities associated with stress; this region is also linked with thermoregulation and energy metabolism.

## Hypothalamic peptides and neurotransmitters

Hypothalamic peptide markers, identifying either the neurotransmitter or its receptor(s), can be used to identify function. Peptide markers have been vital in the study of the orexins, which are specifically located in the posterior hypothalamus. Orexins are known for their role in the regulation of sleep and wakefulness, because their deficiency is associated with the human disease narcolepsy; stimulation of the orexin receptors also evokes sympathetically mediated cardiovascular responses (9).

Neurons of the posterior hypothalamus have multiple transmitters including glutamate, gamma-aminobutyric acid (GABA), and histamine, as well as orexin. Cell groups in the same area, expressing different transmitters, can play different functional roles, including stimulation of eating, metabolism, sympathetic and adrenal activation, locomotion, and/or cortical activation associated with arousal (8). Substances that co-localize with orexin include dynorphin (an endogenous opiate), vesicular glutamate transporter, neuronal activity-related pentraxin (a secreted protein that regulates α-amino-3-hydroxy-5-methyl-4-isoxazolepropionic acid [AMPA] receptor clustering), and protein delta-like 1 homologue (DLK-1) (10). The AMPA receptor is a non-NMDA receptor for glutamate.

Other neurotransmitter systems have been found with similar functional profiles to the orexins. These include the 26RFa/QRFPQRFPR system and neurons expressing agouti-related protein (AgRP). QRFP is a 43-amino acid pyroglutamylated RFamide peptide, also known as 26RFa or P513, belonging to the family of RF amide peptides, which are identified by having the motif Arg-Phe-NH2 at the C-terminal end. It is located in the retrochiasmatic area and arcuate nucleus in the hypothalamus, and regulates arousal in mice (11). It also appears to function as a downstream mediator of the arcuate nucleus to regulate feeding behavior, mood, wakefulness, and activity. Neurons expressing AgRP sense metabolic needs and regulate hunger, making the arcuate nucleus (which has high AgRP expression) the major locus controlling food intake (12).

# Early Neuropathological Studies of the Hypothalamus in SIDS

The studies by Ozand and Tildon 1983 (13) and Sparks and Hunsaker 1991 (2) were performed using homogenates of the hypothalamus, so they did not differentiate amongst the different hypothalamic regions. These studies focused on the serotoninergic and catecholaminergic systems, finding alterations in the levels of their neurotransmitters and activities similar to those reported in the brainstem (14).

Ozand and Tildon found that dopamine hydroxylase (DH) activity was reduced and tyrosine hydroxylase (TH) activity was increased in the hypothalamus and other brain regions, but not in the brainstem (13). Tyrosine hydroxylase is an enzyme fulfilling a rate-limiting step in the production of dopamine, while DH (also known as dopamine β-hydroxylase or DBH) is involved in the breakdown of dopamine. The expected combined effect of these changes would be to increase levels of dopamine. DOPA decarboxylase (also known as aromatic-L-amino-acid decarboxylase or tryptophan decarboxylase) synthesizes dopamine and serotonin; catechol-O-methyltransferase (COMT) degrades several catecholamines. Comparisons were made between 63 SIDS and 22 non-SIDS cases, and for TH, 28 SIDS cases were compared to 20 non-SIDS cases (13). Activity of DOPA decarboxylase and COMT were not different. Subsequent studies have shown that catecholaminergic neurons form a dense network in the paraventricular nucleus (PVN), the supraoptic nucleus (SON), and in the basal part of the infundibulum, including the infundibular nucleus. Fibers in the PVN and SON are thought to be noradrenergic. Dopaminergic neurons stain for both DBH and TH and are the predominant catecholaminergic neuron type in the hypothalamus, situated mainly in the periventricular and medial hypothalamic zones of the pre-optic and tuberal regions, functioning to modulate release of oxytocin and vasopressin (15). The neurophysiology of the region is, however, complex, and TH (dopaminergic) neurons in the arcuate nucleus also have orexigenic action, at least in rats (16).

Sparks and Hunsaker also used homogenates of the hypothalamus, in this case studying a broad range of hypothalamic chemicals, but in smaller numbers of subjects (eight SIDS and six non-SIDS) (2). Tryptophan content was increased and serotonin content was decreased; serotonin receptor binding was increased while imipramine binding was unchanged; MAO was increased without an effect on monoamine oxidase-B; ChAT activity (responsible for production of acetylcholine — ACh) was decreased; and acetylcholinesterase (responsible for breakdown of ACh) activity was unchanged. Put together, the authors concluded that these were indicators of reduced serotonin in the hypothalamus (2). Hypothalamic serotonin receptors are involved in behavioral and physiological changes associated with stress and anxiety (17). Most descriptions of the roles of serotonin in the hypothalamus refer to brainstem projections and regulation of serotoninergic receptors in the hypothalamus, including its roles in cardiovascular and sympathetic responses to stress (17, 18). The observed reduction in ChAT, if translating to reduced cholinergic activity, may have a functional role in energy balance as well as innervation of other neurons in the lateral hypothalamus (19).

The study by Kopp et al. 1992 utilized immunohistochemisty to differentiate changes occurring in specific regions of the hypothalamus, but it included only four SIDS cases (20). They studied somatostatin-releasing inhibitory factor (SRIF), thyrotropin-releasing hormone (TRH), luteinizing hormone-releasing hormone (LHRH, also known as gonadotropin-releasing factor, or GnRH), and delta sleep-inducing peptide (DSIP, which may be linked to glucocorticoid-induced leucine zipper or GILZ). In the SIDS cases, they found dramatic reduction in the fibers expressing these peptides in the periventricular and paraventricular nuclei (20). Co-localization of the two peptides has been confirmed in the ventral hypothalamus (21). Investigations of LHRH most often relate to the hypothalamic-pituitary-gonadal axis, which importantly is active from birth to 6 months of age before being silenced through early childhood (22). DSIP is more widespread in the brain, and while it is likely to be a regulatory peptide of endocrine function, it has been shown to induce release of GnRH and also to reduce the sensitivity of neurons to stimulation (23-25).

## The orexinergic system

Within the hypothalamus, orexinergic neurons sense and regulate metabolism including feeding, stress responses, and control of wakefulness/arousal. We have undertaken several studies focusing on the orexinergic system in SIDS cases. We chose to study the orexinergic system because of its integrative roles in many functions and because orexin is specifically produced and located within the neurons of the hypothalamus, predominantly in the perifornical and lateral hypothalamus at the level of the tuberal hypothalamus (6, 26).

Orexin (Ox) is produced in its pre-pro form (PPO), which is a 131-amino-acid-length gene that cleaves into its subunits A and B (OxA and OxB) (27). From the hypothalamus, orexinergic axons distribute widely throughout the central nervous system, except to the cerebellum. Orexin subsequently induces activity via its only two G-protein coupled receptors, being orexin receptor 1 and 2 (OxR1 and OxR2) (28).

The functions controlled by the hypothalamus, through the orexins, cover many of the hypothesized causes of SIDS. These include some combination of the vulnerability of the infant and the risks or stressors to which they are exposed (29). Orexin activity is also altered by exposure to factors which also underlie SIDS risk, such as maternal cigarette smoking during pregnancy and prone sleep. For example, nicotine exposure generally causes increased orexin expression, and hypoxia (and its variations, including ischemia, which may occur during prone sleep position) tends to cause reduced expression of the orexins but increased expression of the receptors (30).

Early studies in SIDS infants used immunohistochemistry, enzyme activities, and tissue binding, with a focus on the catecholamines; these are summarized in Table 28.1. The patterns seen were of reductions in serotonin (5-HT), ChAT, and dopamine β-hydroxylase (DBH), with increases in monoamine oxidase A (MAO-A), and tyrosine hydroxylase (TH) activity (2, 13, 20). Our studies examined very different neuronal activities.

The orexin peptides were discovered by two groups in 1998 (28, 35), and it was demonstrated that if they were injected into the lateral ventricles or near specific arousal regions such as the locus coeruleus of the pons, they led to increased wakefulness and marked suppression of rapid eye movement (REM) sleep (28, 36, 37). Narcolepsy is caused by loss of orexin neurons in humans; it is associated with severe sleepiness and intrusion of fragments of REM sleep into wakefulness, including dream-like hallucinations and sudden bouts of loss of muscle tone (cataplexy), brought on by emotion. The orexin system is also dysregulated in other, less specific neurodegenerative disorders (38, 39). It was known that narcolepsy was associated with brain lesions in the pre-optic area of the anterior hypothalamus before the neurotransmitter was identified (40).

We accessed human brain tissue from the Coroner and from the NSW Tissue Resource Centre, University of Sydney (Sydney, New South Wales, Australia) in order to evaluate changes in the normal distribution of orexin with ageing, within the tuberal hypothalamus. The expression of orexin was compared amongst four age groups, including infants (<12 months), children (4-10 years), young adults (22-32 years), and older adults (45-60 years). There was a 23% decrease in the percentage of orexin neurons between infants and older adults (p<0.001), and a 10% decrease in older, compared with younger, adults (p<0.03). The 23% fall in the proportion of co-localized OxA and OxB neurons was accompanied by a 25% reduction in the density of these neurons in adults compared with infants and/or children. While the cause of the loss is speculative, it could result in sleep dysregulation in normal ageing, since the loss of orexin neurons is known to cause this effect in other medical disorders (41).

Is orexin also abnormal in SIDS? Amongst 27 SIDS infants compared to 19 non-SIDS cases, there were fewer OxA- and OxB-containing neurons in the hypothalamus. In addition, in SIDS infants, orexin immunoreactivity was decreased by up to 21% compared to non-SIDS. There were also 40-50% fewer OxA and OxB projections to most regions of the brainstem pons, including the raphe and the locus coeruleus. While in piglets we could correlate such changes with exposure to intermittent hypoxia, we found no correlations with risk factors in the infants. For infants, risk exposures were identified from questionnaire information collected at the death scene investigation or were documented in relationship to the location and circumstances of death, including prone sleeping position and cigarette smoke exposure.

Our laboratory studies the brain of newborn piglets exposed to various experimental paradigms in parallel with our studies of human infant brain tissue. The animal studies model exposure to SIDS risk factors, allow comparison to control subjects, and therefore add to the understanding of our findings in SIDS infants (see below). The two experimental paradigms used are of intermittent hypercapnic hypoxia (IHH) and nicotine exposure (Nic): exposure to IHH models obstructive sleep apnea (OSA), or facial entrapment in unsafe sleep environments, while postnatal exposure to nicotine mimics levels seen in infants of smoking mothers. The piglet models therefore explore mechanisms that may underlie the neuropathological lesions in SIDS infants by studying brain changes secondary to noxious insults, rather than underlying vulnerabilities such as genetic defects. In the framework of the Triple Risk Hypothesis for SIDS (42), one can postulate how noxious exposures cause brain changes, or one can postulate that they may cause secondary vulnerabilities.

From a neuropathological perspective, our focus within these piglet models was predominantly of the medulla. Studying various neurotransmitter and growth factor systems provided a way to decipher mechanisms responsible for our findings of increased apoptosis in the medulla of these models (43). We found that the dorsal motor nucleus of the vagus (DMNV) within the medulla repeatedly showed changes for the markers studied, indicating a strong vagal effect of these exposures (44). The markers we have studied include apoptosis, the cholinergic and catecholaminergic systems, serotoninergic, and growth factors (BDNF) (44). As the PVN of the hypothalamus is the only direct forebrain projection to the DMNV (31), this provided us with additional rationale for expanding our studies to the hypothalamus.

The first study of the hypothalamus within our laboratory was in our piglet models of IHH and/or Nic compared to controls, to determine whether the orexin system was affected. The regional distribution of the OxR1 and OxR2 employed qualitative methods, and examined eight hypothalamic nuclei/areas (32). A single IHH exposure led to increased OxR1 and OxR2 protein expression that was region-dependent. Animals in the Nic group showed increased expression of OxR1 and OxR2 which was both receptor- and region-specific. For OxR1 expression, the increase after combined Nic+IHH exposure occurred in all nuclei, except for the tuberal mammillary nucleus, but showed no greater increase than that seen after IHH alone. For OxR2, however, the combined exposure resulted in even greater increases (32).

A follow-up quantitative evaluation of OxA and OxB expression examined the cumulative effects of IHH exposure in the tuberal hypothalamus (33). After one day and two days of exposure to IHH, total OxA and OxB expression decreased by 20% and 40%, respectively, progressing to 50% after four consecutive days of IHH exposure. This progressive decrease in both OxA and OxB indicated that chronic IHH exposure induces progressively greater changes in orexin neuropeptide expression in the hypothalamus. The reduction seen after four days of IHH exposure would be expected to disrupt sleep regulation (33). In addition to noting that these changes were in regions of the hypothalamus known to control arousal and stress responses, physiological studies in the same piglets had shown that these changes correlated with decrease and delay of the animals' arousal responses (34).

## Mechanisms

Three methods were used to examine the possible mechanisms for the reduction in orexin in SIDS infants. First, the studies already described in piglets examined changes in animals exposed to IHH and/or Nic compared to controls. Second, liquid chromatography-Matrix assisted laser desorption/ionization (LC-MALDI) was used to identify proteins (based on peptides) across brain samples. Finally, we evaluated markers of programmed cell death (apoptosis), impaired maturation/structural stability of neurons, neurologic inflammation, and the unfolding protein response (UPR) to evaluate which, if any, of these processes has a role in the decrease of orexin neurons in SIDS infants.

The study in piglets compared OxA and OxB expression in piglets exposed to IHH and/or Nic, to controls (45). Interestingly, Nic exposure was associated with both increased expression of OxA and OxB and an increase in the number of orexin neurons in the central tuberal hypothalamus. As with our first study in piglets, IHH exposure was associated with reduced expression of OxA and OxB in the hypothalamus and pons, although this occurred without changes in neuronal numbers. Combined exposure to Nic and IHH did not prevent the nicotine-induced increases. Thus, although both nicotine and IHH are risk factors for SIDS, they appear to have opposing effects on the expression of OxA and OxB. In terms of possible associations with SIDS, the IHH exposure produced results most closely mimicking our results in SIDS infants.

Our protein studies have been confined to the brainstem so far, rather than the hypothalamus, but they remain relevant to the exploration of mechanisms for the hypothalamic abnormalities. A methodological hurdle was working with formalin fixed tissue, since this is the preferred method for tissue preservation from SIDS autopsies (46). However, proteomic studies have now identified peptides and thereby protein abnormalities in SIDS infants compared to controls. For this technique, only small group numbers are used (six in each group), but differences were identified, affecting proteins involved with molecular function, cellular component organization, biological processes, cellular components, and cytoskeletal protein classes (47). Of these, the expression of three proteins, glial fibrillary acid protein (GFAP), β-tubulin III (TUBB3), and myelin basic protein (MBP), were investigated further at an immunohistochemical level to confirm the proteomic findings, and we found that they were (47). Interestingly, when we examined these exact three markers in the hypothalamus of the SIDS infants, we found their expression not to differ when compared to the non-SIDS controls (48)

(Table 28.1). This indicates that the mechanisms at play within the SIDS brain may be region-dependent.

Our investigation of increased apoptosis and altered UPR in the hypothalamus of our SIDS cohort compared to control cases showed that decreased orexin levels in SIDS infants matched the decrease of dynorphin (48). No differences were found for the markers of apoptosis, so this ruled out a loss of orexin cells due to activation of cell death pathways. However, an accumulation of the UPR markers, phosphorylated proteinkinase RNA-like endoplasmic reticulum kinase (pPERK) and activating transcription factor 4 (ATF4; also known as cAMP-response element binding protein 2 or CREB2), was seen (48), suggesting that decreased orexin expression in SIDS is most likely due to a decrease in translation of orexin. As accumulation of pPERK can inhibit protein translation, this mechanism could affect multiple neuronal groups/pathways rather than just the orexinergic pathway. Since accumulation of pPERK was also found in areas of the pons (locus coeruleus and dorsal raphe), the finding could both indicate a common pathway for loss of protein expression and be responsible for the reduction in other neurotransmitters, such as 5-HT and noradrenaline, which have also been found found in SIDS in these regions.

## Discussion

Failure to arouse contributes to (or perhaps causes) an infant's death in SIDS, since death typically occurs during sleep, in an infant who is apparently healthy. As the orexins are essential for promoting wakefulness and arousal, they are an excellent candidate (pathway) for study. The orexinergic neurons are responsible for maintaining wakefulness, and project to almost every brain region involved in the regulation of wakefulness (49). The orexinergic neurons also participate in "stress" responses with raised heart rate and blood pressure, and in other physiological functions such as feeding, thermogenesis, breathing, and even pain perception (5). However, hypothalamic neurotransmitters other than the orexins are involved in the arousal response, particularly PrRP (Prolactin releasing peptide), creating evidence for hierarchy, redundancy, and feedback in the sleep-regulatory system (50, 51). Thus, further investigation of the hypothalamus in SIDS is warranted in order to add to our already-known findings of the abnormalities reported to date, as summarized in Table 28.1.

While it seems unlikely that a single transmitter defect would lead to failure of the arousal system, orexin is unique in that a deficiency is associated with the human disease narcolepsy. Alternatively, identification of several individual abnormalities may reveal a pattern of defects, or clues to a more generalized process. The abnormal process in SIDS infants may occur throughout the entire brain or throughout a particular system(s), such as the arousal pathways, of the brain. This wider view is important to consider, given the strong evidence for an abnormality in the serotoninergic system of SIDS infants, the role of serotonin in the arousal pathways, and the close inter-relationships between the serotonin and orexin systems (52).

The amount of orexin found in infants was consistent for different groups, both across our studies and in the literature. This applies to both immunoreactivity and neuronal numbers. In addition to comparison with controls, methods to account for whether loss of orexin is due to loss of orexin neurons, or to loss of the transmitter alone, include comparison with other cell types, or evaluation of co-localized transmitters (53, 54). The fairly steady decline in neuron numbers and neuron density with increasing age required that we study groups of infants and children (47) in contrast to other authors who focused on adult disease (54). Several groups have studied the number of orexin neurons in the hypothalamus, although most report cell numbers using stereological techniques, which we were not able to undertake due to the limits of the tissue available. However, use of control cases, including adults, allowed us to make appropriate comparisons with the number of cells per section (55, 56) and cell density (57), where these have been reported.

Comparison of SIDS and non-SIDS cases showed reduced expression of OxA and OxB in the hypothalamus of infants who died from SIDS. The magnitude of the decrease (20%) is not as high as that seen in human narcolepsy, but studies in human brain tissue of narcoleptics have been in adults, with the youngest being 23 years old (57, 58). The changes we saw are of similar magnitude to those seen in other diseases — for example, traumatic brain injury, where there is a reduction of 27% (59). These findings could also indicate involvement of other neurotransmitters released by the same cells (53), although this has not yet been studied in SIDS cases.

In our piglet models, exposure to IHH replicates the reduction in OxA and OxB expression in SIDS infants (33). However, in the piglets we also examined effects on the orexin receptors. Animal models of narcolepsy are attributable to a defect in the gene for the orexin receptor, while studies in human subjects with narcolepsy have implicated the distribution of the orexin receptors and axons with the disease process (57, 60). In contrast to studies in narcolepsy, the orexin receptor showed increased expression after the exposures to IHH and/or nicotine (32), suggesting a compensatory increase, given the reduction in OxA and OxB immunoreactivity after the same IHH exposure (45). This does not detract from the application of previous findings to discussion of the relevance to sudden infant death where it is postulated that neurodevelopment of the control of respiration creates a vulnerable profile in early development. Experimental work supports the hypothesis that abnormalities in the arousal (raphe) system can lead to higher mortality after hypoxia/anoxic insults (61, 62).

The complexity of the hypothalamic pathways, including internal cross-talk, makes it easy to correlate our recent studies with the earlier findings in SIDS infants — for example, the finding of reduced cholinergic synthetic enzymes and the knowledge that hypothalamic neurons involved in energy balance have a cholinergic phenotype (19).

Reduced serotonin content in the hypothalamus could link to low levels of serotonin expression in the brainstem neurons that project to this area (63). It seems likely that as our understanding of these neurotransmitter pathways evolve, so, too, will our ability to link the many abnormalities found.

Other hypothalamic transmitter-receptor systems may also be worthy of future exploration, including the RFamide peptide family (peptides possessing an Arg-Phe-NH2 motif at their C-terminus), which exerts important neuroendocrine, behavioral, sensory, and autonomic functions (64). Five RFamide groups have been identified, including the neuropeptide FF (NPFF) group, the PrRP group, the gonadotropin-inhibitory hormone (GnIH) group (human RFRP), the kisspeptin group (Human KiSS-1), and the 26RFa group (64). Of these, the 26RFa/QRFP—QRFPR system is the most recently identified member of the RFamide peptide family in the hypothalamus. This system has orexinergic activity, which in humans is associated with regulation of food intake and energy homeostasis; but it has also been linked to activity and sleep in other species (65). This same transmitter-receptor system has other roles which are potentially as diverse as pituitary hormone secretion, steroidogenesis, bone formation, nociceptive transmission, and arterial blood pressure (65). The importance of this, apart from suggesting redundancy in the transmitter-receptor systems available to control various functions (such as energy homeostasis and sleep/wakefulness, like the orexins), is that the functions of these peptides and their receptors along with disease models of their dysfunction are still being elucidated.

## Conclusions

The hypothalamus is a hub of neuronal control that oversees many vital functions and receives input from, and has projections to, large areas of the brain, as well as having direct interaction with the bloodstream (66). Recently available techniques for study promise to continue to elucidate various locations and functions of neurons (67). Wide-ranging possibilities are likely to exist for future research, first by exploring systems such as these other transmitters within the hypothalamus, but also by utilizing newer research methods, including the data-mining approaches that first led to the identification of some of these peptides themselves. Abnormalities identified in the hypothalamus of SIDS infants may affect other brain areas directly, through loss of their "controller" functions, or indirectly, if they indicate a common pathology that can also occur in other brain regions. Ongoing research will help refine the insights obtained from our studies to date, with clarification of their importance to the unexpected death of these infants.

# References

1.  Burbridge S, Stewart I, Placzek M. Development of the neuroendocrine hypothalamus. Compr Physiol. 2016;6(2):623-43. https://doi.org/10.1002/cphy.c150023.

2.  Sparks DL, Hunsaker JC 3rd. Sudden infant death syndrome: Altered aminergic-cholinergic synaptic markers in hypothalamus. J Child Neurol. 1991;6(4):335-9. https://doi.org/10.1177/088307389100600409.

3.  Swaab DF. Development of the human hypothalamus. Neurochem Res. 1995;20(5):509-19. https://doi.org/10.1007/BF01694533.

4.  Toni R, Malaguti A, Benfenati F, Martini L. The human hypothalamus: A morpho-functional perspective. J Endocrinol Invest. 2004;27(6 Suppl):73-94.

5.  Graebner AK, Iyer M, Carter ME. Understanding how discrete populations of hypothalamic neurons orchestrate complicated behavioral states. Front Syst Neurosci. 2015;9:111. https://doi.org/10.3389/fnsys.2015.00111.

6.  Saper CB, Lowell BB. The hypothalamus. Curr Biol. 2014;24(23):R1111-16. https://doi.org/10.1016/j.cub.2014.10.023.

7.  Clarke IJ. Hypothalamus as an endocrine organ. Compr Physiol. 2015;5(1):217-53.

8.  Jones BE. Arousal systems. Front Biosci. 2003;8:s438-51. https://doi.org/10.2741/1074.

9.  Carrive P. Orexin, stress and central cardiovascular control. A Link with hypertension? Neurosci Biobehav Rev. 2017;74(Pt B):376-92.

10. Li J, Hu Z, de Lecea L. The hypocretins/orexins: Integrators of multiple physiological functions. Br J Pharmacol. 2014;171(2):332-50. https://doi.org/10.1111/bph.12415.

11. Takayasu S, Sakurai T, Iwasaki S, Teranishi H, Yamanaka A, Williams SC, et al. A neuropeptide ligand of the G protein-coupled receptor GPR103 regulates feeding, behavioral arousal, and blood pressure in mice. Proc Natl Acad Sci USA. 2006;103(19):7438-43. https://doi.org/10.1073/pnas.0602371103.

12. Chartrel N, Picot M, El Medhi M, Arabo A, Berrahmoune H, Alexandre D, et al. The neuropeptide 26RFa (QRFP) and its role in the regulation of energy homeostasis: A mini-review. Front Neurosci. 2016;10:549. https://doi.org/10.3389/fnins.2016.00549.

13. Ozand PT, Tildon JT. Alterations of catecholamine enzymes in several brain regions of victims of sudden infant death syndrome. Life Sci. 1983;32(15):1765-70. https://doi.org/10.1016/0024-3205(83)90840-8.

14. Machaalani R, Waters KA. Neurochemical abnormalities in the brainstem of the sudden infant death syndrome (SIDS). Paediatr Respir Rev. 2014;15(4):293-300. https://doi.org/10.1016/j.prrv.2014.09.008.

15. Dudas B, Baker M, Rotoli G, Grignol G, Bohn MC, Merchenthaler I. Distribution and morphology of the catecholaminergic neural elements in the human hypothalamus. Neuroscience. 2010;171(1):187-95. https://doi.org/10.1016/j.neuroscience.2010.08.050.

16. Zhang X, van den Pol AN. Hypothalamic arcuate nucleus tyrosine hydroxylase neurons play orexigenic role in energy homeostasis. Nat Neurosci. 2016;19(10):1341-7. https://doi.org/10.1038/nn.4372.

17. Horiuchi J, McDowall LM, Dampney RA. Differential control of cardiac and sympathetic vasomotor activity from the dorsomedial hypothalamus. Clin Exp Pharmacol Physiol. 2006;33(12):1265-8. https://doi.org/10.1111/j.1440-1681.2006.04522.x.

18. Versteeg RI, Serlie MJ, Kalsbeek A, la Fleur SE. Serotonin, a possible intermediate between disturbed circadian rhythms and metabolic disease. Neuroscience. 2015;301:155-67. https://doi.org/10.1016/j.neuroscience.2015.05.067.

19. Meister B, Gomuc B, Suarez E, Ishii Y, Durr K, Gillberg L. Hypothalamic proopiomelanocortin (POMC) neurons have a cholinergic phenotype. Eur J Neurosci. 2006;24(10):2731-40. https://doi.org/10.1111/j.1460-9568.2006.05157.x.

20. Kopp N, Najimi M, Champier J, Chigr F, Charnay Y, Epelbaum J, et al. Ontogeny of peptides in human hypothalamus in relation to sudden infant death syndrome (SIDS). Prog Brain Res. 1992;93:167-87; discussion 87-8. https://doi.org/10.1016/S0079-6123(08)64571-9.

21. Vallet PG, Charnay Y, Bouras C. Distribution and colocalization of delta sleep-inducing peptide and luteinizing hormone-releasing hormone in the aged human braIn: An immunohistochemical study. J Chem Neuroanat. 1990;3(3):207-14.

22. Abreu AP, Kaiser UB. Pubertal development and regulation. Lancet Diabetes Endocrinol.2016;4(3):254-64.https://doi.org/10.1016/S2213-8587(15)00418-0.

23. Grigorchuk OS, Umriukhin PE. Neuronal activity in the dorsal hippocampus after lateral hypothalamus stimulation: Effects of delta-sleep-inducing peptide. Bull Exp Biol Med. 2012;153(5):614-16. https://doi.org/10.1007/s10517-012-1779-4.

24. Iyer KS, McCann SM. Delta sleep inducing peptide (DSIP) stimulates the release of LH but not FSH via a hypothalamic site of action in the rat. Brain Res Bull. 1987;19(5):535-8. https://doi.org/10.1016/0361-9230(87)90069-4.

25. Kovalzon VM, Strekalova TV. Delta sleep-inducing peptide (DSIP): A still unresolved riddle. J Neurochem. 2006;97(2):303-9. https://doi.org/10.1111/j.1471-4159.2006.03693.x.

26. Marcus JN, Elmquist JK. Orexin projections and localization of orexin receptos. In: The orexin/hypocretin system: Physiology and pathophysiology. Eds Nishino S, Sakurai T. Totowa, NJ: Humana Press, 2007. p. 21-45.

27. Sakurai T, Moriguchi T, Furuya K, Kajiwara N, Nakamura T, Yanagisawa M, et al. Structure and function of human prepro-orexin gene. J Biol Chem. 1999;274(25):17771-6. https://doi.org/10.1074/jbc.274.25.17771.

28. Sakurai T, Amemiya A, Ishii M, Matsuzaki I, Chemelli RM, Tanaka H, et al. Orexins and orexin receptors: A family of hypothalamic neuropeptides and G protein-coupled receptors that regulate feeding behavior. Cell. 1998;92(5):1 page following 696.

29. Hunt CE, Darnall RA, McEntire BL, Hyma BA. Assigning cause for sudden unexpected infant death. Forensic Sci Med Pathol. 2015;11(2):283-8. https://doi.org/10.1007/s12024-014-9650-8.

30. Machaalani R, Hunt NJ, Waters KA. Effects of changes in energy homeostasis and exposure of noxious insults on the expression of orexin (hypocretin) and its receptors in the brain. Brain Res. 2013;1526:102-22. https://doi.org/10.1016/j.brainres.2013.06.035.

31. Rogers RC, Kita H, Butcher LL, Novin D. Afferent projections to the dorsal motor nucleus of the vagus. Brain Res Bull. 1980;5(4):365-73. https://doi.org/10.1016/S0361-9230(80)80006-2.

32. Hunt NJ, Waters KA, Machaalani R. Orexin receptors in the developing piglet hypothalamus, and effects of nicotine and intermittent hypercapnic hypoxia exposures. Brain Res. 2013;1508:73-82. https://doi.org/10.1016/j.brainres.2013.03.003.

33. Du MK, Hunt NJ, Waters KA, Machaalani R. Cumulative effects of repetitive intermittent hypercapnic hypoxia on orexin in the developing piglet hypothalamus. Int J Dev Neurosci. 2016;48:1-8. https://doi.org/10.1016/j.ijdevneu.2015.10.007.

34. Waters KA, Tinworth KD. Habituation of arousal responses after intermittent hypercapnic hypoxia in piglets. Am J Respir Crit Care Med. 2005;171(11):1305-11. https://doi.org/10.1164/rccm.200405-595OC.

35. van den Pol AN, Gao XB, Obrietan K, Kilduff TS, Belousov AB. Presynaptic and postsynaptic actions and modulation of neuroendocrine neurons by a new hypothalamic peptide, hypocretin/orexin. J Neurosci. 1998;18(19):7962-71.

36. de Lecea L, Kilduff TS, Peyron C, Gao X, Foye PE, Danielson PE, et al. The hypocretins: Hypothalamus-specific peptides with neuroexcitatory activity. Proc Natl Acad Sci USA. 1998;95(1):322-7. https://doi.org/10.1073/pnas.95.1.322.

37. Hagan JJ, Leslie RA, Patel S, Evans ML, Wattam TA, Holmes S, et al. Orexin A activates locus coeruleus cell firing and increases arousal in the rat. Proc Natl Acad Sci USA. 1999;96(19):10911-16. https://doi.org/10.1073/pnas.96.19.10911.

38. Liguori C, Romigi A, Mercuri NB, Nuccetelli M, Izzi F, Albanese M, et al. Cerebrospinal-fluid orexin levels and daytime somnolence in frontotemporal dementia. J Neurol. 2014;261(9):1832-6. https://doi.org/10.1007/s00415-014-7455-z.

39. Liguori C, Romigi A, Nuccetelli M, Zannino S, Sancesario G, Martorana A, et al. Orexinergic system dysregulation, sleep impairment, and cognitive decline in Alzheimer disease. JAMA Neurol. 2014;71(12):1498-505. https://doi.org/10.1001/jamaneurol.2014.2510.

40. De la Herran-Arita AK, Guerra-Crespo M, Drucker-Colin R. Narcolepsy and orexins: An example of progress in sleep research. Front Neurol. 2011;2:26. https://doi.org/10.3389/fneur.2011.00026.

41. Nixon JP, Mavanji V, Butterick TA, Billington CJ, Kotz CM, Teske JA. Sleep disorders, obesity, and aging: The role of orexin. Ageing Res Rev. 2015;20:63-73. https://doi.org/10.1016/j.arr.2014.11.001.

42. Kinney HC, Richerson GB, Dymecki SM, Darnall RA, Nattie EE. The brainstem and serotonin in the sudden infant death syndrome. Annu Rev Pathol. 2009;4:517-50. https://doi.org/10.1146/annurev.pathol.4.110807.092322.

43. Machaalani R, Waters KA. Postnatal nicotine and/or intermittent hypercapnic hypoxia effects on apoptotic markers in the developing piglet brainstem medulla. Neuroscience. 2006;142(1):107-17. https://doi.org/10.1016/j.neuroscience.2006.06.015.

44. Bejjani C, Machaalani R, Waters KA. The dorsal motor nucleus of the vagus (DMNV) in sudden infant death syndrome (SIDS): Pathways leading to apoptosis. Respir Physiol Neurobiol. 2013;185(2):203-10. https://doi.org/10.1016/j.resp.2012.09.001.

45. Hunt NJ, Russell B, Du MK, Waters KA, Machaalani R. Changes in orexinergic immunoreactivity of the piglet hypothalamus and pons after exposure to chronic postnatal nicotine and intermittent hypercapnic hypoxia. Eur J Neurosci. 2016;43(12):1612-22. https://doi.org/10.1111/ejn.13246.

46. Casale V, Oneda R, Lavezzi AM, Matturri L. Optimisation of postmortem tissue preservation and alternative protocol for serotonin transporter gene polymorphisms

amplification in SIDS and SIUD cases. Exp Mol Pathol. 2010;88(1):202-5. https://doi.org/10.1016/j.yexmp.2009.10.003.

47. Hunt NJ, Rodriguez ML, Waters KA, Machaalani R. Changes in orexin (hypocretin) neuronal expression with normal aging in the human hypothalamus. Neurobiol Aging. 2015;36(1):292-300. https://doi.org/10.1016/j.neurobiolaging.2014.08.010.

48. Hunt NJ, Waters KA, Machaalani R. Promotion of the unfolding protein response in orexin/dynorphin neurons in sudden infant death syndrome (SIDS): Elevated pPERK and ATF4 expression. Mol Neurobiol. 2016 [Epub ahead of print]. https://doi.org/10.1007/s12035-016-0234-3.

49. Alexandre C, Andermann ML, Scammell TE. Control of arousal by the orexin neurons. Curr Opin Neurobiol. 2013;23(5):752-9. https://doi.org/10.1016/j.conb.2013.04.008.

50. Dodd GT, Luckman SM. Physiological roles of GPR10 and PrRP signaling. Front Endocrinol (Lausanne). 2013;4:20. https://doi.org/10.3389/fendo.2013.00020.

51. Sorooshyari S, Huerta R, de Lecea L. A framework for quantitative modeling of neural circuits involved in sleep-to-wake transition. Front Neurol. 2015;6:32. https://doi.org/10.3389/fneur.2015.00032.

52. Brown RE, Sergeeva O, Eriksson KS, Haas HL. Orexin A excites serotonergic neurons in the dorsal raphe nucleus of the rat. Neuropharm. 2001;40(3):457-9. https://doi.org/10.1016/S0028-3908(00)00178-7.

53. Blouin AM, Thannickal TC, Worley PF, Baraban JM, Reti IM, Siegel JM. Narp immunostaining of human hypocretin (orexin) neurons: Loss in narcolepsy. Neurology. 2005;65(8):1189-92. https://doi.org/10.1212/01.wnl.0000175219.01544.c8.

54. Thannickal TC, Moore RY, Nienhuis R, Ramanathan L, Gulyani S, Aldrich M, et al. Reduced number of hypocretin neurons in human narcolepsy. Neuron. 2000;27(3):469-74. https://doi.org/10.1016/S0896-6273(00)00058-1.

55. Fronczek R, Overeem S, Lee SY, Hegeman IM, van Pelt J, van Duinen SG, et al. Hypocretin (orexin) loss in Parkinson's disease. Brain. 2007;130(Pt 6):1577-85. https://doi.org/10.1093/brain/awm090.

56. Thannickal TC, Lai YY, Siegel JM. Hypocretin (orexin) cell loss in Parkinson's disease. Brain. 2007;130(Pt 6):1586-95. https://doi.org/10.1093/brain/awm097.

57. Thannickal TC, Siegel JM, Nienhuis R, Moore RY. Pattern of hypocretin (orexin) soma and axon loss, and gliosis, in human narcolepsy. Brain Pathol. 2003;13(3):340-51. https://doi.org/10.1111/j.1750-3639.2003.tb00033.x.

58. Peyron C, Faraco J, Rogers W, Ripley B, Overeem S, Charnay Y, et al. A mutation in a case of early onset narcolepsy and a generalized absence of hypocretin peptides in human narcoleptic brains. Nat Med. 2000;6(9):991-7. https://doi.org/10.1038/79690.

59. Baumann CR, Bassetti CL, Valko PO, Haybaeck J, Keller M, Clark E, et al. Loss of hypocretin (orexin) neurons with traumatic brain injury. Ann Neurol. 2009;66(4):555-9. https://doi.org/10.1002/ana.21836.

60. Liblau RS, Vassalli A, Seifinejad A, Tafti M. Hypocretin (orexin) biology and the pathophysiology of narcolepsy with cataplexy. Lancet Neurol. 2015;14(3):318-28. https://doi.org/10.1016/S1474-4422(14)70218-2.

61. Barrett KT, Dosumu-Johnson RT, Daubenspeck JA, Brust RD, Kreouzis V, Kim JC, et al. Partial raphe dysfunction in neurotransmission is sufficient to increase mortality after anoxic exposures in mice at a critical reriod in postnatal development. J Neurosci. 2016;36(14):3943-53. https://doi.org/10.1523/JNEUROSCI.1796-15.2016.

62. Wong-Riley MT, Liu Q. Neurochemical development of brain stem nuclei involved in the control of respiration. Respir Physiol Neurobiol. 2005;149(1-3):83-98. https://doi.org/10.1016/j.resp.2005.01.011.

63. Kinney HC, Broadbelt KG, Haynes RL, Rognum IJ, Paterson DS. The serotonergic anatomy of the developing human medulla oblongata: Implications for pediatric disorders of homeostasis. J Chem Neuroanat. 2011;41(4):182-99. https://doi.org/10.1016/j.jchemneu.2011.05.004.

64. Ukena K, Vaudry H, Leprince J, Tsutsui K. Molecular evolution and functional characterization of the orexigenic peptide 26RFa and its receptor in vertebrates. Cell Tissue Res. 2011;343(3):475-81. https://doi.org/10.1007/s00441-010-1116-z.

65. Chartrel N, Alonzeau J, Alexandre D, Jeandel L, Alvear-Perez R, Leprince J, et al. The RFamide neuropeptide 26RFa and its role in the control of neuroendocrine functions. Front Neuroendocrinol. 2011;32(4):387-97. https://doi.org/10.1016/j.yfrne.2011.04.001.

66. Lechan RM, Toni R. Functional anatomy of the hypothalamus and pituitary. In: Endotext. Eds De Groot LJ, Chrousos G, Dungan K, et al. South Dartmouth (MA): MDText.com, Inc.; 2000-. Endotext [Internet]. 2016. [Available from: https://www.ncbi.nlm.nih.gov/books/NBK279126/]. Accessed 29 November 2017.

67. Weber F, Dan Y. Circuit-based interrogation of sleep control. Nature. 2016;538(7623):51-9. https://doi.org/10.1038/nature19773.

68. Hunt NJ, Waters KA, Rodriguez ML, Machaalani R. Decreased orexin (hypocretin) immunoreactivity in the hypothalamus and pontine nuclei in sudden infant death syndrome. Acta Neuropathol. 2015;130(2):185-98. https://doi.org/10.1007/s00401-015-1437-9.

Table 28.1: Summary of studies of the hypothalmus in SIDS.
Immunohistochemistry (IHC), Somatostatin-releasing inhibiting factor (SRIF), Luteinizing hormone-releasing hormone (LHRH or GnRH), Dopamine β-hydroxylase (DBH), Tyrosine hydroxylase (TH), Catecholamine-o-methyltransferase (COMT), Monoamine oxidase (MAO), Choline acetyltransferase (ChAT), Orexin A (OxA), Orexin B (OxB), Phosphorylated protein kinase RNA-like endoplasmic reticulum kinase (pPERK), Activating transcription factor 4 (ATF4), Glial fibrillary acid protein (GFAP), Tubulin beta chain 3 (TUBB3), Myelin basic protein (MBP) and Interleukin 1 beta (IL-Iβ).

| | Dataset | Hypothalamus region | Markers studied | Method | Results |
|---|---|---|---|---|---|
| Kopp et al. 1992 (20) | 4 SIDS 4 non-SIDS | Anterior hypothalamus | SRIF, LH-RH | IHC | ↓ LH-RH immunoreactive fibres peri- and para-ventricular nuclei. |
| Sparks and Hunsaker 1991 (2) | 8 SIDS 6 non-SIDS | Homogenized whole hypothalamus | Tryptophan, 5HT, 5-HIAA, ChAT, AChE, H3-imipramine and H3-serotonin binding, MAO-A, MAO-B | Chemical levels, tissue binding, enzyme activities, and protein content | 74%↑ tryptophan 32%↓ serotonin 37%↑ MAO-A 71%↓ ChAT |
| Ozand and Tildon 1983 (13) | 31 SIDS (27 for TH) 21 non-SIDS | Homogenized whole hypothalamus | DBH, TH, DOPA decarboxylase, COMT | Enzyme activities | ↓ DBH ↑ TH |
| Hunt et al. 2015 (68) | 27 SIDS 19 non-SIDS | Tuberal hypothalamus: dorsomedial, perifornical, and lateral hypothalamus at anterior, central, and posterior levels | OxA, OxB | IHC | 19%↓ anterior (5 SIDS, 5 non-SIDS) 11%↓ central (14 SIDS, 9 non-SIDS) 21%↓ posterior (8 SIDS, 5 non-SIDS) |
| Hunt et al. 2016 (48) | 27 SIDS 19 non-SIDS | Same regions as Hunt et al. 2015 (68) | Dyn, c-fos, pPERK, ATF4, Lipo, apoptosis (Caspase-3, 9 and TUNEL) GFAP, MBP, TUBB3, IL-1β, and ATF4 | IHC | 20%↓ OxA & Dyn 35%↑ pPERK 15%↑ ATF4 ↓ OxA correlated with ↑ pPERK/ATF4 |

# 29 Abnormalities of the Hippocampus in Sudden and Unexpected Death in Early Life

Hannah C Kinney, MD[1],
Robin L Haynes, PhD[1],
Dawna D Armstrong, MD[2] and
Richard D Goldstein, MD[3]

[1]Department of Pathology, Boston Children's Hospital and
Harvard Medical School, Boston, USA
[2]Retired Professor Pathology Baylor College of Medicine,
Department of Pathology, Houston, USA
[3]Department of Psychosocial Oncology and Palliative Care, Dana-Farber
Cancer Institute, Department of Medicine, Boston Children's Hospital and
Harvard Medical School, Boston, USA

## Introduction

The terrifying aspect of the sudden infant death syndrome (SIDS) is that it occurs in infants who seem healthy and then die without warning when put down to sleep. SIDS is not typically witnessed and it is surmized that death occurs during sleep, or during one of the many transitions to waking that occur during normal infant sleep-wake cycles (1). Multiple sleep-related mechanisms have been proposed to cause SIDS (1, 2). These mechanisms include suffocation/asphyxiation in the face-down sleep position, central and/or obstructive sleep apnea, impaired-state-dependent responses to hypoxia and/or hypercarbia, inadequate autoresuscitation, defective autonomic regulation of blood pressure or thermal responses, and abnormal arousal to life-threatening challenges during sleep.

In this chapter, we review the hypothesis and the neuropathologic evidence that SIDS is precipitated by a dentate gyrus-related seizure or a limbic-related instability that involves the central homeostatic network (CHN). We begin with an overview of this hypothesis, and then review our neuropathologic evidence for an epileptiform hippocampal lesion in the brain of a subset of SIDS infants and young children (41-50% respectively) who died suddenly and unexpectedly (3-5). We then consider the putative mechanism whereby dentate lesions cause seizures, the role of the hippocampus as part of the CHN in stress responses (such as the face-down sleep position), and the potential interactions of brainstem serotonergic (5-HT) deficits and the hippocampus in the pathogenesis of sudden death in infants. We conclude with further directions for research into the role of the hippocampus in sudden and unexpected death in early life.

## The Limbic Seizure-Related Hypothesis in SIDS

In 1986, Harper suggested that some SIDS deaths may be due to a fatal seizure during sleep that arises in forebrain-limbic-related circuits (6). This hypothesis arose from the recognition of the following inter-related phenomena: limbic regions are particularly susceptible to epileptogenesis; sleep states lower the threshold for seizure; and SIDS is linked to sleep and arousal. Sleep itself is thought to be a precarious state, in part because of the loss of the major "back-up" forebrain systems of waking which influence the final common pathways in the brainstem that mediate central cardiorespiratory function during sleep. Forebrain limbic regions, such as the hippocampus and amygdala, which are part of the CHN, modulate brainstem cardiorespiratory control in a manner influenced by the sleep-waking cycles.

In line with Harper's reasoning we propose that SIDS, or a subset of SIDS, is triggered by a seizure-like or paroxysmal event in unstable electrical circuits of the CHN, some of which originated in and are propagated from the hippocampus. The main evidence is neuropathologic observations that we identify as an epileptiform lesion in the hippocampus, a key structure of the CHN (Figure 29.1); such lesions are present in infants and young children with sleep-related sudden and unexplained death. The lesion is dentate bilamination (DB) (Figure 29.2), a morphological variant of granule cell (GC) dispersion that is recognized virtually exclusively in temporal lobe epilepsy (3).

The presence of DB in cases of SIDS and sudden and unexplained death in childhood (SUDC) suggests a seizure-related mechanism of sudden death, arising from a bout of electrical instability generated from the abnormal dentate gyrus in the CHN. We propose that this electrical instability is precipitated by an exogenous stressor (e.g. hyperthermia or asphyxia), because of the epidemiological link of SIDS deaths to over-bundling and unsafe sleep environments such as the prone sleep position. Clinical seizures with abnormal movements are not usually recognized in infants dying of SIDS,

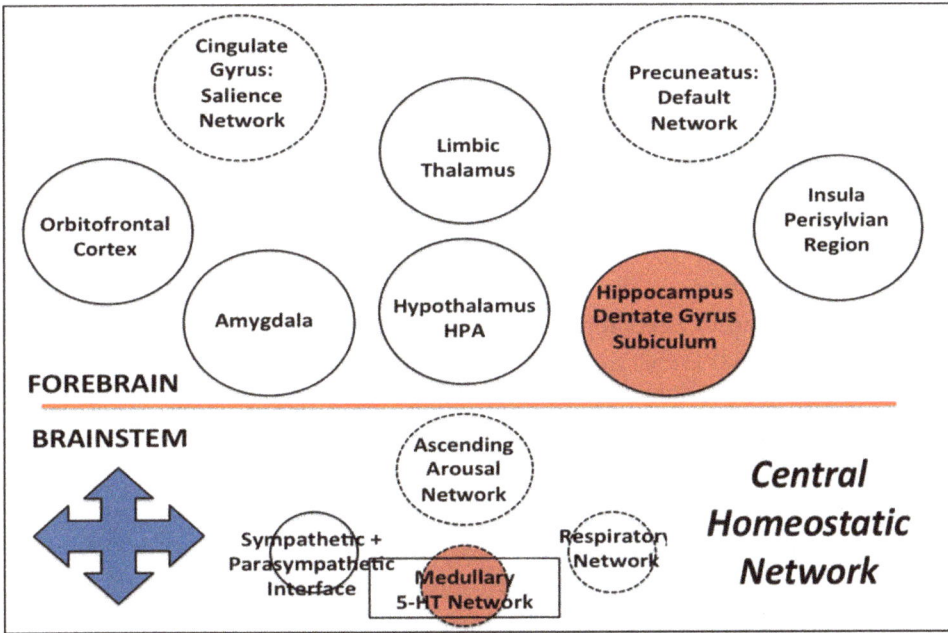

Figure 29.1: Schematic of the putative central homeostatic network with forebrain and brainstem nodes and interconnections. The abnormalities in SIDS reported by our laboratory are colored in red. (Authors' own work.)

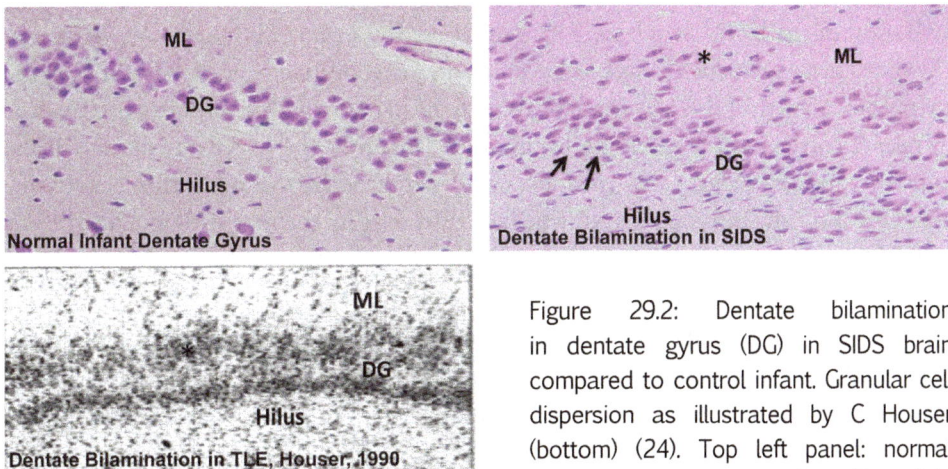

Figure 29.2: Dentate bilamination in dentate gyrus (DG) in SIDS brain compared to control infant. Granular cell dispersion as illustrated by C Houser (bottom) (24). Top left panel: normal dentate gyrus in an infant. Top right panel: granular cell layer with diffuse dispersion as found in temporal lobe epilepsy. There is a row of GCs in one layer (asterisks) separated by a cell-free zone from the main body of GCs. There are immature cells in the subgranular layer (arrows). Bottom panel: dentate gyrus with bilamination (DB) in temporal lobe epilepsy as first defined by Houser (24). (Top and middle panel are reproduced with permission from (32). Bottom panel is reproduced from (24) with permission from Elsevier.)

either before, or at the time of, death. We have reported, however, an infant who was discovered having a seizure during sleep and whose death was deemed unexplained by a complete autopsy (7). Also, approximately 12% of SIDS cases have been associated with antecedent acute life-threatening events (ALTEs), with the ALTEs described as possible seizures in 6-16% (8). It does seem possible that some SIDS and SUDC cases arise from subclinical autonomic seizures during sleep that result in apnea, bradycardia, or other forms of cardiorespiratory dysfunction and sudden death.

The major network in the human brain that copes with stress is the CHN (9). This network comprises ascending and descending interconnections between brainstem nuclei and forebrain limbic regions, including the hippocampus, which together regulate and integrate respiratory, autonomic, immune, neuroendocrine, affective, and cognitive responses to stress during sleep or waking. Although the limbic lobe/system was historically regarded as the neuroanatomic substrate of emotion (10, 11), its role in the regulation of homeostasis has been increasingly recognized. As such, the originally defined sites have been encompassed in the central autonomic network (12-15) or "flight or fight" system of the hypothalamic-pituitary-adrenal axis (HPA) (16, 17). The biomediators of the CHN (e.g. cortisol, sympathetic and parasympathetic transmitters, 5-HT, cytokines, metabolic hormones) operate interactively, down- and up-regulating each other, depending on concentration, anatomic location, and physiological needs.

## The Hippocampus, Regulation of Stress, and the CHN

The hippocampus plays an instrumental role in regulating the HPA (9, 18). Stress involves activation of the CHN to release a cascade of neurotransmitters, hormones, and other chemical messengers that induce behavioral and metabolic changes. A delayed response to stress involves the HPA axis, via activation of the hypothalamic paraventricular nucleus to release corticotrophin-releasing hormone (CRH) into the portal vasculature of the anterior pituitary gland. This stimulates the release of adrenocorticotropic hormone (ACTH) from the pituitary gland, which in turn triggers the release of glucocorticoids from the adrenal cortex.

All types of stress reactions operate through the HPA axis (19, 20). Through the release of glucocorticoids, the HPA axis mobilizes energy reserves in order to ensure that the organism has the resources to prepare for, and meet, a homeostatic challenge (19). The glucocorticoids exert negative feedback, regulating HPA axis activity via its own receptors (glucocorticoid receptors (GRs) and mineralocorticoid receptors (MRs)) in the hippocampus, as well as in the anterior pituitary, hypothalamus, and prefrontal cortex (19). The GRs and MRs are both ligand-gated transcription factors that alter expression of multiple genes (21). The hippocampus has the highest concentration of MRs in the brain. Higher levels of glucocorticoids (those following stress) activate lower-affinity GRs, which promotes expression of a wide variety of genes, and mediates glucocorticoid effects on neural function in the hippocampus (21).

Within the hippocampus, a critical CHN and HPA component is the dentate gyrus. The dentate gyrus is a central region of the hippocampus and is critical to its functions, which include learning and the formation of new memories. Furthermore, it is one of the major regions in the adult CNS with the capacity for constitutive neurogenesis throughout life (22). In humans, neurogenesis takes place in the subgranular zone of the dentate gyrus. Neural progenitor cells migrate from the dentate subgranular zone to the GC layer. The majority of cells are generated early in life, but new dentate GCs arise at a lower rate throughout adulthood and into late life in humans and rodents. Adult-born neurons make up about 6% of the GC layer in rats. These cells integrate into hippocampal circuitry and acquire characteristics of mature GCs, as demonstrated in part through BrdU labeling experiments (23).

Although the hippocampus mediates stress responses via the HPA axis, it is itself especially vulnerable to the deleterious effects of excessive corticoid stimulation in abnormal stress responses. In animal models, chronic stressful experiences (e.g. prolonged immobilization, housing in dominance hierarchies, early maternal separation) can remodel hippocampal neurons and result in changes in gross and microscopic morphology of the hippocampus (21). Animal model studies of the adult hippocampus have revealed mechanisms by which repeated stress causes remodeling of hippocampal circuitry. These include: [1] suppression of neurogenesis, which is ongoing in the young adult dentate gyrus; [2] shortening of dendrites; and [3] loss of spine synapses (21). Stress decreases neurogenesis by stimulating the release of adrenal corticosteroids via the HPA axis (see above); the adrenal corticosterioids then bind to the GC progenitors in the dentate gyrus and decrease cell proliferation. In certain diseases related to stress (e.g. depression or post-traumatic stress syndrome (21)), there is a subsequent decreased volume of the hippocampus.

Replacement of neurons via neurogenesis is one neuroplastic mechanism to protect against and/or to adapt to stress; however, it is also affected by excessive or dysregulated stress itself. Studies have demonstrated that the proliferation of GC precursors and production of new GCs, are dependent on the levels of circulating adrenocortiocoid steroids (20); these hormones inhibit cell proliferation in the dentate gyrus during the early postnatal period and in adulthood. The suppressive action of glucocorticoids on cell proliferation is not direct but occurs through an N-methyl-D-aspartate (NMDA) receptor-dependent excitatory pathway. Stressful experiences, which are known to elevate circulating levels of glucocorticoids and to stimulate hippocampal glutamate release, inhibit the proliferation of GC precursors. However, different experimental paradigms indicate that stress can not only decrease neurogenesis, but also increase it, depending upon the type of stress, the amount, the developmental window, and other factors.

# Hippocampal Pathology in SIDS

## Overview

We have reported developmental abnormalities in the dentate gyrus of the hippocampus in ~40% of SIDS infants dying suddenly, unexpectedly, and without an obvious explanation (3). The developmental abnormalities we observe in the dentate gyrus include GC dispersion and in all cases its variant, DB. The normal dentate gyrus has a compact single layer of closely packed GCs (24) (Figure 29.2). Dentate bilamination is characterized by two layers of GCs, separated by an acellular layer of neuropil. Houser first described dentate bilamination as a part of the pathologic spectrum of GC dispersion observed in temporal lobe epilepsy (TLE) in 1990 (24). Other features of GC dispersion included tight packing of cells and widening of the GC layer, and ectopic GCs in the molecular layer (Figure 29.2). Because the DB and associated GC abnormalities that we observed in the SIDS cases had been previously reported almost exclusively in TLE (24-27), we postulated that in SIDS there may be a potential link between DB (the epileptiform lesion) and seizures. We have therefore investigated this association in SIDS infants using the presence of DB as a potential marker of vulnerability to seizures. In SIDS these seizures could be triggered by stressful homeostatic challenges such as hyperthermia, asphyxia, and/or hypoxia.

## The San Diego cohort of SIDS cases and autopsy controls

In a blinded study we examined the hippocampus for DB in 153 cases of sudden unexpected infant death in the San Diego medical examiner system (3). Because in the USA autopsies of sudden unexpected death in infants (explained and unexplained) are under the legal jurisdiction of the medical examiner's office, the study was necessarily performed utilizing the available archival neuropathological materials in the medical examiner's system. This typically included a single hippocampal section at a random level, and had limited capability for special tissue studies. The objective was to determine if DB was detectable and increased in frequency in, at least, a single random hippocampal section of cases with sudden unexplained infant death. We classified the infant deaths according to a scheme of unexplained (SIDS) versus explained deaths by review of clinical history, circumstances of death, complete autopsy, and death scene investigation; in unexplained deaths these processes did not reveal a known cause of death. Explained deaths were those in which the post-mortem studies revealed a known cause of death, including infection, accident, homicide, or unequivocal asphyxia (defined as documented obstruction of the nose and mouth, or chest constriction upon the death scene investigation). Infants with somatic and/or brain malformations, or known seizure disorders, were excluded. In all cases, information about multiple prenatal, neonatal, and postnatal parameters, including history of seizures, were collected from the clinical and autopsy records. The explained cases served as the controls in this study.

## Clinicopathologic findings in the San Diego cohort of the hippocampal study

In the San Diego cohort we found that the frequency of DB was significantly increased in the unexplained group compared to the explained group. Dentate bilamination was present in 41.2% (47/114) of the unexplained group compared to 7.7% (3/39) in the explained (p<0.001). This lesion was recognized at anterior, mid-, and posterior sections of the hippocampus in the unexplained category. The frequency of clusters of immature cells in the subgranular layer of the dentate gyrus was also significantly increased in the unexplained group (53.5% [61/114]) versus 10.3% (4/39) in the explained group, p<0.001). Immunocytochemical analysis indicated that these immature cells expressed Tuj1, a marker of early neuronal differentiation (3); these cells did not express immunomarkers for reactive astrocytes or activated microglia. The presence of DB was significantly associated with four features which were absent in cases without DB: [1] DB located in the bend of the C-shaped dentate gyrus; [2] clusters of immature cells in the subgranular layer of the dentate gyrus; [3] single ectopic GCs in the dentate gyrus molecular layer; and [4] clusters of ectopic GCs in the dentate gyrus molecular layer (3). There was no effect of increasing postconceptional age upon the frequency of DB, single/clusters of ectopic GCs, or immature cells in the subgranular layer of the dentate gyrus. Of note, in cases in which the right and left side of the hippocampus were available, we observed in some SIDS cases gross hippocampal asymmetry, which also demonstrated microscopic dentate abnormalities. We previously reported (28), for example, the case of a 10-month-old infant boy whose clinical presentation included a sleep-related death: prone position upon discovery, minor illness within two days of death, and no anatomic explanation for sudden death upon systemic autopsy. Nevertheless, neuropathologic examination revealed striking hippocampal asymmetry (Figure 29.3) and DB similar to that reported in cases in the San Diego cohort above.

In the San Diego infant cohort of unexplained (SIDS) and explained (control) cases, we also examined the dentate gyrus, temporal cortex, and white matter for possible linked morphologic profiles. In the unexplained group there was no significant increase in the frequency of acquired features indicative of acute or chronic hypoxic-schemic injury. However, 64.1% (25/39) of the explained group demonstrated acquired features compared to 21.1% (24/114) of the unexplained group (p<0.001). Because ischemia is known to stimulate neurogenesis, we postulated that the frequency of DB with hypoxic features (DB-HI) (e.g. hypereosinophilic GCs with pyknosis, gliosis in dentate gyrus) was not significantly different between the explained (15.4% [6/39]) and unexplained (14.0% [16/114]) groups (p=0.80) with hypoxia-ischemia, and we found this to be the case. The presence of DB-HI was significantly associated with features indicative of acute and/or chronic injury outside of the dentate gyrus (e.g. in the temporal cortex and Ammon's horn), whereas DB was not associated with HI changes. Thus, the morphological profile of linked features differed significantly between DB and DB-HI, indicating distinct entities, with DB almost exclusively found in the unexplained group.

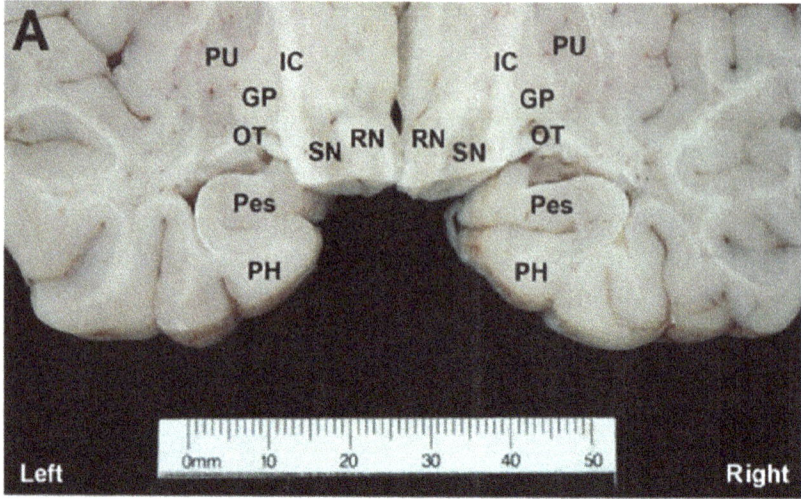

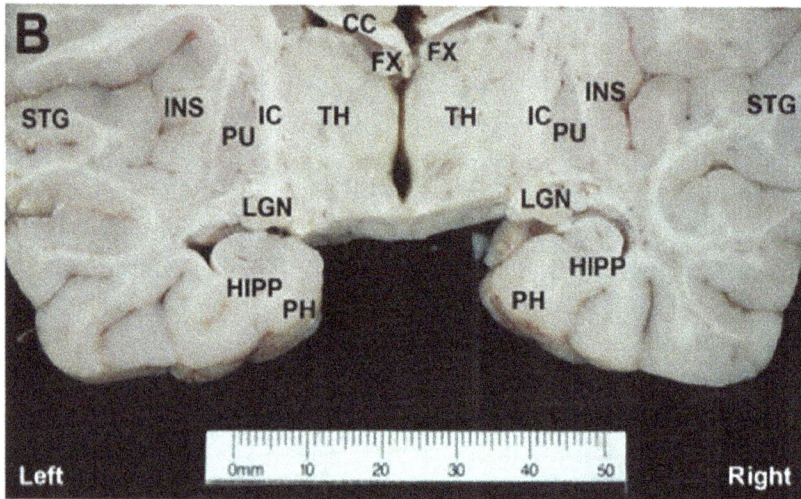

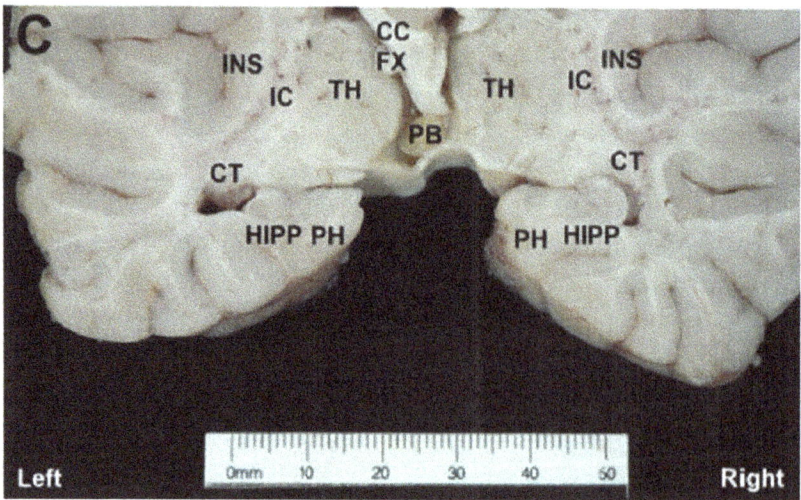

Figure 29.3 (left): Asymmetry of the hippocampus in a 10-month-old with sudden death. The macroscopic abnormalities are restricted to the hippocampus. A: At the anterior level (level of the substantia nigra and red nucleus), the left pes appeared globular and shortened in the mediolateral plane. B: At the mid-level (level of the lateral geniculate nucleus), the left hippocampus was slightly flattened and elongated in the mediolateral plane, and the temporal horn of the lateral ventricle appeared slightly dilated. C: At the posterior level (level of the pineal body and tail of the caudate), the left hippocampus was markedly flattened and appeared smaller than the right side, and the dilatation of the temporal ventricle was increased. The parahippocampal gyri, and superior, middle, and inferior temporal gyri appeared intact. Abbreviations: CC = corpus callosum; CT = tail of the caudate; FX fornix; HIPP = hippocampus; GP = globus pallidus; IC = internal capsule; IN = insula; LGN = lateral geniculate nucleus; OT = optic tract; PB = pineal body; PE = pes of hippocampus; PH = parahippocampal gyrus; PU = putamen; RN = red nucleus of midbrain; SN = substantia nigra of midbrain; TH = thalamus. (Reproduced from (28) with permission from Springer.)

## Defining a clinicopathologic phenotype associated with the subset of SIDS cases with dentate bilamination

We sought to determine whether there is a profile of clinicopathologic features that distinguishes the group of SIDS cases with DB (41.2% [47/114]) compared to that without DB (58.8% [67/114]). The incidence of prematurity (gestational age at birth <37 weeks) was significantly decreased in the unexplained group with DB (10.6% [5/47]) compared to the unexplained group without DB (29.9% [20/67]) (p=0.015). Thus, SIDS cases with DB tended to be born at term, a nonspecific feature clinically in and of itself (3). There were no significant differences in postnatal age, race, gender, or presence of pulmonary edema or intrathoracic petechiae at autopsy.

Due to the debate about the potential role of hypoxia/asphyxia in sudden infant death related to unsafe sleep environments (3), we further subdivided SIDS cases according to an "asphyxia risk profile". Explained deaths were subdivided into those with, or without, acute hypoxic insult as the immediate cause, the former including drowning and intentional suffocation. Unexplained deaths were subdivided into [1] death occurring in the setting of recommended sleep practices, as delineated by the Task Force on SIDS (29); [2] death occurring in the setting of non-recommended sleep practices; and [3] possible suffocation (airway obstruction) by history, but lacking physical evidence on autopsy. Importantly, the dentate abnormalities in this study were present in infants in the unexplained group with both recommended and non-recommended sleep environments, and with and without possible suffocation. In summary, a particular clinicopathologic phenotype, as determined by standard demographic and anatomic or forensic pathology, is not presently linked to SIDS cases with the DB lesion.

An unavoidable limitation of the study of the San Diego infant cohort is the use of control autopsy infants with acute disorders (e.g. infection), whose influence upon dentate gyrus structure is currently unknown. Indeed, we found that DB was present in 7.7% (3/39) of infants dying of explained causes, but without a history of seizures and/or somatic/brain malformations. This suggests that DB is not specific to unexplained death, but rather occurs in the unexplained category with significantly increased frequency (3). Until the etiology and pathogenesis of DB are discovered, the basis of its overlap in explained and unexplained infants remains unknown.

## Hippocampal Pathology in Sudden Unexpected Death Beyond Infancy

A major finding in children dying suddenly and unexpectedly over 1 year without explanation (e.g. SUDC) is hippocampal pathology, first reported by us in SUDC cases of the San Diego SUDC Research Project (30). A final summary of the San Diego database was published in 2015 (4, 5) in a study in which the findings in toto from 2007 to 2015 were collectively reported. We undertook analysis of a retrospective cohort of 151 cases, of which 80% (121/151) were subclassified as SUDC, 11% (16/151) as explained, 7% (10/151) as undetermined, and 3% (4/151) as seizure-related. There were no significant differences between SUDC and explained cases in postnatal, gestational, or postconceptional age, frequency of preterm birth, gender, race, or organ weights. In contrast, 96.7% (117/121) of the SUDC group were discovered during a sleep period compared to 53.3% (8/15) of the explained group (p<0.001). Of the SUDC cases, 48.8% (59/121) had a personal and/or family history of febrile seizures compared to 6.7% (1/15) of the explained group (p<0.001). Of the explained deaths, 56% (9/16) were subclassified as infection, 31% (5/16) cardiac, 6% (1/16) accidental, and 6% (1/16) metabolic. Two of the three cases specifically tested for cardiac channelopathies at autopsy based upon clinical indications had genetic variants in cardiac genes, one of uncertain significance. Two of the four seizure-related deaths were witnessed, with two of the brains from these cases showing generalized malformations. Hippocampal anomalies, including a specific combination we termed Hippocampal Maldevelopment Associated with Sudden Death (HMASD), were found in almost 50% (40/83) of the SUDC cases in which hippocampal sections were available. This study highlights the key role for the hippocampus, febrile seizures, and sleep in SUDC pathophysiology.

In the SUDC San Diego cohort, we characterized in greater detail the hippocampal pathology in 121 cases (4, 5). We performed comparative analysis on these cases, which we classified as one of the following: HMASD, SUDC with febrile seizure phenotype (SUDC-FS) but without hippocampal pathology, SUDC without hippocampal pathology or febrile seizure phenotype, and explained deaths. The frequency of each subgroup was: HMASD 48% (40/83); SUDC-FS 18% (15/83); SUDC 27% (22/83); and explained 7% (6/83). HMASD was characterized clinically by sudden, sleep-related death, term birth, and discovery in the prone position. Key morphologic features of

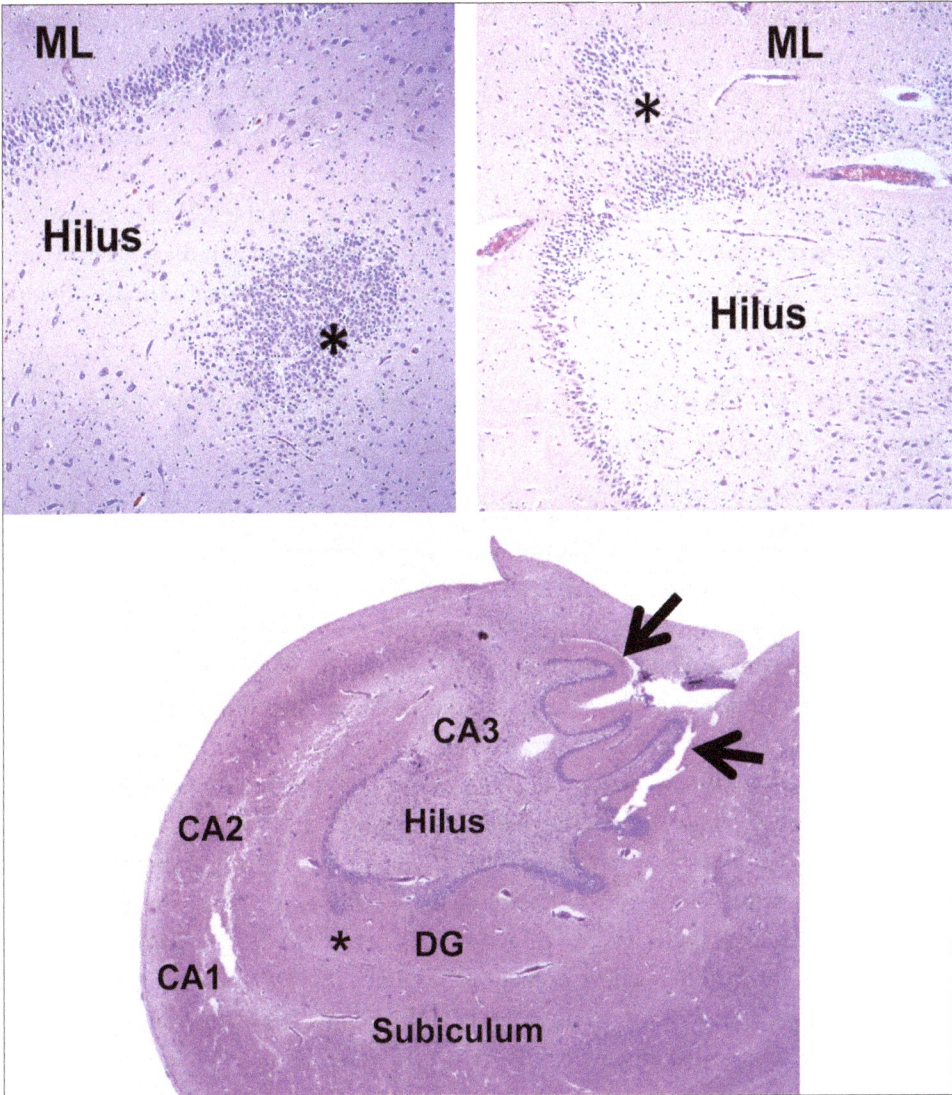

Figure 29.4: Developmental abnormalities in the hippocampus. Top left panel: granule cell heterotopia (asterisks) in hilus of hippocampus in SIDS. Top right panel: granule cell heterotopia (asterisks) in molecular layer of dentate gyrus in SIDS. Lower panel: scalloped shaped hyperconvolution of dentate gyrus in SIDS with excessive convolutions of the GC layer of the dentate gyrus at the medial surface (arrows). A GC heterotopia is in the molecular layer (asterisk). H&E, Whole mount. (Reproduced from (32) with permission from Oxford University Press.)

HMASD were focal GC bilamination of the dentate gyrus with, or without, asymmetry and/or malrotation of the hippocampus associated with significantly increased frequencies of 11 other developmental abnormalities (Figure 29.4). We identified no other distinct phenotype in the unexplained categories, except for an association of febrile seizures without hippocampal maldevelopment. This finding could reflect incomplete sampling of the hippocampus with failure to detect the hippocampal lesion. Alternatively, febrile seizure without hippocampal pathology may indicate that febrile seizures are a risk factor for sudden death without a direct link to anatomically obvious hippocampal pathology.

## Spectrum of Dentate Anomalies before and after One Year of Life (the Age "Cut-off" for SIDS)

We first reported hippocampal abnormalities in separate cohorts of SIDS (3) and SUDC (4, 5, 30, 31) cases. In the SUDC study, in the children between 1 and 6 years of age with hippocampal maldevelopment, 62.5% (25/40) had a personal and/or family history of febrile seizures compared to the population frequency of 3-5% (4, 5). We then asked if the hippocampal anomalies were the same, or similar, in SIDS and SUDC cases. We tested this in a different cohort of 32 SIDS and SUDC brains combined, and reported that in both age groups there was a similar spectrum of anomalies in the formation of the hippocampus and/or subiculum (32). Thus this study defined, for the first time, a unifying neuropathologic entity in sudden unexplained death in pediatrics (SUDP), involving children less than, and older than, 1 year of age. This was characterized by dentate/hippocampal/subicular maldevelopment, an entity we had previously reported separately in SIDS (3) and SUDC cases (4, 5, 30, 31). We have termed this lesion "hippocampal formation maldevelopment in SUDP" (SUDP-HFM), and identified four morphological variants of the disorder: [1] DB and GC anomalies only (Pattern A); [2] DB with hippocampal asymmetry (Pattern B) (Figure 29.5); [3] DB with subicular anomalies (Pattern C) (Figure 29.6); and [4] DB with hippocampal dysplasia (Pattern D) (32). These patterns may prove to be related to specific clinical subtypes, and/or variable genetic and environmental factors involved in the pathogenesis. All patterns display focal DB, with or without asymmetry/malrotation of the hippocampus proper (dentate gyrus and Ammon's horn). The major distinction among them is the presence of abnormal subicular folding (Pattern C) versus the absence of such folding (Patterns A, B, and D). While Patterns A, B, and D were present in all age groups, Pattern C was only observed in children older than 1 year of age. Pattern C also carried an 11-fold increase in risk of personal febrile seizures compared to Patterns A, B, and D combined, and a tendency toward larger head/brain size compared to Patterns A, B, and D combined. This latter observation needs confirmation in larger samples and comparison with parental head circumference data.

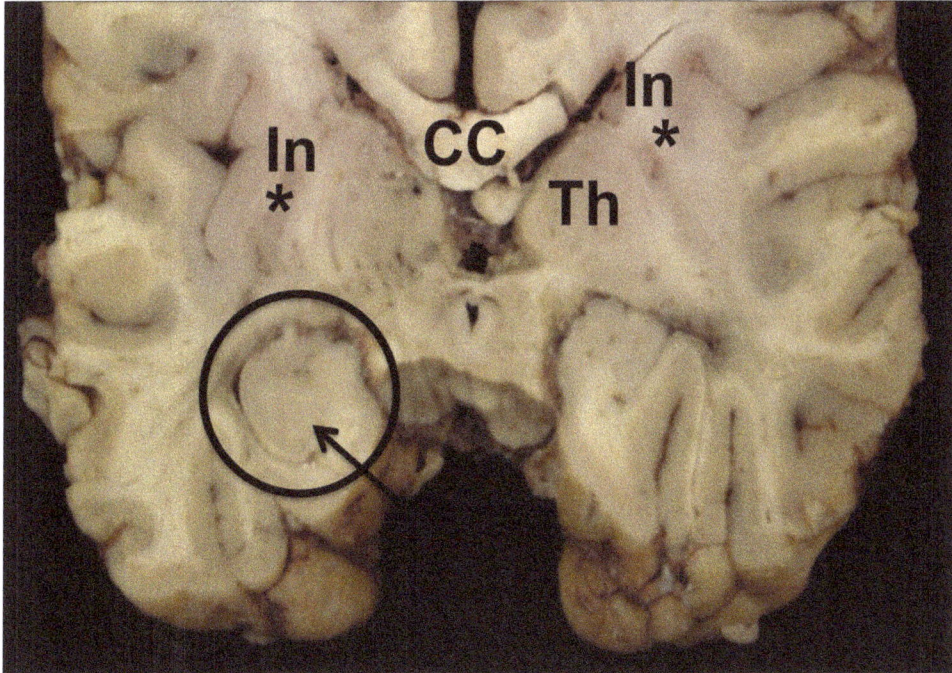

Figure 29.5: Asymmetry of the hippocampus (abnormal globular shape) in toddler with history of seizures and sudden death. Malrotation of the hippocampus proper is notable for a rounded and upright shape (encircled hippocampus). The toddler also has abnormal folding of the subiculum (arrow) and an asymmetric insular cortex (asterisk on each side of the insular cortex). Abbreviations: CC = corpus callosum; In = insula; Th = thalamus. (Reproduced from (32) with permission from Oxford University Press.)

In addition to DB, the brains of the 32 cases of SUDP-HFM exhibited a range of microdysgenetic features in temporal and non-temporal regions. These microdysgenetic features have been shown to be associated with epilepsy (32), and include focal cortical dysplasia, heterotopia, and hamartia. In addition, we found anomalies of derivatives of the embryonic rhombic lip, including hypo- or hyperplasia of the arcuate nucleus, olivary heterotopia and dysplasia, and dispersed GCs in the molecular layer of the cerebellar cortex (32). Although the DB and associated dentate gyral anomalies are the sine qua non of the SUDP-HFM entity that we describe, the presence of developmental pathology in the cerebral cortex and rhombic lip derivatives in the majority of SUDP-HFM cases suggests that this constellation of anomalies could relate to common processes involved in the development of the different regional anlages. It is possible that in some cases these three embryonic anlages are developmentally and functionally linked, and pattern disruptions occur in the genetic regulation of a signaling molecule or transcription factor shared by all three embryonic anlages in SUDP-HM. Many of the abnormalities inside

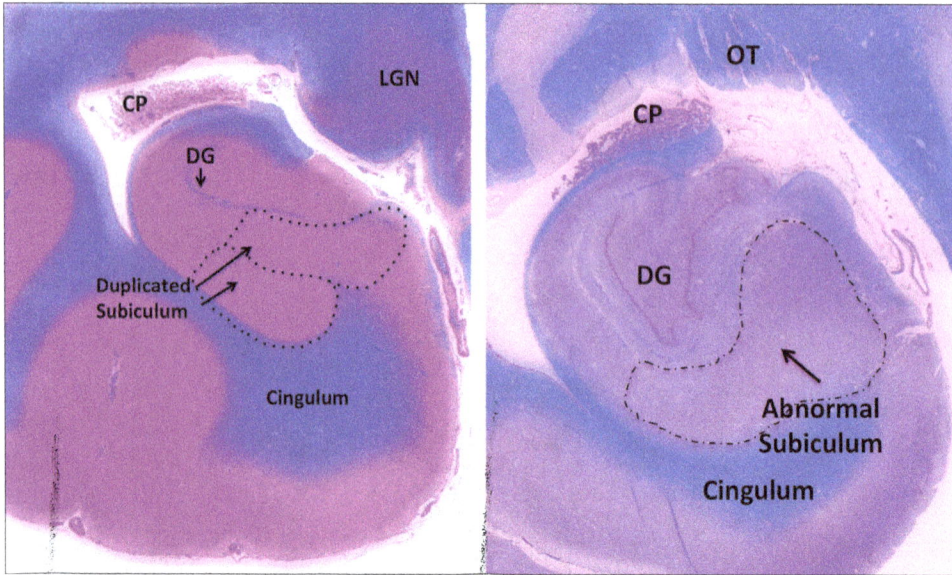

Figure 29.6: Anomalies of the subiculum in two cases of SUDC between the ages of 1 and 6 years. Left panel: duplication of the subiculum is characterized by the "splitting" of CA1 of Ammon's horn into two thick "branches" of subiculum (arrows, enclosed in dashed circles). Whole mount. Right panel: abnormal subicular folding is characterized by an uneven thickness in its shape. Whole mount. Abbreviations: CP = choroid plexus; DG = dentate gyrus; LGN = lateral geniculate nucleus; OT = optic tract. (Reproduced from (32) with permission from Oxford University Press.)

and outside the hippocampus proper are consistent with neuronal migration defects — for example, DB, focal cortical dysplasia, heterotopia, peripheralization of olivary neurons, arcuate nucleus hyperplasia, and dispersed GCs in the molecular layer of the dentate gyrus and cerebellar cortex — suggesting that genetic disturbances in shared migration factors (e.g. reelin) may occur in different parts of the brain.

The association between sudden death with personal febrile seizures in young children likely reflects the developing brain's vulnerability between the ages of 6 postnatal months and 6 years to high fever due to brain maturational factors related to thermal sensitivity, involving the CHN (33). Under 6 months, heightened thermal sensitivity may also be present, but may manifest as putative central autonomic instability and increased risk for sudden unexplained death due to over-bundling in SIDS (33).

In the combined study of infants and children who died suddenly, brain regions, in addition to the hippocampus, were examined for pathology. Of the cases under 1 year of age, 10/13 (77%) had diffuse cerebral white matter gliosis. This declined to 6% (1/17) in young children under 6 years, and to 0% in the two cases over 6 years. The majority of cases in the first year of life had brainstem tegmental gliosis, including the dorsal raphe and olivary gliosis; both of these features were reduced by half in early childhood (32). There was sparing of gliosis and neuronal loss in the thalamus, putamen, caudate, globus pallidus, and amygdala, and relative sparing of the hypothalamus. In the hippocampus there was hilar gliosis in both the infants (0 to less than 1 year, 46% [6/13]) and young children (1 to less than 6 years old, 47% [8/17]), without obvious neuronal loss. There was neither gliosis nor neuronal loss in hippocampal CA1-3 pyramidal neurons in any age group. The degree of myelination was age-appropriate in all forebrain and brainstem regions in which myelin counter-staining with Luxol-fast-blue was available (six infants and nine children over 1 year).

## General autopsy findings

We reviewed the autopsy reports in all 32 cases of SUDP-HFM. In 21 cases, microscopic slides of somatic organs were evaluated. In 20 cases, there was evidence of antigenic stimulation, defined as mucosal or submucosal inflammation and/or increased numbers and prominence of lymphoid follicles with active germinal centers in upper respiratory tract, gastrointestinal tract, splenic white pulp, and/or enlarged lymph nodes. Focal, lymphocytic inflammation was noted in the leptomeninges in 13 of 32 cases, suggesting mild (non-lethal) aseptic meningitis. Microbial cultures were reported as positive for pathogens in 3 of the 20 cases with antigenic stimulation. The presence of antigenic stimulation in somatic organs in most cases may support a role for fever and inflammation in the pathogenesis of sudden death with SUDP-HFM, although it is not an uncommon autopsy finding in young children. In six SUDP-HFM cases, death certificates listed a specific, non-seizure-related cause of death, including respiratory tract infection or sepsis, also evidence of antigenic stimulation. In our cases, in which the listed cause of death was infection or cardiac channelopathy, hippocampal pathology was not recognized by the medical examiner, who concluded that the etiology was non-brain-related. Increased recognition of SUDP-HFM may further clarify the relationship between brain vulnerability and potential triggering or augmentation by infection, genetic susceptibilities to arrhythmias, or other factors.

There was no definitive evidence of terminal/acute or gastric aspiration in the 21 cases. Esophagitis with eosinophils was present in four cases. Pulmonary edema was present in 10/21 (48%) and pulmonary hemorrhage in 14/21 (67%) of cases. These pulmonary pathologies are notably analogous to autopsy features reported in, though not specific to, sudden unexpected death in epilepsy (SUDEP), and are considered to be related to a neurogenic pathogenesis (32). Of nine young child cases with age-appropriate dentition in the autopsy reports, bite marks on the tongue were reported in three cases and equivocally in one, consistent with an acute, terminal seizure.

# The Pathogenesis of Dentate Gyral Abnormalities in SIDS/SUDC

The etiology of DB observed in the dentate gyrus in sudden and unexpected death in early life is unknown. We suggest that DB represents a developmental defect in neuronal proliferation, migration, and/or cell survival in the dentate gyrus related to [1] an unknown teratogen during gestation; [2] abnormalities in the trophic effects of 5-HT (see below); or [3] an unrecognized genetic defect in dentate gyral formation. In the SIDS cases, evidence of proliferation of GC, scalloping, and hyperconvolution of the dentate gyrus suggests an excess number of GCs packed into the undulating configuration of the dentate gyrus, which influences GC dispersion and DB, as evidenced by the excessive clusters of progenitor-like cells in the subgranular layers with markers of immature neurons (e.g. Tuj1). The strong association of DB with other features of maldevelopment in the dentate gyrus (e.g. excessive single or clustered ectopic GCs in the dentate molecular layer and hilus) and clusters of immature cells in its subgranular layer (the zone of GC neurogenesis) supports such a developmental hypothesis.

This is further supported by a lack of acquired inflammation (i.e. reactive astrocytes), activated microglia, and/or apparent neuronal loss. In the San Diego cohort study, the immature cells, labeled by Tuj1, in excessive clusters in the subgranular layer are potentially "stalled" in the subgranular layer due to impaired migration; or, alternatively, they "accumulate" in the subgranular layer due to an abnormally prolonged cell survival, a mechanism suggested in the PET1 knockout mouse with impaired 5-HT cell development (32). The undulations of the dentate gyrus and its molecular layer, particularly in the medial distribution, in Pattern D (hippocampal dysplasia) are reminiscent of the histopathologic dentate findings in the genetically engineered mutant mice which lack the non-receptor tyrosine kinase gene fyn and demonstrate impaired long-term potentiation, spatial learning, seizures, and sudden death (39, 40). The lack of fyn during hippocampal development in this mouse mutant results in an increased number of GCs in the dentate gyrus, giving it a "scalloped" or "dysplastic" appearance, as seen in our Pattern D. The increase in cells was postulated to result from over-proliferation, altered cell fates, or failure of cell death (39). Granule cell production occurs in the human dentate gyrus pre- and postnatally, with stabilization within the first three years (41). Granule cell dispersion has not, however, been observed in normal dentate development; rather, its presence is invariably considered pathologic (41).

We regard the abnormal hippocampus with Patterns A-D as primary developmental lesions because they are not associated with gliosis and/or neuronal loss in the hippocampal formation (HF), except for hilar gliosis (see below). We speculate that abnormal folding of the hippocampus proper (Pattern B), subiculum (Pattern C), and GC and molecular layers of the dentate gyrus (Pattern D) originates as the hippocampus begins to form and fold at the end of the first trimester (32). The embryonic anlage of the HF, the cortical hem, which induces the formation of the hippocampus proper and subiculum within the adjacent cortical neuroepithelium (32), may be at fault in Patterns B, C, and D. Granule cells in the dentate gyrus are generated from stem cells in the subgranular layer throughout life, and integrate into the mature hippocampal circuitry, potentially participating in the formation of new memories (22). Because neurogenesis continues after birth into adulthood (22), Pattern A, consisting of DB only, could arise pre- and/or postnatally. GC dispersion, including DB, is hypothesized to be due to increased proliferation of progenitor cells from the subgranular zone, a defect in neuronal migration upwards from the subgranular zone, and/or inhibition of programmed GC death.

We have examined the cohort histories for possible teratogens that could operate during early gestation (e.g. prenatal exposure to alcohol and cigarette smoke). Patterns A, B, and D combined demonstrated variable frequencies of borderline significance with exposure to prenatal alcohol, which is a known risk factor for SIDS (42), as is prenatal exposure to smoking (43). Pattern C, with abnormal subicular folding, was not associated with these exposures, suggesting that Pattern C may have a distinctive pathogenesis with a developmental vulnerability of the subiculum different from the hippocampus proper — a hypothesis for future testing in larger cohorts with more detailed exposure histories.

## Granule Cell Dispersion in the Dentate Gyrus and its Role in the Genesis of Seizures

The dentate gyrus in the hippocampus is a well-recognized site of epileptogenesis (23), as demonstrated in genetically engineered mouse models in which dentate morphological disorganization is responsible for the origin of seizures, and not secondary to them (44). Granule cell dispersion, however, is also recognized to be secondary to seizures, with seizure activity resulting in the formation of the lesion. Thus, a role for seizures must be considered in the pathogenesis of increased GCs in SIDS cases. Data from rodent models of medial temporal lobe epilepsy show that prolonged seizures acutely increase adult GC neurogenesis (23). In the rat pilocarpine model of temporal lobe epilepsy, as assessed by the expression of Ki-67 (an endogenous cell proliferation marker) or short-pulse bromodeoxyuridine (BrdU) mitotic labeling, the dentate gyrus responds to status epilepticus (SE) by increasing cell proliferation in the subgranular zone (45).

Seizures can also induce other morphological changes in the dentate gyrus that affect dentate function. The epileptic dentate gyrus in human TLE is associated with mossy fiber sprouting, ectopically located GCs, and GCs with very prominent hilar basal dendrites (HBDs), as well as GC dispersion (23). In rodent models of status epilepticus such as the pilocarpine model, hippocampal pathways exhibit structural plasticity analogous to changes reported in humans. After SE, many dentate GCs erroneously migrate into the dentate hilus or through the granular layer into the molecular layer

(23). These ectopic cells are found in rodent models of epilepsy (46), in the epileptic human hippocampus (23), and in the SIDS and SUDC cases of our studies.

One proposed cause of the aberrant migration is loss of the migration guidance cue reelin, which is expressed in the adult rodent hippocampus (23). In epileptic brains, dentate GC dispersion is thought to result in aberrant synaptic connectivity, increasing susceptibility to seizures through hyperexcitability (23). A large body of information supports the hypothesis that cellular abnormalities such as mossy fiber sprouting, ectopic dentate GCs, and HBDs contribute to epileptogenesis in experimental and human TLE. Seizures in TLE have been proposed to result from hyperexcitability due to aberrant excitatory recurrent axon collaterals between GCs in mossy fiber sprouting (23). Additionally, evidence suggests that normal gamma-Aminobutyric acid (GABA) inhibition is diminished by mossy fiber terminals, further contributing to hyperexcitability in mossy fiber sprouting. Hilar ectopic GCs themselves are also thought to be hyperexcitable (23). Timm staining and dynorphin immunoreactivity, as markers for mossy fibers, have demonstrated substantial sprouting in patients with mesial TLE that is considered secondary to chronic seizures (23). Normally, glutamatergic mossy fibers project into the dentate hilus from the GC layer and stratum lucidum of CA3 and synapse with inhibitory interneurons, hilar mossy cells, and CA3 pyramidal cells, but only very rarely with other GCs. Consequently, most GCs normally do not display functional, monosynaptic, recurrent excitation (23).

Overall, there is considerable anatomical and physiological evidence that mossy fiber sprouting creates a positive-feedback, seizure-generating circuit among GCs. In epileptic tissue, sprouted mossy fibers form excitatory synapses with ectopic GCs in the hilus, GC basal dendrites in the hilus, GC somata in the GC layer, and GC apical dendrites in the GC layer and inner molecular layer. Furthermore, mossy fiber sprouting correlates with hilar neuron loss in patients with mesial TLE (23). In our tissue sections, neuronal loss was not always visually apparent, and quantitative studies would be needed to determine subtle loss.

## Speculation about the Mechanism(s) of Sudden Death associated with Dentate Gyral Abnormalities in SIDS/SUDC

The dentate gyral abnormalities are a putative morphological marker of an impaired central homeostatic network (which involves brainstem, forebrain, and limbic systems) which increases the risk of sudden infant death due to instability of modulation of brainstem cardiorespiratory-related nuclei, or to a subclinical autonomic seizure in an infant with a predisposition to epilepsy, not yet manifested as a clinical seizure. We propose that this morphological marker "identifies" a vulnerable infant at risk for sudden death during a critical developmental period (birth to 6 years) when the infant or child meets an exogenous stressor of the Triple Risk model for SIDS and now SUDC (34). The hippocampus is interconnected with other forebrain loci in the limbic

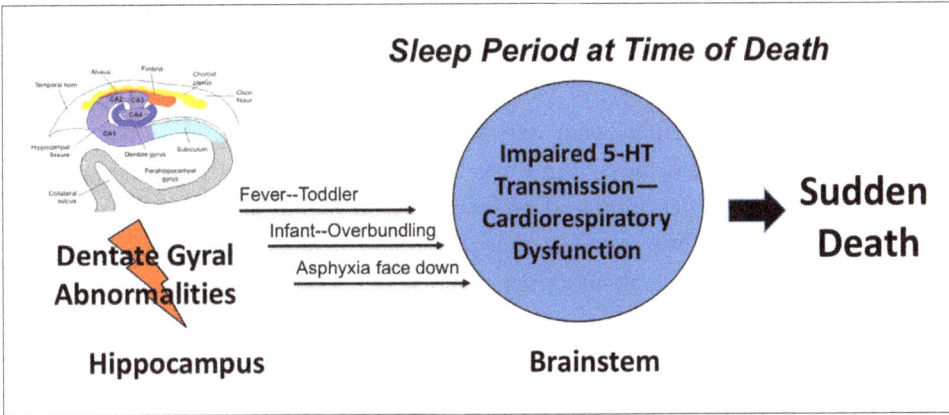

Figure 29.7: Potential mechanism of death in dentate gyral dysplasia with compromised serotonergic pathways in the brainstem. (Authors' own work.)

network (e.g. amygdala, insula, hypothalamus), as well as the brainstem sites which directly mediate respiratory autonomic control. The hippocampus exhibits a striking propensity to seizure generation and propagation, and the seizure discharges in temporal lobe epilepsy, especially, precipitate serious cardiorespiratory events (e.g. apnea and bradycardia (35)). Autonomic seizures are a consideration in sudden infant death, since recurrent episodes of apnea, reported in infants who subsequently die of SIDS (36), may be the sole manifestation of seizures (without movement abnormalities) in infants with temporal lobe pathology (37). The association of seizures (and sudden death during sleep periods) with limbic/hippocampal pathology suggests that sleep state in some way lowers the threshold for epileptogenesis in the limbic system.

The neuropathologic findings in these children provide a plausible mechanism for sudden and unexpected death via an epilepsy-like mechanism. Seizures, known to arise in all hippocampal formation (HF) substructures (32), may be generated in the abnormal hippocampal formation in SUDP-HFM, triggered by stress (e.g. asphyxia or fever) (Figure 29.7). The dentate gyrus is a well-recognized site of epileptogenesis (23) (see below). We speculate that abnormal electrical discharges in the disorganized HF are propagated to regions of the brainstem involved in breathing and/or autonomic function during sleep, leading to lethal disruption of vital functions and sudden death during sleep, when the threshold for epileptogenesis is lowered. We agree with Noebels, who recently coined the term "epilepsy in situ" in SUDC cases with hippocampal maldevelopment as an apt "new term that may be usefully applied to a microscopic epileptiform lesion with or without evidence of actual seizures" (38) (p. 198).

Using the Connectome in living adult volunteers, we have provided evidence for connectivity between the hippocampus and caudal brainstem regions (nodes) that participate in the regulation of homeostasis in the human brain (9). These nodes, and connections between the brainstem and hippocampus and other forebrain limbic-related sites, possibly represent the CHN due to the fact that its nodes regulate not only emotion and autonomic functions, but also homeostatic functions such as respiration (paragigantocellularis lateralis) and arousal (e.g. median and dorsal raphe, and the functions of the locus coeruleus). An important question is why the abnormalities of the HF, arising during gestation and present at birth, manifest themselves as sudden death at different ages. We speculate that the timing is due to the child's individual developmental, environmental, and genetic risk factors, which influence the underlying HF vulnerability.

## Potential Relationship between Brainstem and Hippocampal Abnormalities in the Same Cases

Over the last two decades, our group has provided substantial evidence in four published independent datasets that a subset of SIDS (~40%) is characterized by 5-HT defects. These are located in cardiorespiratory- and arousal-related regions in the medulla oblongata (caudal brainstem) and were identified using neurochemical techniques in frozen brainstem tissue (47-50). In 2015, we reported the novel morphological finding in the dentate gyrus of DB in a major subset of SIDS cases (~40%) in a separate dataset, as described above. It is currently unknown whether the same SIDS cases share hippocampal DB and 5-HT brainstem pathology, or whether each of these problems defines two separate entities currently under the rubric "SIDS". If the hippocampal and brainstem abnormalities are part of one disease process, the presence of GC dispersion in the SIDS cases suggests the possibility that sudden death is the consequence of a seizure generated from the abnormal dentate gyrus. This would be triggered by stress (e.g. asphyxia or over-bundling/hyperthermia) and cannot be compensated by activation of 5-HT pathways in the brainstem, due to the simultaneously defective brainstem-mediated protective responses (e.g. arousal), thereby resulting in death. Importantly, recent experimental evidence suggests that brainstem 5-HT systems are critical in autonomic and respiratory changes during and after seizures arising above the brainstem, with implications for seizure-related sudden death (51).

The vulnerability of the hippocampus among forebrain sites to brainstem 5-HT pathology may reflect its preferential and extensive innervation with known heavy concentrations of 5-HT terminals by the rostral raphe (52). Neuroanatomic interconnections exist between the rostral and caudal 5-HT cell domains (52) and between the caudal 5-HT domain and limbic sites (9), as we have shown in Connectome studies of adult in vivo brains. We propose that the developmental malposition of GCs in SIDS-DB is due to defective brainstem 5-HT cell domains interfering with 5-HT innervation of hippocampal Cajal Retzius (CR) cells. Serotonergic fibers enter the marginal zone of the cerebral cortex before birth, where they influence cortical development through synaptic contacts with these CR cells (53). Perturbation of these early 5-HT contacts with CR cells decreases reelin in the brains of the newborn pups, and the formation of the presubicular cortex is altered (53). This work suggests a mechanism where 5-HT deficiencies involving ascending 5-HT projections in the brainstem during hippocampal development could lead to DB — that is, via decreased 5-HT-mediated production of reelin by the CR cells and secondary migration defects in the GCs that are known to be innervated by CR cells. In regards to 5-HT brainstem pathology in SIDS and its possible link to hippocampal defects, 5-HT is released from nuclei in the rostral raphe in the caudal midbrain and upper pons to play a trophic role in neurogenesis, migration, and neuronal survival in the dentate gyrus in early development (54). Moreover, 5-HT from the rostral raphe helps regulate neurogenesis in the dentate gyrus throughout life. Serotonin dysfunction is implicated in the seizure pathogenesis, and hippocampal abnormalities of 5-HT1A receptor binding have been reported in TLE (55). Thus, the underlying vulnerability in the infant at risk for sudden death may reflect a 5-HT brainstem disorder with deficient projections from the rostral raphe to the hippocampus, or alternatively, brainstem and hippocampus disorders independent from one another. Future research is needed to determine the role of brainstem 5-HT in the dentate disorganization reported here.

## Conclusions

The finding of DB, a distinctive variant of GC dispersion, in the hippocampus of infants and children with sudden unexplained death opens new avenues for research into underlying vulnerabilities of these individuals to sudden death. Given that GC dispersion is a pathologic hallmark of TLE, its presence in the brains of infants and children dying suddenly without explanation raises provocative questions about the possible role of an underlying anatomic anomaly of the hippocampal dentate gyrus in initiating sudden death through epileptogenesis or faulty modulation of the CHN. The identification of this anatomic marker of a potential vulnerability to sudden early death unifies our approach to the investigation of SIDS, SUDC, and SUDEP. The descriptive observation of DB in sudden infant and child death is a potentially critical clue towards guiding both future neuropathologic studies in human youth and mechanistic testing in developmental animal models with consideration of hippocampal-brainstem and CHN interactions. Further research is also needed to investigate the relationship between hippocampal and the previously reported brainstem pathology in sudden infant death.

This study concludes that the presence of DB neuropathology in the HF in sudden unexplained death of infants and children challenges the age-related conventions for separating SIDS and SUDC. SUDP-HFM must be carefully identified in neuropathologic examination of sudden death in infants and children by assessment of both hippocampi in more than one tissue section. We believe it is appropriate to designate SUDP-HFM as a distinct cause of death for the purposes of family counseling, vital statistics, and death certificates. In our opinion, the robustness of the clinicopathologic phenotype, and the biologic plausibility of a fatal seizure-like event triggered by a set of exogenous factors in a critical developmental period, justify this conclusion. The outcomes of our research may lead to an increased understanding of antecedent risk factors for this entity.

# References

1.  Kinney HC, Thach BT. The sudden infant death syndrome. N Engl J Med. 2009;361(8):795-805. https://doi.org/10.1056/NEJMra0803836.

2.  Harper RM, Kinney HC. Potential mechanisms of failure in the sudden infant death syndrome. Curr Pediatr Rev. 2010;6(1):39-47. https://doi.org/10.2174/157339610791317214.

3.  Kinney HC, Cryan JB, Haynes RL, Paterson DS, Haas EA, Mena OJ, et al. Dentate gyrus abnormalities in sudden unexplained death in infants: Morphological marker of underlying brain vulnerability. Acta Neuropathol. 2015;129(1):65-80. https://doi.org/10.1007/s00401-014-1357-0.

4.  Hefti MM, Kinney HC, Cryan JB, Haas EA, Chadwick AE, Crandall LA, et al. Sudden unexpected death in early childhood: General observations in a series of 151 cases: Part 1 of the investigations of the San Diego SUDC Research Project. Forensic Sci Med Pathol. 2016;12(1):4-13. https://doi.org/10.1007/s12024-015-9724-2.

5.  Hefti MM, Cryan JB, Haas EA, Chadwick AE, Crandall LA, Trachtenberg FL, et al. Hippocampal malformation associated with sudden death in early childhood: A neuropathologic study: Part 2 of the investigations of The San Diego SUDC Research Project. Forensic Sci Med Pathol. 2016;12(1):14-25. https://doi.org/10.1007/s12024-015-9731-3.

6.  Harper RM. State-related physiological changes and risk for the sudden infant death syndrome. Aust Paediatr J. 1986;22 Suppl 1:55-8.

7.  Kinney HC, McDonald AG, Minter ME, Berry GT, Poduri A, Goldstein RD. Witnessed sleep-related seizure and sudden unexpected death in infancy: A case report. Forensic Sci Med Pathol. 2013;9(3):418-21. https://doi.org/10.1007/s12024-013-9448-0.

8.  Hewertson J, Poets CF, Samuels MP, Boyd SG, Neville BG, Southall DP. Epileptic seizure-induced hypoxemia in infants with apparent life-threatening events. Pediatrics. 1994;94(2 Pt 1):148-56.

9.  Edlow BL, McNab JA, Witzel T, Kinney HC. The structural Connectome of the human central homeostatic network. Brain Connect. 2016;6(3):187-200. https://doi.org/10.1089/brain.2015.0378.

10. Barger N, Hanson KL, Teffer K, Schenker-Ahmed NM, Semendeferi K. Evidence for evolutionary specialization in human limbic structures. Front Hum Neurosci. 2014;8:277. https://doi.org/10.3389/fnhum.2014.00277.

11. Kaas JH. The evolution of brains from early mammals to humans. Wiley Interdiscip Rev Cogn Sci. 2013;4(1):33-45. https://doi.org/10.1002/wcs.1206.

12. Beissner F, Meissner K, Bar KJ, Napadow V. The autonomic braIn: An activation likelihood estimation meta-analysis for central processing of autonomic function. J Neurosci. 2013;33(25):10503-11. https://doi.org/10.1523/JNEUROSCI.1103-13.2013.

13. Benarroch EE. The central autonomic network: Functional organization, dysfunction, and perspective. Mayo Clin Proc. 1993;68(10):988-1001. https://doi.org/10.1016/S0025-6196(12)62272-1.

14. Saper CB. The central autonomic nervous system: Conscious visceral perception and autonomic pattern generation. Ann Rev Neurosci. 2002;25:433-69. https://doi.org/10.1146/annurev.neuro.25.032502.111311.

15. Mraovitch S, Calando Y. Interactions between limbic, thalamo-striatal-cortical, and central autonomic pathways during epileptic seizure progression. J Comp Neurol. 1999;411(1):145-61. https://doi.org/10.1002/(SICI)1096-9861(19990816)411:1<145::AID-CNE11>3.0.CO;2-1.

16. Ulrich-Lai YM, Herman JP. Neural regulation of endocrine and autonomic stress responses. Nat Rev Neurosci. 2009;10(6):397-409. https://doi.org/10.1038/nrn2647.

17. Nicolaides NC, Kyratzi E, Lamprokostopoulou A, Chrousos GP, Charmandari E. Stress, the stress system and the role of glucocorticoids. Neuroimmunomodulation. 2015;22(1-2):6-19. https://doi.org/10.1159/000362736.

18. van Bodegom M, Homberg JR, Henckens M. Modulation of the hypothalamic-pituitary-adrenal axis by early life stress exposure. Front Cell Neurosci. 2017;11:87. https://doi.org/10.3389/fncel.2017.00087.

19. Herman JP, McKlveen JM, Ghosal S, Kopp B, Wulsin A, Makinson R, et al. Regulation of the hypothalamic-pituitary-adrenocortical stress response. Compr Physiol. 2016;6(2):603-21. https://doi.org/10.1002/cphy.c150015.

20. McEwen BS, Gianaros PJ. Central role of the brain in stress and adaptation: Links to socioeconomic status, health, and disease. Ann NY Acad Sci. 2010;1186:190-222. https://doi.org/10.1111/j.1749-6632.2009.05331.x.

21. McEwen BS, Magarinos AM. Stress effects on morphology and function of the hippocampus. Ann NY Acad Sci. 1997;821:271-84. https://doi.org/10.1111/j.1749-6632.1997.tb48286.x.

22. Aimone JB, Li Y, Lee SW, Clemenson GD, Deng W, Gage FH. Regulation and function of adult neurogenesis: From genes to cognition. Physiol Rev. 2014;94(4):991-1026. https://doi.org/10.1152/physrev.00004.2014.

23. Parent JM, Kron MM. Neurogenesis and epilepsy. In: Jasper's basic mechanisms of the epilepsies. Eds Noebels JL, Avoli M, Rogawski MA, Olsen RW, Delgado-Escueta AV. 4th ed. Bethesda (MD): Oxford University Press, 2012. https://doi.org/10.1093/med/9780199746545.003.0038.

24. Houser CR. Granule cell dispersion in the dentate gyrus of humans with temporal lobe epilepsy. Brain Res. 1990;535(2):195-204. https://doi.org/10.1016/0006-8993(90)91601-C.

25. Armstrong DD. Epilepsy-induced microarchitectural changes in the brain. Pediatr Dev Pathol. 2005;8(6):607-14. https://doi.org/10.1007/s10024-005-0054-3.

26. Armstrong DD. The neuropathology of temporal lobe epilepsy. J Neuropathol Exp Neurol. 1993;52(5):433-43. https://doi.org/10.1097/00005072-199309000-00001.

27. Blumcke I, Kistner I, Clusmann H, Schramm J, Becker AJ, Elger CE, et al. Towards a clinico-pathological classification of granule cell dispersion in human mesial temporal lobe epilepsies. Acta neuropathol. 2009;117(5):535-44. https://doi.org/10.1007/s00401-009-0512-5.

28. Rodriguez ML, McMillan K, Crandall LA, Minter ME, Grafe MR, Poduri A, et al. Hippocampal asymmetry and sudden unexpected death in infancy: A case report. Forensic Sci Med Pathol. 2012;8(4):441-6. https://doi.org/10.1007/s12024-012-9367-5.

29. Task Force on Sudden Infant Death Syndrome, & Moon RY. SIDS and other sleep-related infant deaths: Expansion of recommendations for a safe infant sleeping environment. Pediatrics. 2011;128(5):1030-9. https://doi.org/10.1542/peds.2011-2284.

30. Kinney HC, Armstrong DL, Chadwick AE, Crandall LA, Hilbert C, Belliveau RA, et al. Sudden death in toddlers associated with developmental abnormalities of the hippocampus: A report of five cases. Pediatr Dev Pathol. 2007;10(3):208-23. https://doi.org/10.2350/06-08-0144.1.

31. Kinney HC, Chadwick AE, Crandall LA, Grafe M, Armstrong DL, Kupsky WJ, et al. Sudden death, febrile seizures, and hippocampal and temporal lobe maldevelopment in toddlers: A new entity. Pediatr Dev Pathol. 2009;12(6):455-63. https://doi.org/10.2350/08-09-0542.1.

32. Kinney HC, Poduri AH, Cryan JB, Haynes RL, Teot L, Sleeper LA, et al. Hippocampal formation maldevelopment and sudden unexpected death across the pediatric age spectrum. J Neuropathol Exp Neurol. 2016;75(10):981-97. https://doi.org/10.1093/jnen/nlw075.

33. Hoppenbrouwers T. Sudden infant death syndrome, sleep, and seizures. J Child Neurol. 2015;30(7):904-11. https://doi.org/10.1177/0883073814549243.

34. Filiano JJ, Kinney HC. A perspective on neuropathologic findings in victims of the sudden infant death syndrome: The triple-risk model. Biol Neonate. 1994;65(3-4):194-7. https://doi.org/10.1159/000244052.

35. Moseley B, Bateman L, Millichap JJ, Wirrell E, Panayiotopoulos CP. Autonomic epileptic seizures, autonomic effects of seizures, and SUDEP. Epilepsy Behav. 2013;26(3):375-85. https://doi.org/10.1016/j.yebeh.2012.08.020.

36. Poets CF, Meny RG, Chobanian MR, Bonofiglo RE. Gasping and other cardiorespiratory patterns during sudden infant deaths. Pediatr Res. 1999;45(3):350-4. https://doi.org/10.1203/00006450-199903000-00010.

37. Miyagawa T, Sotero M, Avellino AM, Kuratani J, Saneto RP, Ellenbogen RG, et al. Apnea caused by mesial temporal lobe mass lesions in infants: Report of 3 cases. J Child Neurol. 2007;22(9):1079-83. https://doi.org/10.1177/0883073807306245.

38. Noebels J. Hippocampal abnormalities and sudden childhood death. Forensic Sci Med Pathol. 2016;12(2):198-9. https://doi.org/10.1007/s12024-016-9768-y.

39. Grant SG, O'Dell TJ, Karl KA, Stein PL, Soriano P, Kandel ER. Impaired long-term potentiation, spatial learning, and hippocampal development in fyn mutant mice. Science. 1992;258(5090):1903-10. https://doi.org/10.1126/science.1361685.

40. Kojima N, Ishibashi H, Obata K, Kandel ER. Higher seizure susceptibility and enhanced tyrosine phosphorylation of N-methyl-D-aspartate receptor subunit 2B in fyn transgenic mice. Learn Mem. 1998;5(6):429-45.

41. Insausti R, Cebada-Sanchez S, Marcos P. Postnatal development of the human hippocampal formation. BerlIn: Springer, 2010. https://doi.org/10.1007/978-3-642-03661-3.

42. Iyasu S, Randall LL, Welty TK, Hsia J, Kinney HC, Mandell F, et al. Risk factors for sudden infant death syndrome among northern plains Indians. JAMA. 2002;288(21):2717-23. https://doi.org/10.1001/jama.288.21.2717.

43.  Mitchell EA, Milerad J. Smoking and the sudden infant death syndrome. Rev Environ Health. 2006;21(2):81-103. https://doi.org/10.1515/REVEH.2006.21.2.81.

44.  Pun RY, Rolle IJ, Lasarge CL, Hosford BE, Rosen JM, Uhl JD, et al. Excessive activation of mTOR in postnatally generated granule cells is sufficient to cause epilepsy. Neuron. 2012;75(6):1022-34. https://doi.org/10.1016/j.neuron.2012.08.002.

45.  Parent JM, Yu TW, Leibowitz RT, Geschwind DH, Sloviter RS, Lowenstein DH. Dentate granule cell neurogenesis is increased by seizures and contributes to aberrant network reorganization in the adult rat hippocampus. J Neurosci. 1997;17(10):3727-38.

46.  Parent JM. Adult neurogenesis in the intact and epileptic dentate gyrus. Prog Brain Res. 2007;163:529-40. https://doi.org/10.1016/S0079-6123(07)63028-3.

47.  Panigrahy A, Filiano J, Sleeper LA, Mandell F, Valdes-Dapena M, Krous HF, et al. Decreased serotonergic receptor binding in rhombic lip-derived regions of the medulla oblongata in the sudden infant death syndrome. J Neuropathol Exp Neurol. 2000;59(5):377-84. https://doi.org/10.1093/jnen/59.5.377.

48.  Paterson DS, Trachtenberg FL, Thompson EG, Belliveau RA, Beggs AH, Darnall R, et al. Multiple serotonergic brainstem abnormalities in sudden infant death syndrome. JAMA. 2006;296(17):2124-32. https://doi.org/10.1001/jama.296.17.2124.

49.  Duncan JR, Paterson DS, Hoffman JM, Mokler DJ, Borenstein NS, Belliveau RA, et al. Brainstem serotonergic deficiency in sudden infant death syndrome. JAMA. 2010;303(5):430-7. https://doi.org/10.1001/jama.2010.45.

50.  Kinney HC, Randall LL, Sleeper LA, Willinger M, Belliveau RA, Zec N, et al. Serotonergic brainstem abnormalities in Northern Plains Indians with the sudden infant death syndrome. J Neuropathol Exp Neurol. 2003;62(11):1178-91. https://doi.org/10.1093/jnen/62.11.1178.

51.  Zhan Q, Buchanan GF, Motelow JE, Andrews J, Vitkovskiy P, Chen WC, et al. Impaired serotonergic brainstem function during and after seizures. J Neurosci. 2016;36(9):2711-22. https://doi.org/10.1523/JNEUROSCI.4331-15.2016.

52.  Azmitia EC, Gannon PJ. The primate serotonergic system: A review of human and animal studies and a report on Macaca fascicularis. Adv Neurol. 1986;43:407-68.

53.  Janusonis S, Gluncic V, Rakic P. Early serotonergic projections to Cajal-Retzius cells: Relevance for cortical development. J Neurosci. 2004;24(7):1652-9. https://doi.org/10.1523/JNEUROSCI.4651-03.2004.

54. Djavadian RL. Serotonin and neurogenesis in the hippocampal dentate gyrus of adult mammals. Acta Neurobiol Exp. 2004;64(2):189-200.

55. Savic I, Lindstrom P, Gulyas B, Halldin C, Andree B, Farde L. Limbic reductions of 5-HT1A receptor binding in human temporal lobe epilepsy. Neurology. 2004;62(8):1343-51. https://doi.org/10.1212/01.WNL.0000123696.98166.AF.

# 30 Cytokines, Infection, and Immunity

Siri Hauge Opdal, PhD

*Department of Forensic Sciences, Group of Pediatric Forensic Medicine, Oslo University Hospital, Norway*

## Introduction

Both experimental and observational studies provide evidence indicating that infection and inflammation might play a role in sudden infant death syndrome (SIDS). Indeed, as early as 1889, Paltauf demonstrated mild inflammatory changes in the walls of the bronchioles in SIDS cases (1). In the 1950s the notion of minimal inflammation of the airways in SIDS was again noted, and since then several studies have reported that a large proportion of SIDS victims have signs of infection prior to death (2-5). Several of the factors associated with susceptibility to infection and inflammation have also proven to be risks for SIDS. A mild upper respiratory infection has been reported in about half of SIDS cases in the last days prior to death (6).

Signs of slight infection are often found by microscopic investigations, just as markers of infections and inflammation are often found at autopsy in SIDS. There are several studies indicating that the mucosal immune system is activated in SIDS (7-9). A higher number of IgM immunocytes in the tracheal wall, as well as a higher number of IgA immunocytes in the duodenal mucosa, have been reported in SIDS cases compared to controls (7). It has also been shown that SIDS victims have higher IgG and IgA immunocyte density in the palatine tonsillar compartments than controls (8). Furthermore, a higher number of CD45+ stromal leucocytes, as well as intensified epithelial expression of human leukocyte antigen—antigen D related (HLA-DR) and secretory component, and an increased expression of HLA class I and II have been reported in the salivary glands in SIDS (9). These observations confirm that the immune system is activated in SIDS, probably with release of certain cytokines that are known to up-regulate epithelia expression of HLA-DR and secretory component.

There are a vast number of studies reporting findings of bacteria in SIDS (4, 5, 10-14). It has been reported that there is a higher prevalence of *S. aureus* in nasopharyngeal flora from SIDS, and samples from the intestinal tract in SIDS have shown that *S. aureus* and staphylococcal endotoxins were more prevalent in SIDS compared to samples of feces from healthy controls (10-12). It is suggested that the toxins from *S. aureus* might contribute to SIDS via synergistic interactions with other colonizing species, in particular *E. coli* (4). *E. coli* colonizes the bowel of infants in the first days of life, and both a higher detection rate and a higher variety of serotypes have been reported in SIDS compared to controls (13, 14). Also, detection of *H. pylori* antigen in feces is associated both with SIDS and deaths due to infections (15). This study suggests that *H. pylori* infection in infancy may be involved as the triggering pathogen for sudden death during the first five months after birth. Taken together, it is plausible that common bacterial toxins, together with a viral infection, can cause SIDS in a vulnerable infant (16).

There are also several studies indicating that virus infections may play a role in SIDS, and higher rates of viruses have been isolated in samples from SIDS compared to controls (17-19). The involvement of viruses may be direct, by induction of a cytokine storm upon viral infection, or indirect, through synergistic interactions with bacterial virulence factors and/or immunregulatory polymorphisms. However, so far, no single respiratory virus has been exclusively found in a high proportion of SIDS cases: rather, a range of viruses are found at a higher frequency in SIDS compared to controls.

## Cytokines and Interleukins

The term cytokine defines a large group of small non-structural proteins that are involved in cell signaling. Included in the cytokine family are interleukins (IL), interferons (IFN), chemokines, lymphokines, and tumor necrosis factors (TNF). The cytokines act on target cells by binding to specific receptors, thereby triggering signal transduction pathways within the cell. Cytokines are usually produced in cascades and they act in sequence, as a part of a complex co-ordinated network. Cytokine production is carefully regulated, both intracellularly and extracellularly. So far, IL-1 to IL-38 has been described, in addition to a number of other cytokines.

Cytokines play an important role in the immune system by regulating both the intensity and duration of the immune response. The cytokines may be divided into two groups, according to their function: pro- and anti-inflammatory cytokines. The pro-inflammatory cytokines are those that favor inflammation, the major ones responsible for early responses being IL-1α, IL-1β, IL-6, and TNF-α. In contrast, the anti-inflammatory cytokines counteract various aspects of inflammation, including the production of pro-inflammatory cytokines. Some cytokines may have both pro- and anti-inflammatory activities, dependent on the situation. The balance between the pro- and anti-inflammatory cytokines determines the net effect of an inflammatory response, and a disturbed cytokine homeostasis disables proper function of the immune system.

There is a growing body of evidence indicating that both the risk of acquiring infection and the risk of developing severe complications are determined by host genetic factors (20). These genetic factors include single gene defects with serious consequences, but also genetic variants with subtle effects on the regulation and function of the immune system. Aberrant cytokine production may contribute to pathological processes, and dysregulated cytokine production is involved in the pathogenesis of different inflammatory and autoimmune diseases.

The cytokine genes are highly polymorphic, and a vast number of polymorphisms in each gene have been described. A number of them are of biological significance, either by altering the amino acid sequence of the gene product, or by altering mRNA splicing or stability. Many of the reported polymorphisms are within the 5' and 3' regulatory sequences, and may thus have a significant effect upon transcription.

There are several polymorphisms in each gene that influence the production of any given cytokine, but the results are conflicting as to whether a specific genotype results in higher or lower cytokine production; this is partly due to whether the studies are in vivo or in vitro. The results from in vitro studies differ according to cell type and stimulation used, and results from different assays may be difficult to compare. The results from in vivo studies depend on whether the study group contains individuals with known illnesses or healthy individuals, due to the fact that the immune system of most patients may be in an activated state because of their disease. This may be the fact even if the disease is of a non-infectious cause. In addition, most studies investigate only one or a few single nucleotide polymorphisms (SNP) or microsatellites/variable number of tandem repeat (VNTR) polymorphisms; however, it is most likely the combination of different polymorphisms into haplotypes that influences gene expression.

## Measurements of cytokines and interleukins in SIDS

An early study investigating IL-6 in the cerebral spinal fluid (CSF) found elevated levels in SIDS compared to controls, a finding that was later confirmed in a larger study group (21, 22). About half of the SIDS cases had IL-6 levels in the CSF in the same range as infants dying of severe infections such as meningitis or septicemia, favoring the hypothesis that an overreaction of the immune system to an otherwise harmless infection may be involved in SIDS. It has further been shown that SIDS infants with high IL-6 levels in the CSF have increased expression of both IgA and HLA-DR in the laryngeal mucosa (23, 24). The finding of increased levels of IL-6 in SIDS is interesting in the light of findings of *S. aureus* in these cases, as *S. aureus* toxins are known to be powerful inducers of IL-6. Significantly elevated IL-6 levels have also been reported in the CSF from SIDS cases positive for *H. Pylori* stool antigen (HpSA), compared with HpSA-negative SIDS cases (15). A later study investigating several cytokines in the CSF in German SIDS cases did not find any difference in the IL-6 level between SIDS and controls (25). There may be several reasons for this, including heterogeneity of the cases, the selection of controls, or differences in diagnostic criteria used to set the SIDS diagnosis.

Interleukin 1β (IL-1β) and TNF-α have been measured, both in CSF and serum, from SIDS, but without any significant findings (22, 25). In both studies there was no detectable concentration of IL-1β in a large number of the SIDS cases. The reason for this may be that IL-1β, together with TNF-α, peaks early after stimulation and thereafter rapidly returns to baseline, in contrast to IL-6, which seems to peak later and remain elevated for a longer period of time.

High neuronal IL-1β immunoreactivity has been detected in different parts of the brainstem in SIDS, with a region-specific pattern of cytokine expression in SIDS brains compared to non-SIDS brains (26). An overexpression of IL-1β in the brainstem might contribute to a disturbed homeostatic control of cardiorespiratory and arousal responses, possibly leading to SIDS (27). In addition, an overexpression of IL-2 in vital neural centers in the brainstem have been reported in SIDS, further suggesting that there is a neuro-cytokine connection (28).

The expression of IL-6 receptors (IL-6R) and gp130 (involved in IL-6R signaling) in the brainstem have been investigated in SIDS (29). In this study, the mean IL-6R intensity grade in the arcuate nucleus, which is a major component of the medullary serotonergic system, was significantly higher in the SIDS group than in the controls. The same study also found a positive correlation between IL-6 CSF levels and immunostaining of gp130 in the arcuate nucleus in SIDS (29). This, together with the studies finding elevated levels of ILs in the CSF, indicates a connection between the mucosal immune system and dysfunction of the serotonergic network in the brainstem.

During infection, peripherally cytokines may cross the blood-brain barrier, bind to cytokine receptors on neurons that determine stress responses in the hypothalamus and/or brainstem, and thereby determine sickness behaviors, including blunted arousal and depressed respiration (29). In an infant with an underlying vulnerability in the brainstem, as reported in SIDS (30), a mild infection that initiates a cytokine cascade might trigger sudden death.

# Genes for cytokines and interleukins in SIDS

## Interleukin 6

The pro-inflammatory cytokine IL-6 is an acute phase protein that, among other things, induces B- and T-cell growth and differentiation. This cytokine is an important mediator of fever, and influences the effect of other cytokines. In healthy subjects IL-6 plasma levels are barely detectable, but during the early stages of inflammation there is a massive increase. Due to the rapid plasma clearance of IL-6, the circulating levels of this cytokine are largely regulated at the level of gene expression. IL-6 overexpression plays a fundamental role in the pathogenesis of various inflammatory and autoimmune diseases, B-cell malignancies, multiple myeloma, and Castleman's disease.

The gene encoding IL-6 is located on chromosome 7, and a number of polymorphisms with functional effect have been described. The most frequently studied polymorphism is -174G/C (rs1800795), which is located in the promoter region of the gene. The -174G allele seems to be associated with high IL-6 levels, even though an association between the -174C allele and high IL-6 levels have been reported in neonates (31, 32). Additional polymorphisms in the IL-6 gene promoter are -597G/A (rs1800797), -572G/C (rs1800796), and -373$A_n T_n$; and it is most likely that a combination of the polymorphisms regulate the expression of the gene, rather than the -174G/C polymorphism alone (33).

The first study to investigate this polymorphism in cases of SIDS was a British study, which found that the IL-6 -174GG genotype was more frequent in SIDS cases than in controls (34). This finding has not been confirmed, even though an association with -174GG has been reported in a small group of 19 Australian SIDS cases included in the paper by Moscovis et al. (35) (Table 30.1). These reports, however, only included 25 and 19 SIDS cases respectively; such case numbers are far too low for it to be possible to draw any firm conclusions from them. In total, -174G/C has been investigated in 475 Caucasian SIDS cases and 517 controls (Table 30.1). Pooling the studies, there is no association between this SNP and SIDS (p=0.10), and the most common genotype in both SIDS cases and controls is GC (Table 30.1).

There are few studies that have investigated other SNPs in the IL-6 gene other than -174G/C in cases of SIDS. The -572G/C polymorphism gene was investigated in a Norwegian SIDS cohort, but without any significant findings (36). Another study of European SIDS cases included two additional SNPS in the IL-6 gene — rs1882043 and rs1554606 — but there was no association between these SNPs and SIDS (37).

Table 30.1: Genotype distribution of -174G/C in the IL-6 gene in Caucasian SIDS and control populations.

| Study | Number of SIDS cases/controls | GG | GC | CC | p-value |
|---|---|---|---|---|---|
| Dashash et al. 2006 (34) | 25[1] 136[2] | 18 (72%) 58 (58%) | 4 (16%) 60 (44%) | 3 (12%) 18 (13%) | 0.003[3] |
| Moscovis et al. 2006 (35) | 86 121 | 25 (29%) 51 (42%) | 44 (51%) 50 (41%) | 17 (20%) 20 (17%) | 0.16 |
| Opdal et al. 2007 (38) | 175 71 | 61 (35%) 25 (35%) | 75 (43%) 31 (44%) | 39 (22%) 15 (21%) | 0.98 |
| Fard et al. 2016 (37)4 | 189 189 | 81 (43%) 77 (41%) | 76 (40%) 92 (49%) | 32 (17%) 20 (10%) | 0.11 |
| Total | 475 517 | 185 (39%) 211 (38%) | 199 (42%) 233 (46%) | 91 (19%) 73 (16%) | 0.10 |

[1]SIDS.
[2]Controls.
[3]Chi-square test, 3 x 2 table.
[4]Genotypes taken from Online Resource 4 in the paper by Fard et al. (37).

## Interleukin 10

Interleukin 10 (IL-10) is an important regulatory cytokine that down-regulates the production of pro-inflammatory cytokines and controls the balance between inflammatory and humoral responses. IL-10 also plays an important role in the development of infectious disease, and dysfunction of IL-10 is likely involved in the pathogenesis of allergic disorders and autoimmune diseases.

The gene encoding IL-10 is located on chromosome 1. The gene is highly polymorphic, and a number of promoter and coding region polymorphisms have been described. Several of them are proven to be of biological significance. The polymorphisms investigated most are -1082A/G (rs1800896), -819C/T (rs1800871), and -592A/C (rs1800872), situated in the promoter region of the gene. These generally combine into the haplotypes GCC, ACC, and ATA; the haplotype GTA is extremely rare. In addition, the promoter also contains two microsatellites, termed IL-10R and IL-10G. These two microsatellites combine with the -1082/-819/-592 SNPs to form haplotype families (39).

It has been suggested that between 50% and 75% of the variability in IL-10 secretion is explained by genetic determinants. However, so far it has been difficult to determine the exact relationship between IL-10 genotype and the corresponding cytokine production. When it comes to the SNPs -1082A/G, -819C/T, and -592A/C, it is clear that they influence the expression of the gene, but the same haplotype has been reported to be associated both with high and low IL-10 production. For example, the ATA haplotype has been reported to be associated both with increased plasma IL-10 levels and with low IL-10 mRNA expression in healthy individuals (40, 41), and also with low IL-10 release and higher mortality in critically ill patients (42).

There are several studies that have investigated the three common SNPs in the IL-10 gene promoter in SIDS (37, 43-48). A small study by Summers et al. included 23 SIDS cases and found that the ATA haplotype was associated with SIDS (43). Since then, several studies have been performed to verify this finding, but the results are conflicting. Two studies, which only included a few SIDS cases, have reported an association between the ATA haplotype and the ATA/ATA genotype and SIDS, respectively (45, 47), while others have not (44, 48). However, the studies are in some ways difficult to compare, as not all of them investigate all of the three common promoter SNPs. Three studies that do include all of them are listed in Table 30.2, with a total of 275 SIDS cases and 566 controls. The results from the pooled analysis do not support any association between the promoter polymorphisms or the ATA haplotype and SIDS (p=0.76 and 0.47, respectively) (Table 30.2). The most common haplotype is GCC, found in half of both the SIDS cases and the controls.

Table 30.2: Haplotype distribution of -1082A/G, -819C/T, and -592A/C in the IL-10 gene in Caucasian SIDS and control populations.

| Study | Number of SIDS cases/controls | GCC | ACC | ATA | p-value |
|---|---|---|---|---|---|
| Opdal et al. 2003 (44) | 214[1] 136[2] | 220 (51%) 140 (51%) | 118 (28%) 78 (29%) | 90 (21%) 54 (20%) | 0.91[3] 0.71[4] |
| Koratci et al. 2004[5] (45) | 38 330 | 34 (45%) 336 (51%) | 10 (13%) 163 (25%) | 32 (42%) 161 (24%) | 0.002 0.001 |
| Perskvist et al. 2008 (47) | 23 100 | 23 (50%) 102 (51%) | 9 (20%) 51 (26%) | 14 (30%) 47 (23%) | 0.53 0.33 |
| Total | 275 566 | 277 (50%) 578 (51%) | 137 (25%) 292 (26%) | 136 (25%) 262 (23%) | 0.76 0.47 |

[1]SIDS.
[2]Controls.
[3]Chi square test, 3 x 2 table.
[4]Chi square test, ATA vs GCC/ACC, 2 x 2 table.
[5]This study includes the 23 SIDS cases from Summers et al. 2000 (43).

Several studies investigate -1082G/C or -592A/C separately (see Tables 30.3 and 30.4). From the different studies, the -1082G/C allele frequency could be deduced in 672 SIDS cases and 1,278 controls (Table 30.3). A pooled analysis indicates that this SNP is not associated with SIDS. Regarding the -592A/C polymorphism, the allele frequency could be deduced in 587 SIDS cases and 1,160 controls (Table 30.4). Even though two studies report an association between the -592C allele and SIDS, the pooled analysis does not.

Table 30.3: Allele frequency of -1082A/G in the IL-10 gene in Caucasian SIDS cases and controls.

| Study | Number of SIDS cases/controls | A | G | p-value |
|---|---|---|---|---|
| Opdal et al. 2003 (44) | 214[1] 136[2] | 208 (49%) 132 (49%) | 220 (51%) 140 (51%) | 0.99[3] |
| Koratchi et al. 2004 (45) | 38 330 | 42 (55%) 324 (49%) | 34 (45%) 336 (51%) | 0.31 |
| Moscovis et al. 2004 (46) | 85 118 | 90 (53%) 120 (51%) | 80 (47%) 116 (49%) | 0.68 |
| Perskvist et al. 2008 (47) | 23 100 | 23 (50%) 98 (49%) | 23 (50%) 102 (51%) | 0.9 |
| Courts et al. 2011 (48) | 123 406 | 138 (56%) 490 (60%) | 108 (44%) 322 (40%) | 0.24 |
| Fard et al. 2015 (37) | 189[4] 188 | 186 (49%) 161 (43%) | 192 (51%) 215 (57%) | 0.08 |
| Total | 672 1,278 | 657 (49%) 2,556 (55%) | 687 (51%) 1,150 (45%) | 0.69 |

[1]SIDS.
[2]Controls.
[3]Chi square test, 2 x 2 table.
[4]Genotypes taken from Online Resource 4 in the paper by Fard et al. (37).

Table 30.4: Allele frequency of -592A/C in the IL-10 gene in Caucasian SIDS cases and controls.

| Study | Number of SIDS cases/controls | A | C | p-value |
|---|---|---|---|---|
| Opdal et al. 2003 (44) | 214[1] 136[2] | 90 (21%) 54 (20%) | 338 (79%) 218 (80%) | 0.71[3] |
| Koratchi et al. 2004 (45) | 38 330 | 32 (42%) 161 (24%) | 44 (58%) 499 (76%) | 0.01 |
| Perskvist et al. 2008 (47) | 23 100 | 14 (30%) 47 (24%) | 32 (70%) 153 (77%) | 0.33 |
| Courts et al. 2011 (48) | 123 406 | 69 (28%) 241 (30%) | 177 (72%) 571 (70%) | 0.62 |
| Fard et al. 2015 (37) | 189[4] 188 | 83 (22%) 111 (30%) | 295 (78%) 265 (70%) | 0.018 |
| Total | 587 1,160 | 288 (25%) 614 (27%) | 886 (75%) 1,706 (73%) | 0.22 |

[1]SIDS.
[2]Controls.
[3]Chi square test, 2 x 2 table.
[4]Genotypes taken from Online Resource 4 in the paper by Fard et al. (37).

Only one study has investigated the microsatellites IL-10G and IL-10R in cases of SIDS (44). This study included 214 SIDS cases, and found a significantly higher percentage of the genotype G21/G22 in SIDS compared to controls. Perhaps just as interesting, however, is that several IL-10 haplotypes, including ATA, G21/G22, and G21/G23, were found to be more frequent in cases of sudden unexpected death due to infection than in both death due to SIDS and in controls (44). One might speculate that genetic variation in the IL-10 gene promoter might be of higher importance with regard to sudden unexpected death due to infection than with regard to SIDS, at least in Caucasians.

In addition to variation in the IL-10 gene, four SNPs in the gene encoding the IL-10 receptor IL-10RA, including rs2256111, rs2229113, rs11216666, and rs17121510, have been investigated in SIDS. However, there were no significant findings with regard to differences in genotype frequencies between SIDS cases and controls (37).

Interleukin 1 (IL-1) is a pro-inflammatory cytokine that contributes to the acute phase response. IL-1 has the ability to induce fever, and may also suppress respiration. There are two structurally distinct forms of IL1: IL-1α, which is the acidic form, and IL-1β, which is the neutral form. The IL-1 gene cluster is located on the long arm of chromosome 2, and several polymorphisms have been described, including variable number tandem repeat (VNTR) polymorphisms, dinucleotide repeat polymorphisms, and several SNPs. Another member of the IL-1 family, the IL-1 receptor antagonist IL-1Ra, functions as a specific inhibitor of both IL-1α and IL-1β. Also in this gene several polymorphisms have been described, the most common investigated being an 86 bp VNTR in intron 2. Dysregulation of IL-1 expression is associated with a wide range of inflammatory and autoimmune diseases.

In the gene encoding IL-1α, a VNTR in intron 6 and the +4845G/T (rs17561) polymorphism have been investigated in SIDS (49). When investigating each polymorphism separately, no differences between genotype frequencies between the diagnosis groups and controls were found. However, when combining VNTR and SNP genotypes, there was an association between the gene combinations IL-1α A1A1/+4548TT and SIDS (49). It was reported that the gene expression driven by the IL-1α promoter decreases with increasing numbers of the repeat sequence; thus one might expect the A1A1 genotype to result in relatively high IL-1α production (50). Individuals with the +4548T allele exhibit high efficiency in processing pre-IL-1α, thus facilitating high cellular release of mature IL-1α (51). One could therefore speculate that a genotype with both A1A1 and +4548TT might contribute to a changed expression of IL-1α, creating a disturbance in the immunologic response.

One commonly investigated polymorphism in the IL-1β gene is -511C/T (rs16944), located in the promoter region of the gene. It is known that the T-allele of this SNP gives an increase in LPS-induced IL-1β protein secretion (52). The SNP has been investigated in SIDS, but without any significant findings (49, 53). Other SNPs that have been investigated in the IL-1β gene in cases of SIDS include rs1143643, rs1143634, and rs1143627, all without any significant findings (37).

One commonly investigated polymorphism in the IL-1Ra gene is an 86 bp VNTR in intron 2 of the gene. The VNTR is of functional significance, and it has been shown that the A2 allele is associated with higher plasma levels of IL-1Ra (54). This VNTR has been investigated in several SIDS populations (49, 55, 56), and the A2/A2 haplotype has been reported to be associated with SIDS in a study of sudden unexpected death in infancy (SUDI) due to different causes (55). The same association was found in SIDS infants born during the years with a high SIDS incidence, i.e. 1984 to 1994 (56). The latter might indicate that a major contribution factor to death during the SIDS epidemic was infection. One might speculate that infants with the A2/A2 genotype are more susceptible to a sustained pro-inflammatory response, which may predispose vulnerable infants to death. In addition, several SNPs in the IL-1Ra gene have been investigated in SIDS, including 2018T/C, rs419598, and rs1143627, but without any significant findings (37, 53).

## TNF-α

Tumor necrosis factor alpha (TNF-α) is a transmembrane protein produced as a result of the presence of bacterial toxins. TNF-α acts as a pro-inflammatory cytokine and is an important regulator of immune cells; in addition, it stimulates inflammation and controls viral replication. The gene encoding TNF-α is situated within the HLA region on chromosome 6, and is highly polymorphic. The level of TNF-α production in healthy individuals shows wide and stable variation, with high and low levels producing phenotypes in the population. This indicates a substantial genetic influence on the production of this cytokine. The first step of control in the expression of TNF-α is at the transcriptional level, making SNPs in the promoter region of the gene important.

The most commonly studied TNF-α polymorphism is -308A/G (rs1800629), located in the promoter region of the gene. This SNP has been reported to be associated with a variety of infectious diseases including, among others, cerebral malaria, hepatitis B, and hepatitis C, as well as with death as a result of septic shock (57). The -308A allele is reported to give an increased expression of TNF-α, even though there are several in vivo and in vitro studies that fail to demonstrate any functionality for this SNP (58, 59). Another commonly investigated and putative functional promoter polymorphism is -238G/A (rs5361525). The -238A allele is suggested to be a "low producer" allele, but there are also contradictory findings for this SNP (60, 61).

Both -308A/G and -238G/A have been investigated in several SIDS populations (37, 47, 62, 63). The majority of the results were negative, but an association between -238GG and SIDS was found in a Norwegian study (62), and also an association between -308AA and an Australian subgroup of SIDS (63). The -308A/G SNP has been investigated in 254 SIDS cases and 351 controls (see Table 30.5). However, no association between this SNP and SIDS was determined, and most of the cases had the -308GG genotype.

A Norwegian study investigated four SNPs in the TNF-α promoter, including -1031C/T (rs1799964), -857C/T (rs1799724), -308A/G, and -238A/G. It was found that the SNP profiles -1031CT/-238GG/-857CC/-308GG and -1031TT/-238GG/-857CC/-308AA were more frequent in SIDS than in controls (62). As these SNPs are all located in the promoter region of the gene, it is likely that they influence the expression, and hence TNF-α levels. It is, however, difficult to say whether these profiles lead to higher or lower TNF-α production; either way, they may, depending on the circumstances, possibly contribute to altered immunological homeostasis in SIDS.

Table 30.5: Genotype distribution of -308G/A in the TNF-α gene in Caucasian SIDS cases and controls.

| Study | Number of SIDS cases/controls | GG | GA | AA | p-value |
|---|---|---|---|---|---|
| Perskvist et al. 2008 (47) | 23[1] 100[2] | 18 (78%) 63 (63%) | 5 (22%) 34 (34%) | 0 (0%) 3 (3%) | 0.33[3] 0.16[4] |
| Ferrante et al. 2008 (62) | 142 133 | 101 (71%) 94 (72%) | 37 (26%) 36 (28%) | 4 (3%) 0 (0%) | 0.16 0.83 |
| Moscovis et al. 2015 (63) | 89 118 | 62 (70%) 80 (68%) | 21 (24%) 34 (29%) | 7 (6%) 4 (3%) | 0.57 0.87 |
| Total | 254 351 | 181 (71%) 237 (68%) | 63 (25%) 104 (30%) | 11 (4%) 7 (2%) | 0.24 0.45 |

[1]SIDS.
[2]Controls.
[3]Chi square test, 3 x 2 table.
[4]Chi square test, GG vs GA/AA, 2 x 2 table.

## Interleukin Genotypes and Risk Factors for SIDS

There are several well-known risk factors for SIDS, including prone sleeping position, maternal smoking, unfavorable sleeping environments, and slight infection. However, most infants that are exposed to one, or several, of these will not die. Thus there have to be additional factors present in order for SIDS to occur. One of these factors may very well be an inborn vulnerability in the immune system, inherited as an unfavorable combination of different polymorphisms in genes involved in mediating the immune response. This may be put together in the concept of the fatal triangle in SIDS (see Figure 30.1) (64).

One of the best documented risk factors for SIDS is maternal smoking. The risk of SIDS increases with increased exposure to cigarette smoke (65). It is known that smoking influences cytokine production, and studies indicate that smokers have lower levels of both IL-10, IL-1β, and INF-γ (46, 66, 67). There is also evidence to support the fact that exposure to cigarette smoke alters cytokine responses, more for some genotypes than others (63). The ability of infants to suppress inflammatory responses may be impaired if the levels of pro-inflammatory cytokines are constitutively low due to host genetic factors, and then further reduced by interactions with nicotine due to exposure to maternal smoking. In addition, nicotine exposure may increase the risk for SIDS by giving a greater susceptibility to viral and bacterial infections.

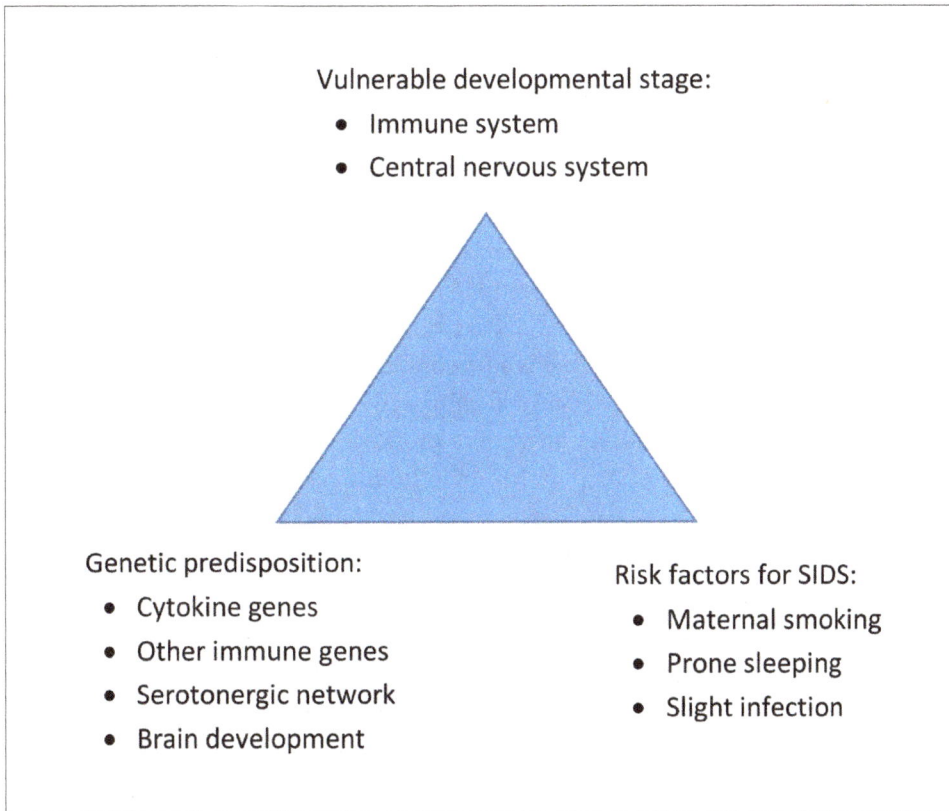

Figure 30.1: The concept of a fatal triangle in SIDS. (Adapted from Rognum and Saugstad 1993 (64).)

It has also been shown that nicotine, in doses within the range of what a child of a smoking mother could receive through environmental tobacco smoke and breastmilk, interferes with autoresuscitation and arousal following normal occurring apnea (27). This situation is seriously aggravated when combined with the presence of IL-1β released during an infection, which may be the situation in a SIDS infant with slight infection prior to death. Thus, in addition to increasing the susceptibility to infections, smoking may increase the risk for SIDS by both suppressing the production of pro-inflammatory cytokines and decreasing arousal.

With regard to IL-10 genotypes and nicotine exposure in SIDS, associations to the IL-10R and IL-10G VNTR in the IL-10 gene (44) have been reported. SIDS cases with smoking mothers had a higher percentage of the R13/R14 genotype and a lower percentage of the G23/G25 genotype, compared to SIDS infants not exposed to smoking. It is, however, difficult to decide whether this is specific to the SIDS group, as there was no information regarding smoking status in the controls.

Another well-known risk factor for SIDS is prone sleeping. A prone position may increase the temperature in the upper airways and also stimulate bacterial colonization and toxin production. Hyperthermia resulting from infection or prone sleeping might trigger events leading to SIDS. It has been shown that nasal temperature in the prone position is increased and may reach the temperature required for toxin production, suggesting that this could be one reason why prone sleeping is a risk factor for SIDS (68).

A few studies have searched for a correlation between being found dead in a prone sleeping position and cytokine genotype (36, 37, 49). In the gene encoding IL-8, the genotypes -251AA/AT and -781CT/TT have been reported to be associated with the prone sleeping position in SIDS. IL-8 is a pro-inflammatory cytokine and an increased production, as reported to be associated with -251A and -781T (69, 70), might represent an additional risk for an infant in a prone sleeping position. An association between genotype and prone sleeping have also been reported for IL-1β; most of the SIDS infants with the -511CC/CT genotypes were found dead in a prone sleeping position (49). In addition, the SNP -174G/C in the IL-6 gene has been found to be associated with a prone sleeping position in SIDS (37).

A study evaluating the correlation between HLA-DR expression in laryngeal mucosa and IL gene variation found that 12 out of 13 SIDS cases with the combination of high HLA-DR expression, prone sleeping position, and signs of infection prior to death had the IL-6 -174CG/CC genotypes (24). Furthermore, the IL-8 SNPs -781 CC/CT and -251 AA/AT genotypes were observed in 93% of SIDS cases with one or more risk factors present, compared to SIDS cases with no risk factors. During the vulnerable developmental periods, certain gene variants may constitute a predisposition for an immunological overreaction to an otherwise harmless event, such as a common cold or prone sleeping position. This fits with the concept of a fatal triangle in SIDS (see Figure 30.1).

## Conclusions

There is convincing evidence that slight infection and an activated immune system are involved in SIDS. One common thread may be the dysregulation of inflammatory responses to apparently mild infections, leading to a cytokine storm that contributes to death. The human immune system is, however, extremely complex, and is controlled by a vast array of genes. While the list of candidate genes for polymorphism analysis in SIDS seems endless, the genes involved in the cytokine network deserve special attention, as they have a powerful effect on the homeostatic balance.

Even though a large number of papers have investigated several of the cytokine genes in SIDS, it has proven difficult to find specific gene variants clearly associated with this syndrome. There is a large discrepancy in the results from different studies. There may be several reasons for this. First, the number of cases in the different studies differ, from as low as 23 (43, 47) to as high as 579 SIDS cases (37). Second, there may be differences in the criteria used to diagnose the cause of death, and there may also be differences in age and sex distribution. Not all studies give this information, which makes the studies difficult to compare. Third, there are differences in the number of controls, from only 71 cases (38) to as many as 1124 (37). Furthermore, the constitution of the control groups differs, from dead infants and dead adults to living healthy controls. Fourth, to assume that the specific genotype of one SNP causes SIDS, or at least is found in almost all cases of SIDS, is an oversimplification. Within each gene there are a large number of SNPs and VNTRs, and together these constitute haplotypes that influence the production of each cytokine. Fifth, external factors such as nicotine exposure interfere with cytokine production and will complicate interpretation of the results. Even if one tries to take smoking into consideration when interpreting the results, the findings may not be entirely accurate if there are parents who do not admit to smoking. Sixth, when measuring cytokine levels in, for instance, serum or CSF, differences in timing of the sample according to the introduction of an infectious agent, such as a virus or bacteria, will highly influence the results.

Adding to the complexity of the situation is the fact that the inflammatory pathway and signaling during infection are diverse, so the contribution from any one component or cytokine is small. The contribution from one SNP in one single gene is even smaller, and might be compensated for or masked by changes in other cytokines, making it hard to prove any significant associations.

It has been shown that there is a rapid development of the mucosal immune system from the second week after birth (71, 72). This implies that in the first weeks and months of life the infant is particularly vulnerable to various stimuli of the immune system. If the infant is exposed to trigger events, such as slight infection, prone sleeping, or maternal smoking, and if the infant also has inborn gene variants and polymorphisms that influence the balance between pro- and anti-inflammatory cytokines, this may lead to death in SIDS. Even small changes in the development of immune responses can turn a minor illness into a lethal event.

Finally, death in SIDS cases may be due to more than one mechanism. It is, however, likely that a dysregulation of inflammatory responses to apparently mild infections is involved in a proportion of SIDS. Genetic variations in cytokine genes are most likely involved, as they contribute to differences in the expression, translation, cellular transport, and secretion of the cytokine. However, it is important to interpret cytokine SNP data with caution and to consider the effects of other genetic, developmental, and environmental influences on the responses.

# References

1. Paltauf A. Plötzlichen Thümustod. Wien Klin Wochenschr 1889 and 1890;II:877 and 172.

2. Werne J, Garrow I. Sudden apparently unexplained death during infancy. I. Pathologic findings in infants found dead. Am J Pathol. 1953;29(4):633-75.

3. Vege A, Ole Rognum T. Sudden infant death syndrome, infection and inflammatory responses. FEMS Immunol Med Microbiol. 2004;42(1):3-10. https://doi.org/10.1016/j.femsim.2004.06.015.

4. Highet AR. An infectious aetiology of sudden infant death syndrome. J Appl Microbiol. 2008;105(3):625-35. https://doi.org/10.1111/j.1365-2672.2008.03747.x.

5. Alfelali M, Khandaker G. Infectious causes of sudden infant death syndrome. Paediatr Respir Rev. 2014;15(4):307-11. https://doi.org/10.1016/j.prrv.2014.09.004.

6. Arnestad M, Andersen M, Vege A, Rognum TO. Changes in the epidemiological pattern of sudden infant death syndrome in southeast Norway, 1984-1998: Implications for future prevention and research. Arch Dis Child. 2001;85(2):108-15. https://doi.org/10.1136/adc.85.2.108.

7. Stoltenberg L, Saugstad OD, Rognum TO. Sudden infant death syndrome victims show local immunoglobulin M response in tracheal wall and immunoglobulin A response in duodenal mucosa. Pediat Res. 1992;31(4 Pt 1):372-5. https://doi.org/10.1203/00006450-199204000-00013.

8. Stoltenberg L, Vege A, Saugstad OD, Rognum TO. Changes in the concentration and distribution of immunoglobulin-producing cells in SIDS palatine tonsils. Pediatr Allergy Immunol. 1995;6(1):48-55. https://doi.org/10.1111/j.1399-3038.1995.tb00258.x.

9. Thrane PS, Rognum TO, Brandtzaeg P. Up-regulated epithelial expression of HLA-DR and secretory component in salivary glands: Reflection of mucosal immunostimulation in sudden infant death syndrome. Pediatr Res. 1994;35(5):625-8. https://doi.org/10.1203/00006450-199405000-00017.

10. Highet AR, Berry AM, Bettelheim KA, Goldwater PN. Gut microbiome in sudden infant death syndrome (SIDS) differs from that in healthy comparison babies and offers an explanation for the risk factor of prone position. Int J Med Microbiol. 2014;304(5-6):735-41. https://doi.org/10.1016/j.ijmm.2014.05.007.

11. Blackwell CC, MacKenzie DA, James VS, Elton RA, Zorgani AA, Weir DM, et al. Toxigenic bacteria and sudden infant death syndrome (SIDS): Nasopharyngeal flora during the first year of life. FEMS Immunol Med Microbiol. 1999;25(1-2):51-8. https://doi.org/10.1111/j.1574-695X.1999.tb01326.x.

12. Highet AR, Goldwater PN. Staphylococcal enterotoxin genes are common in Staphylococcus aureus intestinal flora in sudden infant death syndrome (SIDS) and live comparison infants. FEMS Immunol Med Microbiol. 2009;57(2):151-5. https://doi.org/10.1111/j.1574-695X.2009.00592.x.

13. Pearce JL, Bettelheim KA, Luke RK, Goldwater PN. Serotypes of Escherichia coli in sudden infant death syndrome. J Appl Microbiol. 2010;108(2):731-5. https://doi.org/10.1111/j.1365-2672.2009.04473.x.

14. Weber MA, Klein NJ, Hartley JC, Lock PE, Malone M, Sebire NJ. Infection and sudden unexpected death in infancy: A systematic retrospective case review. Lancet. 2008;371(9627):1848-53. https://doi.org/10.1016/S0140-6736(08)60798-9.

15. Stray-Pedersen A, Vege A, Rognum TO. Helicobacter pylori antigen in stool is associated with SIDS and sudden infant deaths due to infectious disease. Pediatr Res. 2008;64(4):405-10. https://doi.org/10.1203/PDR.0b013e31818095f7.

16. Morris JA. The common bacterial toxins hypothesis of sudden infant death syndrome. FEMS Immunol Med Microbiol. 1999;25(1-2):11-7. https://doi.org/10.1111/j.1574-695X.1999.tb01322.x.

17. Niklasson B, Almqvist PR, Hornfeldt B, Klitz W. Sudden infant death syndrome and Ljungan virus. Forensic Sci Med Pathol. 2009;5(4):274-9. https://doi.org/10.1007/s12024-009-9086-8.

18. Alvarez-Lafuente R, Aguilera B, Suarez-Mier MA, Morentin B, Vallejo G, Gomez J, et al. Detection of human herpesvirus-6, Epstein-Barr virus and cytomegalovirus in formalin-fixed tissues from sudden infant death: A study with quantitative real-time PCR. Forensic Sci Int. 2008;178(2-3):106-11. https://doi.org/10.1016/j.forsciint.2008.02.007.

19. Dettmeyer R, Baasner A, Schlamann M, Padosch SA, Haag C, Kandolf R, et al. Role of virus-induced myocardial affections in sudden infant death syndrome: A prospective postmortem study. Pediatric research. 2004;55(6):947-52. https://doi.org/10.1203/01.pdr.0000127022.45831.54.

20. Kwiatkowski D. Genetic dissection of the molecular pathogenesis of severe infection. Intensive Care Med. 2000;26 Suppl 1:S89-97. https://doi.org/10.1007/s001340051124.

21. Vege A, Rognum TO, Scott H, Aasen AO, Saugstad OD. SIDS cases have increased levels of interleukin-6 in cerebrospinal fluid. Acta Paediatr. 1995;84(2):193-6. https://doi.org/10.1111/j.1651-2227.1995.tb13608.x.

22. Vege A, Rognum TO, Aasen AO, Saugstad OD. Are elevated cerebrospinal fluid levels of IL-6 in sudden unexplained deaths, infectious deaths and deaths

due to heart/lung disease in infants and children due to hypoxia? Acta Paediatr. 1998;87(8):819-24. https://doi.org/10.1111/j.1651-2227.1998.tb01544.x.

23. Vege A, Rognum TO, Anestad G. IL-6 cerebrospinal fluid levels are related to laryngeal IgA and epithelial HLA-DR response in sudden infant death syndrome. Pediatr Res. 1999;45(6):803-9. https://doi.org/10.1203/00006450-199906000-00004.

24. Ferrante L, Opdal SH, Vege A, Rognum TO. Is there any correlation between HLA-DR expression in laryngeal mucosa and interleukin gene variation in sudden infant death syndrome? Acta Paediatr. 2013;102(3):308-13. https://doi.org/10.1111/apa.12107.

25. Vennemann MM, Loddenkotter B, Fracasso T, Mitchell EA, Debertin AS, Larsch KP, et al. Cytokines and sudden infant death. Int J Legal Med. 2012;126(2):279-84. https://doi.org/10.1007/s00414-011-0638-6.

26. Kadhim H, Kahn A, Sebire G. Distinct cytokine profile in SIDS braIn: A common denominator in a multifactorial syndrome? Neurology. 2003;61(9):1256-9. https://doi.org/10.1212/01.WNL.0000092014.14997.47.

27. Froen JF, Akre H, Stray-Pedersen B, Saugstad OD. Adverse effects of nicotine and interleukin-1beta on autoresuscitation after apnea in piglets: Implications for sudden infant death syndrome. Pediatrics. 2000;105(4):E52. https://doi.org/10.1542/peds.105.4.e52.

28. Kadhim H, Deltenre P, de Prez C, Sebire G. Interleukin-2 as a neuromodulator possibly implicated in the physiopathology of sudden infant death syndrome. Neurosci Lett. 2010;480(2):122-6. https://doi.org/10.1016/j.neulet.2010.06.021.

29. Rognum IJ, Haynes RL, Vege A, Yang M, Rognum TO, Kinney HC. Interleukin-6 and the serotonergic system of the medulla oblongata in the sudden infant death syndrome. Acta Neuropathol. 2009;118(4):519-30. https://doi.org/10.1007/s00401-009-0535-y.

30. Kinney HC, Richerson GB, Dymecki SM, Darnall RA, Nattie EE. The brainstem and serotonin in the sudden infant death syndrome. Annu Rev Pathol. 2009;4:517-50. https://doi.org/10.1146/annurev.pathol.4.110807.092322.

31. Fishman D, Faulds G, Jeffery R, Mohamed-Ali V, Yudkin JS, Humphries S, et al. The effect of novel polymorphisms in the interleukin-6 (IL-6) gene on IL-6 transcription and plasma IL-6 levels, and an association with systemic-onset juvenile chronic arthritis. J Clin Invest. 1998;102(7):1369-76. https://doi.org/10.1172/JCI2629.

32. Kilpinen S, Hulkkonen J, Wang XY, Hurme M. The promoter polymorphism of the interleukin-6 gene regulates interleukin-6 production in neonates but not in adults. Eur Cytokine Netw. 2001;12(1):62-8.

33. Terry CF, Loukaci V, Green FR. Cooperative influence of genetic polymorphisms on interleukin 6 transcriptional regulation. J Biol Chem. 2000;275(24):18138-44. https://doi.org/10.1074/jbc.M000379200.

34. Dashash M, Pravica V, Hutchinson IV, Barson AJ, Drucker DB. Association of sudden infant death syndrome with VEGF and IL-6 gene polymorphisms. Hum Immunol. 2006;67(8):627-33. https://doi.org/10.1016/j.humimm.2006.05.002.

35. Moscovis SM, Gordon AE, Al Madani OM, Gleeson M, Scott RJ, Roberts-Thomson J, et al. IL6 G-174C associated with sudden infant death syndrome in a Caucasian Australian cohort. Hum Immunol. 2006;67(10):819-25. https://doi.org/10.1016/j.humimm.2006.07.010.

36. Ferrante L, Opdal SH, Vege A, Rognum T. Cytokine gene polymorphisms and sudden infant death syndrome. Acta Paediatr. 2010;99(3):384-8. https://doi.org/10.1111/j.1651-2227.2009.01611.x.

37. Fard D, Laer K, Rothamel T, Schurmann P, Arnold M, Cohen M, et al. Candidate gene variants of the immune system and sudden infant death syndrome. Int J Legal Med. 2016;130(4):1025-33. https://doi.org/10.1007/s00414-016-1347-y.

38. Opdal SH, Rognum TO. The IL6 -174G/C polymorphism and sudden infant death syndrome. Hum Immunol. 2007;68(6):541-3. https://doi.org/10.1016/j.humimm.2007.02.008.

39. Eskdale J, Keijsers V, Huizinga T, Gallagher G. Microsatellite alleles and single nucleotide polymorphisms (SNP) combine to form four major haplotype families at the human interleukin-10 (IL-10) locus. Genes Immun. 1999;1(2):151-5. https://doi.org/10.1038/sj.gene.6363656.

40. Kilpinen S, Huhtala H, Hurme M. The combination of the interleukin-1alpha (IL-1alpha-889) genotype and the interleukin-10 (IL-10 ATA) haplotype is associated with increased interleukin-10 (IL-10) plasma levels in healthy individuals. Eur Cytokine Netw. 2002;13(1):66-71.

41. Suarez A, Castro P, Alonso R, Mozo L, Gutierrez C. Interindividual variations in constitutive interleukin-10 messenger RNA and protein levels and their association with genetic polymorphisms. Transplantation. 2003;75(5):711-17. https://doi.org/10.1097/01.TP.0000055216.19866.9A.

42. Lowe PR, Galley HF, Abdel-Fattah A, Webster NR. Influence of interleukin-10 polymorphisms on interleukin-10 expression and survival in critically ill patients.

Crit Care Med. 2003;31(1):34-8. https://doi.org/10.1097/00003246-20030100 0-00005.

43. Summers AM, Summers CW, Drucker DB, Hajeer AH, Barson A, Hutchinson IV. Association of IL-10 genotype with sudden infant death syndrome. Hum Immunol. 2000;61(12):1270-3. https://doi.org/10.1016/S0198-8859(00)00183-X.

44. Opdal SH, Opstad A, Vege A, Rognum TO. IL-10 gene polymorphisms are associated with infectious cause of sudden infant death. Hum Immunol. 2003;64(12):1183-9. https://doi.org/10.1016/j.humimm.2003.08.359.

45. Korachi M, Pravica V, Barson AJ, Hutchinson IV, Drucker DB. Interleukin 10 genotype as a risk factor for sudden infant death syndrome: Determination of IL-10 genotype from wax-embedded postmortem samples. FEMS Immunol Med Microbiol. 2004;42(1):125-9. https://doi.org/10.1016/j.femsim.2004.06.008.

46. Moscovis SM, Gordon AE, Al Madani OM, Gleeson M, Scott RJ, Roberts-Thomson J, et al. Interleukin-10 and sudden infant death syndrome. FEMS Immunol Med Microbiol. 2004;42(1):130-8. https://doi.org/10.1016/j.femsim.2004.06.020.

47. Perskvist N, Skoglund K, Edston E, Backstrom G, Lodestad I, Palm U. TNF-alpha and IL-10 gene polymorphisms versus cardioimmunological responses in sudden infant death. Fetal Pediatr Pathol. 2008;27(3):149-65. https://doi.org/10.1080/15513810802077651.

48. Courts C, Madea B. No association of IL-10 promoter SNP -592 and -1082 and SIDS. Forensic Sci Int. 2011;204(1-3):179-81. https://doi.org/10.1016/j.forsciint.2010.06.001.

49. Ferrante L, Opdal SH, Vege A, Rognum TO. IL-1 gene cluster polymorphisms and sudden infant death syndrome. Hum Immunol. 2010;71(4):402-6. https://doi.org/10.1016/j.humimm.2010.01.011.

50. Bailly S, Israel N, Fay M, Gougerot-Pocidalo MA, Duff GW. An intronic polymorphic repeat sequence modulates interleukin-1 alpha gene regulation. Mol Immunol. 1996;33(11-12):999-1006. https://doi.org/10.1016/S0161-5890(96)00042-9.

51. Kawaguchi Y, Tochimoto A, Hara M, Kawamoto M, Sugiura T, Saito S, et al. Contribution of single nucleotide polymorphisms of the IL1A gene to the cleavage of precursor IL-1alpha and its transcription activity. Immunogenetics. 2007;59(6):441-8. https://doi.org/10.1007/s00251-007-0213-y.

52. Hall SK, Perregaux DG, Gabel CA, Woodworth T, Durham LK, Huizinga TW, et al. Correlation of polymorphic variation in the promoter region of the interleukin-1 beta gene with secretion of interleukin-1 beta protein. Arthritis Rheum. 2004;50(6):1976-83. https://doi.org/10.1002/art.20310.

53. Moscovis SM, Gordon AE, Hall ST, Gleeson M, Scott RJ, Roberts-Thomsom J, et al. Interleukin 1-beta responses to bacterial toxins and sudden infant death syndrome. FEMS Immunol Med Microbiol. 2004;42(1):139-45. https://doi.org/10.1016/j.femsim.2004.06.005.

54. Hurme M, Santtila S. IL-1 receptor antagonist (IL-1Ra) plasma levels are co-ordinately regulated by both IL-1Ra and IL-1beta genes. Eur J Immunol. 1998;28(8):2598-602. https://doi.org/10.1002/(SICI)1521-4141(199808)28:08<2598::AID-IMMU2598>3.0.CO;2-K.

55. Highet AR, Berry AM, Goldwater PN. Distribution of interleukin-1 receptor antagonist genotypes in sudden unexpected death in infancy (SUDI); unexplained SUDI have a higher frequency of allele 2. Ann Med. 2010;42(1):64-9. https://doi.org/10.3109/07853890903325360.

56. Highet AR, Gibson CS, Goldwater PN. Variant interleukin 1 receptor antagonist gene alleles in sudden infant death syndrome. Arch Dis Child. 2010;95(12):1009-12. https://doi.org/10.1136/adc.2010.188268.

57. Bayley JP, Ottenhoff TH, Verweij CL. Is there a future for TNF promoter polymorphisms? Genes Immun. 2004;5(5):315-29. https://doi.org/10.1038/sj.gene.6364055.

58. Wilson AG, Symons JA, McDowell TL, McDevitt HO, Duff GW. Effects of a polymorphism in the human tumor necrosis factor alpha promoter on transcriptional activation. Proc Natl Acad Sci USA. 1997;94(7):3195-9. https://doi.org/10.1073/pnas.94.7.3195.

59. Bayley JP, de Rooij H, van den Elsen PJ, Huizinga TW, Verweij CL. Functional analysis of linker-scan mutants spanning the -376, -308, -244, and -238 polymorphic sites of the TNF-alpha promoter. Cytokine. 2001;14(6):316-23. https://doi.org/10.1006/cyto.2001.0902.

60. Kaluza W, Reuss E, Grossmann S, Hug R, Schopf RE, Galle PR, et al. Different transcriptional activity and in vitro TNF-alpha production in psoriasis patients carrying the TNF-alpha 238A promoter polymorphism. J Invest Dermatol. 2000;114(6):1180-3. https://doi.org/10.1046/j.1523-1747.2000.00001.x.

61. Pociot F, D'Alfonso S, Compasso S, Scorza R, Richiardi PM. Functional analysis of a new polymorphism in the human TNF alpha gene promoter. Scand J Immunol. 1995;42(4):501-4. https://doi.org/10.1111/j.1365-3083.1995.tb03686.x.

62. Ferrante L, Opdal SH, Vege A, Rognum TO. TNF-alpha promoter polymorphisms in sudden infant death. Hum Immunol. 2008;69(6):368-73. https://doi.org/10.1016/j.humimm.2008.04.006.

63. Moscovis SM, Gordon AE, Al Madani OM, Gleeson M, Scott RJ, Hall ST, et al. Genetic and environmental factors affecting TNF-alpha responses in relation to sudden infant death syndrome. Front Immunol. 2015;6:374. https://doi.org/10.3389/fimmu.2015.00374.

64. Rognum TO, Saugstad OD. Biochemical and immunological studies in SIDS victims. Clues to understanding the death mechanism. Acta Paediatr Suppl. 1993;82 Suppl 389:82-5. https://doi.org/10.1111/j.1651-2227.1993.tb12886.x.

65. Zhang K, Wang X. Maternal smoking and increased risk of sudden infant death syndrome: A meta-analysis. Leg Med (Tokyo). 2013;15(3):115-21. https://doi.org/10.1016/j.legalmed.2012.10.007.

66. Gordon AE, El Ahmer OR, Chan R, Al Madani OM, Braun JM, Weir DM, et al. Why is smoking a risk factor for sudden infant death syndrome? Child Care Health Dev. 2002;28 Suppl 1:23-5. https://doi.org/10.1046/j.1365-2214.2002.00007.x.

67. Moscovis SM, Gordon AE, Al Madani OM, Gleeson M, Scott RJ, Hall ST, et al. Virus infections and sudden death in infancy: The role of Interferon-gamma. Front Immunol. 2015;6:107. https://doi.org/10.3389/fimmu.2015.00107.

68. Molony N, Blackwell CC, Busuttil A. The effect of prone posture on nasal temperature in children in relation to induction of staphylococcal toxins implicated in sudden infant death syndrome. FEMS Immunol Med Microbiol. 1999;25(1-2):109-13. https://doi.org/10.1111/j.1574-695X.1999.tb01333.x.

69. Tsai YY, Lin JM, Wan L, Lin HJ, Tsai Y, Lee CC, et al. Interleukin gene polymorphisms in age-related macular degeneration. Invest Ophthalmol Vis Sci. 2008;49(2):693-8. https://doi.org/10.1167/iovs.07-0125.

70. Hull J, Thomson A, Kwiatkowski D. Association of respiratory syncytial virus bronchiolitis with the interleukin 8 gene region in UK families. Thorax. 2000;55(12):1023-7. https://doi.org/10.1136/thorax.55.12.1023.

71. Stoltenberg L, Thrane PS, Rognum TO. Development of immune response markers in the trachea in the fetal period and the first year of life. Pediatr Allergy Immunol. 1993;4(1):13-19. https://doi.org/10.1111/j.1399-3038.1993.tb00059.x.

72. Rognum TO, Thrane S, Stoltenberg L, Vege A, Brandtzaeg P. Development of intestinal mucosal immunity in fetal life and the first postnatal months. Pediatr Res. 1992;32(2):145-9. https://doi.org/10.1203/00006450-199208000-00003.

# 31

# The Genetics of Sudden Infant Death Syndrome

Catherine A Brownstein, MPH, PhD,
Annapurna Poduri, MPH, MD,
Richard D Goldstein, MD and
Ingrid A Holm, MPH, MD

*Boston Children's Hospital, Boston, USA*

## Introduction

Despite a decrease in the mortality rates of sudden infant death syndrome (SIDS) over the past decades, SIDS is still one of the leading causes of post-neonatal and infant death. In the United States, 8% of all infant deaths are attributed to SIDS, only behind congenital malformations and chromosomal abnormalities (21%) and disorders relating to prematurity and low birth weight (17%) (1). While efforts have been made to reduce the role of environmental factors, such as sleep environment and smoking, this persistent mortality highlights the importance of intrinsic factors involved in SIDS, including genetic changes that predispose infants to, or are directly responsible for, SIDS (2, 3). In addition, the incidence of SIDS in families where one infant has died from SIDS is increased by over fivefold, providing further evidence of a role for genetic factors (4, 5).

A role for genetic factors in SIDS is consistent with the Triple Risk Model of SIDS, with genetic factors contributing to the "vulnerable infant". The Triple Risk Model hypothesizes that three elements are present for SIDS to occur (6):

1. **Critical developmental period**: Mortality from SIDS clusters during certain ages. Developmental changes in autonomic control co-incide with periods of increased susceptibility to SIDS.

2. **Vulnerable infant**: Understood largely in terms of associated risk factors such as race or exposure to alcohol or tobacco during pregnancy; infants dying from SIDS have been shown to have differences in autonomic responses that impair their ability to respond to challenges in the sleep environment. In addition, genetic conditions, such as a cardiac channelopathy, a metabolic condition, or a seizure disorder, may cause the infant to be vulnerable and at greater risk of SIDS.

3. **Exogenous stressor(s)**: Stressors associated with SIDS include overheating, secondhand tobacco smoke, upper respiratory tract infection, bed sharing, and prone sleeping position (6).

According to the Triple Risk Model, although most babies encounter and survive environmental stressors, a vulnerable infant who becomes challenged during a critical period may not be able to overcome the stressor, leading to SIDS. Thus, SIDS can be seen as representing a severe, lethal phenotype with genetic causes that contribute to the vulnerable infant. Genomic approaches to SIDS attempt to understand genetic mechanisms causing or contributing to this infant vulnerability.

## Genetics of SIDS

By definition, SIDS, as the unexplained death of a seemingly healthy baby less than a year old, is an undiagnosed "disease". As such, it can be approached similarly to other undiagnosed diseases. In clinical medicine, if a living individual presents with an unknown or unexplained disease, the standard practice is to exhaustively investigate until the cause is (hopefully) understood. This process often includes conducting genetic studies. If applicable, family members also undergo genetic testing. Since death in SIDS can be understood as a more extreme phenotype and/or outcome than illness, the same logic and approach should be taken with SIDS as an undiagnosed disease. Genetic studies are crucial in this evaluation, enabling exploration of the role of genes implicated in the etiology of SIDS, ranging from abnormalities in neurotransmitters, neuroanatomy, receptors, growth factors, and apoptotic markers (7). For example, neuroanatomical abnormalities of the hippocampus have been reported in over 40% of SIDS cases in a sample with limited selection bias (8), and the precise mechanisms of these and other neuropathological changes are still unknown and may involve genetic changes.

### Next-generation sequencing

Over the past two decades, targeted genetic studies have led to findings that suggest that genetic answers may be forthcoming (9-15). With the more recent development of next-generation sequencing (NGS) techniques to interrogate patients' genomes, and the increased rate of discovery of causative genetic variants, the ability to identify genes that may play a role in the vulnerability to sudden death in early life, and to provide answers to family, will also likely greatly increase. NGS has already been applied to SIDS in a few studies. In one whole-exome sequencing (WES) study of 161 SIDS infants focused on cardiovascular and metabolic diseases, 20% of cases were found to have variants that might be causal, including 9% with variants in a cardiac channel gene, 7% in a cardiomyopathy gene, and 1% in a metabolic gene (16). Such findings, though preliminary, support the role of NGS in detecting genetic changes that increase the risk for SIDS.

The application of NGS is complicated by the vast amounts of data generated, much of which are, at least currently, unclear. As a result, NGS has resulted in rich datasets of genetic variants of unknown significance (VUSs) discovered in patients, including those with SIDS. A VUS is defined as a genetic variant where the association between the variant and disease is not known. Any particular VUS may turn out to be benign, or may turn out to have variable phenotypic expression, known as *variable penetrance*, depending on the age and/or developmental, environmental, and epigenetic factors in the individual. Consistent with the Triple Risk Model of SIDS, a VUS may contribute to the vulnerability of the infant but be benign in a parent who also carries the variant and survived infancy without incident. The fact that in many cases it may take more than just a pathogenic variant makes interpreting VUSs in SIDS a challenge.

NGS genetic studies in SIDS are further complicated by the fact that it seems unlikely that a single causative pathogenic variant exists in all SIDS cases (17). Instead, it is more likely that a multifactorial genetic model applies to SIDS and that in many cases there are changes in several genes that together predispose an infant to SIDS, in combination with additional risk factors as hypothesized by the Triple Risk Model. As suggested by Opdal et. al. (17), genetic variants in SIDS likely fall into in one of two categories: [1] mutations that cause genetic disorders resulting in death; or [2] polymorphisms that may predispose infants to death during the critical period and in the presence of environmental stressors. To date, genetic studies have focused on the former, and variants in genes that cause a genetic disorder that leads to death have been described. Below we have summarized what is currently known about the genetics of SIDS.

## Metabolic diseases

For years, metabolic diseases have been known to occasionally present as SIDS (18, 19), and studies suggest that metabolic disorders may account for 1% to 2% of SIDS cases (20). Fatty acid oxidation disorders are the most common metabolic disorders to lead to SIDS, and they can present with little or no clinical prodrome (21). Fatty acid oxidation defects have been well studied in SIDS, and medium-chain acyl-CoA dehydrogenase (MCAD) deficiency (20, 22) is the most common inherited disorder of fatty acid metabolism (23). MCAD typically presents in early childhood with a hypoketotic, hypoglycemic crisis, which can be fatal if untreated. With the advent of newborn screening for inborn errors of metabolism, including MCAD, across the United States (US) (24), it has become evident that these conditions are more common than previously thought (25).

Given the focus on MCAD deficiency in sudden infant death, there has been great interest in identifying mutations in the MCAD gene, *ACADM*, in cases presenting as SIDS. In 1991, Ding et al. (26) identified an A985G mutation in *ACADM* in seven families whose infants died of SIDS, although others have not been able to replicate these findings (27). More recently, Lovera et al. (28) found a homozygous frame-shift mutation in a 3-day-old who died with MCAD. To date, there is little evidence for a prominent role for variants in the *ACADM* gene in SIDS, which may be because MCAD deficiency is now detected on newborn screening.

Other metabolic conditions are also of interest. Carnitine palmitoyltransferase (CPT) II is a mitochondrial fatty acid oxidation enzyme critical for energy production. There have been reports of variants in the *CPT2* gene in SIDS, including a homozygous F352C variant (29), and a case who was compound heterozygous for a novel p.L644S variant and the known p.F383Y variant (30). Finally, severe hypoglycemia is a potential cause of death in infants, although it is not clear if genes involved in glucose metabolism are related to SIDS (19).

## Cardiac gene

Another important area of investigation in SIDS is cardiac channelopathies, and it has been suggested that approximately 10% of SIDS cases are due to cardiac channelopathies in some series (11, 31). In a subset of SIDS cases, the cause of death has been identified as a pathogenic variant in one of several genes that disrupt ion channel function (32). These conditions include long QT syndrome, Brugada syndrome, and catecholaminergic polymorphic ventricular tachycardia (CPVT).

Long QT syndrome is an ion channelopathy that increases the risk of ventricular tachycardia and sudden cardiac death (33). Long QT is characterized by a prolonged QT interval on an electrocardiogram (ECG) and polymorphic ventricular arrhythmias. This may cause syncope and sudden death in response to exercise or emotional stress, and can present with a sentinel event of sudden cardiac death in infancy. Genes involved in long QT syndrome include *ANK2, KCNE1, KCNE2, KCNJ2, CACNA1C, CAV3, SCN4B, AKAP9, SNTA1, KCNJ5, CALM1*, and *CALM2* (34). Because variants in these genes have been primarily identified in probands with the condition, the actual penetrance of the genetic changes in families and the general population is often unknown. There are some functional validation studies for many of these variants. For example, in SIDS cases, three variants in the gene for alpha1-syntrophin, *SNTA1*, have been shown to lead to changes in sodium channel properties (35). However, much work is left in understanding the relationship between many of the genetic variants found and their role in SIDS.

Brugada syndrome is characterized by incomplete right bundle-branch block and ST-segment elevations in the anterior precordial leads of an ECG, and is also associated with SIDS (33, 36). Death often occurs during rest or while sleeping, which makes it a likely candidate for SIDS. Genes associated with Brugada syndrome include *ABCC9*, *CACNA1C*, *CACNA2D1*, *CACNB2*, *FGF12*, *GPD1L*, *HCN4*, *KCND2*, *KCND3*, *KCNE5*, *KCNE3*, *KCNH2*, *KCNJ8*, *PKP2*, *RANGRF*, *SCN1B*, *SCN2B*, *SCN3B*, *SCN5A*, *SCN10A*, *SEMA3A*, *SLMAP*, and *TRPM4* (37).

CPVT, which results in potentially lethal arrhythmias typically triggered by stress or exercise, has also been associated with SIDS (33). There may be sudden increases in sympathetic activation during sleep, making CPVT-affected infants susceptible to arrhythmias and subsequently to SIDS (38). Stressors such as pain, hunger, overheating, and infection may provide a mechanism to trigger a lethal cardiac event in an infant who has a genetic mutation in the *RYR2* gene (autosomal-dominant form of CPVT) or mutations in both alleles of the *CASQ2* or *TRDN* genes (where autosomal-recessive mutations may result in CPVT) (39).

Although a growing number of genes have been associated with CPVT, Brugada, and long QT, the involvement of four genes in these disorders is most understood: *KCNQ1*, *KCNH2*, and *SCN5A* in long QT syndrome and/or Brugada syndrome, and *RYR2* and *SCN5A* in CPVT (32). Below we discuss each of these genes in more detail.

## SCN5A

*SCN5A* is associated with Brugada, long QT syndrome, and CPVT (40). The *SCN5A* protein forms a sodium-selective channel through which sodium ions may pass in accordance with their electrochemical gradient. Channel inactivation is regulated by intracellular calcium levels. This protein is found primarily in cardiac muscle and is responsible for the initial upstroke of the action potential in an ECG (40). Pathogenic variants in *SCN5A* are implicated in several reports of SIDS. Schwartz et al. reported a clinically typical instance of "near-SIDS" in an infant who was found to be heterozygous for a missense variant in *SCN5A* (10). Ackerman et al. performed post-mortem mutation analysis of the *SCN5A* gene in 93 cases of SIDS or undetermined infant death and identified missense variants in *SCN5A* in two cases (11). Homozygosity for the *SCN5A* variant S1103Y was identified in three African American autopsy-confirmed cases of SIDS (12).

## KCNQ1

Schwartz et al. identified a de novo, heterozygous pathogenic variant in the *KCNQ1* gene of an infant who died from SIDS (9). They found the same variant in affected members of an unrelated family with long QT syndrome. *KCNQ1* interacts with two other potassium channel proteins, *KCNE1* and *KCNE3*, and is hypothesized to be important in the repolarization phase of the cardiac action potential. Mutations in this gene are associated with hereditary long QT syndrome 1 (also known as Romano-Ward syndrome), Jervell and Lange-Nielsen syndrome, and familial atrial fibrillation (41).

### KCNH2 (hERG1)

The *KCNH2* gene belongs to a large family of potassium channel genes. Mutations in *KCNH2* are associated with SIDS, long QT syndrome, Brugada syndrome, and short QT syndrome (37, 42-45). The *KCNH2* and *KCNE2* proteins interact to form a functional potassium channel. Four alpha subunits, each produced from the *KCNH2* gene, form the structure of each channel. One beta subunit, produced from the *KCNE2* gene, binds to the channel and regulates its activity. Pathogenic variants in *KCNH2* may interfere with the structure or function of the subunit (34).

### RYR2

The *RYR2* protein is part of a family of ryanodine receptors, which form channels that transport positively charged calcium ions within cells. Channels made with the *RYR2* protein are found in cardiac myocytes and are embedded in the sarcoplasmic reticulum. The *RYR2* channel controls the flow of calcium ions out of the sarcoplasmic reticulum (46). Mutations in the *RYR2* gene have been found to cause CPVT and have been associated with SIDS (46, 47). These pathogenic variants alter the structure and/or function of the *RYR2* channel. For example, the R2267H and S4565R variants associated with SIDS enhance the sensitivity of *RYR2* to cytosolic Ca(2+) during β-adrenergic stress (47). Animal models support this association: mice engineered with an R176Q variant have a higher rate of postnatal mortality due to abnormal Ca(2+) release and ectopic activity (48), and mice engineered with an R2474S variant have increased rate of intrauterine lethality (49).

## Genes related to serotonin

Serotonin (5-hydroxytryptamine; 5-HT) is a neurotransmitter in the central and peripheral nervous systems. The serotonergic system plays an important role in brainstem cardiorespiratory and thermoregulatory centers, such as regulating breathing, blood circulation, heart rate, body temperature, and the sleep-wake cycle. There is evidence that 5-HT is involved in SIDS: dysregulated autonomic control and altered neurochemistry have been found in SIDS cases (50-53), and brainstem 5-HT, tryptophan hydroxylase-2 (TPH-2), and 5-HT receptor binding and receptor expression are lower in SIDS cases (54-56). Similar alterations in mouse models have been shown to impair function in arousal pathways, resulting in a decreased tendency to arouse from sleep when challenged during sleep to respond to homeostatic threats (57). Likewise, in an infant, hypoxia or hypercarbia normally trigger autoresuscitation as the infant senses inadequate air intake, and there are reflexive arousal and autonomic responses. In an infant with a brainstem abnormality, however, these protective mechanisms may be less effective, so the child may succumb to SIDS. The relationship of the serotonergic pathway to SIDS has led to much interest in identifying genetic factors that alter the pathway, potentially leading to SIDS. A number of genes involved in the serotonin pathway have been implicated in SIDS [see (58) for a review].

Probably the best-studied gene in the 5-HT pathway is *SLC6A4*, the gene for 5-HT. Following release, 5-HT is actively cleared from synaptic spaces by *SLC6A4*, a high-affinity, Na(+)- and Cl(-)-dependent transporter localized in presynaptic neuronal membranes. Narita et al. examined the long/short promoter polymorphism of the *SLC6A4* gene in Japanese SIDS cases and found an excess of the L/L genotype and L allele in the SIDS group relative to controls (59). Weese-Mayer et al. investigated this variable tandem repeat sequence polymorphism in the promoter region in a cohort of 87 SIDS cases (43 African American and 44 Caucasian) and gender-/ethnicity-matched controls (13). They also found increases in the L/L genotype and the L allele. However, Paterson et al. (60) and others (61) did not find an association between the serotonin transporter (5-HTT) promoter genotype and SIDS. Weese-Mayer et al. also demonstrated that an intron 2 polymorphism (12-repeat allele), which also differentially regulates 5-HTT expression, was associated with increased risk of SIDS in African American but not Caucasian SIDS cases (13), an association that has not been replicated (58, 61-63).

Other genes in the serotonergic pathway have been studied in SIDS with mixed results. These include the Fifth Ewing Variant (*FEV*) which may play a role in the development of the 5-HT neurons (64, 65); *TPH2*, which codes for the rate-limiting enzyme in 5-HT biosynthesis (63); and the MAO-A promoter VNTR (66-68). None of these has been confirmed as contributing to SIDS and thus they are unlikely to play a significant role (58).

## Inflammatory genes

Ferrante et al. showed alterations in expression in a number of genes involved in inflammation in SIDS cases compared to controls, suggesting that changes in genes regulating the inflammatory process may predispose to SIDS (69). Interleukin-10 (IL-10) is an inflammatory cytokine that plays a role in the development of infectious diseases. Lower levels of IL-10 production have been hypothesized to be associated with SIDS (70) and there is evidence for an association between the IL-10 gene ATA promoter haplotype (1082A, -819T, and -592A) and both death due to infectious disease and SIDS (70, 71). Studies have revealed an association between partial deletions of the highly polymorphic C4 gene and mild respiratory infections in infants who have died of SIDS (72). Differences in C4 expression may contribute to differences in immune system response, and therefore susceptibility to infectious and autoimmune diseases that put infants at higher risk of SIDS (72). Variants reported in other immune system genes, including mannose-binding lectin 2 (MBL2), have also been reported to be associated with SIDS (73).

## Genes related to development

Congenital central hypoventilation syndrome (CCHS) is a rare disorder characterized by abnormal control of breathing early on in life. CCHS appears to be an autosomal disorder with variable penetrance (74), and variants in *PHOX2B* have been identified in CCHS (74, 75). *PHOX2B* is involved in the development of the autonomic nervous system, and since SIDS is considered to be due to autonomic dysfunction, *PHOX2B* could be a candidate gene for at least some cases (76, 77). A variation in a polyalanine repeat in exon 3 of the *PHOX2B* gene has been found in some studies to be associated with SIDS (78), although other studies have not shown this association (79, 80). At this time, there is no clear evidence for mutations or polymorphism in *PHOX2B* in SIDS. Other genes involved in the autonomic nervous system have also been studied (81), again without clear associations.

Polymorphisms in genes that affect brain development and have also been associated with SIDS include *PHOX2A*, *RET*, *ECE1*, *TLX3* and *EN1* (81). The role of these findings is not clear.

## Copy number variants in SIDS

There has been at least one study of copy number variants and SIDS in which de novo CNVs were detected in 3 of 27 SIDS cases (82). The role of this finding is unclear.

# The Role of Genes in Sudden Unexplained Death in Epilepsy and SIDS

There is recent evidence for links between SUDEP (sudden unexplained death in epilepsy) and SIDS, and a growing body of literature ties both entities to the serotoninergic pathway (52, 83). SUDEP is the sudden, unexpected, non-traumatic death of individuals with epilepsy with or without evidence of a seizure, in whom post-mortem examination does not reveal a structural or toxicological cause for death. A hypothesized mechanism for SUDEP is that seizures initiate pathogenic signaling between the brain and heart, resulting in lethal cardiac arrhythmias (84, 85). Given that defects in membrane excitability can result in both epilepsy and cardiac arrhythmias, ion channels co-expressed in the brain and heart are leading candidates for SUDEP (85, 86). Selected genes for SUDEP, where a link to SIDS has been hypothesized, include *SCN1A*, *SCN1B*, and *DEPDC5* (14, 87-90).

## SCN1A

*SCN1A* mediates the voltage-dependent sodium ion permeability of excitable membranes. This protein forms a sodium-selective channel through which Na(+) ions may pass in accordance with their electrochemical gradient. The vertebrate sodium channel is a voltage-gated ion channel essential for the generation and propagation of action potentials, mainly in nerve and muscle. Voltage-sensitive sodium channels are heteromeric complexes consisting of a large central pore-forming glycosylated alpha subunit, and two smaller auxiliary beta subunits. The *SCN1A* gene encodes the large alpha subunit, and mutations in this gene have been associated with several epilepsy, convulsion, and migraine disorders (91, 92). Mutations in *SCN1A* can result in both generalized epilepsy with febrile seizures plus (GEFS+) and Dravet syndrome (2, 12). The risk of SUDEP is high in children with Dravet syndrome, which may be due to the frequency and severity of seizures (13). In one published pedigree, one sibling was reported to have Dravet syndrome and the other had a sudden death after a history of febrile seizures — both inherited a pathogenic variant in *SCN1A* from their unaffected father, who was mosaic for the variant (93).

## SCN1B

Voltage-gated sodium channels are heteromeric proteins that function in the generation and propagation of action potentials in muscle and neuronal cells. They are composed of one alpha and two beta subunits, where the alpha subunit provides channel activity and the beta-1 subunit modulates the kinetics of channel inactivation. *SCN1B* encodes a sodium channel beta-1 subunit. Mutations in *SCN1B* are associated with generalized epilepsy with febrile seizures plus, Brugada syndrome, and defects in cardiac conduction (94). A case report has linked the *SCN1B* R214Q variant to the deaths of three individuals, including one female SIDS case (14). This variant has been suggested to be a functional polymorphism that affects the sodium channel current and potassium current (10).

## DEPDC5

Linked to familial epilepsies such as familial temporal lobe epilepsy, epileptic spasms, familial focal epilepsy with variable foci, autosomal dominant nocturnal frontal lobe epilepsy, and cortical dysplasia, pathogenic variants in *DEPDC5* have been reported in SUDEP (90). *DEPDC5*, *NPRL2*, and *NPRL3* encode the GATOR1 (GTPase-activating protein (GAP) activity toward RAGs) subcomplex 1. The GATOR1 and GATOR2 subcomplexes comprise GATOR, which is a critical regulator of the pathway that signals amino acid sufficiency to mTORC1 (95). mTORC1 regulates protein synthesis (95).

## KCNA1 (Kv1.1)

*KCNA1* has been suggested as a SUDEP gene from mouse and human studies (15, 96, 97). Mice bearing Kv1.1 channel pathogenic variants exhibit hippocampal and peripheral nerve hyperexcitability, severe epilepsy characterized by partial and generalized tonic-clonic seizures, and premature death (15, 98). In Kv1.1-deficient mice, the onset of epilepsy at 2-3 weeks of age co-occurs with 25% lethality in homozygotes, suggesting a link between seizures and sudden death (98, 99). In a case report of SUDEP, a 3-year-old proband with severe myoclonic epilepsy of infancy was found to have a combination of de novo single nucleotide polymorphisms (SNPs) and copy number variations (CNVs) in the *SCN1A* and *KCNA1* genes. The combination was determined to result in both the epilepsy and the premature death (96).

## SCN8A

*SCN8A* has also been suggested as a SUDEP gene based on mouse and human studies (15, 96, 97). In fact, the initial epilepsy proband reported with a pathogenic variant in *SCN8A* also had SUDEP (97). Pathogenic variants in *SCN8A* are a cause of early onset severe epilepsy, and have been linked to SUDEP (100). This voltage-dependent sodium channel is a key substrate enabling dendritic excitability (101).

## Conclusions

Evidence suggests likely genomic complexity and a degree of overlap amongst sudden cardiac death, SIDS, and SUDEP. The advent of next-generation sequencing will improve our understanding of the genetics of SIDS, and will result in more answers for families with a family history of sudden or unexplained deaths. However, a Mendelian approach is not likely to explain all cases. Genetic risk factors combined with a critical developmental period and a vulnerable infant are all likely to play a part in most cases. Many important challenges remain in this field and future progress requires collaborative and interdisciplinary research (3).

## References

1.  Matthews TJ, MacDorman MF. Infant mortality statistics from the 2010 period linked birth/infant death data set. National vital statistics reports: Centers for Disease Control and Prevention, National Center for Health Statistics, National Vital Statistics System. 2013;62(8):1-26.

2.    Goldstein RD, Trachtenberg FL, Sens MA, Harty BJ, Kinney HC. Overall postneonatal mortality and rates of SIDS. Pediatrics. 2016;137(1):e20152298. https://doi.org/10.1542/peds.2015-2298.

3.    Goldstein RD, Kinney HC, Willinger M. Sudden unexpected death in fetal life through early childhood. Pediatrics. 2016;137(6):e20154661. https://doi.org/10.1542/peds.2015-4661.

4.    Guntheroth WG, Lohmann R, Spiers PS. Risk of sudden infant death syndrome in subsequent siblings. J Pediatrics. 1990;116(4):520-4. https://doi.org/10.1016/S0022-3476(05)81596-3.

5.    Oyen N, Skjaerven R, Irgens LM. Population-based recurrence risk of sudden infant death syndrome compared with other infant and fetal deaths. Am J Epidemiol. 1996;144(3):300-5. https://doi.org/10.1093/oxfordjournals.aje.a008925.

6.    Filiano JJ, Kinney HC. A perspective on neuropathologic findings in victims of the sudden infant death syndrome: The triple-risk model. Biol Neonate. 1994;65(3-4):194-7. https://doi.org/10.1159/000244052.

7.    Machaalani R, Waters KA. Neurochemical abnormalities in the brainstem of the sudden infant death syndrome (SIDS). Paediatr Respir Rev. 2014;15(4):293-300. https://doi.org/10.1016/j.prrv.2014.09.008.

8.    Kinney HC, Poduri AH, Cryan JB, Haynes RL, Teot L, Sleeper LA, et al. Hippocampal formation maldevelopment and sudden unexpected death across the pediatric age spectrum. J Neuropath Exp Neurol. 2016;75(10):981-97. https://doi.org/10.1093/jnen/nlw075.

9.    Schwartz PJ, Priori SG, Bloise R, Napolitano C, Ronchetti E, Piccinini A, et al. Molecular diagnosis in a child with sudden infant death syndrome. Lancet. 2001;358(9290):1342-3. https://doi.org/10.1016/S0140-6736(01)06450-9.

10.   Schwartz PJ, Priori SG, Dumaine R, Napolitano C, Antzelevitch C, Stramba-Badiale M, et al. A molecular link between the sudden infant death syndrome and the long-QT syndrome. New England J Med. 2000;343(4):262-7. https://doi.org/10.1056/NEJM200007273430405.

11.   Ackerman MJ, Siu BL, Sturner WQ, Tester DJ, Valdivia CR, Makielski JC, et al. Postmortem molecular analysis of SCN5A defects in sudden infant death syndrome. JAMA. 2001;286(18):2264-9. https://doi.org/10.1001/jama.286.18.2264.

12.   Plant LD, Bowers PN, Liu Q, Morgan T, Zhang T, State MW, et al. A common cardiac sodium channel variant associated with sudden infant death in African Americans, SCN5A S1103Y. J Clin Invest. 2006;116(2):430-5. https://doi.org/10.1172/JCI25618.

13. Weese-Mayer DE, Berry-Kravis EM, Maher BS, Silvestri JM, Curran ME, Marazita ML. Sudden infant death syndrome: Association with a promoter polymorphism of the serotonin transporter gene. Am J Med Genet Part A. 2003;117A(3):268-74. https://doi.org/10.1002/ajmg.a.20005.

14. Hu D, Barajas-Martinez H, Medeiros-Domingo A, Crotti L, Veltmann C, Schimpf R, et al. A novel rare variant in SCN1Bb linked to Brugada syndrome and SIDS by combined modulation of Na(v)1.5 and K(v)4.3 channel currents. Heart Rhythm. 2012;9(5):760-9. https://doi.org/10.1016/j.hrthm.2011.12.006.

15. Glasscock E, Yoo JW, Chen TT, Klassen TL, Noebels JL. Kv1.1 potassium channel deficiency reveals brain-driven cardiac dysfunction as a candidate mechanism for sudden unexplained death in epilepsy. J Neurosci. 2010;30(15):5167-75. https://doi.org/10.1523/JNEUROSCI.5591-09.2010.

16. Neubauer J, Lecca MR, Russo G, Bartsch C, Medeiros-Domingo A, Berger W, et al. Post-mortem whole-exome analysis in a large sudden infant death syndrome cohort with a focus on cardiovascular and metabolic genetic diseases. Eur J Hum Genet. 2017;25(4):404-9. https://doi.org/10.1038/ejhg.2016.199.

17. Opdal SH, Rognum TO. Gene variants predisposing to SIDS: Current knowledge. Forensic Sci Med Pathol. 2011;7(1):26-36. https://doi.org/10.1007/s12024-010-9182-9.

18. McConkie-Rosell A, Iafolla AK. Medium-chain acyl CoA dehydrogenase deficiency: Its relationship to SIDS and the impact on genetic counseling. J Genetic Counseling. 1993;2(1):17-27. https://doi.org/10.1007/BF00962557.

19. Opdal SH, Rognum TO. The sudden infant death syndrome gene: Does it exist? Pediatrics. 2004;114(4):e506-12. https://doi.org/10.1542/peds.2004-0683.

20. Pryce JW, Weber MA, Heales S, Malone M, Sebire NJ. Tandem mass spectrometry findings at autopsy for detection of metabolic disease in infant deaths: Postmortem changes and confounding factors. J Clin Pathol. 2011;64(11):1005-9. https://doi.org/10.1136/jclinpath-2011-200218.

21. Keeler AM, Flotte TR. Cell and gene therapy for genetic diseases: Inherited disorders affecting the lung and those mimicking sudden infant death syndrome. Hum Gene Ther. 2012;23(6):548-56. https://doi.org/10.1089/hum.2012.087.

22. Lovera C, Porta F, Caciotti A, Catarzi S, Cassanello M, Caruso U, et al. Sudden unexpected infant death (SUDI) in a newborn due to medium chain acyl CoA dehydrogenase (MCAD) deficiency with an unusual severe genotype. Ital J Pediatr. 2012;38:59. https://doi.org/10.1186/1824-7288-38-59.

23. Yusupov R, Finegold DN, Naylor EW, Sahai I, Waisbren S, Levy HL. Sudden death in medium chain acyl-coenzyme a dehydrogenase deficiency (MCADD)

despite newborn screening. Mol Genet Metab. 2010;101(1):33-9. https://doi.org/10.1016/j.ymgme.2010.05.007.

24. Therrell BL, Padilla CD, Loeber JG, Kneisser I, Saadallah A, Borrajo GJ, et al. Current status of newborn screening worldwide: 2015. Semin Perinatol. 2015;39(3):171-87. https://doi.org/10.1053/j.semperi.2015.03.002.

25. Rosenthal NA, Currier RJ, Baer RJ, Feuchtbaum L, Jelliffe-Pawlowski LL. Undiagnosed metabolic dysfunction and sudden infant death syndrome — A case-control study. Paediatr Perinat Epidemiol. 2015;29(2):151-5. https://doi.org/10.1111/ppe.12175.

26. Ding JH, Roe CR, Iafolla AK, Chen YT. Medium-chain acyl-coenzyme A dehydrogenase deficiency and sudden infant death. New England J Med. 1991;325(1):61-2. https://doi.org/10.1056/NEJM199107043250113.

27. Opdal SH, Vege A, Saugstad OD, Rognum TO. Is the medium-chain acyl-CoA dehydrogenase G985 mutation involved in sudden infant death in Norway? European J Ped. 1995;154(2):166-7. https://doi.org/10.1007/BF01991929.

28. Lovera C, Porta F, Caciotti A, Catarzi S, Cassanello M, Caruso U, et al. Sudden unexpected infant death (SUDI) in a newborn due to medium chain acyl CoA dehydrogenase (MCAD) deficiency with an unusual severe genotype. Ital J Pediatr. 2012;38:59. https://doi.org/10.1186/1824-7288-38-59.

29. Yamamoto T, Tanaka H, Emoto Y, Umehara T, Fukahori Y, Kuriu Y, et al. Carnitine palmitoyltransferase 2 gene polymorphism is a genetic risk factor for sudden unexpected death in infancy. Brain Dev. 2014;36(6):479-83. https://doi.org/10.1016/j.braindev.2013.07.011.

30. Yamamoto T, Tanaka H, Kobayashi H, Okamura K, Tanaka T, Emoto Y, et al. Retrospective review of Japanese sudden unexpected death in infancy: The importance of metabolic autopsy and expanded newborn screening. Mol Genet Metab. 2011;102(4):399-406. https://doi.org/10.1016/j.ymgme.2010.12.004.

31. Tfelt-Hansen J, Winkel BG, Grunnet M, Jespersen T. Cardiac channelopathies and sudden infant death syndrome. Cardiology. 2011;119(1):21-33. https://doi.org/10.1159/000329047.

32. Sarquella-Brugada G, Campuzano O, Cesar S, Iglesias A, Fernandez A, Brugada J, et al. Sudden infant death syndrome caused by cardiac arrhythmias: Only a matter of genes encoding ion channels? Int J Legal Med. 2016;130(2):415-20. https://doi.org/10.1007/s00414-016-1330-7.

33. Franciosi S, Perry FKG, Roston TM, Armstrong KR, Claydon VE, Sanatani S. The role of the autonomic nervous system in arrhythmias and sudden cardiac

death. Auto Neurosci: Basic Clin. 2017;205:1-11. https://doi.org/10.1016/j.autneu.2017.03.005.

34. Alders M, Christiaans I. Long QT syndrome. In: GeneReviews® [internet]. Eds Pagon RA, Adam MP, Ardinger HH, Wallace SE, Amemiya A, Bean LJH, et al. Seattle (WA). 1993. [Available from: https://www-ncbi-nlm-nih-gov.ezp-prod1.hul.harvard.edu/pubmed/20301308]. Accessed 20 August 2017.

35. Cheng J, Van Norstrand DW, Medeiros-Domingo A, Valdivia C, Tan BH, Ye B, et al. Alpha1-syntrophin mutations identified in sudden infant death syndrome cause an increase in late cardiac sodium current. Circ Arrhythm Electrophysiol. 2009;2(6):667-76. https://doi.org/10.1161/CIRCEP.109.891440.

36. Hedley PL, Jorgensen P, Schlamowitz S, Moolman-Smook J, Kanters JK, Corfield VA, et al. The genetic basis of Brugada syndrome: A mutation update. Human Mutation. 2009;30(9):1256-66. https://doi.org/10.1002/humu.21066.

37. Brugada R, Campuzano O, Sarquella-Brugada G, Brugada P, Brugada J, Hong K. Brugada syndrome. In: GeneReviews® [internet]. Eds Pagon RA, Adam MP, Ardinger HH, Wallace SE, Amemiya A, Bean LJH, et al. Seattle (WA). 1993. [Available from: https://www-ncbi-nlm-nih-gov.ezp-prod1.hul.harvard.edu/pubmed/20301690]. Accessed 20 August 2017.

38. Tester DJ, Ackerman MJ. Cardiomyopathic and channelopathic causes of sudden unexplained death in infants and children. Ann Rev Med. 2009;60:69-84. https://doi.org/10.1146/annurev.med.60.052907.103838.

39. Napolitano C, Priori SG, Bloise R. Catecholaminergic Polymorphic Ventricular Tachycardia. In: GeneReviews® [internet]. Eds Pagon RA, Adam MP, Ardinger HH, Wallace SE, Amemiya A, Bean LJH, et al. Seattle (WA). 1993.

40. Zaklyazminskaya E, Dzemeshkevich S. The role of mutations in the SCN5A gene in cardiomyopathies. Biochimica Et Biophysica Acta. 2016;1863(7 Pt B):1799-805. https://doi.org/10.1016/j.bbamcr.2016.02.014.

41. Nakano Y, Shimizu W. Genetics of long-QT syndrome. J Human Genet. 2016;61(1):51-5. https://doi.org/10.1038/jhg.2015.74.

42. Glengarry JM, Crawford J, Morrow PL, Stables SR, Love DR, Skinner JR. Long QT molecular autopsy in sudden infant death syndrome. Arch Dis Child. 2014;99(7):635-40. https://doi.org/10.1136/archdischild-2013-305331.

43. Lee YS, Kwon BS, Kim GB, Oh SI, Bae EJ, Park SS, et al. Long QT syndrome: A Korean single center study. J Korean Med Sci. 2013;28(10):1454-60. https://doi.org/10.3346/jkms.2013.28.10.1454.

44. Wolpert C, Schimpf R, Veltmann C, Giustetto C, Gaita F, Borggrefe M. Clinical characteristics and treatment of short QT syndrome. Expert Rev Cardiovasc Ther. 2005;3(4):611-17. https://doi.org/10.1586/14779072.3.4.611.

45. Nof E, Cordeiro JM, Perez GJ, Scornik FS, Calloe K, Love B, et al. A common single nucleotide polymorphism can exacerbate long-QT type 2 syndrome leading to sudden infant death. Circ Cardiovasc Genet. 2010;3(2):199-206. https://doi.org/10.1161/CIRCGENETICS.109.898569.

46. Kushnir A, Marks AR. The ryanodine receptor in cardiac physiology and disease. Adv Phram. 2010;59:1-30. https://doi.org/10.1016/S1054-3589(10)59001-X.

47. Tester DJ, Dura M, Carturan E, Reiken S, Wronska A, Marks AR, et al. A mechanism for sudden infant death syndrome (SIDS): Stress-induced leak via ryanodine receptors. Heart Rhythm. 2007;4(6):733-9. https://doi.org/10.1016/j.hrthm.2007.02.026.

48. Mathur N, Sood S, Wang S, van Oort RJ, Sarma S, Li N, et al. Sudden infant death syndrome in mice with an inherited mutation in RyR2. Circ Arrhythm Electrophysiol. 2009;2(6):677-85. https://doi.org/10.1161/CIRCEP.109.894683.

49. Lehnart SE, Mongillo M, Bellinger A, Lindegger N, Chen BX, Hsueh W, et al. Leaky Ca2+ release channel/ryanodine receptor 2 causes seizures and sudden cardiac death in mice. J Clin Invest. 2008;118(6):2230-45. https://doi.org/10.1172/JCI35346.

50. Kinney HC. Abnormalities of the brainstem serotonergic system in the sudden infant death syndrome: A review. Pediatr Dev Pathol. 2005;8(5):507-24. https://doi.org/10.1007/s10024-005-0067-y.

51. Kinney HC. Brainstem mechanisms underlying the sudden infant death syndrome: Evidence from human pathologic studies. Dev Psychobiol. 2009;51(3):223-33. https://doi.org/10.1002/dev.20367.

52. Kinney HC, Filiano JJ, White WF. Medullary serotonergic network deficiency in the sudden infant death syndrome: Review of a 15-year study of a single dataset. J Neuropath Exp Neurol. 2001;60(3):228-47. https://doi.org/10.1093/jnen/60.3.228.

53. Kinney HC, Richerson GB, Dymecki SM, Darnall RA, Nattie EE. The brainstem and serotonin in the sudden infant death syndrome. Ann Rev Path. 2009;4:517-50. https://doi.org/10.1146/annurev.pathol.4.110807.092322.

54. Haynes RL, Folkerth RD, Paterson DS, Broadbelt KG, Dan Zaharie S, Hewlett RH, et al. Serotonin receptors in the medulla oblongata of the human fetus and infant: The analytic approach of the international Safe Passage Study. J Neuropath

Exp Neurol. 2016;75(11):1048-57. https://academic.oup.com/jnen/article/75/11/1048/2410957.

55. Broadbelt KG, Rivera KD, Paterson DS, Duncan JR, Trachtenberg FL, Paulo JA, et al. Brainstem deficiency of the 14-3-3 regulator of serotonin synthesis: A proteomics analysis in the sudden infant death syndrome. Mol Cell Proteomics. 2012;11(1):M111 009530.

56. Duncan JR, Paterson DS, Hoffman JM, Mokler DJ, Borenstein NS, Belliveau RA, et al. Brainstem serotonergic deficiency in sudden infant death syndrome. JAMA. 2010;303(5):430-7. https://doi.org/10.1001/jama.2010.45.

57. Kato I, Franco P, Groswasser J, Scaillet S, Kelmanson I, Togari H, et al. Incomplete arousal processes in infants who were victims of sudden death. Am J Resp Critical Care Med. 2003;168(11):1298-303. https://doi.org/10.1164/rccm.200301-134OC.

58. Paterson DS. Serotonin gene variants are unlikely to play a significant role in the pathogenesis of the sudden infant death syndrome. Resp Physiol Neurobiol. 2013;189(2):301-14. https://doi.org/10.1016/j.resp.2013.07.001.

59. Narita N, Narita M, Takashima S, Nakayama M, Nagai T, Okado N. Serotonin transporter gene variation is a risk factor for sudden infant death syndrome in the Japanese population. Pediatrics. 2001;107(4):690-2. https://doi.org/10.1542/peds.107.4.690.

60. Paterson DS, Rivera KD, Broadbelt KG, Trachtenberg FL, Belliveau RA, Holm IA, et al. Lack of association of the serotonin transporter polymorphism with the sudden infant death syndrome in the San Diego Dataset. Pediatr Res. 2010;68(5):409-13. https://doi.org/10.1203/PDR.0b013e3181f2edf0.

61. Haas C, Braun J, Bar W, Bartsch C. No association of serotonin transporter gene variation with sudden infant death syndrome (SIDS) in Caucasians. Legal Med. 2009;11 Suppl 1:S210-12. https://doi.org/10.1016/j.legalmed.2009.01.051.

62. Opdal SH, Vege A, Rognum TO. Serotonin transporter gene variation in sudden infant death syndrome. Acta Paediatr. 2008;97(7):861-5. https://doi.org/10.1111/j.1651-2227.2008.00813.x.

63. Nonnis Marzano F, Maldini M, Filonzi L, Lavezzi AM, Parmigiani S, Magnani C, et al. Genes regulating the serotonin metabolic pathway in the brain stem and their role in the etiopathogenesis of the sudden infant death syndrome. Genomics. 2008;91(6):485-91. https://doi.org/10.1016/j.ygeno.2008.01.010.

64. Broadbelt KG, Barger MA, Paterson DS, Holm IA, Haas EA, Krous HF, et al. Serotonin-related FEV gene variant in the sudden infant death syndrome is

a common polymorphism in the African-American population. Pediatr Res. 2009;66(6):631-5. https://doi.org/10.1203/PDR.0b013e3181bd5a31.

65. Rand CM, Berry-Kravis EM, Zhou L, Fan W, Weese-Mayer DE. Sudden infant death syndrome: Rare mutation in the serotonin system FEV gene. Pediatr Res. 2007;62(2):180-2. https://doi.org/10.1203/PDR.0b013e3180a725a0.

66. Klintschar M, Heimbold C. Association between a functional polymorphism in the MAOA gene and sudden infant death syndrome. Pediatrics. 2012;129(3):e756-61. https://doi.org/10.1542/peds.2011-1642.

67. Courts C, Grabmuller M, Madea B. Monoamine oxidase A gene polymorphism and the pathogenesis of sudden infant death syndrome. J Pediatrics. 2013 Jul;163(1):89-93. https://doi.org/10.1016/j.jpeds.2012.12.072.

68. Filonzi L, Magnani C, Lavezzi AM, Rindi G, Parmigiani S, Bevilacqua G, et al. Association of dopamine transporter and monoamine oxidase molecular polymorphisms with sudden infant death syndrome and stillbirth: New insights into the serotonin hypothesis. Neurogenetics. 2009;10(1):65-72. https://doi.org/10.1007/s10048-008-0149-x.

69. Ferrante L, Rognum TO, Vege A, Nygard S, Opdal SH. Altered gene expression and possible immunodeficiency in cases of sudden infant death syndrome. Pediat Res. 2016;80(1):77-84. https://doi.org/10.1038/pr.2016.45.

70. Opdal SH, Opstad A, Vege A, Rognum TO. IL-10 gene polymorphisms are associated with infectious cause of sudden infant death. Human Immunol. 2003;64(12):1183-9. https://doi.org/10.1016/j.humimm.2003.08.359.

71. Summers AM, Summers CW, Drucker DB, Hajeer AH, Barson A, Hutchinson IV. Association of IL-10 genotype with sudden infant death syndrome. Human Immunol. 2000;61(12):1270-3. https://doi.org/10.1016/S0198-8859(00)00183-X.

72. Prandota J. Possible pathomechanisms of sudden infant death syndrome: Key role of chronic hypoxia, infection/inflammation states, cytokine irregularities, and metabolic trauma in genetically predisposed infants. Am J Therapeutics. 2004;11(6):517-46. https://doi.org/10.1097/01.mjt.0000140648.30948.bd.

73. Fard D, Laer K, Rothamel T, Schurmann P, Arnold M, Cohen M, et al. Candidate gene variants of the immune system and sudden infant death syndrome. Int J Legal Med. 2016;130(4):1025-33. https://doi.org/10.1007/s00414-016-1347-y.

74. Gaultier C, Trang H, Dauger S, Gallego J. Pediatric disorders with autonomic dysfunction: What role for PHOX2B? Pediatr Res. 2005;58(1):1-6. Epub 2005 May 18. https://doi.org/10.1203/01.PDR.0000166755.29277.C4.

75. Gaultier C, Amiel J, Dauger S, Trang H, Lyonnet S, Gallego J, et al. Genetics and early disturbances of breathing control. Pediatr Res. 2004;55(5):729-33. https://doi.org/10.1203/01.PDR.0000115677.78759.C5.

76. Rand CM, Patwari PP, Carroll MS, Weese-Mayer DE. Congenital central hypoventilation syndrome and sudden infant death syndrome: Disorders of autonomic regulation. Semin Pediatr Neurol. 2013 Mar;20(1):44-55. https://doi.org/10.1016/j.spen.2013.01.005.

77. Weese-Mayer DE, Berry-Kravis EM, Ceccherini I, Rand CM. Congenital central hypoventilation syndrome (CCHS) and sudden infant death syndrome (SIDS): Kindred disorders of autonomic regulation. Respir Physiol Neurobiol. 2008;164(1-2):38-48. https://doi.org/10.1016/j.resp.2008.05.011.

78. Liebrechts-Akkerman G, Liu F, Lao O, Ooms AH, van Duijn K, Vermeulen M, et al. PHOX2B polyalanine repeat length is associated with sudden infant death syndrome and unclassified sudden infant death in the Dutch population. Int J Legal Med. 2014;128(4):621-9. https://doi.org/10.1007/s00414-013-0962-0.

79. Poetsch M, Todt R, Vennemann M, Bajanowski T. That's not it, either — Neither polymorphisms in PHOX2B nor in MIF are involved in sudden infant death syndrome (SIDS). Int J Legal Med. 2015;129(5):985-9. https://doi.org/10.1007/s00414-015-1213-3.

80. Kijima K, Sasaki A, Niki T, Umetsu K, Osawa M, Matoba R, et al. Sudden infant death syndrome is not associated with the mutation of PHOX2B gene, a major causative gene of congenital central hypoventilation syndrome. Tohoku J Exp Med. 2004;203(1):65-8. https://doi.org/10.1620/tjem.203.65.

81. Weese-Mayer DE, Berry-Kravis EM, Zhou L, Maher BS, Curran ME, Silvestri JM, et al. Sudden infant death syndrome: Case-control frequency differences at genes pertinent to early autonomic nervous system embryologic development. Pediatr Res. 2004;56(3):391-5. https://doi.org/10.1203/01.PDR.0000136285.91048.4A.

82. Toruner GA, Kurvathi R, Sugalski R, Shulman L, Twersky S, Pearson PG, et al. Copy number variations in three children with sudden infant death. Clin Genet. 2009;76(1):63-8. https://doi.org/10.1111/j.1399-0004.2009.01161.x.

83. Richerson GB, Buchanan GF. The serotonin axis: Shared mechanisms in seizures, depression, and SUDEP. Epilepsia. 2011;52 Suppl 1:28-38. https://doi.org/10.1111/j.1528-1167.2010.02908.x.

84. Jehi L, Najm IM. Sudden unexpected death in epilepsy: Impact, mechanisms, and prevention. Cleveland Clin J Med. 2008;75 Suppl 2:S66-70. https://doi.org/10.3949/ccjm.75.Suppl_2.S66.

85. Ravindran K, Powell KL, Todaro M, O'Brien TJ. The pathophysiology of cardiac dysfunction in epilepsy. Epilepsy research. 2016 Nov;127:19-29. https://doi.org/10.1016/j.eplepsyres.2016.08.007.

86. Aiba I, Noebels JL. Spreading depolarization in the brainstem mediates sudden cardiorespiratory arrest in mouse SUDEP models. Sci Translational Med. 2015;7(282):282ra46. https://doi.org/10.1126/scitranslmed.aaa4050.

87. Le Gal F, Korff CM, Monso-Hinard C, Mund MT, Morris M, Malafosse A, et al. A case of SUDEP in a patient with Dravet syndrome with SCN1A mutation. Epilepsia. 2010;51(9):1915-18. https://doi.org/10.1111/j.1528-1167.2010.02691.x.

88. Ramadan W, Patel N, Anazi S, Kentab AY, Bashiri FA, Hamad MH, et al. Confirming the recessive inheritance of SCN1B mutations in developmental epileptic encephalopathy. Clin Genet. 2017;Feb 20 [Epub ahead of print]. https://doi.org/10.1111/cge.12999.

89. Bagnall RD, Crompton DE, Petrovski S, Lam L, Cutmore C, Garry SI, et al. Exome-based analysis of cardiac arrhythmia, respiratory control, and epilepsy genes in sudden unexpected death in epilepsy. Ann Neurol. 2016;79(4):522-34. https://doi.org/10.1002/ana.24596.

90. Nascimento FA, Borlot F, Cossette P, Minassian BA, Andrade DM. Two definite cases of sudden unexpected death in epilepsy in a family with a DEPDC5 mutation. Neurol Genet. 2015;1(4):e28. https://doi.org/10.1212/NXG.0000000000000028.

91. Wei F, Yan LM, Su T, He N, Lin ZJ, Wang J, et al. Ion channel genes and epilepsy: Functional alteration, pathogenic potential, and mechanism of epilepsy. Neurosci Bull. 2017;33(4):455-77. https://doi.org/10.1007/s12264-017-0134-1.

92. Sutherland HG, Griffiths LR. Genetics of migraine: Insights into the molecular basis of migraine disorders. Headache. 2017;57(4):537-69. https://doi.org/10.1111/head.13053.

93. Halvorsen M, Petrovski S, Shellhaas R, Tang Y, Crandall L, Goldstein D, et al. Mosaic mutations in early-onset genetic diseases. Genet Med. 2016;18(7):746-9. https://doi.org/10.1038/gim.2015.155.

94. Tan BH, Pundi KN, van Norstrand DW, Valdivia CR, Tester DJ, Medeiros-Domingo A, et al. Sudden infant death syndrome-associated mutations in the sodium channel beta subunits. Heart Rhythm. 2010;7(6):771-8. https://doi.org/10.1016/j.hrthm.2010.01.032.

95. Bar-Peled L, Chantranupong L, Cherniack AD, Chen WW, Ottina KA, Grabiner BC, et al. A Tumor suppressor complex with GAP activity for the Rag GTPases

that signal amino acid sufficiency to mTORC1. Science. 2013;340(6136):1100-6. https://doi.org/10.1126/science.1232044.

96. Klassen TL, Bomben VC, Patel A, Drabek J, Chen TT, Gu W, et al. High-resolution molecular genomic autopsy reveals complex sudden unexpected death in epilepsy risk profile. Epilepsia. 2014 Feb;55(2):e6-12. https://doi.org/10.1111/epi.12489.

97. Veeramah KR, O'Brien JE, Meisler MH, Cheng X, Dib-Hajj SD, Waxman SG, et al. De novo pathogenic SCN8A mutation identified by whole-genome sequencing of a family quartet affected by infantile epileptic encephalopathy and SUDEP. Am J Human Genet. 2012;90(3):502-10. https://doi.org/10.1016/j.ajhg.2012.01.006.

98. Glasscock E, Qian J, Yoo JW, Noebels JL. Masking epilepsy by combining two epilepsy genes. Nature Neurosci. 2007;10(12):1554-8. https://doi.org/10.1038/nn1999.

99. Smart SL, Lopantsev V, Zhang CL, Robbins CA, Wang H, Chiu SY, et al. Deletion of the K(V)1.1 potassium channel causes epilepsy in mice. Neuron. 1998;20(4):809-19. https://doi.org/10.1016/S0896-6273(00)81018-1.

100. Poduri A. The expanding SCN8A-related epilepsy phenotype. Epilepsy Curr. 2015;15(6):333-4. https://doi.org/10.5698/1535-7511-15.6.333.

101. Lorincz A, Nusser Z. Molecular identity of dendritic voltage-gated sodium channels. Science. 2010;328(5980):906-9. https://doi.org/10.1126/science.1187958.

# 32

# Biomarkers of Sudden Infant Death Syndrome (SIDS) Risk and SIDS Death

Robin L Haynes, PhD

*Department of Pathology, Boston Children's Hospital and Harvard Medical School, Boston, USA*

## Introduction

Sudden infant death syndrome (SIDS) is defined as the sudden death of an infant less than 1 year of age that remains unexplained after a complete autopsy and death scene investigation (1). Typically, SIDS is associated with a sleep period and with risk factors in the sleep environment — for example, prone/face-down sleep, bed sharing, soft bedding, and over-bundling (2-4). Despite national safe sleep campaigns, SIDS remains the leading cause of post-neonatal infant mortality in the United States, with an overall rate of 0.40 SIDS deaths per 1,000 live births (5).

SIDS is a complex heterogeneous disorder that presents in seemingly healthy infants as death — sudden and unexplained. For the family, it comes without warning, devastating all of those in and surrounding the family. For the medical examiner, it comes with the challenge of distinguishing the SIDS death from other sudden and unexpected deaths in infancy, those associated with accidental asphyxia (e.g. accidental suffocation while bed sharing), unidentified infection, or trauma. An ultimate goal in SIDS research is to identify specific biomarkers of SIDS risk which can be used to prevent a SIDS death from occurring (via successful intervention), thus alleviating the burden to the family; or, if the death does occur, to identify a readily accessible biomarker of SIDS death, thus alleviating the burden of the medical examiner adjudicating the death. In this chapter we will address the concept of biomarkers of SIDS, biomarkers of a SIDS death, and biomarkers of SIDS risk.

Biomarkers, defined as objective indicators of a pathologic process, medical condition, or medical state, can be presented in many different forms or types of measurements. They can be biochemical biomarkers with a distinct signature of a single metabolite or group of metabolites specific to a disease process, genomic biomarkers defined as a DNA or RNA characteristic associated with a pathogenic process, or biomarkers which utilize physiological tests (e.g. heart rate and blood pressure) to identify or predict a disease state or disease risk. There have been several studies reporting physiological biomarkers (apnea, cardiac rate abnormalities, and arousal deficits) in infants who subsequently died of SIDS (6-10). Likewise, there have been genetic studies reporting on the potential association of genetic alterations with SIDS death (11-25). In this chapter, however, we will focus solely on peripheral biochemical (metabolite or protein) markers taken in readily accessible fluid which have been reported on in SIDS and which have furthered our understanding of the processes underlying a SIDS death.

The discussion of biomarkers in this chapter is divided into two distinct categories: [1] post-mortem biomarkers which have provided insight into pathological mechanisms of SIDS death and which have potential to distinguish a SIDS death from other types of sudden and unexpected infant death at autopsy; and [2] maternal/infant biomarkers which have been identified as potentially associated with a risk of SIDS death. It is important to note that different studies present conflicting data on the utility of certain biomarkers in SIDS. The biomarkers below are discussed with reference to the studies that both support and refute their use. It is also important to note that at this time there is no clinically available biochemical biomarker of SIDS. The intent of the discussion below, however, is to provide insight into the current landscape of research within this area.

## Post-mortem Biomarkers of SIDS

### Post-mortem biomarker related to serotonin neurotransmission

Serotonin (5-HT), a neurotransmitter produced from the essential amino acid tryptophan, mediates a large variety of functions both peripherally and centrally. Within the central nervous system (CNS), 5-HT is produced from the sequential reactions of tryptophan hydroxylase 2 (TPH2) and 5-hydroxyl-L-tryptophan decarboxylase (AADC). The production of CNS 5-HT is restricted to TPH2-expressing neurons within the brainstem, including within the pons and midbrain (the "rostral" 5-HT system) and the medulla oblongata (the "caudal" 5-HT system). While the rostral 5-HT system projects to the cortex, thalamus, hypothalamus, basal ganglia, hippocampus, and amygdala, and plays a significant role in cognition, waking, and mood, the caudal 5-HT system projects to sites within the brainstem and spinal cord and plays a significant role in homeostasis, respiratory, and autonomic regulation (26). Early in brain development, prior to the maturation of the 5-HT rostral and caudal systems, 5-HT plays a significant role as a trophic factor influencing processes such as cell division, differentiation, migration, and synaptogenesis (27, 28). Outside of the CNS, peripheral 5-HT is produced by tryptophan hydroxylase 1 (TPH1) expressing cells (enterochromaffin cells, EC) of the gut which are scattered within the gastrointestinal (GI) tract epithelium and produce approximately 90-95% of the total body 5-HT. Functions of peripheral 5-HT include platelet aggregation, GI motility, and metabolic homeostasis, including regulation of glucose homeostasis, gluconeogenesis, mobilization of free fatty acids, and browning of white adipose tissue (29-32).

Relative to SIDS, studies of 5-HT within the CNS specifically within the medullary (caudal) brainstem 5-HT network have shown multiple abnormalities in SIDS infants compared to autopsy controls (e.g. infant deaths of known cause). These abnormalities, along with evidence supporting the role of the brainstem in respiratory and autonomic regulation, sleep, and arousal (functions found to be subclinically defective in infants who subsequently die of SIDS (6-10)), provide rationale for the brainstem hypothesis in SIDS. This hypothesis suggests that the cause of death in a subset of SIDS cases relates to brainstem abnormalities in the neuroregulation of cardiorespiratory control (33, 34). The medullary 5-HT network is comprised of nuclei that contain 5-HT-producing neurons (raphe obscurus, magnus, and pallidus; extra-raphe: gigantocellularis, paragigantocellularis lateralis, and intermediate reticular zone) and nuclei that receive 5-HT projections and mediate respiratory and autonomic responses (e.g. hypoglossal nuclei, nucleus of the solitary tract, and dorsal motor nucleus of the vagus, the latter two nuclei directly part of the autonomic nervous system). In SIDS cases compared to controls, reported 5-HT defects include significantly decreased levels of 5-HT (~26%) in two of two 5-HT-producing nuclei (raphe obscurus and paragigantocellularis) sampled (p<0.05) (35), decreased TPH2 (~22%) in the medullary raphe (35) (p=0.03), and an increased density of 5-HT neurons in the raphe and extra-raphe nuclei (up to a 50% increase; p<0.001) (36). In addition, significant decreases in $5HT_{1A}$ receptor binding, as determined by tissue autoradiography, have been reported in nuclei that contain 5-HT cell bodies and receive 5-HT cell projections within the medulla (up to a 50% decrease; p<0.001) (35-38). The finding of 5-HT receptor abnormalities is supported by immunocytochemistry showing a significant decrease in 5-HT receptor expression ($5\text{-HT}_{1A}$ and $5\text{-HT}_{2A}$) in medullary nuclei of SIDS infants compared to controls (39). Together, these data suggest CNS, specifically brainstem, abnormalities in 5-HT synthesis, 5-HT neuronal development, and 5-HT signaling (via 5-HT receptor binding) in a subset of SIDS infants.

In terms of biomarkers, recent progress has been made in identifying abnormalities in peripheral levels of 5-HT in SIDS cases. In a study of 61 SIDS cases and 15 non-SIDS autopsy controls, serum 5-HT levels, as measured by enzyme-linked immunosorbent assay (ELISA) and high-pressure liquid chromatography (HPLC), were found to be significantly elevated (average increase of 95%) in SIDS cases compared to controls (40) (Table 32.1, Figure 32.1A and B). These controls included cases dying acutely from accidental asphyxia (e.g. crib accidents), acquired lung disease, unsuspected congenital heart disease, and accidental head trauma. There was no statistically significant difference in the ratio of 5-HT to 5-hydroxyindoleacetic acid (5-HIAA) (a breakdown product of 5-HT) between the two groups, suggesting that the increase in serum 5-HT in SIDS does not reflect a decreased breakdown of 5-HT itself (40). "High" serum 5-HT was defined post hoc as greater than two standard deviations above the mean of the controls, as determined by ELISA ($\geq$211.8 ng/ml), and "normative" serum 5-HT as below this cut-off (<211.8 ng/ml). The percentage of SIDS cases with high serum 5-HT was 31% (19/61). There was no significant association of serum 5-HT levels with any known risk factor for SIDS (including male sex, prematurity, discovery in the prone position, and illness within 48 hours), or with the genotype of the serotonin transporter (5-HTT) promoter polymorphisms (5-HTTLPR) [SS, SL, or LL], or with the type of nutrition prior to death (breastmilk or formula-fed) (40). There was no effect of post-mortem interval or storage interval on levels of serum 5-HT (Figure 32.1C and D) (40).

While this study provides the first evidence of an abnormality in peripheral levels of 5-HT in SIDS cases, the source(s) of this increase is currently unknown. One possibility includes increased production of 5-HT by gut EC cells, potentially mediated by microbiota residing in the gut and known to influence host EC production of 5-HT (41, 42). Another possibility includes increased production of 5-HT by pulmonary neuroendocrine cells (PNEC) and neuroepithelial bodies (NEBs) of the lung, which function as airway oxygen/carbon dioxide sensors and release 5-HT in a dose-dependent manner in response to hypoxia (43, 44). Hyperplasia and hypertrophy of PNEC/NEB within the lungs of infants dying of SIDS have been reported, and secretory products of these PNEC/NEB cells have been proposed previously as a potential biological marker of SIDS (44). Also unknown are the relationship between the serum and brainstem 5-HT abnormalities in SIDS, and whether elevated serum 5-HT and specific brainstem 5-HT abnormalities co-exist in a single subset of SIDS cases or whether two SIDS subsets exist, independent of the other, one with abnormalities in peripheral 5-HT and the other with abnormalities in central 5-HT. Despite these unanswered questions, measures of serum 5-HT may ultimately prove to be a forensic biomarker at autopsy to distinguish SIDS infants from other infants dying of sudden unexpected deaths, and to identify SIDS infants with central 5-HT abnormalities. Finally, these studies form the foundation of future research involving prospectively collected serum samples in apparently well infants to determine whether blood 5-HT levels can be used to predict the subsequent occurrence of SIDS.

Table 32.1: Serum data for 5-HT in SIDS cases compared to controls, adjusted for post-conceptional age (40). ELISA = enzyme-linked immunosorbent assay; HPLC = high-pressure liquid chromatography.

| | | SIDS;<br>Mean (SE) (ng/ml); n | Controls;<br>Mean (SE) (ng/ml); n | p-value | % in SIDS |
|---|---|---|---|---|---|
| 5-HT | ELISA | 177.2 (15.1); 61 | 91.1 (30.6); 15 | **0.014** | 95% |
| 5-HT | HPLC | 114.6 (13.7); 45 | 52.4 (26.5); 12 | **0.04** | 119% |

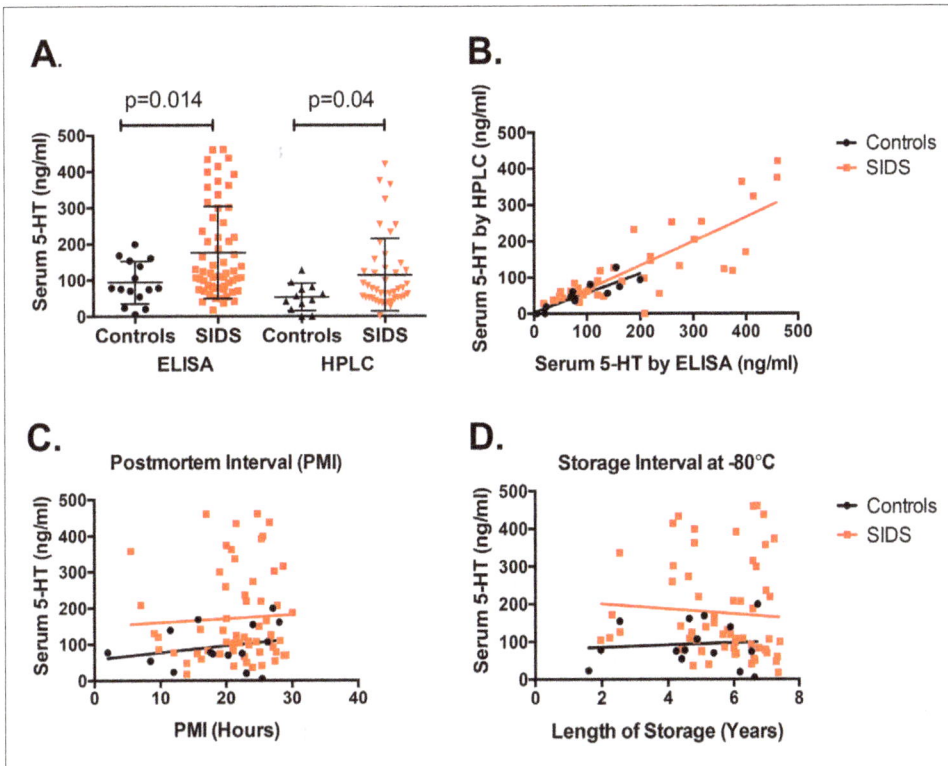

Figure 32.1: Serum 5-HT levels in SIDS and non-SIDS autopsy controls.
A. There is a significant increase in serum 5-HT levels in SIDS compared to controls as determined by ELISA (p=0.014) and HPLC (p=0.04).
B. Serum 5-HT levels obtained by ELISA and HPLC show significant correlation in SIDS cases [Spearman correlation of 0.84 (p<0.001)] and controls [Spearman correlation of 0.87 (p<0.001)]. There is no significant effect of (C) post-mortem interval or of (D) storage interval at -80 °C on the levels of serum 5-HT in control or SIDS infants.

## Post-mortem biomarkers related to hypoxia

Physiological evidence suggests that infants who subsequently die of SIDS have episodes of bradycardia and/or apnea days, or weeks, prior to their death (6, 45), thus implicating a role for hypoxia and/or chronic intermittent hypoxia in the pathogenesis of SIDS. Certain tissue changes further support a role for hypoxia in SIDS, i.e. brainstem gliosis, as originally reported by Naeye et al. (46), and the presence of hyperplasia of PNEC/NEB cells, as reported by Cutz et al. (44). In addition to tissue markers of hypoxia, metabolite and protein markers suggestive of hypoxia have also been identified in various fluids in SIDS cases at autopsy and are presented below as potential biomarkers of hypoxia in SIDS death.

### Hypoxanthine

Hypoxanthine is a metabolite formed during purine catabolism and an intermediate in the purine salvage pathway. During hypoxia there is an accelerated breakdown of the purine adenosine monophosphate (AMP) as cells try to maintain energy state. As AMP breaks down during hypoxia, hypoxanthine accumulates. Increased hypoxanthine concentrations in plasma, urine, cerebrospinal fluid, amniotic fluid, and vitreous humor have been reported in various studies as significantly higher in hypoxic individuals, including hypoxic infants, compared to non-hypoxic individuals (as reviewed in (47)). Animal studies have confirmed the use of hypoxanthine as a biomarker of hypoxia (47), with increased significance in models of intermittent hypoxia as opposed to continuous hypoxia (48). In SIDS, this marker has been examined in multiple studies in the vitreous humor taken at autopsy. It was initially shown by Rognum et al. to be increased in the vitreous humor of 32 SIDS cases compared to 15 controls dying of various causes (49) (Table 32.2). This finding was replicated in a larger cohort of SIDS (n=73) and controls (n=23) with hypoxanthine levels corrected for potential post-mortem changes (50).

Other studies on hypoxanthine in SIDS, involving various ways of correcting for post-mortem changes, utilizing various groups of control infants, and analyzing hypoxanthine using different methods, have reported opposing results on the utility of hypoxanthine as a biomarker for hypoxia in SIDS infants (51, 52). In SIDS cases (n=50) compared to non-SIDS controls (n=41), Belonje et al. found no difference in vitreous humor levels of hypoxanthine (51), while Carpenter et al. found no difference in vitreous humor or cerebrospinal fluid levels of hypoxanthine in SIDS cases compared to cases dying of known causes of death (non-cardiac or pulmonary related causes of death) (SIDS, n=68 or 45, respectively; non-SIDS, n=38 or 21, respectively) (52) (Table 32.2).

To avoid incorrectly correcting for post-mortem changes, and to investigate potential confounding factors such as prone sleep and age of the infant (and corresponding size of the eye), Opdal et al. undertook a large study examining different categories of SIDS (i.e. with or without resuscitation, with or without prior infection, prone vs supine sleep), infectious death controls, controls dying of heart/lung disease, and violent deaths (53).

After matching all cases for post-mortem interval, hypoxanthine was confirmed to be increased in SIDS cases (n=82) compared to violent death infants (n=13) and infants dying from heart and lung disease (n=17) (53). There was no difference in SIDS cases compared to infectious death controls (n=22), nor were there differences among SIDS cases associated with time of death, infection, or sleep position (53) (Table 32.2). Taken together, these various studies suggest that hypoxanthine levels in the vitreous humor taken at autopsy may be utilized as a biomarker for intermittent hypoxic events prior to death in SIDS cases. They also suggest the potential use of hypoxanthine levels to differentiate a SIDS death from other infant deaths involving accidents and trauma.

Table 32.2: Studies examining hypoxanthine (Hx) at autopsy. Studies with positive results supporting the use of the biomarker are shaded. Studies with negative, conflicting results remain in white. Percent differences were determined from the data reported in the article. Hx = hypoxanthine; PM = post-mortem.

| Fluid | SIDS | Controls — Post-mortem | Conclusions | Author (Ref) |
|---|---|---|---|---|
| Vitreous Humor | n=32 | Group 1; n=8 Trauma, drowning, hanging<br><br>Group 2; n=7 Neonates dying suddenly without known hypoxia | Hx levels are significantly increased in SIDS compared to Group 1 controls (222%; p<0.001) and to Group 2 controls (617%; p<0.001). | Rognum (49) |
| Vitreous Humor | n=73 | Group 1; n=17 Violent death<br><br>Group 2; n=6 Neonates dying suddenly without known hypoxemia | Hx levels are significantly increased in SIDS compared to Group 1 controls (932%; p<0.01) and to Group 2 controls (p<0.01), adjusted for PM changes. | Rognum (50) |
| Vitreous Humor | n=82 | Group 1; n=22 Infectious disease<br><br>Group 2; n=17 Heart/lung disease<br><br>Group 3; n=13 Violent death | Hx levels are significantly increased in SIDS compared to Group 2 controls (45%; p<0.01) and to Group 3 controls (90%; p<0.01). There is no difference in SIDS compared to Group 1 controls. Subjects are matched for PM interval. | Opdal (53) |

| Vitreous Humor | n=50 | Group 1; n=5<br>Acute sudden death<br><br>Group 2; n=36<br>Non-SIDS (other causes of death) | Hx levels are not significantly different between SIDS compared to Group 2 controls. Group 1 controls are lower than SIDS and Group 2 controls. | Belonje (51) |
|---|---|---|---|---|
| Vitreous Humor | n=68 | Group 1; n=13<br>Cardiac or pulmonary<br><br>Group 2; n=38<br>Other explained causes of death | Hx levels are not significantly different between SIDS compared to Group 2 controls. | Carpenter (52) |
| | | | Hx levels are statistically increased in SIDS compared to Group 1 controls (52%: $p=0.007$). | |
| Cerebro-spinal fluid | n=45 | Group 1; n=9<br>Cardiac or pulmonary<br><br>Group 2; n=21<br>Other explained causes of death | Hx levels are not significantly different between SIDS compared to controls. | Carpenter (52) |

## Fetal hemoglobin

The protein hemoglobin is an iron-containing oxygen transport protein that is present in red blood cells and responsible for delivering oxygen to tissues throughout the body. In the adult, hemoglobin binds to oxygen in the lungs whereas in the fetus, fetal hemoglobin binds to oxygen in the placenta, specifically from the maternal circulation. The structure of hemoglobin is a heterotetramer protein consisting of two alpha chains and two non-alpha chains, with the non-alpha chains differing depending on whether the hemoglobin is the fetal form ($\alpha2\gamma2$) or the adult form ($\alpha2\beta2$). While the binding mechanism of the fetal and adult forms are the same, the affinity of the fetal form of hemoglobin for oxygen is much greater than that of the adult form, thus allowing fetal hemoglobin to more readily extract oxygen from the maternal circulation. After birth and through the first five to six months of life, the infant switches from the synthesis of fetal hemoglobin to adult hemoglobin (54, 55). However, under certain conditions, including chronic lung disease in infants (56), hypoxia in nonhuman primates (57), and hypoxemia in children with congenital cyanotic heart disease (54), increases in the amount of fetal hemoglobin have been reported and have been suggested as a marker of inadequate tissue oxygenation.

A number of studies have examined the potential of fetal hemoglobin at autopsy as a potential diagnostic post-mortem biomarker for SIDS but have reported conflicting results. In 1987, Giulian et al. reported a significant elevation of fetal hemoglobin in

59 SIDS cases compared to 40 non-SIDS controls, matched for post-conceptional age (58) (Table 32.3). This elevation was postulated by Giulian to be due to a delay in the switch from fetal hemoglobin to adult hemoglobin (58). Supporting this original finding are two additional studies reporting elevated levels of fetal hemoglobin in SIDS infants compared to infants dying of known causes (59, 60) and compared to living, healthy controls (59) (Table 32.3). These data were suggested to provide evidence of an underlying condition in SIDS resulting from chronic hypoxemia (59). Refuting the observations above are studies showing no significant difference in fetal hemoglobin in SIDS compared to controls (61-64) (Table 32.3).

The conflicting results across the different studies are likely due to several factors including methodology of analysis, criteria for diagnosis of SIDS, different controls for comparison, and different analysis of age as a cofounding factor. Despite the disputed role of fetal hemoglobin as a post-mortem marker for SIDS, evidence from prospective studies of SIDS risk suggests an inverse relationship of adult hemoglobin levels measured at birth and a subsequent risk of SIDS death. These data will be discussed under the section "Infant Biomarkers of SIDS Risk". It is important to note that levels of total hemoglobin cannot be accurately determined after death (65), and therefore the relationship between low total hemoglobin, anemia, and SIDS death cannot be quantitated. However, the fact that the peak incidence of SIDS co-incides with the nadir in the physiologic anemia of infancy (66) is possibly suggestive of such a relationship (65).

Table 32.3: Studies examining fetal hemoglobin (HbF) at autopsy. Studies with positive results supporting the use of the biomarker are shaded. Studies with negative, conflicting results remain in white. Percent differences were determined from the data reported in the article. *SID group includes SIDS, infection, and genetic/metabolic abnormalities. PCA = postconceptional age; HbF = fetal hemoglobin; Hb = hemoglobin; PM = post-mortem; SID = sudden infant death.

| Fluid | SIDS | Controls | Conclusions | Author (Ref) |
|-------|------|----------|-------------|--------------|
| Blood | n=59 | Combined controls; n=40<br>• n=32 Living<br>• n=8 PM | HbF is significantly increased in SIDS compared to controls at ages <50 PC weeks (20%; p=0.005) and at ages >50 PC weeks (152%; p=0.0005). | Giulian (58) |
| Blood | n=54 | Combined controls; n=39<br>• n=22 Living<br>• n=17 PM | The percent of HbF relative to total Hb was significantly elevated in SIDS compared to controls, adjusting for PCA (p=0.015). | Gilbert-Barness (59) |

| Blood | n=47 | Combined controls; n=50<br>• n=17 Living<br>• n=33 PM | HbF is significantly increased in SIDS compared to gestational age-matched controls (44%; p<0.001). | Perry (60) |
|-------|------|------|------|------|
| Blood | n=67 | Combined control; n=102<br>• n=80 Living<br>• n=22 PM | HbF levels are not significantly different in SIDS compared to controls. | Zielke (61) |
| Blood | n=19 | n=266 Living infant controls | HbF and total Hb levels are not significantly different in SIDS compared to controls. | Cheron (62) |
| Blood | n=77 | n=30 PM controls | HbF levels are not significantly different in SIDS compared to controls. | Krous (63) |
| Blood | n=135 SID* (including 51 SIDS deaths) | n=570 Living infant controls | Full term SIDS infants show significantly elevated HbF levels compared to age-matched controls (p<0.001).<br><br>Elevations in HbF were found in SIDS infants as well as other SIDS infants with known causes of death (i.e. infections). | Fagan (64) |

## Post-mortem biomarker related to infection

Mild infection has been noted in approximately half of SIDS cases prior to death (67), with evidence of infection coming from post-mortem microbiology and autopsy indication of inflammatory reactions. The role of infection in SIDS is described elsewhere in this book and is therefore not emphasized here. However, with regard to biomarkers of SIDS, it is important to note the role of cytokines as a potential biomarker of immunologic activity and possible dysfunction. Cytokines are small proteins produced and released from various cell types including immune cells (i.e. mast cells, B lymphocytes, and T lymphocytes) and glial cells within the brain (astrocytes and microglia). While cytokines are important in host response to infection, they can also become dysregulated and can contribute to the pathogenesis of a disease process. One cytokine, interleukin-6 (IL-6), is of particular interest given its identification in the cerebrospinal fluid (CSF) of SIDS infants (68, 69). IL-6 acts as a pro-inflammatory cytokine and is an important mediator of fever, crossing the blood-brain barrier and affecting the body's temperature set-point in the hypothalamus (70). Given that the IL-6 receptor shows widespread distribution throughout brainstem nuclei of the medulla (71), it likely plays a role in the co-ordination of brainstem responses to infectious challenges. Interestingly, IL-6 has also been shown to play a role in epigenetic modification of certain genes implicated in diseases such as anxiety (72) and cancer (73, 74). Vege et al. reported an overall increased level of IL-6 in the CSF of infants dying of SIDS (n=20) compared to infants dying from violent deaths (n=5), but an overall decreased level of IL-6 in SIDS infants compared to infectious deaths (n=7) (68) (Table 32.4). Although there was no correlation between IL-6 levels and the presence, or absence, of clinical symptoms of infection prior to death, there was a subpopulation of SIDS cases that overlapped with the infectious death cases (68). In a larger dataset, Vege et al. confirmed the intermediate position of IL-6 levels in SIDS infants with SIDS infants (n=50) showing higher IL6 levels than violent deaths (n=8), but overall lower IL-6 levels than infectious deaths (n=18) and deaths due to heart/lung disease (n=22) (69) (Table 32.4). High levels of CSF IL-6 in SIDS infants were found to be associated with a peripheral immune response, as determined by IgA immunocytes in the laryngeal mucosa and epiglottis (75). Taken together, the high levels of CSF IL-6 may serve as a biomarker for a significant immunological activation in a subpopulation of SIDS infants. Given that this immunological response is often disproportionate with clinical symptoms of infection, high levels of CSF IL-6 in SIDS infants may also serve as a biomarker of over-activation of the immunologic response to moderate stimuli. Of note, the finding of increased IL-6 levels in CSF of SIDS infants, compared to other causes of death with and without infection, was not confirmed in a subsequent study by Vennemann et al., possibly due to heterogeneity of cases with infection and/or diagnostic criteria for SIDS classification (76) (Table 32.4).

Table 32.4: Studies examining cytokines (IL-6) at autopsy. Studies with positive results supporting the use of the biomarker are shaded. Studies with negative, conflicting results remain in white. Percent differences were determined from the data reported in the article.

| Fluid | SIDS | Controls — Postmortem | Conclusions | Author (Ref) |
|-------|------|------------------------|-------------|--------------|
| CSF | n=20 | Group 1; n=7 Infectious deaths<br><br>Group 2; n=5 Violent deaths | IL-6 levels are significantly higher in SIDS compared to violent deaths (p<0.02).<br><br>IL-6 levels are significantly lower (82%) in SIDS compared to infectious deaths (p<0.02).<br><br>There is no difference in SIDS cases with infectious symptoms and those without infectious symptoms. | Vege (68) |

| CSF | n=50 | Group 1; n=18 Infectious deaths<br><br>Group 2; n=8 Violent deaths<br><br>Group 3; n=22 Cases with heart/lung disease<br><br>Group 4; n=9 Borderline SIDS | IL-6 levels are significantly higher in SIDS compared to violent deaths (p=0.004).<br><br>IL-6 levels are significantly lower (96%) in SIDS compared to infectious deaths (p=0.006) and heart/lung disease (95%) (p=0.002). | Vege (69) |
|---|---|---|---|---|
| CSF and Serum | n=20, SIDS without infection<br><br>n=78, SIDS with minor infection | Group 1; n=13 Explained natural death due to infection<br><br>Group 2; n=8 Unnatural deaths (i.e. suffocation, drowning) | IL-6 levels in CSF and serum are not significantly different between SIDS with and without infection or between SIDS and controls. | Venne-mann (76) |

## Post-mortem biomarker related to mast cell degranulation

Mast cells are a type of granulocyte residing in most tissue and preferentially located at the interfaces between host and environment (e.g. skin, mucosa of the GI tract, and lungs). They play a key role in the inflammatory process through the induced release of inflammatory mediators from their storage granules. These mediators include serine proteases (tryptase and chymase), monoamines (histamine and serotonin), proteoglycans (heparin and chondroitin sulfate proteoglycans), and lipid-derived signaling molecules (prostaglandins and leukotrienes). While mast cells are most highly recognized for their role in allergic reactions and anaphylaxis, they are increasingly being appreciated for their role in innate immune responses and in regulation of tissue homeostasis, the latter of which includes regulation of epithelial permeability, smooth muscle contraction and peristalsis, bronchoconstriction, blood flow, and wound healing (77). In an allergic reaction, mast cell activation is mediated via antigen-specific immunoglobulin E (IgE), which binds to its cell surface receptor, FceR1, and leads to crosslinking and aggregation of FceR1 on the surface of mast cells. This subsequently triggers the release of the biologically active compounds listed above (78). Under non-allergic inflammatory and physiological conditions, mast cell activation is mediated by many different non-IgE mechanisms, including binding of toll-like receptor (TLR) ligands to TLRs widely expressed on mast cells, receptor-mediated binding of neuropeptides (corticotrophin-releasing hormone, nerve growth factor, and brain-derived neurotrophic factor), cytokines, chemokines, and adenosine (79). Given the important role that mast cells have under pathological and physiological conditions, a marker by which mast cell activation can be measured is crucial in understanding the involvement of mast cells under these different conditions. The protease tryptase is one such marker.

Tryptases are a family of proteases present in large amounts in mast cell secretory granules. Although basophils also contain and release tryptase, their levels of tryptase are approximately 100 times less than that of mast cells and therefore are not considered significant contributors to tryptase levels (80). There are two types of tryptases, α-tryptase, classified as αI and αII, and β-tryptase, classified as βI, βII, and βIII. The inactive α-protrypase is secreted constitutively from mast cells and is the major form found in the blood. The β-tryptase is stored in secretory granules and is secreted upon mast cell activation and degranulation (81). Tryptase levels in biological fluids are used as markers of mast cell number and activation, with β-tryptases being elevated in subjects with systemic anaphylaxis.

Studies have reported contradictory findings regarding serum levels of tryptase in SIDS (82-87), in part due to differences in detection method and antibody specificity. The α- and β-tryptase forms share 90% sequence identity, and detection of specific tryptase forms is difficult and highly dependent on the methodology used (81). Serum tryptase levels have been reported as elevated in SIDS in four different studies. Using a radioimmunoassay, Platt et al. examined serum levels of tryptase in SIDS cases (n=50) compared to control infants dying from known causes (n=15) and found significantly higher levels of tryptase in SIDS cases, with 40% of SIDS showing tryptase levels above the threshold chosen to indicate pre-mortem mast cell activation (82) (Table 32.5). In the study by Holgate et al. using a radioimmunoassay recognizing both α- and β-tryptase, elevated tryptase was reported in 82 unexplained deaths compared to 24 explained deaths (83) (Table 32.5).

The increases seen by Pratt and Holgate were suggested to support a previously proposed anaphylaxis hypothesis that SIDS infants develop an allergic sensitivity to cow's milk and that death occurs by regurgitation of recently ingested cow's milk into the airways (88-90). In 1999, Edston et al. examined predominately SIDS cases but divided them based on a low-tryptase group (<10 ug/ml) and a high-tryptase group (>10 ug/ml). High tryptase was reported in 40% of SIDS infants tested (n=16/40) (85). To address the anaphylaxis hypothesis, Edston et al also examined total IgE, an immunoglobin increased in the blood with allergic disease. While IgE was increased above clinical reference values in 33% (n=10/30) of the SIDS cases, there was no association between tryptase and IgE levels, and thus this study did not support the anaphylaxis hypothesis in SIDS death (85).

In 2001, Buckley et al. examined serum from SIDS and controls using two different methods, one recognizing predominately β-tryptase, the other with equal sensitivity to α- and β-tryptase (86) (Table 32.5). A significant increase in β-tryptase was reported in SIDS, supporting an increase in mast cell activation and degranulation in SIDS. There was no evidence of an increase in α-tryptase, the variant secreted constitutively from mast cells, suggesting that SIDS is not associated with mast cell hyperplasia (86). In contradiction to the studies described above are two studies by Nishio et al. and Hagan et al., which report no significant difference in tryptase between SIDS and controls (84, 87) (Table 32.5). It is important to note that Hagan et al. used frozen blood separated into serum after thaw, a potential confounder to the results.

In summary, of the results reported above, most available data on SIDS show increased levels of tryptase in a subpopulation of SIDS compared to controls with no associated increase in IgE. This supports a role for a non-IgE-mediated mast cell degranulation in SIDS, not related to anaphylaxis, but rather associated with other non-IgE mechanisms, i.e. potential activation via TLRs, neuropeptides, cytokines, and/or chemokines (79).

Table 32.5: Studies examining tryptase at autopsy. Studies with positive results supporting the use of the biomarker are shaded. Studies with negative, conflicting results remain in white. Percent differences were determined from the data reported in the article. PC = post-conceptional.

| Fluid | SIDS | Controls — Post-mortem | Conclusions | Author (Ref) |
|---|---|---|---|---|
| Serum | n=50 | n=15 Controls dying of known causes | Tryptase levels are significantly higher in SIDS infants compared to controls (464%; p=0.0004). Detection of primarily β-tryptase. | Platt (82) |
| Serum | n=56 SIDS from one clinical site n=26 SIDS from a second clinical site | n=24 Controls dying of known causes | Tryptase levels are significantly higher in both SIDS groups compared to controls (51% and 61%; p=0.03 and p=0.02, respectively). Detection of α- and β-tryptase. | Holgate (83) |
| Serum | n=32[a], 33[b] | n=31[a], 23[b] Controls dying of known causes | [a]Detection of β-tryptase shows significantly higher levels in SIDS compared to controls (p<0.05). [b]Detection of α- and β-tryptase shows no significant difference in SIDS compared to controls. | Buckley (86) |

| Blood-<br>(serum<br>separated<br>after<br>thaw) | n=51 | n=13<br>Controls dying<br>of known causes | There is no difference between<br>the frequency of detectable<br>tryptase levels among SIDS<br>and controls.<br><br>Detection of primarily<br>β-tryptase. | Hagan<br>(84) |
|---|---|---|---|---|
| Serum | n=21 | n=14<br>Controls dying<br>of known causes | There is no difference between<br>SIDS and controls in α- and<br>β-tryptase levels.<br><br>Detection of α- and<br>β-tryptase. | Nishio<br>(87) |

## Biomarkers of SIDS Risk

### Maternal biomarkers of SIDS risk

#### Maternal alpha-fetoprotein

Alpha-fetoprotein is a member of the albumin gene family and is thought to be the fetal form of serum albumin. While alpha-fetoprotein is postulated to serve roles similar to other members of the albumin family (e.g. transport of various ligands and oxygen free radical scavenging), its exact biological function remains relatively unclear. During fetal life, plasma levels of alpha-fetoprotein are highly abundant but then decrease rapidly after birth until adult levels are reached by two years of life (91). During pregnancy, alpha-fetoprotein produced by the fetus crosses the placenta and fetal membranes and appears in maternal serum (91). Prior to the now common use of fetal ultrasound investigation, maternal levels of alpha-fetoprotein in the serum and amniotic fluid were common screening methods for congenital anomalies, including neural tube defects, omphalocele, gastroschisis, and fetal bowel obstructions (91, 92). These defects commonly present with increased levels of maternal alpha-fetoprotein, while decreased levels of maternal alpha-fetoprotein are associated with an increased risk of Down Syndrome (93). High levels of maternal serum alpha-fetoprotein during the second trimester are also associated with the risk of stillbirth in normally formed infants and serve as a biochemical predictor of the risk of unexplained stillbirth (94, 95).

In 2004, Smith et al. sought to show a relationship between unexplained stillbirth and SIDS by examining the association of second-trimester maternal serum levels of alpha-fetoprotein and the subsequent risk of SIDS (96). In the study, a prenatal-screening database from western Scotland was linked to databases of maternity, perinatal death and birth, and death certification recorded from 1980 to 2001. Prenatal screening measurements of alpha-fetoprotein taken at 15 and 21 weeks of gestation were used and cases (n=214,532 women) were divided into quintiles based on increasing maternal

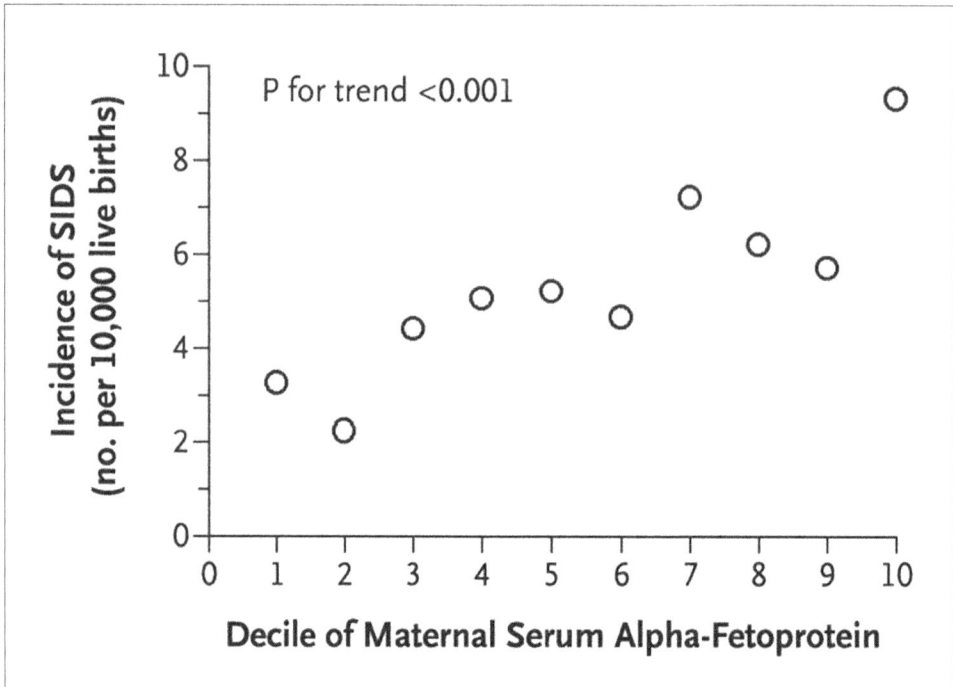

Figure 32.2: Incidence of SIDS within a population of infants divided into 10 groups (deciles) based on maternal alpha-fetoprotein measured in the second trimester of pregnancy. There is a linear trend of increasing incidence of SIDS with increasing alpha-fetoprotein decile. Data was generated from a prenatal-screening database for women in western Scotland with databases of maternity, perinatal death, and birth/death certifications. (Reproduced with permission from (96).)

levels of alpha-fetoprotein. The incidence of SIDS increased significantly across quintiles with an incidence of 2.7/10,000 births among the lowest quintile compared to 7.5/10,000 births among the highest quintile (p for trend <0.001) (Figure 32.2). After adjusting for birth weight and gestational age at delivery, each of which varies inversely with the risk of SIDS, a significant association between alpha-fetoprotein and risk for SIDS was determined with the odds ratio of SIDS death increasing significantly with increasing quintiles (p for trend = 0.01). The odds ratio of SIDS death was 2.2 (95% confidence interval, 1.1 to 4.3) at the highest quintile compared to 1.7 (95% confidence interval, 0.8 to 3.5) at the lowest quintile (96). The association of high levels of alpha-fetoprotein with SIDS risk was cited by the authors to reflect the role of the intrauterine environment, specifically the role of placental dysfunction during pregnancy (96). This is based on the concept that elevated maternal serum levels of alpha-fetoprotein in the absence of fetal abnormalities indicate an increase in placental permeability and thus a defect in placental functions (94). Studies examining further the relationship between SIDS risk and maternal alpha-fetoprotein have yet to be reported.

## Infant biomarkers of SIDS risk

### Fetal hemoglobin

In the earlier section on post-mortem biomarkers of SIDS death, we describe studies examining blood levels of fetal hemoglobin in SIDS infants compared to control infants with various known causes of death. Although these studies show conflicting data on the use of fetal hemoglobin as a post-mortem biomarker for SIDS death, the concept of abnormalities in fetal versus adult levels of hemoglobin has been tested in the living infant in regard to risk of SIDS death. In 2003, Bard et al. prospectively examined levels of $[\gamma/(\gamma+\beta)]$-globin mRNA in normal healthy infants (n=37) compared to infants being monitored at home after an apparent life-threatening event (ALTE) and considered at risk for SIDS (n=35) (97). Levels of $[\gamma/(\gamma+\beta)]$-globin mRNA significantly correlate with levels of fetal hemoglobin synthesis (98), and thus represent an alternative means to examine the potential of fetal hemoglobin as a biomarker of SIDS risk. As previously stated, an increase in fetal hemoglobin in infancy is suggestive of hypoxia and/or hypoxemia (54, 56, 57), with the synthesis of fetal hemoglobin thought to be a result of an erythropoietic response to oxygen insufficiency (99). In the study, Bard et al. found significant increases in the $[\gamma/(\gamma+\beta)]$-globin mRNA levels in the ALTE group compared to the controls at two different age intervals, 42 to 45 post-conceptional weeks (55.2+/-17.4% compared to 42.6+/-13.7%, p=0.03) and 46 to 49 post-conceptional weeks (33.9+/-14% compared to 23.6+/- 9.8%, p=0.02). Other age intervals tested up to approximately 60 post-conceptional weeks were not significantly different. While the exact cause of the increased fetal hemoglobin in the ALTE infants is unknown, Bard et al. suggest a release of immature red cells into the circulation due to stress-induced erythropoiesis or possibly a decrease or delay in the switch from fetal to adult hemoglobin (97). Both could potentially result from repeated but undetected episodes of hypoxemia. Of note, chronic intermittent hypoxia is hypothesized to play a role in the pathogenesis of SIDS in some cases (34). Given that the study by Bard et al. does not prospectively follow the ALTE infants to look for associations between abnormal fetal hemoglobin and incidence of SIDS death, the significance of the increased fetal hemoglobin during the observed time frame is unknown. It does, however, support the role of hypoxia/hypoxemia in infants known to be at risk for SIDS death.

### Adult hemoglobin

With regard to hemoglobin levels, the studies discussed thus far look at abnormally high levels of fetal hemoglobin and its relationship to SIDS death/risk. In 2004, Richardson et al. provided data supporting the concept of abnormal hemoglobin in SIDS, but did so by providing evidence of abnormally low levels of adult hemoglobin

(100). In the population-based study, Richardson et al. followed up 3.2 million infants enrolled in California's Newborn Screening program from 1990 to 1997 in order to identify deaths attributed to SIDS, looking at the association between incidence of SIDS and adult levels of hemoglobin in the first hours after birth. Of the 3,242,606 infants, there were 2,425 deaths attributed to SIDS (74.8 per 100,000 live births). SIDS infants were categorized based on adult levels of hemoglobin at birth and put into quintiles. After adjusting for sex, race/ethnicity, maternal age, maternal education, maternal smoking, preeclampsia, intrauterine growth restriction, and gestational age, the risk for SIDS was estimated to be 2.15-fold greater for infants in the lowest quintile (i.e. the lowest levels of adult hemoglobin) (100). This decrease in adult hemoglobin represents a true decrease in the fraction of adult hemoglobin, rather than a decrease in total hemoglobin levels (100). The study by Richardson et al. suggests that the low levels of adult hemoglobin in SIDS infants reflect an underlying chronic pathological condition or developmental impairment in processes such as cardiorespiratory control. Alternatively, low adult hemoglobin may reflect adverse prenatal conditions, such as maternal smoking and/or drinking (100). Unknown in this study is the persistence of this decrease in adult hemoglobin after birth and closer to the time of death. However, the post-mortem studies described above suggesting increased fetal hemoglobin at autopsy support a persistence of the hemoglobin abnormality, at least in some SIDS cases (58-60).

## Conclusions

As previously stated, there are no known biochemical biomarkers consistently used to identify SIDS infants at autopsy or to identify SIDS risk in living infants. While several of the biomarkers discussed above show potential, their use as forensic or clinical biomarkers requires critical steps, including validation in additional, oftentimes larger, datasets to access the reliability, sensitivity, and specificity of the biomarker. With regard to a forensic biomarker, this requirement proves difficult, given the relatively low incidence of SIDS death and the low availability of SIDS and non-SIDS autopsy tissue. This difficulty is exacerbated by the shift in nomenclature and the increasing movement away from calling a sudden and unexpected death a "SIDS death" to the increasingly used "sudden unexpected infant death (SUID)" or alternatively "cause unknown" (101). A death ruled as SIDS falls under the broader category of SUID, which includes deaths where evidence suggests a role for positional asphyxia or accidental overlay associated with bed sharing during a sleep period. Even after a thorough death scene investigation, the differentiation between a death due to SIDS and a death involving an asphyxia event is difficult, leaving a blurred distinction between the two and a possible misdiagnosis. A single biomarker specific to SIDS, or, more likely, a profile of multiple biomarkers specific to SIDS may allow for distinction between the two possible diagnoses. With regard to a biomarker of SIDS risk, validation requires very large prospective studies of living infants, collection of accessible fluids, and follow-up to determine incidence of SIDS death. Given that SIDS is likely a heterogeneous disorder due to multiple causes, a single biomarker will only identify a subset of infants at risk for SIDS, with this subset related to the biomarker-specific pathogenesis (e.g. SIDS related to 5-HT abnormalities). Despite the very difficult nature of biomarker studies in SIDS, the importance lies in the potential ability to identify abnormalities in SIDS infants, to better define pathogenic mechanisms involved in SIDS, and to identify infants or a subset of infants who are at risk of SIDS death and who may benefit from preventative strategies.

## Acknowledgments

The author thanks Dr Hannah C Kinney, Dr Eugene E Nattie, Dr Richard D Goldstein, Dr Alan D Michelson, and Jacob B Cotton for critical readings of this chapter.

## References

1.  Krous HF, Beckwith JB, Byard RW, Rognum TO, Bajanowski T, Corey T, et al. Sudden infant death syndrome and unclassified sudden infant deaths: A definitional and diagnostic approach. Pediatrics. 2004;114(1):234-8 https://doi.org/10.1542/peds.114.1.234.

2.  Willinger M, Hoffman HJ, Hartford RB. Infant sleep position and risk for sudden infant death syndrome: Report of meeting held January 13 and 14, 1994, National Institutes of Health, Bethesda, MD. Pediatrics. 1994;93(5):814-19. https://doi.org/10.1097/00006205-199407000-00006.

3.  American Academy of Pediatrics AAP Task Force on infant positioning and SIDS: Positioning and SIDS. Pediatrics. 1992;89(6 Pt 1):1120-6.

4.  Trachtenberg FL, Haas EA, Kinney HC, Stanley C, Krous HF. Risk factor changes for sudden infant death syndrome after initiation of Back-to-Sleep campaign. Pediatrics. 2012;129(4):630-8. https://doi.org/10.1542/peds.2011-1419.

5.  Matthews TJ, MacDorman MF, Thoma ME. Infant mortality statistics from the 2013 period linked birth/infant death data set. Natl Vital Stat Rep. 2015;64(9):1-30.

6.  Sridhar R, Thach BT, Kelly DH, Henslee JA. Characterization of successful and failed autoresuscitation in human infants, including those dying of SIDS. Pediatr Pulmonol. 2003;36(2):113-22. https://doi.org/10.1002/ppul.10287.

7.  Meny RG, Carroll JL, Carbone MT, Kelly DH. Cardiorespiratory recordings from infants dying suddenly and unexpectedly at home. Pediatrics. 1994;93(1):44-9.

8.  Franco P, Szliwowski H, Dramaix M, Kahn A. Decreased autonomic responses to obstructive sleep events in future victims of sudden infant death syndrome. Pediatr Res. 1999;46(1):33-9. https://doi.org/10.1203/00006450-199907000-00006.

9.  Schechtman VL, Lee MY, Wilson AJ, Harper RM. Dynamics of respiratory patterning in normal infants and infants who subsequently died of the sudden infant death syndrome. Pediatr Res. 1996;40(4):571-7. https://doi.org/10.1203/00006450-199610000-00010.

10. Kahn A, Groswasser J, Rebuffat E, Sottiaux M, Blum D, Foerster M, et al. Sleep and cardiorespiratory characteristics of infant victims of sudden death: A prospective case-control study. Sleep. 1992;15(4):287-92. https://doi.org/10.1093/sleep/15.4.287.

11. Ioakeimidis NS, Papamitsou T, Meditskou S, Iakovidou-Kritsi Z. Sudden infant death syndrome due to long QT syndrome: A brief review of the genetic substrate and prevalence. J Biol Res (Thessalon). 2017;24:6. https://doi.org/10.1186/s40709-017-0063-1.

12. Neubauer J, Lecca MR, Russo G, Bartsch C, Medeiros-Domingo A, Berger W, et al. Post-mortem whole-exome analysis in a large sudden infant death syndrome cohort with a focus on cardiovascular and metabolic genetic diseases. Eur J Hum Genet. 2017;25(4):404-9. https://doi.org/10.1038/ejhg.2016.199.

13. Laer K, Dork T, Vennemann M, Rothamel T, Klintschar M. Polymorphisms in genes of respiratory control and sudden infant death syndrome. Int J Legal Med. 2015;129(5):977-84. https://doi.org/10.1007/s00414-015-1232-0.

14. Winkel BG, Yuan L, Olesen MS, Sadjadieh G, Wang Y, Risgaard B, et al. The role of the sodium current complex in a nonreferred nationwide cohort of sudden infant death syndrome. Heart Rhythm. 2015;12(6):1241-9. https://doi.org/10.1016/j.hrthm.2015.03.013.

15. Ferrante L, Opdal SH. Sudden infant death syndrome and the genetics of inflammation. Front Immunol. 2015;6:63. https://doi.org/10.3389/fimmu.2015.00063.

16. Poetsch M, Nottebaum BJ, Wingenfeld L, Frede S, Vennemann M, Bajanowski T. Impact of sodium/proton exchanger 3 gene variants on sudden infant death syndrome. J Pediatr. 2010;156(1):44-8 e1.

17. Courts C, Madea B. Significant association of TH01 allele 9.3 and SIDS. J Forensic Sci. 2011;56(2):415-17. https://doi.org/10.1111/j.1556-4029.2010.01670.x.

18. Opdal SH, Vege A, Rognum TO. Serotonin transporter gene variation in sudden infant death syndrome. Acta Paediatr. 2008;97(7):861-5. https://doi.org/10.1111/j.1651-2227.2008.00813.x.

19. Paterson DS, Rivera KD, Broadbelt KG, Trachtenberg FL, Belliveau RA, Holm IA, et al. Lack of association of the serotonin transporter polymorphism with the sudden infant death syndrome in the San Diego Dataset. Pediatr Res. 2010;68(5):409-13. https://doi.org/10.1203/PDR.0b013e3181f2edf0.

20. Hu D, Barajas-Martinez H, Medeiros-Domingo A, Crotti L, Veltmann C, Schimpf R, et al. A novel rare variant in SCN1Bb linked to Brugada syndrome and SIDS by combined modulation of Na(v)1.5 and K(v)4.3 channel currents. Heart Rhythm. 2012;9(5):760-9. https://doi.org/10.1016/j.hrthm.2011.12.006.

21. Tfelt-Hansen J, Winkel BG, Grunnet M, Jespersen T. Cardiac channelopathies and sudden infant death syndrome. Cardiology. 2011;119(1):21-33. https://doi.org/10.1159/000329047.

22. Ferrante L, Opdal SH, Vege A, Rognum T. Cytokine gene polymorphisms and sudden infant death syndrome. Acta Paediatr. 2010;99(3):384-8. https://doi.org/10.1111/j.1651-2227.2009.01611.x.

23. Highet AR, Gibson CS, Goldwater PN. Variant interleukin 1 receptor antagonist gene alleles in sudden infant death syndrome. Arch Dis Child. 2010;95(12):1009-12. https://doi.org/10.1136/adc.2010.188268.

24. Klintschar M, Heimbold C. Association between a functional polymorphism in the MAOA gene and sudden infant death syndrome. Pediatrics. 2012;129(3):e756-61. https://doi.org/10.1542/peds.2011-1642.

25. Paterson DS. Serotonin gene variants are unlikely to play a significant role in the pathogenesis of the sudden infant death syndrome. Respir Physiol Neurobiol. 2013;189(2):301-14. https://doi.org/10.1016/j.resp.2013.07.001.

26. Kinney HC, Broadbelt KG, Haynes RL, Rognum IJ, Paterson DS. The serotonergic anatomy of the developing human medulla oblongata: Implications for pediatric disorders of homeostasis. J Chem Neuroanat. 2011;41(4):182-99. https://doi.org/10.1016/j.jchemneu.2011.05.004.

27. Brummelte S, Mc Glanaghy E, Bonnin A, Oberlander TF. Developmental changes in serotonin signaling: Implications for early brain function, behavior and adaptation. Neuroscience. 2017;342:212-31. https://doi.org/10.1016/j.neuroscience.2016.02.037.

28. Gaspar P, Cases O, Maroteaux L. The developmental role of serotonIn: News from mouse molecular genetics. Nat Rev Neurosci. 2003;4(12):1002-12. https://doi.org/10.1038/nrn1256.

29. Martin AM, Young RL, Leong L, Rogers GB, Spencer NJ, Jessup CF, et al. The diverse metabolic roles of peripheral serotonin. Endocrinology. 2017;158(5):1049-63. https://doi.org/10.1210/en.2016-1839.

30. Crane JD, Palanivel R, Mottillo EP, Bujak AL, Wang H, Ford RJ, et al. Inhibiting peripheral serotonin synthesis reduces obesity and metabolic dysfunction by promoting brown adipose tissue thermogenesis. Nat Med. 2015;21(2):166-72. https://doi.org/10.1038/nm.3766.

31. Watanabe H, Akasaka D, Ogasawara H, Sato K, Miyake M, Saito K, et al. Peripheral serotonin enhances lipid metabolism by accelerating bile acid turnover. Endocrinology. 2010;151(10):4776-86. https://doi.org/10.1210/en.2009-1349.

32. Sumara G, Sumara O, Kim JK, Karsenty G. Gut-derived serotonin is a multifunctional determinant to fasting adaptation. Cell Metab. 2012;16(5):588-600. https://doi.org/10.1016/j.cmet.2012.09.014.

33. Hunt CE, Brouillette RT. Sudden infant death syndrome: 1987 perspective. J Pediatr. 1987;110(5):669-78. https://doi.org/10.1016/S0022-3476(87)80001-X.

34. Kinney HC, Richerson GB, Dymecki SM, Darnall RA, Nattie EE. The brainstem and serotonin in the sudden infant death syndrome. Annu Rev Pathol. 2009;4:517-50. https://doi.org/10.1146/annurev.pathol.4.110807.092322.

35. Duncan JR, Paterson DS, Hoffman JM, Mokler DJ, Borenstein NS, Belliveau RA, et al. Brainstem serotonergic deficiency in sudden infant death syndrome. JAMA. 2010;303(5):430-7. https://doi.org/10.1001/jama.2010.45.

36. Paterson DS, Trachtenberg FL, Thompson EG, Belliveau RA, Beggs AH, Darnall R, et al. Multiple serotonergic brainstem abnormalities in sudden infant death syndrome. JAMA. 2006;296(17):2124-32. https://doi.org/10.1001/jama.296.17.2124.

37. Kinney HC, Randall LL, Sleeper LA, Willinger M, Belliveau RA, Zec N, et al. Serotonergic brainstem abnormalities in Northern Plains Indians with the sudden infant death syndrome. J Neuropathol Exp Neurol. 2003;62(11):1178-91. https://doi.org/10.1093/jnen/62.11.1178.

38. Panigrahy A, Filiano J, Sleeper LA, Mandell F, Valdes-Dapena M, Krous HF, et al. Decreased serotonergic receptor binding in rhombic lip-derived regions of the medulla oblongata in the sudden infant death syndrome. J Neuropathol Exp Neurol. 2000;59(5):377-84. https://doi.org/10.1093/jnen/59.5.377.

39. Ozawa Y, Okado N. Alteration of serotonergic receptors in the brain stems of human patients with respiratory disorders. Neuropediatrics. 2002;33(3):142-9. https://doi.org/10.1055/s-2002-33678.

40. Haynes RL, Frelinger AL, Giles EK, Goldstein RD, Tran H, Kozakewich HP, et al. High serum serotonin in sudden infant death syndrome. PNAS. 2017;114(29):7695-700. https://doi.org/10.1073/pnas.1617374114.

41. Reigstad CS, Salmonson CE, Rainey JF 3rd, Szurszewski JH, Linden DR, Sonnenburg JL, et al. Gut microbes promote colonic serotonin production through an effect of short-chain fatty acids on enterochromaffin cells. FASEB J. 2015;29(4):1395-403. https://doi.org/10.1096/fj.14-259598.

42. Yano JM, Yu K, Donaldson GP, Shastri GG, Ann P, Ma L, et al. Indigenous bacteria from the gut microbiota regulate host serotonin biosynthesis. Cell. 2015;161(2):264-76. https://doi.org/10.1016/j.cell.2015.02.047.

43. Livermore S, Zhou Y, Pan J, Yeger H, Nurse CA, Cutz E. Pulmonary neuroepithelial bodies are polymodal airway sensors: Evidence for $CO_2$/H+ sensing. Am J Physiol Lung Cell Mol Physiol. 2015;308(8):L807-15. https://doi.org/10.1152/ajplung.00208.2014.

44. Cutz E, Perrin DG, Pan J, Haas EA, Krous HF. Pulmonary neuroendocrine cells and neuroepithelial bodies in sudden infant death syndrome: Potential markers of airway chemoreceptor dysfunction. Pediatr Dev Pathol. 2007;10(2):106-16. https://doi.org/10.2350/06-06-0113.1.

45. Poets CF, Meny RG, Chobanian MR, Bonofiglo RE. Gasping and other cardiorespiratory patterns during sudden infant deaths. Pediatr Res. 1999;45(3):350-4. https://doi.org/10.1203/00006450-199903000-00010.

46. Naeye RL. Brain-stem and adrenal abnormalities in the sudden-infant-death syndrome. Am J Clin Pathol. 1976;66(3):526-30. https://doi.org/10.1093/ajcp/66.3.526.

47. Saugstad OD. Hypoxanthine as an indicator of hypoxia: Its role in health and disease through free radical production. Pediatr Res. 1988;23(2):143-50. https://doi.org/10.1203/00006450-198802000-00001.

48. Stoltenberg L, Rootwelt T, Oyasaeter S, Rognum TO, Saugstad OD. Hypoxanthine, xanthine, and uric acid concentrations in plasma, cerebrospinal fluid, vitreous humor, and urine in piglets subjected to intermittent versus continuous hypoxemia. Pediatr Res. 1993;34(6):767-71. https://doi.org/10.1203/00006450-199312000-00013.

49. Rognum TO, Saugstad OD, Oyasaeter S, Olaisen B. Elevated levels of hypoxanthine in vitreous humor indicate prolonged cerebral hypoxia in victims of sudden infant death syndrome. Pediatrics. 1988;82(4):615-18.

50. Rognum TO, Saugstad OD. Hypoxanthine levels in vitreous humor: Evidence of hypoxia in most infants who died of sudden infant death syndrome. Pediatrics. 1991;87(3):306-10.

51. Belonje PC, Wilson GR, Siroka SA. High postmortem concentrations of hypoxanthine and urate in the vitreous humor of infants are not confined to cases of sudden infant death syndrome. S Afr Med J. 1996;86(7):827-8.

52. Carpenter KH, Bonham JR, Worthy E, Variend S. Vitreous humour and cerebrospinal fluid hypoxanthine concentration as a marker of pre-mortem hypoxia in SIDS. J Clin Pathol. 1993;46(7):650-3. https://doi.org/10.1136/jcp.46.7.650.

53. Opdal SH, Rognum TO, Vege A, Saugstad OD. Hypoxanthine levels in vitreous humor: A study of influencing factors in sudden infant death syndrome. Pediatr Res. 1998;44(2):192-6. https://doi.org/10.1203/00006450-199808000-00009.

54. Bard H, Fouron JC, Gagnon C, Gagnon J. Hypoxemia and increased fetal hemoglobin synthesis. J Pediatr. 1994;124(6):941-3. https://doi.org/10.1016/S0022-3476(05)83188-9.

55. Davis LR. Changing blood picture in sickle-cell anaemia from shortly after birth to adolescence. J Clin Pathol. 1976;29(10):898-901. https://doi.org/10.1136/jcp.29.10.898.

56. Bard H, Prosmanne J. Elevated levels of fetal hemoglobin synthesis in infants with bronchopulmonary dysplasia. Pediatrics. 1990;86(2):193-6.

57. DeSimone J, Biel SI, Heller P. Stimulation of fetal hemoglobin synthesis in baboons by hemolysis and hypoxia. PNAS USA. 1978;75(6):2937-40. https://doi.org/10.1073/pnas.75.6.2937.

58. Giulian GG, Gilbert EF, Moss RL. Elevated fetal hemoglobin levels in sudden infant death syndrome. N Engl J Med. 1987;316(18):1122-6. https://doi.org/10.1056/NEJM198704303161804.

59. Gilbert-Barness E, Kenison K, Carver J. Fetal hemoglobin and sudden infant death syndrome. Arch Pathol Lab Med. 1993;117(2):177-9.

60. Perry GW, Vargas-Cuba R, Vertes RP. Fetal hemoglobin levels in sudden infant death syndrome. Arch Pathol Lab Med. 1997;121(10):1048-54.

61. Zielke HR, Meny RG, O'Brien MJ, Smialek JE, Kutlar F, Huisman TH, et al. Normal fetal hemoglobin levels in the sudden infant death syndrome. N Engl J Med. 1989;321(20):1359-64. https://doi.org/10.1056/NEJM198911163212003.

62. Cheron G, Bachoux I, Maier M, Massonneau M, Peltier JY, Girot R. Fetal hemoglobin in sudden infant death syndrome. N Engl J Med. 1989;320(15):1011-12. https://doi.org/10.1056/NEJM198904133201513.

63. Krous HF, Haas EA, Chadwick AE, Masoumi H, Stanley C, Perry GW. Hemoglobin F in sudden infant death syndrome: A San Diego SIDS/SUDC Research Project report. J Forensic Leg Med. 2007;14(8):456-60. https://doi.org/10.1016/j.jflm.2006.11.005.

64. Fagan DG, Walker A. Haemoglobin F levels in sudden infant deaths. Br J Haematol. 1992;82(2):422-30. https://doi.org/10.1111/j.1365-2141.1992.tb06440.x.

65. Poets CF, Samuels MP, Wardrop CA, Picton-Jones E, Southall DP. Reduced haemoglobin levels in infants presenting with apparent life-threatening events — A retrospective investigation. Acta Paediatr. 1992;81(4):319-21. https://doi.org/10.1111/j.1651-2227.1992.tb12234.x.

66. Grether JK, Schulman J. Sudden infant death syndrome and birth weight. J Pediatr. 1989;114(4 Pt 1):561-7. https://doi.org/10.1016/S0022-3476(89)80694-8.

67. Kinney HC, Thach BT. The sudden infant death syndrome. N Engl J Med. 2009;361(8):795-805. https://doi.org/10.1056/NEJMra0803836.

68. Vege A, Rognum TO, Scott H, Aasen AO, Saugstad OD. SIDS cases have increased levels of interleukin-6 in cerebrospinal fluid. Acta Paediatr. 1995;84(2):193-6. https://doi.org/10.1111/j.1651-2227.1995.tb13608.x.

69. Vege A, Rognum TO, Aasen AO, Saugstad OD. Are elevated cerebrospinal fluid levels of IL-6 in sudden unexplained deaths, infectious deaths and deaths due to heart/lung disease in infants and children due to hypoxia? Acta Paediatr. 1998;87(8):819-24. https://doi.org/10.1111/j.1651-2227.1998.tb01544.x.

70. Kluger MJ, Kozak W, Leon LR, Soszynski D, Conn CA. Cytokines and fever. Neuroimmunomodulation. 1995;2(4):216-23. https://doi.org/10.1159/000097199.

71. Rognum IJ, Haynes RL, Vege A, Yang M, Rognum TO, Kinney HC. Interleukin-6 and the serotonergic system of the medulla oblongata in the sudden infant death syndrome. Acta Neuropathol. 2009;118(4):519-30. https://doi.org/10.1007/s00401-009-0535-y.

72. Murphy TM, O'Donovan A, Mullins N, O'Farrelly C, McCann A, Malone K. Anxiety is associated with higher levels of global DNA methylation and altered expression of epigenetic and interleukin-6 genes. Psychiatr Genet. 2015;25(2):71-8. https://doi.org/10.1097/YPG.0000000000000055.

73. Rokavec M, Oner MG, Hermeking H. Inflammation-induced epigenetic switches in cancer. Cell Mol Life Sci. 2016;73(1):23-39. https://doi.org/10.1007/s00018-015-2045-5.

74. Gasche JA, Hoffmann J, Boland CR, Goel A. Interleukin-6 promotes tumorigenesis by altering DNA methylation in oral cancer cells. Int J Cancer. 2011;129(5):1053-63. https://doi.org/10.1002/ijc.25764.

75. Vege A, Rognum TO, Anestad G. IL-6 cerebrospinal fluid levels are related to laryngeal IgA and epithelial HLA-DR response in sudden infant death syndrome. Pediatr Res. 1999;45(6):803-9. https://doi.org/10.1203/00006450-199906000-00004.

76. Vennemann MM, Loddenkotter B, Fracasso T, Mitchell EA, Debertin AS, Larsch KP, et al. Cytokines and sudden infant death. Int J Legal Med. 2012;126(2):279-84. https://doi.org/10.1007/s00414-011-0638-6.

77. Bischoff SC. Role of mast cells in allergic and non-allergic immune responses: Comparison of human and murine data. Nat Rev Immunol. 2007;7(2):93-104. https://doi.org/10.1038/nri2018.

78. Galli SJ, Tsai M. IgE and mast cells in allergic disease. Nat Med. 2012;18(5):693-704. https://doi.org/10.1038/nm.2755.

79. Yu Y, Blokhuis BR, Garssen J, Redegeld FA. Non-IgE mediated mast cell activation. Eur J Pharmacol. 2016;778:33-43. https://doi.org/10.1016/j.ejphar.2015.07.017.

80. Foster B, Schwartz LB, Devouassoux G, Metcalfe DD, Prussin C. Characterization of mast-cell tryptase-expressing peripheral blood cells as basophils. J Allergy Clin Immunol. 2002;109(2):287-93. https://doi.org/10.1067/mai.2002.121454.

81. Payne V, Kam PC. Mast cell tryptase: A review of its physiology and clinical significance. Anaesthesia. 2004;59(7):695-703. https://doi.org/10.1111/j.1365-2044.2004.03757.x.

82. Platt MS, Yunginger JW, Sekula-Perlman A, Irani AM, Smialek J, Mirchandani HG, et al. Involvement of mast cells in sudden infant death syndrome. J Allergy Clin Immunol. 1994;94(2 Pt 1):250-6. https://doi.org/10.1053/ai.1994.v94.a56337.

83. Holgate ST, Walters C, Walls AF, Lawrence S, Shell DJ, Variend S, et al. The anaphylaxis hypothesis of sudden infant death syndrome (SIDS): Mast cell degranulation in cot death revealed by elevated concentrations of tryptase in serum. Clin Exp Allergy. 1994;24(12):1115-22. https://doi.org/10.1111/j.1365-2222.1994.tb03316.x.

84. Hagan LL, Goetz DW, Revercomb CH, Garriott J. Sudden infant death syndrome: A search for allergen hypersensitivity. Ann Allergy Asthma Immunol. 1998;80(3):227-31. https://doi.org/10.1016/S1081-1206(10)62962-6.

85. Edston E, Gidlund E, Wickman M, Ribbing H, van Hage-Hamsten M. Increased mast cell tryptase in sudden infant death — Anaphylaxis, hypoxia

or artefact? Clin Exp Allergy. 1999;29(12):1648-54. https://doi.org/10.1046/j.1365-2222.1999.00679.x.

86. Buckley MG, Variend S, Walls AF. Elevated serum concentrations of beta-tryptase, but not alpha-tryptase, in sudden infant death syndrome (SIDS). An investigation of anaphylactic mechanisms. Clin Exp Allergy. 2001;31(11):1696-704. https://doi.org/10.1046/j.1365-2222.2001.01213.x.

87. Nishio H, Suzuki K. Serum tryptase levels in sudden infant death syndrome in forensic autopsy cases. Forensic Sci Int. 2004;139(1):57-60. https://doi.org/10.1016/j.forsciint.2003.09.011.

88. Coombs RR, Holgate ST. Allergy and cot death: With special focus on allergic sensitivity to cows' milk and anaphylaxis. Clin Exp Allergy. 1990;20(4):359-66. https://doi.org/10.1111/j.1365-2222.1990.tb02794.x.

89. Parish WE, Barrett AM, Coombs RR, Gunther M, Camps FE. Hypersensitivity to milk and sudden death in infancy. Lancet. 1960;2(7160):1106-10. https://doi.org/10.1016/S0140-6736(60)92187-5.

90. Parish WE, Richards CB, France NE, Coombs RR. Further investigations on the hypothesis that some cases of cot-death are due to a modified anaphylactic reaction to cow's milk. Int Arch Allergy Appl Immunol. 1964;24:215-43. https://doi.org/10.1159/000229462.

91. Schieving JH, de Vries M, van Vugt JM, Weemaes C, van Deuren M, Nicolai J, et al. Alpha-fetoprotein, a fascinating protein and biomarker in neurology. Eur J Paediatr Neurol. 2014;18(3):243-8. https://doi.org/10.1016/j.ejpn.2013.09.003.

92. Mizejewski GJ. Levels of alpha-fetoprotein during pregnancy and early infancy in normal and disease states. Obstet Gynecol Surv. 2003;58(12):804-26. https://doi.org/10.1097/01.OGX.0000099770.97668.18.

93. Kronquist KE, Dreazen E, Keener SL, Nicholas TW, Crandall BF. Reduced fetal hepatic alpha-fetoprotein levels in Down's syndrome. Prenat Diagn. 1990;10(11):739-51. https://doi.org/10.1002/pd.1970101108.

94. Waller DK, Lustig LS, Smith AH, Hook EB. Alpha-fetoproteIn: A biomarker for pregnancy outcome. Epidemiology. 1993;4(5):471-6. https://doi.org/10.1097/00001648-199309000-00014.

95. Smith GC. Screening and prevention of stillbirth. Best Pract Res Clin Obstet Gynaecol. 2017;38:71-82. https://doi.org/10.1016/j.bpobgyn.2016.08.002.

96. Smith GC, Wood AM, Pell JP, White IR, Crossley JA, Dobbie R. Second-trimester maternal serum levels of alpha-fetoprotein and the subsequent risk of sudden infant

death syndrome. N Engl J Med. 2004;351(10):978-86. https://doi.org/10.1056/
NEJMoa040963.

97. Bard H, Cote A, Praud JP, Infante-Rivard C, Gagnon C. Fetal hemoglobin
    synthesis determined by γ-mRNA/γ -mRNA + β-mRNA quantitation in infants
    at risk for sudden infant death syndrome being monitored at home for apnea.
    Pediatrics. 2003;112(4):e285. https://doi.org/10.1542/peds.112.4.e285.

98. Bard H, Widness JA, Ziegler EE, Gagnon C, Peri KG. The proportions of G
    gamma- and A gamma-globins in the fetal hemoglobin synthesized in preterm and
    term infants. Pediatr Res. 1995;37(3):361-4. https://doi.org/10.1203/00006450-
    199503000-00018.

99. Bard H. Hypoxemia and increased fetal hemoglobin synthesis during the perinatal
    period. Semin Perinatol. 1992;16(3):191-5.

100. Richardson DB, Wing S, Lorey F, Hertz-Picciotto I. Adult hemoglobin levels
     at birth and risk of sudden infant death syndrome. Arch Pediatr Adolesc Med.
     2004;158(4):366-71. https://doi.org/10.1001/archpedi.158.4.366.

101. Goldstein RD, Trachtenberg FL, Sens MA, Harty BJ, Kinney HC. Overall
     postneonatal mortality and rates of SIDS. Pediatrics. 2016;137(1):1-10. https://
     doi.org/10.1542/peds.2015-2298.

# 33 Animal Models: Illuminating the Pathogenesis of Sudden Infant Death Syndrome

Aihua Li, MD[1],
Robert A Darnall, MD[1,2],
Susan Dymecki, MD[3], PhD and
James C Leiter, MD[1]

[1]Department of Molecular and Systems Biology,
Geisel School of Medicine at Dartmouth, Lebanon, USA
[2]Department of Pediatrics, Geisel School of Medicine at
Dartmouth, Lebanon, USA
[3]Department of Genetics, Harvard Medical School, Boston, USA

## Introduction

Three research areas derived from human studies of epidemiology, pathology, and sleep in infants have made contributions to our understanding of sudden infant death syndrome (SIDS). Epidemiological studies of infants who died of SIDS have identified a variety of risk factors associated with increased and decreased risk of SIDS (1-7), including prone sleeping position (8, 9), maternal cigarette smoking during pregnancy, and heat stress in the infant, often related to overheated environments, excessive bed clothing, or other unsafe sleeping practices (8, 10, 11). Additional risk factors include a recent upper respiratory tract infection, bed sharing, prematurity, and intrauterine and/or postnatal hypoxic stress.

Similar progress in understanding the origins of SIDS has been made by pathologists analysing the brains of infants who died and were classified as SIDS. Analyses of brain tissue from these infants have consistently revealed a high prevalence of abnormalities in the brainstem serotoninergic system including an increased number of serotonergic neurons, a higher proportion of serotonergic neurons displaying immature morphology, decreased tissue levels of serotonin (5-HT) and its synthetic enzyme, tryptophan hydroxylase 2 (TPH2), and decreased 5-HT receptor binding intensity both in serotonergic nuclei themselves and in several nuclei that are important in cardiorespiratory control (9, 12-16). Similar serotonin system deficits have been described in infants who died of asphyxia (17). There has been persistent speculation that infants who died of SIDS suffered from hypoxia (i.e. low oxygen levels) at some time preceding death (18-22), and hypoxia appeared to delay maturation of the brain in infants who died of SIDS (19-21, 23, 24).

Finally, sleep studies in the infants who subsequently died of SIDS have revealed a sequence of repetitive episodes of hypoxia preceding, or following, apnea and/or bradycardia, followed by autoresuscitative efforts to restore normal breathing and arouse from sleep (25-28). Death occurred when the autoresuscitation or arousal following prolonged apnea failed to restore regular breathing and adequate oxygenation. Many infants experienced sequences of multiple hypoxic apneic events from which they recovered, only to succumb to a final event in which autoresuscitation and/or arousal failed.

## The Triple Risk Model of SIDS — A Guide to Animal Studies

The Triple Risk Model posits a sequence of events leading to death, triggered during sleep when a vulnerable infant is exposed to an exogenous stressor during a critical period of development (29). The Triple Risk model has been immensely useful in structuring experimental approaches to studying SIDS. The risk factors for SIDS and the associated serotonergic defects observed in SIDS cases can all be seen as triggering events or vulnerabilities that contribute to apnea or failed autoresuscitation and arousal. However, the model has limitations: it describes associations among three classes of variables, but it posits no causal relationships and no neurophysiological mechanisms. Therefore, a major goal of animal studies has been to suggest plausible physiological mechanisms for vulnerabilities, exogenous stressors, and critical developmental events as they are reflected in the important epidemiological, pathological, and behavioral elements previously associated with SIDS. Animal studies permit experimental interventions, manipulations of neurotransmitter levels, and selection of relatively immature animals so that the observations made in human studies can be connected mechanistically to physiological responses that may plausibly lead to the sudden death of an infant.

The animal studies discussed in this chapter, which owe a genuine debt to the Triple Risk Model, will be discussed in the context of a two-step hypothesis in which SIDS occurs in infants who, first, have an unusual propensity for prolonged reflex apneas and hypoxia, and, second, lack adequate mechanisms to terminate apneas and/or restore regular, eupneic breathing (30). Apneas in SIDS have been attributed to three oxygen-conserving reflexes: the dive reflex, the laryngeal chemoreflex, or primary hypoxic apnea, with or without mechanical or obstructive asphyxiation. All these reflex apneic mechanisms originate from cranial nerves and elicit behaviors that preserve oxygen; and all are particularly prominent in infants (30). In terms of the second step of this hypothesis, both autoresuscitation and arousal responses are thought to be abnormal in infants who died of SIDS (31-34). As a consequence, a large number of animal studies have tested the hypothesis that risk factors for SIDS, hypoxic responses, and especially deficient serotonergic function modify apnea propensity, autoresuscitation, or arousal responses and increase the likelihood of SIDS and asphyxial deaths.

## The Role of Apneagenic Reflexes in SIDS

### The diving reflex

Wolf was among the first to suggest that an "over exuberant oxygen conserving reflex" might contribute to SIDS (35). There are two interesting aspects to his idea. First is the idea that apneagenic oxygen-conserving reflexes may initiate a process ending in a sudden infant death; second, there is the idea that in certain infants, the reflex is over-exuberant and might either be elicited by relatively mild and apparently innocuous stimuli, or, when elicited by appropriate stimuli, might be particularly long-lasting.

The possibility that the diving reflex might contribute to SIDS was investigated in monkeys aged postnatal day (P) 0 to 3 months by occluding the nose, or placing a cold, moist, non-occlusive stimulus on the face, or by inserting the face directly into cold water (36). The investigators immediately confronted a problem, as eliciting the dive reflex in awake animals caused marked excitation and arousal of the animal. Therefore, subsequent studies were conducted under anesthesia. Still, even under anesthesia, a number of animals had excitatory responses when the diving reflex was elicited. When the diving reflex was successfully elicited in infant monkeys, it caused prolonged apneas and bradycardias, especially if the reflex was elicited during sleep or if it was "abnormally" sensitive. The dive reflex seemed to diminish in strength as the animals grew older. The authors concluded that the diving reflex was possibly associated with SIDS.

Subsequently, there has been additional speculation that the dive response contributes to SIDS (37, 38), but French et al. (36) are the only researchers to have conducted animal studies to examine the diving reflex as a precursor of SIDS. The diving reflex was allegedly the origin of apnea and a SIDS death in a baby, but the actual report of the death does not describe any stimulation of the trigeminal area, no wet or cold stimulation, and no obstruction of the nose (39). It seems more likely that reflex apnea was generated by an internal and unseen stimulus, such as hypoxia or the laryngeal chemoreflex, based on the limited information given in the report.

In summary, the dive reflex, which is elicited by cold, wet, occlusive stimuli in the area of the nose, lacks face validity. SIDS generally occurs in a warm environment that is not wet. Moreover, the requirement of anesthesia to elicit the reflex in monkeys is significant for two reasons: anesthesia may enhance the inhibitory effects of reflex apnea, and covering the face or occluding the nose usually stimulates a struggle and stimulates ventilation. The idea that facial covering inhibits breathing, with or without cold, wet stimuli, is not consistent with the observations in monkeys. Thus, the diving reflex seems to be a possible, but unlikely, contributor to SIDS based on the animal studies available.

## The laryngeal chemoreflex

The laryngeal chemoreflex (LCR) is elicited when fluid with a low chloride content or low pH enters the larynx (40-43). The LCR is made up of behaviors that prevent aspiration of fluids into the upper airway, clear the offending fluids from the airway, and preserve oxygen delivery to vital organs (Figure 33.1) (41, 44-46). Manifestations of the LCR seem to evolve over the course of development: swallowing and apnea are prominent in preterm infants, and swallowing remains in full term neonates, but the duration of apnea declines during this period of development, and coughing may emerge as a more prominent element of the response in adult animals (47). Arousal from sleep is common, but not universal, when the reflex is elicited; arousals tend to be less frequent during active sleep (48, 49). The LCR is frequently elicited in the normal course of neonatal life. Many investigators have suggested that the LCR is the first step in a process that starts with respiratory inhibition and apnea, and ends with failed termination of apnea, failed restoration of regular breathing, and failed arousal, leading to SIDS and asphyxial deaths in human infants (30, 41, 47, 50, 51).

### Risk factors for SIDS and the LCR — Presynaptic mechanisms in the nucleus of the solitary tract

#### Impact of thermal stress

SIDS is often associated with heat stress (53-58), though there is some disagreement about this (59). Moreover, Guntheroth and Spiers (55) emphasized that the danger of the prone sleeping position may relate more to heat stress than to asphyxia, since prone infants lose heat more slowly than supine infants, both from the body surface and via the respiratory tract (60).

Elevated body temperature in dogs enhanced laryngeal adduction induced by superior laryngeal nerve (SLN) stimulation, which mimics the effect of eliciting the LCR (44). Therefore, we tested the hypothesis that increased body temperature would also be associated with prolongation of the LCR in piglets (61). We modeled thermal stress by increasing body temperature in decerebrate, neonatal piglets aged P3 to P15. Although thermal stress has been identified as a risk factor for SIDS, this does not necessarily mean that thermally stressed infants who died of SIDS had an elevated body temperature. Nonetheless, we hypothesized that thermal stress, by enhancing the LCR, may increase the likelihood of prolonged apneas that result ultimately in sudden death in neonates. We elicited the LCR by injecting 0.1 ml of water into the larynx through a

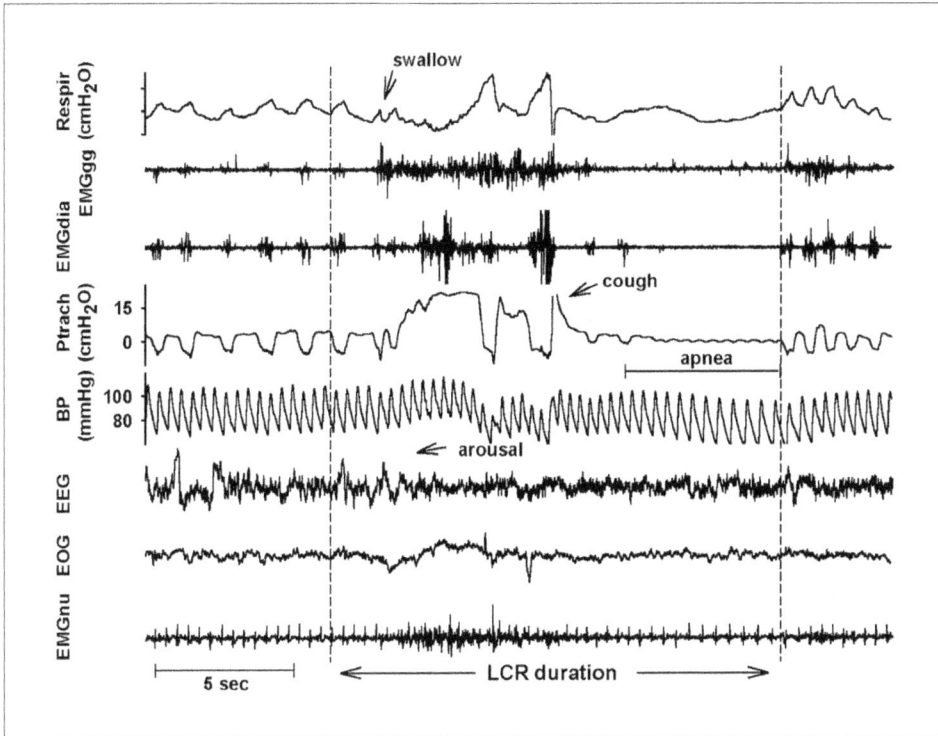

Figure 33.1: An example of the laryngeal chemoreflex. LCR elicited in piglets by injecting 0.05 ml of water (first vertical dashed line) during non-rapid eye movement (NREM) sleep while 1 mM muscimol was dialyzed into the rostral ventral medulla. Respiration (Respir; obtained from the plethysmograph), genioglossal electromyographic (EMG; EMGgg), diaphragmatic EMG (EMGdia), tracheal pressure (Ptrach), blood pressure (BP), EEG, electrooculographic (EOG), and nuchal EMG (EMGnu) activity are shown in the tracings. Note the occurrence of a swallow, which was associated with a characteristic negative Ptrach deflection and a burst of EMGgg activity that interrupted the EMGdia. Coughing was detected by the increase in EMGdia activity that preceded forceful expiratory activity, which was indicated by the increase in Ptrach. Apneas, defined as periods without breathing that lasted longer than the last two breaths preceding the injection of fluid into the larynx, were also associated with cessation of EMGdia activity and respiratory pressure fluctuations in the Ptrach record. Arousals were identified from the occurrence of body movements, opening of the eyes, increased EMGnu activity, and increased fast activity in the EEG signal, in this case from high amplitude and low frequency to low amplitude and fast frequency (from NREM sleep to wakefulness). The two vertical dashed lines mark the length of the LCR. (Reproduced with permission from (52).)

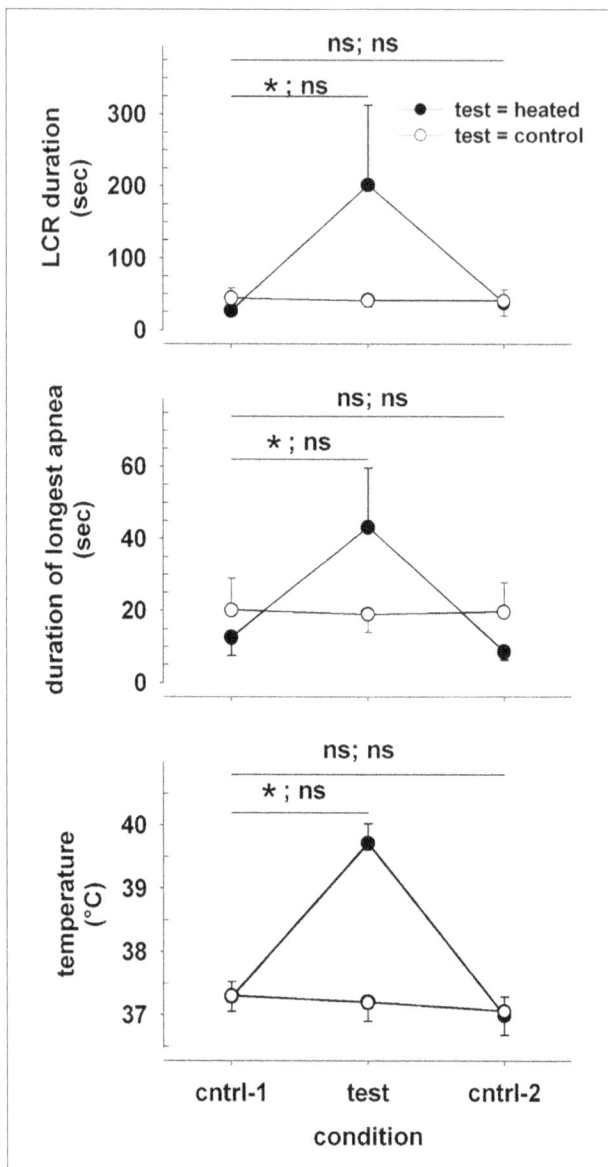

Figure 33.2: Average duration of the laryngeal chemoreflex, duration of the longest apnea, and rectal temperature in decerebrate, ventilated piglets. Values are means ±SE. • = results from animals in which body temperature was elevated during the test period (n = 12); o = results from the time-control animals in which body temperature was constant throughout (n = 5). Statistical comparisons (indicated by the horizontal lines above each graph) were made with respect to the first control period (cntrl-1), and the results of this comparison among the test animals are presented first. Hence, the LCR and apnea durations were significantly longer during the test period compared with control (*p<0.05), but there were no changes in these variables in the time-control animals when the same comparisons were made. (ns = not significant; cntrl-2 = second control period.) (Reproduced with permission from (61).)

catheter passed through one side of the nose, and then found that by elevating the body temperature ~2.5 °C the LCR was significantly prolonged (Figure 33.2).

*The effect of elevated body temperature is centrally mediated*

In a subsequent study, we recorded the electrical activity within the superior laryngeal nerve of individual afferent fibers that respond to water stimulation. We found that the peripheral afferent fibers were not themselves thermally sensitive in the range of body temperatures that we studied (62). However, focally warming the area in and around the nucleus of the nucleus of the solitary tract (NTS) by ~2.0 °C with a thermode prolonged the LCR, even though body temperature was held constant at ~38 °C (63). Moreover, the effect was specific to the NTS, since warming another area of the brainstem did not prolong the LCR. Thus, thermal prolongation of the LCR seems to originate in the central nervous system (CNS) from an elevated temperature in the region of the NTS.

*The impact of transient receptor potential vanilloid-1 receptors*

We next turned to the question of determining the nature of the thermally sensitive process within the NTS that prolongs the LCR. It is well established that transient receptor potential vanilloid-1 (TRPV1) receptors, which are ligand-gated ion channels, are thermally sensitive, and TRPV1 receptors are found in the NTS (64, 65). The usual temperature range over which TRPV1 channels are activated in isolation is >42 °C (66). However, TRPV1 channel activation in the NTS, which enhances asynchronous release of glutamate following visceral afferent stimulation, was thermally modulated by temperatures between 25-38 °C (67), temperatures well within the range of normal body temperatures. Moreover, spontaneous glutamatergic excitatory post-synaptic currents (currents occurring in the absence of visceral afferent activation) were strongly influenced by TRPV1 channel activity, and TRPV1 activity in this setting had a thermal range of 30-42 °C (68). The function of TRPV1 channels is also modified by other factors that may be relevant to SIDS. In addition to thermal activation of TRPV1 channels, reduced pH (for example during hypercapnia), bradykinin (perhaps related to co-existing infection or inflammation), and nicotine all appear to enhance TRPV1 sensitivity (69).

Therefore, we tested the hypothesis that TRPV1 receptors mediate the thermal prolongation of the LCR originating in the NTS (70). We studied the LCR in decerebrate piglets aged P4 to P7 and micro-injected drugs into the NTS as we changed body temperature. 5'iodoresiniferatoxin is an antagonist of TRPV1 receptors, and focal, bilateral injection of 5'iodoresiniferatoxin into the NTS prevented the thermal prolongation of the LCR, even though body temperature was elevated by approximately 2.7 °C. Resiniferatoxin is a TRPV1 agonist, and bilateral micro-injections of resiniferatoxin in the caudal NTS significantly increased the duration of the LCR, even though body temperature was not elevated. Thus, a TRPV1 antagonist micro-injected into the NTS blocked the hyperthermic prolongation of the LCR, and a TRPV1 agonist increased the duration of the LCR without any change in body temperature. Thus,

TRPV1 receptors may mediate all, or part, of the thermal prolongation of the LCR, at least in piglets.

TRPV1 channels are expressed presynaptically on visceral afferent C-fibers within the NTS (64, 71, 72). When activated, TRPV1 channels within the presynaptic membrane seem to amplify glutamate release, presumably by making more calcium available to enhance vesicular release of the neurotransmitter and amplify glutamate release at second-order neurons in the NTS. Since prone infants (particularly those who are over-blanketed and/or who have their faces in the bedclothes) lose heat more slowly than supine infants do, both from the body surface and via the respiratory tract (60), and since thermal stress is a risk factor for SIDS, it seems plausible that the risk factor of thermal stress may increase the likelihood of prolonged apneas that result ultimately in sudden death in neonates by enhancing the activity of presynaptic TRPV1 receptors in the NTS.

*Upper respiratory tract infections and inflammation — A role for interleukin 1-β*

A recent history of an upper respiratory tract infection (URI) is also a risk factor for SIDS (73, 74), and viral infections, particularly respiratory syncytial virus infections, may prolong reflex apneas in newborn lambs (75, 76). The effect of recent URIs depends on the synthesis and release of inflammatory cytokines (77, 78), and these inflammatory mediators are either transmitted retrograde from the larynx into the CNS through the superior laryngeal nerves or made locally within the CNS itself (75, 76, 79). In anesthetized piglets, endotoxin administration prolonged apneas elicited by laryngeal stimulation with acidic water, and systemic administration of interleukin-1β (IL-1β) prolonged apnea induced by ammonia introduced into the larynx (80). In neither of the foregoing studies was body temperature allowed to rise, although both endotoxin and IL-1β are pyrogenic. TRPV1 channels are sensitized by inflammatory mediators. To test the hypothesis that inflammatory mediators might prolong the LCR, we studied decerebrate piglets P3 to P7 days of age, combining treatment of IL-1β with elevated body temperature, and assessed the impact of these interventions on the duration of the LCR (81). We also tested the effect of IL-1β in the presence of the mixed cyclooxygenase-1 and -2 inhibitor, indomethacin, to determine whether IL-1β-dependent effects on the LCR are mediated by IL-1β itself, or by downstream mediators such as prostaglandin E2 (PGE2) (82). Indomethacin alone did not interfere with the thermal prolongation of the LCR. In contrast, IL-1β given systemically dramatically prolonged the LCR, even when body temperature was normal. Moreover, IL-1β amplified the thermal prolongation of the LCR. Treatment with indomethacin blocked the amplifying effect of IL-1β on the LCR, but left the normal thermal prolongation of the LCR intact. Elevated levels of IL-1β led to increased synthesis of IL-6 levels — a cytokine pyrogen in its own right (82, 83). IL-6 treatment prolonged the LCR under normothermic conditions and significantly amplified the thermal prolongation of the LCR, and treatment with indomethacin completely blocked these effects of IL-6 treatment.

As noted above, we have already identified presynaptic TRPV1 receptors in the NTS as the likely mediator of the thermal prolongation of the LCR, and non-thermal stimuli, many of which are inflammatory mediators (including IL-1β and IL-6), may also modify the activity of TRPV1 channels, irrespective of temperature (84, 85) and potentiate TRPV1 activation (86). These cytokines stimulate the synthesis and release of eicosanoids such as $PGE_2$ (87), which leads to activation of protein kinase A (85, 88) and phosphorylation of TRPV1. Phosphorylation of TRPV1 enhances both its conductance and calcium entry into the cell (89), which leads to greater release of glutamate (90). We believe that these same processes are active in C-fiber vagal sensory neurons that terminate in the NTS. Thus, IL-1β and IL-6 may increase $PGE_2$ in the NTS, thereby sensitizing TRPV1 channels, amplifying the potency of thermal information, and enhancing thermal prolongation of the LCR by virtue of increased glutamate release from the C-fiber afferents onto second order neurons in the NTS mediating the LCR.

The effects of IL-1β and elevated body temperature were interactive, meaning that the combined effect of these interventions was greater than the sum of the interventions. IL-1β treatment created a thermal reflex hyperalgesia in which TRPV1 receptors were responsive to stimuli that would normally be innocuous. This amplification of TRPV1 activity can be seen as a form of reflex allodynia analogous to thermal hyperalgesia in peripheral nerves following central pain sensitization (85, 88, 91, 92). Thus, cytokine-related sensitization of the LCR could lead to profound apnea in infants with a history of recent URIs following normally innocuous laryngeal stimulation at body temperatures that need not be elevated. TRPV1 channel activity may provide a common molecular mechanism for the epidemiological association of SIDS associated with thermal stress and recent infections.

## Inhibitory pre- and post-synaptic mechanisms in the NTS

### Gamma-aminobutyric acid inhibition in the NTS and the LCR

Blocking gamma-aminobutyric acid (GABA) receptors shortened the duration of laryngeal apnea induced by electrical stimulation of the superior laryngeal nerve in normothermic decerebrate neonatal piglets (93). Therefore, we tested the hypothesis that blocking GABAergic neurotransmission would prevent the thermal prolongation of the apnea that followed SLN stimulation (94). We studied decerebrate piglets aged P3 to P15, and we stimulated the SLN for 10 seconds during the initial phase of inspiration to elicit apnea. Elevating body temperature by ~2 °C increased the duration of the apnea following SLN stimulation. The effect was reversible once body temperature was returned to the normal, control levels. Systemic administration of gabazine or bicuculline (both $GABA_A$ receptor antagonists) prevented the thermal prolongation of the apnea that followed SLN stimulation. The $GABA_A$ receptor antagonists did not, however, shorten the duration of the baseline normothermic apnea that followed SLN stimulation. The failure to alter the normothermic apnea duration following SLN stimulation suggests that GABA is not the primary element in generating apnea (we think this is a glutamatergic process originating from second order neurons in the NTS), but the thermal prolongation of apnea following SLN stimulation did depend on a thermally mediated GABAergic process. In a subsequent study, we tested the hypothesis that the thermally mediated GABAergic process resided within the NTS (95). We studied decerebrate piglets ranging in age from P3 to P13, and we dialyzed gabazine unilaterally into the dorsal medulla in the region of the NTS. Rather than using SLN stimulation, we elicited the LCR by injecting 0.1 ml of water into the larynx to elicit the LCR. Much like administration of systemic bicuculline, gabazine focally dialyzed into the NTS blocked the thermal prolongation of the LCR without altering the normothermic duration of the LCR.

*A GABAergic interaction with TRPV1*

Having determined that TRPV1 mediated the thermal prolongation of the LCR, we investigated the role of GABAergic mechanisms on TRPV1-mediated prolongation of the LCR. We tested the hypothesis that bicuculline could block prolongation of the LCR following micro-injection of a TRPV1 agonist, resiniferatoxin, into the NTS. We studied decerebrate piglets aged P4 to P7, and we administered bicuculline intravenously before and after resiniferatoxin was micro-injected into the NTS. When resiniferatoxin was given first, the LCR was prolonged, even though the body temperature remained normal. Subsequent treatment with bicuculline blocked the effect of resiniferatoxin, and the LCR was no different from the control values in these animals. When bicuculline was given first, resiniferatoxin micro-injections into the NTS did not prolong the LCR duration. Thus, $GABA_A$ receptor antagonists blocked both the thermally mediated and the TRPV1-mediated prolongation of the LCR. This is consistent with the hypothesis that TRPV1 channels within, or close to, the NTS mediate thermal prolongation of the LCR, and there is a GABAergic process that contributes to the thermally mediated amplification of the LCR.

*Presynaptic modulation of GABAergic activity*

Activation of presynaptic adenosine $A_{2A}$ (Ad-$A_{2A}$) receptors seems to enhance GABA release (96-98). An adenosine agonist injected into the cistern of decerebrate piglets enhanced apnea elicited by SLN stimulation. This effect was mediated by Ad-$A_{2A}$ receptors, and the effect of Ad-$A_{2A}$ receptor activation was blocked by $GABA_A$ antagonists (99). Moreover, Ad-$A_{2A}$ antagonists shortened the duration of the LCR, which was attributed to blockade of the Ad-$A_{2A}$ receptors on GABAergic neurons in the medulla (100-102). The site of Ad-$A_{2A}$ action within the brainstem was not further explored in these studies, and to address this issue, we studied the interactions among Ad-$A_{2A}$ agonists and antagonists, $GABA_A$ receptor antagonists, and the thermal prolongation of the LCR (103). We studied decerebrate piglets aged P4 to P13 days and micro-injected

SCH-58261, an Ad-A$_{2A}$ antagonist, into the NTS. Blocking Ad-A$_{2A}$ receptors focally in the NTS reversed the thermal prolongation of the LCR in decerebrate piglets, but focal administration of Ad-A$_{2A}$ did not alter the LCR under normothermic conditions. Ad-A$_{2A}$ has been identified presynaptically on GABAergic and glutamatergic neurons. On GABAergic neurons, activation of Ad-A$_{2A}$ receptors enhances GABA release (96-98). Thus, thermal prolongation of the LCR may depend on GABAergic and adenosinergic mechanisms specifically in the region of the NTS.

The apparent role of GABA in the thermal prolongation of the LCR led us to test the hypotheses that [1] activation of GABA receptors in the NTS should prolong the LCR even when body temperature is not elevated; [2] activation of Ad-A$_{2A}$ receptors should prolong the LCR in the absence of any elevation of body temperature; and [3] Ad-A$_{2A}$-receptor-dependent normothermic prolongation of the LCR within the NTS should be prevented by blocking GABA$_A$ receptors (104). We studied decerebrate piglets aged between P3 to P8 days. Nipecotic acid blocks reuptake of GABA by GABA transporter proteins and may, at higher concentrations, directly activate GABA$_A$ receptors (105). We injected nipecotic acid unilaterally into the caudal NTS and found that the LCR duration increased more than twofold, even at normal body temperatures. When we focally micro-injected CGS-21680, an Ad-A$_{2A}$ receptor agonist, into the NTS, the LCR duration was prolonged, but the response was more variable than either the response to hyperthermia in the same animals or the response to nipecotic acid. To confirm that CGS-21680 treatment increased the duration of the LCR by modulation of extracellular GABA levels, we combined CGS-21680 with systemic administration of bicuculline, an antagonist of GABA$_A$ receptors. Bicuculline treatment alone did not alter the normothermic duration of the LCR, but the CGS-21680-mediated prolongation of the LCR was reversed after bicuculline treatment. Thus, CGS-21680 treatment during normothermia significantly increased the LCR duration, and bicuculline occluded the effect of CGS-21680 treatment, regardless of the order of treatment.

Based on the foregoing studies of both GABAergic and adenosinergic modulation of the LCR, and thermal prolongation of the LCR, it is our hypothesis that hyperthermia augments GABAergic neurotransmission within the NTS when the LCR is elicited, and activation of Ad-A$_{2A}$ receptors during hyperthermic conditions amplifies GABA release within the NTS. The results of these studies have been clear, but identification of the mechanism and site of action of these agents within the NTS is difficult. Within the NTS, there are second order neurons that are stimulated by sensory afferents (and some of these second order neurons are GABAergic), and there are many GABAergic interneurons in the NTS. Hence, there may be GABAergic inhibition of GABAergic second order neurons (a net excitatory influence) and GABAergic inhibition of glutamatergic second order neurons (an inhibitory or disfacilitatory influence).

As a consequence, it is difficult to dissect the synaptic mechanisms associated with experimental manipulation of GABA and GABA receptors. One possible scenario is that the second order neurons that elicit apnea and the LCR, which we believe are glutamatergic, are normally inhibited by eupneic breathing — the inappropriate emergence of apnea would disrupt the normal functions of eupnea. Therefore, we can imagine a reciprocal inhibitory relationship between apnea and eupnea, so that each activity inhibits the other, a supposition that is consistent with the observation that eupnea and apnea are mutually exclusive. Thus, when the LCR is elicited, in addition to activation of glutamatergic second order neurons that elicit the apnea, there are parallel inhibitory GABAergic processes acting on second order neurons within the NTS that normally drive or support eupnea, such as pump neurons, second order neurons receiving information from the carotid body, or $CO_2$-sensitive neurons within the NTS. To the extent that these eupnea-promoting processes, which must be inhibited to allow apnea to occur, were not inhibited following blockade of GABA receptors or Ad-A$_{2A}$ receptors in the NTS, the duration of LCR would tend to be shortened by the early re-emergence of eupnea. This is speculation, but the adenosinergic and GABAergic processes that we identified beg for a more complete explanation at the level of synaptic interactions within the NTS.

### Serotonin and the LCR

The NTS is among the regions of the brainstem where 5-HT receptor binding deficiencies have been observed in infants who died of SIDS (9, 106). The NTS receives projections from serotonergic neurons in the caudal raphe nuclei, and neurons in the NTS express 5-HT 1A, 1B, 2A, 3, 4, and 7 receptors (107-110). As discussed below, 5-HT makes an important contribution to autoresuscitation and arousal responses following apneas, and we wondered if 5-HT was also part of the recovery process from the apnea itself. Therefore, we tested the hypothesis that augmenting levels of serotonergic signaling in the brainstem of immature rats, particularly in the caudal NTS, would reduce the duration of the LCR (111).

To test this hypothesis, we elicited the LCR in anesthetized neonatal rats aged P9 to P17 before, and after, treatment with a variety of serotonergic agonists and antagonists. When 5-HT was micro-injected directly into the NTS, the LCR was significantly shortened. This effect cannot be attributed to 5-HT$_{1A}$ receptors, which are reduced in infants who died of SIDS (9), or to 5-HT$_2$ receptors, which are ubiquitous in the brainstem, since agonists of these receptor types did not modify the duration of the LCR. In contrast, 5-HT$_3$ receptors are present in the NTS and found presynaptically on C-fiber afferents. To assess the role of 5-HT$_3$ receptors in the serotonin-mediated shortening of the LCR, we elicited the LCR in animals that received either bilateral micro-injections of 24 mM 1-(3-chlorophenyl)-biguanide HCl (CPG), a 5-HT$_3$ agonist, or saline alone. The LCR duration was shortened significantly in the CPG-treated group, but not in the vehicle-treated group.

Most of the central 5-HT$_3$ expression appears to be presynaptic on glutamatergic vagal afferents, but, given the idea that the second order neurons mediating the LCR are glutamatergic (112-114), it is difficult to imagine how greater activity of these second order neurons could shorten the LCR. Therefore, we speculated that $5\text{-HT}_3$ receptors mediating the LCR shortening are presynaptic receptors on vagal afferent fibers synapsing on to GABAergic interneurons in the NTS, and that $5\text{-HT}_3$ activation increases synaptic calcium levels and enhances GABA release onto the second order glutamatergic neurons mediating the LCR, thereby inhibiting them and terminating the apnea (111). GABAergic neurons are ubiquitous in the NTS, and many of these neurons are interneurons within the NTS — ideally suited, when activated, to inhibit the activity of other second order neurons within the NTS. Therefore, it is our hypothesis that C-fiber afferents are segregated into at least two classes: one population targets excitatory glutamatergic neurons, while the other population targets GABAergic neurons. This supposition will require electrophysiological confirmation.

## Caudal raphe serotonin and the LCR

The foregoing studies raise the question: where does the 5-HT targeting the $5\text{-HT}_3$ receptors come from? The raphe pallidus and raphe obscurus send many projections to the NTS, and these projections enter the NTS near its rostral extent but travel to projection sites caudally beyond the obex (115). Therefore, we tested the hypothesis that activation of neurons within the caudal raphe would shorten the LCR in rat pups by a serotonergic mechanism involving $5\text{-HT}_3$ receptors located in the NTS (116). We studied anesthetized rat pups ranging in age from P9 to P17. We made micro-injections into the commissural region of the NTS and into the caudal raphe. Micro-injection of α-amino-3-hydroxy-5-methyl-4-isoxazolepropionic acid (AMPA), a glutamate agonist, into the caudal raphe significantly shortened the LCR duration. The results of this experiment indicate that activation of neurons within the caudal raphe can shorten the LCR duration, but there are both serotonergic and non-serotonergic neurons in the caudal raphe, and the response to AMPA injection cannot be attributed to any specific neuronal type based on these findings. Therefore, we micro-injected ondansetron, a selective $5\text{-HT}_3$ receptor antagonist, bilaterally in the NTS to determine whether blocking $5\text{-HT}_3$ receptors would prevent the shortening of the LCR mediated by AMPA injected into the caudal raphe. Vehicle micro-injections into the NTS did not alter the ability of AMPA micro-injected into the caudal raphe to shorten the duration of the LCR following injection of water into the larynx (Figure 33.3). In contrast, AMPA micro-injected into the caudal raphe had no significant effect on the LCR duration in animals given bilateral micro-injections of ondansetron into the NTS. Thus, AMPA-mediated activation of serotonergic neurons within the caudal raphe leads to release of 5-HT in the NTS where it interacts with $5\text{-HT}_3$ receptors to shorten the LCR.

The raphe obscurus is the most likely nuclear origin for the neurons that were excited by AMPA. The raphe obscurus is located in the midline and extends rostrocaudally through a large extent of the medulla from the vicinity of the facial nucleus to the obex. Even though the micro-injection sites were concentrated in the region of the raphe

**A**

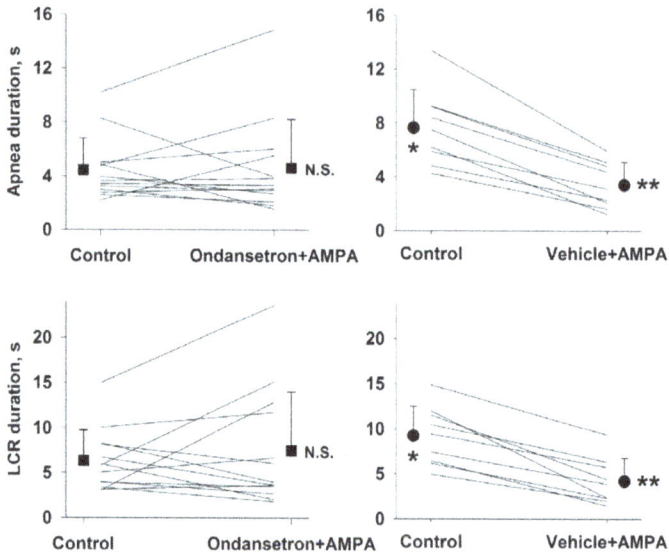

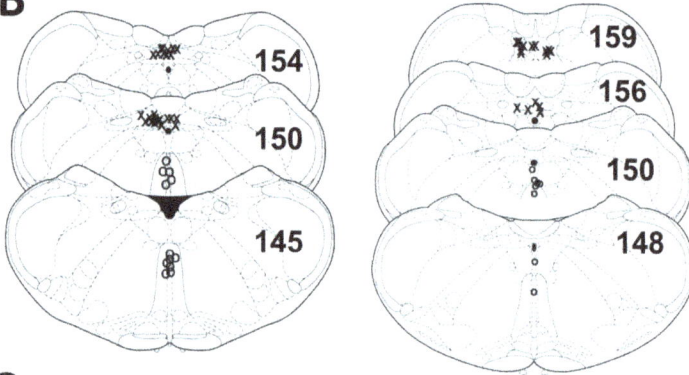

**B**

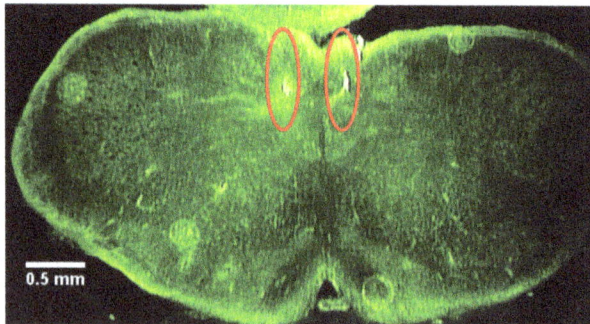

**C**

SIDS — SUDDEN INFANT AND EARLY CHILDHOOD DEATH

Figure 33.3 (left): The effect of focal injection of 50 nL of 100 uM s-AMPA into raphe obscurus after bilateral injection of 50 nL of ondansetron or 50 nL of vehicle into the NTS. (A) Response to injections on apnea or LCR duration. The sites of micro-injections into both the NTS ("X") and the caudal raphe ("O") are shown in the anatomical schematic figures in the middle panel. The plate number from Paxinos and Watson (117) is indicated on each schematic section. A representative photomicrograph of a single section though the NTS is shown to demonstrate how the sites of micro-injection were identified by the presence of fluorescent microbeads (C). (n.s. = not statistically significant from the pretreatment control condition; * = p<0.05.) (Reproduced with permission from (116).)

obscurus, we suspect that other caudal raphe nuclei containing serotonergic neurons (i.e. the raphe magnus and raphe pallidus, which also send projections to the NTS (118)) may also play a role in terminating apneas and restoring eupnea.

We believe that terminating apnea is an essential first step in restoring eupnea. The reflex apnea elicited by the LCR has been called post-inspiratory apneusis, and until the apparently excitatory effects of apnea producing second order neurons in the NTS on post-inspiratory neurons are terminated, eupnea cannot be restored. Thus, two things must occur to allow the restoration of normal breathing following elicitation of the LCR (and likely other apneas). First, the apnea-generating second order neurons in the NTS must be inhibited or disfacilitated, and second, other respiratory neurons that usually sustain eupnea must be activated. Termination of severe apneas also relies on autoresuscitation (119), which occurs when brain oxygen levels get so low that gasping emerges. This is followed by restoration of eupnea and arousal if gasping restores oxygenation. We believe that gasping, autoresuscitation, termination of apnea, restoration of eupnea, and arousal are mechanistically separable processes (120). Inherent to this description of the sequence of autoresuscitation, restoration of eupnea, and arousal is the idea that the recovery from apnea begins caudally in the brainstem and moves rostrally to completion when cortical arousal and wakefulness are achieved. Serotonin, arising in the caudal raphe, seems to provide important organizing inputs along the entire caudal to rostral axis of the autoresuscitation to arousal process. In the context of our two-step hypothesis of SIDS, 5-HT may have a variety of beneficial effects. Serotonin may terminate reflex apneas by activating 5-HT$_3$ receptors in the NTS; it may participate in restoring eupnea by acting on 5-HT$_2$ and 5-HT$_4$ receptors in the ventral medulla (121, 122); it may aid in autoresuscitation as experimentally augmenting serotonergic function restored effective autoresuscitation in 5-HT-deficient mice (123); and it may be associated with arousal from sleep (124), the state in which SIDS appears to occur most commonly.

Cortical arousal depends on an ascending arousal system that originates in the rostral pons and includes the parabrachial nucleus, which projects to the basal forebrain, which in turn projects to the cortex (125). The parabrachial nucleus seems to be an important integration site of arousing stimuli related to hypercapnia, which accompanies prolonged apneas (126). The parabrachial nucleus also receives serotonergic inputs from the raphe nuclei, including the dorsal raphe (127, 128); and serotonergic inputs interacting with 5-HT$_{2A}$ receptors are required for arousal from hypercapnia (129, 130). Since systemic administration of 5-HT$_{2A}$ agonists restored the arousal response in transgenic mice lacking serotonergic neurons, the restoration of arousal does not seem to depend on the hypercapnic sensitivity of serotonergic neurons (126). Thus rostral serotonergic projections from the caudal raphe may have at least three separable functions, each associated with a different set of serotonergic receptor subtypes, and each associated with a different target region of the brain.

### Modifications to the LCR by hypercapnia and hypoxia

#### Hypercapnia and the LCR

Apnea is accompanied by hypoxia and hypercapnia, which get worse the longer the apnea persists. Moreover, sleep recordings of infants who died of SIDS reveal antecedent hypoxia before respiration ceases. Therefore, we studied the interactions of hypoxia and hypercapnia with the LCR to see if either of these conditions made the LCR more "exuberant", as Wolf first suggested for the diving reflex (35). We first examined the effect of modifying the sensitivity of the respiratory system to carbon dioxide ($CO_2$). We studied the LCR in intact piglets, aged P3 to P16, and dialyzed muscimol (a GABA$_A$ agonist that inhibits the activity of many neurons) into the rostroventral medulla (RVM), in order to assess the impact of decreased ventilatory $CO_2$ sensitivity on the duration of the LCR during wakefulness and sleep. The RVM includes many of the nuclei in which decreased neurotransmitter receptor binding was found in infants dying of the SIDS, and the RVM in piglets may be homologous with parts of the arcuate nucleus in humans. Inhibition of neurons within the RVM following dialysis of 10 mM muscimol reduced the ventilatory response to 5% inhaled $CO_2$ in neonatal piglets during wakefulness and non-rapid eye movement (NREM) sleep (131). Cooling of the ventral medullary surface enhanced respiratory inhibition following superior laryngeal nerve stimulation in anesthetized piglets (132). Therefore, we tested the hypothesis that muscimol dialysis in the RVM would enhance the inhibitory action of the LCR on respiration in neonatal piglets. The LCR elicited by water was prolonged during sleep, particularly during REM sleep; muscimol dialyzed into the RVM prolonged the LCR elicited by water injected into the larynx. Arousal from sleep in piglets was significantly more likely after injecting water rather than saline into the larynx, unlike human infants, in whom arousal is equally likely following water or saline instilled above the larynx (133). Arousal in the piglets was also more likely from NREM sleep than REM sleep.

In general, there is an inverse relationship between the duration of the LCR and respiratory drive in unanesthetized animals; and the progressive prolongation of the reflex from wakefulness to NREM sleep and then to REM sleep might reflect the state-related reduction in the respiratory drive to breathe. The sleep-state-related changes in ventilation are also correlated with sleep-state-related changes in $CO_2$

chemosensitivity (131): the ventilatory response to $CO_2$ is least during REM sleep, intermediate in NREM sleep, and slightly greater during wakefulness. Furthermore, the duration of the LCR was reduced in anesthetized humans (134) and anesthetized piglets (135) during exposure to hypercapnia, and hypercapnia blunted the inhibition of ventilation associated with superior laryngeal stimulate in anesthetized piglets (132). Thus, the mechanism of action of muscimol to prolong the LCR may be correlated with reduced sensitivity to $CO_2$.

While muscimol dialyzed into the RVM prolonged the LCR, it did not modify the arousal response to LCR stimulation. This implies that the neurons in the RVM that were inhibited by muscimol did not play a significant role in the arousal response to the LCR. This is interesting, as the arousal response seems to be more dependent on 5-HT derived from medullary neurons than on the $CO_2$ sensitivity of these serotonergic neurons (126).

We also examined the influence of hypocapnia, mild hypercapnia, and hypoxia on the LCR in decerebrate piglets artificially ventilated at a constant frequency and tidal volume with controlled gas mixtures. We examined the influence of hypocapnia and hypercapnia to test both whether hypocapnia would prolong the LCR and whether hypercapnia would shorten the LCR, as has been reported in unanesthetized animals (132, 135). We elicited the LCR by injecting 0.1 ml of water into the larynx. Mild hypocapnia ($\sim$4% $CO_2$) tended to prolong the LCR, and eliciting the LCR under mildly hypercapnic conditions (end-tidal $CO_2$ = $\sim$6%) reduced the duration of the LCR compared to eucapnic or hypocapnic conditions in the same animal. The duration of the LCR was inversely related to the end-tidal $CO_2$ concentration in these experiments, which is consistent with the idea that increasing respiratory drive acts to reduce the inhibitory effectiveness of the laryngeal protective reflex. Lawson (135) also found that the duration of phrenic apnea following electrical stimulation of the SLN was greater under hypocapnic conditions than it was under hypercapnic conditions in anesthetized, vagotomized, paralyzed, ventilated piglets. Litmanovitz et al. (132) reported similar responses of the diaphragm EMG in anesthetized, spontaneously breathing piglets. Bongianni et al. (136) found a comparable response of phrenic activity during hypocapnia in anesthetized adult cats, but did not find a shortening of reflex apnea under hypercapnic conditions.

To result in apnea, an inhibitory reflex must overcome the individual's underlying drive to breathe. Thus it is not surprising that when respiratory drive is reduced by hypocapnia (135) or general anesthesia (42, 137), laryngeal reflex apnea may be long-lasting and occasionally fatal. In contrast, hypercapnia (132, 138), exercise (139), and aminophylline (42) increase the drive to breathe, and these interventions shorten the duration of the LCR. We find little evidence that hypercapnia contributes to the onset of apnea or apneic prolongation, and little support for the idea that the hypercapnic aspects of rebreathing may enhance asphyxial stress, as some have suggested (140, 141). Hypercapnia seems to provide consistent excitatory drive to breathe that stabilizes respiratory activity, shortens apnea duration, shortens the duration of the LCR, and leads to arousal. Hypoxia, however, is more likely to promote and enhance apnea in neonates.

## Hypoxia and the LCR

Hypoxia may prolong the LCR in anesthetized piglets and exacerbate the apnea and bradycardia associated with the reflex (142), but other studies, also in piglets, suggest that hypoxia shortened apnea duration (143) following electrical stimulation of the superior laryngeal nerve in decerebrate piglets (144). However, it prolongs the apnea associated with laryngeal infusion of water in infants (145). It is appealingly simple to suggest that the duration of the LCR is inversely related to the level of respiratory drive, but the reality is more complicated. In newborns, breathing is stimulated by hypoxic activation of the peripheral chemoreceptors (146), but ventilation is depressed by the direct action of hypoxia on brain function (147). The duality of hypoxic effects on respiratory activity is apparent in the time-dependent, biphasic respiratory response to sustained hypoxia — early ventilatory stimulation is followed by ventilatory depression, particularly in newborns and infants (148, 149). With respect to the LCR, hypoxia becomes progressively more severe as the apneic time becomes prolonged; by contrast, the partial pressure of arterial $CO_2$ only rises to approach the value in mixed venous blood (150). There is a complex asymmetry of effect of developing hypoxia and hypercapnia during an apnea: the initial excitatory effects of hypoxia quickly pass and the adverse inhibitory effects of hypoxia grow as the apnea persists, but the arousing, excitatory effects of hypercapnia are more limited and develop only slowly as the apnea persists.

When we studied the impact of hypoxia on the duration of the LCR in decerebrate piglets, we found that among piglets exposed to 10% or 12% hypoxia during each test period, the LCR duration and the longest apnea elicited by intralaryngeal water increased during hypoxic exposure in some animals and tended to increase as the hypoxic exposure lengthened. This is consistent with roll-off of the hypoxic respiratory stimulation in early stages of the apnea and central depression that developed as the apnea associated with the LCR persisted, but the data were more variable than during hypercapnia and not statistically significant (151).

Other investigators have found similarly mixed results with respect to hypoxic effects on the duration of the LCR. The duration of apnea following intralaryngeal water instillation has generally been shortened by acute hypoxia (152-154), although not significantly at all ages. The apneic response to laryngeal stimulation during acute hypoxia may be attenuated by carotid chemoreceptor-mediated ventilatory drive, but may be enhanced by the attendant hypocapnia (153). The apneas that predominate early in life can be long-lasting and can result in repeated episodes of profound hypoxemia and hypercapnia. As hypoxemia is itself an inhibitor of respiratory drive in neonates (155), it is possible that LCR-induced apnea could lead to a downward spiral of increasing hypoxic inhibition that ultimately leads to death, especially if serotonergic arousal responses are deficient (30, 111, 116). Wennergren and colleagues (145) measured the apneic responses to intralaryngeal water instillation in 12 human infants during normoxia and mild hypoxia (usually 15% fractional inspired oxygen; FIO$_2$). The average apneic duration was 2.6 seconds in normoxia and 5.3 seconds in hypoxia (p<0.01). Strikingly, one 4-week-old boy had 15 seconds of apnea during normoxia, which increased to 30 seconds during hypoxia; this child died unexpectedly six weeks later, with a diagnosis of SIDS.

## Risk factors for SIDS reflected in the LCR

### Maternal tobacco smoke exposure increases the duration of the LCR

Maternal tobacco smoke exposure during pregnancy is a well-recognized risk factor for SIDS. Therefore, we combined two epidemiological risk factors for SIDS (maternal smoking and thermal stress) in rat pups to test the hypothesis that maternal exposure to cigarette smoke during pregnancy would enhance the thermal prolongation of the LCR (156). We exposed pregnant dams starting on the third day of pregnancy to combined mainstream and side-stream cigarette smoke generated by a Teague model TE-10z smoking machine for four hours a day, five days a week, to achieve a moderate level of maternal smoke exposure. Mothers of rat pups in the control group were exposed to clean air in the same room. The pups were studied at intervals between the postnatal ages of 4 and 15 days (P4 and P15). The rat pups were anesthetized with urethane and chloralose, and the LCR was elicited by instilling small volumes of water into the larynx. Hyperthermia prolonged the LCR duration significantly more in the smoke-exposed pups compared to the control animals. Under baseline conditions, before the pups were made hyperthermic, both measures of the LCR were most prolonged in the youngest animals and then diminished slightly, but significantly, as postnatal age increased (see Figure 33.4). There was no significant difference in the age-related normothermic baseline response pattern between the two treatment groups. Thus, maternal smoke exposure alone had no effect on the LCR under baseline conditions and no effect on the age-related shortening of the LCR.

However, the thermal prolongation of the LCR was exaggerated in the young pups exposed to cigarette smoke during pregnancy. Thus, gestational smoke exposure of mother rats enhanced the hyperthermic prolongation of the LCR in the youngest pups, but this effect waned with age and was not apparent by day P15. The results of this study confirm our earlier report (157) that the duration of the LCR was enhanced by mild hyperthermia in young rat pups, as previously shown in piglets (61, 63, 95, 103), and that the enhancement was greatest in the youngest animals studied. The age-related response pattern is consistent with previous reports in other species that the duration and manifestation of the LCR diminish as animals mature (40, 42, 158-160).

The demonstration that maternal smoke exposure in rats increases the duration of reflex apnea in the offspring may provide an important mechanistic link between the LCR, thermal stress, maternal cigarette smoking, and the pathogenesis of SIDS. These

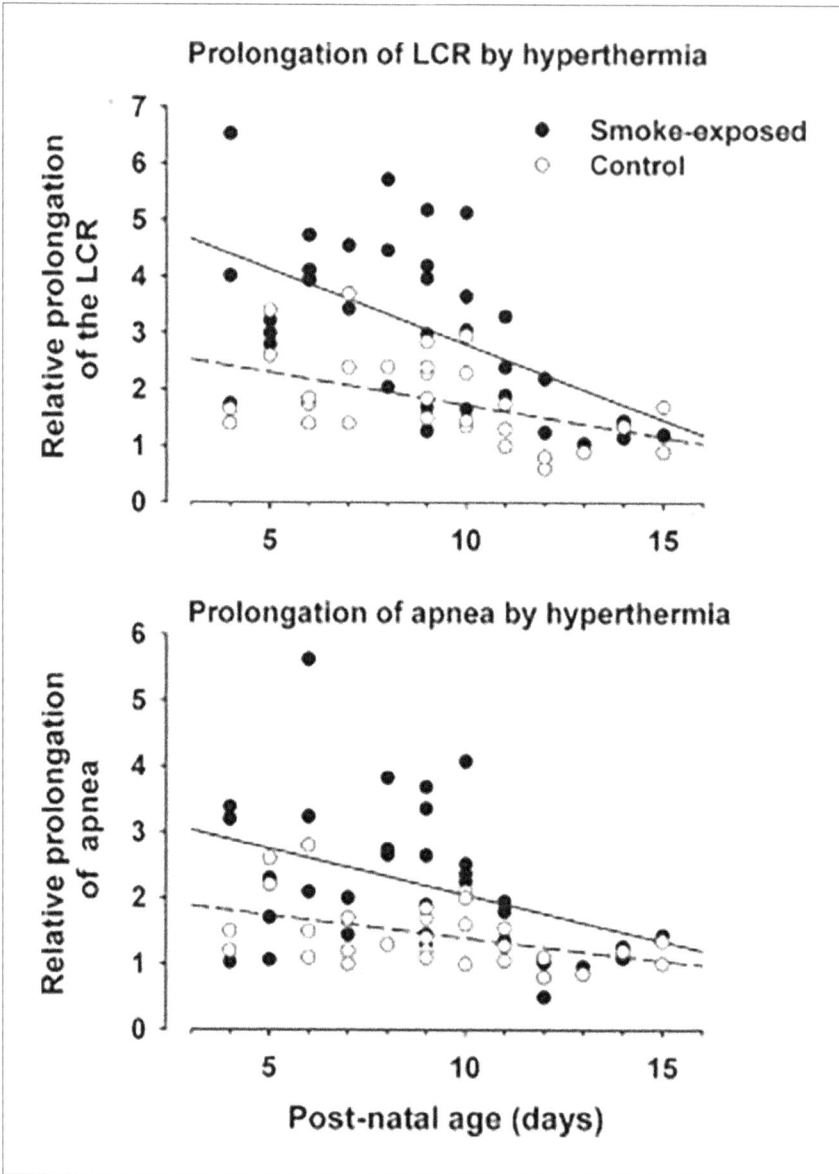

Figure 33.4: Maternal smoking increases the laryngeal chemoreflex. Prolongation of the LCR (upper panel) and the longest associated apnea (lower panel) by hyperthermia as a function of age in pups of dams exposed during gestation to cigarette smoke (•) and controls (o). Each point indicates the ratio of the average of hyperthermic tests to the average of control and recovery tests for one animal. The regression lines for exposed (solid lines) and control (dashed lines) animals are significantly different in each panel, indicating that the hyperthermic prolongation of the LCR and the longest associated apnea are both exaggerated in the younger animals by maternal exposure to cigarette smoke during pregnancy. (Reproduced with permission from (156).)

findings suggest that, insofar as maternal cigarette smoke exposure enhances the risk of reflex apnea, it does so through a thermally sensitive process (which, based on previous studies, is likely to involve TRPV1 receptors).

*Gestational nicotine exposure enhances thermal prolongation of the LCR*

The effect of maternal cigarette smoke exposure on the LCR in rat pups raises the question: what component of cigarette smoke is responsible for the effects on the LCR in neonatal rats? Therefore, we worked to determine whether nicotine administration to pregnant rats would alter the LCR or its hyperthermic exaggeration in the pups. In this study, pregnant Sprague-Dawley rats on the third day of gestation (G3) were anesthetized briefly with halothane, and an osmotic minipump was implanted subcutaneously in the interscapular region. The pumps provided a dose of nicotine that averaged 6.5 mg/kg per day. Both nicotine-treated and control animals delivered their pups on G21, and the pups were kept with the dams and studied at intervals between P4 and P12. The LCR was significantly prolonged when body temperature was increased in both control and nicotine-exposed rat pups. However, the duration of the LCR was significantly longer in the nicotine-exposed animals compared to the control animals, and the thermal prolongation of the LCR was significantly enhanced in the nicotine-exposed animals. Under normothermic conditions, the LCR duration was longest in the youngest animals and diminished significantly with age.

These results are consistent with previous studies. Nicotine administered directly to neonatal lambs (154) and piglets (77) prolonged and accentuated the LCR. In mechanistic terms, stimulation of nicotinic acetylcholine receptors on presynaptic nerve terminals increases GABA release by brainstem neurons (161). Elevation of GABA, or its agonists, increases the density and activity of $GABA_A$ receptors in intact brain (162) and cultured cells (163). Thus, as proposed by Luo and associates (164), prenatal (or early postnatal) nicotine exposure may lead to an up-regulation of brainstem GABA release and/or the density of $GABA_A$ receptors, enhancing the GABAergic inhibition of breathing elicited by the LCR and/or its exaggeration during hyperthermia (93-95). Thus it seems likely that maternal cigarette smoke exposure and intrauterine nicotine exposure enhance thermal prolongation of the LCR through a GABAergic mechanism.

## Autoresuscitation in SIDS: A model for animal studies

Autoresuscitation represents a final defense against hypoxia sufficient to depress respiratory activity in neonates (165). Autoresuscitation occurs when early defense mechanisms (e.g. arousal) are absent or when they fail to terminate hypoxia apnea (50, 165, 166). Gasping is critical in autoresuscitation during apnea in human infants (166-168), and failure to autoresuscitate may play a role in some, or many, SIDS deaths, even though there is no failure of gasping in the great majority of SIDS deaths (50). Human studies suggest that autoresuscitation by hypoxic gasping is impaired to some degree in infants who died of SIDS compared to infants dying from other causes (25, 26, 50, 169).

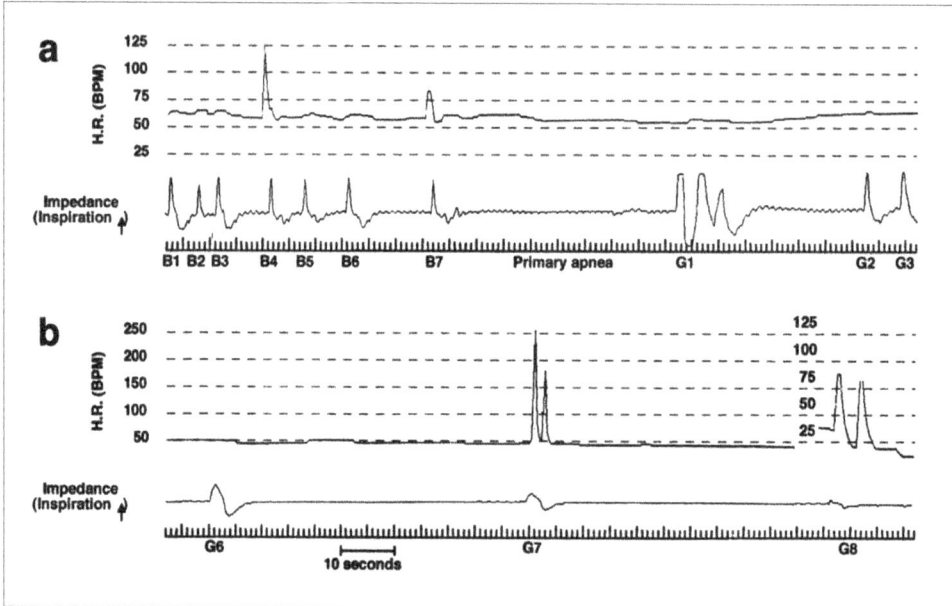

Figure 33.5: Two segments of event recordings, uninterrupted by artificial resuscitation efforts in an infant diagnosed as having SIDS.
A. Onset of apnea and gasping. Hyperpneic breaths (B1-B7) are followed by 35 seconds of "primary" apnea. Gasps (G1-G3) follow "primary" apnea. G1 is a "triple" gasp. Note similarity in wave configuration between hyperpneic breaths and gasps (B7-G2). Onset of hypoxic gasping is defined by occurrence of primary apnea, in accordance with past studies in animal models (see text).
B. Terminal gasps. This section of tracing occurs about 10 minutes after onset of primary apnea. Note decreasing amplitude and altered configuration of these terminal gasps. G8 is last gasp. (Reproduced with permission from (25).)

In human infants, severe hypoxia and asphyxia can be induced by rebreathing, obstructive apnea, upper airway compression in the facedown position, or reflex apnea (25, 27, 33, 140, 170-172). If hypoxia is sustained, cortical activity in the CNS is depressed, and most brainstem-mediated reflexes cease to function. Profound brainstem hypoxia triggers a set of emergency reflexes which elicit intermittent hypoxic gasps that, in the absence of compromised lung or cardiovascular function, provide sufficient oxygen to the brain to restore normal cardiorespiratory function. A typical autoresuscitation response to asphyxia or severe hypoxia includes four stages: [1] hyperpneic breaths; [2] primary hypoxic apnea; [3] gasping; and then, if autoresuscitation is unsuccessful, [4] terminal apnea (Figure 33.5). If autoresuscitation is successful, there is restoration of eupnea and reversal of bradycardia (25, 34, 173, 174). Infants who subsequently died of SIDS often had episodes of tachycardia and bradycardia for hours or days before death, along with recurrent hypoxic episodes and frequent gasping, suggesting that recurrent autoresuscitation events occurred until a final autoresuscitation failed (25, 169). Therefore, the inability to autoresuscitate from severe hypoxia and asphyxia is a common mechanism preceding death in SIDS (25, 30, 33, 141, 169, 175).

Failure to autoresuscitate from profound hypoxia may result from a lack of reflex responses that normally protect infants from the profound hypoxia associated with apnea (140, 170). These deficits in cardiorespiratory and autonomic control have been associated with abnormalities in the brain 5-HT system that have been documented in a majority of SIDS cases studied (9, 14, 15, 106).

Studies of autoresuscitation are rare in humans, and the information gleaned from studies in human infants is based on observation alone. Therefore, animal studies have been used to study the properties of autoresuscitation, cardiorespiratory recovery, and arousal responses from repetitive severe hypoxia or asphyxia. These studies have tested the hypothesis that impaired neurotransmitter function adversely affects the capacity to autoresuscitate from profound hypoxia. The studies have been carried out in animals at ages that reflect the occurrence of SIDS in humans, which are generally P7 to P15 in rat pups. In addition, these animal studies have permitted investigators to identify the possible "predictors of risks" and evaluate the potential rescue or preventative treatments that might be used in infants at risk for SIDS.

Most of these animal studies have focused on the deficiency of central 5-HT systems due to this being the most consist pathological finding in human infants who died of SIDS (176, 177) and asphyxia (17). In neonatal rodents, a loss of brainstem 5-HT in utero, or in the early postnatal period, compromises anoxia-induced gasping and the recovery of normal heart rates and breathing following the re-oxygenation initiated by gasping (123, 178-180).

In many animal studies (171, 180-182), autoresuscitation was tested by applying single or multiple episodes of anoxic gas (97% $N_2$/3% $CO_2$) to animals until primary apnea occurred (when the animal was not breathing and had been motionless for 5 seconds), at which point the gas was changed back to room air. Thus, when gasping developed, each animal was able to inhale room air and restore normal levels of oxygenation. Multiple episodes of anoxia were repeated at ~5-minute intervals from the time that respiratory rate and heart rate returned to ≥60% of baseline (171, 180). The number of autoresuscitative episodes varied depending on the study, and 4-15 serial autoresuscitative trials were common in recent studies (180, 183).

## Autoresuscitation in 5-HT-deficient transgenic neonatal animals

Transgenic mice with deficient 5-HT during the prenatal period have been used to determine whether the neonates born with prenatal 5-HT deficiency have abnormal autoresuscitation during the postnatal period (123, 178, 179, 183). *Pet-1* transcription deficient (*Pet-1*[-/-]) rat pups lack ~90% of their 5-HT content in the brainstem due to a 60-70% loss of 5-HT-producing neurons in CNS (179, 184). The *Pet-1*[-/-] rat pups exhibit spontaneous bradycardias in room air at P5 and P12 (185) and delayed gasping in response to a single episode of anoxia at P4.5 and P9.5 (178, 179). The failed autoresuscitative episodes were characterized by impaired gasping and failed restoration of heart rate (Figure 33.6) (179), a phenotype that mimics the pattern of autoresuscitative dysfunction seen in recordings from infants who died of SIDS (25, 26, 169). Pet-1 transcription factor is critical to induce brain 5-HT synthesis and 5-HT reuptake and co-ordinates post-mitotic expression of genes necessary for maturation of 5-HT neurons (184, 186). Disruption of gene expression patterns in Pet-1$^{-/-}$ 5-HT neurons blocks functional maturation of 5-HT neurons and results in reduced innervation of the usual serotonergic target fields (184, 186).

The question whether the observed autoresuscitation defects in Pet-1$^{-/-}$ mice were due specifically to a loss of 5-HT content, or to a loss of normal 5-HT neurons, in the CNS was addressed with several new transgenic mouse lines. In Pet1::Flpe-silenced and Slc6a4::cre-silenced transgenic mice, exocytic 5-HT release was impaired via conditional expression of the tetanus toxin light chain (tox) in raphe neurons expressing serotonergic drivers Pet1 or Slc6a4 (183). In both transgenic mouse models, Pet1 expression was normal, but ~35% and 75% of raphe neurons no longer expressed TPH2 in Pet1::Flpe-silenced and Slc6a4::cre-silenced animals, respectively. Silencing these fractions of raphe neurons in both models resulted in excessive mortality following exposure to repetitive anoxia at ages P5 and P8 due to severe defects in gasping and heart rate recovery (183). Similar failure of autoresuscitation was found in global TPH2 knockout mice (Tph$^{-/-}$), which lack more than 95% of brainstem 5-HT due to lack of the 5-HT synthetic enzyme (123). Restoration of 5-HT levels in the brainstem, following injection of 5-hydryoxytryptophan (5-HTP), a TPH2 and 5-HT precursor, significantly improved survival rates following repetitive anoxia episodes. Treatment with 5-HTP shortened the gasp latency and shortened the time to achieve effective cardiorespiratory recovery (123).

In summary, normal concentrations of central 5-HT are essential for normal autoresuscitation and spontaneous cardiorespiratory recovery from episodes of severe anoxia and primary apnea. Prenatal loss of 5-HT in the CNS can lead to compromised gasping and failed autoresuscitation in developing animals at a postnatal age in rats that seems to correspond to the peak incidence of SIDS in human infants. Thus the serotonergic defects identified in infants who died of SIDS and asphyxia may be responsible for the ineffective autoresuscitative efforts observed in sleep recordings of infants who died of SIDS.

### The effect of deficient 5-HT in the post-natal period on autoresuscitation

Investigators have also addressed the impact of 5-HT deficiency acquired after birth on autoresuscitation to assess its impact during this critical period of development. Pharmacological lesions of 5-HT neurons during the first week of life (P2-P3) were

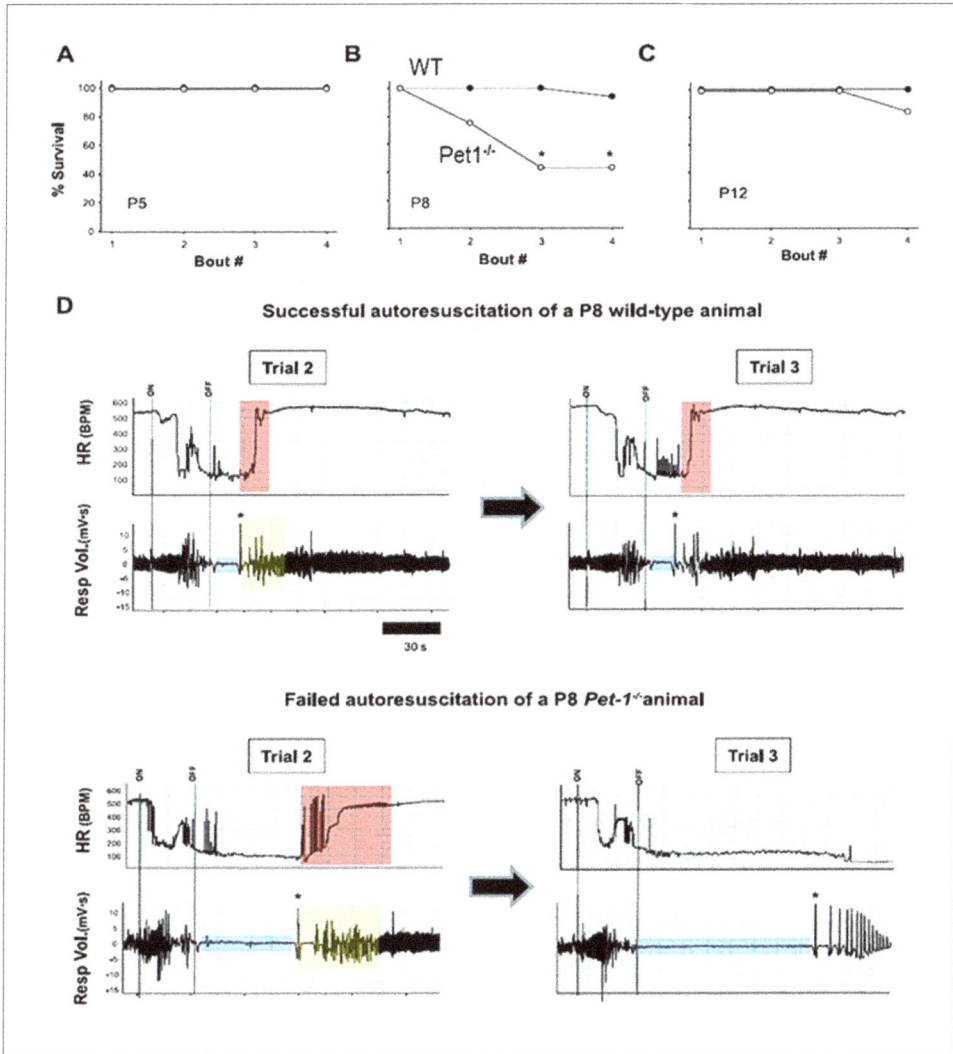

Figure 33.6: Autoresuscitation in a seretonin difeciency mouse model. *Pet-1⁻/⁻* mice (open circle) have highest autoresuscitation failure rate in response to episodic anoxia at P8 (B); compare to wild-type littermates (WT; dark circle). D = typical heart rate (HR) and respiratory volume (Resp Vol.) traces from a single WT animal (top) and a *Pet-1⁻/⁻* animal (bottom). Beginning (ON) and end (OFF) of anoxia is indicated by vertical lines. Despite robust gasping (first gasp indicated by *), the time required for the *Pet-1⁻/⁻* animal to recover 90% of the prehypoxic heart rate during the second trial is ~ three times that of the wild-type animal (compare region of heart rate trace shaded red for each animal), and completely fails during the third trial. Duration of hypoxic apnea (blue bar) and the time required to recover a normal breathing pattern (yellow bar) are also considerably longer in the *Pet-1⁻/⁻* animal. BPM = beats/min. (Reproduced with permission from (179).)

created by intracisternal injection of 5,7-dihydroxytryptamine (5,7-DHT), which resulted in an ~80% reduction of 5-HT content in the medulla and significantly impaired autoresuscitation in rat pups aged P7-P10 (180). The pups were exposed to a sequence of 15 episodes of anoxia, and only 25% of these 5-HT-deficient animals survived all 15 episodes, compared to 79% of control littermates. The 5,7-DHT treatment delayed the onset of gasping, delayed recovery of heart rate from hypoxia-induced bradycardia, and delayed recovery of eupnea following the primary hypoxic apnea (180). Depletion of brain 5-HT for a day during the second week of life (P8 to P13) via multiple systemic injections of 6-fluorotryptophan (6FL), a serotonin synthesis inhibitor, resulted in ~70% loss of 5-HT in the brainstem and also severely impaired autoresuscitation.

The failure of autoresuscitation in this model was characterized by a progressive deterioration of blood pressure and heart rate recovery during each successive episode of anoxia, despite the normal onset of gasping following the primary hypoxic apnea and a normal duration of gasping efforts (187). Thus normal concentrations of 5-HT in CNS are critical for the initiation of gasping and restoration of heart rate in response to anoxia during the first week of life and for maintenance and restoration of heart rate and blood pressure during the second week of life. Postnatal loss of 5-HT is sufficient both to compromise autoresuscitation in response to repeated episodes of environmental anoxia and to impair gasping, heart rate, and blood pressure recovery in response to repetitive episodes of anoxia. The fact that the loss of 5-HT in the postnatal period had similar effects on the process of resuscitation as the effect of prevention of formation of serotonin starting during embryogenesis in transgenic animals indicates that 5-HT itself is the key element in successful recovery from prolonged hypoxic and apneic episodes.

## Mechanisms underlying 5-HT deficiency and autoresuscitation during development

Gasping is generated by neurons within the pre-Bötzinger complex (188-191), which are disinhibited by profound hypoxia and which have a discharge pattern that is influenced by 5-HT (121, 192, 193). Studies in conscious 5-HT-deficient animals suggest that gasp initiation may occur without 5-HT; however, 5-HT is essential both for the maintenance of normal and sustained gasping and for the restoration of normal cardiorespiratory function following hypoxia and primary apnea during the first two weeks of life (123, 178-180, 183, 185, 187, 194). These findings are consistent with earlier studies in brain slices and brainstem-perfused preparations in which 5-HT was found to play a role in generation and maintenance of the respiratory rhythm (121, 195-197).

The role of 5-HT in autoresuscitation also appears to be age-dependent. In 5-HT-deficient rat and mouse pups, the age range of P8 to P13 appears to be a critical developmental period during which a brainstem 5-HT deficiency increases the risk of death during episodes of anoxia (123, 179, 180, 183, 185, 187). It is interesting that even transgenic animals with a severe and sustained lack of 5-HT cease to have problems with autoresuscitation as they mature. Some other aspects of development, which do not require 5-HT, must emerge, either as a normal part of the increasing complexity of brain development or as part of some compensatory response to 5-HT deficiency that stabilizes respiratory function, decreases the frequency of occurrence of hypoxic apneic episodes, and decreases the risk of death. These serotonin-deficient animals appear to outgrow the risk of death following hypoxic apneic episodes at an approximately similar developmental stage as the incidence of SIDS declines in human infants at risk of SIDS. Human infants retain the capacity to synthesize 5-HT, and if infants at risk for SIDS have large numbers of immature serotonergic neurons (9), these neurons may mature and produce normal levels of 5-HT, perhaps at the time that the risk of SIDS begins to decline, although such a process cannot explain the decline in autoresuscitative dysfunction in transgenic animals lacking 5-HT. The resolution of both spontaneous respiratory instability and the risk of apneic death in transgenic animals as these transgenic animals mature (178, 198, 199), suggests that the dominant effects of deficient 5-HT are due to 5-HT as a neurotransmitter and not 5-HT as a neuromodulator of trophic factors for other neurotransmitter systems.

Prenatal exposures to alcohol and cigarette smoke have a direct effect on neurotransmitter systems that are critical to homeostatic control in the developing human brain (200). Exposure to these substances also decreased the number of successful autoresuscitations in P1-P2 and P5-P6 pups (201). In rat pups born to mothers fed a tryptophan-deficient diet, the rat pups had a minor 5-HT deficiency in the medulla, and perinatal nicotine exposure impaired autoresuscitation in these rat pups at P10 (202). This suggests that an existing underlying vulnerability (i.e. 5-HT deficiency) and an exogenous stressor (i.e. nicotine) can adversely affect the ability to autoresuscitate from severe hypoxia and asphyxia in neonates at a critical age.

Further evidence of the importance of 5-HT as a neurotransmitter has emerged from efforts to treat the respiratory instability and deficient autoresuscitation responses to anoxia with deficient 5-HT (123, 179, 180). Treating 5-HT-deficient *Pet-1-/-* mice with caffeine (1, 5 and 10 mg/kg) can restore proper autoresuscitation (Figure 33.7) and increase the survival rate in response to repetitive anoxia (203). Restoration of 5-HT levels in the brainstem by supplying exogenous 5-HT in TPH2-deficient mice improved autoresuscitation success (123). Caffeine can increase brainstem 5-HT level in adult rats (204) and promote 5-HT-dependent respiratory long-term facilitation (205, 206). However, the cellular mechanisms through which caffeine restored autoresuscitation and promoted survival in these 5-HT-deficient mice may be more complex. It is likely that multiple neurotransmitters and neurotransmitter systems are involved in autoresuscitation. For example, adenosine and Ad-A$_1$ or Ad-A$_{2A}$-receptor receptors; glutamate and N-methyl-D-aspartate (NMDA) receptors; cholinergic receptors and GABA and GABA$_A$ receptors (207-210); and adenosine antagonists may decrease GABAergic function and increase glutamatergic function. Both may also foster successful autoresuscitation (100, 101, 210, 211). Nevertheless, the dominant finding

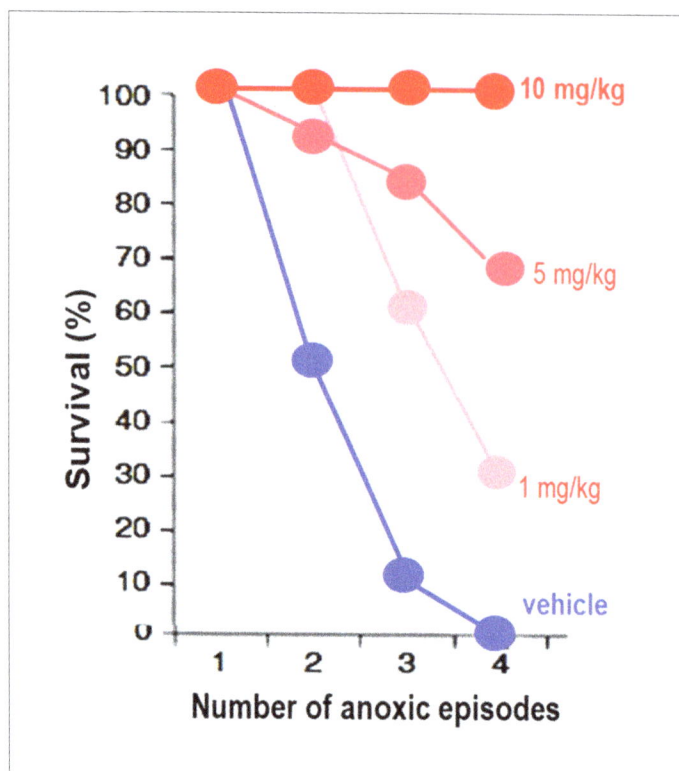

Figure 33.7: Caffeine administration in *Pet-1⁻/⁻* rodents. Caffeine dose-dependence hastens the onset of gasping, recovery of breathing, and restoration of heart rate in *Pet-1⁻/⁻* rodents, thereby improving survival across asphyxial episodes. (Adapted from Figure 1 in (203).)

in studies of animals with 5-HT deficiency, regardless of cause, is that normal central 5-HT levels are essential to maintain normal autoresuscitation and cardiorespiratory response to repetitive severe hypoxia and asphyxia in neonates. It seems inescapable that 5-HT deficiency represents an essential vulnerability in infants at risk for SIDS and infants with this vulnerability will have greater difficulty responding to apneic and hypoxic events, especially during sleep, when arousal is such an important part of responding to hypoxia (212).

## Arousal Responses

### Arousal and SIDS

Arousal failure has been implicated in the pathogenesis of SIDS for at least three decades (213-216). The usual definition of "arousal" or "awakening" from sleep involves a constellation of physiologic responses including increases in heart rate, blood pressure, and muscle tone; a sustained inspiratory effort or breathing pause; and activation of the EEG. Thach and colleagues have described a stereotypical sequence of arousal events in human infants that begins with an augmented breath, followed by a startle with changes in heart rate, followed by EEG changes. This sequence of arousal events is similar in quiet (NREM) sleep (QS) and active (REM) sleep (AS) (217, 218). Similar stereotypical changes, either occurring spontaneously or in response to hypoxia and/or hypercapnia, have been observed in piglets and rodent pups and have been the basis for arousal identification in the developing mammal (219-221). Autonomic or subcortical components of the arousal response involving changes in heart rate, blood pressure, and upper airway control may serve to provide cardiovascular support to a full cortical arousal, or maintain airway patency, particularly during obstructive apnea, without fully disrupting sleep (222, 223).

In a study of spontaneous arousals in piglets identified both behaviorally and with a wavelet analysis, we determined that when EEG changes were accompanied by heart rate and/or blood pressure changes, the autonomic changes always preceded the EEG changes (221). From these data, it is tempting to hypothesize that spontaneous arousals originate in the brainstem. The EEG and heart rate changes and their temporal relationships in piglets and human infants are strikingly similar. Figure 33.8 shows

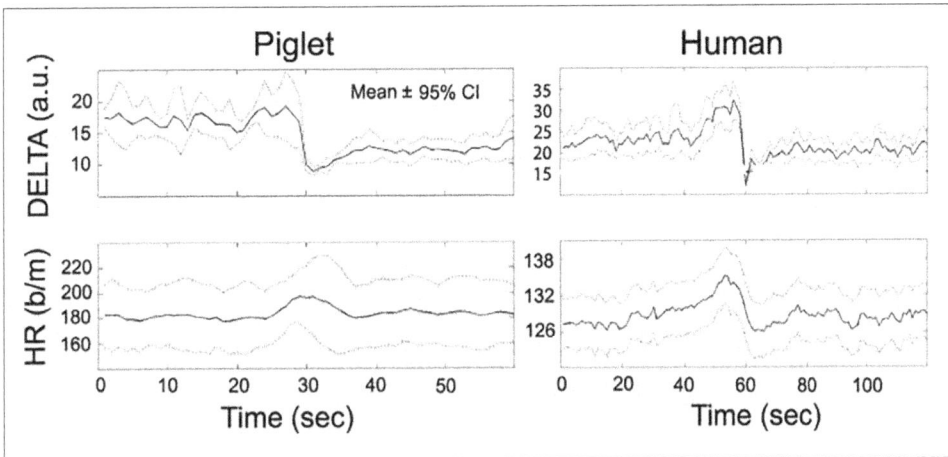

Figure 33.8: Delta activity and heart rate activity during spontaneous arousals in the piglet and human infant. Values of delta activity (1-4 Hz) derived from wavelet analyses (upper panels) and heart rate (lower panels) are ensemble averages triggered on the heart rate peak derived from 75 spontaneous arousals in five piglets (left panels) and 73 spontaneous arousals in a single 3-month-old infant (right panels). Values shown are means ±95% confidence intervals. Note that the increase in heart rate precedes the fall in delta power. HR = heart rate; DELTA = delta power or activity. (Adapted from (224).)

changes in EEG delta power and heart rate in 75 spontaneous arousals in five piglets compared to 73 arousals in a single 3-month-old infant (224).

## Arousal to hypoxia in developing animals

In contrast to findings in human infants where arousal is blunted during QS, newborn and young animals exhibit delayed or impaired arousal during AS. Studies in newborn calves (225) and lambs (226, 227) show that the arousal response to hypoxia occurs at a lower oxygen saturation ($SaO_2$) during AS. In more altricial species, including mice and rats, pups transition rapidly between QS, AS, and wakefulness, and there is no state-related electro-cortical activity discernible before ~P11 (228, 229). Thus it is not possible to study hypoxia-related arousal separately during QS and AS in these species. This continues to become difficult to study until sleep cycling becomes less frequent. In these models, arousal is most often detected using behavioral criteria, sometimes with the addition of neck EMG (230, 231).

We examined arousal using behavioral criteria in response to 5% oxygen in P5, P15, and P25 rat pups. In all cases the change to hypoxia occurred when the animal was in a state of "quiet immobility" or putative QS. Mean arousal latencies ranged from 20 to 26 seconds for the three ages, and mean $SaO_2$ at arousal was between 91% and 93%. Importantly, however, after the onset of hypoxia but before arousal, sleep transitioned to AS (evidenced by behavioral criteria) nearly 100% of the time at P5, and 50% of the time at P15. Neither arousal latencies nor $SaO_2$ at arousal were different among the three ages. In all cases, arousal latencies in response to hypoxia were shorter than the interval between spontaneous arousals (220).

In human infants, arousal to wakefulness in response to hypercapnia appears to be more robust than to hypoxia and does not seem to be affected by age at least from 1 to 13 weeks postnatal age (232). In tracheotomized lambs, the probability of arousal in response to hypercapnia was greater during QS compared to AS (233, 234). Another study in lambs showed that arousal latencies during hyperoxic hypercapnia were significantly longer in AS (58±17 seconds) compared to QS (21±10 sec) (235). In P15 rat pups, during putative QS, we found that arousal latency in response to 8% $CO_2$ in room air was 34.7±2.3 seconds, and that the $CO_2$ arousal threshold was 4.4±0.3%) (236).

## Intermittent hypoxia and arousal habituation

Both premature and full term newborn infants, and children with obstructive sleep apnea (OBS), are frequently exposed to intermittent hypoxia (IH) and re-oxygenation, and this adversely affects executive function and cognition (237-239). In animal studies, exposure to IH in the neonatal period results in long-lasting effects, which include adverse effects on cardiorespiratory control (240, 241), neuropathologic and neurocognitive deficits (242-245), reduced neuronal integrity (246), and apoptosis (247-249).

The first description of "arousal habituation" in response to acute intermittent hypoxia (AIH) in newborn animals was provided in 1988 by Fewell and colleagues (250). Since these initial reports, habituation of the arousal response to AIH has been described in the newborns of several species. In piglets, arousal habituation occurs in response to as few as four repeated exposures to hypoxia/hypercapnia. Arousal latencies increased over the four trials and when tested again four days later, the increase in latency was more pronounced, suggesting the presence of both short- and long-term habituation (251). In very young newborn mice (P4), progressive lengthening of arousal latency occurred during eight trials of hypoxia (5% $O_2$) (252).

Habituation of arousal in response to AIH depends on age. We reported the arousal response to eight 3-minute exposures to 5% $O_2$ in P5, P15, and P25 rat pups (220). Arousal latencies were significantly shorter than the time between spontaneous arousals at all ages. Habituation was more robust in P15 and P25 pups compared to P5 animals measured as the slope of arousal latency across trials. In addition, if $O_2$ was switched back to room air immediately upon arousal after three to four trials, the habituation process reversed and arousal latencies approached those observed in trial 1, suggesting that the interval between hypoxia exposure contributes to this phenomenon. Figure 33.9 shows plots of arousal latency during eight trials of hypoxia in rat pups at three developmental ages.

Progressive blunting of arousal during hypoxia could be explained by inhibitory biochemical processes with relatively long-term constants such that a relatively long exposure to hypoxia and a relatively short recovery time would result in progressive cumulative inhibition between exposures. This is consistent with our results showing that if the hypoxia period is shortened and the recovery period between exposures is lengthened, there is gradual recovery of arousal latencies toward baseline values (see Figure 33.9).

Acute hypoxemia is associated with increases in the extracellular concentration of both excitatory and inhibitory neurotransmitters and/or neuromodulators in the brainstem, including opioids, glutamate, GABA, taurine, adenosine, and 5-HT (253-256). Blockade of opioid receptors did not reverse arousal habituation associated with repeated hypoxia exposure in newborn lambs (257). Adenosine is a ubiquitous nucleoside that is released from cells into the extracellular space when oxygen supply no longer matches oxygen needs (258), and it is a potential candidate that could directly inhibit excitatory neurons involved in arousal via $A_1$ receptors, or that could indirectly inhibit these neurons by acting on excitatory adenosine $A_{2A}$ receptors located on GABAergic neurons.

We explored the possible role of GABA in arousal habituation in response to AIH (236). We found in P15 to P25 rat pups that the local application of muscimol, a $GABA_A$ receptor agonist, into the medullary raphe, caused a progressive prolongation of arousal latency during four repeated trials of hypoxia compared to controls. Similarly,

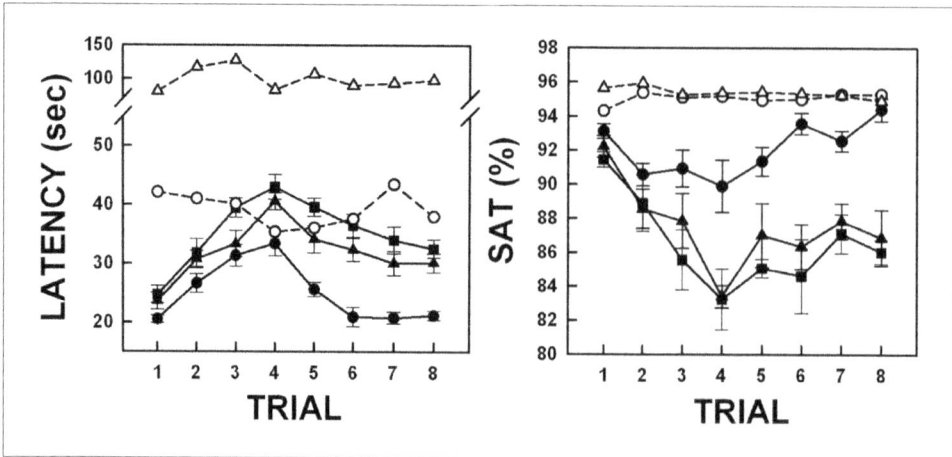

Figure 33.9: Arousal latency and SaO$_2$ at arousal in response to repeated exposure to 5% oxygen in P5, P15, and P25 rat pups. Arousal latencies are shown in the left panel and SaO$_2$ (SAT) at arousal in the right panel. For the first three trials, each animal was exposed to 3 minutes of 5% oxygen interspersed with 6 minutes of normoxia. Starting with the fourth trial, hypoxia was switched to room air immediately upon arousal. The filled symbols are data from pups exposed to hypoxia. The open symbols represent the times between spontaneous arousals and the SaO$_2$ at spontaneous arousal. P5 hypoxia = closed circles; P5 spontaneous arousal rate = open circles; P15 hypoxia = closed triangles; P15 spontaneous arousals = open triangles; P25 hypoxia = closed squares; P25 spontaneous arousals not shown. Arousal habituation is illustrated by the progressive lengthening of arousal latencies and progressive decrease in SaO$_2$ across trials of hypoxia. Note that arousal latencies progressively increased over the first four trials of hypoxia (habituation). When the hypoxia duration was decreased and the recovery time increased by switching to room air at arousal, there was a "reversal" of habituation. All values are expressed as means ±SEM. (Adapted from (220).)

blocking GABA reuptake with the GABA transporter (GAT) antagonist nipecotic acid increased habituation compared to controls. Finally, local application of bicuculline, a GABA$_A$ receptor antagonist, resulted in a dramatic reduction in habituation. Muscimol would be expected to inhibit the activity of all neurons expressing GABA$_A$ receptors, and therefore would produce a generalized inhibition of medullary raphe neuronal activity, thus reducing excitatory input to midbrain arousal centers. Nipecotic acid, with a high affinity for GAT1 and GAT3, would be expected to block the reuptake of GABA into both neurons (GAT1) and glia (GAT3) (259, 260). Our results suggest that inhibiting reuptake of ambient GABA enhances arousal habituation. Blocking GABA$_A$ receptors with bicuculline did not shorten mean arousal latency compared to controls, but resulted in an elimination of habituation. Together these data indicate that neurons

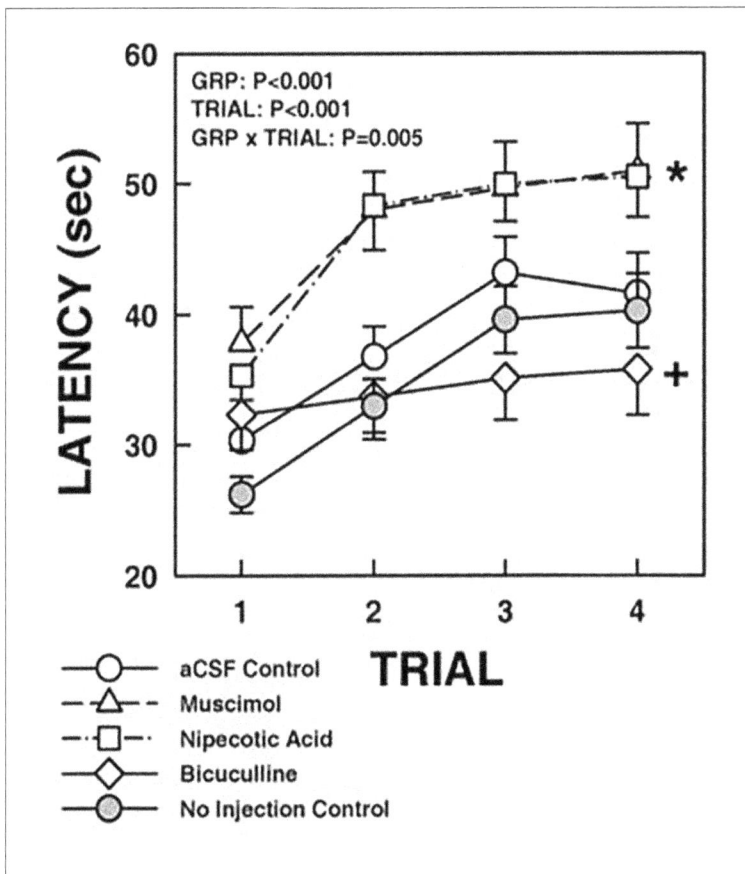

Figure 33.10: Arousal latency over the course of four exposures to 10% breathing after local application into the medullary raphe of aCSF, muscimol, nipecotic acid, and bicuculline. Under isofluorane anesthesia, neurochemicals were micro-injected directly into the medullary raphe in the rostrocaudal dimensions of the facial nucleus in P15-P25 rat pups. After recovery (~30 minutes) pups were exposed to four 3-minute periods of 10% oxygen interspersed with 6 minutes of normoxia. The arousal responses after aCSF and no-injection controls (no anesthesia, surgery, or injections) are represented by open and grey circles, respectively. Note that the response after aCSF is almost identical to that in non-injected controls. Muscimol (GABA$_A$ receptor agonist) and nipecotic acid (GABA reuptake inhibitor) are shown as open triangles and squares respectively. Note the increase in arousal latency. The results after bicuculline (GABA$_A$ receptor antagonist) are shown as open diamonds. Note that in all of the other conditions, there is significant habituation (progressive increase in arousal latency over the four hypoxia exposures). After bicuculline application, habituation is abolished. These data suggest that the progressive increase in arousal latency during repeated hypoxia exposures is secondary to increasing levels of ambient GABA, and that GABA$_A$ receptor activation is necessary for habituation to occur. All values are expressed as means ±SEM. (Reproduced with permission from (236).)

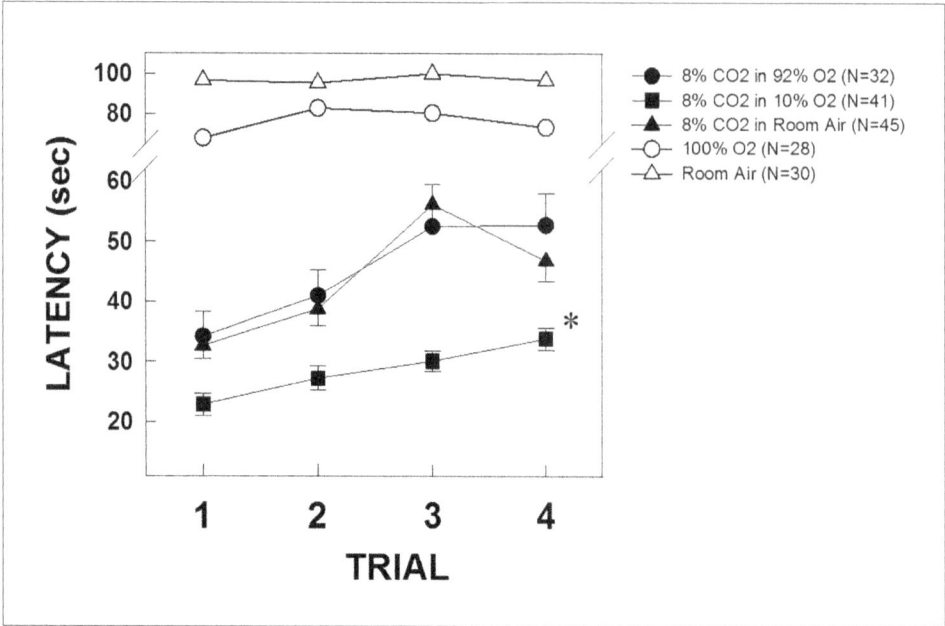

Figure 33.11: Habituation in response to repeated exposure to four exposures to 8% $CO_2$. Open figures illustrate latency to spontaneous arousal in room air (open triangles) or 100% oxygen (open circles). Closed triangles are latencies during exposures to 8% $CO_2$ in room air. Closed circles are latencies during exposure to 8% $CO_2$ combined with 93% oxygen in an attempt to silence the CB component of the arousal response. Closed squares are latencies during exposure to 8% $CO_2$ combined with 10% oxygen (combined hypercapnia and hypoxia). Note that during exposures to $CO_2$, all of the latencies were significantly shorter than spontaneous latencies in either room air or 100% oxygen, and that hypercapnia combined with hypoxia produced the shortest arousal latencies, significantly different from those during exposures to $CO_2$ in room air or in 92% oxygen. All values are means ±SEM. (Authors' own work.)

in the medullary raphe contribute to arousal habituation through the progressive accumulation of GABA, and that activation of medullary raphe $GABA_A$ receptors is necessary for arousal habituation (Figure 33.10).

Arousal habituation also occurs with combined hypoxia-hypercapnia (251). There are only a few studies investigating the effects of repeated $CO_2$ exposure on arousal. At least one study in lambs showed that many repeated exposures to $CO_2$ (one exposure during each change in sleep state) resulted in little or no habituation of the arousal response measured as the probability of arousal (233). However, we determined arousal latency in P9 to P20 rat pups in response to repeated exposures to 8% $CO_2$ (four exposures over ~20 minutes, all during putative QS; n=45). In other experiments, we measured arousal latency exposed to 8% $CO_2$ combined with 92% oxygen (n=32) to minimize the carotid body (CB) response to $CO_2$ and combined with 10% oxygen (n=41) to explore the arousal response to combined hypoxia/hypercapnia (asphyxia). These arousal responses were compared to spontaneous arousal latencies in room air (RA) (n=30) and in 100% oxygen (n=28) (Figure 33.11). As expected, the spontaneous arousal latencies for pups in RA and in 100% oxygen were consistently longer than in pups exposed to $CO_2$ in RA or combinations of $CO_2$ with 92% or 10% oxygen (p<0.001). Significant arousal habituation occurred (p<0.001) in response to repeated exposures to $CO_2$, similar to that which occurs in response to hypoxia. Arousal latencies and habituation were similar in pups exposed to $CO_2$ in RA and $CO_2$ in 92% oxygen, suggesting that, at least in infant and young rat pups, the CB plays a minimal role in the arousal response to $CO_2$. Finally, arousal latencies were significantly shorter in pups exposed to the combination of hypercapnia and hypoxia, indicating that the arousal response to $CO_2$ and hypoxia is at least additive (236).

## Role of brainstem serotonergic mechanisms in arousal

We have used two approaches to examine the role of 5-HT in arousal and arousal habituation. The first involved direct injection, into the medullary raphe, of 5,7-DHT a neuronal toxin specific for 5-HT neurons (when noradrenergic uptake is blocked with desiprimine). P2 rat pups were injected with 5,7-DHT into the cisterna magnum, which results in an 80% reduction in medullary 5-HT neurons, and were then studied at P5, P15, and P25. Compared to pups injected with artificial CSF, or those which were injected with 5,7-DHT but had limited neuronal destruction, pups injected with 5,7-DHT with significant medullary neuronal destruction, at all three ages, had longer arousal latencies and a reduced respiratory rate response to hypoxia. Thus destruction of medullary 5-HT neurons resulted in a generalized blunting of arousal with little or no effect on arousal habituation (Figure 33.12) (124).

Our second approach involved examining mice lacking ~70% of their 5-HT neurons (*Pet-1*$^{-/-}$). Pups were exposed at P6-P10 to four episodes of hypoxia during sleep to illicit an arousal response. Arousal, heart rate, and respiratory rate responses of *Pet-1*$^{-/-}$ mice pups were compared to responses of Null (WT + HET) pups. The time to arousal from the onset of hypoxia (latency) was measured during four hypoxia exposures, while heart rate, respiratory rate, and chamber oxygen concentration were continuously monitored. Arousal latencies in *Pet-1*$^{-/-}$ pups were significantly longer and arousal habituation was more robust compared to the latencies and habituation in the Null pups. In addition, *Pet-1*$^{-/-}$ pups had lower metabolic rates, heart rate, and respiratory rate compared to Null pups (Figure 33.13). The results of these two approaches indicate that 5-HT neurons modulate arousal and perhaps arousal habituation in response to hypoxia (261).

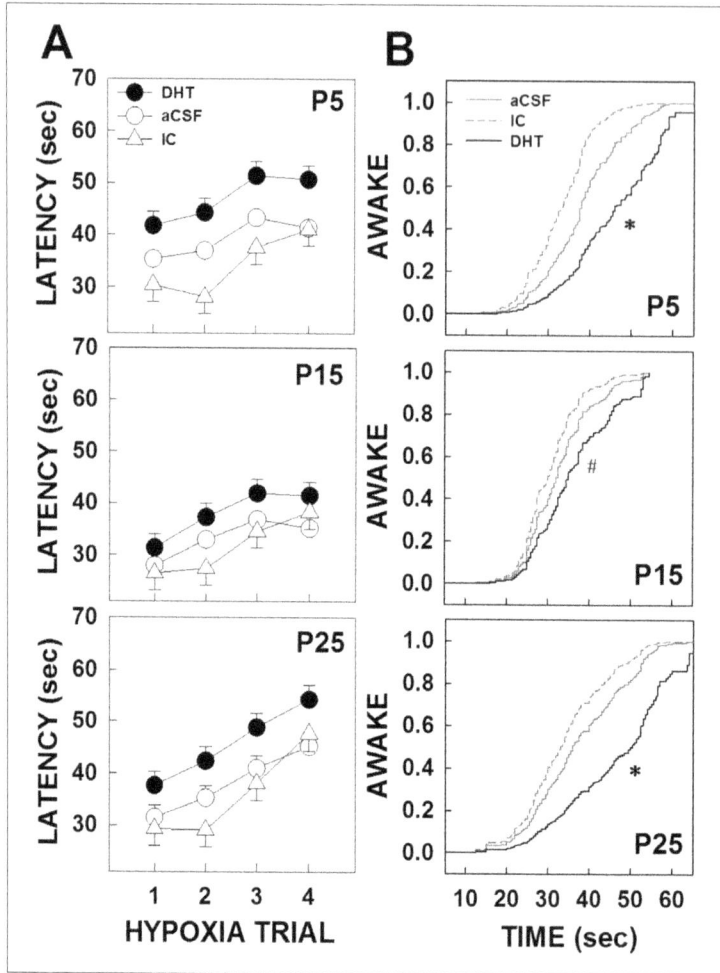

Figure 33.12: Arousal latencies across four repeated hypoxia trials at P5, P15, and P25 after treatment with DHT. Pups were exposed to four episodes of hypoxia (10% $O_2$) begun in quiet sleep, and the latency to subsequent behavioral arousal determined. Latencies of pups with loss of 5-HT neurons after DHT administration (closed circles) were compared with those in pups injected with aCSF (open circles) and those injected with DHT but without a significant reduction of medullary 5-HT neurons (open triangles). Latency increased with successive trials (habituation) in all treatment groups (p<0.001). The mean arousal latency was greatest in the DHT pups at P5 and P25. Values are expressed as the mean ±SEM. B = Cox regression analysis showing the proportion of pups awake at various times after the onset of hypoxia. For any given time, the probability of being awake was lower in the DHT groups compared with the controls at all ages. For example, at P25, forty seconds after the onset of hypoxia, 60-75% of the control pups had aroused in contrast to only 33% of the DHT-treated pups. Consistent with our mixed model analysis, the effects of DHT were more prominent at P5 (*p<0.001) and P25 (*p<0.001) compared with P15 pups (#p=0.039). (Adapted from (124).)

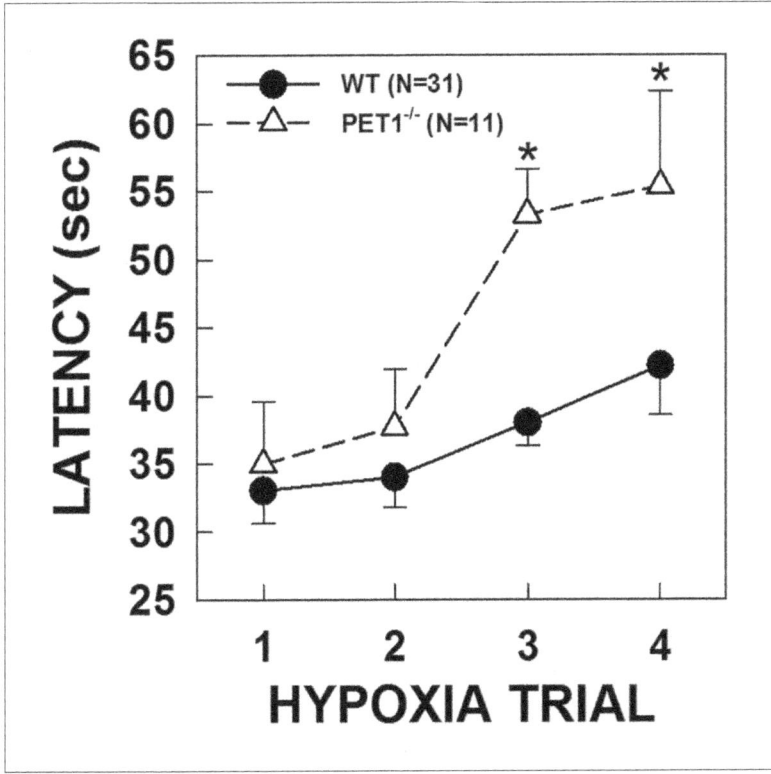

Figure 33.13: A comparison of arousal latencies during four exposures to 10% oxygen in *PET⁻ᐟ⁻* and control mice. Pups were exposed at P6-P10 to four episodes of hypoxia during sleep to illicit an arousal response. The time to arousal from the onset of hypoxia (latency) was measured during four hypoxia exposures. Arousal latencies in *Pet-1⁻ᐟ⁻* pups (open triangles, dashed lines) were significantly longer compared to the latencies in the Null pups (closed circles, solid lines) and arousal habituation was more apparent in the *Pet-1⁻ᐟ⁻* pups. Values are expressed as means ±SEM. Overall, there was a main effect of group (p=0.032) and Trial (p<0.001). Latencies were significantly longer during trials 3 and 4 (asterisk). (Authors' own work.)

## Arousal in response to $CO_2$ in adult rats is 5-HT-dependent

In adult mice, arousal to $CO_2$ appears to be dependent on the presence of 5-HT neurons, which have been shown to be chemosensitive after P12 (262, 263). Mice hemizygous for ePet1-Cre and homozygous for floxed Lmx1b (Lmx1b$^{f/f/p}$), which have no 5-HT neurons, fail to arouse to $CO_2$ but seem to arouse normally to hypoxia, sound, and an air puff (129). These mice were only tested during NREM sleep, however. It is unknown whether 5-HT neurons play such a role during REM sleep, since they are normally silent during this state (264). In addition, these findings are in contrast to our findings in rat pups that either destruction of medullary 5-HT neurons or a genetically engineered lack of 5-HT neurons decreases the ability to arouse in response to repeated exposures to hypoxia (124, 261). The reason for this discrepancy is unclear, but it may be that the newborn and young pup rely more on serotonergic input to arousal during hypoxia than does the adult.

## Brainstem arousal mechanisms

Carotid body chemoreceptors are the primary sites for the detection of hypoxia and to a lesser extent, hypercapnia, both of which in the infant reflexively increase ventilation. Although active in the fetus, the CB becomes more sensitive to hypoxia after birth, temporally associated with an abrupt increase in the partial pressure of $O_2$ and sympathetic activity. From both in vitro and in vivo studies in animals, it appears evident that the strength of the CB reflexes to hypoxia continues to increase with maturation over the first two to three weeks of life, apparently regardless of the maturity of the species at birth (265-268). The time over which CB reflexes mature is less clear in human infants and estimates range from a few days to 10 weeks (269, 270). Several lines of evidence also support the idea that the CB also plays an important role in behavioral arousal in response to hypoxia. In adult dogs, removal of the CB greatly delays arousal co-incident with a reduced ventilatory response to hypoxia (271) or airway occlusion (272). Similarly, in lambs, denervation of the CB reduces arousal probability in response to both rapidly developing hypoxia and airway obstruction (235, 273). Moreover, in these studies, baseline blood pressure and heart rate increased after CB denervation in QS, whereas during AS only blood pressure was increased. After CB denervation, when arousal did occur, the increase in respiratory rate in response to rapidly developing hypoxemia was eliminated and the increase in blood pressure and heart rate was greatly exaggerated (227, 235). Evidence for a role of CB chemoreception in arousal in response to $CO_2$ is less clear, and preferential stimulation of central chemoreceptors appears to be sufficient to cause arousal (274). In a study in lambs, CB denervation decreased the arousal response to $CO_2$ in lambs (234). However, our observations in P9 to P20 rat pups showed that during putative QS, arousal latencies were similar with 8% $CO_2$ in room air and 8% $CO_2$ in 92% oxygen (34.7±2.3 vs 35.3±4.1 seconds) (Figure 33.11). Similarly, $CO_2$ arousal thresholds were similar (4.38±0.28 vs 4.28±0.35%) (236). Also, in adult rodents without any 5-HT neurons, there is only a minimal arousal response to $CO_2$ (129), suggesting that pathways from the CB to arousal networks that did not involve 5-HT were only minimally contributing to arousal. Overall, these data indicate that there may be significant species and age differences in the role of the CB in arousal during hypercapnia.

Although the CB and/or central chemoreceptor stimulation contribute to arousal from sleep in response to hypoxia and hypercapnia, the specific mechanisms have not been fully elucidated. It remains unclear whether arousal results from a direct stimulation of arousal networks or whether arousal networks are indirectly stimulated either from, or as part of, brainstem respiratory networks proportional to respiratory drive or from mechanoreceptor stimuli arising from the ventilatory apparatus during breathing (275). Neurons located in the retrotrapezoid nucleus (RTN), medullary raphe, NTS, and locus coeruleus (LC), and certain astrocytes located on the ventral surface of the brainstem have been found to respond directly to $CO_2$ or acidification (276). Although activation of neurons in these regions usually results in changes in ventilation, some central chemoreceptors have no apparent effect on respiration and may be involved in maintaining vigilance (276). In contrast, hypoxia is generally thought to have an inhibitory effect on most CNS neurons, and the "biphasic" ventilatory response to hypoxia is thought to be the sum of CB excitation and delayed CNS inhibition. However, certain groups of neurons, including those located in the C1 region, are directly activated by hypoxia and could also act as central chemoreceptors (277). There are several lines of evidence indicating that the RTN may be particularly important in both the ventilatory and the arousal response to hypercapnia and asphyxia (278, 279). In addition to their direct activation by pH/$CO_2$, RTN neurons also receive inputs from the CBs via the NTS (280), respiratory networks, lung stretch receptors, and hypothalamic orexinergic neurons (281), and are activated by raphe 5-HT neurons (282). Importantly, RTN glutamatergic neurons project to neurons in the lateral parabrachial nucleus (PB), major components of the ascending arousal system that project to the basal forebrain, lateral hypothalamus, midline thalamus, and cerebral cortex (126).

Our findings that arousal in response to repeated episodes of hypoxia is influenced by both medullary raphe 5-HT and GABAergic mechanisms suggest that the medullary raphe either lies in an arousal pathway or modulates other ascending arousal pathways activated by hypoxia. This idea is supported by observations that [1] there are direct projections from midline serotonergic neurons to the RTN, a major region for convergence of arousal-related inputs (283); [2] long-term facilitation associated with exposure to AIH requires the activation of medullary 5-HT neurons that project to the spinal cord (284, 285); [3] stimulation of the carotid sinus nerves induces FOS-like protein (a marker of neuronal activation) in regions of the medullary raphe (286); and [4] multi-array extracellular recordings show that midline raphe neurons are critical components of a larger raphe-ponto-medullary network of neurons with respiratory-related activity that responds to peripheral chemoreceptor stimulation in concert with the entire network (287). Figure 33.14 illustrates the various possible pathways that promote waking during exposure to hypoxia, hypercapnia, or asphyxia.

Sleep state plays a major role in arousal but is highly species-dependent. Whereas newborn and adult mammals appear to have depressed arousal during AS, the opposite occurs in human infants, where the probability of arousal in response to hypoxia is increased during AS and depressed during QS. There are other state-related effects on physiological control systems where the human infant appears to be an outlier in the mammalian world. For example, in most small mammals, REM or AS is associated with an attenuation of thermoregulation. Thus brown fat metabolism, shivering, and sweating are all suspended during REM (288, 289). In the human infant, however, thermoregulation is preserved during REM sleep, and may even be more effective (290-292).

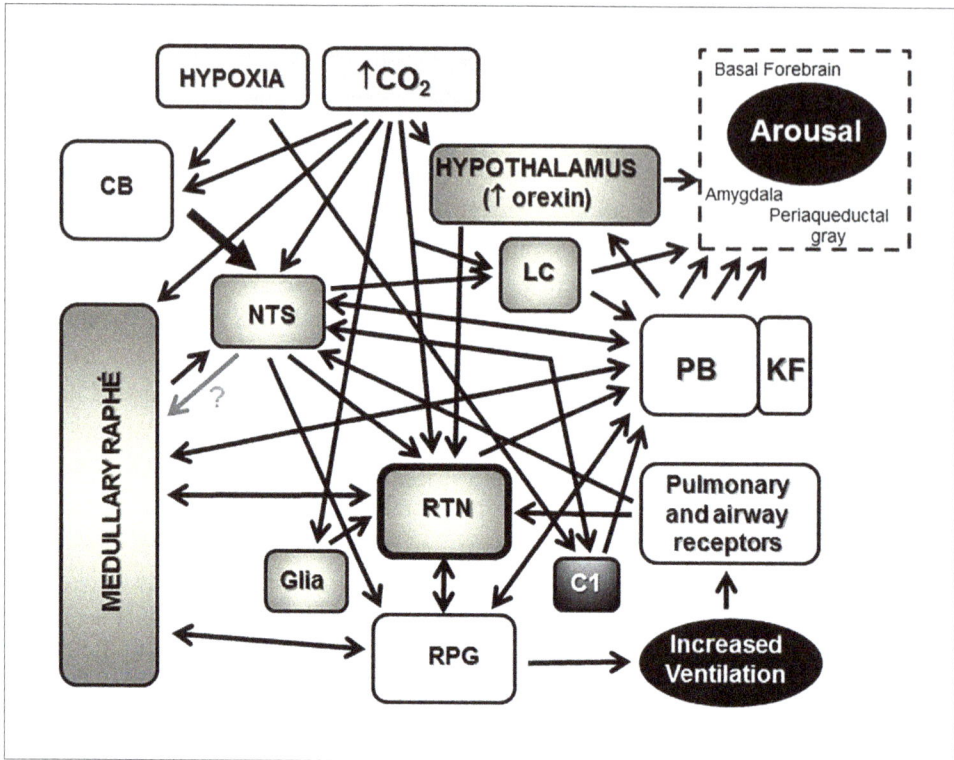

Figure 33.14: Potential arousal pathways in response to hypoxia and/or hypercapnia. The lightly shaded areas are the stimuli (i.e. hypoxia and hypercapnia). The darker shaded areas are regions that are known to be responsive to $CO_2$ exposure (potential $CO_2$ chemoreceptors). The black areas are the major responses, increased ventilation and arousal. Arrows represent known projections from various regions. (Authors' own work.)

## Arousal and epidemiological risk factors for SIDS

Smoking during pregnancy is a major preventable risk factor for SIDS (293) and 5-6-month-old infants born to mothers who smoke have longer arousal latencies in response to breathing 15% oxygen compared to infants born to non-smoking mothers (294). Nicotine, a well-characterized component in cigarette smoke, has been largely used in animal experiments. Nicotine exposure during pregnancy alters nicotine receptor (nAChR) expression and receptor binding in the fetal and infant medullae (200, 295-298). In newborn lambs, arousal to 10% oxygen was delayed and occurred at a lower $SaO_2$ after a short-term IV infusion of nicotine compared to lambs treated similarly after an infusion of normal saline (299). We recently examined arousal and arousal habituation during AIH in rat pups continuously prenatally exposed to nicotine (PNE) and a tryptophan-deficient diet (TDD), which results in a mild serotonergic deficiency in the pups. From E4 to P10, pregnant dams that received a normal control diet (CD) or a TDD received either normal saline (NS) or nicotine (NIC) (6 mg/kg/day), continuously delivered by a subcutaneously implanted osmotic pump. The NIC dose corresponded to about 0.5-1 pack of cigarettes a day in human smokers. Four groups of litters were studied: CD/NS, CD/NIC, TDD/NS, and TDD/NIC. P7 and P13 pups from each litter were evaluated for arousal and arousal habituation in response to AIH. At P13, but not at P7, arousal latencies were longer in the CD/NIC pups compared to the CD/NS and TD/NS pups. Arousal latencies for the TD/NIC pups fell between those of the CD/NIC and the CD/NS pups, but were not significantly different from the other three groups. We concluded that PNE impairs arousal in response to hypoxia, whereas arousal is not affected by a mild 5-HT deficiency, compared to a more severe 5-HT deficiency (see above). There were no effects of either prenatal nicotine or a mild 5-HT deficiency on arousal habituation (300). Figure 33.15 illustrates the effect of PNE on arousal and arousal habituation.

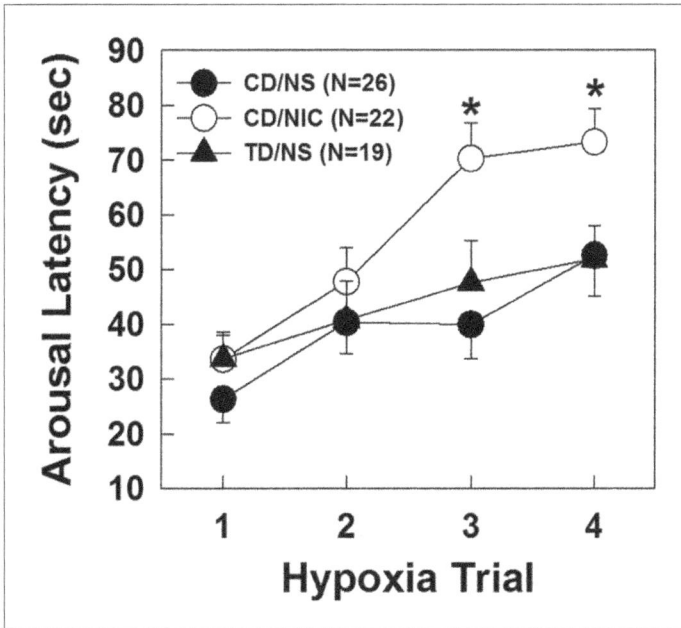

Figure 33.15: Arousal latencies to four episodes of 10% oxygen in 15-day-old pups after prenatal exposure to nicotine and a tryptophan-deficient diet. Dams were exposed to a combination of either a control diet (CD) or tryptophan-deficient diet (TD) and either nicotine (NIC) or normal saline (NS). NIC and NS were delivered continuously with a surgically implanted osmotic pump. Pups exposed prenatally to the combination of a CD and NIC (open circles) had significantly longer arousal latencies in response to hypoxia than either a CD combined with NS (closed circles) or a TD combined with NS (closed triangles). The combination of NIC and a TD (not shown for clarity) produced latencies in response to hypoxia that were midway between CD/NIC and CD/NS or TD/NS and were not significantly different from any of the other groups. All values are means ±SEM. (Authors' own work.)

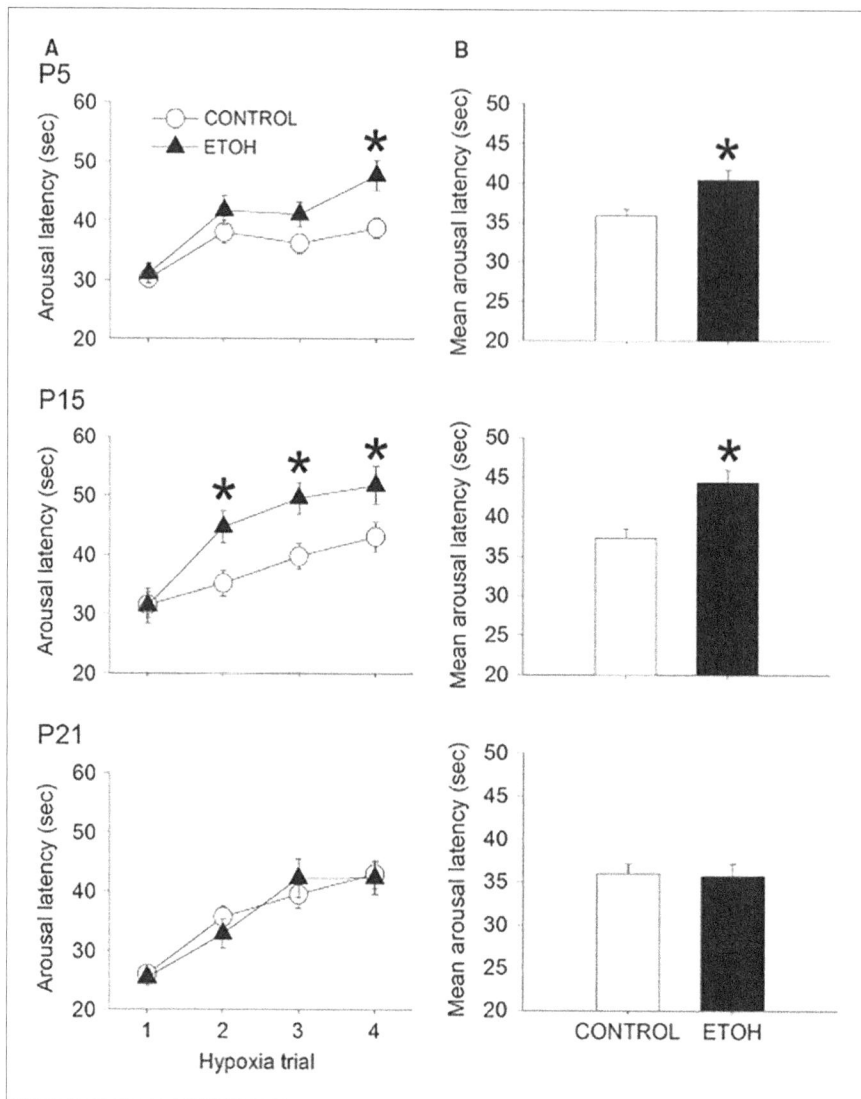

Figure 33.16: The effect of prenatal alcohol exposure on arousal in response to four exposures to 10% oxygen.

A. Arousal latencies of pups exposed to prenatal alcohol (closed triangles) and controls (open circles) during four trials of hypoxia.

B. The mean arousal latencies (averaged over the four trials of hypoxia) of pups exposed to prenatal alcohol (black bars) compared to controls (open bars). Values are expressed as means ±SEM and asterisks indicate significance at least at $p<0.05$. Previous physiological studies have focused on the role of reduced excitatory respiratory reflexes (e.g. ventilatory responses to hypoxia and hypercapnia) in the pathogenesis of SIDS (213, 302), and the current study emphasizes that enhanced activity of inhibitory neurotransmitters and inhibitory reflexes may also increase the likelihood of SIDS. (Authors' own work.)

Prenatal alcohol exposure (PAE) increases the risk for SIDS (3), but little is known about the effect of PAE on arousal or arousal habituation in response to hypoxia. We recently examined the effects of PAE in rat pups on arousal and arousal habituation in response to hypoxia. Since arousal and arousal habituation is modulated by GABAergic and serotonergic mechanisms (124, 236), we also wanted to examine whether any effects of PAE were enhanced or inhibited by manipulating brainstem GABAergic neurons by direct medullary injections of aCSF, nipecotic acid (NIP), and gabazine (GABA$_A$ receptor antagonist). Finally, we wanted to determine whether PAE altered brainstem concentrations of various neurotransmitters, including 5-HT and GABA. Pregnant dams were fed either an alcohol-containing diet (ETOH), a calorically matched non-alcohol-containing liquid diet (PF), or a standard chow diet (CHOW). Our main finding was that compared to control pups (PF and CHOW combined) arousal latency was increased at P15 and P21 and brainstem GABA concentrations were elevated at P21. NIP injections into control animals resulted in arousal latencies similar in magnitude to those in ETOH pups after aCSF injections. NIP-injected ETOH pups had no further increases in arousal latencies. We concluded that PAE impairs arousal and this is mediated or modulated by GABAergic mechanisms. We found no effect of PAE on arousal habituation (Figure 33.16) (301).

## Conclusions

We found that reflex apneas, hypoxic apnea, autoresuscitation, and arousal — the essential features recorded from infants who died of SIDS — are all modified in animal studies by risk factors associated with SIDS. Moreover, instead of describing these associations using the descriptive terms of the Triple Risk Model of SIDS, we have advanced to talking about specific molecular mechanisms, specific neurotransmitters, and specific pathways within the brain. These include TRPV1 receptors, 5-HT$_3$ receptors, 5-HT, GABA and adenosine, the NTS, the caudal raphe nuclei, the rostral ventral medulla, and the parabrachial nucleus.

Animal studies have illuminated the mechanistic underpinnings of the Triple Risk Model and focused investigators' attention on two aspects of the pathogenesis of SIDS. First, it seems likely that infants who die of SIDS have an unusual propensity for respiratory inhibition by reflex apneas and hypoxia; second, they have a markedly reduced capacity to recover from these apneic, hypoxic events through the processes of autoresuscitation and arousal. Autoresuscitation and arousal from sleep are major defense mechanisms in infants against hypoxia and/or hypercapnia during rebreathing, airway obstruction, and apnea. The combination of autoresuscitation and subcortical and cortical arousal allows the infant to move out of a dangerous situation and mount an appropriate physiological response. The areas of the brainstem that have been found to be abnormal in many infants who died of SIDS and asphyxia are involved in the apnea generation, autoresuscitation, apnea termination, restoration of eupnea, and arousal processes, all of which seem to be mechanistically and neurophysiologically separable processes. Moreover, autoresuscitation, apnea termination, restoration of eupnea, and arousal processes are all influenced by medullary 5-HT mechanisms in which each process is associated with a specific set of 5-HT receptors and specific regions of the brainstem. Prenatal and postnatal exposure to hypoxia may enhance the propensity for apnea and may reduce the capacity for autoresuscitation, and repeated exposure to hypoxia causes a progressive blunting of arousal (arousal habituation) that involves a medullary raphe GABAergic mechanisms. The CBs and central chemoreceptors contribute heavily to apnea termination, autoresuscitation, and arousal in response to hypoxia and hypercapnia.

Whether CBs and/or central chemoreceptor stimulation directly stimulates the important restorative processes or whether this is done indirectly through respiratory networks remains unclear, but some combination is likely. That the medullary raphe contributes to the processes of apnea termination, autoresuscitation, restoration of eupnea, and arousal in response to apnea and hypoxia has important implications for infants at risk for SIDS and asphyxia. Up to 70% of these infants have decreased medullary raphe 5-HT and TPH2 levels, which may result in a loss or decrease in an important excitatory input to the apnea-terminating, eupnea-generating, and autoresuscitative and arousal processes. Medullary GABAergic mechanisms also enhance apnea generation and arousal habituation, which may increase the propensity for prolonged apnea and failed arousal when infants are repeatedly exposed to hypoxia in utero, during repetitive apneas, or in asphyxiating sleeping environments. Important preventable risk factors for SIDS, including prenatal nicotine and alcohol exposure, also enhance the likelihood of apnea and impair autoresuscitation and arousal. Animal studies have identified specific mechanisms promoting SIDS and asphyxia, and in so doing, these studies also point to future interventions and possible therapies to prevent SIDS and asphyxia.

# References

1. L'Hoir MP, Engelberts AC, van Well CTJ, Westers P, Mellenbergh GJ, Wolters WHG, et al. Case-control study of the current validity of previously described risk factors of SIDS in the Netherlands. Arch Dis Child. 1998;79:386-93. https://doi.org/10.1136/adc.79.5.386.

2. Paris CA, Remler R, Daling JR. Risk factors for sudden infant death syndrome: Changes associated with sleep position recommendations. J Pediatr. 2001;139:771-7. https://doi.org/10.1067/mpd.2001.118568.

3.  Iyasu S, Randall LL, Welty TK, Hsia J, Kinney HC, Mandell F, et al. Risk factors for sudden infant death syndrome among northern plains Indians. JAMA. 2002;288:2717-23. https://doi.org/10.1001/jama.288.21.2717.

4.  Kahn A, Sawaguchi T, Sawaguchi A, Groswasser J, Franco P, Scaillet S, et al. Sudden infant deaths: From epidemiology to physiology. Foren Sci Intern. 2002;130S:S8-S20. https://doi.org/10.1016/S0379-0738(02)00134-2.

5.  Li DK, Wi S. Maternal pre-eclampsia/eclampsia and the risk of sudden infant death syndrome in offspring. Paediatr Perinat Epidemiol. 2000;14(2):141-4. https://doi.org/10.1046/j.1365-3016.2000.00245.x.

6.  Malloy MH. Prematurity and sudden infant death syndrome: United States 2005-2007. J Perinatol. 2013;33(6):470-5. https://doi.org/10.1038/jp.2012.158.

7.  Trachtenberg FL, Haas EA, Kinney HC, Stanley C, Krous HF. Risk factor changes for sudden infant death syndrome after initiation of back-to-sleep campaign. Pediatrics. 2012;129(4):630-8. https://doi.org/10.1542/peds.2011-1419.

8.  Blair PS, Fleming PJ, Bensley D, Smith I, Bacon C, Taylor E, et al. Smoking and the sudden infant death syndrome: Results from 1993-5 case-control study for confidential inquiry into still births and deaths in infancy. BMJ. 1996;313:195-8. https://doi.org/10.1136/bmj.313.7051.195.

9.  Paterson DS, Trachtenberg FL, Thompson EG, Belliveau RA, Beggs AH, Darnall RA, et al. Multiple serotonergic brainstem abnormalities in the sudden infant death syndrome. JAMA. 2006;296:2124-32. https://doi.org/10.1001/jama.296.17.2124.

10. Mitchell EA, Ford RPK, Stewart AK, Taylor BJ, Becroft DMO, Thompson JMD, et al. Smoking and the sudden infant death syndrome. Pediatrics. 1993;91:893-6.

11. Anderson ME, Johnson DC, Batal HA. Sudden infant death syndrome and prenatal maternal smoking: Rising attributed risk in the back to sleep era. BMC Med. 2005;11:3-4. https://doi.org/10.1186/1741-7015-3-4.

12. Kinney HC, Filiano JJ, Sleeper LA, Mandell F, Valdes-Dapena M, White WF. Decreased muscarinic receptor binding in the arcuate nucleus in sudden infant death syndrome. Science. 1995;269:1446-50. https://doi.org/10.1126/science.7660131.

13. Panigrahy A, Filiano JJ, Sleeper LA, Mandell F, Valdes-Dapena M, Krous HF, et al. Decreased kainate receptor binding in the arcuate nucleus of the sudden infant death syndrome. J Neuropathol Exp Neurol. 1997;56(11):1253-61. https://doi.org/10.1097/00005072-199711000-00010.

14. Panigrahy A, Filiano JJ, Sleeper LA, Mandell F, Valdes-Dapena M, Krous HF, et al. Decreased serotonergic receptor binding in rhombic lip-derived regions of the medulla oblongata in the sudden infant death syndrome. J Neuropathol Exp Neurol. 2000;59:377-84. https://doi.org/10.1093/jnen/59.5.377.

15. Duncan JR, Paterson DS, Hoffman JM, Mokler DJ, Borenstein NS, Belliveau RA, et al. Brainstem serotonergic deficiency in sudden infant death syndrome. JAMA. 2010;303:430-7. https://doi.org/10.1001/jama.2010.45.

16. Kinney HC, Randall LL, Sleeper LA, Willinger M, Belliveau RA, Zec N, et al. Serotonergic brainstem abnormalities in northern plains Indians with the sudden infant death syndrome. J Neuropath Exp Neurol. 2003;62:1178-91. https://doi.org/10.1093/jnen/62.11.1178.

17. Randall BB, Paterson DS, Haas EA, Broadbelt KG, Duncan JR, Mena OJ, et al. Potential asphyxia and brainstem abnormalities in sudden and unexpected death in infants. Pediatrics. 2013;132(6):e1616-25. https://doi.org/10.1542/peds.2013-0700.

18. Naeye RL. Sudden infant death. Sci Am. 1980;242:56-62. https://doi.org/10.1038/scientificamerican0480-56.

19. Naeye RL, Ladis B, Drage JS. Sudden infant death syndrome. A prospective study. Am J Dis Child. 1976;130:1207-10. https://doi.org/10.1001/archpedi.1976.02120120041005.

20. Kinney HC, Burger PC, Harrell FE Jr., Hudson RP Jr. Reactive gliosis in the medulla oblongota of victims of the sudden infant death syndrome. Pediatrics. 1983;72:181-7.

21. Kinney HC, Filiano JJ, Harper RM. The neuropathology of the sudden infant death syndrome. A review. J Neuropathol Exp Neurol. 1992;51:115-26. https://doi.org/10.1097/00005072-199203000-00001.

22. Valdes-Dapena M. Sudden infant death syndrome. Morphology update for forensic pathologists — 1985. Forensic Sci Int. 1986;30(2-3):177-86. https://doi.org/10.1016/0379-0738(86)90012-5.

23. Becker LE. Neural maturational delay as a link in the chain of events leading to SIDS. The Canadian journal of neurological sciences/Le J Canadien Des Sciences Neurologiques. 1990;17(4):361-71. https://doi.org/10.1017/S0317167100030894.

24. Quattrochi JJ, McBride PT, Yates AJ. Brainstem immaturity in sudden infant death syndrome: A quantitative rapid golgi study of dendritic spines in 95 infants. Brain Res. 1985;325:39-48. https://doi.org/10.1016/0006-8993(85)90300-2.

25. Sridhar R, Thach BT, Kelly DH, Henslee JA. Characterization of successful and failed autoresuscitation in human infants. Pediatr Pulmonol. 2003;36:113-22. https://doi.org/10.1002/ppul.10287.

26. Meny RG, Carroll JL, Carbone MT, Kelly DH. Cardiorespiratory recordings from infants dying suddenly and unexpectedly at home. Pediatrics. 1994;93:44-9.

27. Poets CF. Apparent life-threatening events and sudden infant death on a monitor. Paediatr Resp Rev. 2004;5 Suppl A:S383-6.

28. Poets CF, Samuels MP, Noyes JP, Hewertson J, Hartmann H, Holder A, et al. Home event recordings of oxygenation, breathing movements, and heart rate and rhythm in infants with recurrent life-threatening events. J Pediatr. 1993;123(5):693-701. https://doi.org/10.1016/S0022-3476(05)80842-X.

29. Filiano JJ, Kinney HC. A perspective on neuropathological findings in victims of the sudden infant death syndrome: The triple-risk model. Biol Neonate. 1994;65:194-7. https://doi.org/10.1159/000244052.

30. Leiter JC, Böhm I. Mechanisms of pathogenesis in the sudden infant death syndrome (SIDS). Respir Physiol Neurobiol. 2007;159:127-38. https://doi.org/10.1016/j.resp.2007.05.014.

31. Hunt CE, Brouillette RT. Sudden infant death syndrome: 1987 perspective. J Pediatrics. 1987;110:669-78. https://doi.org/10.1016/S0022-3476(87)80001-X.

32. Franco P, Kato I, Richardson HL, Yang JS, Montemitro E, Horne RS. Arousal from sleep mechanisms in infants. Sleep Med. 2010;11(7):603-14. https://doi.org/10.1016/j.sleep.2009.12.014.

33. Thach B. Tragic and sudden death. Potential and proven mechanisms causing sudden infant death syndrome. EMBO Rep. 2008;9(2):114-18. https://doi.org/10.1038/sj.embor.7401163.

34. Fewell JE. Protective responses of the newborn to hypoxia. Respir Physiol Neurobiol. 2005;149(1-3):243-55. https://doi.org/10.1016/j.resp.2005.05.006.

35. Wolf S. Sudden death and the oxygen-conserving reflex. Am Heart J. 1966;71(6):840-1. https://doi.org/10.1016/0002-8703(66)90609-0.

36. French JW, Morgan BC, Guntheroth WG. Infant monkeys — A model for crib death. Am J Dis Child. 1972;123(5):480-4. https://doi.org/10.1001/archpedi.1972.02110110108011.

37. Lobban CDR. The oxygen-conserving dive reflex re-examined as the principal contributing factor in sudden infant death. Medical Hypoth. 1995;44:273-7. https://doi.org/10.1016/0306-9877(95)90179-5.

38. Singh GP, Chowdhury T, Bindu B, Schaller B. Sudden infant death syndrome — Role of trigeminocardiac reflex: A review. Front Neurol. 2016;7:221. https://doi.org/10.3389/fneur.2016.00221.

39. Matturri L, Ottaviani G, Lavezzi AM. Sudden infant death triggered by dive reflex. J Clin Path. 2005;58(1):77-80. https://doi.org/10.1136/jcp.2004.020867.

40. Boggs DF, Bartlett D Jr. Chemical specificity of a laryngeal apneic reflex in puppies. J Appl Physiol. 1982;53:455-62.

41. Downing SE, Lee JC. Laryngeal chemosensitivity: A possible mechanism of sudden infant death. Pediatrics. 1975;55:640-9.

42. Lee JC, Stoll BJ, Downing SE. Properties of the laryngeal chemoreflex in neonatal piglets. Am J Physiol. 1977;233:R30-R6.

43. St Hilaire M, Nsegbe E, Gagnon-Gervais K, Samson N, Moreau-Bussière F, Fortier P-H, et al. Laryngeal chemoreflexes induced by acid, water and saline in non-sedated newborn lambs during quiet sleep. J Appl Physiol. 2005;102:1429-38.

44. Haraguchi S, Fung RQ, Sasaki R. Effect of hyperthermia on the laryngeal closure reflex. Implications in the sudden infant death syndrome. Ann Otol Rhinol Laryngol. 1983;92:24-8. https://doi.org/10.1177/000348948309200106.

45. Sasaki CT. Development of laryngeal function: Etiologic significance in the sudden infant death syndrome. The Laryngoscope. 1979;89:1964-82. https://doi.org/10.1288/00005537-197912000-00010.

46. Grogaard J, Lindstrom DP, Stahlman MT, Marchal F, Sundell H. The cardiovascular response to laryngeal water administration in young lambs. J Dev Physiol. 1982;4:353-70.

47. Thach BT. Maturation and transformation of reflexes that protect the laryngeal airway from liquid aspiration from fetal to adult life. Am J Med. 2001;111(8):69-77. https://doi.org/10.1016/S0002-9343(01)00860-9.

48. Page M, Jeffery HE, Marks V, Post EJ, Wood AKW. Mechanisms of airway protection after pharyngeal fluid infusion in healthy sleeping piglets. J Appl Physiol. 1995;78:1942-9.

49. Sullivan CE, Murphy E, Kozar LF, Phillipson EA. Waking and ventilatory responses to laryngeal stimulation in sleeping dogs. J Appl Physiol. 1978;45:681-9.

50. Thach BT. The role of respiratory control disorders in SIDS. Respir Physiol Neurobiol. 2005;149:343-53. https://doi.org/10.1016/j.resp.2005.06.011.

51. Page M, Jeffery HE. The role of gastro-oesophageal reflux in the aetiology of SIDS. Early Hum Dev. 2000;59:127-49. https://doi.org/10.1016/S0378-3782(00)00093-1.

52. van der Velde L, Curran A, Filiano JJ, Darnall RA, Bartlett D Jr., Leiter JC. Prolongation of the laryngeal chemoreflex after inhibition of the rostroventral medulla in piglets: A role in SIDS? J Appl Physiol. 2003;94:1883-95. https://doi.org/10.1152/japplphysiol.01103.2002.

53. Blair PS, Mitchell EA, Heckstall-Smith EMA, Fleming PJ. Head covering — A major modifiable risk factor for sudden infant death syndrome: A systematic review. Arch Dis Child. 2008;93:778-83. https://doi.org/10.1136/adc.2007.136366.

54. Kleemann WJ, Schlaud M, Fieguth A, Hiller AS, Rothämel T, Tröger HD. Body and head position, covering of the head by bedding and risk of sudden infant death (SID). Int J Legal Med. 1998;112:22-6. https://doi.org/10.1007/s004140050192.

55. Guntheroth WG, Spiers PS. Thermal stress in sudden infant death: Is there an ambiguity with the rebreathing hypothesis? Pediatrics. 2001;107:693-8. https://doi.org/10.1542/peds.107.4.693.

56. Williams SM, Taylor BJ, Mitchell EA. Sudden infant death syndrome: Insulation from bedding and clothing and its effect modifiers. Int J Epidemiol. 1996;25:366-75. https://doi.org/10.1093/ije/25.2.366.

57. Fleming PJ, Gilbert R, Azaz Y, Berry PJ, Rudd PT, Stewart A, et al. Interaction between bedding and sleeping position in the SIDS: A population based case-control study. BMJ. 1990;301:85-9. https://doi.org/10.1136/bmj.301.6743.85.

58. Ponsonby A-L, Dwyer T, Couper D, Cochrane JA. Association between use of a quilt and sudden infant death syndrome: Case-control study. BMJ. 1998;316:195-6. https://doi.org/10.1136/bmj.316.7126.195.

59. Sheers-Masters JR, Schootman M, Thach BT. Heat stress and sudden infant death syndrome incidence: A United States population epidemiologic study. Pediatrics. 2004;113:e586-92. https://doi.org/10.1542/peds.113.6.e586.

60. Bolton DPG, Nelson EAS, Taylor BJ, Weatherall IL. Thermal balance in infants. J Appl Physiol. 1996;80:2234-42.

61. Curran AK, Xia L, Leiter JC, Bartlett D Jr. Elevated body temperature enhances the laryngeal chemoreflex in decerebrate piglets. J Appl Physiol. 2005;98:780-6. https://doi.org/10.1152/japplphysiol.00906.2004.

62. Xia L, Leiter JC, Bartlett D Jr. Laryngeal water receptors are insensitive to body temperature in neonatal piglets. Respir Physiol Neurobiol. 2005;150:82-6. https://doi.org/10.1016/j.resp.2005.05.021.

63. Xia L, Damon TA, Leiter JC, Bartlett D Jr. Focal warming of the nucleus of the solitary tract prolongs the laryngeal chemoreflex in decerebrate piglets. J Appl Physiol. 2007;102:54-62. https://doi.org/10.1152/japplphysiol.00720.2006.

64. Mezey A, Toth ZE, Cortright DN, Arzubi MK, Krause JE, Elde R, et al. Distribution of mRNA for vanilloid receptor subtype 1 (VR1), and VR1-like immunoreactivity, in the central nervous system of the rat and human. Proc Natl Acad Sci. 2000;97:3655-60. https://doi.org/10.1073/pnas.97.7.3655.

65. Guo A, Vulchanova L, Wang J, Li X, Elde R. Immunocytochemical localization of the vanilloid receptor 1 (VR1): Relationship to neuropeptides, the P2X3 purinoceptor and IB4 binding sites. Eur J Neurosci. 1999;11:946-58. https://doi.org/10.1046/j.1460-9568.1999.00503.x.

66. Caterina MJ. Transient receptor potential ion channels as participants in thermosensation and thermoregulation. Am J Physiol. 2007;292:R64-R76.

67. Peters JH, McDougall SJ, Fawley JA, Smith SM, Andresen MC. Primary afferent activation of thermosensitive TRPV1 triggers asynchronous glutamate release at central neurons. Neuron. 2010;65:657-69. https://doi.org/10.1016/j.neuron.2010.02.017.

68. Shoudai K, Peters JH, McDougall SJ, Fawley JA, Andresen MC. Thermally active TRPV 1 tonically drives central spontaneous glutamate release. J Neurosci. 2010;30:14470-5. https://doi.org/10.1523/JNEUROSCI.2557-10.2010.

69. Venkatachalam K, Montell C. TRP channels. Annu Rev Biochem. 2007;76:387-417. https://doi.org/10.1146/annurev.biochem.75.103004.142819.

70. Xia L, Bartlett D Jr., Leiter JC. TRPV 1 channels in the nucleus of the solitary tract mediate thermal prolongation of the LCR in decerebrate piglets. Respir Physiol Neurobiol. 2011;176:21-31. https://doi.org/10.1016/j.resp.2011.01.008.

71. Patterson LM, Zheng H, Ward SM, Berthoud H-R. Vanilloid receptor (VR1) expression in vagal afferent neurons innervating the gastrointestinal tract. Cell Tissue Res. 2003;311:277-87.

72. Sun H, Li D-P, Chen S-R, Hittelman WN, Pan H-L. Sensing of blood pressure increase by transient receptor potential vanilloid 1 receptors on baroreceptors. J Pharmacol Exp Therap. 2009;331:851-9. https://doi.org/10.1124/jpet.109.160473.

73. Steinschneider A. Prolonged apnea and the sudden infant death syndrome: Clinical and laboratory observations. Pediatrics. 1972;50(4):646-54.

74. Dalveit AK, Irgens LM, Øyen N, Skjaerven R, Markstad T, Wennergren G. Circadian variations in sudden infant death syndrome: Associations with maternal smoking, sleeping position and infections. The Nordic Epidemiological SIDS study. Acta Paediatr. 2003;92:1007-13. https://doi.org/10.1111/j.1651-2227.2003.tb02567.x.

75. Lindgren C, Grogaard J. Reflex apnoea response and inflammatory mediators in infants with respiratory tract infection. Acta Paediatr. 1996;85:798-803. https://doi.org/10.1111/j.1651-2227.1996.tb14154.x.

76. Lindgren C, Jing L, Graham B, Grogaard J, Sundell H. Respiratory syncytial virus infection reinforces reflex apnea in young lambs. Pediatri Res. 1992;31:381-5. https://doi.org/10.1203/00006450-199204000-00015.

77. Frøen JF, Akre H, Stray-Pedersen B, Saugstad OD. Adverse effects of nicotine and interleukin-1beta on autoresuscitation after apnea in piglets: Implications for sudden infant death syndrome. Pediatrics. 2000;105:E52. https://doi.org/10.1542/peds.105.4.e52.

78. Frøen JF, Akre H, Stray-Pedersen B, Saugstad OD. Prolonged apneas and hypoxia mediated by nicotine and endotoxin in piglets. Biol Neonat. 2002;81:119-25. https://doi.org/10.1159/000047196.

79. Thach BT. The brainstem and vulnerability to sudden infant death syndrome. Neurol. 2003;61:1170-1. https://doi.org/10.1212/WNL.61.9.1170.

80. Stoltenberg L, Sundar T, Almaas R, Storm H, Rognumm TO, Saugstad OD. Changes in apnea and autoresuscitation in piglets after intravenous and intrathecal interleukin-1 beta injection. J Perinat Med. 1994;22:421-32. https://doi.org/10.1515/jpme.1994.22.5.421.

81. Xia L, Bartlett D Jr., Leiter JC. Interleukin-1beta and interleukin-6 enhance thermal prolongation of the LCR in decerebrate piglets. Respir Physiol Neurobiol. 2016;230:44-53. https://doi.org/10.1016/j.resp.2016.05.006.

82. Dinarello CA. Infection, fever, and exogenous and endogenous pyrogens: Some concepts have changed. J Endotoxin Res. 2004;10(4):201-22.

83. Tsakiri N, Kimber I, Rothwell NJ, Pinteaux E. Interleukin-1-induced interleukin-6 synthesis is mediated by the neutral sphingomyelinase/Src kinase pathway in neurones. Br J Pharmacol. 2008;153(4):775-83. https://doi.org/10.1038/sj.bjp.0707610.

84. Jia Y, Lee LY. Role of TRPV receptors in respiratory diseases. Biochim Biophys Acta. 2007;1772(8):915-27. https://doi.org/10.1016/j.bbadis.2007.01.013.

85. Premkumar LS, Abooj M. TRP channels and analgesia. Life Sci. 2013;92(8-9):415-24. https://doi.org/10.1016/j.lfs.2012.08.010.

86. Schaible HG. Nociceptive neurons detect cytokines in arthritis. Arthritis Res Ther. 2014;16(5):470. https://doi.org/10.1186/s13075-014-0470-8.

87. Hwang SW, Cho H, Lee S-Y, Kang C-J, Jung JY, Cho S, et al. Direct activation of capsaicin receptors by products of lipoxygenases: Endogenous capsaicin-like

substances. Proc Natl Acad Sci. 2000;97:6155-60. https://doi.org/10.1073/pnas.97.11.6155.

88. Kawabata A. Prostaglandin e2 and pain — An update. Biol Pharm Bull. 2011;34(8):1170-3. https://doi.org/10.1248/bpb.34.1170.

89. Jeske NA, Diogenes A, Ruparel NB, Fehrenbacher JC, Henry M, Akopian AN, et al. A-kinase anchoring protein mediates TRPV thermal hyperalgesia through PKA phosphorylation of TRPV. Pain. 2008;138(3):604-16. https://doi.org/10.1016/j.pain.2008.02.022.

90. Sekiyama N, Mizuta S, Hori A, Kobayashi S. Prostaglandin e2 facilitates excitatory synaptic transmission in the nucleus tractus solitarii of rats. Neurosci Lett. 1995;188(2):101-4. https://doi.org/10.1016/0304-3940(95)11407-N.

91. Matta JA, Ahern GP. TRPV and synaptic transmission. Curr Pharm Biotechnol. 2011;12(1):95-101. https://doi.org/10.2174/138920111793937925.

92. Grace PM, Hutchinson MR, Maier SF, Watkins LR. Pathological pain and the neuroimmune interface. Nat Rev Immunol. 2014;14(4):217-31. https://doi.org/10.1038/nri3621.

93. Abu-Shaweesh JM, Dreshaj IA, Haxhiu MA, Martin RJ. Central GABAergic mechanisms are involved in apnea induced by SLN stimulation in piglets. J Appl Physiol. 2001;90:1570-6.

94. Böhm I, Xia L, Leiter JC, Bartlett D Jr. GABAergic processes mediate thermal prolongation of laryngeal reflex apnea in decerebrate piglets. Respir Physiol Neurobiol. 2007;156:229-33. https://doi.org/10.1016/j.resp.2006.10.005.

95. Xia L, Damon T, Niblock MM, Bartlett D Jr., Leiter JC. Unilateral microdialysis of gabazine in the dorsal medulla reverses thermal prolongation of the laryngeal chemoreflex in decerebrate piglets. J Appl Physiol. 2007;103:1864-72. https://doi.org/10.1152/japplphysiol.00524.2007.

96. Hong Z-Y, Huang Z-L, Qu W-M, Eguchi N, Urade Y, Hayaishi O. An adenosine $A_{2A}$ receptor agonist induces sleep by increasing GABA release in the tuberomammillary nucleus to inhibit histaminergic systems in rats. J Neurochem. 2005;92:1542-9. https://doi.org/10.1111/j.1471-4159.2004.02991.x.

97. Phillis JW. Inhibitory action of CGS 21680 on cerebral cortical neurons is antagonized by bicuculline and picrotoxin — Is GABA involved? Brain Res. 1998;807:193-8. https://doi.org/10.1016/S0006-8993(98)00756-2.

98. Ochi M, Koga K, Kurokawa M, Kase H, Nakamura J-I, Kuwana Y. Systemic administration of adenosine $A_{2A}$ receptor antagonist reverses increased GABA release in the globus pallidus of unilateral 6-hydroxydopamine-lesioned rats:

A microdialysis study. Neurosci. 2000;100:53-62. https://doi.org/10.1016/S0306-4522(00)00250-5.

99. Abu-Shaweesh JM. Activation of central adenosine $A_{2A}$ receptors enhances superior laryngeal nerve stimulation-induced apnea in piglets via a GABAergic pathway. J Appl Physiol. 2007;103:1205-11. https://doi.org/10.1152/japplphysiol.01420.2006.

100. Wilson CG, Martin RJ, Jaber M, Abu-Shaweesh JM, Jafri A, Haxhiu MA, et al. Adenosine $A_{2A}$ receptors interact with GABAergic pathways to modulate respiration in neonatal piglets. Respir Physiol Neurobiol. 2004;141:201-11. https://doi.org/10.1016/j.resp.2004.04.012.

101. Martin RJ, Wilson CG, Abu-Shaweesh JM, Haxhiu MA. Role of inhibitory neurotransmitter interactions in the pathogenesis of neonatal apnea: Implications for management. Semin Perinatol. 2004;28:273-8. https://doi.org/10.1053/j.semperi.2004.08.004.

102. Mayer CA, Haxhiu MA, Martin RJ, Wilson CG. Adenosine $A_{2A}$ receptors mediate GABAergic inhibition of respiration in rats. J Appl Physiol. 2006;100:91-7. https://doi.org/10.1152/japplphysiol.00459.2005.

103. Xia L, Bartlett D Jr., Leiter JC. An adenosine $A_{2A}$ antagonist injected in the NTS reverses thermal prolongation of the ICR in decerebrate piglets. Respir Physiol Neurobiol. 2008;164:358-65. https://doi.org/10.1016/j.resp.2008.08.002.

104. Duy MP, Xia L, Bartlett D Jr., Leiter JC. An adenosine $A_{2A}$ agonist injected in the NTS prolongs the ICR by a GABAergic mechanism in decerebrate piglets. Exp Physiol. 2010;95:774-87. https://doi.org/10.1113/expphysiol.2010.052647.

105. Barrett-Jolley R. Nipecotic acid directly activates $GABA_A$-like ion channels. Brit J Pharm. 2001;133:673-8. https://doi.org/10.1038/sj.bjp.0704128.

106. Machaalani R, Say M, Waters KA. Serotonergic receptor 1a in the sudden infant death syndrome brainstem medulla and associations with clinical risk factors. Acta Neuropathol. 2009;117:257-65. https://doi.org/10.1007/s00401-008-0468-x.

107. Liu Q, Wong-Riley MTT. Postnatal changes in the expressions of serotonin 1a, 1b, and 2a receptors in ten brain stem nuclei of the rat: Implication for a sensitive period. Neurosci. 2010;165:61-78. https://doi.org/10.1016/j.neuroscience.2009.09.078.

108. Varnas K, Halldin C, Hall H. Autoradiographic distribution of serotonin transporters and receptor subtypes in human brain. Hum Brain Mapp. 2004;22(3):246-60. https://doi.org/10.1002/hbm.20035.

109. Dergacheva O, Kamendi H, Wang X, Pinol RM, Frank J, Jameson H, et al. The role of 5-$HT_3$ and other excitatory receptors in central cardiorespiratory

responses to hypoxia: Implications for sudden infant death syndrome. Pediatr Res. 2009;65(6):625-30. https://doi.org/10.1203/PDR.0b013e3181a16e9c.

110. Gustafson EL, Durkin MM, Bard JA, Zgombick J, Branchek TA. A receptor autoradiographic and in situ hybridization analysis of the distribution of the 5-HT$_7$ receptor in rat brain. Br J Pharmacol. 1996;117(4):657-66. https://doi.org/10.1111/j.1476-5381.1996.tb15241.x.

111. Donnelly WT, Bartlett D Jr., Leiter JC. Serotonin in the solitary tract nucleus shortens the laryngeal chemoreflex in anesthetized neonatal rats. Exp Physiol. 2016;in press. https://doi.org/10.1113/EP085716.

112. Remmers JE, Richter DW, Ballantyne D, Bainton CR, Klein JP. Reflex prolongation of stage I of expiration. Pflügers Arch. 1986;407:190-8. https://doi.org/10.1007/BF00580675.

113. Czyzyk-Krzeska MF, Lawson EE. Synaptic events in ventral respiratory neurones during apnoea induced by laryngeal nerve stimulation in neonatal piglet. J Physiol. 1991;436:131-47. https://doi.org/10.1113/jphysiol.1991.sp018543.

114. Kubin L, Alheid GF, Zuperku EJ, McCrimmon DR. Central pathways of pulmonary and lower airway vagal afferents. J Appl Physiol. 2006;101:618-27. https://doi.org/10.1152/japplphysiol.00252.2006.

115. Palkovits M, Mezey E, Eskay RL, Brownstein MJ. Innervation of the nucleus of the solitary tract and the dorsal vagal nucleus by thyrotropin-releasing hormone-containing raphe neurons. Brain Res. 1986;373(1-2):246-51. https://doi.org/10.1016/0006-8993(86)90338-0.

116. Donnelly WT, Bartlett D Jr., Leiter JC. Activation of serotonergic neurons in the medullary caudal raphe shortens the laryngeal chemoreflex in anaesthetized neonatal rats. Exp Physiol. 2017;102(8):1007-18. https://doi.org/10.1113/EP086082.

117. Paxinos G, Watson C. The rat brain in stereotaxic coordinates. 4th ed. San Diego, CA: Academic Press, 1998.

118. Thor KB, Blitz-Seibert A, Hlke CJ. Discrete localization of high-density 5-HT$_{1A}$ binding sites in the midline raphe and parapyramidal region of the ventral medulla oblongata of the rat. Neurosci Lett. 1990;108:249-54. https://doi.org/10.1016/0304-3940(90)90649-T.

119. Guntheroth WG, Kawabori I. Hypoxic apnea and gasping. J Clin Invest. 1975;56:1371-7. https://doi.org/10.1172/JCI108217.

120. Leiter JC. Serotonin, gasping, autoresuscitation and sids — A contrarian view. J Appl Physiol. 2009;106(6):1761-2. https://doi.org/10.1152/japplphysiol.00329.2009.

121. St John WM, Leiter JC. Maintenance of gasping and restoration of eupnea after hypoxia is impaired following blockers of α-1 adrenergic receptors and serotonin 5HT2 receptors. J Appl Physiol. 2008;104:665-73. https://doi.org/10.1152/japplphysiol.00599.2007.

122. Ptak K, Yamanishi T, Aungst J, Milescu LS, Zhang R, Richerson GB, et al. Raphe neurons stimulate respiratory circuit activity by multiple mechanisms via endogenously released serotonin and substance P. J Neurosci. 2009;29(12):3720-37. https://doi.org/10.1523/JNEUROSCI.5271-08.2009.

123. Chen J, Magnusson J, Karsenty G, Cummings KJ. Time- and age-dependent effects of serotonin on gasping and autoresuscitation in neonatal mice. J Appl Physiol. 2013;114(12):1668-76. https://doi.org/10.1152/japplphysiol.00003.2013.

124. Darnall RA, Schneider RW, Tobia CM, Commons KG. Eliminating medullary 5-HT neurons delays arousal and decreases the respiratory response to repeated episodes of hypoxia in neonatal rat pups. J Appl Physiol. 2016;120(5):514-25. https://doi.org/10.1152/japplphysiol.00560.2014.

125. Fuller PM, Sherman D, Pedersen NP, Saper CB, Lu J. Reassessment of the structural basis of the ascending arousal system. J Comp Neurol. 2011;519(5):933-56. https://doi.org/10.1002/cne.22559.

126. Kaur S, Pedersen NP, Yokota S, Hur EE, Fuller PM, Lazarus M, et al. Glutamatergic signaling from the parabrachial nucleus plays a critical role in hypercapnic arousal. J Neurosci. 2013;33(18):7627-40. https://doi.org/10.1523/JNEUROSCI.0173-13.2013.

127. Miller RL, Stein MK, Loewy AD. Serotonergic inputs to FOXP2 neurons of the pre-locus coeruleus and parabrachial nuclei that project to the ventral tegmental area. Neuroscience. 2011;193:229-40. https://doi.org/10.1016/j.neuroscience.2011.07.008.

128. Bang SJ, Jensen P, Dymecki SM, Commons KG. Projections and interconnections of genetically defined serotonin neurons in mice. European J Neurosci. 2012;35(1):85-96. https://doi.org/10.1111/j.1460-9568.2011.07936.x.

129. Buchanan GF, Richerson GB. Central serotonin neurons are required for arousal to $CO_2$. Proc Natl Acad Sci USA. 2010;107(37):16354-9. https://doi.org/10.1073/pnas.1004587107.

130. Buchanan GF, Smith HR, MacAskill A, Richerson GB. 5-HT$_{2A}$ receptor activation is necessary for $CO_2$-induced arousal. J Neurophysiol. 2015;114(1):233-43. https://doi.org/10.1152/jn.00213.2015.

131. Curran AK, Darnall RA, Filiano JJ, Li A, Nattie EE. Muscimol dialysis in the rostral ventral medulla reduces the ventilatory response to $CO_2$ in awake and sleeping piglets. J Appl Physiol. 2001;90:971-80.

132. Litmanovitz I, Dreshaj I, Miller MJ, Haxhiu MA, Martin RJ. Central chemosensitivity affects respiratory muscle responses to laryngeal stimulation in the piglet. J Appl Physiol. 1994;76:403-8.

133. Davies AM, Koenig JS, Thach BT. Upper airway chemoreflex responses to saline and water in preterm infants. J Appl Physiol. 1988;64:1412-20.

134. Nishino T, Hiraga K, Honda Y. Inhibitory effects of $CO_2$ on airway defensive reflexes in enflurane-anesthetized humans. J Appl Physiol. 1989;66:2642-6.

135. Lawson EE. Recovery from central apnea: Effect of stimulus duration and end-tidal $CO_2$ partial pressure. J Appl Physiol. 1982;53:105-9.

136. Bongianni F, Corda M, Fontana GA, Pantaleo T. Excitatory and depressant respiratory responses to chemical stimulation of the rostral ventrolateral medulla in the cat. Acta Physiol Scand. 1993;148:315-25. https://doi.org/10.1111/j.1748-1716.1993.tb09562.x.

137. Richardson MA, Adams J. Fatal apnea in piglets by way of laryngeal chemoreflex: Postmortem findings as anatomic correlates of sudden infant death syndrome in the human infant. The Laryngoscope. 2005;115:1163-9. https://doi.org/10.1097/01.MLG.0000165458.52991.1B.

138. Sasaki CT, Hundal JS, Wadie M, Woo JS, Rosenblatt W. Modulating effects of hypoxia and hypercarbia on glottic closing force. Ann Otology Rhinology Laryngology. 2009;118(2):148-53. https://doi.org/10.1177/000348940911800211.

139. Haouzi P, Bayaert C, Gille JP, Chalon B, Marchal F. Laryngeal reflex apnea is blunted during and after hindlimb muscle contraction in sheep. Am J Physiol. 1997;272:R586-R92.

140. Kemp JS, Kowalski RM, Burch PM, Graham MA, Thach BT. Unintentional suffocation by rebreathing: A death scene and physiologic investigation of a possible cause of sudden infant death. J Pediatr. 1993;122:874-80. https://doi.org/10.1016/S0022-3476(09)90010-5.

141. Kinney HC, Thach BT. The sudden infant death syndrome. New England J Med. 2009;361(8):795-805. https://doi.org/10.1056/NEJMra0803836.

142. Lanier B, Richardson MA, Cummings C. Effect of hypoxia on laryngeal reflex apnea — Implications for sudden infant death. Otolaryngol Head Neck Surg. 1983;91:597. https://doi.org/10.1177/019459988309100602.

143. Woodson GE, Brauel G. Arterial chemoreceptor influences on the laryngeal chemoreflex. Otolaryngol Head Neck Surg. 1992;107:775-82. https://doi.org/10.1177/019459988910700612.1.

144. Darnall RA. Hypoxia decreases apnea produced by stimulation of superior laryngeal nerves in decerebrate piglets. Pediatr Res. 1993;33:321A.

145. Wennergren G, Hertzberg T, Milerad J, Bjure J, Lagercrantz H. Hypoxia reinforces laryngeal reflex bradycardia in infants. Acta Paediatr Scand. 1989;78:11-17. https://doi.org/10.1111/j.1651-2227.1989.tb10879.x.

146. Kumar P. Systemic effects resulting from carotid body stimulation — Invited article. In: Arterial chemoreceptors. Advances in experimental medicine and biology. Eds Gonzalez C, Nurse CA, Peers C. Vol. 648. Dordrecht: Springer, 2009. p. 223-33. https://doi.org/10.1007/978-90-481-2259-2_26.

147. Bissonnette JM. Mechanisms regulating hypoxic respiratory depression during fetal and postnatal life. Am J Physiol Regul Integr Comp Physiol. 2000;278(6):R1391-400.

148. Powell FL, Milsom WK, Mitchell GS. Time domains of the hypoxic ventilatory response. Respir Physiol. 1998;112:123-34. https://doi.org/10.1016/S0034-5687(98)00026-7.

149. Cohen G, Malcolm G, Henderson-Smart D. Ventilatory response of the newborn infant to mild hypoxia. Pediatric Pulmonology. 1997;24(3):163-72. https://doi.org/10.1002/(SICI)1099-0496(199709)24:3<163::AID-PPUL1>3.0.CO;2-O.

150. Sasse SA, Berry RB, Nguyen TK, Light RW, Mahutte CK. Arterial blood gas changes during breath-holding from functional residual capacity. Chest. 1996;110(4):958-64. https://doi.org/10.1378/chest.110.4.958.

151. Xia L, Leiter JC, Bartlett D Jr. Laryngeal reflex apnea in neonates: Effects of $CO_2$ and the tangled influence of hypoxia. Resp Physiol Neurobiol. 2013;186(1):109-13. https://doi.org/10.1016/j.resp.2013.01.004.

152. Sladek M, Grogaard RA, Parker RA, Sundell HW. Prolonged hypoxemia enhances and acute hypoxia attenuates laryngeal reflex apnea in youg lambs. Pediatr Res. 1993;34:813-20. https://doi.org/10.1203/00006450-199312000-00024.

153. Milerad J, Hertzberg T, Wennergren G, Lagercrantz H. Respiratory and arousal responses to hypoxia in apnoeic infants reinvestigated. European J Pediatr. 1989;148(6):565-70. https://doi.org/10.1007/BF00441560.

154. Sundell HW, Karmo H, Milerad J. Impaired cardiorespiratory recovery after laryngeal stimulation in nicotine-exposed young lambs. Pediatr Res. 2003;53:104-12. https://doi.org/10.1203/00006450-200301000-00018.

155. Saetta M, Mortola JP. Interaction of hypoxic and hypercapnic stimuli on breathing pattern in the newborn rat. J Appl Physiol (1985). 1987;62(2):506-12.

156. Xia L, Crane-Godreau MA, Leiter JC, Bartlett D Jr. Gestational cigarette smoke exposure and hyperthermic enhancement of laryngeal chemoreflex in rat pups. Respir Physiol Neurobiol. 2009;165:161-6. https://doi.org/10.1016/j. resp.2008.11.004.

157. Xia L, Leiter JC, Bartlett D Jr. Laryngeal apnea in rat pups: Effects of age and body temperature. J Appl Physiol. 2008;104:269-74. https://doi.org/10.1152/ japplphysiol.00721.2007.

158. Storey AT, Johnson P. Laryngeal water receptors initiating apnea in the lamb. Exp Neurol. 1975;47:42-55. https://doi.org/10.1016/0014-4886(75)90235-6.

159. Sutton D, Taylor EM, Lindeman RC. Prolonged apnea in infant monkeys resulting from stimulation of superior laryngeal nerve. Pediatrics. 1978;61:519-27.

160. Abu-Shaweesh JM. Maturation of respiratory reflex responses in the fetus and neonate. Semin Neonatol. 2004;9:169-80. https://doi.org/10.1016/j. siny.2003.09.003.

161. Bertolino M, Keller KJ, Vicini S, Gillis RA. Nicotinic receptor mediates spontaneous GABA release in the rat dorsal motor nucleus of the vagus. Neurosci. 1997;79:671-81. https://doi.org/10.1016/S0306-4522(97)00026-2.

162. Sykes C, Prestwich S, Horton R. Chronic administration of the GABA-transaminase inhibitor ethanolamine O-sulfate leads to up-regulation of GABA binding sites. Biochem Pharmacol. 1984;33:387-93. https://doi.org/10.1016/0006-2952(84)9 0230-2.

163. Pericic D, Strac DS, Jembrek MJ, Rajcan I. Prolonged exposure to gama-aminobutyric acid up-regulated stably expressed recombinant alpha 1 beta 2 gamma 2s $GABA_A$ receptors. Eur J Pharmacol. 2003;482:117-25. https://doi. org/10.1016/j.ejphar.2003.10.023.

164. Luo Z, Costy-Bennett S, Fregosi RF. Prenatal nicotine exposure increases the strength of $GABA_A$ receptor-mediated inhibition of respiratory rhythm in neonates. J Physiol (Lond). 2004;561:387-93. https://doi.org/10.1113/ jphysiol.2004.062927.

165. Guntheroth WG. Crib death. Lancet. 1983;1(8320):352. https://doi.org/10.1016/ S0140-6736(83)91651-3.

166. Thach BT. Sleep apnea in infancy and childhood. Med Clin North Am. 1985;69(6):1289-315. https://doi.org/10.1016/S0025-7125(16)30988-9.

167. Peiper A. [apnea]. Monatsschrift fur Kinderheilkunde. Uber die Schnappatmung. 1953;101(2):58-9.

168. Stevens LH. Sudden unexplained death in infancy. Amer J Dis Child. 1965;110:243-7. https://doi.org/10.1001/archpedi.1965.02090030257004.

169. Poets CF, Meny RG, Chobanian MR, Bonofiglo RE. Gasping and other cardiorespiratory patterns during sudden infant death. Pediatr Res. 1999;45:350-4. https://doi.org/10.1203/00006450-199903000-00010.

170. Mitchell EA, Thach BT, Thompson JMD, Williams S. Changing infants' sleep position increases risk of sudden infant death syndrome. Arch Pedaitr Adolesc Med. 1999;153:1136-41. https://doi.org/10.1001/archpedi.153.11.1136.

171. Fewell JE, Smith FG. Perinatal nicotine exposure impairs ability of newborn rats to autoresuscitate from apnea during hypoxia. J Appl Physiol. 1998;85(6):2066-74.

172. Shannon DC, Kelly DH. SIDS and near-SIDS. New England J Med. 1983;306:959-65, 1022-8. https://doi.org/10.1056/NEJM198204223061604.

173. Godfrey S. Blood gases during asphyxia and resuscitation of fetal and newborn rabbits. Respir Physiol. 1968;4(3):309-21. https://doi.org/10.1016/0034-5687(68)90037-6.

174. Lawson EE, Thach BT. Respiratory patterns during progressive asphyxia in newborn rabbits. J Appl Physiol: Respir, Enviro Exerc Physio. 1977;43(3):468-74.

175. Fewell JE, Smith FG, Ng VKY, Wong VH, Wang YT. Postnatal age influences the ability of rats to autoresuscitate from hypoxic-induced apnea. Am J Physiol. 2000;279:R39-R46.

176. Kinney HC, Richerson GB, Dymecki SM, Darnall RA, Nattie EE. The brainstem and serotonin in the sudden infant death syndrome. Ann Rev Path. 2009;4:517-50. https://doi.org/10.1146/annurev.pathol.4.110807.092322.

177. Kinney HC, Broadbelt KG, Haynes RL, Rognum IJ, Paterson DS. The serotonergic anatomy of the developing human medulla oblongata: Implications for pediatric disorders of homeostasis. J Chem Neuroanat. 2011;41(4):182-99. https://doi.org/10.1016/j.jchemneu.2011.05.004.

178. Erikson JT, Sposato BC. Autoresuscitation responses to hypoxia-induced apnea are delayed in newborn 5-HT-deficient *Pet-1* homozygous mice. J Appl Physiol. 2009;106(6):1785-92. https://doi.org/10.1152/japplphysiol.90729.2008.

179. Cummings KJ, Commons KG, Hewitt JC, Daubenspeck JA, Li A, Kinney HC, et al. Failed heart rate recovery at a critical age in 5-HT-deficient mice exposed to episodic anoxia: Implications for SIDS. J Appl Physiol. 2011;111(3):825-33. https://doi.org/10.1152/japplphysiol.00336.2011.

180. Cummings KJ, Hewitt JC, Li A, Daubenspeck JA, Nattie EE. Postnatal loss of brainstem serotonin neurones compromises the ability of neonatal rats to survive episodic severe hypoxia. J Physiol. 2011;589(Pt 21):5247-56. https://doi.org/10.1113/jphysiol.2011.214445.

181. Gershan WM, Jacobi MS, Thach BT. Mechanisms underlying induced autoresuscitation failure in BALB/c and SWR mice. J Appl Physiol. 1992;72(2):677-85.

182. Cummings KJ, Frappell PB. Breath-to-breath hypercapnic response in neonatal rats: Temperature dependency of the chemoreflexes and potential implications for breathing stability. Am J Physiol Regul Integr Comp Physiol. 2009;297(1):R124-34. https://doi.org/10.1152/ajpregu.91011.2008.

183. Barrett KT, Dosumu-Johnson RT, Daubenspeck JA, Brust RD, Kreouzis V, Kim JC, et al. Partial raphe dysfunction in neurotransmission is sufficient to increase mortality after anoxic exposures in mice at a critical period in postnatal development. J Neuroscie. 2016;36(14):3943-53. https://doi.org/10.1523/JNEUROSCI.1796-15.2016.

184. Hendricks TJ, Fyodorov DV, Wegman LJ, Leluth NB, Pehek EA, Yamamoto B, et al. *Pet-1* ETS gene plays a critical role in 5-HT neuron development and is required for normal anxiety-like and aggressive behavior. Neuron. 2003;37:233-47. https://doi.org/10.1016/S0896-6273(02)01167-4.

185. Cummings KJ, Li A, Deneris ES, Nattie EE. Bradycardia in serotonin-deficient *Pet-1*$^{-/-}$ mice: Influence of respiratory dysfunction and hyperthermia over the first 2 postnatal weeks. Am J Physiol Regul Integr Comp Physiol. 2010;298(5):R1333-42. https://doi.org/10.1152/ajpregu.00110.2010.

186. Wyler SC, Spencer WC, Green NH, Rood BD, Crawford L, Craige C, et al. *Pet-1* switches transcriptional targets postnatally to regulate maturation of serotonin neuron excitability. The Journal of Neuroscience : The Official Journal of the Society for Neuroscience. 2016;36(5):1758-74. https://doi.org/10.1523/JNEUROSCI.3798-15.2016.

187. Yang HT, Cummings KJ. Brain stem serotonin protects blood pressure in neonatal rats exposed to episodic anoxia. J Appl Physiol. 2013;115(12):1733-41. https://doi.org/10.1152/japplphysiol.00970.2013.

188. Lieske SP, Thoby-Brisson M, Telgkamp P, Ramirez JM. Reconfiguration of the neural network controlling multiple breathing patterns: Eupnea, sighs and gasps [see comment]. Nature Neurosci. 2000;3(6):600-7. https://doi.org/10.1038/75776.

189. Paton JFR, Abdala AP, Koizumi H, Smith JC, St John WM. Respiratory rhythm generation during gasping depends on persistent sodium current. Nat Neurosci. 2006;9:311-13. https://doi.org/10.1038/nn1650.

190. Huang Q, Zhou D, St John WM. Lesions of regions for in vitro ventilatory genesis eliminate gasping but not eupnea. Respir Physiol. 1997;107:111-23. https://doi.org/10.1016/S0034-5687(96)02513-3.

191. St John WM. Medullary regions for neurogenesis of gasping: Noeud vital or noeuds vitals? J Appl Physiol. 1996;81:1865-77.

192. Pena F, Ramirez JM. Endogenous activation of serotonin-2A receptors is required for respiratory rhythm generation in vitro. J Neurosci. 2002;22(24):11055-64.

193. Harvey PJ, Li X, Li Y, Bennett DJ. 5-HT$_2$ receptor activation facilitates a persistent sodium current and repetitive firing in spinal motoneurons of rats with and without chronic spinal cord injury. J Neurophysiol. 2006;96:1158-70. https://doi.org/10.1152/jn.01088.2005.

194. Cummings KJ, Li A, Nattie EE. Brainstem serotonin deficiency in the neonatal period: Autonomic dysregulation during mild cold stress. J Physiol. 2011;589(Pt 8):2055-64. https://doi.org/10.1113/jphysiol.2010.203679.

195. Tryba AK, Pe-a F, Ramirez J-M. Gasping activity in vitro: A rhythm dependent on 5-HT$_{2A}$ receptors. J Neurosci. 2006;26(10):2623-34. https://doi.org/10.1523/JNEUROSCI.4186-05.2006.

196. Toppin VAL, Harris MB, Kober AM, Leiter JC, St John WM. Persistence of eupnea and gasping following blockade of both serotonin type 1 and 2 receptors in the in situ juvenile rat preparation. J Appl Physiol. 2007;103:220-7. https://doi.org/10.1152/japplphysiol.00071.2007.

197. St John WM. Noeud vital for breathing in the brainstem: Gasping — yes; eupnea — doubtful. Philos Trans R Soc Lond B Biol Sci. 2009;364(1529):2625-33. https://doi.org/10.1098/rstb.2009.0080.

198. Hodges MR, Tattersall GT, Harris MB, McEvoy SD, Richerson DN, Deneris ES, et al. Defects in breathing and thermoregulation in mice with near-complete absence of central serotonin neurons. J Neurosci. 2008;28:2495-505. https://doi.org/10.1523/JNEUROSCI.4729-07.2008.

199. Hodges MR, Wehner M, Aungst J, Smith JC, Richerson GB. Transgenic mice lacking serotonin neurons have severe apnea and high mortality during development. J Neurosci. 2009;29:10341-9. https://doi.org/10.1523/JNEUROSCI.1963-09.2009.

200. Duncan JR, Randall LL, Belliveau RA, Trachtenberg FL, Randall B, Habbe D, et al. The effect of maternal smoking and drinking during pregnancy upon $^3$H-nicotine receptor brainstem binding in infants dying of the sudden infant death syndrome: Initial observations in a high risk population. Brain Path. 2008;18(1):21-31. https://doi.org/10.1111/j.1750-3639.2007.00093.x.

201. Fewell JE, Smith FG, Ng VK. Prenatal exposure to nicotine impairs protective responses of rat pups to hypoxia in an age-dependent manner. Respir Physiol. 2001;127(1):61-73. https://doi.org/10.1016/S0034-5687(01)00232-8.

202. Lee S, Nattie EE. Prenatal and early postnatal nicotine exposure adversely affects autoresuscitation in serotonin deficient rats. FASEB J. 2015;29(1):861.5.

203. Cummings KJ, Commons KG, Trachtenberg FL, Li A, Kinney HC, Nattie EE. Caffeine improves the ability of serotonin-deficient (*Pet-1*$^{-/-}$) mice to survive episodic asphyxia. Pediatr Res. 2013;73(1):38-45. https://doi.org/10.1038/pr.2012.142.

204. Berkowitz BA, Spector S. The effect of caffeine and theophylline on the disposition of brain serotonin in the rat. European J Pharmacol. 1971;16(3):322-5. https://doi.org/10.1016/0014-2999(71)90034-3.

205. Julien CA, Joseph V, Bairam A. Caffeine reduces apnea frequency and enhances ventilatory long-term facilitation in rat pups raised in chronic intermittent hypoxia. Pediatr Res. 2010;68(2):105-11. https://doi.org/10.1203/PDR.0b013e3181e5bc78.

206. Mitchell GS, Baker TL, Nanda SA, Fuller DD, Zabka AG, Hodgeman BA, et al. Invited review: Intermittent hypoxia and respiratory plasticity. J Appl Physiol (1985). 2001;90(6):2466-75.

207. Slotkin TA, Epps TA, Stenger ML, Sawyer KJ, Seidler FJ. Cholinergic receptors in heart and brainstem of rats exposed to nicotine during development: Implications for hypoxia tolerance and perinatal mortality. Brain Res Devel Brain Res. 1999;113(1-2):1-12. https://doi.org/10.1016/S0165-3806(98)00173-4.

208. Waters KA, Machaalani R. NMDA receptors in the developing brain and effects of noxious insults. Neuro-Signals. 2004;13:162-74. https://doi.org/10.1159/000077523.

209. Fewell JE, Lun R. Adenosine A1-receptor blockade impairs the ability of rat pups to autoresuscitate from primary apnea during repeated exposure to hypoxia. Physiol Reports. 2015;3(8):e12458. https://doi.org/10.14814/phy2.12458.

210. Zaidi SIA, Jafri A, Martin RJ, Haxhui MA. Adenosine A$_{2A}$ receptors are expressed by GABAergic neurons of medulla oblongata in developing rat. Brain Res. 2006;1071:42-53. https://doi.org/10.1016/j.brainres.2005.11.077.

211. Atik A, Harding R, de Matteo R, Kondos-Devcic D, Cheong J, Doyle LW, et al. Caffeine for apnea of prematurity: Effects on the developing brain. Neurotoxicology. 2017;58:94-102. https://doi.org/10.1016/j.neuro.2016.11.012.

212. Phillipson EA, Sullivan C. Arousal: The forgotten response to respiratory stimuli. Am Rev Respir Dis. 1978;118:807-9.

213. Hunt CE. Abnormal hypercarbic and hypoxic sleep arousal responses in near-miss SIDS infants. Pediatr Res. 1981;15:1462-4. https://doi.org/10.1203/00006450-198111000-00015.

214. McCulloch K, Brouillette RT, Guzzetta AJ, Hunt CE. Arousal responses in near-miss sudden infant death syndrome and in normal infants. J Pediatrics. 1982;101:911-17. https://doi.org/10.1016/S0022-3476(82)80009-7.

215. Harper RM, Bandler R. Finding the failure mechanism in sudden infant death syndrome. Nature Med. 1998;4:157-8. https://doi.org/10.1038/nm0298-157.

216. Kahn A, Groswasser J, Franco P, Scaillet S, Sawaguchi T, Kelmanson I, et al. Sudden infant deaths: Arousal as a survival mechanism. Sleep medicine. 2002;3 Suppl 2:S11-14. https://doi.org/10.1016/S1389-9457(02)00157-0.

217. McNamara F, Lijowska AS, Thach BT. Spontaneous arousal activity in infants during NREM and REM sleep. J Physiol (Lond). 2002;538:263-9. https://doi.org/10.1113/jphysiol.2001.012507.

218. McNamara F, Wulbrand H, Thach BT. Characteristics of the infant arousal response. J Appl Physiol. 1998;85:2314-21.

219. Dauger S, Aizenfisz S, Renolleau S, Durand E, Vardon G, Gaultier C, et al. Arousal response to hypoxia in newborn mice. Respir Physiol. 2001;128(2):235-40. https://doi.org/10.1016/S0034-5687(01)00303-6.

220. Darnall RA, McWilliams S, Schneider RW, Tobia CM. Reversible blunting of arousal from sleep in response to intermittent hypoxia in the developing rat. J Appl Physiol. 2010;109(6):1686-96. https://doi.org/10.1152/japplphysiol.00076.2010.

221. BuSha BF, Leiter JC, Curran A, Li A, Nattie EE, Darnall RA. Spontaneous arousals during quiet sleep in piglets: A visual and wavelet-based analysis. Sleep. 2001;24:499-513. https://doi.org/10.1093/sleep/24.5.499.

222. Horner RL. Autonomic consequences of arousal from sleep: Mechanisms and implications. Sleep. 1996;19(10 Suppl):S193-5. https://doi.org/10.1093/sleep/19.suppl_10.S193.

223. Horne RS, Parslow PM, Harding R. Postnatal development of ventilatory and arousal responses to hypoxia in human infants. Respir Physiol Neurobiol. 2005;149(1-3):257-71. https://doi.org/10.1016/j.resp.2005.03.006.

224. Ariagno R, Mirmiran M, Darnall RA. Arousals in infants during the first year of life: Argument for new definitions and criteria. In: Awakening and sleep-wake cycle across development. Eds Salzarulo P, Ficca G. Philadelphia: John Benjamins Publishing Company, 2002. p. 63-78. https://doi.org/10.1075/aicr.38.06ari.

225. Jeffery HE, Read DJ. Ventilatory responses of newborn calves to progressive hypoxia in quiet and active sleep. J Appl Physiol. 1980;48(5):892-5.

226. Henderson-Smart DJ, Read DJ. Ventilatory responses to hypoxaemia during sleep in the newborn. J Devel Physiol. 1979;1(3):195-208.

227. Fewell JE, Baker SB. Arousal from sleep during rapidly developing hypoxemia in lambs. Pediatr Res. 1987;22(4):471-7. https://doi.org/10.1203/00006450-19871 0000-00023.

228. Frank MG, Heller HC. Development of REM and slow wave sleep in the rat. Am J Physiol. 1997;272:R1792-R9.

229. Seelke AM, Blumberg MS. The microstructure of active and quiet sleep as cortical delta activity emerges in infant rats. Sleep. 2008;31(5):691-9. https://doi.org/10.1093/sleep/31.5.691.

230. Balbir A, Lande B, Fitzgerald RS, Polotsky V, Mitzner W, Shirahata M. Behavioral and respiratory characteristics during sleep in neonatal DBA/2J and A/J mice. Brain Res. 2008;1241:84-91. https://doi.org/10.1016/j.brainres.2008.09.008.

231. Blumberg MS, Kalrson KÆ, Seelke AMH, Mohns EJ. The ontogeny of mammalain sleep: A response to Frank and Heller (2003). J Sleep Res. 2005;14:91-101. https://doi.org/10.1111/j.1365-2869.2004.00430_1.x.

232. Dunne KP, Fox GP, O'Regan M, Matthews TG. Arousal responses in babies at risk of sudden infant death syndrome at different postnatal ages. Ir Med J. 1992;85:10-22.

233. Johnston RV, Grant DA, Wilkinson MH, Walker AM. The effects of repeated exposure to hypercapnia on arousal and cardiorespiratory responses during sleep in lambs. J Physiol. 2007;582(Pt 1):369-78. https://doi.org/10.1113/jphysiol.2007.132415.

234. Fewell JE, Kondo CS, Dascalu V, Filyk SC. Influence of carotid-denervation on the arousal and cardiopulmonary responses to alveolar hypercapnia in lambs. J Devel Physiol. 1989;12(4):193-9.

235. Fewell JE, Kondo CS, Dascalu V, Filyk SC. Influence of carotid denervation on the arousal and cardiopulmonary response to rapidly developing hypoxemia in lambs. Pediatr Res. 1989;25:473-7. https://doi.org/10.1203/00006450-1989050 00-00009.

236. Darnall RA, Schneider RW, Tobia CM, Zemel BM. Arousal from sleep in response to intermittent hypoxia in rat pups is modulated by medullary raphe GABAergic mechanisms. Am J Physiol Regul Integr Comp Physiol. 2012;302(5):R551-60. https://doi.org/10.1152/ajpregu.00506.2011.

237. Gottlieb DJ, Chase C, Vezina RM, Heeren TC, Corwin MJ, Auerbach SH, et al. Sleep-disordered breathing symptoms are associated with poorer cognitive function in 5-year-old children. J Pediatr. 2004;145(4):458-64. https://doi.org/10.1016/j.jpeds.2004.05.039.

238. Hunt CE, Corwin MJ, Baird T, Tinsley LR, Palmer P, Ramanathan R, et al. Cardiorespiratory events detected by home memory monitoring and one-year neurodevelopmental outcome. J Pediatr. 2004;145(4):465-71. https://doi.org/10.1016/j.jpeds.2004.05.045.

239. Bass JL, Corwin M, Gozal D, Moore C, Nishida H, Parker S, et al. The effect of chronic or intermittent hypoxia on cognition in childhood: A review of the evidence. Pediatrics. 2004;114(3):805-16. https://doi.org/10.1542/peds.2004-0227.

240. Gozal D, Reeves SR, Row BW, Neville JJ, Guo SZ, Lipton AJ. Respiratory effects of gestational intermittent hypoxia in the developing rat. Am J Resp Crit Care Med. 2003;167(11):1540-7. https://doi.org/10.1164/rccm.200208-963OC.

241. Martin RJ, Wang K, Koroglu O, di Fiore J, Kc P. Intermittent hypoxic episodes in preterm infants: Do they matter? Neonatology. 2011;100(3):303-10. https://doi.org/10.1159/000329922.

242. Nagata N, Saji M, Ito T, Ikeno S, Takahashi H, Terakawa N. Repetitive intermittent hypoxia-ischemia and brain damage in neonatal rats. Brain & Devel. 2000;22(5):315-20. https://doi.org/10.1016/S0387-7604(00)00123-6.

243. Neubauer JA. Invited review: Physiological and pathophysiological responses to intermittent hypoxia. J Appl Physiol. 2001;90(4):1593-9.

244. Prabhakar NR. Oxygen sensing during intermittent hypoxia: Cellular and molecular mechanisms. J Appl Physiol. 2001;90(5):1986-94.

245. Feldman JL, Mitchell C, Nattie EE. Breathing: Rhythmicity, plasticity, chemosensitivity. Annu Rev Neurosci. 2003;26:239-66. https://doi.org/10.1146/annurev.neuro.26.041002.131103.

246. Douglas RM, Miyasaka N, Takahashi K, Latuszek-Barrantes A, Haddad GG, Hetherington HP. Chronic intermittent but not constant hypoxia decreases NAA/CR ratios in neonatal mouse hippocampus and thalamus. Am J Physiol Regul Integr Comp Physiol. 2007;292(3):R1254-9. https://doi.org/10.1152/ajpregu.00404.2006.

247. Machaalani R, Waters KA. Postnatal nicotine and/or intermittent hypercapnic hypoxia effects on apoptotic markers in the developing piglet brainstem medulla. Neuroscience. 2006;142(1):107-17. https://doi.org/10.1016/j.neuroscience.2006.06.015.

248. Ratner V, Kishkurno SV, Slinko SK, Sosunov SA, Sosunov AA, Polin RA, et al. The contribution of intermittent hypoxemia to late neurological handicap in mice with hyperoxia-induced lung injury. Neonatology. 2007;92(1):50-8. https://doi.org/10.1159/000100086.

249. Ryan S, McNicholas WT. Inflammatory cardiovascular risk markers in obstructive sleep apnoea syndrome. Cardiovasc Hematol Agents Med Chem. 2009;7(1):76-81. https://doi.org/10.2174/187152509787047685.

250. Fewell JE, Williams BJ, Szabo JS, Taylor BJ. Influence of repeated upper airway obstruction on the arousal and cardiopulmonary response to upper airway obstruction in lambs. Pediatr Res. 1988;23(2):191-5. https://doi.org/10.1203/00006450-198802000-00013.

251. Waters KA, Tinworth KD. Habituation of arousal responses after intermittent hypercapnic hypoxia in piglets. Am J Respir Crit Care Med. 2005;171:1305-11. https://doi.org/10.1164/rccm.200405-595OC.

252. Durand E, Lofaso F, Dauger S, Vardon G, Gaultier C, Gallego J. Intermittent hypoxia induces transient arousal delay in newborn mice. J Appl Physiol (1985). 2004;96(3):1216-22; discussion 196.

253. Hehre DA, Devia CJ, Bancalari E, Suguihara C. Brainstem amino acid neurotransmitters and ventilatory response to hypoxia in piglets. Pediatr Res. 2008;63(1):46-50. https://doi.org/10.1203/PDR.0b013e31815b4421.

254. Hoop B, Beagle JL, Maher TJ, Kazemi H. Brainstem amino acid neurotransmitters and hypoxic ventilatory response. Respir Physiol. 1999;118(2-3):117-29. https://doi.org/10.1016/S0034-5687(99)00072-9.

255. Richter DW, Schmidt-Garcon P, Pierrefiche O, Bischoff AM, Lalley PM. Neurotransmitters and neuromodulators controlling the hypoxic respiratory response in anaesthetized cats. J Physiol. 1999;514:567-78. https://doi.org/10.1111/j.1469-7793.1999.567ae.x.

256. Tabata M, Kurosawa H, Kikuchi Y, Hida W, Ogawa H, Okabe S, et al. Role of GABA within the nucleus tractus solitarii in the hypoxic ventilatory decline of awake rats. Am J Physiol Regul Integr Comp Physiol. 2001;281(5):R1411-19.

257. Konduri GG, Fewell JE. Naloxone does not alter the arousal response decrement after repeated exposure to hypoxemia during sleep in lambs. Pediatr Res. 1992;32(2):222-5. https://doi.org/10.1203/00006450-199208000-00019.

258. Darnall RA, Bruce RD. Effects of adenosine and xanthine derivatives on breathing during acute hypoxia in the anesthetized newborn piglet. Pediatr Pulmon. 1987;3:110-16. https://doi.org/10.1002/ppul.1950030213.

259. Gether U, Andersen PH, Larsson OM, Schousboe A. Neurotransmitter transporters: Molecular function of important drug targets. Trends Pharm Sci. 2006;27(7):375-83. https://doi.org/10.1016/j.tips.2006.05.003.

260. Kristensen AS, Andersen J, Jorgensen TN, Sorensen L, Eriksen J, Loland CJ, et al. *Slc6* neurotransmitter transporters: Structure, function, and regulation. Pharmacol Rev. 2011;63(3):585-640. https://doi.org/10.1124/pr.108.000869.

261. Darnall RA, Schneider RW, Tobia CM, Webster CA, Zemel BM, Cummings KJ, et al. *Pet1* knockout mouse pups have impaired arousal in response to intermittent hypoxia: Implications for the sudden infant death syndrome (SIDS). Society for Neuroscience. 2011;286.12/SS8.

262. Hodges MR, Richerson GB. The role of medullary serotonin (5-HT) neurons in respiratory control: Contributions to eupneic ventilation, $CO_2$ chemoreception, and thermoregulation. J Appl Physiol. 2010;108(5):1425-32. https://doi.org/10.1152/japplphysiol.01270.2009.

263. Hodges MR, Richerson GB. Medullary serotonin neurons and their roles in central respiratory chemoreception. Respir Physiol Neurobiol. 2010;173(3):256-63. https://doi.org/10.1016/j.resp.2010.03.006.

264. Jacobs BL, Fornal CA. Activity of serotonergic neurons in behaving animals. Neuropsychopharn. 1999;21:9S-15S. https://doi.org/10.1016/S0893-133X(99)00012-3.

265. Gauda EB, Carroll JL, Donnelly DF. Developmental maturation of chemosensitivity to hypoxia of peripheral arterial chemoreceptors — Invited article. Adv Exp Med Biol. 2009;648:243-55. https://doi.org/10.1007/978-90-481-2259-2_28.

266. Kholwadwala D, Donnelly DF. Maturation of carotid chemoreceptor sensitivity to hypoxia: In vitro studies in the newborn rat. J Physiol (Lond). 1992;453:461-73. https://doi.org/10.1113/jphysiol.1992.sp019239.

267. Bamford OS, Carroll JL. Dynamic ventilatory responses in rats: Normal development and effects of prenatal nicotine exposure. Respir Physiol. 1999;117:29-40. https://doi.org/10.1016/S0034-5687(99)00054-7.

268. Carroll JL, Fitzgerald RS. Carotid chemoreceptor responses to hypoxia and hypercapnia in developing kittens. Adv Exp Med Biol. 1993;337:387-91. https://doi.org/10.1007/978-1-4615-2966-8_54.

269. Sovik S, Lossius K, Eriksen M, Grogaard J, Walloe L. Development of oxygen sensitivity in infants of smoking and non-smoking mothers. Early Human Devel. 1999;56(2-3):217-32. https://doi.org/10.1016/S0378-3782(99)00048-1.

270. Calder NA, Williams BA, Kumar P, Hanson MA. The respiratory response of healthy term infants to breath-by-breath alternations in inspired oxygen at two postnatal ages. Pediatr Res. 1994;35(3):321-4. https://doi.org/10.1203/0000645 0-199403000-00008.

271. Bowes G, Townsend ER, Kozar LF, Bromley SM, Phillipson EA. Effect of carotid body denervation on arousal response to hypoxia in sleeping dogs. J Appl Physiol Respir Environ Exerc Physiol. 1981;51(1):40-5.

272. Bowes G, Townsend ER, Bromley SM, Kozar LF, Phillipson EA. Role of the carotid body and of afferent vagal stimuli in the arousal response to airway occlusion in sleeping dogs. Am Rev Respir Dis. 1981;123(6):644-7.

273. Fewell JE, Taylor BJ, Kondo CS, Dascalu V, Filyk SC. Influence of carotid denervation on the arousal and cardiopulmonary responses to upper airway obstruction in lambs. Pediatr Res. 1990;28(4):374-8. https://doi.org/10.1203/0 0006450-199010000-00014.

274. Phillipson EA, Kozar LF, Rebuck AS, Murphy E. Ventilatory and waking responses to $CO_2$ in sleeping dogs. Am Rev Respir Dis. 1977;115(2):251-9.

275. Gleeson K, Zwillich CW. Adenosine stimulation, ventilation, and arousal from sleep. Am Rev Respir Dis. 1992;145(2 Pt 1):453-7. https://doi.org/10.1164/ ajrccm/145.2_Pt_1.453.

276. Guyenet PG, Abbott SB. Chemoreception and asphyxia-induced arousal. Respir Physiol Neurobiol. 2013;188(3):333-43. https://doi.org/10.1016/j. resp.2013.04.011.

277. Guyenet PG, Brown DL. Unit activity in nucleus paragigantocellularis lateralis during cerebral ischemia in the rat. Brain Res. 1986;364(2):301-14. https://doi.or g/10.1016/0006-8993(86)90843-7.

278. Guyenet PG, Stornetta RL, Bayliss DA. Central respiratory chemoreception. J Comp Neurol. 2010;518(19):3883-906. https://doi.org/10.1002/cne.22435.

279. Mulkey DK, Wenker IC. Astrocyte chemoreceptors: Mechanisms of H+ sensing by astrocytes in the retrotrapezoid nucleus and their possible contribution to respiratory drive. Exp Physiol. 2011;96(4):400-6. https://doi.org/10.1113/ expphysiol.2010.053140.

280. Takakura ACT, Moreira TS, Colombari E, West GH, Stornetta RL, Guyenet PG. Peripheral chemoreceptor inputs to retrotrapezoid nucleus (RTN) $CO_2$-sensitive

neurons in rats. J Phsyiol. 2006;572:503-23. https://doi.org/10.1113/jphysiol.2005.103788.

281. Williams RH, Jensen LT, Verkhratsky A, Fugger L, Burdakov D. Control of hypothalamic orexin neurons by acid and $CO_2$. Proc Natl Acad Sci. 2007;104:10685-90. https://doi.org/10.1073/pnas.0702676104.

282. Mulkey DK, Rosin DL, West GB, Takakura AC, Moreira TS, Bayliss DA, et al. Serotonergic neurons activate chemosensitive retrotrapezoid nucleus neurons by a pH-independent mechanism. J Neurosci. 2007;27:14128-38. https://doi.org/10.1523/JNEUROSCI.4167-07.2007.

283. Brust RD, Corcoran AE, Richerson GB, Nattie E, Dymecki SM. Functional and developmental identification of a molecular subtype of brain serotonergic neuron specialized to regulate breathing dynamics. Cell Rep. 2014;9(6):2152-65. https://doi.org/10.1016/j.celrep.2014.11.027.

284. Baker-Herman TL, Mitchell GS. Phrenic long-term facilitation requires spinal serotonin receptor activation and protein synthesis. J Neurosci. 2002;22(14):6239-46.

285. Baker TL, Mitchell GS. Episodic but not continuous hypoxia elicits long-term facilitation of phrenic motor output in rats. J Physiol. 2000;529:215-19. https://doi.org/10.1111/j.1469-7793.2000.00215.x.

286. Erickson JT, Millhorn DE. Fos-like protein is induced in neurons of the medulla oblongata after stimulation of the carotid sinus nerve in awake and anesthetized rats. Brain Res. 1991;567(1):11-24. https://doi.org/10.1016/0006-8993(91)91430-9.

287. Nuding SC, Segers LS, Shannon R, O'Connor R, Morris KF, Lindsey BG. Central and peripheral chemoreceptors evoke distinct responses in simultaneously recorded neurons of the raphe-pontomedullary respiratory network. Philos Trans R Soc Lond B Biol Sci. 2009;364(1529):2501-16. https://doi.org/10.1098/rstb.2009.0075.

288. Parmeggiani PL, Rabini C. Shivering and panting during sleep. Brain Res. 1967;6:789-91. https://doi.org/10.1016/0006-8993(67)90139-4.

289. Parmeggiani PL, Zamboni G, Cianici T, Calasso M. Absense of themoregulatory vasomotor responses during fast wave sleep in cats. Electroenceph Clin Neurophys. 1977;42:372-80. https://doi.org/10.1016/0013-4694(77)90173-0.

290. Darnall RA, Ariagno RL. The effect of sleep state on active thermoregulation in the premature infant. Pediatr Res. 1982;16:512-14. https://doi.org/10.1203/00006450-198207000-00002.

291. Stothers JK, Warner RM. Oxygen consumption of the new-born infant in a cool environment, measured with regard to sleep state [proceedings]. J Physiol. 1977;272(1):16P-7P.

292. Stothers JK, Warner RM. Oxygen consumption and sleep state in the new-born [proceedings]. J Physiol. 1977;269(1):57P-8P.

293. Moon RY, & Task Force On Sudden Infant Death S. SIDS and other sleep-related infant deaths: Evidence base for 2016 updated recommendations for a safe infant sleeping environment. Pediatrics. 2016;138(5):e20162940. https://doi.org/10.1542/peds.2016-2940.

294. Parslow PM, Cranage SM, Adamson TM, Harding R, Horne RSC. Arousal and ventilatory responses to hypoxia in sleeping infants: Effects of maternal smoking. Respir Physiol Neurobiol. 2004;140:77-87. https://doi.org/10.1016/j.resp.2004.01.004.

295. Duncan JR, Garland M, Stark RI, Myers MM, Fifer WP, Mokler DJ, et al. Prenatal nicotine exposure selectively affects nicotinic receptor expression in primary and associative visual cortices of the fetal baboon. Brain Path. 2015;25(2):171-81. https://doi.org/10.1111/bpa.12165.

296. Duncan JR, Garland M, Myers MM, Fifer WP, Yang M, Kinney HC, et al. Prenatal nicotine-exposure alters fetal autonomic activity and medullary neurotransmitter receptors: Implications for sudden infant death syndrome. J Appl Physiol. 2009;107(5):1579-90. https://doi.org/10.1152/japplphysiol.91629.2008.

297. Frank MG, Srere H, Ledezma C, O'Hara B, Heller HC. Prenatal nicotine alters vigilance states and AChR gene expression in the neonatal rat: Implications for SIDS. Am J Physiol Regul Integr Comp Physiol. 2001;280(4):R1134-40.

298. Nachmanoff DB, Panigrahy A, Filiano JJ, Mandell F, Sleeper LA, Valdes-Dapena M, et al. Brainstem $^3$H-nicotine receptor binding in the sudden infant death syndrome. J Neuropath Exp Neurol. 1998;57:1018-25. https://doi.org/10.1097/00005072-199811000-00004.

299. Hafstrom O. Nicotine delays arousal during hypoxemia in lambs. Pediatr Res. 2000;47:646-52. https://doi.org/10.1203/00006450-200005000-00015.

300. Sirieix CM, Lee S, Darnall RA. Effect of prenatal nicotine exposure and serotonin deficiency on arousal to hypoxia in rat pups. FASEB J. 2015;29:861.3.

301. Sirieix CM, Tobia CM, Schneider RW, Darnall RA. Impaired arousal in rat pups with prenatal alcohol exposure is modulated by GABAergic mechanisms. Physiol Rep. 2015;3(6):e12424. https://doi.org/10.14814/phy2.12424.

302. Hunt CE. The cardiorespiratory control hypothesis for sudden infant death syndrome. Clinics Perinatol. 1992;19:757-71.

This book is available as a free fully-searchable ebook from
**www.adelaide.edu.au/press**